HEALTH CARE STATE RANKINGS
2002

Health Care in the 50 United States

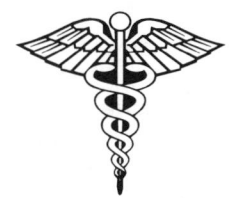

Kathleen O'Leary Morgan and Scott Morgan, Editors

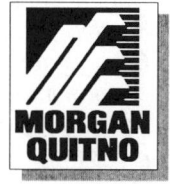

MORGAN QUITNO

Morgan Quitno Press
© Copyright 2002, All Rights Reserved

512 East 9th Street, P.O. Box 1656
Lawrence, KS 66044-8656
USA
800-457-0742 or 785-841-3534
www.statestats.com
Tenth Edition

© Copyright 2002 by
Morgan Quitno Corporation
512 East 9th Street, P.O. Box 1656
Lawrence, Kansas   66044-8656

800-457-0742 or 785-841-3534
www.statetats.com

ISBN: 0-7401-0039-4
ISSN: 1065-1403

Health Care State Rankings 2002 sells for $54.95 ($5.00 shipping) and is only available in paper binding. For those who prefer ranking information tailored to a particular state, we also offer *Health Care State Perspectives*, state-specific reports for each of the 50 states. These individual guides provide information on a state's data and rank for each of the categories featured in the national *Health Care State Rankings* volume. Perspectives sell for $19.00 or $9.50 if ordered with *Health Care State Rankings*. If crime statistics are your interest, please ask about our annual *Crime State Rankings* ($54.95 paper). If you are interested in city and metropolitan crime data, we offer *City Crime Rankings* ($42.95 paper). For a general view of the states, please ask about our annual *State Rankings* reference book ($54.95 paper) or our monthly *State Statistical Trends* ($299 a year). All of our data sets are also available in machine readable format. Shipping and handling is $5.00 per order.

Tenth Edition
Printed in the United States of America
April 2002

PREFACE

Are you looking for up-to-date state health information? Chances are *Health Care State Rankings 2002* has it. This huge collection of state health care information features statistics on births and reproductive health, deaths, disease, insurance and finance, health care providers, facilities and physical fitness. Find out which state has the highest teen birth rate. Discover how much your state government spends on hospitals and health programs. In all, more than 500 tables of state comparisons give you the information you need for virtually every aspect of health care in the 50 United States.

Important Notes About *Health Care State Rankings 2002*

Health Care State Rankings 2002 presents information from government and private sector sources in one user-friendly volume. Our goal in publishing this book is to translate complicated and often convoluted health care data into usable state comparisons. Most tables were updated from last year's book, some were deleted and others are new. A number of tables in the Finance Chapter are "repeats." The Centers For Medicare and Medicaid Services (formerly known as the Health Care Financing Administration) released its updated state health care expenditures last year and will not revise those numbers again for two to four years.

We make every effort to present the data in *Health Care State Rankings 2002* as simply and straightforwardly as possible. Source information and other pertinent footnotes are clearly shown at the bottom of each page. National totals, rates and percentages are prominently displayed at the top of each table. Every other line is shaded in gray for easier reading. In addition, numerous information-finding tools are provided: a thorough table of contents, table listings at the beginning of each chapter, a roster of sources with addresses and phone numbers, a detailed index and a chapter thumb index.

For the ease of our readers, the numbers shown in *Health Care State Rankings* require no additional calculations to convert them from millions, thousands, etc. All states are ranked on a high to low basis, with any ties among the states listed alphabetically for a given ranking. Negative numbers are shown in parentheses "( )." For tables with national totals (as opposed to rates, per capitas, etc.) a separate column is included showing what percent of the national total each individual state's total represents. This column is headed by "% of USA." This percentage figure is particularly interesting when compared with a state's share of the nation's population for a particular year (provided in an appendix).

For those who need information for just one state, check out our *Health Care State Perspective* series of publications. These 21-page comb bound reports feature data and ranking information for an individual state, as reported in *Health Care State Rankings 2002*. (For example

California Health Care about the state of Calif quick reference guides through the entire *He* searching for informatic *Care State Perspectives* a copy of *Health Care* quick reference guides information, please call

Other Books From Mo

In addition to our company offers thr The first of these, *State* view of the states. Statis are featured, includ government finance, he social welfare, energy compilation of state crin *Rankings 2002*. This v user-friendly statistics o expenditures, correction: arrests and offenses. Fo area statistics, *City Crin* metropolitan areas and c (approx. 300 cities). N changes in crime rates ov for all major crime cate 2000 crime data are feat

City Crime Ra *Rankings* and *Crime* available for $54.95. (p data aficionados, the ii available CD-ROM. Tl searchable PDF version data in .dbf, Excel and A sets are $154.95 for each the *City Crime Rankings*

State Statistical journal that examines ch the 50 United States. Ea on a different subject ar graphics and commentar For further information publications, please call check out our web site at

Finally, many th and health care industry with the development, de Your guidance is invalu readers. We always suggestions, so please gi drop us a note with your i

second year annual Health second place by Iowa whic also makes a the least hea third year i Louisiana in

Each yea objective rep some basic determine w State. While indisputable, interesting s states are doi

Methodolog

The He awarded base year 2002 o book, *Healtl* generally hea groups: thos which a high that measure was taken in were weight above.) Thi below the n average, the Dangerous C

The tabl Congratulati

POSITIVE (+)	
1.	Births of Lo
2.	Teenage Bi
3.	Percent of l
4.	Age-Adjus
5.	Infant Mort
6.	Age-Adjus
7.	Age-Adjus
8.	Percent of l
9.	Health Care
10.	Per Capita
11.	Estimated l

HICH STATE IS HEALTHIEST?

Vermont is on a health kick. After years of second place finishes, the Green Mountain State finally grabbed the title as Healthiest State for the first time last year. It seems to like it there, as Vermont has held on for a nd is the winner of our tenth est State Award. Repeating its finish was Minnesota, followed moved up to third. Mississippi repeat appearance, bringing up hy end of the rankings for the a row. It is preceded by 9th and New Mexico in 48th.

we take a step back from our rting of health statistics, feed gures into our computer and ich is the nation's Healthiest we never claim our findings are ve do believe they provide an tistical match-up of how the g with regard to health care.

lthiest State designation is 1 on 21 factors chosen from the lition of our annual reference

2002 HEALTHIEST STATE AWARD

RANK	STATE	SUM	'01	RANK	STATE	SUM	'01
1	Vermont	16.26	1	26	Wisconsin	3.26	24
2	Minnesota	15.91	2	27	Michigan	2.64	27
3	Iowa	15.78	5	28	Indiana	0.33	29
4	New Hampshire	15.54	3	29	Alaska	(0.17)	37
5	Nebraska	14.42	6	30	West Virginia	(1.21)	30
6	Hawaii	13.56	4	31	Illinois	(1.25)	32
7	North Dakota	12.24	9	32	Oklahoma	(1.69)	36
8	Connecticut	11.02	14	33	Kentucky	(1.71)	31
9	Massachusetts	10.83	10	34	North Carolina	(2.19)	35
10	Utah	10.42	12	35	Arizona	(2.59)	28
11	Maine	10.40	8	36	Tennessee	(2.86)	39
12	Kansas	8.84	7	37	Maryland	(3.81)	33
13	California	8.39	17	38	New York	(4.22)	34
14	Washington	8.13	11	39	Missouri	(4.50)	38
15	New Jersey	8.09	16	40	Arkansas	(5.94)	40
16	Rhode Island	7.15	15	41	Georgia	(7.51)	41
17	Montana	6.91	13	42	Texas	(7.93)	42
18	Oregon	6.81	18	43	Delaware	(8.96)	43
19	Virginia	5.74	18	44	Florida	(9.56)	44
20	South Dakota	4.77	23	45	South Carolina	(10.19)	49
21	Colorado	4.12	21	46	Nevada	(11.78)	46
22	Idaho	3.88	26	47	Alabama	(13.53)	47
23	Pennsylvania	3.74	20	48	New Mexico	(16.07)	45
24	Ohio	3.63	22	49	Louisiana	(17.25)	48
25	Wyoming	3.61	25	50	Mississippi	(18.59)	50

Care State Rankings. These factors reflect access to health care providers, affordability of health care and a thy population (see box below.) All 21 factors are the same as last year. The 21 factors were divided into two that are "negative" for which a high ranking would be considered bad for a state, and those that are "positive" for ranking would be considered good for a state. Rates for each of the 21 factors were processed through a formula how a state compares to the national average for a given category. The positive and negative nature of each factor account as part of the formula. Once these computations were made, the factors then were weighted (factors 1 equally.) These weighted scores were then added together to get a state's final score ("SUM" on the table way, states are assessed based on how they stack up against the national average. The end result is that the farther ional average a state's health ranking is, the lower (and less healthy) it ranks. The farther above the national higher (and healthier) a state ranks. This same methodology was used for our Dangerous State and Safest/ y Awards.

above shows how each state fared in the 2002 Healthiest State Award as well as its placement in 2001. ns to the citizens of Vermont. We wish you continued good health!

THE EDITORS

ND NEGATIVE (-) FACTORS CONSIDERED:

Birthweight as a Percent of All Births (Table 13) -
1 Rate (Table 27) -
others Receiving Late or No Prenatal Care (Table 53) -
1 Death Rate (Table 81) -
ity Rate (Table 87) -
1 Death Rate by Malignant Neoplasms (Table 155) -
1 Death Rate by Suicide (Table 176) -
pulation Not Covered by Health Insurance (Table 237) -
Expenditures as a Percent of Gross State Product (Table 280) -
ersonal Health Expenditures (Table 283) -
te of New Cancer Cases (Table 354) -

12. AIDS Rate (Table 378) -
13. Sexually Transmitted Disease Rate (Table 413) -
14. Percent of Population Lacking Access to Primary Care (Table 442) -
15. Percent of Adults Who Are Binge Drinkers (Table 501) -
16. Percent of Adults Who Smoke (Table 503) -
17. Percent of Adults Overweight or Obese (Table 506) -
18. Number of Days in Past Month When Physical Health was "Not Good" (Table 509) -
19. Beds in Community Hospitals per 100,000 Population (Table 202) +
20. Percent of Children Aged 19-35 Months Fully Immunized (Table 411) +
21. Safety Belt Usage Rate (Table 512) +

TABLE OF CONTENTS

I. Births and Reproductive Health

1   Births in 2000
2   Birth Rate in 2000
3   Births in 1999
4   Birth Rate in 1999
5   Birth Rate in 1990
6   Birth Rate in 1980
7   Fertility Rate in 2000
8   Births to White Women in 2000
9   White Births as a Percent of All Births in 2000
10   Births to Black Women in 2000
11   Black Births as a Percent of All Births in 2000
12   Births of Low Birthweight in 2000
13   Births of Low Birthweight as a Percent of All Births in 2000
14   Births of Low Birthweight to White Women in 2000
15   Births of Low Birthweight to White Women as a Percent of All Births to White Women in 2000
16   Births of Low Birthweight to Black Women in 2000
17   Births of Low Birthweight to Black Women as a Percent of All Births to Black Women in 2000
18   Births to Unmarried Women in 2000
19   Births to Unmarried Women as a Percent of All Births in 2000
20   Births to Unmarried White Women in 2000
21   Births to Unmarried White Women as a Percent of All Births to White Women in 2000
22   Births to Unmarried Black Women in 2000
23   Births to Unmarried Black Women as a Percent of All Births to Black Women in 2000
24   Births to Teenage Mothers in 2000
25   Teenage Birth Rate in 2000
26   Births to Teenage Mothers in 1999
27   Teenage Birth Rate in 1999
28   Births to Teenage Mothers as a Percent of Births in 1999
29   Births to White Teenage Mothers in 1999
30   White Teenage Birth Rate in 1999
31   Births to White Teenage Mothers as a Percent of White Births in 1999
32   Births to Black Teenage Mothers in 1999
33   Black Teenage Birth Rate in 1999
34   Births to Black Teenage Mothers as a Percent of Black Births in 1999
35   Pregnancy Rate for 15 to 19 Year Old Women in 1997
36   Percent Change in Pregnancy Rate for 15 to 19 Year Old Women: 1992 to 1997
37   Births to Teenage Mothers in 1990
38   Teenage Birth Rate in 1990
39   Percent Change in Teenage Birth Rate: 1990 to 1999
40   Births to Teenage Mothers in 1980
41   Teenage Birth Rate in 1980
42   Births to Women 35 to 54 Years Old in 1999
43   Births to Women 35 to 54 Years Old as a Percent of All Births in 1999
44   Births by Vaginal Delivery in 1999
45   Percent of Births by Vaginal Delivery in 1999
46   Births by Cesarean Delivery in 1999
47   Percent of Births by Cesarean Delivery in 1999
48   Percent Change in Rate of Cesarean Births: 1995 to 1999
49   Percent of Vaginal Births After a Cesarean (VBAC) in 1999
50   Percent of Mothers Beginning Prenatal Care in First Trimester in 2000
51   Percent of White Mothers Beginning Prenatal Care in First Trimester in 2000
52   Percent of Black Mothers Beginning Prenatal Care in First Trimester in 2000
53   Percent of Mothers Receiving Late or No Prenatal Care in 1999
54   Percent of White Mothers Receiving Late or No Prenatal Care in 1999
55   Percent of Black Mothers Receiving Late or No Prenatal Care in 1999
56   Percent of Mothers Who Smoked During Pregnancy in 1999
57   Percent of Teenage Mothers Who Smoked During Pregnancy in 1999
58   Percent of Births Attended by Midwives in 1999

TABLE OF CONTENTS (continued)

Abortions

59   Reported Legal Abortions in 1997
60   Reported Legal Abortions per 1,000 Live Births in 1997
61   Reported Legal Abortions per 1,000 Women Ages 15 to 44 in 1997
62   Percent of Legal Abortions Obtained by Out-Of-State Residents in 1997
63   Percent of Reported Legal Abortions Obtained by White Women in 1997
64   Percent of Reported Legal Abortions Obtained by Black Women in 1997
65   Percent of Reported Legal Abortions Obtained by Married Women in 1997
66   Percent of Reported Legal Abortions Obtained by Unmarried Women in 1997
67   Reported Legal Abortions Obtained by Teenagers in 1997
68   Percent of Reported Legal Abortions Obtained by Teenagers in 1997
69   Reported Legal Abortions Obtained by Teenagers 17 Years and Younger in 1997
70   Percent of Reported Legal Abortions Obtained by Teenagers 17 Years and Younger in 1997
71   Percent of Teenage Abortions Obtained by Teenagers 17 Years and Younger in 1997
72   Reported Legal Abortions Performed at 12 Weeks or Less of Gestation in 1997
73   Percent of Reported Legal Abortions Performed at 12 Weeks or Less of Gestation in 1997
74   Reported Legal Abortions Performed at or After 21 Weeks of Gestation in 1997
75   Percent of Reported Legal Abortions Performed at or After 21 Weeks of Gestation in 1997

II. Deaths

76   Deaths in 2000
77   Death Rate in 2000
78   Births to Deaths Ratio in 2000
79   Deaths in 1999
80   Death Rate in 1999
81   Age-Adjusted Death Rate in 1999
82   Death Rate in 1990
83   Death Rate in 1980
84   Infant Deaths in 2000
85   Infant Mortality Rate in 2000
86   Infant Deaths in 1999
87   Infant Mortality Rate in 1999
88   Infant Mortality Rate in 1990
89   Infant Mortality Rate in 1980
90   Percent Change in Infant Mortality Rate: 1990 to 1999
91   Percent Change in Infant Mortality Rate: 1980 to 1999
92   White Infant Deaths in 1999
93   White Infant Mortality Rate in 1999
94   Black Infant Deaths in 1999
95   Black Infant Mortality Rate in 1999
96   Percent Change in White Infant Mortality Rate: 1990 to 1999
97   Percent Change in Black Infant Mortality Rate: 1990 to 1999
98   Neonatal Deaths in 1999
99   Neonatal Death Rate in 1999
100   White Neonatal Deaths in 1999
101   White Neonatal Death Rate in 1999
102   Black Neonatal Deaths in 1999
103   Black Neonatal Death Rate in 1999
104   Deaths by AIDS Through 1999
105   Deaths by AIDS in 1999
106   Death Rate by AIDS in 1999
107   Age-Adjusted Death Rate by AIDS in 1999
108   Estimated Deaths by Cancer in 2002
109   Estimated Death Rate by Cancer in 2002
110   Age-Adjusted Death Rate by Cancer for Males in 1998
111   Age-Adjusted Death Rate by Cancer for Females in 1998
112   Estimated Deaths by Female Breast Cancer in 2002
113   Estimated Death Rate by Female Breast Cancer in 2002
114   Estimated Deaths by Colon and Rectum Cancer in 2002
115   Estimated Death Rate by Colon and Rectum Cancer in 2002
116   Estimated Deaths by Leukemia in 2002

TABLE OF CONTENTS (continued)

117 Estimated Death Rate by Leukemia in 2002
118 Estimated Deaths by Liver Cancer in 2002
119 Estimated Death Rate by Liver Cancer in 2002
120 Estimated Deaths by Lung Cancer in 2002
121 Estimated Death Rate by Lung Cancer in 2002
122 Estimated Deaths by Non-Hodgkin's Lymphoma in 2002
123 Estimated Death Rate by Non-Hodgkin's Lymphoma in 2002
124 Estimated Deaths by Pancreatic Cancer in 2002
125 Estimated Death Rate by Pancreatic Cancer in 2002
126 Estimated Deaths by Prostate Cancer in 2002
127 Estimated Death Rate by Prostate Cancer in 2002
128 Estimated Deaths by Ovarian Cancer in 2002
129 Estimated Death Rate by Ovarian Cancer in 2002
130 Estimated Deaths by Brain Cancer in 2002
131 Estimated Death Rate by Brain Cancer in 2002
132 Deaths by Alzheimer's Disease in 1999
133 Death Rate by Alzheimer's Disease in 1999
134 Age-Adjusted Death Rate by Alzheimer's Disease in 1999
135 Deaths by Atherosclerosis in 1999
136 Death Rate by Atherosclerosis in 1999
137 Age-Adjusted Death Rate by Atherosclerosis in 1999
138 Deaths by Cerebrovascular Diseases in 1999
139 Death Rate by Cerebrovascular Diseases in 1999
140 Age-Adjusted Death Rate by Cerebrovascular Diseases in 1999
141 Deaths by Chronic Liver Disease and Cirrhosis in 1999
142 Death Rate by Chronic Liver Disease and Cirrhosis in 1999
143 Age-Adjusted Death Rate by Chronic Liver Disease and Cirrhosis in 1999
144 Deaths by Chronic Lower Respiratory Diseases in 1999
145 Death Rate by Chronic Lower Respiratory Diseases in 1999
146 Age-Adjusted Death Rate by Chronic Lower Respiratory Diseases in 1999
147 Deaths by Diabetes Mellitus in 1999
148 Death Rate by Diabetes Mellitus in 1999
149 Age-Adjusted Death Rate by Diabetes Mellitus in 1999
150 Deaths by Diseases of the Heart in 1999
151 Death Rate by Diseases of the Heart in 1999
152 Age-Adjusted Death Rate by Diseases of the Heart in 1999
153 Deaths by Malignant Neoplasms in 1999
154 Death Rate by Malignant Neoplasms in 1999
155 Age-Adjusted Death Rate by Malignant Neoplasms in 1999
156 Deaths by Pneumonia and Influenza in 1999
157 Death Rate by Pneumonia and Influenza in 1999
158 Age-Adjusted Death Rate by Pneumonia and Influenza in 1999
159 Deaths by Tuberculosis in 1999
160 Death Rate by Tuberculosis in 1999
161 Age-Adjusted Death Rate by Tuberculosis in 1999
162 Deaths by Injury in 1999
163 Death Rate by Injury in 1999
164 Age-Adjusted Death Rate by Injury in 1999
165 Deaths by Accidents in 1999
166 Death Rate by Accidents in 1999
167 Age-Adjusted Death Rate by Accidents in 1999
168 Deaths by Motor Vehicle Accidents in 1999
169 Death Rate by Motor Vehicle Accidents in 1999
170 Age-Adjusted Death Rate by Motor Vehicle Accidents in 1999
171 Deaths by Homicide in 1999
172 Death Rate by Homicide in 1999
173 Age-Adjusted Death Rate by Homicide in 1999
174 Deaths by Suicide in 1999
175 Death Rate by Suicide in 1999
176 Age-Adjusted Death Rate by Suicide in 1999
177 Years Lost by Premature Death in 1999
178 Years Lost by Premature Death from Cancer in 1999
179 Years Lost by Premature Death from Heart Disease in 1999
180 Years Lost by Premature Death from Homicide in 1999

TABLE OF CONTENTS (continued)

181   Years Lost by Premature Death from Suicide in 1999
182   Years Lost by Premature Death from Unintentional Injuries in 1999
183   Alcohol-Induced Deaths in 1999
184   Death Rate by Alcohol-Induced Deaths in 1999
185   Age-Adjusted Death Rate by Alcohol-Induced Deaths in 1999
186   Drug-Induced Deaths in 1999
187   Death Rate from Drug-Induced Deaths in 1999
188   Age-Adjusted Death Rate from Drug-Induced Deaths in 1999
189   Occupational Fatalities in 2000
190   Occupational Fatality Rate in 2000

III. Facilities

191   Community Hospitals in 2000
192   Rate of Community Hospitals in 2000
193   Community Hospitals per 1,000 Square Miles in 2000
194   Community Hospitals in Urban Areas in 2000
195   Percent of Community Hospitals in Urban Areas in 2000
196   Community Hospitals in Rural Areas in 2000
197   Percent of Community Hospitals in Rural Areas in 2000
198   Nongovernment Not-For-Profit Hospitals in 2000
199   Investor-Owned (For-Profit) Hospitals in 2000
200   State and Local Government-Owned Hospitals in 2000
201   Beds in Community Hospitals in 2000
202   Rate of Beds in Community Hospitals in 2000
203   Average Number of Beds per Community Hospital in 2000
204   Admissions to Community Hospitals in 2000
205   Inpatient Days in Community Hospitals in 2000
206   Average Daily Census in Community Hospitals in 2000
207   Average Stay in Community Hospitals in 2000
208   Occupancy Rate in Community Hospitals in 2000
209   Outpatient Visits to Community Hospitals in 2000
210   Emergency Outpatient Visits to Community Hospitals in 2000
211   Surgical Operations in Community Hospitals in 2000
212   Medicare and Medicaid Certified Facilities in 2002
213   Medicare and Medicaid Certified Hospitals in 2002
214   Beds in Medicare and Medicaid Certified Hospitals in 2002
215   Medicare and Medicaid Certified Children's Hospitals in 2002
216   Beds in Medicare and Medicaid Certified Children's Hospitals in 2002
217   Medicare and Medicaid Certified Rehabilitation Hospitals in 2002
218   Beds in Medicare and Medicaid Certified Rehabilitation Hospitals in 2002
219   Medicare and Medicaid Certified Psychiatric Hospitals in 2002
220   Beds in Medicare and Medicaid Certified Psychiatric Hospitals in 2002
221   Medicare and Medicaid Certified Community Mental Health Centers in 2002
222   Medicare and Medicaid Certified Outpatient Physical Therapy Facilities in 2002
223   Medicare and Medicaid Certified Rural Health Clinics in 2002
224   Medicare and Medicaid Certified Home Health Agencies in 2002
225   Medicare and Medicaid Certified Hospices in 2002
226   Hospice Patients in Residential Facilities in 2002
227   Medicare and Medicaid Certified Nursing Care Facilities in 2002
228   Beds in Medicare and Medicaid Certified Nursing Care Facilities in 2002
229   Rate of Beds in Medicare and Medicaid Certified Nursing Care Facilities in 2002
230   Nursing Home Occupancy Rate in 1999
231   Nursing Home Resident Rate in 1999
232   Nursing Home Population 85 Years Old and Older in 1999
233   Health Care Establishments in 1999
234   Offices and Clinics of Doctors of Medicine in 1997
235   Offices and Clinics of Dentists in 1997

TABLE OF CONTENTS (continued)

IV. Finance

236 Persons Not Covered by Health Insurance in 2000
237 Percent of Population Not Covered by Health Insurance in 2000
238 Persons Covered by Health Insurance in 2000
239 Percent of Population Covered by Health Insurance in 2000
240 Persons Not Covered by Health Insurance in 1996
241 Percent of Population Not Covered by Health Insurance in 1996
242 Change in Number of Persons Uninsured: 1996 to 2000
243 Percent Change in Number of Uninsured: 1996 to 2000
244 Change in Percent of Population Uninsured: 1996 to 2000
245 Percent of Children Not Covered by Health Insurance in 2000
246 State Children's Health Insurance Program Enrollment in 2001
247 Percent Change in State Children's Health Insurance Program Enrollment: 2000 to 2001
248 Percent of Children Enrolled in State Children's Health Insurance Program in 2001
249 Percent of Population Covered by Private Health Insurance in 2000
250 Percent of Population Covered by Employment-Based Private Health Insurance in 2000
251 Percent of Population Covered by Government Health Insurance in 2000
252 Percent of Population Covered by Military Health Insurance in 2000
253 Health Maintenance Organizations (HMOs) in 2001
254 Enrollees in Health Maintenance Organizations (HMOs) in 2001
255 Percent Change in Enrollees in Health Maintenance Organizations (HMOs): 2000 to 2001
256 Percent of Population Enrolled in Health Maintenance Organizations (HMOs) in 2001
257 Percent of Insured Population Enrolled in Health Maintenance Organizations (HMOs) in 2001
258 Medicare Enrollees in 2000
259 Medicare Benefit Payments in 2000
260 Medicare Payments per Enrollee in 2000
261 Percent of Population Enrolled in Medicare in 2000
262 Medicare Managed Care Enrollees in 2001
263 Percent of Medicare Enrollees in Managed Care Programs in 2001
264 Percent of Medicare Benefits Paid Through Managed Care in 2000
265 Percent of Medicare Benefits Paid Through Fee for Service Plans in 2000
266 Medicare Physicians in 1999
267 Percent of Physicians Participating in Medicare in 1999
268 Medicaid Enrollment in 2000
269 Percent of Population Enrolled in Medicaid in 2000
270 Percent of Children Covered by Medicaid in 2000
271 Medicaid Enrollment in 1999
272 Medicaid Expenditures in 1999
273 Percent Change in Medicaid Expenditures: 1997 to 1999
274 Medicaid Expenditures per Enrollee in 1999
275 Percent Change in Expenditures per Medicaid Enrollee: 1997 to 1999
276 Medicaid Managed Care Enrollment in 2000
277 Percent of Medicaid Enrollees in Managed Care in 2000
278 Federal Medicaid Matching Fund Rate for 2002
279 Personal Health Care Expenditures in 1998
280 Health Care Expenditures as a Percent of Gross State Product in 1998
281 Percent Change in Personal Health Care Expenditures: 1990 to 1998
282 Average Annual Change in Expenditures for Personal Health Care: 1990 to 1998
283 Per Capita Personal Health Care Expenditures in 1998
284 Percent Change in Per Capita Expenditures for Personal Health Care: 1990 to 1998
285 Average Annual Change in Per Capita Expenditures for Personal Health Care: 1990 to 1998
286 Per Capita Medicare Expenditures for Personal Health Care in 1998
287 Per Capita Medicaid Expenditures for Personal Health Care in 1998
288 Expenditures for Hospital Care in 1998
289 Percent of Total Personal Health Care Expenditures Spent on Hospital Care in 1998
290 Percent Change in Expenditures for Hospital Care: 1990 to 1998
291 Average Annual Change in Expenditures for Hospital Care: 1990 to 1998
292 Per Capita Expenditures for Hospital Care in 1998
293 Percent Change in Per Capita Expenditures for Hospital Care: 1990 to 1998
294 Average Annual Change in Per Capita Expenditures for Hospital Care: 1990 to 1998
295 Per Capita Medicare Expenditures for Hospital Care in 1998
296 Per Capita Medicaid Expenditures for Hospital Care in 1998

TABLE OF CONTENTS (continued)

297   Expenditures for Physician and Other Professional Services in 1998
298   Percent of Total Personal Health Care Expenditures Spent on Physician and Other Professional Services in 1998
299   Percent Change in Expenditures for Physician and Other Professional Services: 1990 to 1998
300   Average Annual Change in Expenditures for Physician and Other Professional Services: 1990 to 1998
301   Per Capita Expenditures for Physician and Other Professional Services in 1998
302   Percent Change in Per Capita Expenditures for Physician and Other Professional Services: 1990 to 1998
303   Average Annual Change in Per Capita Expenditures for Physician Services: 1990 to 1998
304   Per Capita Medicare Expenditures for Physician Services in 1998
305   Per Capita Medicaid Expenditures for Physician Services in 1998
306   Expenditures for Prescription Drugs in 1998
307   Percent of Total Personal Health Care Expenditures Spent on Prescription Drugs in 1998
308   Percent Change in Expenditures for Prescription Drugs: 1990 to 1998
309   Average Annual Change in Expenditures for Prescription Drugs: 1990 to 1998
310   Per Capita Expenditures for Prescription Drugs in 1998
311   Percent Change in Per Capita Expenditures for Prescription Drugs: 1990 to 1998
312   Average Annual Change in Per Capita Expenditures for Prescription Drugs: 1990 to 1998
313   Expenditures for Dental Services in 1998
314   Percent of Total Personal Health Care Expenditures Spent on Dental Services in 1998
315   Average Annual Change in Expenditures for Dental Services: 1990 to 1998
316   Per Capita Expenditures for Dental Services in 1998
317   Per Capita Medicaid Expenditures for Dental Services in 1998
318   Expenditures for Other Personal Health Care Services in 1998
319   Percent of Total Personal Health Care Expenditures Spent on Other Personal Health Care Services in 1998
320   Average Annual Change in Expenditures for Other Personal Health Care Services: 1990 to 1998
321   Per Capita Expenditures for Other Personal Health Care Services in 1998
322   Expenditures for Home Health Care in 1998
323   Percent of Total Personal Health Care Expenditures Spent on Home Health Care in 1998
324   Average Annual Change in Expenditures for Home Health Care: 1990 to 1998
325   Per Capita Expenditures for Home Health Care in 1998
326   Per Capita Medicare Expenditures for Home Health Care in 1998
327   Per Capita Medicaid Expenditures for Home Health Care in 1998
328   Expenditures for Over-the-Counter Drugs and Other Medical Non-Durables in 1998
329   Percent of Total Personal Health Care Expenditures Spent on Over-the-Counter Drugs and Other Medical Non-Durables in 1998
330   Average Annual Change in Expenditures for Over-the-Counter Drugs and Other Medical Non-Durables: 1990 to 1998
331   Per Capita Expenditures for Over-the-Counter Drugs and Other Medical Non-Durables in 1998
332   Expenditures for Vision Products and Other Medical Durables in 1998
333   Percent of Total Personal Health Care Expenditures Spent on Vision Products and Other Medical Durables in 1998
334   Average Annual Change in Expenditures for Vision Products and Other Medical Durables: 1990 to 1998
335   Per Capita Expenditures for Vision Products and Other Medical Durables in 1998
336   Expenditures for Nursing Home Care in 1998
337   Percent of Total Personal Health Care Expenditures Spent on Nursing Home Care in 1998
338   Average Annual Change in Expenditures for Nursing Home Care: 1990 to 1998
339   Per Capita Expenditures for Nursing Home Care in 1998
340   Per Capita Medicare Expenditures for Nursing Home Care in 1998
341   Per Capita Medicaid Expenditures for Nursing Home Care in 1998
342   Estimated State Funds from the Tobacco Settlement Through 2025
343   State Government Expenditures for Health Programs in 1999
344   Per Capita State Government Expenditures for Health Programs in 1999
345   State Government Expenditures for Hospitals in 1999
346   Per Capita State Government Expenditures for Hospitals in 1999
347   Payroll of Health Care Establishments in 1999
348   Average Pay per Health Care Establishment Employee in 1999
349   Receipts per Health Service Establishment in 1997
350   Receipts per Hospital in 1997
351   Receipts per Office or Clinic of Doctors of Medicine in 1997
352   Receipts per Office or Clinic of Dentists in 1997

TABLE OF CONTENTS (continued)

V. Incidence of Disease

353 Estimated New Cancer Cases in 2002
354 Estimated Rate of New Cancer Cases in 2002
355 Age-Adjusted Rate of New Cancer Cases for Males in 1998
356 Age-Adjusted Rate of New Cancer Cases for Females in 1998
357 Estimated New Cases of Bladder Cancer in 2002
358 Estimated Rate of New Bladder Cancer Cases in 2002
359 Estimated New Female Breast Cancer Cases in 2002
360 Estimated Rate of New Female Breast Cancer Cases in 2002
361 Percent of Women 40 and Older Who Have Ever Had a Mammogram: 2000
362 Estimated New Colon and Rectum Cancer Cases in 2002
363 Estimated Rate of New Colon and Rectum Cancer Cases in 2002
364 Estimated New Leukemia Cases in 2002
365 Estimated Rate of New Leukemia Cases in 2002
366 Estimated New Lung Cancer Cases in 2002
367 Estimated Rate of New Lung Cancer Cases in 2002
368 Estimated New Non-Hodgkin's Lymphoma Cases in 2002
369 Estimated Rate of New Non-Hodgkin's Lymphoma Cases in 2002
370 Estimated New Prostate Cancer Cases in 2002
371 Estimated Rate of New Prostate Cancer Cases in 2002
372 Estimated New Skin Melanoma Cases in 2002
373 Estimated Rate of New Skin Melanoma Cases in 2002
374 Estimated New Cervical Cancer Cases in 2002
375 Estimated Rate of New Cervical Cancer Cases in 2002
376 Percent of Women 18 Years Old and Older Who Had a Pap Smear Within the Past Three Years: 2000
377 AIDS Cases Reported in 2001
378 AIDS Rate in 2001
379 AIDS Cases Reported Through June 2001
380 AIDS Cases in Children 12 Years and Younger Through June 2001
381 E-Coli Cases Reported in 2001
382 E-Coli Rate in 2001
383 German Measles (Rubella) Cases Reported in 2001
384 German Measles (Rubella) Rate in 2001
385 Hepatitis A and B Cases Reported in 2001
386 Hepatitis A and B Rate in 2001
387 Hepatitis C Cases Reported in 2001
388 Hepatitis C Rate in 2001
389 Legionellosis Cases Reported in 2001
390 Legionellosis Rate in 2001
391 Lyme Disease Cases in 2001
392 Lyme Disease Rate in 2001
393 Malaria Cases Reported in 2001
394 Malaria Rate in 2001
395 Measles (Rubeola) Cases Reported in 2001
396 Measles (Rubeola) Rate in 2001
397 Meningococcal Infections Reported in 2001
398 Meningococcal Infection Rate in 2001
399 Mumps Cases Reported in 2001
400 Mumps Rate in 2001
401 Rabies (Animal) Cases Reported in 2001
402 Rabies (Animal) Rate in 2001
403 Salmonellosis Cases Reported in 2001
404 Salmonellosis Rate in 2001
405 Shigellosis Cases Reported in 2001
406 Shigellosis Rate in 2001
407 Tuberculosis Cases Reported in 2001
408 Tuberculosis Rate in 2001
409 Whooping Cough (Pertussis) Cases Reported in 2001
410 Whooping Cough (Pertussis) Rate in 2001
411 Percent of Children Aged 19 to 35 Months Fully Immunized in 2000
412 Sexually Transmitted Diseases in 2000
413 Sexually Transmitted Disease Rate in 2000
414 Chancroid Cases in 2000

TABLE OF CONTENTS (continued)

415   Chancroid Rate in 2000
416   Chlamydia Cases Reported in 2000
417   Chlamydia Rate in 2000
418   Gonorrhea Cases Reported in 2000
419   Gonorrhea Rate in 2000
420   Syphilis Cases Reported in 2000
421   Syphilis Rate in 2000

VI. Providers

422   Physicians in 2000
423   Male Physicians in 2000
424   Female Physicians in 2000
425   Percent of Physicians Who Are Female: 2000
426   Physicians Under 35 Years Old in 2000
427   Percent of Physicians Under 35 Years Old in 2000
428   Physicians 35 to 44 Years Old in 2000
429   Physicians 45 to 54 Years Old in 2000
430   Physicians 55 to 64 Years Old in 2000
431   Physicians 65 Years Old and Older in 2000
432   Percent of Physicians 65 Years Old and Older in 2000
433   Federal Physicians in 2000
434   Rate of Federal Physicians in 2000
435   Nonfederal Physicians in 2000
436   Rate of Nonfederal Physicians in 2000
437   Nonfederal Physicians in Patient Care in 2000
438   Rate of Nonfederal Physicians in Patient Care in 2000
439   Physicians in Primary Care in 2000
440   Rate of Physicians in Primary Care in 2000
441   Percent of Physicians in Primary Care in 2000
442   Percent of Population Lacking Access to Primary Care in 2001
443   Nonfederal Physicians in General/Family Practice in 2000
444   Rate of Nonfederal Physicians in General/Family Practice in 2000
445   Percent of Nonfederal Physicians Who Are Specialists in 2000
446   Nonfederal Physicians in Medical Specialties in 2000
447   Rate of Nonfederal Physicians in Medical Specialties in 2000
448   Nonfederal Physicians in Internal Medicine in 2000
449   Rate of Nonfederal Physicians in Internal Medicine in 2000
450   Nonfederal Physicians in Pediatrics in 2000
451   Rate of Nonfederal Physicians in Pediatrics in 2000
452   Nonfederal Physicians in Surgical Specialties in 2000
453   Rate of Nonfederal Physicians in Surgical Specialties in 2000
454   Nonfederal Physicians in General Surgery in 2000
455   Rate of Nonfederal Physicians in General Surgery in 2000
456   Nonfederal Physicians in Obstetrics and Gynecology in 2000
457   Rate of Nonfederal Physicians in Obstetrics and Gynecology in 2000
458   Nonfederal Physicians in Ophthalmology in 2000
459   Rate of Nonfederal Physicians in Ophthalmology in 2000
460   Nonfederal Physicians in Orthopedic Surgery in 2000
461   Rate of Nonfederal Physicians in Orthopedic Surgery in 2000
462   Nonfederal Physicians in Plastic Surgery in 2000
463   Rate of Nonfederal Physicians in Plastic Surgery in 2000
464   Nonfederal Physicians in Other Specialties in 2000
465   Rate of Nonfederal Physicians in Other Specialties in 2000
466   Nonfederal Physicians in Anesthesiology in 2000
467   Rate of Nonfederal Physicians in Anesthesiology in 2000
468   Nonfederal Physicians in Psychiatry in 2000
469   Rate of Nonfederal Physicians in Psychiatry in 2000
470   Percent of Population Lacking Access to Mental Health Care in 2001
471   International Medical School Graduates Practicing in the U.S. in 2000
472   Rate of International Medical School Graduates Practicing in the U.S. in 2000
473   International Medical School Graduates as a Percent of Nonfederal Physicians in 2000
474   Osteopathic Physicians in 2002

TABLE OF CONTENTS (continued)

475 Rate of Osteopathic Physicians in 2002
476 Podiatric Physicians in 1999
477 Rate of Podiatric Physicians in 1999
478 Doctors of Chiropractic in 2000
479 Rate of Doctors of Chiropractic in 2000
480 Physician Assistants in Clinical Practice in 2002
481 Rate of Physician Assistants in Clinical Practice in 2002
482 Registered Nurses in 2000
483 Rate of Registered Nurses in 2000
484 Dentists in 1998
485 Rate of Dentists in 1998
486 Percent of Population Lacking Access to Dental Care in 2001
487 Employment in Health Care in 1999

VII. Physical Fitness

488 Users of Exercise Equipment in 2000
489 Participants in Golf in 2000
490 Participants in Running/Jogging in 2000
491 Participants in Swimming in 2000
492 Participants in Tennis in 2000
493 Alcohol Consumption in 1998
494 Adult Per Capita Alcohol Consumption in 1998
495 Apparent Beer Consumption in 1998
496 Adult Per Capita Beer Consumption in 1998
497 Wine Consumption in 1998
498 Adult Per Capita Wine Consumption in 1998
499 Distilled Spirits Consumption in 1998
500 Adult Per Capita Apparent Distilled Spirits Consumption in 1998
501 Percent of Adults Who Are Binge Drinkers: 1999
502 Percent of Adults Who Drink and Drive: 1999
503 Percent of Adults Who Smoke: 2000
504 Percent of Males Who Smoke: 2000
505 Percent of Women Who Smoke: 2000
506 Percent of Adults Overweight or Obese: 2000
507 Percent of Adults Who Have Not Had Their Blood Pressure Checked in the Past Two Years: 1999
508 Percent of Adults Who Have Not Been Tested in Past Year for HIV: 2000
509 Number of Days in Past Month When Physical Health was "Not Good": 2000
510 Number of Days in Past Month When Mental Health was "Not Good": 2000
511 Percent of Population Who are Illicit Drug Users: 1999
512 Safety Belt Usage Rate in 2000

VIII. Appendix

A-1 Population in 2001
A-2 Population in 2000 Census
A-3 Male Population in 2000
A-4 Female Population in 2000
A-5 Population in 1998

IX. Sources

X. Index

I. BIRTHS AND REPRODUCTIVE HEALTH

1   Births in 2000
2   Birth Rate in 2000
3   Births in 1999
4   Birth Rate in 1999
5   Birth Rate in 1990
6   Birth Rate in 1980
7   Fertility Rate in 2000
8   Births to White Women in 2000
9   White Births as a Percent of All Births in 2000
10 Births to Black Women in 2000
11 Black Births as a Percent of All Births in 2000
12 Births of Low Birthweight in 2000
13 Births of Low Birthweight as a Percent of All Births in 2000
14 Births of Low Birthweight to White Women in 2000
15 Births of Low Birthweight to White Women as a Percent of All Births to White Women in 2000
16 Births of Low Birthweight to Black Women in 2000
17 Births of Low Birthweight to Black Women as a Percent of All Births to Black Women in 2000
18 Births to Unmarried Women in 2000
19 Births to Unmarried Women as a Percent of All Births in 2000
20 Births to Unmarried White Women in 2000
21 Births to Unmarried White Women as a Percent of All Births to White Women in 2000
22 Births to Unmarried Black Women in 2000
23 Births to Unmarried Black Women as a Percent of All Births to Black Women in 2000
24 Births to Teenage Mothers in 2000
25 Teenage Birth Rate in 2000
26 Births to Teenage Mothers in 1999
27 Teenage Birth Rate in 1999
28 Births to Teenage Mothers as a Percent of Births in 1999
29 Births to White Teenage Mothers in 1999
30 White Teenage Birth Rate in 1999
31 Births to White Teenage Mothers as a Percent of White Births in 1999
32 Births to Black Teenage Mothers in 1999
33 Black Teenage Birth Rate in 1999
34 Births to Black Teenage Mothers as a Percent of Black Births in 1999
35 Pregnancy Rate for 15 to 19 Year Old Women in 1997
36 Percent Change in Pregnancy Rate for 15 to 19 Year Old Women: 1992 to 1997
37 Births to Teenage Mothers in 1990
38 Teenage Birth Rate in 1990
39 Percent Change in Teenage Birth Rate: 1990 to 1999
40 Births to Teenage Mothers in 1980
41 Teenage Birth Rate in 1980
42 Births to Women 35 to 54 Years Old in 1999
43 Births to Women 35 to 54 Years Old as a Percent of All Births in 1999
44 Births by Vaginal Delivery in 1999
45 Percent of Births by Vaginal Delivery in 1999
46 Births by Cesarean Delivery in 1999
47 Percent of Births by Cesarean Delivery in 1999
48 Percent Change in Rate of Cesarean Births: 1995 to 1999
49 Percent of Vaginal Births After a Cesarean (VBAC) in 1999
50 Percent of Mothers Beginning Prenatal Care in First Trimester in 2000
51 Percent of White Mothers Beginning Prenatal Care in First Trimester in 2000
52 Percent of Black Mothers Beginning Prenatal Care in First Trimester in 2000
53 Percent of Mothers Receiving Late or No Prenatal Care in 1999
54 Percent of White Mothers Receiving Late or No Prenatal Care in 1999
55 Percent of Black Mothers Receiving Late or No Prenatal Care in 1999
56 Percent of Mothers Who Smoked During Pregnancy in 1999
57 Percent of Teenage Mothers Who Smoked During Pregnancy in 1999
58 Percent of Births Attended by Midwives in 1999

I. BIRTHS AND REPRODUCTIVE HEALTH (CONTINUED)

Abortions

59   Reported Legal Abortions in 1997
60   Reported Legal Abortions per 1,000 Live Births in 1997
61   Reported Legal Abortions per 1,000 Women Ages 15 to 44 in 1997
62   Percent of Legal Abortions Obtained by Out-Of-State Residents in 1997
63   Percent of Reported Legal Abortions Obtained by White Women in 1997
64   Percent of Reported Legal Abortions Obtained by Black Women in 1997
65   Percent of Reported Legal Abortions Obtained by Married Women in 1997
66   Percent of Reported Legal Abortions Obtained by Unmarried Women in 1997
67   Reported Legal Abortions Obtained by Teenagers in 1997
68   Percent of Reported Legal Abortions Obtained by Teenagers in 1997
69   Reported Legal Abortions Obtained by Teenagers 17 Years and Younger in 1997
70   Percent of Reported Legal Abortions Obtained by Teenagers 17 Years and Younger in 1997
71   Percent of Teenage Abortions Obtained by Teenagers 17 Years and Younger in 1997
72   Reported Legal Abortions Performed at 12 Weeks or Less of Gestation in 1997
73   Percent of Reported Legal Abortions Performed at 12 Weeks or Less of Gestation in 1997
74   Reported Legal Abortions Performed at or After 21 Weeks of Gestation in 1997
75   Percent of Reported Legal Abortions Performed at or After 21 Weeks of Gestation in 1997

Births in 2000

National Total = 4,064,948 Live Births*

RANK	STATE	BIRTHS	% of USA
23	Alabama	63,317	1.6%
46	Alaska	10,026	0.2%
13	Arizona	85,274	2.1%
33	Arkansas	38,031	0.9%
1	California	531,832	13.1%
22	Colorado	65,434	1.6%
30	Connecticut	43,154	1.1%
43	Delaware	11,050	0.3%
4	Florida	204,152	5.0%
8	Georgia	132,711	3.3%
39	Hawaii	17,544	0.4%
38	Idaho	20,371	0.5%
5	Illinois	185,066	4.6%
12	Indiana	87,111	2.1%
32	Iowa	38,545	0.9%
31	Kansas	39,690	1.0%
24	Kentucky	56,197	1.4%
20	Louisiana	67,964	1.7%
41	Maine	13,603	0.3%
18	Maryland	74,341	1.8%
14	Massachusetts	81,650	2.0%
7	Michigan	136,273	3.4%
21	Minnesota	67,393	1.7%
29	Mississippi	44,106	1.1%
17	Missouri	76,456	1.9%
44	Montana	10,964	0.3%
36	Nebraska	24,650	0.6%
34	Nevada	30,910	0.8%
40	New Hampshire	14,613	0.4%
10	New Jersey	115,071	2.8%
35	New Mexico	27,238	0.7%
3	New York	258,036	6.3%
9	North Carolina	120,249	3.0%
47	North Dakota	7,696	0.2%
NA	Ohio**	NA	NA
26	Oklahoma	49,905	1.2%
28	Oregon	45,800	1.1%
6	Pennsylvania	146,243	3.6%
42	Rhode Island	12,493	0.3%
25	South Carolina	56,116	1.4%
45	South Dakota	10,354	0.3%
16	Tennessee	79,630	2.0%
2	Texas	366,841	9.0%
27	Utah	47,368	1.2%
48	Vermont	6,497	0.2%
11	Virginia	98,907	2.4%
15	Washington	81,033	2.0%
37	West Virginia	20,912	0.5%
19	Wisconsin	69,428	1.7%
49	Wyoming	6,247	0.2%

RANK	STATE	BIRTHS	% of USA
1	California	531,832	13.1%
2	Texas	366,841	9.0%
3	New York	258,036	6.3%
4	Florida	204,152	5.0%
5	Illinois	185,066	4.6%
6	Pennsylvania	146,243	3.6%
7	Michigan	136,273	3.4%
8	Georgia	132,711	3.3%
9	North Carolina	120,249	3.0%
10	New Jersey	115,071	2.8%
11	Virginia	98,907	2.4%
12	Indiana	87,111	2.1%
13	Arizona	85,274	2.1%
14	Massachusetts	81,650	2.0%
15	Washington	81,033	2.0%
16	Tennessee	79,630	2.0%
17	Missouri	76,456	1.9%
18	Maryland	74,341	1.8%
19	Wisconsin	69,428	1.7%
20	Louisiana	67,964	1.7%
21	Minnesota	67,393	1.7%
22	Colorado	65,434	1.6%
23	Alabama	63,317	1.6%
24	Kentucky	56,197	1.4%
25	South Carolina	56,116	1.4%
26	Oklahoma	49,905	1.2%
27	Utah	47,368	1.2%
28	Oregon	45,800	1.1%
29	Mississippi	44,106	1.1%
30	Connecticut	43,154	1.1%
31	Kansas	39,690	1.0%
32	Iowa	38,545	0.9%
33	Arkansas	38,031	0.9%
34	Nevada	30,910	0.8%
35	New Mexico	27,238	0.7%
36	Nebraska	24,650	0.6%
37	West Virginia	20,912	0.5%
38	Idaho	20,371	0.5%
39	Hawaii	17,544	0.4%
40	New Hampshire	14,613	0.4%
41	Maine	13,603	0.3%
42	Rhode Island	12,493	0.3%
43	Delaware	11,050	0.3%
44	Montana	10,964	0.3%
45	South Dakota	10,354	0.3%
46	Alaska	10,026	0.2%
47	North Dakota	7,696	0.2%
48	Vermont	6,497	0.2%
49	Wyoming	6,247	0.2%
NA	Ohio**	NA	NA
	District of Columbia	7,666	0.2%

*Source: U.S. Department of Health and Human Services, National Center for Health Statistics
"National Vital Statistics Reports" (Vol. 49, No. 5, July 24, 2001)*
*Data are preliminary estimates by state of residence.
**Not available.

Birth Rate in 2000

National Rate = 14.8 Live Births per 1,000 Population*

ALPHA ORDER			RANK ORDER		
RANK	STATE	RATE	RANK	STATE	RATE
22	Alabama	14.4	1	Utah	21.9
6	Alaska	16.1	2	Texas	18.0
3	Arizona	17.5	3	Arizona	17.5
17	Arkansas	14.8	4	Georgia	16.7
8	California	15.8	5	Nevada	16.4
8	Colorado	15.8	6	Alaska	16.1
39	Connecticut	13.1	7	Idaho	16.0
21	Delaware	14.5	8	California	15.8
37	Florida	13.3	8	Colorado	15.8
4	Georgia	16.7	8	Mississippi	15.8
15	Hawaii	14.9	11	New Mexico	15.6
7	Idaho	16.0	12	Louisiana	15.5
14	Illinois	15.2	12	North Carolina	15.5
20	Indiana	14.6	14	Illinois	15.2
36	Iowa	13.4	15	Hawaii	14.9
15	Kansas	14.9	15	Kansas	14.9
27	Kentucky	14.1	17	Arkansas	14.8
12	Louisiana	15.5	17	Nebraska	14.8
49	Maine	10.8	17	Oklahoma	14.8
25	Maryland	14.2	20	Indiana	14.6
38	Massachusetts	13.2	21	Delaware	14.5
34	Michigan	13.7	22	Alabama	14.4
29	Minnesota	14.0	22	Tennessee	14.4
8	Mississippi	15.8	24	South Carolina	14.3
32	Missouri	13.9	25	Maryland	14.2
43	Montana	12.3	25	Virginia	14.2
17	Nebraska	14.8	27	Kentucky	14.1
5	Nevada	16.4	27	New York	14.1
46	New Hampshire	12.0	29	Minnesota	14.0
29	New Jersey	14.0	29	New Jersey	14.0
11	New Mexico	15.6	29	South Dakota	14.0
27	New York	14.1	32	Missouri	13.9
12	North Carolina	15.5	32	Washington	13.9
44	North Dakota	12.2	34	Michigan	13.7
NA	Ohio**	NA	34	Oregon	13.7
17	Oklahoma	14.8	36	Iowa	13.4
34	Oregon	13.7	37	Florida	13.3
44	Pennsylvania	12.2	38	Massachusetts	13.2
42	Rhode Island	12.5	39	Connecticut	13.1
24	South Carolina	14.3	39	Wisconsin	13.1
29	South Dakota	14.0	41	Wyoming	13.0
22	Tennessee	14.4	42	Rhode Island	12.5
2	Texas	18.0	43	Montana	12.3
1	Utah	21.9	44	North Dakota	12.2
48	Vermont	10.9	44	Pennsylvania	12.2
25	Virginia	14.2	46	New Hampshire	12.0
32	Washington	13.9	47	West Virginia	11.6
47	West Virginia	11.6	48	Vermont	10.9
39	Wisconsin	13.1	49	Maine	10.8
41	Wyoming	13.0	NA	Ohio**	NA
				District of Columbia	14.8

Source: U.S. Department of Health and Human Services, National Center for Health Statistics
   "National Vital Statistics Reports" (Vol. 49, No. 5, July 24, 2001)
*Data are preliminary estimates by state of residence.
**Not available.

Births in 1999

National Total = 3,959,417 Births*

ALPHA ORDER					RANK ORDER			
RANK	STATE	BIRTHS	% of USA		RANK	STATE	BIRTHS	% of USA
24	Alabama	62,122	1.6%		1	California	518,508	13.1%
47	Alaska	9,950	0.3%		2	Texas	349,245	8.8%
14	Arizona	81,145	2.0%		3	New York	255,612	6.5%
34	Arkansas	36,729	0.9%		4	Florida	197,023	5.0%
1	California	518,508	13.1%		5	Illinois	182,068	4.6%
23	Colorado	62,167	1.6%		6	Ohio	152,584	3.9%
30	Connecticut	43,310	1.1%		7	Pennsylvania	145,347	3.7%
45	Delaware	10,676	0.3%		8	Michigan	133,607	3.4%
4	Florida	197,023	5.0%		9	Georgia	126,717	3.2%
9	Georgia	126,717	3.2%		10	New Jersey	114,105	2.9%
40	Hawaii	17,038	0.4%		11	North Carolina	113,795	2.9%
39	Idaho	19,872	0.5%		12	Virginia	95,469	2.4%
5	Illinois	182,068	4.6%		13	Indiana	86,031	2.2%
13	Indiana	86,031	2.2%		14	Arizona	81,145	2.0%
33	Iowa	37,558	0.9%		15	Massachusetts	80,939	2.0%
32	Kansas	38,782	1.0%		16	Washington	79,586	2.0%
26	Kentucky	54,403	1.4%		17	Tennessee	77,803	2.0%
21	Louisiana	67,136	1.7%		18	Missouri	75,432	1.9%
42	Maine	13,616	0.3%		19	Maryland	71,967	1.8%
19	Maryland	71,967	1.8%		20	Wisconsin	68,208	1.7%
15	Massachusetts	80,939	2.0%		21	Louisiana	67,136	1.7%
8	Michigan	133,607	3.4%		22	Minnesota	65,970	1.7%
22	Minnesota	65,970	1.7%		23	Colorado	62,167	1.6%
31	Mississippi	42,684	1.1%		24	Alabama	62,122	1.6%
18	Missouri	75,432	1.9%		25	South Carolina	54,948	1.4%
44	Montana	10,785	0.3%		26	Kentucky	54,403	1.4%
37	Nebraska	23,907	0.6%		27	Oklahoma	49,010	1.2%
35	Nevada	29,362	0.7%		28	Utah	46,290	1.2%
41	New Hampshire	14,041	0.4%		29	Oregon	45,204	1.1%
10	New Jersey	114,105	2.9%		30	Connecticut	43,310	1.1%
36	New Mexico	27,191	0.7%		31	Mississippi	42,684	1.1%
3	New York	255,612	6.5%		32	Kansas	38,782	1.0%
11	North Carolina	113,795	2.9%		33	Iowa	37,558	0.9%
48	North Dakota	7,639	0.2%		34	Arkansas	36,729	0.9%
6	Ohio	152,584	3.9%		35	Nevada	29,362	0.7%
27	Oklahoma	49,010	1.2%		36	New Mexico	27,191	0.7%
29	Oregon	45,204	1.1%		37	Nebraska	23,907	0.6%
7	Pennsylvania	145,347	3.7%		38	West Virginia	20,728	0.5%
43	Rhode Island	12,366	0.3%		39	Idaho	19,872	0.5%
25	South Carolina	54,948	1.4%		40	Hawaii	17,038	0.4%
46	South Dakota	10,524	0.3%		41	New Hampshire	14,041	0.4%
17	Tennessee	77,803	2.0%		42	Maine	13,616	0.3%
2	Texas	349,245	8.8%		43	Rhode Island	12,366	0.3%
28	Utah	46,290	1.2%		44	Montana	10,785	0.3%
49	Vermont	6,567	0.2%		45	Delaware	10,676	0.3%
12	Virginia	95,469	2.4%		46	South Dakota	10,524	0.3%
16	Washington	79,586	2.0%		47	Alaska	9,950	0.3%
38	West Virginia	20,728	0.5%		48	North Dakota	7,639	0.2%
20	Wisconsin	68,208	1.7%		49	Vermont	6,567	0.2%
50	Wyoming	6,129	0.2%		50	Wyoming	6,129	0.2%
						District of Columbia	7,522	0.2%

Source: U.S. Department of Health and Human Services, National Center for Health Statistics
"National Vital Statistics Reports" (Vol. 49, No. 1, April 17, 2001)
*Final data by state of residence.

Birth Rate in 1999

National Rate = 14.5 Live Births per 1,000 Population*

ALPHA ORDER

RANK ORDER

RANK	STATE	RATE		RANK	STATE	RATE
22	Alabama	14.2		1	Utah	21.7
6	Alaska	16.1		2	Texas	17.4
3	Arizona	17.0		3	Arizona	17.0
18	Arkansas	14.4		4	Georgia	16.3
8	California	15.6		5	Nevada	16.2
12	Colorado	15.3		6	Alaska	16.1
37	Connecticut	13.2		7	Idaho	15.9
22	Delaware	14.2		8	California	15.6
40	Florida	13.0		8	New Mexico	15.6
4	Georgia	16.3		10	Louisiana	15.4
18	Hawaii	14.4		10	Mississippi	15.4
7	Idaho	15.9		12	Colorado	15.3
13	Illinois	15.0		13	Illinois	15.0
17	Indiana	14.5		14	North Carolina	14.9
38	Iowa	13.1		15	Kansas	14.6
15	Kansas	14.6		15	Oklahoma	14.6
33	Kentucky	13.7		17	Indiana	14.5
10	Louisiana	15.4		18	Arkansas	14.4
50	Maine	10.9		18	Hawaii	14.4
28	Maryland	13.9		18	South Dakota	14.4
38	Massachusetts	13.1		21	Nebraska	14.3
36	Michigan	13.5		22	Alabama	14.2
30	Minnesota	13.8		22	Delaware	14.2
10	Mississippi	15.4		22	Tennessee	14.2
30	Missouri	13.8		25	South Carolina	14.1
44	Montana	12.2		26	New Jersey	14.0
21	Nebraska	14.3		26	New York	14.0
5	Nevada	16.2		28	Maryland	13.9
47	New Hampshire	11.7		28	Virginia	13.9
26	New Jersey	14.0		30	Minnesota	13.8
8	New Mexico	15.6		30	Missouri	13.8
26	New York	14.0		30	Washington	13.8
14	North Carolina	14.9		33	Kentucky	13.7
45	North Dakota	12.1		34	Ohio	13.6
34	Ohio	13.6		34	Oregon	13.6
15	Oklahoma	14.6		36	Michigan	13.5
34	Oregon	13.6		37	Connecticut	13.2
45	Pennsylvania	12.1		38	Iowa	13.1
43	Rhode Island	12.5		38	Massachusetts	13.1
25	South Carolina	14.1		40	Florida	13.0
18	South Dakota	14.4		40	Wisconsin	13.0
22	Tennessee	14.2		42	Wyoming	12.8
2	Texas	17.4		43	Rhode Island	12.5
1	Utah	21.7		44	Montana	12.2
49	Vermont	11.1		45	North Dakota	12.1
28	Virginia	13.9		45	Pennsylvania	12.1
30	Washington	13.8		47	New Hampshire	11.7
48	West Virginia	11.5		48	West Virginia	11.5
40	Wisconsin	13.0		49	Vermont	11.1
42	Wyoming	12.8		50	Maine	10.9
					District of Columbia	14.5

Source: U.S. Department of Health and Human Services, National Center for Health Statistics
        "National Vital Statistics Reports" (Vol. 49, No. 5, July 24, 2001)
*Final data by state of residence.

Birth Rate in 1990

National Rate = 16.7 Births per 1,000 Population*

ALPHA ORDER

RANK	STATE	RATE
26	Alabama	15.7
1	Alaska	21.6
4	Arizona	18.8
29	Arkansas	15.5
3	California	20.6
20	Colorado	16.2
38	Connecticut	15.2
15	Delaware	16.7
32	Florida	15.4
9	Georgia	17.4
6	Hawaii	18.5
18	Idaho	16.3
10	Illinois	17.1
28	Indiana	15.6
48	Iowa	14.2
26	Kansas	15.7
43	Kentucky	14.8
10	Louisiana	17.1
49	Maine	14.1
13	Maryland	16.8
32	Massachusetts	15.4
16	Michigan	16.5
29	Minnesota	15.5
12	Mississippi	16.9
29	Missouri	15.5
45	Montana	14.5
32	Nebraska	15.4
8	Nevada	18.0
22	New Hampshire	15.8
22	New Jersey	15.8
7	New Mexico	18.1
16	New York	16.5
22	North Carolina	15.8
45	North Dakota	14.5
32	Ohio	15.4
39	Oklahoma	15.1
39	Oregon	15.1
45	Pennsylvania	14.5
39	Rhode Island	15.1
13	South Carolina	16.8
22	South Dakota	15.8
32	Tennessee	15.4
5	Texas	18.6
2	Utah	21.1
44	Vermont	14.7
21	Virginia	16.1
18	Washington	16.3
50	West Virginia	12.6
42	Wisconsin	14.9
32	Wyoming	15.4

RANK ORDER

RANK	STATE	RATE
1	Alaska	21.6
2	Utah	21.1
3	California	20.6
4	Arizona	18.8
5	Texas	18.6
6	Hawaii	18.5
7	New Mexico	18.1
8	Nevada	18.0
9	Georgia	17.4
10	Illinois	17.1
10	Louisiana	17.1
12	Mississippi	16.9
13	Maryland	16.8
13	South Carolina	16.8
15	Delaware	16.7
16	Michigan	16.5
16	New York	16.5
18	Idaho	16.3
18	Washington	16.3
20	Colorado	16.2
21	Virginia	16.1
22	New Hampshire	15.8
22	New Jersey	15.8
22	North Carolina	15.8
22	South Dakota	15.8
26	Alabama	15.7
26	Kansas	15.7
28	Indiana	15.6
29	Arkansas	15.5
29	Minnesota	15.5
29	Missouri	15.5
32	Florida	15.4
32	Massachusetts	15.4
32	Nebraska	15.4
32	Ohio	15.4
32	Tennessee	15.4
32	Wyoming	15.4
38	Connecticut	15.2
39	Oklahoma	15.1
39	Oregon	15.1
39	Rhode Island	15.1
42	Wisconsin	14.9
43	Kentucky	14.8
44	Vermont	14.7
45	Montana	14.5
45	North Dakota	14.5
45	Pennsylvania	14.5
48	Iowa	14.2
49	Maine	14.1
50	West Virginia	12.6
	District of Columbia	19.5

Source: U.S. Department of Health and Human Services, National Center for Health Statistics
"Monthly Vital Statistics Report" (Vol. 41, No. 9, Supplement, February 25, 1993)
*Final data by state of residence.

Birth Rate in 1980

National Rate = 15.9 Births per 1,000 Population*

<table>
<tr><td colspan="3">ALPHA ORDER</td><td colspan="3">RANK ORDER</td></tr>
<tr><td>RANK</td><td>STATE</td><td>RATE</td><td>RANK</td><td>STATE</td><td>RATE</td></tr>
<tr><td>27</td><td>Alabama</td><td>16.3</td><td>1</td><td>Utah</td><td>28.6</td></tr>
<tr><td>2</td><td>Alaska</td><td>23.7</td><td>2</td><td>Alaska</td><td>23.7</td></tr>
<tr><td>11</td><td>Arizona</td><td>18.4</td><td>3</td><td>Wyoming</td><td>22.5</td></tr>
<tr><td>27</td><td>Arkansas</td><td>16.3</td><td>4</td><td>Idaho</td><td>21.4</td></tr>
<tr><td>18</td><td>California</td><td>17.0</td><td>5</td><td>New Mexico</td><td>20.0</td></tr>
<tr><td>15</td><td>Colorado</td><td>17.2</td><td>6</td><td>Louisiana</td><td>19.5</td></tr>
<tr><td>50</td><td>Connecticut</td><td>12.5</td><td>7</td><td>South Dakota</td><td>19.2</td></tr>
<tr><td>33</td><td>Delaware</td><td>15.8</td><td>7</td><td>Texas</td><td>19.2</td></tr>
<tr><td>45</td><td>Florida</td><td>13.5</td><td>9</td><td>Mississippi</td><td>19.0</td></tr>
<tr><td>19</td><td>Georgia</td><td>16.9</td><td>10</td><td>Hawaii</td><td>18.8</td></tr>
<tr><td>10</td><td>Hawaii</td><td>18.8</td><td>11</td><td>Arizona</td><td>18.4</td></tr>
<tr><td>4</td><td>Idaho</td><td>21.4</td><td>11</td><td>North Dakota</td><td>18.4</td></tr>
<tr><td>20</td><td>Illinois</td><td>16.6</td><td>13</td><td>Montana</td><td>18.1</td></tr>
<tr><td>30</td><td>Indiana</td><td>16.1</td><td>14</td><td>Nebraska</td><td>17.4</td></tr>
<tr><td>24</td><td>Iowa</td><td>16.4</td><td>15</td><td>Colorado</td><td>17.2</td></tr>
<tr><td>15</td><td>Kansas</td><td>17.2</td><td>15</td><td>Kansas</td><td>17.2</td></tr>
<tr><td>27</td><td>Kentucky</td><td>16.3</td><td>15</td><td>Oklahoma</td><td>17.2</td></tr>
<tr><td>6</td><td>Louisiana</td><td>19.5</td><td>18</td><td>California</td><td>17.0</td></tr>
<tr><td>41</td><td>Maine</td><td>14.6</td><td>19</td><td>Georgia</td><td>16.9</td></tr>
<tr><td>43</td><td>Maryland</td><td>14.2</td><td>20</td><td>Illinois</td><td>16.6</td></tr>
<tr><td>49</td><td>Massachusetts</td><td>12.7</td><td>20</td><td>Minnesota</td><td>16.6</td></tr>
<tr><td>34</td><td>Michigan</td><td>15.7</td><td>20</td><td>Nevada</td><td>16.6</td></tr>
<tr><td>20</td><td>Minnesota</td><td>16.6</td><td>20</td><td>South Carolina</td><td>16.6</td></tr>
<tr><td>9</td><td>Mississippi</td><td>19.0</td><td>24</td><td>Iowa</td><td>16.4</td></tr>
<tr><td>30</td><td>Missouri</td><td>16.1</td><td>24</td><td>Oregon</td><td>16.4</td></tr>
<tr><td>13</td><td>Montana</td><td>18.1</td><td>24</td><td>Washington</td><td>16.4</td></tr>
<tr><td>14</td><td>Nebraska</td><td>17.4</td><td>27</td><td>Alabama</td><td>16.3</td></tr>
<tr><td>20</td><td>Nevada</td><td>16.6</td><td>27</td><td>Arkansas</td><td>16.3</td></tr>
<tr><td>39</td><td>New Hampshire</td><td>14.9</td><td>27</td><td>Kentucky</td><td>16.3</td></tr>
<tr><td>47</td><td>New Jersey</td><td>13.2</td><td>30</td><td>Indiana</td><td>16.1</td></tr>
<tr><td>5</td><td>New Mexico</td><td>20.0</td><td>30</td><td>Missouri</td><td>16.1</td></tr>
<tr><td>44</td><td>New York</td><td>13.6</td><td>32</td><td>Wisconsin</td><td>15.9</td></tr>
<tr><td>42</td><td>North Carolina</td><td>14.4</td><td>33</td><td>Delaware</td><td>15.8</td></tr>
<tr><td>11</td><td>North Dakota</td><td>18.4</td><td>34</td><td>Michigan</td><td>15.7</td></tr>
<tr><td>34</td><td>Ohio</td><td>15.7</td><td>34</td><td>Ohio</td><td>15.7</td></tr>
<tr><td>15</td><td>Oklahoma</td><td>17.2</td><td>36</td><td>Vermont</td><td>15.4</td></tr>
<tr><td>24</td><td>Oregon</td><td>16.4</td><td>37</td><td>Tennessee</td><td>15.1</td></tr>
<tr><td>46</td><td>Pennsylvania</td><td>13.4</td><td>37</td><td>West Virginia</td><td>15.1</td></tr>
<tr><td>48</td><td>Rhode Island</td><td>12.9</td><td>39</td><td>New Hampshire</td><td>14.9</td></tr>
<tr><td>20</td><td>South Carolina</td><td>16.6</td><td>40</td><td>Virginia</td><td>14.7</td></tr>
<tr><td>7</td><td>South Dakota</td><td>19.2</td><td>41</td><td>Maine</td><td>14.6</td></tr>
<tr><td>37</td><td>Tennessee</td><td>15.1</td><td>42</td><td>North Carolina</td><td>14.4</td></tr>
<tr><td>7</td><td>Texas</td><td>19.2</td><td>43</td><td>Maryland</td><td>14.2</td></tr>
<tr><td>1</td><td>Utah</td><td>28.6</td><td>44</td><td>New York</td><td>13.6</td></tr>
<tr><td>36</td><td>Vermont</td><td>15.4</td><td>45</td><td>Florida</td><td>13.5</td></tr>
<tr><td>40</td><td>Virginia</td><td>14.7</td><td>46</td><td>Pennsylvania</td><td>13.4</td></tr>
<tr><td>24</td><td>Washington</td><td>16.4</td><td>47</td><td>New Jersey</td><td>13.2</td></tr>
<tr><td>37</td><td>West Virginia</td><td>15.1</td><td>48</td><td>Rhode Island</td><td>12.9</td></tr>
<tr><td>32</td><td>Wisconsin</td><td>15.9</td><td>49</td><td>Massachusetts</td><td>12.7</td></tr>
<tr><td>3</td><td>Wyoming</td><td>22.5</td><td>50</td><td>Connecticut</td><td>12.5</td></tr>
<tr><td></td><td></td><td></td><td></td><td>District of Columbia</td><td>14.7</td></tr>
</table>

Source: U.S. Department of Health and Human Services, National Center for Health Statistics
"Vital Statistics of the United States, 1980" and "Monthly Vital Statistics Report"
*Live births by state of residence.

Fertility Rate in 2000

National Rate = 67.6 Live Births per 1,000 Women 15 to 44 Years Old*

ALPHA ORDER			RANK ORDER		
RANK	STATE	RATE	RANK	STATE	RATE
26	Alabama	65.0	1	Utah	94.5
5	Alaska	75.0	2	Arizona	84.4
2	Arizona	84.4	3	Texas	80.8
15	Arkansas	69.5	4	Nevada	80.0
12	California	70.6	5	Alaska	75.0
7	Colorado	73.1	6	Idaho	74.8
38	Connecticut	61.3	7	Colorado	73.1
32	Delaware	63.5	8	New Mexico	72.7
20	Florida	66.9	9	Hawaii	72.3
11	Georgia	71.4	10	North Carolina	71.5
9	Hawaii	72.3	11	Georgia	71.4
6	Idaho	74.8	12	California	70.6
15	Illinois	69.5	13	Mississippi	70.3
22	Indiana	66.3	14	Oklahoma	70.1
28	Iowa	64.5	15	Arkansas	69.5
17	Kansas	69.3	15	Illinois	69.5
30	Kentucky	63.8	17	Kansas	69.3
18	Louisiana	69.2	18	Louisiana	69.2
48	Maine	49.5	19	Nebraska	68.9
36	Maryland	62.0	20	Florida	66.9
42	Massachusetts	59.2	21	South Dakota	66.8
36	Michigan	62.0	22	Indiana	66.3
31	Minnesota	63.6	23	Oregon	65.8
13	Mississippi	70.3	24	New Jersey	65.5
29	Missouri	64.0	25	Tennessee	65.2
38	Montana	61.3	26	Alabama	65.0
19	Nebraska	68.9	27	New York	64.8
4	Nevada	80.0	28	Iowa	64.5
47	New Hampshire	52.3	29	Missouri	64.0
24	New Jersey	65.5	30	Kentucky	63.8
8	New Mexico	72.7	31	Minnesota	63.6
27	New York	64.8	32	Delaware	63.5
10	North Carolina	71.5	33	South Carolina	63.3
43	North Dakota	58.8	34	Washington	63.2
NA	Ohio**	NA	35	Wyoming	62.7
14	Oklahoma	70.1	36	Maryland	62.0
23	Oregon	65.8	36	Michigan	62.0
44	Pennsylvania	58.2	38	Connecticut	61.3
45	Rhode Island	58.0	38	Montana	61.3
33	South Carolina	63.3	40	Virginia	61.2
21	South Dakota	66.8	41	Wisconsin	60.5
25	Tennessee	65.2	42	Massachusetts	59.2
3	Texas	80.8	43	North Dakota	58.8
1	Utah	94.5	44	Pennsylvania	58.2
49	Vermont	48.8	45	Rhode Island	58.0
40	Virginia	61.2	46	West Virginia	56.0
34	Washington	63.2	47	New Hampshire	52.3
46	West Virginia	56.0	48	Maine	49.5
41	Wisconsin	60.5	49	Vermont	48.8
35	Wyoming	62.7	NA	Ohio**	NA
				District of Columbia	63.0

Source: U.S. Department of Health and Human Services, National Center for Health Statistics
   "National Vital Statistics Reports" (Vol. 49, No. 5, July 24, 2001)
*Data are preliminary estimates by state of residence.
**Not available.

Births to White Women in 2000

National Total = 3,202,932 Live Births to White Women*

<u>ALPHA ORDER</u>

RANK	STATE	BIRTHS	% of USA
24	Alabama	42,075	1.3%
46	Alaska	6,394	0.2%
12	Arizona	74,765	2.3%
32	Arkansas	29,249	0.9%
1	California	429,516	13.4%
19	Colorado	59,679	1.9%
29	Connecticut	36,118	1.1%
44	Delaware	8,010	0.3%
4	Florida	150,614	4.7%
9	Georgia	84,813	2.6%
49	Hawaii	4,018	0.1%
38	Idaho	19,710	0.6%
5	Illinois	142,729	4.5%
11	Indiana	76,279	2.4%
28	Iowa	36,153	1.1%
31	Kansas	35,320	1.1%
21	Kentucky	50,351	1.6%
27	Louisiana	38,169	1.2%
40	Maine	13,185	0.4%
22	Maryland	45,569	1.4%
15	Massachusetts	68,571	2.1%
7	Michigan	107,433	3.4%
20	Minnesota	58,738	1.8%
34	Mississippi	23,558	0.7%
16	Missouri	63,169	2.0%
42	Montana	9,476	0.3%
36	Nebraska	22,293	0.7%
33	Nevada	26,095	0.8%
39	New Hampshire	14,077	0.4%
10	New Jersey	84,254	2.6%
35	New Mexico	22,902	0.7%
3	New York	183,010	5.7%
8	North Carolina	86,393	2.7%
45	North Dakota	6,729	0.2%
NA	Ohio**	NA	NA
26	Oklahoma	38,899	1.2%
25	Oregon	41,694	1.3%
6	Pennsylvania	121,249	3.8%
41	Rhode Island	10,803	0.3%
30	South Carolina	35,338	1.1%
43	South Dakota	8,431	0.3%
17	Tennessee	61,237	1.9%
2	Texas	313,424	9.8%
23	Utah	44,912	1.4%
47	Vermont	6,363	0.2%
13	Virginia	71,173	2.2%
14	Washington	68,679	2.1%
37	West Virginia	20,017	0.6%
18	Wisconsin	59,899	1.9%
48	Wyoming	5,865	0.2%

<u>RANK ORDER</u>

RANK	STATE	BIRTHS	% of USA
1	California	429,516	13.4%
2	Texas	313,424	9.8%
3	New York	183,010	5.7%
4	Florida	150,614	4.7%
5	Illinois	142,729	4.5%
6	Pennsylvania	121,249	3.8%
7	Michigan	107,433	3.4%
8	North Carolina	86,393	2.7%
9	Georgia	84,813	2.6%
10	New Jersey	84,254	2.6%
11	Indiana	76,279	2.4%
12	Arizona	74,765	2.3%
13	Virginia	71,173	2.2%
14	Washington	68,679	2.1%
15	Massachusetts	68,571	2.1%
16	Missouri	63,169	2.0%
17	Tennessee	61,237	1.9%
18	Wisconsin	59,899	1.9%
19	Colorado	59,679	1.9%
20	Minnesota	58,738	1.8%
21	Kentucky	50,351	1.6%
22	Maryland	45,569	1.4%
23	Utah	44,912	1.4%
24	Alabama	42,075	1.3%
25	Oregon	41,694	1.3%
26	Oklahoma	38,899	1.2%
27	Louisiana	38,169	1.2%
28	Iowa	36,153	1.1%
29	Connecticut	36,118	1.1%
30	South Carolina	35,338	1.1%
31	Kansas	35,320	1.1%
32	Arkansas	29,249	0.9%
33	Nevada	26,095	0.8%
34	Mississippi	23,558	0.7%
35	New Mexico	22,902	0.7%
36	Nebraska	22,293	0.7%
37	West Virginia	20,017	0.6%
38	Idaho	19,710	0.6%
39	New Hampshire	14,077	0.4%
40	Maine	13,185	0.4%
41	Rhode Island	10,803	0.3%
42	Montana	9,476	0.3%
43	South Dakota	8,431	0.3%
44	Delaware	8,010	0.3%
45	North Dakota	6,729	0.2%
46	Alaska	6,394	0.2%
47	Vermont	6,363	0.2%
48	Wyoming	5,865	0.2%
49	Hawaii	4,018	0.1%
NA	Ohio**	NA	NA
	District of Columbia	2,325	0.1%

Source: U.S. Department of Health and Human Services, National Center for Health Statistics
"National Vital Statistics Reports" (Vol. 49, No. 5, July 24, 2001)
Preliminary data by state of residence. By race of mother.
**Not available.*

White Births as a Percent of All Births in 2000

National Percent = 78.8% of Live Births*

RANK	STATE	PERCENT
42	Alabama	66.5
44	Alaska	63.8
14	Arizona	87.7
34	Arkansas	76.9
30	California	80.8
9	Colorado	91.2
26	Connecticut	83.7
38	Delaware	72.5
36	Florida	73.8
43	Georgia	63.9
49	Hawaii	22.9
3	Idaho	96.8
33	Illinois	77.1
15	Indiana	87.6
8	Iowa	93.8
13	Kansas	89.0
12	Kentucky	89.6
47	Louisiana	56.2
2	Maine	96.9
46	Maryland	61.3
25	Massachusetts	84.0
31	Michigan	78.8
17	Minnesota	87.2
48	Mississippi	53.4
28	Missouri	82.6
19	Montana	86.4
11	Nebraska	90.4
23	Nevada	84.4
4	New Hampshire	96.3
37	New Jersey	73.2
24	New Mexico	84.1
41	New York	70.9
40	North Carolina	71.8
16	North Dakota	87.4
NA	Ohio**	NA
32	Oklahoma	77.9
10	Oregon	91.0
27	Pennsylvania	82.9
18	Rhode Island	86.5
45	South Carolina	63.0
29	South Dakota	81.4
34	Tennessee	76.9
21	Texas	85.4
6	Utah	94.8
1	Vermont	97.9
39	Virginia	72.0
22	Washington	84.8
5	West Virginia	95.7
20	Wisconsin	86.3
7	Wyoming	93.9

RANK	STATE	PERCENT
1	Vermont	97.9
2	Maine	96.9
3	Idaho	96.8
4	New Hampshire	96.3
5	West Virginia	95.7
6	Utah	94.8
7	Wyoming	93.9
8	Iowa	93.8
9	Colorado	91.2
10	Oregon	91.0
11	Nebraska	90.4
12	Kentucky	89.6
13	Kansas	89.0
14	Arizona	87.7
15	Indiana	87.6
16	North Dakota	87.4
17	Minnesota	87.2
18	Rhode Island	86.5
19	Montana	86.4
20	Wisconsin	86.3
21	Texas	85.4
22	Washington	84.8
23	Nevada	84.4
24	New Mexico	84.1
25	Massachusetts	84.0
26	Connecticut	83.7
27	Pennsylvania	82.9
28	Missouri	82.6
29	South Dakota	81.4
30	California	80.8
31	Michigan	78.8
32	Oklahoma	77.9
33	Illinois	77.1
34	Arkansas	76.9
34	Tennessee	76.9
36	Florida	73.8
37	New Jersey	73.2
38	Delaware	72.5
39	Virginia	72.0
40	North Carolina	71.8
41	New York	70.9
42	Alabama	66.5
43	Georgia	63.9
44	Alaska	63.8
45	South Carolina	63.0
46	Maryland	61.3
47	Louisiana	56.2
48	Mississippi	53.4
49	Hawaii	22.9
NA	Ohio**	NA

District of Columbia 30.3

Source: Morgan Quitno Press using data from U.S. Dept. of Health and Human Services, Nat'l Center for Health Statistics "National Vital Statistics Reports" (Vol. 49, No. 5, July 24, 2001)
*Preliminary data by state of residence. By race of mother.
**Not available.

Births to Black Women in 2000

National Total = 619,970 Live Births to Black Women*

ALPHA ORDER

RANK	STATE	BIRTHS	% of USA
14	Alabama	20,515	3.3%
40	Alaska	466	0.1%
30	Arizona	2,789	0.4%
21	Arkansas	8,031	1.3%
5	California	34,856	5.6%
28	Colorado	3,032	0.5%
24	Connecticut	5,143	0.8%
31	Delaware	2,633	0.4%
2	Florida	47,390	7.6%
3	Georgia	44,066	7.1%
39	Hawaii	472	0.1%
46	Idaho	75	0.0%
6	Illinois	34,243	5.5%
19	Indiana	9,500	1.5%
34	Iowa	1,243	0.2%
29	Kansas	2,869	0.5%
23	Kentucky	5,155	0.8%
8	Louisiana	28,375	4.6%
43	Maine	112	0.0%
9	Maryland	24,918	4.0%
20	Massachusetts	8,101	1.3%
10	Michigan	24,346	3.9%
26	Minnesota	3,935	0.6%
15	Mississippi	19,906	3.2%
18	Missouri	11,465	1.8%
48	Montana	46	0.0%
33	Nebraska	1,376	0.2%
32	Nevada	2,383	0.4%
42	New Hampshire	182	0.0%
12	New Jersey	21,003	3.4%
38	New Mexico	499	0.1%
1	New York	54,729	8.8%
7	North Carolina	29,342	4.7%
45	North Dakota	82	0.0%
NA	Ohio**	NA	NA
25	Oklahoma	4,829	0.8%
36	Oregon	1,023	0.2%
13	Pennsylvania	20,646	3.3%
35	Rhode Island	1,112	0.2%
16	South Carolina	19,741	3.2%
44	South Dakota	106	0.0%
17	Tennessee	16,916	2.7%
4	Texas	40,969	6.6%
41	Utah	332	0.1%
49	Vermont	32	0.0%
11	Virginia	22,507	3.6%
27	Washington	3,496	0.6%
37	West Virginia	775	0.1%
22	Wisconsin	6,494	1.0%
47	Wyoming	57	0.0%

RANK ORDER

RANK	STATE	BIRTHS	% of USA
1	New York	54,729	8.8%
2	Florida	47,390	7.6%
3	Georgia	44,066	7.1%
4	Texas	40,969	6.6%
5	California	34,856	5.6%
6	Illinois	34,243	5.5%
7	North Carolina	29,342	4.7%
8	Louisiana	28,375	4.6%
9	Maryland	24,918	4.0%
10	Michigan	24,346	3.9%
11	Virginia	22,507	3.6%
12	New Jersey	21,003	3.4%
13	Pennsylvania	20,646	3.3%
14	Alabama	20,515	3.3%
15	Mississippi	19,906	3.2%
16	South Carolina	19,741	3.2%
17	Tennessee	16,916	2.7%
18	Missouri	11,465	1.8%
19	Indiana	9,500	1.5%
20	Massachusetts	8,101	1.3%
21	Arkansas	8,031	1.3%
22	Wisconsin	6,494	1.0%
23	Kentucky	5,155	0.8%
24	Connecticut	5,143	0.8%
25	Oklahoma	4,829	0.8%
26	Minnesota	3,935	0.6%
27	Washington	3,496	0.6%
28	Colorado	3,032	0.5%
29	Kansas	2,869	0.5%
30	Arizona	2,789	0.4%
31	Delaware	2,633	0.4%
32	Nevada	2,383	0.4%
33	Nebraska	1,376	0.2%
34	Iowa	1,243	0.2%
35	Rhode Island	1,112	0.2%
36	Oregon	1,023	0.2%
37	West Virginia	775	0.1%
38	New Mexico	499	0.1%
39	Hawaii	472	0.1%
40	Alaska	466	0.1%
41	Utah	332	0.1%
42	New Hampshire	182	0.0%
43	Maine	112	0.0%
44	South Dakota	106	0.0%
45	North Dakota	82	0.0%
46	Idaho	75	0.0%
47	Wyoming	57	0.0%
48	Montana	46	0.0%
49	Vermont	32	0.0%
NA	Ohio**	NA	NA
	District of Columbia	5,155	0.8%

Source: U.S. Department of Health and Human Services, National Center for Health Statistics
   "National Vital Statistics Reports" (Vol. 49, No. 5, July 24, 2001)
*Preliminary data by state of residence. By race of mother.
**Not available.

Black Births as a Percent of All Births in 2000

National Percent = 15.3% of Live Births*

ALPHA ORDER

RANK	STATE	PERCENT
6	Alabama	32.4
32	Alaska	4.6
36	Arizona	3.3
13	Arkansas	21.1
29	California	6.6
32	Colorado	4.6
19	Connecticut	11.9
8	Delaware	23.8
9	Florida	23.2
5	Georgia	33.2
38	Hawaii	2.7
48	Idaho	0.4
14	Illinois	18.5
21	Indiana	10.9
37	Iowa	3.2
28	Kansas	7.2
25	Kentucky	9.2
2	Louisiana	41.8
45	Maine	0.8
4	Maryland	33.5
22	Massachusetts	9.9
16	Michigan	17.9
30	Minnesota	5.8
1	Mississippi	45.1
17	Missouri	15.0
48	Montana	0.4
31	Nebraska	5.6
27	Nevada	7.7
41	New Hampshire	1.2
15	New Jersey	18.3
40	New Mexico	1.8
11	New York	21.2
7	North Carolina	24.4
42	North Dakota	1.1
NA	Ohio**	NA
23	Oklahoma	9.7
39	Oregon	2.2
18	Pennsylvania	14.1
26	Rhode Island	8.9
3	South Carolina	35.2
43	South Dakota	1.0
11	Tennessee	21.2
20	Texas	11.2
46	Utah	0.7
47	Vermont	0.5
10	Virginia	22.8
34	Washington	4.3
35	West Virginia	3.7
24	Wisconsin	9.4
44	Wyoming	0.9

RANK ORDER

RANK	STATE	PERCENT
1	Mississippi	45.1
2	Louisiana	41.8
3	South Carolina	35.2
4	Maryland	33.5
5	Georgia	33.2
6	Alabama	32.4
7	North Carolina	24.4
8	Delaware	23.8
9	Florida	23.2
10	Virginia	22.8
11	New York	21.2
11	Tennessee	21.2
13	Arkansas	21.1
14	Illinois	18.5
15	New Jersey	18.3
16	Michigan	17.9
17	Missouri	15.0
18	Pennsylvania	14.1
19	Connecticut	11.9
20	Texas	11.2
21	Indiana	10.9
22	Massachusetts	9.9
23	Oklahoma	9.7
24	Wisconsin	9.4
25	Kentucky	9.2
26	Rhode Island	8.9
27	Nevada	7.7
28	Kansas	7.2
29	California	6.6
30	Minnesota	5.8
31	Nebraska	5.6
32	Alaska	4.6
32	Colorado	4.6
34	Washington	4.3
35	West Virginia	3.7
36	Arizona	3.3
37	Iowa	3.2
38	Hawaii	2.7
39	Oregon	2.2
40	New Mexico	1.8
41	New Hampshire	1.2
42	North Dakota	1.1
43	South Dakota	1.0
44	Wyoming	0.9
45	Maine	0.8
46	Utah	0.7
47	Vermont	0.5
48	Idaho	0.4
48	Montana	0.4
NA	Ohio**	NA

District of Columbia   67.2

Source: Morgan Quitno Press using data from U.S. Dept. of Health and Human Services, Nat'l Center for Health Statistics
"National Vital Statistics Reports" (Vol. 49, No. 5, July 24, 2001)
*Preliminary data by state of residence. By race of mother.
**Not available.

Births of Low Birthweight in 2000

National Total = 308,936 Live Births*

ALPHA ORDER

RANK	STATE	BIRTHS	% of USA
16	Alabama	6,205	2.0%
46	Alaska	561	0.2%
17	Arizona	5,969	1.9%
28	Arkansas	3,271	1.1%
1	California	32,974	10.7%
20	Colorado	5,496	1.8%
29	Connecticut	3,193	1.0%
40	Delaware	950	0.3%
4	Florida	16,332	5.3%
6	Georgia	11,413	3.7%
39	Hawaii	1,316	0.4%
38	Idaho	1,365	0.4%
5	Illinois	14,620	4.7%
14	Indiana	6,446	2.1%
33	Iowa	2,351	0.8%
31	Kansas	2,739	0.9%
22	Kentucky	4,721	1.5%
13	Louisiana	7,000	2.3%
43	Maine	816	0.3%
15	Maryland	6,393	2.1%
19	Massachusetts	5,797	1.9%
8	Michigan	10,766	3.5%
26	Minnesota	3,909	1.3%
23	Mississippi	4,675	1.5%
18	Missouri	5,811	1.9%
44	Montana	680	0.2%
37	Nebraska	1,676	0.5%
34	Nevada	2,226	0.7%
41	New Hampshire	921	0.3%
10	New Jersey	8,860	2.9%
35	New Mexico	2,179	0.7%
3	New York	19,869	6.4%
9	North Carolina	10,582	3.4%
48	North Dakota	493	0.2%
NA	Ohio**	NA	NA
27	Oklahoma	3,693	1.2%
32	Oregon	2,565	0.8%
7	Pennsylvania	11,261	3.6%
42	Rhode Island	899	0.3%
21	South Carolina	5,443	1.8%
45	South Dakota	642	0.2%
12	Tennessee	7,326	2.4%
2	Texas	26,779	8.7%
30	Utah	3,126	1.0%
49	Vermont	396	0.1%
11	Virginia	7,814	2.5%
24	Washington	4,538	1.5%
36	West Virginia	1,736	0.6%
25	Wisconsin	4,513	1.5%
47	Wyoming	519	0.2%

RANK ORDER

RANK	STATE	BIRTHS	% of USA
1	California	32,974	10.7%
2	Texas	26,779	8.7%
3	New York	19,869	6.4%
4	Florida	16,332	5.3%
5	Illinois	14,620	4.7%
6	Georgia	11,413	3.7%
7	Pennsylvania	11,261	3.6%
8	Michigan	10,766	3.5%
9	North Carolina	10,582	3.4%
10	New Jersey	8,860	2.9%
11	Virginia	7,814	2.5%
12	Tennessee	7,326	2.4%
13	Louisiana	7,000	2.3%
14	Indiana	6,446	2.1%
15	Maryland	6,393	2.1%
16	Alabama	6,205	2.0%
17	Arizona	5,969	1.9%
18	Missouri	5,811	1.9%
19	Massachusetts	5,797	1.9%
20	Colorado	5,496	1.8%
21	South Carolina	5,443	1.8%
22	Kentucky	4,721	1.5%
23	Mississippi	4,675	1.5%
24	Washington	4,538	1.5%
25	Wisconsin	4,513	1.5%
26	Minnesota	3,909	1.3%
27	Oklahoma	3,693	1.2%
28	Arkansas	3,271	1.1%
29	Connecticut	3,193	1.0%
30	Utah	3,126	1.0%
31	Kansas	2,739	0.9%
32	Oregon	2,565	0.8%
33	Iowa	2,351	0.8%
34	Nevada	2,226	0.7%
35	New Mexico	2,179	0.7%
36	West Virginia	1,736	0.6%
37	Nebraska	1,676	0.5%
38	Idaho	1,365	0.4%
39	Hawaii	1,316	0.4%
40	Delaware	950	0.3%
41	New Hampshire	921	0.3%
42	Rhode Island	899	0.3%
43	Maine	816	0.3%
44	Montana	680	0.2%
45	South Dakota	642	0.2%
46	Alaska	561	0.2%
47	Wyoming	519	0.2%
48	North Dakota	493	0.2%
49	Vermont	396	0.1%
NA	Ohio**	NA	NA
	District of Columbia	905	0.3%

Source: Morgan Quitno Press using data from U.S. Dept. of Health and Human Services, Nat'l Center for Health Statistics
"National Vital Statistics Reports" (Vol. 49, No. 5, July 24, 2001)
*Births of less than 2,500 grams (5 pounds 8 ounces). Preliminary data by state of residence. Calculated by the editors by multiplying total number of births by percent of such births reported as being low birthweight.
**Not available.

Births of Low Birthweight as a Percent of All Births in 2000

National Percent = 7.6% of Live Births*

ALPHA ORDER				RANK ORDER		
RANK	STATE	PERCENT		RANK	STATE	PERCENT
3	Alabama	9.8		1	Mississippi	10.6
47	Alaska	5.6		2	Louisiana	10.3
32	Arizona	7.0		3	Alabama	9.8
7	Arkansas	8.6		4	South Carolina	9.7
40	California	6.2		5	Tennessee	9.2
11	Colorado	8.4		6	North Carolina	8.8
25	Connecticut	7.4		7	Arkansas	8.6
7	Delaware	8.6		7	Delaware	8.6
15	Florida	8.0		7	Georgia	8.6
7	Georgia	8.6		7	Maryland	8.6
24	Hawaii	7.5		11	Colorado	8.4
35	Idaho	6.7		11	Kentucky	8.4
17	Illinois	7.9		13	West Virginia	8.3
25	Indiana	7.4		13	Wyoming	8.3
43	Iowa	6.1		15	Florida	8.0
33	Kansas	6.9		15	New Mexico	8.0
11	Kentucky	8.4		17	Illinois	7.9
2	Louisiana	10.3		17	Michigan	7.9
45	Maine	6.0		17	Virginia	7.9
7	Maryland	8.6		20	New Jersey	7.7
31	Massachusetts	7.1		20	New York	7.7
17	Michigan	7.9		20	Pennsylvania	7.7
46	Minnesota	5.8		23	Missouri	7.6
1	Mississippi	10.6		24	Hawaii	7.5
23	Missouri	7.6		25	Connecticut	7.4
40	Montana	6.2		25	Indiana	7.4
34	Nebraska	6.8		25	Oklahoma	7.4
29	Nevada	7.2		28	Texas	7.3
39	New Hampshire	6.3		29	Nevada	7.2
20	New Jersey	7.7		29	Rhode Island	7.2
15	New Mexico	8.0		31	Massachusetts	7.1
20	New York	7.7		32	Arizona	7.0
6	North Carolina	8.8		33	Kansas	6.9
38	North Dakota	6.4		34	Nebraska	6.8
NA	Ohio**	NA		35	Idaho	6.7
25	Oklahoma	7.4		36	Utah	6.6
47	Oregon	5.6		37	Wisconsin	6.5
20	Pennsylvania	7.7		38	North Dakota	6.4
29	Rhode Island	7.2		39	New Hampshire	6.3
4	South Carolina	9.7		40	California	6.2
40	South Dakota	6.2		40	Montana	6.2
5	Tennessee	9.2		40	South Dakota	6.2
28	Texas	7.3		43	Iowa	6.1
36	Utah	6.6		43	Vermont	6.1
43	Vermont	6.1		45	Maine	6.0
17	Virginia	7.9		46	Minnesota	5.8
47	Washington	5.6		47	Alaska	5.6
13	West Virginia	8.3		47	Oregon	5.6
37	Wisconsin	6.5		47	Washington	5.6
13	Wyoming	8.3		NA	Ohio**	NA
					District of Columbia	11.8

Source: U.S. Department of Health and Human Services, National Center for Health Statistics
    "National Vital Statistics Reports" (Vol. 49, No. 5, July 24, 2001)
*Estimates based on preliminary data by state of residence. Births of less than 2,500 grams (5 pounds 8 ounces).
**Not available.

Births of Low Birthweight to White Women in 2000

National Total = 208,191 Live Births*

<table>
<tr><td colspan="4">ALPHA ORDER</td><td colspan="4">RANK ORDER</td></tr>
<tr><td>RANK</td><td>STATE</td><td>BIRTHS</td><td>% of USA</td><td>RANK</td><td>STATE</td><td>BIRTHS</td><td>% of USA</td></tr>
<tr><td>21</td><td>Alabama</td><td>3,282</td><td>1.6%</td><td>1</td><td>California</td><td>24,053</td><td>11.6%</td></tr>
<tr><td>48</td><td>Alaska</td><td>313</td><td>0.2%</td><td>2</td><td>Texas</td><td>20,686</td><td>9.9%</td></tr>
<tr><td>12</td><td>Arizona</td><td>5,084</td><td>2.4%</td><td>3</td><td>New York</td><td>12,262</td><td>5.9%</td></tr>
<tr><td>32</td><td>Arkansas</td><td>2,077</td><td>1.0%</td><td>4</td><td>Florida</td><td>9,941</td><td>4.8%</td></tr>
<tr><td>1</td><td>California</td><td>24,053</td><td>11.6%</td><td>5</td><td>Illinois</td><td>9,135</td><td>4.4%</td></tr>
<tr><td>14</td><td>Colorado</td><td>4,774</td><td>2.3%</td><td>6</td><td>Pennsylvania</td><td>8,124</td><td>3.9%</td></tr>
<tr><td>28</td><td>Connecticut</td><td>2,456</td><td>1.2%</td><td>7</td><td>Michigan</td><td>6,876</td><td>3.3%</td></tr>
<tr><td>43</td><td>Delaware</td><td>569</td><td>0.3%</td><td>8</td><td>North Carolina</td><td>6,134</td><td>2.9%</td></tr>
<tr><td>4</td><td>Florida</td><td>9,941</td><td>4.8%</td><td>9</td><td>Georgia</td><td>5,598</td><td>2.7%</td></tr>
<tr><td>9</td><td>Georgia</td><td>5,598</td><td>2.7%</td><td>10</td><td>New Jersey</td><td>5,477</td><td>2.6%</td></tr>
<tr><td>49</td><td>Hawaii</td><td>213</td><td>0.1%</td><td>11</td><td>Indiana</td><td>5,111</td><td>2.5%</td></tr>
<tr><td>38</td><td>Idaho</td><td>1,321</td><td>0.6%</td><td>12</td><td>Arizona</td><td>5,084</td><td>2.4%</td></tr>
<tr><td>5</td><td>Illinois</td><td>9,135</td><td>4.4%</td><td>13</td><td>Tennessee</td><td>4,776</td><td>2.3%</td></tr>
<tr><td>11</td><td>Indiana</td><td>5,111</td><td>2.5%</td><td>14</td><td>Colorado</td><td>4,774</td><td>2.3%</td></tr>
<tr><td>31</td><td>Iowa</td><td>2,133</td><td>1.0%</td><td>15</td><td>Virginia</td><td>4,626</td><td>2.2%</td></tr>
<tr><td>29</td><td>Kansas</td><td>2,296</td><td>1.1%</td><td>16</td><td>Massachusetts</td><td>4,594</td><td>2.2%</td></tr>
<tr><td>18</td><td>Kentucky</td><td>3,927</td><td>1.9%</td><td>17</td><td>Missouri</td><td>4,169</td><td>2.0%</td></tr>
<tr><td>25</td><td>Louisiana</td><td>2,825</td><td>1.4%</td><td>18</td><td>Kentucky</td><td>3,927</td><td>1.9%</td></tr>
<tr><td>40</td><td>Maine</td><td>791</td><td>0.4%</td><td>19</td><td>Washington</td><td>3,640</td><td>1.7%</td></tr>
<tr><td>24</td><td>Maryland</td><td>2,916</td><td>1.4%</td><td>20</td><td>Wisconsin</td><td>3,474</td><td>1.7%</td></tr>
<tr><td>16</td><td>Massachusetts</td><td>4,594</td><td>2.2%</td><td>21</td><td>Alabama</td><td>3,282</td><td>1.6%</td></tr>
<tr><td>7</td><td>Michigan</td><td>6,876</td><td>3.3%</td><td>22</td><td>Minnesota</td><td>3,231</td><td>1.6%</td></tr>
<tr><td>22</td><td>Minnesota</td><td>3,231</td><td>1.6%</td><td>23</td><td>Utah</td><td>2,964</td><td>1.4%</td></tr>
<tr><td>34</td><td>Mississippi</td><td>1,861</td><td>0.9%</td><td>24</td><td>Maryland</td><td>2,916</td><td>1.4%</td></tr>
<tr><td>17</td><td>Missouri</td><td>4,169</td><td>2.0%</td><td>25</td><td>Louisiana</td><td>2,825</td><td>1.4%</td></tr>
<tr><td>42</td><td>Montana</td><td>578</td><td>0.3%</td><td>26</td><td>Oklahoma</td><td>2,684</td><td>1.3%</td></tr>
<tr><td>37</td><td>Nebraska</td><td>1,427</td><td>0.7%</td><td>27</td><td>South Carolina</td><td>2,544</td><td>1.2%</td></tr>
<tr><td>35</td><td>Nevada</td><td>1,748</td><td>0.8%</td><td>28</td><td>Connecticut</td><td>2,456</td><td>1.2%</td></tr>
<tr><td>39</td><td>New Hampshire</td><td>887</td><td>0.4%</td><td>29</td><td>Kansas</td><td>2,296</td><td>1.1%</td></tr>
<tr><td>10</td><td>New Jersey</td><td>5,477</td><td>2.6%</td><td>30</td><td>Oregon</td><td>2,251</td><td>1.1%</td></tr>
<tr><td>33</td><td>New Mexico</td><td>1,878</td><td>0.9%</td><td>31</td><td>Iowa</td><td>2,133</td><td>1.0%</td></tr>
<tr><td>3</td><td>New York</td><td>12,262</td><td>5.9%</td><td>32</td><td>Arkansas</td><td>2,077</td><td>1.0%</td></tr>
<tr><td>8</td><td>North Carolina</td><td>6,134</td><td>2.9%</td><td>33</td><td>New Mexico</td><td>1,878</td><td>0.9%</td></tr>
<tr><td>46</td><td>North Dakota</td><td>431</td><td>0.2%</td><td>34</td><td>Mississippi</td><td>1,861</td><td>0.9%</td></tr>
<tr><td>NA</td><td>Ohio**</td><td>NA</td><td>NA</td><td>35</td><td>Nevada</td><td>1,748</td><td>0.8%</td></tr>
<tr><td>26</td><td>Oklahoma</td><td>2,684</td><td>1.3%</td><td>36</td><td>West Virginia</td><td>1,601</td><td>0.8%</td></tr>
<tr><td>30</td><td>Oregon</td><td>2,251</td><td>1.1%</td><td>37</td><td>Nebraska</td><td>1,427</td><td>0.7%</td></tr>
<tr><td>6</td><td>Pennsylvania</td><td>8,124</td><td>3.9%</td><td>38</td><td>Idaho</td><td>1,321</td><td>0.6%</td></tr>
<tr><td>41</td><td>Rhode Island</td><td>702</td><td>0.3%</td><td>39</td><td>New Hampshire</td><td>887</td><td>0.4%</td></tr>
<tr><td>27</td><td>South Carolina</td><td>2,544</td><td>1.2%</td><td>40</td><td>Maine</td><td>791</td><td>0.4%</td></tr>
<tr><td>44</td><td>South Dakota</td><td>497</td><td>0.2%</td><td>41</td><td>Rhode Island</td><td>702</td><td>0.3%</td></tr>
<tr><td>13</td><td>Tennessee</td><td>4,776</td><td>2.3%</td><td>42</td><td>Montana</td><td>578</td><td>0.3%</td></tr>
<tr><td>2</td><td>Texas</td><td>20,686</td><td>9.9%</td><td>43</td><td>Delaware</td><td>569</td><td>0.3%</td></tr>
<tr><td>23</td><td>Utah</td><td>2,964</td><td>1.4%</td><td>44</td><td>South Dakota</td><td>497</td><td>0.2%</td></tr>
<tr><td>47</td><td>Vermont</td><td>382</td><td>0.2%</td><td>45</td><td>Wyoming</td><td>487</td><td>0.2%</td></tr>
<tr><td>15</td><td>Virginia</td><td>4,626</td><td>2.2%</td><td>46</td><td>North Dakota</td><td>431</td><td>0.2%</td></tr>
<tr><td>19</td><td>Washington</td><td>3,640</td><td>1.7%</td><td>47</td><td>Vermont</td><td>382</td><td>0.2%</td></tr>
<tr><td>36</td><td>West Virginia</td><td>1,601</td><td>0.8%</td><td>48</td><td>Alaska</td><td>313</td><td>0.2%</td></tr>
<tr><td>20</td><td>Wisconsin</td><td>3,474</td><td>1.7%</td><td>49</td><td>Hawaii</td><td>213</td><td>0.1%</td></tr>
<tr><td>45</td><td>Wyoming</td><td>487</td><td>0.2%</td><td>NA</td><td>Ohio**</td><td>NA</td><td>NA</td></tr>
<tr><td></td><td></td><td></td><td></td><td></td><td>District of Columbia</td><td>172</td><td>0.1%</td></tr>
</table>

Source: Morgan Quitno Press using data from U.S. Dept. of Health and Human Services, Nat'l Center for Health Statistics
 "National Vital Statistics Reports" (Vol. 49, No. 5, July 24, 2001)
*Births of less than 2,500 grams (5 pounds 8 ounces).   Preliminary data by state of residence. Calculated by the editors by multiplying total number of births to white women by percent of births to white women reported as being low birthweight.
**Not available.

Births of Low Birthweight to White Women
As a Percent of All Births to White Women in 2000
National Percent = 6.5% of Live Births to White Women*

ALPHA ORDER

RANK	STATE	PERCENT
6	Alabama	7.8
49	Alaska	4.9
15	Arizona	6.8
11	Arkansas	7.1
44	California	5.6
3	Colorado	8.0
15	Connecticut	6.8
11	Delaware	7.1
23	Florida	6.6
23	Georgia	6.6
47	Hawaii	5.3
17	Idaho	6.7
32	Illinois	6.4
17	Indiana	6.7
41	Iowa	5.9
28	Kansas	6.5
6	Kentucky	7.8
9	Louisiana	7.4
39	Maine	6.0
32	Maryland	6.4
17	Massachusetts	6.7
32	Michigan	6.4
45	Minnesota	5.5
5	Mississippi	7.9
23	Missouri	6.6
38	Montana	6.1
32	Nebraska	6.4
17	Nevada	6.7
37	New Hampshire	6.3
28	New Jersey	6.5
2	New Mexico	8.2
17	New York	6.7
11	North Carolina	7.1
32	North Dakota	6.4
NA	Ohio**	NA
14	Oklahoma	6.9
46	Oregon	5.4
17	Pennsylvania	6.7
28	Rhode Island	6.5
10	South Carolina	7.2
41	South Dakota	5.9
6	Tennessee	7.8
23	Texas	6.6
23	Utah	6.6
39	Vermont	6.0
28	Virginia	6.5
47	Washington	5.3
3	West Virginia	8.0
43	Wisconsin	5.8
1	Wyoming	8.3

RANK ORDER

RANK	STATE	PERCENT
1	Wyoming	8.3
2	New Mexico	8.2
3	Colorado	8.0
3	West Virginia	8.0
5	Mississippi	7.9
6	Alabama	7.8
6	Kentucky	7.8
6	Tennessee	7.8
9	Louisiana	7.4
10	South Carolina	7.2
11	Arkansas	7.1
11	Delaware	7.1
11	North Carolina	7.1
14	Oklahoma	6.9
15	Arizona	6.8
15	Connecticut	6.8
17	Idaho	6.7
17	Indiana	6.7
17	Massachusetts	6.7
17	Nevada	6.7
17	New York	6.7
17	Pennsylvania	6.7
23	Florida	6.6
23	Georgia	6.6
23	Missouri	6.6
23	Texas	6.6
23	Utah	6.6
28	Kansas	6.5
28	New Jersey	6.5
28	Rhode Island	6.5
28	Virginia	6.5
32	Illinois	6.4
32	Maryland	6.4
32	Michigan	6.4
32	Nebraska	6.4
32	North Dakota	6.4
37	New Hampshire	6.3
38	Montana	6.1
39	Maine	6.0
39	Vermont	6.0
41	Iowa	5.9
41	South Dakota	5.9
43	Wisconsin	5.8
44	California	5.6
45	Minnesota	5.5
46	Oregon	5.4
47	Hawaii	5.3
47	Washington	5.3
49	Alaska	4.9
NA	Ohio**	NA

District of Columbia 7.4

Source: U.S. Department of Health and Human Services, National Center for Health Statistics
"National Vital Statistics Reports" (Vol. 49, No. 5, July 24, 2001)
*Estimates based on preliminary data by state of residence. Births of less than 2,500 grams (5 pounds 8 ounces).
**Not available.

Births of Low Birthweight to Black Women in 2000

National Total = 79,976 Live Births*

<table>
<tr><td colspan="4">ALPHA ORDER</td><td colspan="4">RANK ORDER</td></tr>
<tr><td>RANK</td><td>STATE</td><td>BIRTHS</td><td>% of USA</td><td>RANK</td><td>STATE</td><td>BIRTHS</td><td>% of USA</td></tr>
<tr><td>11</td><td>Alabama</td><td>2,913</td><td>3.6%</td><td>1</td><td>New York</td><td>6,239</td><td>7.8%</td></tr>
<tr><td>39</td><td>Alaska</td><td>55</td><td>0.1%</td><td>2</td><td>Florida</td><td>5,829</td><td>7.3%</td></tr>
<tr><td>29</td><td>Arizona</td><td>357</td><td>0.4%</td><td>3</td><td>Georgia</td><td>5,596</td><td>7.0%</td></tr>
<tr><td>20</td><td>Arkansas</td><td>1,100</td><td>1.4%</td><td>4</td><td>Texas</td><td>5,203</td><td>6.5%</td></tr>
<tr><td>7</td><td>California</td><td>4,008</td><td>5.0%</td><td>5</td><td>Illinois</td><td>4,828</td><td>6.0%</td></tr>
<tr><td>26</td><td>Colorado</td><td>449</td><td>0.6%</td><td>6</td><td>Louisiana</td><td>4,058</td><td>5.1%</td></tr>
<tr><td>25</td><td>Connecticut</td><td>607</td><td>0.8%</td><td>7</td><td>California</td><td>4,008</td><td>5.0%</td></tr>
<tr><td>31</td><td>Delaware</td><td>348</td><td>0.4%</td><td>8</td><td>North Carolina</td><td>3,991</td><td>5.0%</td></tr>
<tr><td>2</td><td>Florida</td><td>5,829</td><td>7.3%</td><td>9</td><td>Michigan</td><td>3,530</td><td>4.4%</td></tr>
<tr><td>3</td><td>Georgia</td><td>5,596</td><td>7.0%</td><td>10</td><td>Maryland</td><td>3,190</td><td>4.0%</td></tr>
<tr><td>40</td><td>Hawaii</td><td>49</td><td>0.1%</td><td>11</td><td>Alabama</td><td>2,913</td><td>3.6%</td></tr>
<tr><td>NA</td><td>Idaho**</td><td>NA</td><td>NA</td><td>12</td><td>Virginia</td><td>2,813</td><td>3.5%</td></tr>
<tr><td>5</td><td>Illinois</td><td>4,828</td><td>6.0%</td><td>13</td><td>South Carolina</td><td>2,803</td><td>3.5%</td></tr>
<tr><td>19</td><td>Indiana</td><td>1,188</td><td>1.5%</td><td>14</td><td>Mississippi</td><td>2,787</td><td>3.5%</td></tr>
<tr><td>35</td><td>Iowa</td><td>145</td><td>0.2%</td><td>14</td><td>Pennsylvania</td><td>2,787</td><td>3.5%</td></tr>
<tr><td>30</td><td>Kansas</td><td>350</td><td>0.4%</td><td>16</td><td>New Jersey</td><td>2,667</td><td>3.3%</td></tr>
<tr><td>23</td><td>Kentucky</td><td>706</td><td>0.9%</td><td>17</td><td>Tennessee</td><td>2,470</td><td>3.1%</td></tr>
<tr><td>6</td><td>Louisiana</td><td>4,058</td><td>5.1%</td><td>18</td><td>Missouri</td><td>1,513</td><td>1.9%</td></tr>
<tr><td>NA</td><td>Maine**</td><td>NA</td><td>NA</td><td>19</td><td>Indiana</td><td>1,188</td><td>1.5%</td></tr>
<tr><td>10</td><td>Maryland</td><td>3,190</td><td>4.0%</td><td>20</td><td>Arkansas</td><td>1,100</td><td>1.4%</td></tr>
<tr><td>21</td><td>Massachusetts</td><td>867</td><td>1.1%</td><td>21</td><td>Massachusetts</td><td>867</td><td>1.1%</td></tr>
<tr><td>9</td><td>Michigan</td><td>3,530</td><td>4.4%</td><td>22</td><td>Wisconsin</td><td>864</td><td>1.1%</td></tr>
<tr><td>27</td><td>Minnesota</td><td>425</td><td>0.5%</td><td>23</td><td>Kentucky</td><td>706</td><td>0.9%</td></tr>
<tr><td>14</td><td>Mississippi</td><td>2,787</td><td>3.5%</td><td>24</td><td>Oklahoma</td><td>623</td><td>0.8%</td></tr>
<tr><td>18</td><td>Missouri</td><td>1,513</td><td>1.9%</td><td>25</td><td>Connecticut</td><td>607</td><td>0.8%</td></tr>
<tr><td>NA</td><td>Montana**</td><td>NA</td><td>NA</td><td>26</td><td>Colorado</td><td>449</td><td>0.6%</td></tr>
<tr><td>33</td><td>Nebraska</td><td>179</td><td>0.2%</td><td>27</td><td>Minnesota</td><td>425</td><td>0.5%</td></tr>
<tr><td>32</td><td>Nevada</td><td>307</td><td>0.4%</td><td>28</td><td>Washington</td><td>374</td><td>0.5%</td></tr>
<tr><td>NA</td><td>New Hampshire**</td><td>NA</td><td>NA</td><td>29</td><td>Arizona</td><td>357</td><td>0.4%</td></tr>
<tr><td>16</td><td>New Jersey</td><td>2,667</td><td>3.3%</td><td>30</td><td>Kansas</td><td>350</td><td>0.4%</td></tr>
<tr><td>38</td><td>New Mexico</td><td>65</td><td>0.1%</td><td>31</td><td>Delaware</td><td>348</td><td>0.4%</td></tr>
<tr><td>1</td><td>New York</td><td>6,239</td><td>7.8%</td><td>32</td><td>Nevada</td><td>307</td><td>0.4%</td></tr>
<tr><td>8</td><td>North Carolina</td><td>3,991</td><td>5.0%</td><td>33</td><td>Nebraska</td><td>179</td><td>0.2%</td></tr>
<tr><td>NA</td><td>North Dakota**</td><td>NA</td><td>NA</td><td>34</td><td>Rhode Island</td><td>146</td><td>0.2%</td></tr>
<tr><td>NA</td><td>Ohio**</td><td>NA</td><td>NA</td><td>35</td><td>Iowa</td><td>145</td><td>0.2%</td></tr>
<tr><td>24</td><td>Oklahoma</td><td>623</td><td>0.8%</td><td>36</td><td>West Virginia</td><td>120</td><td>0.2%</td></tr>
<tr><td>37</td><td>Oregon</td><td>112</td><td>0.1%</td><td>37</td><td>Oregon</td><td>112</td><td>0.1%</td></tr>
<tr><td>14</td><td>Pennsylvania</td><td>2,787</td><td>3.5%</td><td>38</td><td>New Mexico</td><td>65</td><td>0.1%</td></tr>
<tr><td>34</td><td>Rhode Island</td><td>146</td><td>0.2%</td><td>39</td><td>Alaska</td><td>55</td><td>0.1%</td></tr>
<tr><td>13</td><td>South Carolina</td><td>2,803</td><td>3.5%</td><td>40</td><td>Hawaii</td><td>49</td><td>0.1%</td></tr>
<tr><td>NA</td><td>South Dakota**</td><td>NA</td><td>NA</td><td>41</td><td>Utah</td><td>42</td><td>0.1%</td></tr>
<tr><td>17</td><td>Tennessee</td><td>2,470</td><td>3.1%</td><td>NA</td><td>Idaho**</td><td>NA</td><td>NA</td></tr>
<tr><td>4</td><td>Texas</td><td>5,203</td><td>6.5%</td><td>NA</td><td>Maine**</td><td>NA</td><td>NA</td></tr>
<tr><td>41</td><td>Utah</td><td>42</td><td>0.1%</td><td>NA</td><td>Montana**</td><td>NA</td><td>NA</td></tr>
<tr><td>NA</td><td>Vermont**</td><td>NA</td><td>NA</td><td>NA</td><td>New Hampshire**</td><td>NA</td><td>NA</td></tr>
<tr><td>12</td><td>Virginia</td><td>2,813</td><td>3.5%</td><td>NA</td><td>North Dakota**</td><td>NA</td><td>NA</td></tr>
<tr><td>28</td><td>Washington</td><td>374</td><td>0.5%</td><td>NA</td><td>Ohio**</td><td>NA</td><td>NA</td></tr>
<tr><td>36</td><td>West Virginia</td><td>120</td><td>0.2%</td><td>NA</td><td>South Dakota**</td><td>NA</td><td>NA</td></tr>
<tr><td>22</td><td>Wisconsin</td><td>864</td><td>1.1%</td><td>NA</td><td>Vermont**</td><td>NA</td><td>NA</td></tr>
<tr><td>NA</td><td>Wyoming**</td><td>NA</td><td>NA</td><td>NA</td><td>Wyoming**</td><td>NA</td><td>NA</td></tr>
<tr><td></td><td></td><td></td><td></td><td></td><td>District of Columbia</td><td>717</td><td>0.9%</td></tr>
</table>

Source: Morgan Quitno Press using data from U.S. Dept. of Health and Human Services, Nat'l Center for Health Statistics "National Vital Statistics Reports" (Vol. 49, No. 5, July 24, 2001)

Births of less than 2,500 grams (5 pounds 8 ounces). Preliminary data by state of residence. Calculated by the editors by multiplying total number of births to black women by percent of births to black women reported as being low birthweight.

**Insufficient data.*

Births of Low Birthweight to Black Women
As a Percent of All Births to Black Women in 2000
National Percent = 12.9% of Live Births to Black Women*

<table>
<tr><td colspan="3">ALPHA ORDER</td><td colspan="3">RANK ORDER</td></tr>
<tr><td>RANK</td><td>STATE</td><td>PERCENT</td><td>RANK</td><td>STATE</td><td>PERCENT</td></tr>
<tr><td>6</td><td>Alabama</td><td>14.2</td><td>1</td><td>West Virginia</td><td>15.5</td></tr>
<tr><td>32</td><td>Alaska</td><td>11.9</td><td>2</td><td>Colorado</td><td>14.8</td></tr>
<tr><td>22</td><td>Arizona</td><td>12.8</td><td>3</td><td>Tennessee</td><td>14.6</td></tr>
<tr><td>10</td><td>Arkansas</td><td>13.7</td><td>4</td><td>Michigan</td><td>14.5</td></tr>
<tr><td>35</td><td>California</td><td>11.5</td><td>5</td><td>Louisiana</td><td>14.3</td></tr>
<tr><td>2</td><td>Colorado</td><td>14.8</td><td>6</td><td>Alabama</td><td>14.2</td></tr>
<tr><td>33</td><td>Connecticut</td><td>11.8</td><td>6</td><td>South Carolina</td><td>14.2</td></tr>
<tr><td>15</td><td>Delaware</td><td>13.2</td><td>8</td><td>Illinois</td><td>14.1</td></tr>
<tr><td>30</td><td>Florida</td><td>12.3</td><td>9</td><td>Mississippi</td><td>14.0</td></tr>
<tr><td>24</td><td>Georgia</td><td>12.7</td><td>10</td><td>Arkansas</td><td>13.7</td></tr>
<tr><td>41</td><td>Hawaii</td><td>10.4</td><td>10</td><td>Kentucky</td><td>13.7</td></tr>
<tr><td>NA</td><td>Idaho**</td><td>NA</td><td>12</td><td>North Carolina</td><td>13.6</td></tr>
<tr><td>8</td><td>Illinois</td><td>14.1</td><td>13</td><td>Pennsylvania</td><td>13.5</td></tr>
<tr><td>27</td><td>Indiana</td><td>12.5</td><td>14</td><td>Wisconsin</td><td>13.3</td></tr>
<tr><td>34</td><td>Iowa</td><td>11.7</td><td>15</td><td>Delaware</td><td>13.2</td></tr>
<tr><td>31</td><td>Kansas</td><td>12.2</td><td>15</td><td>Missouri</td><td>13.2</td></tr>
<tr><td>10</td><td>Kentucky</td><td>13.7</td><td>17</td><td>Rhode Island</td><td>13.1</td></tr>
<tr><td>5</td><td>Louisiana</td><td>14.3</td><td>18</td><td>Nebraska</td><td>13.0</td></tr>
<tr><td>NA</td><td>Maine**</td><td>NA</td><td>18</td><td>New Mexico</td><td>13.0</td></tr>
<tr><td>22</td><td>Maryland</td><td>12.8</td><td>20</td><td>Nevada</td><td>12.9</td></tr>
<tr><td>39</td><td>Massachusetts</td><td>10.7</td><td>20</td><td>Oklahoma</td><td>12.9</td></tr>
<tr><td>4</td><td>Michigan</td><td>14.5</td><td>22</td><td>Arizona</td><td>12.8</td></tr>
<tr><td>38</td><td>Minnesota</td><td>10.8</td><td>22</td><td>Maryland</td><td>12.8</td></tr>
<tr><td>9</td><td>Mississippi</td><td>14.0</td><td>24</td><td>Georgia</td><td>12.7</td></tr>
<tr><td>15</td><td>Missouri</td><td>13.2</td><td>24</td><td>New Jersey</td><td>12.7</td></tr>
<tr><td>NA</td><td>Montana**</td><td>NA</td><td>24</td><td>Texas</td><td>12.7</td></tr>
<tr><td>18</td><td>Nebraska</td><td>13.0</td><td>27</td><td>Indiana</td><td>12.5</td></tr>
<tr><td>20</td><td>Nevada</td><td>12.9</td><td>27</td><td>Utah</td><td>12.5</td></tr>
<tr><td>NA</td><td>New Hampshire**</td><td>NA</td><td>27</td><td>Virginia</td><td>12.5</td></tr>
<tr><td>24</td><td>New Jersey</td><td>12.7</td><td>30</td><td>Florida</td><td>12.3</td></tr>
<tr><td>18</td><td>New Mexico</td><td>13.0</td><td>31</td><td>Kansas</td><td>12.2</td></tr>
<tr><td>36</td><td>New York</td><td>11.4</td><td>32</td><td>Alaska</td><td>11.9</td></tr>
<tr><td>12</td><td>North Carolina</td><td>13.6</td><td>33</td><td>Connecticut</td><td>11.8</td></tr>
<tr><td>NA</td><td>North Dakota**</td><td>NA</td><td>34</td><td>Iowa</td><td>11.7</td></tr>
<tr><td>NA</td><td>Ohio**</td><td>NA</td><td>35</td><td>California</td><td>11.5</td></tr>
<tr><td>20</td><td>Oklahoma</td><td>12.9</td><td>36</td><td>New York</td><td>11.4</td></tr>
<tr><td>37</td><td>Oregon</td><td>10.9</td><td>37</td><td>Oregon</td><td>10.9</td></tr>
<tr><td>13</td><td>Pennsylvania</td><td>13.5</td><td>38</td><td>Minnesota</td><td>10.8</td></tr>
<tr><td>17</td><td>Rhode Island</td><td>13.1</td><td>39</td><td>Massachusetts</td><td>10.7</td></tr>
<tr><td>6</td><td>South Carolina</td><td>14.2</td><td>39</td><td>Washington</td><td>10.7</td></tr>
<tr><td>NA</td><td>South Dakota**</td><td>NA</td><td>41</td><td>Hawaii</td><td>10.4</td></tr>
<tr><td>3</td><td>Tennessee</td><td>14.6</td><td>NA</td><td>Idaho**</td><td>NA</td></tr>
<tr><td>24</td><td>Texas</td><td>12.7</td><td>NA</td><td>Maine**</td><td>NA</td></tr>
<tr><td>27</td><td>Utah</td><td>12.5</td><td>NA</td><td>Montana**</td><td>NA</td></tr>
<tr><td>NA</td><td>Vermont**</td><td>NA</td><td>NA</td><td>New Hampshire**</td><td>NA</td></tr>
<tr><td>27</td><td>Virginia</td><td>12.5</td><td>NA</td><td>North Dakota**</td><td>NA</td></tr>
<tr><td>39</td><td>Washington</td><td>10.7</td><td>NA</td><td>Ohio**</td><td>NA</td></tr>
<tr><td>1</td><td>West Virginia</td><td>15.5</td><td>NA</td><td>South Dakota**</td><td>NA</td></tr>
<tr><td>14</td><td>Wisconsin</td><td>13.3</td><td>NA</td><td>Vermont**</td><td>NA</td></tr>
<tr><td>NA</td><td>Wyoming**</td><td>NA</td><td>NA</td><td>Wyoming**</td><td>NA</td></tr>
<tr><td></td><td></td><td></td><td></td><td>District of Columbia</td><td>13.9</td></tr>
</table>

Source: U.S. Department of Health and Human Services, National Center for Health Statistics
"National Vital Statistics Reports" (Vol. 49, No. 5, July 24, 2001)
*Estimates based on preliminary data by state of residence. Births of less than 2,500 grams (5 pounds 8 ounces).
**Insufficient data.

Births to Unmarried Women in 2000

National Total = 1,345,498 Live Births*

ALPHA ORDER

RANK ORDER

RANK	STATE	BIRTHS	% of USA
20	Alabama	21,718	1.6%
46	Alaska	3,309	0.2%
10	Arizona	33,513	2.5%
29	Arkansas	13,577	1.0%
1	California	173,377	12.9%
27	Colorado	16,359	1.2%
30	Connecticut	12,558	0.9%
42	Delaware	4,199	0.3%
4	Florida	78,190	5.8%
6	Georgia	49,103	3.6%
38	Hawaii	5,649	0.4%
39	Idaho	4,400	0.3%
5	Illinois	63,848	4.7%
13	Indiana	30,315	2.3%
34	Iowa	10,793	0.8%
32	Kansas	11,510	0.9%
25	Kentucky	17,365	1.3%
12	Louisiana	31,060	2.3%
41	Maine	4,231	0.3%
17	Maryland	25,722	1.9%
21	Massachusetts	21,637	1.6%
8	Michigan	45,515	3.4%
24	Minnesota	17,387	1.3%
23	Mississippi	20,289	1.5%
16	Missouri	26,454	2.0%
45	Montana	3,377	0.3%
36	Nebraska	6,705	0.5%
33	Nevada	11,128	0.8%
43	New Hampshire	3,609	0.3%
11	New Jersey	33,256	2.5%
31	New Mexico	12,393	0.9%
3	New York	93,667	7.0%
9	North Carolina	40,043	3.0%
47	North Dakota	2,178	0.2%
NA	Ohio**	NA	NA
26	Oklahoma	16,868	1.3%
28	Oregon	13,786	1.0%
7	Pennsylvania	47,821	3.6%
40	Rhode Island	4,285	0.3%
19	South Carolina	22,334	1.7%
44	South Dakota	3,469	0.3%
15	Tennessee	27,472	2.0%
2	Texas	110,786	8.2%
35	Utah	8,147	0.6%
48	Vermont	1,832	0.1%
14	Virginia	29,573	2.2%
18	Washington	22,851	1.7%
37	West Virginia	6,650	0.5%
22	Wisconsin	20,342	1.5%
49	Wyoming	1,799	0.1%

RANK	STATE	BIRTHS	% of USA
1	California	173,377	12.9%
2	Texas	110,786	8.2%
3	New York	93,667	7.0%
4	Florida	78,190	5.8%
5	Illinois	63,848	4.7%
6	Georgia	49,103	3.6%
7	Pennsylvania	47,821	3.6%
8	Michigan	45,515	3.4%
9	North Carolina	40,043	3.0%
10	Arizona	33,513	2.5%
11	New Jersey	33,256	2.5%
12	Louisiana	31,060	2.3%
13	Indiana	30,315	2.3%
14	Virginia	29,573	2.2%
15	Tennessee	27,472	2.0%
16	Missouri	26,454	2.0%
17	Maryland	25,722	1.9%
18	Washington	22,851	1.7%
19	South Carolina	22,334	1.7%
20	Alabama	21,718	1.6%
21	Massachusetts	21,637	1.6%
22	Wisconsin	20,342	1.5%
23	Mississippi	20,289	1.5%
24	Minnesota	17,387	1.3%
25	Kentucky	17,365	1.3%
26	Oklahoma	16,868	1.3%
27	Colorado	16,359	1.2%
28	Oregon	13,786	1.0%
29	Arkansas	13,577	1.0%
30	Connecticut	12,558	0.9%
31	New Mexico	12,393	0.9%
32	Kansas	11,510	0.9%
33	Nevada	11,128	0.8%
34	Iowa	10,793	0.8%
35	Utah	8,147	0.6%
36	Nebraska	6,705	0.5%
37	West Virginia	6,650	0.5%
38	Hawaii	5,649	0.4%
39	Idaho	4,400	0.3%
40	Rhode Island	4,285	0.3%
41	Maine	4,231	0.3%
42	Delaware	4,199	0.3%
43	New Hampshire	3,609	0.3%
44	South Dakota	3,469	0.3%
45	Montana	3,377	0.3%
46	Alaska	3,309	0.2%
47	North Dakota	2,178	0.2%
48	Vermont	1,832	0.1%
49	Wyoming	1,799	0.1%
NA	Ohio**	NA	NA
	District of Columbia	4,623	0.3%

Source: Morgan Quitno Press using data from U.S. Dept. of Health and Human Services, Nat'l Center for Health Statistics
"National Vital Statistics Reports" (Vol. 49, No. 5, July 24, 2001)
*Preliminary data by state of residence. Calculated by the editors by multiplying total number of births by reported percent of births to unmarried women.
**Not available.

Births to Unmarried Women as a Percent of All Births in 2000

National Percent = 33.1% of Live Births*

<table>
<tr><td colspan="3">ALPHA ORDER</td><td colspan="3">RANK ORDER</td></tr>
<tr><td>RANK</td><td>STATE</td><td>PERCENT</td><td>RANK</td><td>STATE</td><td>PERCENT</td></tr>
<tr><td>17</td><td>Alabama</td><td>34.3</td><td>1</td><td>Mississippi</td><td>46.0</td></tr>
<tr><td>23</td><td>Alaska</td><td>33.0</td><td>2</td><td>Louisiana</td><td>45.7</td></tr>
<tr><td>5</td><td>Arizona</td><td>39.3</td><td>3</td><td>New Mexico</td><td>45.5</td></tr>
<tr><td>11</td><td>Arkansas</td><td>35.7</td><td>4</td><td>South Carolina</td><td>39.8</td></tr>
<tr><td>25</td><td>California</td><td>32.6</td><td>5</td><td>Arizona</td><td>39.3</td></tr>
<tr><td>46</td><td>Colorado</td><td>25.0</td><td>6</td><td>Florida</td><td>38.3</td></tr>
<tr><td>35</td><td>Connecticut</td><td>29.1</td><td>7</td><td>Delaware</td><td>38.0</td></tr>
<tr><td>7</td><td>Delaware</td><td>38.0</td><td>8</td><td>Georgia</td><td>37.0</td></tr>
<tr><td>6</td><td>Florida</td><td>38.3</td><td>9</td><td>New York</td><td>36.3</td></tr>
<tr><td>8</td><td>Georgia</td><td>37.0</td><td>10</td><td>Nevada</td><td>36.0</td></tr>
<tr><td>26</td><td>Hawaii</td><td>32.2</td><td>11</td><td>Arkansas</td><td>35.7</td></tr>
<tr><td>48</td><td>Idaho</td><td>21.6</td><td>12</td><td>Indiana</td><td>34.8</td></tr>
<tr><td>15</td><td>Illinois</td><td>34.5</td><td>13</td><td>Maryland</td><td>34.6</td></tr>
<tr><td>12</td><td>Indiana</td><td>34.8</td><td>13</td><td>Missouri</td><td>34.6</td></tr>
<tr><td>42</td><td>Iowa</td><td>28.0</td><td>15</td><td>Illinois</td><td>34.5</td></tr>
<tr><td>36</td><td>Kansas</td><td>29.0</td><td>15</td><td>Tennessee</td><td>34.5</td></tr>
<tr><td>29</td><td>Kentucky</td><td>30.9</td><td>17</td><td>Alabama</td><td>34.3</td></tr>
<tr><td>2</td><td>Louisiana</td><td>45.7</td><td>17</td><td>Rhode Island</td><td>34.3</td></tr>
<tr><td>28</td><td>Maine</td><td>31.1</td><td>19</td><td>Oklahoma</td><td>33.8</td></tr>
<tr><td>13</td><td>Maryland</td><td>34.6</td><td>20</td><td>South Dakota</td><td>33.5</td></tr>
<tr><td>44</td><td>Massachusetts</td><td>26.5</td><td>21</td><td>Michigan</td><td>33.4</td></tr>
<tr><td>21</td><td>Michigan</td><td>33.4</td><td>22</td><td>North Carolina</td><td>33.3</td></tr>
<tr><td>45</td><td>Minnesota</td><td>25.8</td><td>23</td><td>Alaska</td><td>33.0</td></tr>
<tr><td>1</td><td>Mississippi</td><td>46.0</td><td>24</td><td>Pennsylvania</td><td>32.7</td></tr>
<tr><td>13</td><td>Missouri</td><td>34.6</td><td>25</td><td>California</td><td>32.6</td></tr>
<tr><td>30</td><td>Montana</td><td>30.8</td><td>26</td><td>Hawaii</td><td>32.2</td></tr>
<tr><td>43</td><td>Nebraska</td><td>27.2</td><td>27</td><td>West Virginia</td><td>31.8</td></tr>
<tr><td>10</td><td>Nevada</td><td>36.0</td><td>28</td><td>Maine</td><td>31.1</td></tr>
<tr><td>47</td><td>New Hampshire</td><td>24.7</td><td>29</td><td>Kentucky</td><td>30.9</td></tr>
<tr><td>37</td><td>New Jersey</td><td>28.9</td><td>30</td><td>Montana</td><td>30.8</td></tr>
<tr><td>3</td><td>New Mexico</td><td>45.5</td><td>31</td><td>Texas</td><td>30.2</td></tr>
<tr><td>9</td><td>New York</td><td>36.3</td><td>32</td><td>Oregon</td><td>30.1</td></tr>
<tr><td>22</td><td>North Carolina</td><td>33.3</td><td>33</td><td>Virginia</td><td>29.9</td></tr>
<tr><td>39</td><td>North Dakota</td><td>28.3</td><td>34</td><td>Wisconsin</td><td>29.3</td></tr>
<tr><td>NA</td><td>Ohio**</td><td>NA</td><td>35</td><td>Connecticut</td><td>29.1</td></tr>
<tr><td>19</td><td>Oklahoma</td><td>33.8</td><td>36</td><td>Kansas</td><td>29.0</td></tr>
<tr><td>32</td><td>Oregon</td><td>30.1</td><td>37</td><td>New Jersey</td><td>28.9</td></tr>
<tr><td>24</td><td>Pennsylvania</td><td>32.7</td><td>38</td><td>Wyoming</td><td>28.8</td></tr>
<tr><td>17</td><td>Rhode Island</td><td>34.3</td><td>39</td><td>North Dakota</td><td>28.3</td></tr>
<tr><td>4</td><td>South Carolina</td><td>39.8</td><td>40</td><td>Vermont</td><td>28.2</td></tr>
<tr><td>20</td><td>South Dakota</td><td>33.5</td><td>40</td><td>Washington</td><td>28.2</td></tr>
<tr><td>15</td><td>Tennessee</td><td>34.5</td><td>42</td><td>Iowa</td><td>28.0</td></tr>
<tr><td>31</td><td>Texas</td><td>30.2</td><td>43</td><td>Nebraska</td><td>27.2</td></tr>
<tr><td>49</td><td>Utah</td><td>17.2</td><td>44</td><td>Massachusetts</td><td>26.5</td></tr>
<tr><td>40</td><td>Vermont</td><td>28.2</td><td>45</td><td>Minnesota</td><td>25.8</td></tr>
<tr><td>33</td><td>Virginia</td><td>29.9</td><td>46</td><td>Colorado</td><td>25.0</td></tr>
<tr><td>40</td><td>Washington</td><td>28.2</td><td>47</td><td>New Hampshire</td><td>24.7</td></tr>
<tr><td>27</td><td>West Virginia</td><td>31.8</td><td>48</td><td>Idaho</td><td>21.6</td></tr>
<tr><td>34</td><td>Wisconsin</td><td>29.3</td><td>49</td><td>Utah</td><td>17.2</td></tr>
<tr><td>38</td><td>Wyoming</td><td>28.8</td><td>NA</td><td>Ohio**</td><td>NA</td></tr>
<tr><td></td><td></td><td></td><td></td><td>District of Columbia</td><td>60.3</td></tr>
</table>

Source: U.S. Department of Health and Human Services, National Center for Health Statistics
  "National Vital Statistics Reports" (Vol. 49, No. 5, July 24, 2001)
*Estimates based on preliminary data by state of residence.
**Not available.

Births to Unmarried White Women in 2000

National Total = 867,995 Live Births*

RANK	STATE	BIRTHS	% of USA
32	Alabama	7,616	0.9%
48	Alaska	1,496	0.2%
7	Arizona	27,663	3.2%
33	Arkansas	7,371	0.8%
1	California	141,311	16.3%
18	Colorado	14,263	1.6%
29	Connecticut	8,885	1.0%
43	Delaware	2,275	0.3%
4	Florida	44,732	5.2%
11	Georgia	19,337	2.2%
49	Hawaii	687	0.1%
38	Idaho	4,139	0.5%
5	Illinois	36,967	4.3%
9	Indiana	22,884	2.6%
27	Iowa	9,544	1.1%
28	Kansas	9,148	1.1%
20	Kentucky	13,444	1.5%
25	Louisiana	9,695	1.1%
39	Maine	4,061	0.5%
24	Maryland	10,207	1.2%
15	Massachusetts	16,046	1.8%
8	Michigan	27,073	3.1%
21	Minnesota	13,216	1.5%
37	Mississippi	5,112	0.6%
14	Missouri	17,119	2.0%
42	Montana	2,407	0.3%
36	Nebraska	5,373	0.6%
30	Nevada	8,768	1.0%
40	New Hampshire	3,491	0.4%
12	New Jersey	18,957	2.2%
26	New Mexico	9,573	1.1%
3	New York	53,256	6.1%
10	North Carolina	19,438	2.2%
47	North Dakota	1,575	0.2%
NA	Ohio**	NA	NA
23	Oklahoma	10,931	1.3%
22	Oregon	12,341	1.4%
6	Pennsylvania	31,403	3.6%
41	Rhode Island	3,338	0.4%
31	South Carolina	8,128	0.9%
44	South Dakota	2,108	0.2%
16	Tennessee	15,003	1.7%
2	Texas	84,624	9.7%
34	Utah	7,366	0.8%
45	Vermont	1,794	0.2%
17	Virginia	14,946	1.7%
13	Washington	18,406	2.1%
35	West Virginia	6,045	0.7%
19	Wisconsin	14,136	1.6%
46	Wyoming	1,601	0.2%

RANK	STATE	BIRTHS	% of USA
1	California	141,311	16.3%
2	Texas	84,624	9.7%
3	New York	53,256	6.1%
4	Florida	44,732	5.2%
5	Illinois	36,967	4.3%
6	Pennsylvania	31,403	3.6%
7	Arizona	27,663	3.2%
8	Michigan	27,073	3.1%
9	Indiana	22,884	2.6%
10	North Carolina	19,438	2.2%
11	Georgia	19,337	2.2%
12	New Jersey	18,957	2.2%
13	Washington	18,406	2.1%
14	Missouri	17,119	2.0%
15	Massachusetts	16,046	1.8%
16	Tennessee	15,003	1.7%
17	Virginia	14,946	1.7%
18	Colorado	14,263	1.6%
19	Wisconsin	14,136	1.6%
20	Kentucky	13,444	1.5%
21	Minnesota	13,216	1.5%
22	Oregon	12,341	1.4%
23	Oklahoma	10,931	1.3%
24	Maryland	10,207	1.2%
25	Louisiana	9,695	1.1%
26	New Mexico	9,573	1.1%
27	Iowa	9,544	1.1%
28	Kansas	9,148	1.1%
29	Connecticut	8,885	1.0%
30	Nevada	8,768	1.0%
31	South Carolina	8,128	0.9%
32	Alabama	7,616	0.9%
33	Arkansas	7,371	0.8%
34	Utah	7,366	0.8%
35	West Virginia	6,045	0.7%
36	Nebraska	5,373	0.6%
37	Mississippi	5,112	0.6%
38	Idaho	4,139	0.5%
39	Maine	4,061	0.5%
40	New Hampshire	3,491	0.4%
41	Rhode Island	3,338	0.4%
42	Montana	2,407	0.3%
43	Delaware	2,275	0.3%
44	South Dakota	2,108	0.2%
45	Vermont	1,794	0.2%
46	Wyoming	1,601	0.2%
47	North Dakota	1,575	0.2%
48	Alaska	1,496	0.2%
49	Hawaii	687	0.1%
NA	Ohio**	NA	NA
	District of Columbia	581	0.1%

Source: Morgan Quitno Press using data from U.S. Dept. of Health and Human Services, Nat'l Center for Health Statistics
"National Vital Statistics Reports" (Vol. 49, No. 5, July 24, 2001)
*Preliminary data by state of residence. Calculated by the editors by multiplying total number of births to white women by percent of such births reported as being to unmarried white women.
**Not available.

Births to Unmarried White Women
As a Percent of All Births to White Women in 2000
National Percent = 27.1% of Live Births*

RANK	STATE	PERCENT
47	Alabama	18.1
35	Alaska	23.4
2	Arizona	37.0
26	Arkansas	25.2
4	California	32.9
33	Colorado	23.9
30	Connecticut	24.6
12	Delaware	28.4
9	Florida	29.7
39	Georgia	22.8
48	Hawaii	17.1
45	Idaho	21.0
21	Illinois	25.9
8	Indiana	30.0
20	Iowa	26.4
21	Kansas	25.9
19	Kentucky	26.7
24	Louisiana	25.4
6	Maine	30.8
43	Maryland	22.4
35	Massachusetts	23.4
26	Michigan	25.2
40	Minnesota	22.5
44	Mississippi	21.7
16	Missouri	27.1
24	Montana	25.4
32	Nebraska	24.1
3	Nevada	33.6
29	New Hampshire	24.8
40	New Jersey	22.5
1	New Mexico	41.8
11	New York	29.1
40	North Carolina	22.5
35	North Dakota	23.4
NA	Ohio**	NA
14	Oklahoma	28.1
10	Oregon	29.6
21	Pennsylvania	25.9
5	Rhode Island	30.9
38	South Carolina	23.0
28	South Dakota	25.0
31	Tennessee	24.5
17	Texas	27.0
49	Utah	16.4
13	Vermont	28.2
45	Virginia	21.0
18	Washington	26.8
7	West Virginia	30.2
34	Wisconsin	23.6
15	Wyoming	27.3

RANK	STATE	PERCENT
1	New Mexico	41.8
2	Arizona	37.0
3	Nevada	33.6
4	California	32.9
5	Rhode Island	30.9
6	Maine	30.8
7	West Virginia	30.2
8	Indiana	30.0
9	Florida	29.7
10	Oregon	29.6
11	New York	29.1
12	Delaware	28.4
13	Vermont	28.2
14	Oklahoma	28.1
15	Wyoming	27.3
16	Missouri	27.1
17	Texas	27.0
18	Washington	26.8
19	Kentucky	26.7
20	Iowa	26.4
21	Illinois	25.9
21	Kansas	25.9
21	Pennsylvania	25.9
24	Louisiana	25.4
24	Montana	25.4
26	Arkansas	25.2
26	Michigan	25.2
28	South Dakota	25.0
29	New Hampshire	24.8
30	Connecticut	24.6
31	Tennessee	24.5
32	Nebraska	24.1
33	Colorado	23.9
34	Wisconsin	23.6
35	Alaska	23.4
35	Massachusetts	23.4
35	North Dakota	23.4
38	South Carolina	23.0
39	Georgia	22.8
40	Minnesota	22.5
40	New Jersey	22.5
40	North Carolina	22.5
43	Maryland	22.4
44	Mississippi	21.7
45	Idaho	21.0
45	Virginia	21.0
47	Alabama	18.1
48	Hawaii	17.1
49	Utah	16.4
NA	Ohio**	NA
	District of Columbia	25.0

Source: U.S. Department of Health and Human Services, National Center for Health Statistics
"National Vital Statistics Reports" (Vol. 49, No. 5, July 24, 2001)
*Data are preliminary estimates by state of residence. By race of mother.
**Not available.

Births to Unmarried Black Women in 2000

National Total = 424,679 Live Births*

ALPHA ORDER				RANK ORDER			
RANK	STATE	BIRTHS	% of USA	RANK	STATE	BIRTHS	% of USA
15	Alabama	13,971	3.3%	1	New York	36,942	8.7%
39	Alaska	212	0.0%	2	Florida	31,988	7.5%
30	Arizona	1,726	0.4%	3	Georgia	29,304	6.9%
20	Arkansas	6,007	1.4%	4	Illinois	26,127	6.2%
6	California	21,785	5.1%	5	Texas	25,114	5.9%
32	Colorado	1,565	0.4%	6	California	21,785	5.1%
24	Connecticut	3,436	0.8%	7	Louisiana	20,941	4.9%
29	Delaware	1,867	0.4%	8	North Carolina	19,307	4.5%
2	Florida	31,988	7.5%	9	Michigan	17,724	4.2%
3	Georgia	29,304	6.9%	10	Pennsylvania	15,691	3.7%
41	Hawaii	113	0.0%	11	Maryland	15,125	3.6%
44	Idaho	36	0.0%	12	Mississippi	14,949	3.5%
4	Illinois	26,127	6.2%	13	Virginia	14,134	3.3%
19	Indiana	7,220	1.7%	14	South Carolina	13,996	3.3%
34	Iowa	920	0.2%	15	Alabama	13,971	3.3%
27	Kansas	1,988	0.5%	16	New Jersey	13,610	3.2%
23	Kentucky	3,773	0.9%	17	Tennessee	12,230	2.9%
7	Louisiana	20,941	4.9%	18	Missouri	8,851	2.1%
43	Maine	49	0.0%	19	Indiana	7,220	1.7%
11	Maryland	15,125	3.6%	20	Arkansas	6,007	1.4%
22	Massachusetts	4,771	1.1%	21	Wisconsin	5,332	1.3%
9	Michigan	17,724	4.2%	22	Massachusetts	4,771	1.1%
26	Minnesota	2,385	0.6%	23	Kentucky	3,773	0.9%
12	Mississippi	14,949	3.5%	24	Connecticut	3,436	0.8%
18	Missouri	8,851	2.1%	25	Oklahoma	3,361	0.8%
47	Montana	20	0.0%	26	Minnesota	2,385	0.6%
33	Nebraska	926	0.2%	27	Kansas	1,988	0.5%
31	Nevada	1,606	0.4%	28	Washington	1,870	0.4%
42	New Hampshire	70	0.0%	29	Delaware	1,867	0.4%
16	New Jersey	13,610	3.2%	30	Arizona	1,726	0.4%
38	New Mexico	297	0.1%	31	Nevada	1,606	0.4%
1	New York	36,942	8.7%	32	Colorado	1,565	0.4%
8	North Carolina	19,307	4.5%	33	Nebraska	926	0.2%
NA	North Dakota**	NA	NA	34	Iowa	920	0.2%
NA	Ohio**	NA	NA	35	Rhode Island	696	0.2%
25	Oklahoma	3,361	0.8%	36	Oregon	660	0.2%
36	Oregon	660	0.2%	37	West Virginia	585	0.1%
10	Pennsylvania	15,691	3.7%	38	New Mexico	297	0.1%
35	Rhode Island	696	0.2%	39	Alaska	212	0.0%
14	South Carolina	13,996	3.3%	40	Utah	176	0.0%
44	South Dakota	36	0.0%	41	Hawaii	113	0.0%
17	Tennessee	12,230	2.9%	42	New Hampshire	70	0.0%
5	Texas	25,114	5.9%	43	Maine	49	0.0%
40	Utah	176	0.0%	44	Idaho	36	0.0%
NA	Vermont**	NA	NA	44	South Dakota	36	0.0%
13	Virginia	14,134	3.3%	46	Wyoming	22	0.0%
28	Washington	1,870	0.4%	47	Montana	20	0.0%
37	West Virginia	585	0.1%	NA	North Dakota**	NA	NA
21	Wisconsin	5,332	1.3%	NA	Ohio**	NA	NA
46	Wyoming	22	0.0%	NA	Vermont**	NA	NA
					District of Columbia	4,011	0.9%

Source: Morgan Quitno Press using data from U.S. Dept. of Health and Human Services, Nat'l Center for Health Statistics
"National Vital Statistics Reports" (Vol. 49, No. 5, July 24, 2001)
*Preliminary data by state of residence. Calculated by the editors by multiplying total number of births to black women by percent of such births reported as being to unmarried black women.
**Insufficient data.

Births to Unmarried Black Women
As a Percent of All Births to Black Women in 2000
National Percent = 68.5% of Live Births*

ALPHA ORDER

RANK	STATE	PERCENT
18	Alabama	68.1
41	Alaska	45.6
31	Arizona	61.9
8	Arkansas	74.8
30	California	62.5
39	Colorado	51.6
23	Connecticut	66.8
14	Delaware	70.9
19	Florida	67.5
24	Georgia	66.5
47	Hawaii	23.9
40	Idaho	48.0
3	Illinois	76.3
4	Indiana	76.0
9	Iowa	74.0
17	Kansas	69.3
11	Kentucky	73.2
10	Louisiana	73.8
42	Maine	43.8
33	Maryland	60.7
36	Massachusetts	58.9
12	Michigan	72.8
34	Minnesota	60.6
7	Mississippi	75.1
2	Missouri	77.2
43	Montana	43.5
22	Nebraska	67.3
21	Nevada	67.4
45	New Hampshire	38.5
26	New Jersey	64.8
35	New Mexico	59.5
19	New York	67.5
25	North Carolina	65.8
NA	North Dakota**	NA
NA	Ohio**	NA
16	Oklahoma	69.6
27	Oregon	64.5
4	Pennsylvania	76.0
29	Rhode Island	62.6
14	South Carolina	70.9
46	South Dakota	34.0
13	Tennessee	72.3
32	Texas	61.3
38	Utah	52.9
NA	Vermont**	NA
28	Virginia	62.8
37	Washington	53.5
6	West Virginia	75.5
1	Wisconsin	82.1
44	Wyoming	38.6

RANK ORDER

RANK	STATE	PERCENT
1	Wisconsin	82.1
2	Missouri	77.2
3	Illinois	76.3
4	Indiana	76.0
4	Pennsylvania	76.0
6	West Virginia	75.5
7	Mississippi	75.1
8	Arkansas	74.8
9	Iowa	74.0
10	Louisiana	73.8
11	Kentucky	73.2
12	Michigan	72.8
13	Tennessee	72.3
14	Delaware	70.9
14	South Carolina	70.9
16	Oklahoma	69.6
17	Kansas	69.3
18	Alabama	68.1
19	Florida	67.5
19	New York	67.5
21	Nevada	67.4
22	Nebraska	67.3
23	Connecticut	66.8
24	Georgia	66.5
25	North Carolina	65.8
26	New Jersey	64.8
27	Oregon	64.5
28	Virginia	62.8
29	Rhode Island	62.6
30	California	62.5
31	Arizona	61.9
32	Texas	61.3
33	Maryland	60.7
34	Minnesota	60.6
35	New Mexico	59.5
36	Massachusetts	58.9
37	Washington	53.5
38	Utah	52.9
39	Colorado	51.6
40	Idaho	48.0
41	Alaska	45.6
42	Maine	43.8
43	Montana	43.5
44	Wyoming	38.6
45	New Hampshire	38.5
46	South Dakota	34.0
47	Hawaii	23.9
NA	North Dakota**	NA
NA	Ohio**	NA
NA	Vermont**	NA
	District of Columbia	77.8

Source: U.S. Department of Health and Human Services, National Center for Health Statistics
"National Vital Statistics Reports" (Vol. 49, No. 5, July 24, 2001)
Data are preliminary estimates by state of residence. By race of mother.
**Insufficient data.*

Births to Teenage Mothers in 2000

National Total = 468,990 Live Births*

ALPHA ORDER				RANK ORDER			
RANK	STATE	BIRTHS	% of USA	RANK	STATE	BIRTHS	% of USA
16	Alabama	9,727	2.1%	1	California	55,463	11.8%
45	Alaska	1,162	0.2%	2	Texas	54,315	11.6%
11	Arizona	12,018	2.6%	3	Florida	25,166	5.4%
27	Arkansas	6,400	1.4%	4	New York	20,783	4.4%
1	California	55,463	11.8%	5	Illinois	20,714	4.4%
24	Colorado	7,550	1.6%	6	Ohio	18,455	3.9%
36	Connecticut	3,277	0.7%	7	Georgia	17,994	3.8%
41	Delaware	1,330	0.3%	8	North Carolina	15,353	3.3%
3	Florida	25,166	5.4%	9	Pennsylvania	14,177	3.0%
7	Georgia	17,994	3.8%	10	Michigan	14,122	3.0%
40	Hawaii	1,788	0.4%	11	Arizona	12,018	2.6%
39	Idaho	2,349	0.5%	12	Tennessee	11,458	2.4%
5	Illinois	20,714	4.4%	13	Louisiana	11,269	2.4%
14	Indiana	10,846	2.3%	14	Indiana	10,846	2.3%
35	Iowa	3,788	0.8%	15	Missouri	9,852	2.1%
31	Kansas	4,706	1.0%	16	Alabama	9,727	2.1%
23	Kentucky	7,775	1.7%	17	Virginia	9,630	2.1%
13	Louisiana	11,269	2.4%	18	South Carolina	8,382	1.8%
42	Maine	1,273	0.3%	19	Washington	8,127	1.7%
25	Maryland	7,202	1.5%	20	New Jersey	8,087	1.7%
29	Massachusetts	5,308	1.1%	21	Mississippi	8,028	1.7%
10	Michigan	14,122	3.0%	22	Oklahoma	7,780	1.7%
28	Minnesota	5,495	1.2%	23	Kentucky	7,775	1.7%
21	Mississippi	8,028	1.7%	24	Colorado	7,550	1.6%
15	Missouri	9,852	2.1%	25	Maryland	7,202	1.5%
43	Montana	1,268	0.3%	26	Wisconsin	6,977	1.5%
38	Nebraska	2,477	0.5%	27	Arkansas	6,400	1.4%
34	Nevada	3,861	0.8%	28	Minnesota	5,495	1.2%
47	New Hampshire	995	0.2%	29	Massachusetts	5,308	1.1%
20	New Jersey	8,087	1.7%	30	Oregon	5,094	1.1%
32	New Mexico	4,655	1.0%	31	Kansas	4,706	1.0%
4	New York	20,783	4.4%	32	New Mexico	4,655	1.0%
8	North Carolina	15,353	3.3%	33	Utah	4,146	0.9%
49	North Dakota	786	0.2%	34	Nevada	3,861	0.8%
6	Ohio	18,455	3.9%	35	Iowa	3,788	0.8%
22	Oklahoma	7,780	1.7%	36	Connecticut	3,277	0.7%
30	Oregon	5,094	1.1%	37	West Virginia	2,839	0.6%
9	Pennsylvania	14,177	3.0%	38	Nebraska	2,477	0.5%
44	Rhode Island	1,258	0.3%	39	Idaho	2,349	0.5%
18	South Carolina	8,382	1.8%	40	Hawaii	1,788	0.4%
46	South Dakota	1,155	0.2%	41	Delaware	1,330	0.3%
12	Tennessee	11,458	2.4%	42	Maine	1,273	0.3%
2	Texas	54,315	11.6%	43	Montana	1,268	0.3%
33	Utah	4,146	0.9%	44	Rhode Island	1,258	0.3%
50	Vermont	521	0.1%	45	Alaska	1,162	0.2%
17	Virginia	9,630	2.1%	46	South Dakota	1,155	0.2%
19	Washington	8,127	1.7%	47	New Hampshire	995	0.2%
37	West Virginia	2,839	0.6%	48	Wyoming	840	0.2%
26	Wisconsin	6,977	1.5%	49	North Dakota	786	0.2%
48	Wyoming	840	0.2%	50	Vermont	521	0.1%
					District of Columbia	1,057	0.2%

Source: Morgan Quitno Press using data from U.S. Dept. of Health and Human Services, Nat'l Center for Health Statistics
unpublished data
*Live births to women under the age of 15 to 19 years old.

Teenage Birth Rate in 2000

National Rate = 48.5 Births per 1,000 15 to 19 Year Old Women*

ALPHA ORDER

RANK	STATE	RATE
7	Alabama	62.9
28	Alaska	42.4
3	Arizona	69.1
4	Arkansas	68.5
21	California	48.5
19	Colorado	49.2
43	Connecticut	31.9
16	Delaware	51.6
15	Florida	52.6
6	Georgia	64.2
25	Hawaii	45.1
27	Idaho	43.1
18	Illinois	49.5
17	Indiana	50.3
41	Iowa	34.7
24	Kansas	45.3
14	Kentucky	55.3
9	Louisiana	62.1
46	Maine	28.7
29	Maryland	41.6
48	Massachusetts	27.1
33	Michigan	39.2
45	Minnesota	29.6
1	Mississippi	72.0
20	Missouri	48.8
38	Montana	35.8
36	Nebraska	37.2
8	Nevada	62.2
50	New Hampshire	23.4
44	New Jersey	31.7
5	New Mexico	66.2
39	New York	35.6
13	North Carolina	59.9
47	North Dakota	28.2
23	Ohio	45.6
12	Oklahoma	60.1
26	Oregon	43.2
40	Pennsylvania	35.2
34	Rhode Island	38.4
11	South Carolina	60.6
36	South Dakota	37.2
10	Tennessee	61.5
2	Texas	69.2
32	Utah	40.0
49	Vermont	24.1
30	Virginia	40.8
35	Washington	38.2
22	West Virginia	46.4
42	Wisconsin	34.5
30	Wyoming	40.8

RANK ORDER

RANK	STATE	RATE
1	Mississippi	72.0
2	Texas	69.2
3	Arizona	69.1
4	Arkansas	68.5
5	New Mexico	66.2
6	Georgia	64.2
7	Alabama	62.9
8	Nevada	62.2
9	Louisiana	62.1
10	Tennessee	61.5
11	South Carolina	60.6
12	Oklahoma	60.1
13	North Carolina	59.9
14	Kentucky	55.3
15	Florida	52.6
16	Delaware	51.6
17	Indiana	50.3
18	Illinois	49.5
19	Colorado	49.2
20	Missouri	48.8
21	California	48.5
22	West Virginia	46.4
23	Ohio	45.6
24	Kansas	45.3
25	Hawaii	45.1
26	Oregon	43.2
27	Idaho	43.1
28	Alaska	42.4
29	Maryland	41.6
30	Virginia	40.8
30	Wyoming	40.8
32	Utah	40.0
33	Michigan	39.2
34	Rhode Island	38.4
35	Washington	38.2
36	Nebraska	37.2
36	South Dakota	37.2
38	Montana	35.8
39	New York	35.6
40	Pennsylvania	35.2
41	Iowa	34.7
42	Wisconsin	34.5
43	Connecticut	31.9
44	New Jersey	31.7
45	Minnesota	29.6
46	Maine	28.7
47	North Dakota	28.2
48	Massachusetts	27.1
49	Vermont	24.1
50	New Hampshire	23.4
	District of Columbia	80.7

Source: U.S. Department of Health and Human Services, National Center for Health Statistics
"National Vital Statistics Reports" (Vol. 50, No. 5, February 12, 2002)
*By mother's residence.

Births to Teenage Mothers in 1999

National Total = 476,050 Live Births*

<table>
<tr><td colspan="4">ALPHA ORDER</td><td colspan="4">RANK ORDER</td></tr>
<tr><td>RANK</td><td>STATE</td><td>BIRTHS</td><td>% of USA</td><td>RANK</td><td>STATE</td><td>BIRTHS</td><td>% of USA</td></tr>
<tr><td>17</td><td>Alabama</td><td>9,850</td><td>2.1%</td><td>1</td><td>California</td><td>56,635</td><td>11.9%</td></tr>
<tr><td>46</td><td>Alaska</td><td>1,123</td><td>0.2%</td><td>2</td><td>Texas</td><td>54,367</td><td>11.4%</td></tr>
<tr><td>11</td><td>Arizona</td><td>11,789</td><td>2.5%</td><td>3</td><td>Florida</td><td>24,912</td><td>5.2%</td></tr>
<tr><td>27</td><td>Arkansas</td><td>6,434</td><td>1.4%</td><td>4</td><td>New York</td><td>21,489</td><td>4.5%</td></tr>
<tr><td>1</td><td>California</td><td>56,635</td><td>11.9%</td><td>5</td><td>Illinois</td><td>21,417</td><td>4.5%</td></tr>
<tr><td>24</td><td>Colorado</td><td>7,251</td><td>1.5%</td><td>6</td><td>Ohio</td><td>18,710</td><td>3.9%</td></tr>
<tr><td>36</td><td>Connecticut</td><td>3,386</td><td>0.7%</td><td>7</td><td>Georgia</td><td>18,027</td><td>3.8%</td></tr>
<tr><td>41</td><td>Delaware</td><td>1,384</td><td>0.3%</td><td>8</td><td>North Carolina</td><td>15,049</td><td>3.2%</td></tr>
<tr><td>3</td><td>Florida</td><td>24,912</td><td>5.2%</td><td>9</td><td>Pennsylvania</td><td>14,604</td><td>3.1%</td></tr>
<tr><td>7</td><td>Georgia</td><td>18,027</td><td>3.8%</td><td>10</td><td>Michigan</td><td>14,547</td><td>3.1%</td></tr>
<tr><td>40</td><td>Hawaii</td><td>1,759</td><td>0.4%</td><td>11</td><td>Arizona</td><td>11,789</td><td>2.5%</td></tr>
<tr><td>39</td><td>Idaho</td><td>2,396</td><td>0.5%</td><td>12</td><td>Tennessee</td><td>11,723</td><td>2.5%</td></tr>
<tr><td>5</td><td>Illinois</td><td>21,417</td><td>4.5%</td><td>13</td><td>Louisiana</td><td>11,538</td><td>2.4%</td></tr>
<tr><td>14</td><td>Indiana</td><td>11,189</td><td>2.4%</td><td>14</td><td>Indiana</td><td>11,189</td><td>2.4%</td></tr>
<tr><td>34</td><td>Iowa</td><td>3,948</td><td>0.8%</td><td>15</td><td>Missouri</td><td>10,006</td><td>2.1%</td></tr>
<tr><td>31</td><td>Kansas</td><td>4,920</td><td>1.0%</td><td>16</td><td>Virginia</td><td>9,935</td><td>2.1%</td></tr>
<tr><td>22</td><td>Kentucky</td><td>8,045</td><td>1.7%</td><td>17</td><td>Alabama</td><td>9,850</td><td>2.1%</td></tr>
<tr><td>13</td><td>Louisiana</td><td>11,538</td><td>2.4%</td><td>18</td><td>South Carolina</td><td>8,467</td><td>1.8%</td></tr>
<tr><td>42</td><td>Maine</td><td>1,313</td><td>0.3%</td><td>19</td><td>Washington</td><td>8,441</td><td>1.8%</td></tr>
<tr><td>25</td><td>Maryland</td><td>7,238</td><td>1.5%</td><td>20</td><td>New Jersey</td><td>8,282</td><td>1.7%</td></tr>
<tr><td>28</td><td>Massachusetts</td><td>5,524</td><td>1.2%</td><td>21</td><td>Mississippi</td><td>8,200</td><td>1.7%</td></tr>
<tr><td>10</td><td>Michigan</td><td>14,547</td><td>3.1%</td><td>22</td><td>Kentucky</td><td>8,045</td><td>1.7%</td></tr>
<tr><td>29</td><td>Minnesota</td><td>5,503</td><td>1.2%</td><td>23</td><td>Oklahoma</td><td>7,850</td><td>1.6%</td></tr>
<tr><td>21</td><td>Mississippi</td><td>8,200</td><td>1.7%</td><td>24</td><td>Colorado</td><td>7,251</td><td>1.5%</td></tr>
<tr><td>15</td><td>Missouri</td><td>10,006</td><td>2.1%</td><td>25</td><td>Maryland</td><td>7,238</td><td>1.5%</td></tr>
<tr><td>43</td><td>Montana</td><td>1,249</td><td>0.3%</td><td>26</td><td>Wisconsin</td><td>7,194</td><td>1.5%</td></tr>
<tr><td>38</td><td>Nebraska</td><td>2,470</td><td>0.5%</td><td>27</td><td>Arkansas</td><td>6,434</td><td>1.4%</td></tr>
<tr><td>35</td><td>Nevada</td><td>3,777</td><td>0.8%</td><td>28</td><td>Massachusetts</td><td>5,524</td><td>1.2%</td></tr>
<tr><td>47</td><td>New Hampshire</td><td>997</td><td>0.2%</td><td>29</td><td>Minnesota</td><td>5,503</td><td>1.2%</td></tr>
<tr><td>20</td><td>New Jersey</td><td>8,282</td><td>1.7%</td><td>30</td><td>Oregon</td><td>5,492</td><td>1.2%</td></tr>
<tr><td>32</td><td>New Mexico</td><td>4,753</td><td>1.0%</td><td>31</td><td>Kansas</td><td>4,920</td><td>1.0%</td></tr>
<tr><td>4</td><td>New York</td><td>21,489</td><td>4.5%</td><td>32</td><td>New Mexico</td><td>4,753</td><td>1.0%</td></tr>
<tr><td>8</td><td>North Carolina</td><td>15,049</td><td>3.2%</td><td>33</td><td>Utah</td><td>4,253</td><td>0.9%</td></tr>
<tr><td>49</td><td>North Dakota</td><td>703</td><td>0.1%</td><td>34</td><td>Iowa</td><td>3,948</td><td>0.8%</td></tr>
<tr><td>6</td><td>Ohio</td><td>18,710</td><td>3.9%</td><td>35</td><td>Nevada</td><td>3,777</td><td>0.8%</td></tr>
<tr><td>23</td><td>Oklahoma</td><td>7,850</td><td>1.6%</td><td>36</td><td>Connecticut</td><td>3,386</td><td>0.7%</td></tr>
<tr><td>30</td><td>Oregon</td><td>5,492</td><td>1.2%</td><td>37</td><td>West Virginia</td><td>3,044</td><td>0.6%</td></tr>
<tr><td>9</td><td>Pennsylvania</td><td>14,604</td><td>3.1%</td><td>38</td><td>Nebraska</td><td>2,470</td><td>0.5%</td></tr>
<tr><td>44</td><td>Rhode Island</td><td>1,222</td><td>0.3%</td><td>39</td><td>Idaho</td><td>2,396</td><td>0.5%</td></tr>
<tr><td>18</td><td>South Carolina</td><td>8,467</td><td>1.8%</td><td>40</td><td>Hawaii</td><td>1,759</td><td>0.4%</td></tr>
<tr><td>45</td><td>South Dakota</td><td>1,175</td><td>0.2%</td><td>41</td><td>Delaware</td><td>1,384</td><td>0.3%</td></tr>
<tr><td>12</td><td>Tennessee</td><td>11,723</td><td>2.5%</td><td>42</td><td>Maine</td><td>1,313</td><td>0.3%</td></tr>
<tr><td>2</td><td>Texas</td><td>54,367</td><td>11.4%</td><td>43</td><td>Montana</td><td>1,249</td><td>0.3%</td></tr>
<tr><td>33</td><td>Utah</td><td>4,253</td><td>0.9%</td><td>44</td><td>Rhode Island</td><td>1,222</td><td>0.3%</td></tr>
<tr><td>50</td><td>Vermont</td><td>549</td><td>0.1%</td><td>45</td><td>South Dakota</td><td>1,175</td><td>0.2%</td></tr>
<tr><td>16</td><td>Virginia</td><td>9,935</td><td>2.1%</td><td>46</td><td>Alaska</td><td>1,123</td><td>0.2%</td></tr>
<tr><td>19</td><td>Washington</td><td>8,441</td><td>1.8%</td><td>47</td><td>New Hampshire</td><td>997</td><td>0.2%</td></tr>
<tr><td>37</td><td>West Virginia</td><td>3,044</td><td>0.6%</td><td>48</td><td>Wyoming</td><td>845</td><td>0.2%</td></tr>
<tr><td>26</td><td>Wisconsin</td><td>7,194</td><td>1.5%</td><td>49</td><td>North Dakota</td><td>703</td><td>0.1%</td></tr>
<tr><td>48</td><td>Wyoming</td><td>845</td><td>0.2%</td><td>50</td><td>Vermont</td><td>549</td><td>0.1%</td></tr>
<tr><td></td><td></td><td></td><td></td><td></td><td>District of Columbia</td><td>1,076</td><td>0.2%</td></tr>
</table>

*Source: U.S. Dept of Health & Human Services, National Center for Health Statistics
(unpublished data)*
Live births to women age 15 to 19 years old by state of residence.

Teenage Birth Rate in 1999

National Rate = 49.6 Births per 1,000 Teenage Women*

ALPHA ORDER				RANK ORDER		
RANK	STATE	RATE		RANK	STATE	RATE
8	Alabama	62.8		1	Mississippi	72.5
30	Alaska	41.8		2	Texas	70.1
3	Arizona	69.6		3	Arizona	69.6
4	Arkansas	68.1		4	Arkansas	68.1
19	California	50.7		5	New Mexico	67.4
21	Colorado	48.4		6	Georgia	65.1
43	Connecticut	33.3		7	Nevada	64.1
15	Delaware	54.3		8	Alabama	62.8
16	Florida	53.5		8	Louisiana	62.8
6	Georgia	65.1		10	Tennessee	62.7
26	Hawaii	43.8		11	South Carolina	60.8
27	Idaho	43.7		12	Oklahoma	60.5
18	Illinois	51.1		13	North Carolina	59.5
17	Indiana	51.6		14	Kentucky	56.4
40	Iowa	35.8		15	Delaware	54.3
23	Kansas	47.4		16	Florida	53.5
14	Kentucky	56.4		17	Indiana	51.6
8	Louisiana	62.8		18	Illinois	51.1
46	Maine	29.8		19	California	50.7
29	Maryland	42.6		20	Missouri	49.6
47	Massachusetts	28.7		21	Colorado	48.4
31	Michigan	40.5		22	West Virginia	47.9
45	Minnesota	30.0		23	Kansas	47.4
1	Mississippi	72.5		24	Oregon	46.5
20	Missouri	49.6		25	Ohio	46.0
42	Montana	35.1		26	Hawaii	43.8
37	Nebraska	37.0		27	Idaho	43.7
7	Nevada	64.1		28	Virginia	42.7
50	New Hampshire	24.0		29	Maryland	42.6
44	New Jersey	32.8		30	Alaska	41.8
5	New Mexico	67.4		31	Michigan	40.5
37	New York	37.0		32	Wyoming	40.4
13	North Carolina	59.5		33	Utah	40.2
48	North Dakota	27.7		34	Washington	40.1
25	Ohio	46.0		35	Rhode Island	38.2
12	Oklahoma	60.5		36	South Dakota	37.6
24	Oregon	46.5		37	Nebraska	37.0
39	Pennsylvania	36.2		37	New York	37.0
35	Rhode Island	38.2		39	Pennsylvania	36.2
11	South Carolina	60.8		40	Iowa	35.8
36	South Dakota	37.6		41	Wisconsin	35.7
10	Tennessee	62.7		42	Montana	35.1
2	Texas	70.1		43	Connecticut	33.3
33	Utah	40.2		44	New Jersey	32.8
49	Vermont	25.7		45	Minnesota	30.0
28	Virginia	42.7		46	Maine	29.8
34	Washington	40.1		47	Massachusetts	28.7
22	West Virginia	47.9		48	North Dakota	27.7
41	Wisconsin	35.7		49	Vermont	25.7
32	Wyoming	40.4		50	New Hampshire	24.0
					District of Columbia	83.5

Source: U.S. Department of Health and Human Services, National Center for Health Statistics
   "National Vital Statistics Reports" (Vol. 49, No. 1, April 17, 2001)
*Women aged 15 to 19 years old.

Births to Teenage Mothers as a Percent of Births in 1999

National Percent = 12.0% of Live Births*

ALPHA ORDER

RANK	STATE	PERCENT
6	Alabama	15.9
28	Alaska	11.3
12	Arizona	14.5
2	Arkansas	17.5
30	California	10.9
26	Colorado	11.7
47	Connecticut	7.8
17	Delaware	13.0
21	Florida	12.6
13	Georgia	14.2
36	Hawaii	10.3
23	Idaho	12.1
25	Illinois	11.8
17	Indiana	13.0
33	Iowa	10.5
20	Kansas	12.7
10	Kentucky	14.8
4	Louisiana	17.2
41	Maine	9.6
38	Maryland	10.1
50	Massachusetts	6.8
30	Michigan	10.9
46	Minnesota	8.3
1	Mississippi	19.2
15	Missouri	13.3
27	Montana	11.6
36	Nebraska	10.3
19	Nevada	12.9
49	New Hampshire	7.1
48	New Jersey	7.3
2	New Mexico	17.5
44	New York	8.4
16	North Carolina	13.2
42	North Dakota	9.2
22	Ohio	12.3
5	Oklahoma	16.0
23	Oregon	12.1
39	Pennsylvania	10.0
40	Rhode Island	9.9
8	South Carolina	15.4
29	South Dakota	11.2
9	Tennessee	15.1
7	Texas	15.6
42	Utah	9.2
44	Vermont	8.4
35	Virginia	10.4
32	Washington	10.6
11	West Virginia	14.7
33	Wisconsin	10.5
14	Wyoming	13.8

RANK ORDER

RANK	STATE	PERCENT
1	Mississippi	19.2
2	Arkansas	17.5
2	New Mexico	17.5
4	Louisiana	17.2
5	Oklahoma	16.0
6	Alabama	15.9
7	Texas	15.6
8	South Carolina	15.4
9	Tennessee	15.1
10	Kentucky	14.8
11	West Virginia	14.7
12	Arizona	14.5
13	Georgia	14.2
14	Wyoming	13.8
15	Missouri	13.3
16	North Carolina	13.2
17	Delaware	13.0
17	Indiana	13.0
19	Nevada	12.9
20	Kansas	12.7
21	Florida	12.6
22	Ohio	12.3
23	Idaho	12.1
23	Oregon	12.1
25	Illinois	11.8
26	Colorado	11.7
27	Montana	11.6
28	Alaska	11.3
29	South Dakota	11.2
30	California	10.9
30	Michigan	10.9
32	Washington	10.6
33	Iowa	10.5
33	Wisconsin	10.5
35	Virginia	10.4
36	Hawaii	10.3
36	Nebraska	10.3
38	Maryland	10.1
39	Pennsylvania	10.0
40	Rhode Island	9.9
41	Maine	9.6
42	North Dakota	9.2
42	Utah	9.2
44	New York	8.4
44	Vermont	8.4
46	Minnesota	8.3
47	Connecticut	7.8
48	New Jersey	7.3
49	New Hampshire	7.1
50	Massachusetts	6.8
	District of Columbia	14.3

Source: Morgan Quitno Press using data from U.S. Dept of Health & Human Services, National Center for Health Statistics
(unpublished data)
*Live births to women age 15 to 19 years old by state of residence.

Births to White Teenage Mothers in 1999

National Total = 337,888 Live Births*

ALPHA ORDER				RANK ORDER			
RANK	STATE	BIRTHS	% of USA	RANK	STATE	BIRTHS	% of USA
20	Alabama	5,314	1.6%	1	California	47,559	14.1%
47	Alaska	558	0.2%	2	Texas	45,494	13.5%
8	Arizona	10,041	3.0%	3	Florida	15,619	4.6%
25	Arkansas	4,295	1.3%	4	Ohio	13,660	4.0%
1	California	47,559	14.1%	5	New York	13,620	4.0%
17	Colorado	6,475	1.9%	6	Illinois	13,069	3.9%
37	Connecticut	2,501	0.7%	7	Pennsylvania	10,165	3.0%
45	Delaware	754	0.2%	8	Arizona	10,041	3.0%
3	Florida	15,619	4.6%	9	Michigan	9,587	2.8%
10	Georgia	9,575	2.8%	10	Georgia	9,575	2.8%
50	Hawaii	202	0.1%	11	Indiana	8,951	2.6%
38	Idaho	2,299	0.7%	12	North Carolina	8,794	2.6%
6	Illinois	13,069	3.9%	13	Tennessee	7,960	2.4%
11	Indiana	8,951	2.6%	14	Missouri	7,360	2.2%
32	Iowa	3,568	1.1%	15	Washington	7,132	2.1%
28	Kansas	4,102	1.2%	16	Kentucky	6,914	2.0%
16	Kentucky	6,914	2.0%	17	Colorado	6,475	1.9%
23	Louisiana	4,828	1.4%	18	Oklahoma	5,679	1.7%
40	Maine	1,273	0.4%	19	Virginia	5,587	1.7%
35	Maryland	3,087	0.9%	20	Alabama	5,314	1.6%
26	Massachusetts	4,236	1.3%	21	Oregon	5,015	1.5%
9	Michigan	9,587	2.8%	22	Wisconsin	4,916	1.5%
31	Minnesota	3,986	1.2%	23	Louisiana	4,828	1.4%
33	Mississippi	3,160	0.9%	24	New Jersey	4,770	1.4%
14	Missouri	7,360	2.2%	25	Arkansas	4,295	1.3%
43	Montana	946	0.3%	26	Massachusetts	4,236	1.3%
39	Nebraska	2,022	0.6%	27	South Carolina	4,155	1.2%
34	Nevada	3,109	0.9%	28	Kansas	4,102	1.2%
41	New Hampshire	979	0.3%	29	New Mexico	4,028	1.2%
24	New Jersey	4,770	1.4%	30	Utah	3,991	1.2%
29	New Mexico	4,028	1.2%	31	Minnesota	3,986	1.2%
5	New York	13,620	4.0%	32	Iowa	3,568	1.1%
12	North Carolina	8,794	2.6%	33	Mississippi	3,160	0.9%
49	North Dakota	536	0.2%	34	Nevada	3,109	0.9%
4	Ohio	13,660	4.0%	35	Maryland	3,087	0.9%
18	Oklahoma	5,679	1.7%	36	West Virginia	2,854	0.8%
21	Oregon	5,015	1.5%	37	Connecticut	2,501	0.7%
7	Pennsylvania	10,165	3.0%	38	Idaho	2,299	0.7%
42	Rhode Island	974	0.3%	39	Nebraska	2,022	0.6%
27	South Carolina	4,155	1.2%	40	Maine	1,273	0.4%
46	South Dakota	748	0.2%	41	New Hampshire	979	0.3%
13	Tennessee	7,960	2.4%	42	Rhode Island	974	0.3%
2	Texas	45,494	13.5%	43	Montana	946	0.3%
30	Utah	3,991	1.2%	44	Wyoming	786	0.2%
48	Vermont	540	0.2%	45	Delaware	754	0.2%
19	Virginia	5,587	1.7%	46	South Dakota	748	0.2%
15	Washington	7,132	2.1%	47	Alaska	558	0.2%
36	West Virginia	2,854	0.8%	48	Vermont	540	0.2%
22	Wisconsin	4,916	1.5%	49	North Dakota	536	0.2%
44	Wyoming	786	0.2%	50	Hawaii	202	0.1%
					District of Columbia	115	0.0%

Source: U.S. Dept of Health & Human Services, National Center for Health Statistics
    (unpublished data)
Live births to women age 15 to 19 years old by state of residence.

White Teenage Birth Rate in 1999

National Rate = 34.0 Births per 1,000 White Teenage Women*

ALPHA ORDER				RANK ORDER		
RANK	STATE	RATE		RANK	STATE	RATE
6	Alabama	50.8		1	Arkansas	57.4
32	Alaska	29.0		2	Tennessee	53.7
16	Arizona	39.6		3	Kentucky	53.2
1	Arkansas	57.4		4	Mississippi	53.0
41	California	25.2		5	Oklahoma	52.0
30	Colorado	29.9		6	Alabama	50.8
48	Connecticut	16.1		7	Georgia	49.3
24	Delaware	35.7		8	West Virginia	47.1
17	Florida	39.5		9	South Carolina	46.9
7	Georgia	49.3		10	Louisiana	45.6
49	Hawaii	14.7		11	Nevada	45.3
21	Idaho	38.2		12	Indiana	44.6
35	Illinois	27.5		13	North Carolina	43.0
12	Indiana	44.6		14	Missouri	42.0
27	Iowa	31.8		15	Texas	41.9
20	Kansas	38.3		16	Arizona	39.6
3	Kentucky	53.2		17	Florida	39.5
10	Louisiana	45.6		18	Oregon	38.7
31	Maine	29.4		19	Ohio	38.6
37	Maryland	26.6		20	Kansas	38.3
47	Massachusetts	17.9		21	Idaho	38.2
29	Michigan	30.4		22	New Mexico	37.7
45	Minnesota	21.0		23	Wyoming	37.4
4	Mississippi	53.0		24	Delaware	35.7
14	Missouri	42.0		25	Utah	33.0
33	Montana	28.8		26	Washington	32.6
34	Nebraska	28.6		27	Iowa	31.8
11	Nevada	45.3		28	Virginia	31.1
43	New Hampshire	23.5		29	Michigan	30.4
50	New Jersey	13.5		30	Colorado	29.9
22	New Mexico	37.7		31	Maine	29.4
46	New York	20.5		32	Alaska	29.0
13	North Carolina	43.0		33	Montana	28.8
44	North Dakota	22.5		34	Nebraska	28.6
19	Ohio	38.6		35	Illinois	27.5
5	Oklahoma	52.0		36	South Dakota	27.0
18	Oregon	38.7		37	Maryland	26.6
40	Pennsylvania	25.5		38	Vermont	26.1
39	Rhode Island	25.7		39	Rhode Island	25.7
9	South Carolina	46.9		40	Pennsylvania	25.5
36	South Dakota	27.0		41	California	25.2
2	Tennessee	53.7		42	Wisconsin	24.2
15	Texas	41.9		43	New Hampshire	23.5
25	Utah	33.0		44	North Dakota	22.5
38	Vermont	26.1		45	Minnesota	21.0
28	Virginia	31.1		46	New York	20.5
26	Washington	32.6		47	Massachusetts	17.9
8	West Virginia	47.1		48	Connecticut	16.1
42	Wisconsin	24.2		49	Hawaii	14.7
23	Wyoming	37.4		50	New Jersey	13.5
					District of Columbia**	NA

Source: U.S. Department of Health and Human Services, National Center for Health Statistics
"National Vital Statistics Reports" (Vol. 49, No. 10, September 25, 2001)
*Women aged 15 to 19 years old.
**Insufficient data.

Births to White Teenage Mothers as a Percent of White Births in 1999

National Percent = 10.8% of White Live Births*

ALPHA ORDER

RANK	STATE	PERCENT
11	Alabama	12.7
37	Alaska	8.5
7	Arizona	14.1
3	Arkansas	15.1
22	California	11.3
21	Colorado	11.4
46	Connecticut	6.9
29	Delaware	9.8
25	Florida	10.6
19	Georgia	11.8
50	Hawaii	5.0
15	Idaho	12.0
31	Illinois	9.3
16	Indiana	11.9
27	Iowa	10.1
16	Kansas	11.9
6	Kentucky	14.2
12	Louisiana	12.6
30	Maine	9.6
45	Maryland	7.0
48	Massachusetts	6.2
33	Michigan	9.1
46	Minnesota	6.9
8	Mississippi	13.9
19	Missouri	11.8
27	Montana	10.1
31	Nebraska	9.3
13	Nevada	12.4
44	New Hampshire	7.2
49	New Jersey	5.7
1	New Mexico	17.7
43	New York	7.3
23	North Carolina	10.8
42	North Dakota	8.0
23	Ohio	10.8
4	Oklahoma	14.7
14	Oregon	12.1
38	Pennsylvania	8.4
35	Rhode Island	9.0
16	South Carolina	11.9
36	South Dakota	8.6
10	Tennessee	13.3
2	Texas	15.3
33	Utah	9.1
40	Vermont	8.3
41	Virginia	8.2
26	Washington	10.5
5	West Virginia	14.4
38	Wisconsin	8.4
9	Wyoming	13.7

RANK ORDER

RANK	STATE	PERCENT
1	New Mexico	17.7
2	Texas	15.3
3	Arkansas	15.1
4	Oklahoma	14.7
5	West Virginia	14.4
6	Kentucky	14.2
7	Arizona	14.1
8	Mississippi	13.9
9	Wyoming	13.7
10	Tennessee	13.3
11	Alabama	12.7
12	Louisiana	12.6
13	Nevada	12.4
14	Oregon	12.1
15	Idaho	12.0
16	Indiana	11.9
16	Kansas	11.9
16	South Carolina	11.9
19	Georgia	11.8
19	Missouri	11.8
21	Colorado	11.4
22	California	11.3
23	North Carolina	10.8
23	Ohio	10.8
25	Florida	10.6
26	Washington	10.5
27	Iowa	10.1
27	Montana	10.1
29	Delaware	9.8
30	Maine	9.6
31	Illinois	9.3
31	Nebraska	9.3
33	Michigan	9.1
33	Utah	9.1
35	Rhode Island	9.0
36	South Dakota	8.6
37	Alaska	8.5
38	Pennsylvania	8.4
38	Wisconsin	8.4
40	Vermont	8.3
41	Virginia	8.2
42	North Dakota	8.0
43	New York	7.3
44	New Hampshire	7.2
45	Maryland	7.0
46	Connecticut	6.9
46	Minnesota	6.9
48	Massachusetts	6.2
49	New Jersey	5.7
50	Hawaii	5.0

District of Columbia   6.8

Source: Morgan Quitno Press using data from U.S. Dept of Health & Human Services, National Center for Health Statistics (unpublished data)

*Live births to women age 15 to 19 years old by state of residence.

Births to Black Teenage Mothers in 1999

National Total = 121,166 Live Births*

ALPHA ORDER					RANK ORDER			
RANK	STATE		BIRTHS	% of USA	RANK	STATE		BIRTHS	% of USA

RANK	STATE	BIRTHS	% of USA	RANK	STATE	BIRTHS	% of USA
12	Alabama	4,481	3.7%	1	Florida	8,993	7.4%
40	Alaska	75	0.1%	2	Texas	8,397	6.9%
30	Arizona	593	0.5%	3	Georgia	8,315	6.9%
21	Arkansas	2,061	1.7%	4	Illinois	8,158	6.7%
8	California	5,639	4.7%	5	New York	7,361	6.1%
32	Colorado	531	0.4%	6	Louisiana	6,585	5.4%
26	Connecticut	831	0.7%	7	North Carolina	5,675	4.7%
29	Delaware	614	0.5%	8	California	5,639	4.7%
1	Florida	8,993	7.4%	9	Mississippi	4,969	4.1%
3	Georgia	8,315	6.9%	10	Ohio	4,916	4.1%
42	Hawaii	41	0.0%	11	Michigan	4,668	3.9%
46	Idaho	12	0.0%	12	Alabama	4,481	3.7%
4	Illinois	8,158	6.7%	13	Pennsylvania	4,272	3.5%
20	Indiana	2,164	1.8%	14	South Carolina	4,249	3.5%
35	Iowa	275	0.2%	15	Virginia	4,202	3.5%
28	Kansas	700	0.6%	16	Maryland	4,048	3.3%
23	Kentucky	1,093	0.9%	17	Tennessee	3,674	3.0%
6	Louisiana	6,585	5.4%	18	New Jersey	3,378	2.8%
43	Maine	19	0.0%	19	Missouri	2,520	2.1%
16	Maryland	4,048	3.3%	20	Indiana	2,164	1.8%
25	Massachusetts	1,050	0.9%	21	Arkansas	2,061	1.7%
11	Michigan	4,668	3.9%	22	Wisconsin	1,755	1.4%
27	Minnesota	757	0.6%	23	Kentucky	1,093	0.9%
9	Mississippi	4,969	4.1%	24	Oklahoma	1,063	0.9%
19	Missouri	2,520	2.1%	25	Massachusetts	1,050	0.9%
50	Montana	5	0.0%	26	Connecticut	831	0.7%
34	Nebraska	329	0.3%	27	Minnesota	757	0.6%
33	Nevada	470	0.4%	28	Kansas	700	0.6%
47	New Hampshire	11	0.0%	29	Delaware	614	0.5%
18	New Jersey	3,378	2.8%	30	Arizona	593	0.5%
39	New Mexico	105	0.1%	31	Washington	552	0.5%
5	New York	7,361	6.1%	32	Colorado	531	0.4%
7	North Carolina	5,675	4.7%	33	Nevada	470	0.4%
44	North Dakota	13	0.0%	34	Nebraska	329	0.3%
10	Ohio	4,916	4.1%	35	Iowa	275	0.2%
24	Oklahoma	1,063	0.9%	36	Oregon	185	0.2%
36	Oregon	185	0.2%	37	West Virginia	180	0.1%
13	Pennsylvania	4,272	3.5%	38	Rhode Island	144	0.1%
38	Rhode Island	144	0.1%	39	New Mexico	105	0.1%
14	South Carolina	4,249	3.5%	40	Alaska	75	0.1%
44	South Dakota	13	0.0%	41	Utah	51	0.0%
17	Tennessee	3,674	3.0%	42	Hawaii	41	0.0%
2	Texas	8,397	6.9%	43	Maine	19	0.0%
41	Utah	51	0.0%	44	North Dakota	13	0.0%
49	Vermont	7	0.0%	44	South Dakota	13	0.0%
15	Virginia	4,202	3.5%	46	Idaho	12	0.0%
31	Washington	552	0.5%	47	New Hampshire	11	0.0%
37	West Virginia	180	0.1%	47	Wyoming	11	0.0%
22	Wisconsin	1,755	1.4%	49	Vermont	7	0.0%
47	Wyoming	11	0.0%	50	Montana	5	0.0%
					District of Columbia	956	0.8%

Source: U.S. Dept of Health & Human Services, National Center for Health Statistics
(unpublished data)
*Live births to women age 15 to 19 years old by state of residence.

Black Teenage Birth Rate in 1999

National Rate = 81.0 Births per 1,000 Black Teenage Women*

ALPHA ORDER				RANK ORDER		
RANK	STATE	RATE		RANK	STATE	RATE
19	Alabama	83.2		1	Wisconsin	122.9
34	Alaska	66.7		2	Minnesota	109.9
26	Arizona	74.9		3	Illinois	105.2
8	Arkansas	96.5		4	Delaware	99.8
39	California	58.4		5	Kansas	97.6
32	Colorado	67.4		6	Nebraska	97.5
33	Connecticut	67.1		7	Indiana	97.2
4	Delaware	99.8		8	Arkansas	96.5
18	Florida	83.5		9	Iowa	95.5
17	Georgia	84.4		10	Mississippi	95.0
41	Hawaii	31.0		11	Pennsylvania	93.6
NA	Idaho**	NA		12	Missouri	92.0
3	Illinois	105.2		13	Tennessee	90.6
7	Indiana	97.2		14	Louisiana	89.7
9	Iowa	95.5		15	Ohio	88.6
5	Kansas	97.6		16	Kentucky	85.3
16	Kentucky	85.3		17	Georgia	84.4
14	Louisiana	89.7		18	Florida	83.5
NA	Maine**	NA		19	Alabama	83.2
28	Maryland	73.0		20	Oklahoma	82.9
31	Massachusetts	68.0		21	Nevada	81.6
24	Michigan	79.8		22	South Carolina	80.5
2	Minnesota	109.9		23	North Carolina	80.2
10	Mississippi	95.0		24	Michigan	79.8
12	Missouri	92.0		25	Texas	76.0
NA	Montana**	NA		26	Arizona	74.9
6	Nebraska	97.5		27	Virginia	73.8
21	Nevada	81.6		28	Maryland	73.0
NA	New Hampshire**	NA		29	New Jersey	72.6
29	New Jersey	72.6		30	West Virginia	71.7
40	New Mexico	50.4		31	Massachusetts	68.0
38	New York	59.3		32	Colorado	67.4
23	North Carolina	80.2		33	Connecticut	67.1
NA	North Dakota**	NA		34	Alaska	66.7
15	Ohio	88.6		35	Rhode Island	66.2
20	Oklahoma	82.9		36	Oregon	64.5
36	Oregon	64.5		37	Washington	60.7
11	Pennsylvania	93.6		38	New York	59.3
35	Rhode Island	66.2		39	California	58.4
22	South Carolina	80.5		40	New Mexico	50.4
NA	South Dakota**	NA		41	Hawaii	31.0
13	Tennessee	90.6		NA	Idaho**	NA
25	Texas	76.0		NA	Maine**	NA
NA	Utah**	NA		NA	Montana**	NA
NA	Vermont**	NA		NA	New Hampshire**	NA
27	Virginia	73.8		NA	North Dakota**	NA
37	Washington	60.7		NA	South Dakota**	NA
30	West Virginia	71.7		NA	Utah**	NA
1	Wisconsin	122.9		NA	Vermont**	NA
NA	Wyoming**	NA		NA	Wyoming**	NA
					District of Columbia	127.8

Source: U.S. Department of Health and Human Services, National Center for Health Statistics
   "National Vital Statistics Reports" (Vol. 49, No. 10, September 25, 2001)
*Women aged 15 to 19 years old.
**Insufficient data.

Births to Black Teenage Mothers as a Percent of Black Births in 1999

National Percent = 20.0% of Black Live Births*

ALPHA ORDER			RANK ORDER		
RANK	STATE	PERCENT	RANK	STATE	PERCENT
14	Alabama	22.7	1	Wisconsin	27.0
37	Alaska	16.3	2	Arkansas	26.7
20	Arizona	21.2	3	Nebraska	25.7
2	Arkansas	26.7	4	Mississippi	25.6
39	California	15.7	5	Kansas	24.5
32	Colorado	18.3	6	Louisiana	24.2
40	Connecticut	15.6	7	West Virginia	23.9
13	Delaware	22.8	8	Illinois	23.8
26	Florida	19.9	9	Iowa	23.6
27	Georgia	19.7	10	Ohio	23.4
49	Hawaii	8.9	11	Indiana	23.2
40	Idaho	15.6	12	Oklahoma	22.9
8	Illinois	23.8	13	Delaware	22.8
11	Indiana	23.2	14	Alabama	22.7
9	Iowa	23.6	15	Missouri	22.4
5	Kansas	24.5	16	South Carolina	22.2
18	Kentucky	22.0	16	Tennessee	22.2
6	Louisiana	24.2	18	Kentucky	22.0
33	Maine	17.9	19	Texas	21.6
35	Maryland	16.5	20	Arizona	21.2
48	Massachusetts	12.7	21	Nevada	21.1
28	Michigan	19.4	21	New Mexico	21.1
30	Minnesota	18.8	23	Pennsylvania	20.7
4	Mississippi	25.6	24	Oregon	20.4
15	Missouri	22.4	25	North Carolina	20.0
46	Montana	14.3	26	Florida	19.9
3	Nebraska	25.7	27	Georgia	19.7
21	Nevada	21.1	28	Michigan	19.4
50	New Hampshire	7.9	29	Utah	18.9
38	New Jersey	15.8	30	Minnesota	18.8
21	New Mexico	21.1	31	Virginia	18.7
47	New York	13.7	32	Colorado	18.3
25	North Carolina	20.0	33	Maine	17.9
42	North Dakota	15.1	34	Vermont	17.5
10	Ohio	23.4	35	Maryland	16.5
12	Oklahoma	22.9	36	Washington	16.4
24	Oregon	20.4	37	Alaska	16.3
23	Pennsylvania	20.7	38	New Jersey	15.8
44	Rhode Island	14.9	39	California	15.7
16	South Carolina	22.2	40	Connecticut	15.6
45	South Dakota	14.6	40	Idaho	15.6
16	Tennessee	22.2	42	North Dakota	15.1
19	Texas	21.6	42	Wyoming	15.1
29	Utah	18.9	44	Rhode Island	14.9
34	Vermont	17.5	45	South Dakota	14.6
31	Virginia	18.7	46	Montana	14.3
36	Washington	16.4	47	New York	13.7
7	West Virginia	23.9	48	Massachusetts	12.7
1	Wisconsin	27.0	49	Hawaii	8.9
42	Wyoming	15.1	50	New Hampshire	7.9
				District of Columbia	16.9

Source: Morgan Quitno Press using data from U.S. Dept of Health & Human Services, National Center for Health Statistics
   (unpublished data)
*Live births to women age 15 to 19 years old by state of residence.

Pregnancy Rate for 15 to 19 Year Old Women in 1997

National Rate = 71.3 Births and Abortions per 1,000 Women 15-19 Years Old*

ALPHA ORDER

RANK ORDER

RANK	STATE	RATE	RANK	STATE	RATE
9	Alabama	83.1	1	Delaware	107.9
29	Alaska	57.9	2	Georgia	92.0
8	Arizona	83.7	3	Texas	91.6
5	Arkansas	85.7	4	Nevada	90.5
NA	California**	NA	5	Arkansas	85.7
25	Colorado	63.3	6	North Carolina	85.6
22	Connecticut	66.1	7	New Mexico	84.9
1	Delaware	107.9	8	Arizona	83.7
NA	Florida**	NA	9	Alabama	83.1
2	Georgia	92.0	9	Tennessee	83.1
19	Hawaii	69.7	11	New York	82.9
40	Idaho	47.2	12	Mississippi	81.1
NA	Illinois**	NA	13	Louisiana	78.3
22	Indiana	66.1	14	Rhode Island	76.9
NA	Iowa**	NA	15	South Carolina	75.0
17	Kansas	73.8	16	Oregon	74.7
20	Kentucky	69.4	17	Kansas	73.8
13	Louisiana	78.3	18	Washington	70.1
42	Maine	46.2	19	Hawaii	69.7
33	Maryland	55.0	20	Kentucky	69.4
30	Massachusetts	56.9	21	Ohio	68.7
27	Michigan	59.8	22	Connecticut	66.1
41	Minnesota	47.1	22	Indiana	66.1
12	Mississippi	81.1	24	Virginia	65.7
26	Missouri	60.7	25	Colorado	63.3
31	Montana	56.7	26	Missouri	60.7
35	Nebraska	53.3	27	Michigan	59.8
4	Nevada	90.5	28	West Virginia	58.7
NA	New Hampshire**	NA	29	Alaska	57.9
32	New Jersey	55.3	30	Massachusetts	56.9
7	New Mexico	84.9	31	Montana	56.7
11	New York	82.9	32	New Jersey	55.3
6	North Carolina	85.6	33	Maryland	55.0
44	North Dakota	40.6	34	Pennsylvania	54.4
21	Ohio	68.7	35	Nebraska	53.3
NA	Oklahoma**	NA	36	Utah	48.8
16	Oregon	74.7	36	Vermont	48.8
34	Pennsylvania	54.4	38	Wisconsin	48.6
14	Rhode Island	76.9	39	South Dakota	47.6
15	South Carolina	75.0	40	Idaho	47.2
39	South Dakota	47.6	41	Minnesota	47.1
9	Tennessee	83.1	42	Maine	46.2
3	Texas	91.6	43	Wyoming	44.5
36	Utah	48.8	44	North Dakota	40.6
36	Vermont	48.8	NA	California**	NA
24	Virginia	65.7	NA	Florida**	NA
18	Washington	70.1	NA	Illinois**	NA
28	West Virginia	58.7	NA	Iowa**	NA
38	Wisconsin	48.6	NA	New Hampshire**	NA
43	Wyoming	44.5	NA	Oklahoma**	NA

District of Columbia 211.9

Source: Morgan Quitno Press using data from US Dept of Health & Human Serv's, Centers for Disease Control-Prevention
"Abortion Surveillance-United States, 1997" (Morbidity Mortality Weekly Report, Vol. 49, No. SS-11, 12/08/00)
*The sum of live births and legal induced abortions per 1,000 women aged 15-19 years old. Births by state of residence, abortions by state of occurrence. Miscarriages are not included in these rates. National rate includes only states reporting abortions and births.
**Not available.

Percent Change in Pregnancy Rate for 15 to 19 Year Old Women: 1992 to 1997

National Percent Change = 10.5% Decrease*

ALPHA ORDER

RANK	STATE	PERCENT CHANGE
5	Alabama	(10.8)
NA	Alaska**	NA
27	Arizona	(19.1)
1	Arkansas	(5.5)
NA	California**	NA
33	Colorado	(20.7)
NA	Connecticut**	NA
NA	Delaware**	NA
NA	Florida**	NA
11	Georgia	(13.9)
29	Hawaii	(19.3)
35	Idaho	(20.9)
NA	Illinois**	NA
4	Indiana	(8.4)
NA	Iowa**	NA
17	Kansas	(15.2)
16	Kentucky	(15.1)
18	Louisiana	(15.4)
20	Maine	(16.3)
40	Maryland	(28.5)
25	Massachusetts	(18.1)
38	Michigan	(25.0)
14	Minnesota	(14.7)
30	Mississippi	(19.5)
36	Missouri	(22.2)
28	Montana	(19.2)
19	Nebraska	(15.9)
13	Nevada	(14.6)
NA	New Hampshire**	NA
33	New Jersey	(20.7)
21	New Mexico	(16.6)
12	New York	(14.2)
26	North Carolina	(18.2)
39	North Dakota	(25.1)
3	Ohio	(7.9)
NA	Oklahoma**	NA
2	Oregon	(7.8)
37	Pennsylvania	(24.1)
10	Rhode Island	(12.7)
15	South Carolina	(14.8)
31	South Dakota	(19.9)
7	Tennessee	(11.6)
8	Texas	(11.7)
9	Utah	(12.2)
41	Vermont	(29.0)
22	Virginia	(16.8)
24	Washington	(17.6)
6	West Virginia	(11.2)
32	Wisconsin	(20.1)
23	Wyoming	(17.1)

RANK ORDER

RANK	STATE	PERCENT CHANGE
1	Arkansas	(5.5)
2	Oregon	(7.8)
3	Ohio	(7.9)
4	Indiana	(8.4)
5	Alabama	(10.8)
6	West Virginia	(11.2)
7	Tennessee	(11.6)
8	Texas	(11.7)
9	Utah	(12.2)
10	Rhode Island	(12.7)
11	Georgia	(13.9)
12	New York	(14.2)
13	Nevada	(14.6)
14	Minnesota	(14.7)
15	South Carolina	(14.8)
16	Kentucky	(15.1)
17	Kansas	(15.2)
18	Louisiana	(15.4)
19	Nebraska	(15.9)
20	Maine	(16.3)
21	New Mexico	(16.6)
22	Virginia	(16.8)
23	Wyoming	(17.1)
24	Washington	(17.6)
25	Massachusetts	(18.1)
26	North Carolina	(18.2)
27	Arizona	(19.1)
28	Montana	(19.2)
29	Hawaii	(19.3)
30	Mississippi	(19.5)
31	South Dakota	(19.9)
32	Wisconsin	(20.1)
33	Colorado	(20.7)
33	New Jersey	(20.7)
35	Idaho	(20.9)
36	Missouri	(22.2)
37	Pennsylvania	(24.1)
38	Michigan	(25.0)
39	North Dakota	(25.1)
40	Maryland	(28.5)
41	Vermont	(29.0)
NA	Alaska**	NA
NA	California**	NA
NA	Connecticut**	NA
NA	Delaware**	NA
NA	Florida**	NA
NA	Illinois**	NA
NA	Iowa**	NA
NA	New Hampshire**	NA
NA	Oklahoma**	NA

District of Columbia 1.7

Source: Morgan Quitno Press using data from US Dept of Health & Human Serv's, Centers for Disease Control-Prevention "Abortion Surveillance-United States, 1997" (Morbidity Mortality Weekly Report, Vol. 49, No. SS-11, 12/08/00)
*The sum of live births and legal induced abortions per 1,000 women aged 15-19 years old. Births by state of residence, abortions by state of occurrence. Miscarriages are not included in these rates. National rate includes only states reporting abortions and births.
**Not available.

Births to Teenage Mothers in 1990

National Total = 521,826 Live Births*

ALPHA ORDER

RANK	STATE	BIRTHS	% of USA
15	Alabama	11,252	2.2%
47	Alaska	1,142	0.2%
19	Arizona	9,612	1.8%
27	Arkansas	7,011	1.3%
1	California	69,712	13.4%
28	Colorado	5,975	1.1%
33	Connecticut	4,038	0.8%
44	Delaware	1,277	0.2%
3	Florida	27,017	5.2%
8	Georgia	18,369	3.5%
39	Hawaii	2,122	0.4%
40	Idaho	2,009	0.4%
5	Illinois	24,967	4.8%
12	Indiana	12,335	2.4%
34	Iowa	3,989	0.8%
31	Kansas	4,722	0.9%
20	Kentucky	9,349	1.8%
13	Louisiana	12,270	2.4%
41	Maine	1,857	0.4%
23	Maryland	8,143	1.6%
26	Massachusetts	7,266	1.4%
7	Michigan	20,312	3.9%
29	Minnesota	5,342	1.0%
21	Mississippi	8,909	1.7%
16	Missouri	11,227	2.2%
43	Montana	1,331	0.3%
38	Nebraska	2,352	0.5%
37	Nevada	2,663	0.5%
45	New Hampshire	1,258	0.2%
17	New Jersey	10,068	1.9%
32	New Mexico	4,367	0.8%
4	New York	26,608	5.1%
10	North Carolina	16,506	3.2%
49	North Dakota	793	0.2%
6	Ohio	22,690	4.3%
24	Oklahoma	7,590	1.5%
30	Oregon	5,084	1.0%
9	Pennsylvania	18,216	3.5%
42	Rhode Island	1,564	0.3%
18	South Carolina	9,721	1.9%
46	South Dakota	1,172	0.2%
11	Tennessee	12,928	2.5%
2	Texas	48,302	9.3%
36	Utah	3,707	0.7%
50	Vermont	702	0.1%
14	Virginia	11,353	2.2%
22	Washington	8,397	1.6%
35	West Virginia	3,976	0.8%
25	Wisconsin	7,281	1.4%
48	Wyoming	943	0.2%

RANK ORDER

RANK	STATE	BIRTHS	% of USA
1	California	69,712	13.4%
2	Texas	48,302	9.3%
3	Florida	27,017	5.2%
4	New York	26,608	5.1%
5	Illinois	24,967	4.8%
6	Ohio	22,690	4.3%
7	Michigan	20,312	3.9%
8	Georgia	18,369	3.5%
9	Pennsylvania	18,216	3.5%
10	North Carolina	16,506	3.2%
11	Tennessee	12,928	2.5%
12	Indiana	12,335	2.4%
13	Louisiana	12,270	2.4%
14	Virginia	11,353	2.2%
15	Alabama	11,252	2.2%
16	Missouri	11,227	2.2%
17	New Jersey	10,068	1.9%
18	South Carolina	9,721	1.9%
19	Arizona	9,612	1.8%
20	Kentucky	9,349	1.8%
21	Mississippi	8,909	1.7%
22	Washington	8,397	1.6%
23	Maryland	8,143	1.6%
24	Oklahoma	7,590	1.5%
25	Wisconsin	7,281	1.4%
26	Massachusetts	7,266	1.4%
27	Arkansas	7,011	1.3%
28	Colorado	5,975	1.1%
29	Minnesota	5,342	1.0%
30	Oregon	5,084	1.0%
31	Kansas	4,722	0.9%
32	New Mexico	4,367	0.8%
33	Connecticut	4,038	0.8%
34	Iowa	3,989	0.8%
35	West Virginia	3,976	0.8%
36	Utah	3,707	0.7%
37	Nevada	2,663	0.5%
38	Nebraska	2,352	0.5%
39	Hawaii	2,122	0.4%
40	Idaho	2,009	0.4%
41	Maine	1,857	0.4%
42	Rhode Island	1,564	0.3%
43	Montana	1,331	0.3%
44	Delaware	1,277	0.2%
45	New Hampshire	1,258	0.2%
46	South Dakota	1,172	0.2%
47	Alaska	1,142	0.2%
48	Wyoming	943	0.2%
49	North Dakota	793	0.2%
50	Vermont	702	0.1%
	District of Columbia	2,030	0.4%

Source: U.S. Department of Health and Human Services, Centers for Disease Control and Prevention
   "Surveillance for Pregnancy and Birth Rates Among Teenagers" (MMWR, Vol. 42, No. SS-6, 12/17/93)
*Women aged 15 to 19 years old.

Teenage Birth Rate in 1990

National Rate = 59.9 Live Births per 1,000 Teenage Women*

ALPHA ORDER			RANK ORDER		
RANK	STATE	RATE	RANK	STATE	RATE
11	Alabama	71.0	1	Mississippi	81.0
17	Alaska	65.3	2	Arkansas	80.1
4	Arizona	75.5	3	New Mexico	78.2
2	Arkansas	80.1	4	Arizona	75.5
12	California	70.6	4	Georgia	75.5
28	Colorado	54.5	6	Texas	75.3
45	Connecticut	38.8	7	Louisiana	74.2
28	Delaware	54.5	8	Nevada	73.3
13	Florida	69.1	9	Tennessee	72.3
4	Georgia	75.5	10	South Carolina	71.3
20	Hawaii	61.2	11	Alabama	71.0
33	Idaho	50.6	12	California	70.6
18	Illinois	62.9	13	Florida	69.1
22	Indiana	58.6	14	Kentucky	67.6
43	Iowa	40.5	14	North Carolina	67.6
26	Kansas	56.1	16	Oklahoma	66.8
14	Kentucky	67.6	17	Alaska	65.3
7	Louisiana	74.2	18	Illinois	62.9
40	Maine	43.0	19	Missouri	62.8
30	Maryland	53.2	20	Hawaii	61.2
48	Massachusetts	35.1	21	Michigan	59.0
21	Michigan	59.0	22	Indiana	58.6
46	Minnesota	36.3	23	Ohio	57.9
1	Mississippi	81.0	24	West Virginia	57.3
19	Missouri	62.8	25	Wyoming	56.3
35	Montana	48.4	26	Kansas	56.1
42	Nebraska	42.3	27	Oregon	54.6
8	Nevada	73.3	28	Colorado	54.5
50	New Hampshire	33.0	28	Delaware	54.5
43	New Jersey	40.5	30	Maryland	53.2
3	New Mexico	78.2	31	Washington	53.1
39	New York	43.6	32	Virginia	52.9
14	North Carolina	67.6	33	Idaho	50.6
47	North Dakota	35.4	34	Utah	48.5
23	Ohio	57.9	35	Montana	48.4
16	Oklahoma	66.8	36	South Dakota	46.8
27	Oregon	54.6	37	Pennsylvania	44.9
37	Pennsylvania	44.9	38	Rhode Island	43.9
38	Rhode Island	43.9	39	New York	43.6
10	South Carolina	71.3	40	Maine	43.0
36	South Dakota	46.8	41	Wisconsin	42.6
9	Tennessee	72.3	42	Nebraska	42.3
6	Texas	75.3	43	Iowa	40.5
34	Utah	48.5	43	New Jersey	40.5
49	Vermont	34.0	45	Connecticut	38.8
32	Virginia	52.9	46	Minnesota	36.3
31	Washington	53.1	47	North Dakota	35.4
24	West Virginia	57.3	48	Massachusetts	35.1
41	Wisconsin	42.6	49	Vermont	34.0
25	Wyoming	56.3	50	New Hampshire	33.0
				District of Columbia	93.1

Source: U.S. Department of Health and Human Services, Centers for Disease Control and Prevention
"Surveillance for Pregnancy and Birth Rates Among Teenagers" (MMWR, Vol. 42, No. SS-6, 12/17/93)
*Women aged 15 to 19 years old.

Percent Change in Teenage Birth Rate: 1990 to 1999

National Percent Change = 17.2% Decrease*

ALPHA ORDER

RANK	STATE	PERCENT CHANGE
7	Alabama	(11.5)
50	Alaska	(36.0)
3	Arizona	(7.8)
21	Arkansas	(15.0)
45	California	(28.2)
6	Colorado	(11.2)
18	Connecticut	(14.2)
1	Delaware	(0.4)
40	Florida	(22.6)
16	Georgia	(13.8)
47	Hawaii	(28.4)
15	Idaho	(13.6)
31	Illinois	(18.8)
9	Indiana	(11.9)
8	Iowa	(11.6)
24	Kansas	(15.5)
27	Kentucky	(16.6)
23	Louisiana	(15.4)
48	Maine	(30.7)
36	Maryland	(19.9)
30	Massachusetts	(18.2)
49	Michigan	(31.4)
29	Minnesota	(17.4)
5	Mississippi	(10.5)
38	Missouri	(21.0)
44	Montana	(27.5)
11	Nebraska	(12.5)
12	Nevada	(12.6)
43	New Hampshire	(27.3)
32	New Jersey	(19.0)
16	New Mexico	(13.8)
22	New York	(15.1)
10	North Carolina	(12.0)
39	North Dakota	(21.8)
37	Ohio	(20.6)
4	Oklahoma	(9.4)
20	Oregon	(14.8)
34	Pennsylvania	(19.4)
13	Rhode Island	(13.0)
19	South Carolina	(14.7)
35	South Dakota	(19.7)
14	Tennessee	(13.3)
2	Texas	(6.9)
28	Utah	(17.1)
41	Vermont	(24.4)
33	Virginia	(19.3)
42	Washington	(24.5)
26	West Virginia	(16.4)
25	Wisconsin	(16.2)
45	Wyoming	(28.2)

RANK ORDER

RANK	STATE	PERCENT CHANGE
1	Delaware	(0.4)
2	Texas	(6.9)
3	Arizona	(7.8)
4	Oklahoma	(9.4)
5	Mississippi	(10.5)
6	Colorado	(11.2)
7	Alabama	(11.5)
8	Iowa	(11.6)
9	Indiana	(11.9)
10	North Carolina	(12.0)
11	Nebraska	(12.5)
12	Nevada	(12.6)
13	Rhode Island	(13.0)
14	Tennessee	(13.3)
15	Idaho	(13.6)
16	Georgia	(13.8)
16	New Mexico	(13.8)
18	Connecticut	(14.2)
19	South Carolina	(14.7)
20	Oregon	(14.8)
21	Arkansas	(15.0)
22	New York	(15.1)
23	Louisiana	(15.4)
24	Kansas	(15.5)
25	Wisconsin	(16.2)
26	West Virginia	(16.4)
27	Kentucky	(16.6)
28	Utah	(17.1)
29	Minnesota	(17.4)
30	Massachusetts	(18.2)
31	Illinois	(18.8)
32	New Jersey	(19.0)
33	Virginia	(19.3)
34	Pennsylvania	(19.4)
35	South Dakota	(19.7)
36	Maryland	(19.9)
37	Ohio	(20.6)
38	Missouri	(21.0)
39	North Dakota	(21.8)
40	Florida	(22.6)
41	Vermont	(24.4)
42	Washington	(24.5)
43	New Hampshire	(27.3)
44	Montana	(27.5)
45	California	(28.2)
45	Wyoming	(28.2)
47	Hawaii	(28.4)
48	Maine	(30.7)
49	Michigan	(31.4)
50	Alaska	(36.0)

District of Columbia (10.3)

Source: Morgan Quitno Press using data from U.S. Department of Health and Human Services
    "National Vital Statistics Reports" (Vol. 49, No. 1, April 17, 2001)
    "Surveillance for Pregnancy and Birth Rates Among Teenagers" (MMWR, Vol. 42, No. SS-6, 12/17/93)
*Women aged 15 to 19 years old.

Births to Teenage Mothers in 1980

National Total = 562,330 Live Births*

ALPHA ORDER					RANK ORDER			
RANK	STATE	BIRTHS	% of USA		RANK	STATE	BIRTHS	% of USA
15	Alabama	13,096	2.3%		1	California	56,138	10.0%
49	Alaska	1,123	0.2%		2	Texas	50,125	8.9%
25	Arizona	8,235	1.5%		3	Illinois	29,798	5.3%
26	Arkansas	8,060	1.4%		4	New York	28,206	5.0%
1	California	56,138	10.0%		5	Ohio	26,567	4.7%
29	Colorado	6,592	1.2%		6	Florida	24,042	4.3%
36	Connecticut	4,408	0.8%		7	Pennsylvania	22,029	3.9%
45	Delaware	1,572	0.3%		8	Michigan	20,401	3.6%
6	Florida	24,042	4.3%		9	Georgia	19,137	3.4%
9	Georgia	19,137	3.4%		10	Louisiana	16,504	2.9%
40	Hawaii	2,085	0.4%		11	North Carolina	16,192	2.9%
38	Idaho	2,645	0.5%		12	Indiana	15,331	2.7%
3	Illinois	29,798	5.3%		13	Tennessee	13,792	2.5%
12	Indiana	15,331	2.7%		14	Missouri	13,312	2.4%
31	Iowa	5,962	1.1%		15	Alabama	13,096	2.3%
30	Kansas	6,090	1.1%		16	Kentucky	12,559	2.2%
16	Kentucky	12,559	2.2%		17	Virginia	12,138	2.2%
10	Louisiana	16,504	2.9%		18	New Jersey	11,904	2.1%
39	Maine	2,522	0.4%		19	Mississippi	11,079	2.0%
23	Maryland	8,885	1.6%		20	South Carolina	10,282	1.8%
27	Massachusetts	7,765	1.4%		21	Oklahoma	10,206	1.8%
8	Michigan	20,401	3.6%		22	Wisconsin	9,220	1.6%
28	Minnesota	7,048	1.3%		23	Maryland	8,885	1.6%
19	Mississippi	11,079	2.0%		24	Washington	8,495	1.5%
14	Missouri	13,312	2.4%		25	Arizona	8,235	1.5%
43	Montana	1,761	0.3%		26	Arkansas	8,060	1.4%
37	Nebraska	3,313	0.6%		27	Massachusetts	7,765	1.4%
41	Nevada	2,048	0.4%		28	Minnesota	7,048	1.3%
47	New Hampshire	1,475	0.3%		29	Colorado	6,592	1.2%
18	New Jersey	11,904	2.1%		30	Kansas	6,090	1.1%
34	New Mexico	4,758	0.8%		31	Iowa	5,962	1.1%
4	New York	28,206	5.0%		32	West Virginia	5,911	1.1%
11	North Carolina	16,192	2.9%		33	Oregon	5,731	1.0%
48	North Dakota	1,304	0.2%		34	New Mexico	4,758	0.8%
5	Ohio	26,567	4.7%		35	Utah	4,594	0.8%
21	Oklahoma	10,206	1.8%		36	Connecticut	4,408	0.8%
33	Oregon	5,731	1.0%		37	Nebraska	3,313	0.6%
7	Pennsylvania	22,029	3.9%		38	Idaho	2,645	0.5%
46	Rhode Island	1,502	0.3%		39	Maine	2,522	0.4%
20	South Carolina	10,282	1.8%		40	Hawaii	2,085	0.4%
42	South Dakota	1,797	0.3%		41	Nevada	2,048	0.4%
13	Tennessee	13,792	2.5%		42	South Dakota	1,797	0.3%
2	Texas	50,125	8.9%		43	Montana	1,761	0.3%
35	Utah	4,594	0.8%		44	Wyoming	1,634	0.3%
50	Vermont	1,024	0.2%		45	Delaware	1,572	0.3%
17	Virginia	12,138	2.2%		46	Rhode Island	1,502	0.3%
24	Washington	8,495	1.5%		47	New Hampshire	1,475	0.3%
32	West Virginia	5,911	1.1%		48	North Dakota	1,304	0.2%
22	Wisconsin	9,220	1.6%		49	Alaska	1,123	0.2%
44	Wyoming	1,634	0.3%		50	Vermont	1,024	0.2%
						District of Columbia	1,933	0.3%

Source: U.S. Department of Health and Human Services, National Center for Health Statistics
"Vital Statistics of the United States, 1980" (Vol. I-Natality, issued 1984)
*Births to women age 15 to 19 years old.

Teenage Birth Rate in 1980

National Rate = 53.0 Live Births per 1,000 Teenage Women*

ALPHA ORDER

RANK	STATE	RATE
10	Alabama	68.3
15	Alaska	64.4
12	Arizona	65.5
5	Arkansas	74.5
25	California	53.3
31	Colorado	49.9
49	Connecticut	30.5
28	Delaware	51.2
18	Florida	58.5
8	Georgia	71.9
30	Hawaii	50.7
17	Idaho	59.5
24	Illinois	55.8
21	Indiana	57.5
39	Iowa	43.0
23	Kansas	56.8
7	Kentucky	72.3
3	Louisiana	76.0
34	Maine	47.4
38	Maryland	43.4
50	Massachusetts	28.1
37	Michigan	45.0
44	Minnesota	35.4
1	Mississippi	83.7
20	Missouri	57.8
32	Montana	48.5
36	Nebraska	45.1
18	Nevada	58.5
47	New Hampshire	33.6
45	New Jersey	35.2
9	New Mexico	71.8
46	New York	34.8
21	North Carolina	57.5
40	North Dakota	41.7
27	Ohio	52.5
4	Oklahoma	74.6
29	Oregon	50.9
41	Pennsylvania	40.5
48	Rhode Island	33.0
14	South Carolina	64.8
26	South Dakota	52.6
16	Tennessee	64.1
6	Texas	74.3
13	Utah	65.2
42	Vermont	39.5
33	Virginia	48.3
35	Washington	46.7
11	West Virginia	67.8
42	Wisconsin	39.5
2	Wyoming	78.7

RANK ORDER

RANK	STATE	RATE
1	Mississippi	83.7
2	Wyoming	78.7
3	Louisiana	76.0
4	Oklahoma	74.6
5	Arkansas	74.5
6	Texas	74.3
7	Kentucky	72.3
8	Georgia	71.9
9	New Mexico	71.8
10	Alabama	68.3
11	West Virginia	67.8
12	Arizona	65.5
13	Utah	65.2
14	South Carolina	64.8
15	Alaska	64.4
16	Tennessee	64.1
17	Idaho	59.5
18	Florida	58.5
18	Nevada	58.5
20	Missouri	57.8
21	Indiana	57.5
21	North Carolina	57.5
23	Kansas	56.8
24	Illinois	55.8
25	California	53.3
26	South Dakota	52.6
27	Ohio	52.5
28	Delaware	51.2
29	Oregon	50.9
30	Hawaii	50.7
31	Colorado	49.9
32	Montana	48.5
33	Virginia	48.3
34	Maine	47.4
35	Washington	46.7
36	Nebraska	45.1
37	Michigan	45.0
38	Maryland	43.4
39	Iowa	43.0
40	North Dakota	41.7
41	Pennsylvania	40.5
42	Vermont	39.5
42	Wisconsin	39.5
44	Minnesota	35.4
45	New Jersey	35.2
46	New York	34.8
47	New Hampshire	33.6
48	Rhode Island	33.0
49	Connecticut	30.5
50	Massachusetts	28.1
	District of Columbia	62.4

Source: U.S. Department of Health and Human Services, Centers for Disease Control and Prevention
   "Surveillance for Pregnancy and Birth Rates Among Teenagers" (MMWR, Vol. 42, No. SS-6, 12/17/93)
*Women aged 15 to 19 years old.

Births to Women 35 to 54 Years Old in 1999

National Total = 521,732 Live Births*

ALPHA ORDER

RANK	STATE	BIRTHS	% of USA
27	Alabama	5,240	1.0%
44	Alaska	1,373	0.3%
17	Arizona	8,934	1.7%
38	Arkansas	2,732	0.5%
1	California	80,779	15.5%
19	Colorado	8,733	1.7%
20	Connecticut	8,631	1.7%
46	Delaware	1,346	0.3%
4	Florida	27,012	5.2%
12	Georgia	13,945	2.7%
37	Hawaii	2,789	0.5%
41	Idaho	1,863	0.4%
5	Illinois	25,165	4.8%
21	Indiana	8,341	1.6%
30	Iowa	4,132	0.8%
29	Kansas	4,340	0.8%
28	Kentucky	4,716	0.9%
24	Louisiana	5,906	1.1%
42	Maine	1,735	0.3%
13	Maryland	12,559	2.4%
9	Massachusetts	16,780	3.2%
10	Michigan	16,286	3.1%
16	Minnesota	9,642	1.8%
34	Mississippi	3,060	0.6%
22	Missouri	8,121	1.6%
45	Montana	1,361	0.3%
36	Nebraska	2,826	0.5%
33	Nevada	3,451	0.7%
39	New Hampshire	2,376	0.5%
6	New Jersey	22,697	4.4%
35	New Mexico	2,898	0.6%
2	New York	46,112	8.8%
14	North Carolina	12,179	2.3%
49	North Dakota	892	0.2%
8	Ohio	17,547	3.4%
31	Oklahoma	4,066	0.8%
25	Oregon	5,658	1.1%
7	Pennsylvania	21,446	4.1%
40	Rhode Island	1,952	0.4%
26	South Carolina	5,400	1.0%
47	South Dakota	1,152	0.2%
23	Tennessee	7,364	1.4%
3	Texas	35,161	6.7%
32	Utah	4,059	0.8%
48	Vermont	1,084	0.2%
11	Virginia	14,430	2.8%
15	Washington	11,170	2.1%
43	West Virginia	1,671	0.3%
18	Wisconsin	8,773	1.7%
50	Wyoming	587	0.1%

RANK ORDER

RANK	STATE	BIRTHS	% of USA
1	California	80,779	15.5%
2	New York	46,112	8.8%
3	Texas	35,161	6.7%
4	Florida	27,012	5.2%
5	Illinois	25,165	4.8%
6	New Jersey	22,697	4.4%
7	Pennsylvania	21,446	4.1%
8	Ohio	17,547	3.4%
9	Massachusetts	16,780	3.2%
10	Michigan	16,286	3.1%
11	Virginia	14,430	2.8%
12	Georgia	13,945	2.7%
13	Maryland	12,559	2.4%
14	North Carolina	12,179	2.3%
15	Washington	11,170	2.1%
16	Minnesota	9,642	1.8%
17	Arizona	8,934	1.7%
18	Wisconsin	8,773	1.7%
19	Colorado	8,733	1.7%
20	Connecticut	8,631	1.7%
21	Indiana	8,341	1.6%
22	Missouri	8,121	1.6%
23	Tennessee	7,364	1.4%
24	Louisiana	5,906	1.1%
25	Oregon	5,658	1.1%
26	South Carolina	5,400	1.0%
27	Alabama	5,240	1.0%
28	Kentucky	4,716	0.9%
29	Kansas	4,340	0.8%
30	Iowa	4,132	0.8%
31	Oklahoma	4,066	0.8%
32	Utah	4,059	0.8%
33	Nevada	3,451	0.7%
34	Mississippi	3,060	0.6%
35	New Mexico	2,898	0.6%
36	Nebraska	2,826	0.5%
37	Hawaii	2,789	0.5%
38	Arkansas	2,732	0.5%
39	New Hampshire	2,376	0.5%
40	Rhode Island	1,952	0.4%
41	Idaho	1,863	0.4%
42	Maine	1,735	0.3%
43	West Virginia	1,671	0.3%
44	Alaska	1,373	0.3%
45	Montana	1,361	0.3%
46	Delaware	1,346	0.3%
47	South Dakota	1,152	0.2%
48	Vermont	1,084	0.2%
49	North Dakota	892	0.2%
50	Wyoming	587	0.1%
	District of Columbia	1,260	0.2%

Source: Morgan Quitno Press using data from U.S. Dept of Health & Human Services, National Center for Health Statistics
(unpublished data)
*By state of residence.

Births to Women 35 to 54 Years Old as a Percent of All Births in 1999

National Percent = 13.2% of Live Births*

ALPHA ORDER

RANK	STATE	PERCENT	RANK	STATE	PERCENT
46	Alabama	8.4	1	Massachusetts	20.7
16	Alaska	13.8	2	Connecticut	19.9
30	Arizona	11.0	2	New Jersey	19.9
49	Arkansas	7.4	4	New York	18.0
10	California	15.6	5	Maryland	17.5
14	Colorado	14.0	6	New Hampshire	16.9
2	Connecticut	19.9	7	Vermont	16.5
21	Delaware	12.6	8	Hawaii	16.4
18	Florida	13.7	9	Rhode Island	15.8
30	Georgia	11.0	10	California	15.6
8	Hawaii	16.4	11	Virginia	15.1
42	Idaho	9.4	12	Pennsylvania	14.8
16	Illinois	13.8	13	Minnesota	14.6
39	Indiana	9.7	14	Colorado	14.0
30	Iowa	11.0	14	Washington	14.0
29	Kansas	11.2	16	Alaska	13.8
45	Kentucky	8.7	16	Illinois	13.8
43	Louisiana	8.8	18	Florida	13.7
20	Maine	12.7	19	Wisconsin	12.9
5	Maryland	17.5	20	Maine	12.7
1	Massachusetts	20.7	21	Delaware	12.6
24	Michigan	12.2	21	Montana	12.6
13	Minnesota	14.6	23	Oregon	12.5
50	Mississippi	7.2	24	Michigan	12.2
34	Missouri	10.8	25	Nebraska	11.8
21	Montana	12.6	25	Nevada	11.8
25	Nebraska	11.8	27	North Dakota	11.7
25	Nevada	11.8	28	Ohio	11.5
6	New Hampshire	16.9	29	Kansas	11.2
2	New Jersey	19.9	30	Arizona	11.0
35	New Mexico	10.7	30	Georgia	11.0
4	New York	18.0	30	Iowa	11.0
35	North Carolina	10.7	33	South Dakota	10.9
27	North Dakota	11.7	34	Missouri	10.8
28	Ohio	11.5	35	New Mexico	10.7
47	Oklahoma	8.3	35	North Carolina	10.7
23	Oregon	12.5	37	Texas	10.1
12	Pennsylvania	14.8	38	South Carolina	9.8
9	Rhode Island	15.8	39	Indiana	9.7
38	South Carolina	9.8	40	Wyoming	9.6
33	South Dakota	10.9	41	Tennessee	9.5
41	Tennessee	9.5	42	Idaho	9.4
37	Texas	10.1	43	Louisiana	8.8
43	Utah	8.8	43	Utah	8.8
7	Vermont	16.5	45	Kentucky	8.7
11	Virginia	15.1	46	Alabama	8.4
14	Washington	14.0	47	Oklahoma	8.3
48	West Virginia	8.1	48	West Virginia	8.1
19	Wisconsin	12.9	49	Arkansas	7.4
40	Wyoming	9.6	50	Mississippi	7.2
				District of Columbia	16.8

Source: Morgan Quitno Press using data from U.S. Dept of Health & Human Services, National Center for Health Statistics
(unpublished data)
*By state of residence.

Births by Vaginal Delivery in 1999

National Total = 3,088,345 Live Births*

ALPHA ORDER

RANK	STATE	BIRTHS	% of USA
24	Alabama	46,716	1.5%
45	Alaska	8,477	0.3%
14	Arizona	66,701	2.2%
34	Arkansas	27,400	0.9%
1	California	400,807	13.0%
22	Colorado	51,412	1.7%
30	Connecticut	34,215	1.1%
46	Delaware	8,221	0.3%
4	Florida	150,132	4.9%
9	Georgia	99,219	3.2%
40	Hawaii	14,687	0.5%
38	Idaho	16,434	0.5%
5	Illinois	145,472	4.7%
13	Indiana	68,395	2.2%
33	Iowa	30,084	1.0%
32	Kansas	30,560	1.0%
25	Kentucky	41,727	1.4%
23	Louisiana	49,144	1.6%
42	Maine	10,689	0.3%
20	Maryland	55,271	1.8%
16	Massachusetts	62,809	2.0%
8	Michigan	105,550	3.4%
21	Minnesota	53,502	1.7%
31	Mississippi	31,031	1.0%
18	Missouri	59,063	1.9%
44	Montana	8,757	0.3%
37	Nebraska	18,647	0.6%
35	Nevada	22,961	0.7%
41	New Hampshire	11,247	0.4%
11	New Jersey	84,095	2.7%
36	New Mexico	22,732	0.7%
3	New York	195,288	6.3%
10	North Carolina	87,964	2.8%
48	North Dakota	6,149	0.2%
6	Ohio	122,983	4.0%
28	Oklahoma	37,199	1.2%
29	Oregon	36,886	1.2%
7	Pennsylvania	114,969	3.7%
43	Rhode Island	9,831	0.3%
26	South Carolina	41,651	1.3%
47	South Dakota	8,177	0.3%
17	Tennessee	59,130	1.9%
2	Texas	266,125	8.6%
27	Utah	38,884	1.3%
49	Vermont	5,490	0.2%
12	Virginia	74,752	2.4%
15	Washington	64,544	2.1%
39	West Virginia	15,587	0.5%
19	Wisconsin	56,613	1.8%
50	Wyoming	4,928	0.2%

RANK ORDER

RANK	STATE	BIRTHS	% of USA
1	California	400,807	13.0%
2	Texas	266,125	8.6%
3	New York	195,288	6.3%
4	Florida	150,132	4.9%
5	Illinois	145,472	4.7%
6	Ohio	122,983	4.0%
7	Pennsylvania	114,969	3.7%
8	Michigan	105,550	3.4%
9	Georgia	99,219	3.2%
10	North Carolina	87,964	2.8%
11	New Jersey	84,095	2.7%
12	Virginia	74,752	2.4%
13	Indiana	68,395	2.2%
14	Arizona	66,701	2.2%
15	Washington	64,544	2.1%
16	Massachusetts	62,809	2.0%
17	Tennessee	59,130	1.9%
18	Missouri	59,063	1.9%
19	Wisconsin	56,613	1.8%
20	Maryland	55,271	1.8%
21	Minnesota	53,502	1.7%
22	Colorado	51,412	1.7%
23	Louisiana	49,144	1.6%
24	Alabama	46,716	1.5%
25	Kentucky	41,727	1.4%
26	South Carolina	41,651	1.3%
27	Utah	38,884	1.3%
28	Oklahoma	37,199	1.2%
29	Oregon	36,886	1.2%
30	Connecticut	34,215	1.1%
31	Mississippi	31,031	1.0%
32	Kansas	30,560	1.0%
33	Iowa	30,084	1.0%
34	Arkansas	27,400	0.9%
35	Nevada	22,961	0.7%
36	New Mexico	22,732	0.7%
37	Nebraska	18,647	0.6%
38	Idaho	16,434	0.5%
39	West Virginia	15,587	0.5%
40	Hawaii	14,687	0.5%
41	New Hampshire	11,247	0.4%
42	Maine	10,689	0.3%
43	Rhode Island	9,831	0.3%
44	Montana	8,757	0.3%
45	Alaska	8,477	0.3%
46	Delaware	8,221	0.3%
47	South Dakota	8,177	0.3%
48	North Dakota	6,149	0.2%
49	Vermont	5,490	0.2%
50	Wyoming	4,928	0.2%
	District of Columbia	5,852	0.2%

Source: Morgan Quitno Press using data from U.S. Dept of Health & Human Services, National Center for Health Statistics
"National Vital Statistics Reports" (Vol. 49, No. 1, April 17, 2001)
*By state of residence. Includes VBACs (vaginal births after cesarean).

Percent of Births by Vaginal Delivery in 1999

National Percent = 78.0% of Live Births*

ALPHA ORDER

RANK ORDER

RANK	STATE	PERCENT
45	Alabama	75.2
2	Alaska	85.2
9	Arizona	82.2
47	Arkansas	74.6
34	California	77.3
7	Colorado	82.7
23	Connecticut	79.0
36	Delaware	77.0
40	Florida	76.2
27	Georgia	78.3
1	Hawaii	86.2
7	Idaho	82.7
19	Illinois	79.9
20	Indiana	79.5
17	Iowa	80.1
25	Kansas	78.8
38	Kentucky	76.7
49	Louisiana	73.2
26	Maine	78.5
37	Maryland	76.8
33	Massachusetts	77.6
23	Michigan	79.0
12	Minnesota	81.1
50	Mississippi	72.7
27	Missouri	78.3
11	Montana	81.2
31	Nebraska	78.0
30	Nevada	78.2
17	New Hampshire	80.1
48	New Jersey	73.7
4	New Mexico	83.6
39	New York	76.4
34	North Carolina	77.3
15	North Dakota	80.5
14	Ohio	80.6
43	Oklahoma	75.9
10	Oregon	81.6
22	Pennsylvania	79.1
20	Rhode Island	79.5
44	South Carolina	75.8
32	South Dakota	77.7
42	Tennessee	76.0
40	Texas	76.2
3	Utah	84.0
4	Vermont	83.6
27	Virginia	78.3
12	Washington	81.1
45	West Virginia	75.2
6	Wisconsin	83.0
16	Wyoming	80.4

RANK	STATE	PERCENT
1	Hawaii	86.2
2	Alaska	85.2
3	Utah	84.0
4	New Mexico	83.6
4	Vermont	83.6
6	Wisconsin	83.0
7	Colorado	82.7
7	Idaho	82.7
9	Arizona	82.2
10	Oregon	81.6
11	Montana	81.2
12	Minnesota	81.1
12	Washington	81.1
14	Ohio	80.6
15	North Dakota	80.5
16	Wyoming	80.4
17	Iowa	80.1
17	New Hampshire	80.1
19	Illinois	79.9
20	Indiana	79.5
20	Rhode Island	79.5
22	Pennsylvania	79.1
23	Connecticut	79.0
23	Michigan	79.0
25	Kansas	78.8
26	Maine	78.5
27	Georgia	78.3
27	Missouri	78.3
27	Virginia	78.3
30	Nevada	78.2
31	Nebraska	78.0
32	South Dakota	77.7
33	Massachusetts	77.6
34	California	77.3
34	North Carolina	77.3
36	Delaware	77.0
37	Maryland	76.8
38	Kentucky	76.7
39	New York	76.4
40	Florida	76.2
40	Texas	76.2
42	Tennessee	76.0
43	Oklahoma	75.9
44	South Carolina	75.8
45	Alabama	75.2
45	West Virginia	75.2
47	Arkansas	74.6
48	New Jersey	73.7
49	Louisiana	73.2
50	Mississippi	72.7

District of Columbia 77.8

Source: Morgan Quitno Press using data from U.S. Dept of Health & Human Services, National Center for Health Statistics
"National Vital Statistics Reports" (Vol. 49, No. 1, April 17, 2001)
*By state of residence. Includes VBACs (vaginal births after cesarean).

Births by Cesarean Delivery in 1999

National Total = 871,072 Live Cesarean Births*

ALPHA ORDER					RANK ORDER			
RANK	STATE		BIRTHS	% of USA	RANK	STATE	BIRTHS	% of USA
19	Alabama		15,406	1.8%	1	California	117,701	13.5%
48	Alaska		1,473	0.2%	2	Texas	83,120	9.5%
21	Arizona		14,444	1.7%	3	New York	60,324	6.9%
29	Arkansas		9,329	1.1%	4	Florida	46,891	5.4%
1	California		117,701	13.5%	5	Illinois	36,596	4.2%
28	Colorado		10,755	1.2%	6	Pennsylvania	30,378	3.5%
30	Connecticut		9,095	1.0%	7	New Jersey	30,010	3.4%
43	Delaware		2,455	0.3%	8	Ohio	29,601	3.4%
4	Florida		46,891	5.4%	9	Michigan	28,057	3.2%
10	Georgia		27,498	3.2%	10	Georgia	27,498	3.2%
44	Hawaii		2,351	0.3%	11	North Carolina	25,831	3.0%
39	Idaho		3,438	0.4%	12	Virginia	20,717	2.4%
5	Illinois		36,596	4.2%	13	Tennessee	18,673	2.1%
16	Indiana		17,636	2.0%	14	Massachusetts	18,130	2.1%
33	Iowa		7,474	0.9%	15	Louisiana	17,992	2.1%
32	Kansas		8,222	0.9%	16	Indiana	17,636	2.0%
23	Kentucky		12,676	1.5%	17	Maryland	16,696	1.9%
15	Louisiana		17,992	2.1%	18	Missouri	16,369	1.9%
40	Maine		2,927	0.3%	19	Alabama	15,406	1.8%
17	Maryland		16,696	1.9%	20	Washington	15,042	1.7%
14	Massachusetts		18,130	2.1%	21	Arizona	14,444	1.7%
9	Michigan		28,057	3.2%	22	South Carolina	13,297	1.5%
24	Minnesota		12,468	1.4%	23	Kentucky	12,676	1.5%
26	Mississippi		11,653	1.3%	24	Minnesota	12,468	1.4%
18	Missouri		16,369	1.9%	25	Oklahoma	11,811	1.4%
46	Montana		2,028	0.2%	26	Mississippi	11,653	1.3%
36	Nebraska		5,260	0.6%	27	Wisconsin	11,595	1.3%
35	Nevada		6,401	0.7%	28	Colorado	10,755	1.2%
41	New Hampshire		2,794	0.3%	29	Arkansas	9,329	1.1%
7	New Jersey		30,010	3.4%	30	Connecticut	9,095	1.0%
38	New Mexico		4,459	0.5%	31	Oregon	8,318	1.0%
3	New York		60,324	6.9%	32	Kansas	8,222	0.9%
11	North Carolina		25,831	3.0%	33	Iowa	7,474	0.9%
47	North Dakota		1,490	0.2%	34	Utah	7,406	0.9%
8	Ohio		29,601	3.4%	35	Nevada	6,401	0.7%
25	Oklahoma		11,811	1.4%	36	Nebraska	5,260	0.6%
31	Oregon		8,318	1.0%	37	West Virginia	5,141	0.6%
6	Pennsylvania		30,378	3.5%	38	New Mexico	4,459	0.5%
42	Rhode Island		2,535	0.3%	39	Idaho	3,438	0.4%
22	South Carolina		13,297	1.5%	40	Maine	2,927	0.3%
45	South Dakota		2,347	0.3%	41	New Hampshire	2,794	0.3%
13	Tennessee		18,673	2.1%	42	Rhode Island	2,535	0.3%
2	Texas		83,120	9.5%	43	Delaware	2,455	0.3%
34	Utah		7,406	0.9%	44	Hawaii	2,351	0.3%
50	Vermont		1,077	0.1%	45	South Dakota	2,347	0.3%
12	Virginia		20,717	2.4%	46	Montana	2,028	0.2%
20	Washington		15,042	1.7%	47	North Dakota	1,490	0.2%
37	West Virginia		5,141	0.6%	48	Alaska	1,473	0.2%
27	Wisconsin		11,595	1.3%	49	Wyoming	1,201	0.1%
49	Wyoming		1,201	0.1%	50	Vermont	1,077	0.1%
						District of Columbia	1,670	0.2%

Source: Morgan Quitno Press using data from U.S. Dept of Health & Human Services, National Center for Health Statistics "National Vital Statistics Reports" (Vol. 49, No. 1, April 17, 2001)
*By state of residence.

Percent of Births by Cesarean Delivery in 1999

National Percent = 22.0% of Live Births*

ALPHA ORDER				RANK ORDER		
RANK	**STATE**	**PERCENT**		**RANK**	**STATE**	**PERCENT**
5	Alabama	24.8		1	Mississippi	27.3
49	Alaska	14.8		2	Louisiana	26.8
42	Arizona	17.8		3	New Jersey	26.3
4	Arkansas	25.4		4	Arkansas	25.4
16	California	22.7		5	Alabama	24.8
43	Colorado	17.3		5	West Virginia	24.8
27	Connecticut	21.0		7	South Carolina	24.2
15	Delaware	23.0		8	Oklahoma	24.1
10	Florida	23.8		9	Tennessee	24.0
22	Georgia	21.7		10	Florida	23.8
50	Hawaii	13.8		10	Texas	23.8
43	Idaho	17.3		12	New York	23.6
32	Illinois	20.1		13	Kentucky	23.3
30	Indiana	20.5		14	Maryland	23.2
33	Iowa	19.9		15	Delaware	23.0
26	Kansas	21.2		16	California	22.7
13	Kentucky	23.3		16	North Carolina	22.7
2	Louisiana	26.8		18	Massachusetts	22.4
25	Maine	21.5		19	South Dakota	22.3
14	Maryland	23.2		20	Nebraska	22.0
18	Massachusetts	22.4		21	Nevada	21.8
27	Michigan	21.0		22	Georgia	21.7
38	Minnesota	18.9		22	Missouri	21.7
1	Mississippi	27.3		22	Virginia	21.7
22	Missouri	21.7		25	Maine	21.5
40	Montana	18.8		26	Kansas	21.2
20	Nebraska	22.0		27	Connecticut	21.0
21	Nevada	21.8		27	Michigan	21.0
33	New Hampshire	19.9		29	Pennsylvania	20.9
3	New Jersey	26.3		30	Indiana	20.5
46	New Mexico	16.4		30	Rhode Island	20.5
12	New York	23.6		32	Illinois	20.1
16	North Carolina	22.7		33	Iowa	19.9
36	North Dakota	19.5		33	New Hampshire	19.9
37	Ohio	19.4		35	Wyoming	19.6
8	Oklahoma	24.1		36	North Dakota	19.5
41	Oregon	18.4		37	Ohio	19.4
29	Pennsylvania	20.9		38	Minnesota	18.9
30	Rhode Island	20.5		38	Washington	18.9
7	South Carolina	24.2		40	Montana	18.8
19	South Dakota	22.3		41	Oregon	18.4
9	Tennessee	24.0		42	Arizona	17.8
10	Texas	23.8		43	Colorado	17.3
48	Utah	16.0		43	Idaho	17.3
46	Vermont	16.4		45	Wisconsin	17.0
22	Virginia	21.7		46	New Mexico	16.4
38	Washington	18.9		46	Vermont	16.4
5	West Virginia	24.8		48	Utah	16.0
45	Wisconsin	17.0		49	Alaska	14.8
35	Wyoming	19.6		50	Hawaii	13.8
					District of Columbia	22.2

Source: U.S. Department of Health and Human Services, National Center for Health Statistics
"National Vital Statistics Reports" (Vol. 49, No. 1, April 17, 2001)
*By state of residence.

Percent Change in Rate of Cesarean Births: 1995 to 1999

National Percent Change = 5.8% Increase*

ALPHA ORDER

RANK ORDER

RANK	STATE	PERCENT CHANGE		RANK	STATE	PERCENT CHANGE
22	Alabama	6.0		1	Minnesota	16.0
34	Alaska	2.8		2	Nebraska	14.6
22	Arizona	6.0		3	Colorado	13.8
42	Arkansas	(0.8)		4	Nevada	13.5
11	California	10.2		5	Tennessee	13.2
3	Colorado	13.8		6	New Jersey	12.9
15	Connecticut	9.4		7	South Dakota	12.1
19	Delaware	7.0		8	Rhode Island	11.4
13	Florida	9.7		9	Washington	10.5
35	Georgia	2.4		10	Wisconsin	10.4
50	Hawaii	(25.4)		11	California	10.2
11	Idaho	10.2		11	Idaho	10.2
38	Illinois	1.0		13	Florida	9.7
43	Indiana	(1.0)		14	Wyoming	9.5
19	Iowa	7.0		15	Connecticut	9.4
18	Kansas	7.6		16	Massachusetts	8.7
24	Kentucky	5.9		17	South Carolina	8.0
45	Louisiana	(1.5)		18	Kansas	7.6
35	Maine	2.4		19	Delaware	7.0
28	Maryland	5.5		19	Iowa	7.0
16	Massachusetts	8.7		21	Pennsylvania	6.1
33	Michigan	3.4		22	Alabama	6.0
1	Minnesota	16.0		22	Arizona	6.0
30	Mississippi	5.4		24	Kentucky	5.9
24	Missouri	5.9		24	Missouri	5.9
46	Montana	(1.6)		26	Oklahoma	5.7
2	Nebraska	14.6		26	Oregon	5.7
4	Nevada	13.5		28	Maryland	5.5
41	New Hampshire	(0.5)		28	West Virginia	5.5
6	New Jersey	12.9		30	Mississippi	5.4
49	New Mexico	(9.4)		31	North Carolina	4.6
32	New York	4.0		32	New York	4.0
31	North Carolina	4.6		33	Michigan	3.4
38	North Dakota	1.0		34	Alaska	2.8
43	Ohio	(1.0)		35	Georgia	2.4
26	Oklahoma	5.7		35	Maine	2.4
26	Oregon	5.7		37	Virginia	1.9
21	Pennsylvania	6.1		38	Illinois	1.0
8	Rhode Island	11.4		38	North Dakota	1.0
17	South Carolina	8.0		40	Texas	0.8
7	South Dakota	12.1		41	New Hampshire	(0.5)
5	Tennessee	13.2		42	Arkansas	(0.8)
40	Texas	0.8		43	Indiana	(1.0)
47	Utah	(1.8)		43	Ohio	(1.0)
47	Vermont	(1.8)		45	Louisiana	(1.5)
37	Virginia	1.9		46	Montana	(1.6)
9	Washington	10.5		47	Utah	(1.8)
28	West Virginia	5.5		47	Vermont	(1.8)
10	Wisconsin	10.4		49	New Mexico	(9.4)
14	Wyoming	9.5		50	Hawaii	(25.4)

District of Columbia   0.9

Source: Morgan Quitno Press using data from U.S. Dept of Health & Human Services, National Center for Health Statistics "National Vital Statistics Reports" (Vol. 49, No. 1, April 17, 2001) and unpublished data.
*By state of residence.

Percent of Vaginal Births After a Cesarean (VBAC) in 1999

National Percent = 23.4% of Live Births to Women Who Have Had a Cesarean*

ALPHA ORDER				RANK ORDER		
RANK	STATE	PERCENT		RANK	STATE	PERCENT
40	Alabama	19.1		1	New Hampshire	36.3
5	Alaska	32.8		2	Vermont	35.7
35	Arizona	22.7		3	Utah	35.5
47	Arkansas	15.5		4	Idaho	33.4
46	California	16.3		5	Alaska	32.8
12	Colorado	31.0		6	Hawaii	32.4
22	Connecticut	27.6		6	Oregon	32.4
17	Delaware	28.8		8	Ohio	32.2
42	Florida	18.7		9	North Dakota	31.8
36	Georgia	21.6		10	Montana	31.7
6	Hawaii	32.4		10	Wisconsin	31.7
4	Idaho	33.4		12	Colorado	31.0
17	Illinois	28.8		13	New Mexico	30.9
29	Indiana	24.6		14	Pennsylvania	30.5
21	Iowa	28.2		15	New Jersey	30.0
39	Kansas	19.9		16	New York	29.3
37	Kentucky	21.5		17	Delaware	28.8
50	Louisiana	11.3		17	Illinois	28.8
32	Maine	23.5		17	Washington	28.8
26	Maryland	26.0		20	Massachusetts	28.3
20	Massachusetts	28.3		21	Iowa	28.2
34	Michigan	22.8		22	Connecticut	27.6
27	Minnesota	25.7		23	Wyoming	26.9
49	Mississippi	13.8		24	Rhode Island	26.6
28	Missouri	25.5		24	Virginia	26.6
10	Montana	31.7		26	Maryland	26.0
31	Nebraska	23.9		27	Minnesota	25.7
43	Nevada	18.5		28	Missouri	25.5
1	New Hampshire	36.3		29	Indiana	24.6
15	New Jersey	30.0		30	North Carolina	24.0
13	New Mexico	30.9		31	Nebraska	23.9
16	New York	29.3		32	Maine	23.5
30	North Carolina	24.0		33	South Dakota	23.0
9	North Dakota	31.8		34	Michigan	22.8
8	Ohio	32.2		35	Arizona	22.7
41	Oklahoma	18.9		36	Georgia	21.6
6	Oregon	32.4		37	Kentucky	21.5
14	Pennsylvania	30.5		38	Tennessee	21.0
24	Rhode Island	26.6		39	Kansas	19.9
45	South Carolina	17.9		40	Alabama	19.1
33	South Dakota	23.0		41	Oklahoma	18.9
38	Tennessee	21.0		42	Florida	18.7
48	Texas	15.4		43	Nevada	18.5
3	Utah	35.5		44	West Virginia	18.4
2	Vermont	35.7		45	South Carolina	17.9
24	Virginia	26.6		46	California	16.3
17	Washington	28.8		47	Arkansas	15.5
44	West Virginia	18.4		48	Texas	15.4
10	Wisconsin	31.7		49	Mississippi	13.8
23	Wyoming	26.9		50	Louisiana	11.3
					District of Columbia	27.3

Source: U.S. Department of Health and Human Services, National Center for Health Statistics
   "National Vital Statistics Reports" (Vol. 49, No. 1, April 17, 2001)
*Vaginal births after a cesarean delivery as a percent of all births to women with a previous cesarean delivery giving birth in 1999.

Percent of Mothers Beginning Prenatal Care in First Trimester in 2000

National Percent = 83.2% of Mothers*

ALPHA ORDER			RANK ORDER		
RANK	STATE	PERCENT	RANK	STATE	PERCENT
29	Alabama	82.8	1	New Hampshire	91.1
40	Alaska	80.1	2	Rhode Island	91.0
47	Arizona	76.5	3	Connecticut	89.5
41	Arkansas	79.7	4	Massachusetts	89.3
21	California	84.5	5	Maine	88.7
38	Colorado	80.7	6	Vermont	88.4
3	Connecticut	89.5	7	Iowa	88.2
17	Delaware	85.3	8	Missouri	87.8
24	Florida	83.7	9	Georgia	86.9
9	Georgia	86.9	9	Kansas	86.9
15	Hawaii	85.5	11	Kentucky	86.8
36	Idaho	80.9	12	Maryland	86.4
32	Illinois	82.4	13	North Dakota	86.3
35	Indiana	81.1	14	West Virginia	86.1
7	Iowa	88.2	15	Hawaii	85.5
9	Kansas	86.9	16	Pennsylvania	85.4
11	Kentucky	86.8	17	Delaware	85.3
25	Louisiana	83.3	18	Minnesota	85.2
5	Maine	88.7	18	Virginia	85.2
12	Maryland	86.4	20	North Carolina	84.6
4	Massachusetts	89.3	21	California	84.5
22	Michigan	84.2	22	Michigan	84.2
18	Minnesota	85.2	22	Wisconsin	84.2
33	Mississippi	81.3	24	Florida	83.7
8	Missouri	87.8	25	Louisiana	83.3
25	Montana	83.3	25	Montana	83.3
27	Nebraska	83.2	27	Nebraska	83.2
48	Nevada	74.5	28	Tennessee	83.1
1	New Hampshire	91.1	29	Alabama	82.8
38	New Jersey	80.7	30	Washington	82.7
49	New Mexico	68.6	30	Wyoming	82.7
36	New York	80.9	32	Illinois	82.4
20	North Carolina	84.6	33	Mississippi	81.3
13	North Dakota	86.3	33	Oregon	81.3
NA	Ohio**	NA	35	Indiana	81.1
44	Oklahoma	79.3	36	Idaho	80.9
33	Oregon	81.3	36	New York	80.9
16	Pennsylvania	85.4	38	Colorado	80.7
2	Rhode Island	91.0	38	New Jersey	80.7
43	South Carolina	79.4	40	Alaska	80.1
46	South Dakota	78.7	41	Arkansas	79.7
28	Tennessee	83.1	42	Utah	79.5
45	Texas	78.8	43	South Carolina	79.4
42	Utah	79.5	44	Oklahoma	79.3
6	Vermont	88.4	45	Texas	78.8
18	Virginia	85.2	46	South Dakota	78.7
30	Washington	82.7	47	Arizona	76.5
14	West Virginia	86.1	48	Nevada	74.5
22	Wisconsin	84.2	49	New Mexico	68.6
30	Wyoming	82.7	NA	Ohio**	NA
				District of Columbia	75.3

Source: U.S. Department of Health and Human Services, National Center for Health Statistics
   "National Vital Statistics Reports" (Vol. 49, No. 5, July 24, 2001)
*Preliminary data by state of residence.
**Not available.

Percent of White Mothers Beginning Prenatal Care in First Trimester in 2000

National Percent = 85.0% of White Mothers*

ALPHA ORDER

RANK	STATE	PERCENT
16	Alabama	88.1
33	Alaska	84.2
47	Arizona	77.0
38	Arkansas	82.7
32	California	84.4
44	Colorado	81.0
5	Connecticut	90.6
17	Delaware	87.8
24	Florida	86.8
7	Georgia	89.8
8	Hawaii	89.6
43	Idaho	81.2
29	Illinois	85.0
38	Indiana	82.7
13	Iowa	88.7
19	Kansas	87.6
19	Kentucky	87.6
6	Louisiana	90.5
10	Maine	88.9
4	Maryland	90.8
3	Massachusetts	90.9
23	Michigan	87.2
19	Minnesota	87.6
11	Mississippi	88.8
9	Missouri	89.4
27	Montana	86.1
30	Nebraska	84.5
48	Nevada	75.1
2	New Hampshire	91.4
30	New Jersey	84.5
49	New Mexico	70.1
33	New York	84.2
18	North Carolina	87.7
11	North Dakota	88.8
NA	Ohio**	NA
41	Oklahoma	81.6
41	Oregon	81.6
19	Pennsylvania	87.6
1	Rhode Island	91.9
35	South Carolina	84.1
40	South Dakota	82.6
28	Tennessee	86.0
46	Texas	78.8
45	Utah	80.5
14	Vermont	88.6
15	Virginia	88.2
37	Washington	83.4
25	West Virginia	86.7
26	Wisconsin	86.6
36	Wyoming	83.5

RANK ORDER

RANK	STATE	PERCENT
1	Rhode Island	91.9
2	New Hampshire	91.4
3	Massachusetts	90.9
4	Maryland	90.8
5	Connecticut	90.6
6	Louisiana	90.5
7	Georgia	89.8
8	Hawaii	89.6
9	Missouri	89.4
10	Maine	88.9
11	Mississippi	88.8
11	North Dakota	88.8
13	Iowa	88.7
14	Vermont	88.6
15	Virginia	88.2
16	Alabama	88.1
17	Delaware	87.8
18	North Carolina	87.7
19	Kansas	87.6
19	Kentucky	87.6
19	Minnesota	87.6
19	Pennsylvania	87.6
23	Michigan	87.2
24	Florida	86.8
25	West Virginia	86.7
26	Wisconsin	86.6
27	Montana	86.1
28	Tennessee	86.0
29	Illinois	85.0
30	Nebraska	84.5
30	New Jersey	84.5
32	California	84.4
33	Alaska	84.2
33	New York	84.2
35	South Carolina	84.1
36	Wyoming	83.5
37	Washington	83.4
38	Arkansas	82.7
38	Indiana	82.7
40	South Dakota	82.6
41	Oklahoma	81.6
41	Oregon	81.6
43	Idaho	81.2
44	Colorado	81.0
45	Utah	80.5
46	Texas	78.8
47	Arizona	77.0
48	Nevada	75.1
49	New Mexico	70.1
NA	Ohio**	NA
	District of Columbia	85.5

Source: U.S. Department of Health and Human Services, National Center for Health Statistics
"National Vital Statistics Reports" (Vol. 49, No. 5, July 24, 2001)
Preliminary data by state of residence.
**Not available.*

Percent of Black Mothers Beginning Prenatal Care in First Trimester in 2000

National Percent = 74.2% of Black Mothers*

<table>
<tr><td colspan="3">ALPHA ORDER</td><td colspan="3">RANK ORDER</td></tr>
<tr><td>RANK</td><td>STATE</td><td>PERCENT</td><td>RANK</td><td>STATE</td><td>PERCENT</td></tr>
<tr><td>33</td><td>Alabama</td><td>72.0</td><td>1</td><td>Hawaii</td><td>89.3</td></tr>
<tr><td>6</td><td>Alaska</td><td>81.4</td><td>2</td><td>Montana</td><td>86.7</td></tr>
<tr><td>25</td><td>Arizona</td><td>74.0</td><td>3</td><td>Rhode Island</td><td>86.0</td></tr>
<tr><td>42</td><td>Arkansas</td><td>69.1</td><td>4</td><td>Connecticut</td><td>82.1</td></tr>
<tr><td>5</td><td>California</td><td>81.9</td><td>5</td><td>California</td><td>81.9</td></tr>
<tr><td>22</td><td>Colorado</td><td>75.2</td><td>6</td><td>Alaska</td><td>81.4</td></tr>
<tr><td>4</td><td>Connecticut</td><td>82.1</td><td>7</td><td>Georgia</td><td>81.1</td></tr>
<tr><td>14</td><td>Delaware</td><td>77.4</td><td>8</td><td>Massachusetts</td><td>79.4</td></tr>
<tr><td>28</td><td>Florida</td><td>73.6</td><td>9</td><td>Kansas</td><td>79.1</td></tr>
<tr><td>7</td><td>Georgia</td><td>81.1</td><td>10</td><td>Missouri</td><td>79.0</td></tr>
<tr><td>1</td><td>Hawaii</td><td>89.3</td><td>11</td><td>Kentucky</td><td>78.7</td></tr>
<tr><td>25</td><td>Idaho</td><td>74.0</td><td>12</td><td>North Dakota</td><td>78.0</td></tr>
<tr><td>34</td><td>Illinois</td><td>71.3</td><td>13</td><td>Maryland</td><td>77.7</td></tr>
<tr><td>44</td><td>Indiana</td><td>68.3</td><td>14</td><td>Delaware</td><td>77.4</td></tr>
<tr><td>14</td><td>Iowa</td><td>77.4</td><td>14</td><td>Iowa</td><td>77.4</td></tr>
<tr><td>9</td><td>Kansas</td><td>79.1</td><td>16</td><td>New Hampshire</td><td>76.7</td></tr>
<tr><td>11</td><td>Kentucky</td><td>78.7</td><td>17</td><td>Oregon</td><td>76.3</td></tr>
<tr><td>28</td><td>Louisiana</td><td>73.6</td><td>18</td><td>Texas</td><td>76.1</td></tr>
<tr><td>20</td><td>Maine</td><td>75.9</td><td>19</td><td>Virginia</td><td>76.0</td></tr>
<tr><td>13</td><td>Maryland</td><td>77.7</td><td>20</td><td>Maine</td><td>75.9</td></tr>
<tr><td>8</td><td>Massachusetts</td><td>79.4</td><td>20</td><td>North Carolina</td><td>75.9</td></tr>
<tr><td>40</td><td>Michigan</td><td>70.1</td><td>22</td><td>Colorado</td><td>75.2</td></tr>
<tr><td>43</td><td>Minnesota</td><td>68.8</td><td>23</td><td>Washington</td><td>74.9</td></tr>
<tr><td>31</td><td>Mississippi</td><td>72.4</td><td>24</td><td>Vermont</td><td>74.2</td></tr>
<tr><td>10</td><td>Missouri</td><td>79.0</td><td>25</td><td>Arizona</td><td>74.0</td></tr>
<tr><td>2</td><td>Montana</td><td>86.7</td><td>25</td><td>Idaho</td><td>74.0</td></tr>
<tr><td>45</td><td>Nebraska</td><td>68.0</td><td>27</td><td>Wyoming</td><td>73.7</td></tr>
<tr><td>46</td><td>Nevada</td><td>66.0</td><td>28</td><td>Florida</td><td>73.6</td></tr>
<tr><td>16</td><td>New Hampshire</td><td>76.7</td><td>28</td><td>Louisiana</td><td>73.6</td></tr>
<tr><td>48</td><td>New Jersey</td><td>64.1</td><td>30</td><td>Pennsylvania</td><td>72.7</td></tr>
<tr><td>47</td><td>New Mexico</td><td>65.9</td><td>31</td><td>Mississippi</td><td>72.4</td></tr>
<tr><td>34</td><td>New York</td><td>71.3</td><td>32</td><td>Tennessee</td><td>72.2</td></tr>
<tr><td>20</td><td>North Carolina</td><td>75.9</td><td>33</td><td>Alabama</td><td>72.0</td></tr>
<tr><td>12</td><td>North Dakota</td><td>78.0</td><td>34</td><td>Illinois</td><td>71.3</td></tr>
<tr><td>NA</td><td>Ohio**</td><td>NA</td><td>34</td><td>New York</td><td>71.3</td></tr>
<tr><td>37</td><td>Oklahoma</td><td>70.7</td><td>36</td><td>South Carolina</td><td>70.9</td></tr>
<tr><td>17</td><td>Oregon</td><td>76.3</td><td>37</td><td>Oklahoma</td><td>70.7</td></tr>
<tr><td>30</td><td>Pennsylvania</td><td>72.7</td><td>38</td><td>South Dakota</td><td>70.5</td></tr>
<tr><td>3</td><td>Rhode Island</td><td>86.0</td><td>39</td><td>West Virginia</td><td>70.3</td></tr>
<tr><td>36</td><td>South Carolina</td><td>70.9</td><td>40</td><td>Michigan</td><td>70.1</td></tr>
<tr><td>38</td><td>South Dakota</td><td>70.5</td><td>41</td><td>Wisconsin</td><td>69.9</td></tr>
<tr><td>32</td><td>Tennessee</td><td>72.2</td><td>42</td><td>Arkansas</td><td>69.1</td></tr>
<tr><td>18</td><td>Texas</td><td>76.1</td><td>43</td><td>Minnesota</td><td>68.8</td></tr>
<tr><td>49</td><td>Utah</td><td>56.0</td><td>44</td><td>Indiana</td><td>68.3</td></tr>
<tr><td>24</td><td>Vermont</td><td>74.2</td><td>45</td><td>Nebraska</td><td>68.0</td></tr>
<tr><td>19</td><td>Virginia</td><td>76.0</td><td>46</td><td>Nevada</td><td>66.0</td></tr>
<tr><td>23</td><td>Washington</td><td>74.9</td><td>47</td><td>New Mexico</td><td>65.9</td></tr>
<tr><td>39</td><td>West Virginia</td><td>70.3</td><td>48</td><td>New Jersey</td><td>64.1</td></tr>
<tr><td>41</td><td>Wisconsin</td><td>69.9</td><td>49</td><td>Utah</td><td>56.0</td></tr>
<tr><td>27</td><td>Wyoming</td><td>73.7</td><td>NA</td><td>Ohio**</td><td>NA</td></tr>
<tr><td></td><td></td><td></td><td></td><td>District of Columbia</td><td>70.2</td></tr>
</table>

Source: U.S. Department of Health and Human Services, National Center for Health Statistics
*   "National Vital Statistics Reports" (Vol. 49, No. 5, July 24, 2001)*
Preliminary data by state of residence.
**Not available.*

Percent of Mothers Receiving Late or No Prenatal Care in 1999

National Percent = 3.8% of Mothers*

ALPHA ORDER

RANK	STATE	PERCENT
15	Alabama	3.7
6	Alaska	4.8
2	Arizona	7.0
6	Arkansas	4.8
28	California	3.2
11	Colorado	4.3
46	Connecticut	2.0
20	Delaware	3.6
25	Florida	3.4
41	Georgia	2.5
35	Hawaii	2.9
14	Idaho	3.9
13	Illinois	4.1
15	Indiana	3.7
45	Iowa	2.2
35	Kansas	2.9
40	Kentucky	2.6
15	Louisiana	3.7
48	Maine	1.8
30	Maryland	3.1
43	Massachusetts	2.4
20	Michigan	3.6
38	Minnesota	2.7
20	Mississippi	3.6
38	Missouri	2.7
33	Montana	3.0
35	Nebraska	2.9
3	Nevada	6.7
49	New Hampshire	1.5
8	New Jersey	4.7
1	New Mexico	10.0
5	New York	5.1
33	North Carolina	3.0
46	North Dakota	2.0
23	Ohio	3.5
12	Oklahoma	4.2
15	Oregon	3.7
26	Pennsylvania	3.3
50	Rhode Island	1.4
8	South Carolina	4.7
30	South Dakota	3.1
23	Tennessee	3.5
4	Texas	5.5
10	Utah	4.4
41	Vermont	2.5
28	Virginia	3.2
30	Washington	3.1
43	West Virginia	2.4
26	Wisconsin	3.3
15	Wyoming	3.7

RANK ORDER

RANK	STATE	PERCENT
1	New Mexico	10.0
2	Arizona	7.0
3	Nevada	6.7
4	Texas	5.5
5	New York	5.1
6	Alaska	4.8
6	Arkansas	4.8
8	New Jersey	4.7
8	South Carolina	4.7
10	Utah	4.4
11	Colorado	4.3
12	Oklahoma	4.2
13	Illinois	4.1
14	Idaho	3.9
15	Alabama	3.7
15	Indiana	3.7
15	Louisiana	3.7
15	Oregon	3.7
15	Wyoming	3.7
20	Delaware	3.6
20	Michigan	3.6
20	Mississippi	3.6
23	Ohio	3.5
23	Tennessee	3.5
25	Florida	3.4
26	Pennsylvania	3.3
26	Wisconsin	3.3
28	California	3.2
28	Virginia	3.2
30	Maryland	3.1
30	South Dakota	3.1
30	Washington	3.1
33	Montana	3.0
33	North Carolina	3.0
35	Hawaii	2.9
35	Kansas	2.9
35	Nebraska	2.9
38	Minnesota	2.7
38	Missouri	2.7
40	Kentucky	2.6
41	Georgia	2.5
41	Vermont	2.5
43	Massachusetts	2.4
43	West Virginia	2.4
45	Iowa	2.2
46	Connecticut	2.0
46	North Dakota	2.0
48	Maine	1.8
49	New Hampshire	1.5
50	Rhode Island	1.4
	District of Columbia	9.3

Source: U.S. Department of Health and Human Services, National Center for Health Statistics
"National Vital Statistics Reports" (Vol. 49, No. 1, April 17, 2001)
*Final data by state of residence. "Late" means care begun in third trimester.

Percent of White Mothers Receiving Late or No Prenatal Care in 1999

National Percent = 3.2% of White Mothers*

ALPHA ORDER

RANK	STATE	PERCENT
29	Alabama	2.4
7	Alaska	3.9
2	Arizona	6.8
9	Arkansas	3.8
16	California	3.2
5	Colorado	4.2
43	Connecticut	1.8
19	Delaware	2.9
23	Florida	2.6
43	Georgia	1.8
38	Hawaii	2.1
9	Idaho	3.8
18	Illinois	3.0
14	Indiana	3.3
38	Iowa	2.1
21	Kansas	2.7
29	Kentucky	2.4
41	Louisiana	1.9
46	Maine	1.7
41	Maryland	1.9
40	Massachusetts	2.0
23	Michigan	2.6
35	Minnesota	2.2
46	Mississippi	1.7
35	Missouri	2.2
33	Montana	2.3
26	Nebraska	2.5
3	Nevada	6.7
48	New Hampshire	1.4
14	New Jersey	3.3
1	New Mexico	9.5
7	New York	3.9
35	North Carolina	2.2
49	North Dakota	1.3
21	Ohio	2.7
13	Oklahoma	3.5
11	Oregon	3.6
23	Pennsylvania	2.6
50	Rhode Island	1.1
17	South Carolina	3.1
43	South Dakota	1.8
26	Tennessee	2.5
4	Texas	5.4
6	Utah	4.1
29	Vermont	2.4
33	Virginia	2.3
19	Washington	2.9
29	West Virginia	2.4
26	Wisconsin	2.5
11	Wyoming	3.6

RANK ORDER

RANK	STATE	PERCENT
1	New Mexico	9.5
2	Arizona	6.8
3	Nevada	6.7
4	Texas	5.4
5	Colorado	4.2
6	Utah	4.1
7	Alaska	3.9
7	New York	3.9
9	Arkansas	3.8
9	Idaho	3.8
11	Oregon	3.6
11	Wyoming	3.6
13	Oklahoma	3.5
14	Indiana	3.3
14	New Jersey	3.3
16	California	3.2
17	South Carolina	3.1
18	Illinois	3.0
19	Delaware	2.9
19	Washington	2.9
21	Kansas	2.7
21	Ohio	2.7
23	Florida	2.6
23	Michigan	2.6
23	Pennsylvania	2.6
26	Nebraska	2.5
26	Tennessee	2.5
26	Wisconsin	2.5
29	Alabama	2.4
29	Kentucky	2.4
29	Vermont	2.4
29	West Virginia	2.4
33	Montana	2.3
33	Virginia	2.3
35	Minnesota	2.2
35	Missouri	2.2
35	North Carolina	2.2
38	Hawaii	2.1
38	Iowa	2.1
40	Massachusetts	2.0
41	Louisiana	1.9
41	Maryland	1.9
43	Connecticut	1.8
43	Georgia	1.8
43	South Dakota	1.8
46	Maine	1.7
46	Mississippi	1.7
48	New Hampshire	1.4
49	North Dakota	1.3
50	Rhode Island	1.1
	District of Columbia	5.5

Source: U.S. Department of Health and Human Services, National Center for Health Statistics
"National Vital Statistics Reports" (Vol. 49, No. 1, April 17, 2001)
*Final data by state of residence. "Late" means care begun in third trimester.

Percent of Black Mothers Receiving Late or No Prenatal Care in 1999

National Percent = 6.6% of Black Mothers*

ALPHA ORDER				RANK ORDER		
RANK	STATE	PERCENT		RANK	STATE	PERCENT
19	Alabama	6.3		1	New Jersey	10.8
NA	Alaska**	NA		2	New Mexico	10.4
16	Arizona	6.7		3	Utah	9.8
7	Arkansas	8.3		4	Illinois	8.7
36	California	3.9		4	New York	8.7
18	Colorado	6.4		6	Wisconsin	8.6
38	Connecticut	3.7		7	Arkansas	8.3
25	Delaware	5.9		8	Michigan	8.2
22	Florida	6.0		8	Ohio	8.2
36	Georgia	3.9		10	Nevada	8.1
NA	Hawaii**	NA		11	Pennsylvania	8.0
NA	Idaho**	NA		12	South Carolina	7.7
4	Illinois	8.7		13	Indiana	7.3
13	Indiana	7.3		14	Tennessee	7.1
31	Iowa	5.1		15	Nebraska	6.9
33	Kansas	4.7		16	Arizona	6.7
32	Kentucky	4.9		16	Minnesota	6.7
19	Louisiana	6.3		18	Colorado	6.4
NA	Maine**	NA		19	Alabama	6.3
28	Maryland	5.7		19	Louisiana	6.3
29	Massachusetts	5.4		21	Texas	6.2
8	Michigan	8.2		22	Florida	6.0
16	Minnesota	6.7		22	Oklahoma	6.0
25	Mississippi	5.9		22	Virginia	6.0
25	Missouri	5.9		25	Delaware	5.9
NA	Montana**	NA		25	Mississippi	5.9
15	Nebraska	6.9		25	Missouri	5.9
10	Nevada	8.1		28	Maryland	5.7
NA	New Hampshire**	NA		29	Massachusetts	5.4
1	New Jersey	10.8		30	North Carolina	5.3
2	New Mexico	10.4		31	Iowa	5.1
4	New York	8.7		32	Kentucky	4.9
30	North Carolina	5.3		33	Kansas	4.7
NA	North Dakota**	NA		34	Washington	4.4
8	Ohio	8.2		35	West Virginia	4.3
22	Oklahoma	6.0		36	California	3.9
39	Oregon	3.4		36	Georgia	3.9
11	Pennsylvania	8.0		38	Connecticut	3.7
39	Rhode Island	3.4		39	Oregon	3.4
12	South Carolina	7.7		39	Rhode Island	3.4
NA	South Dakota**	NA		NA	Alaska**	NA
14	Tennessee	7.1		NA	Hawaii**	NA
21	Texas	6.2		NA	Idaho**	NA
3	Utah	9.8		NA	Maine**	NA
NA	Vermont**	NA		NA	Montana**	NA
22	Virginia	6.0		NA	New Hampshire**	NA
34	Washington	4.4		NA	North Dakota**	NA
35	West Virginia	4.3		NA	South Dakota**	NA
6	Wisconsin	8.6		NA	Vermont**	NA
NA	Wyoming**	NA		NA	Wyoming**	NA
					District of Columbia	11.1

Source: U.S. Department of Health and Human Services, National Center for Health Statistics
    "National Vital Statistics Reports" (Vol. 49, No. 1, April 17, 2001)
Final data by state of residence. "Late" means care begun in third trimester.
**Insufficient data.*

Percent of Mothers Who Smoked During Pregnancy in 1999

National Percent = 12.6% of Mothers

ALPHA ORDER

RANK	STATE	PERCENT
26	Alabama	12.8
11	Alaska	18.0
47	Arizona	7.4
7	Arkansas	18.7
NA	California*	NA
36	Colorado	10.5
44	Connecticut	8.3
26	Delaware	12.8
37	Florida	10.3
42	Georgia	9.2
46	Hawaii	7.6
29	Idaho	12.7
33	Illinois	11.4
4	Indiana	20.9
10	Iowa	18.2
25	Kansas	13.2
2	Kentucky	24.5
39	Louisiana	10.1
8	Maine	18.3
40	Maryland	9.8
34	Massachusetts	10.8
18	Michigan	16.0
31	Minnesota	11.8
30	Mississippi	12.6
8	Missouri	18.3
13	Montana	17.5
20	Nebraska	15.1
32	Nevada	11.7
19	New Hampshire	15.2
37	New Jersey	10.3
34	New Mexico	10.8
41	New York	9.3
23	North Carolina	14.3
5	North Dakota	19.2
6	Ohio	18.8
12	Oklahoma	17.9
21	Oregon	14.5
14	Pennsylvania	17.2
24	Rhode Island	13.8
26	South Carolina	12.8
NA	South Dakota*	NA
15	Tennessee	17.1
48	Texas	6.9
45	Utah	8.1
17	Vermont	16.5
43	Virginia	9.0
22	Washington	14.4
1	West Virginia	26.1
15	Wisconsin	17.1
3	Wyoming	21.0

RANK ORDER

RANK	STATE	PERCENT
1	West Virginia	26.1
2	Kentucky	24.5
3	Wyoming	21.0
4	Indiana	20.9
5	North Dakota	19.2
6	Ohio	18.8
7	Arkansas	18.7
8	Maine	18.3
8	Missouri	18.3
10	Iowa	18.2
11	Alaska	18.0
12	Oklahoma	17.9
13	Montana	17.5
14	Pennsylvania	17.2
15	Tennessee	17.1
15	Wisconsin	17.1
17	Vermont	16.5
18	Michigan	16.0
19	New Hampshire	15.2
20	Nebraska	15.1
21	Oregon	14.5
22	Washington	14.4
23	North Carolina	14.3
24	Rhode Island	13.8
25	Kansas	13.2
26	Alabama	12.8
26	Delaware	12.8
26	South Carolina	12.8
29	Idaho	12.7
30	Mississippi	12.6
31	Minnesota	11.8
32	Nevada	11.7
33	Illinois	11.4
34	Massachusetts	10.8
34	New Mexico	10.8
36	Colorado	10.5
37	Florida	10.3
37	New Jersey	10.3
39	Louisiana	10.1
40	Maryland	9.8
41	New York	9.3
42	Georgia	9.2
43	Virginia	9.0
44	Connecticut	8.3
45	Utah	8.1
46	Hawaii	7.6
47	Arizona	7.4
48	Texas	6.9
NA	California*	NA
NA	South Dakota*	NA
	District of Columbia	3.8

Source: U.S. Department of Health and Human Services, National Center for Health Statistics
"National Vital Statistics Reports" (Vol. 49, No. 7, August 28, 2001)
*Not available.

Percent of Teenage Mothers Who Smoked During Pregnancy in 1999

National Percent = 18.0% of Teenage Mothers*

ALPHA ORDER				RANK ORDER		
RANK	STATE	PERCENT		RANK	STATE	PERCENT
36	Alabama	15.2		1	Vermont	38.2
13	Alaska	27.4		2	West Virginia	36.8
48	Arizona	8.3		3	Maine	36.6
24	Arkansas	22.2		4	North Dakota	35.2
NA	California**	NA		5	New Hampshire	35.1
32	Colorado	16.3		6	Kentucky	35.0
37	Connecticut	15.0		7	Wyoming	33.1
30	Delaware	17.2		8	Iowa	32.4
40	Florida	13.4		9	Montana	30.9
45	Georgia	12.3		10	Indiana	30.3
42	Hawaii	13.1		11	Ohio	28.4
22	Idaho	22.9		12	Wisconsin	27.9
33	Illinois	16.0		13	Alaska	27.4
10	Indiana	30.3		14	Missouri	27.0
8	Iowa	32.4		15	Pennsylvania	26.3
28	Kansas	19.3		16	Washington	25.6
6	Kentucky	35.0		17	Oregon	25.2
46	Louisiana	10.8		18	Nebraska	25.1
3	Maine	36.6		19	Minnesota	24.9
39	Maryland	14.4		20	Michigan	24.2
26	Massachusetts	21.2		21	Oklahoma	23.8
20	Michigan	24.2		22	Idaho	22.9
19	Minnesota	24.9		23	Rhode Island	22.5
43	Mississippi	12.7		24	Arkansas	22.2
14	Missouri	27.0		25	Tennessee	21.5
9	Montana	30.9		26	Massachusetts	21.2
18	Nebraska	25.1		27	Utah	19.9
40	Nevada	13.4		28	Kansas	19.3
5	New Hampshire	35.1		29	North Carolina	18.5
31	New Jersey	16.5		30	Delaware	17.2
44	New Mexico	12.5		31	New Jersey	16.5
35	New York	15.7		32	Colorado	16.3
29	North Carolina	18.5		33	Illinois	16.0
4	North Dakota	35.2		34	South Carolina	15.8
11	Ohio	28.4		35	New York	15.7
21	Oklahoma	23.8		36	Alabama	15.2
17	Oregon	25.2		37	Connecticut	15.0
15	Pennsylvania	26.3		38	Virginia	14.9
23	Rhode Island	22.5		39	Maryland	14.4
34	South Carolina	15.8		40	Florida	13.4
NA	South Dakota**	NA		40	Nevada	13.4
25	Tennessee	21.5		42	Hawaii	13.1
47	Texas	8.7		43	Mississippi	12.7
27	Utah	19.9		44	New Mexico	12.5
1	Vermont	38.2		45	Georgia	12.3
38	Virginia	14.9		46	Louisiana	10.8
16	Washington	25.6		47	Texas	8.7
2	West Virginia	36.8		48	Arizona	8.3
12	Wisconsin	27.9		NA	California**	NA
7	Wyoming	33.1		NA	South Dakota**	NA
					District of Columbia	3.8

Source: U.S. Department of Health and Human Services, National Center for Health Statistics
  "National Vital Statistics Reports" (Vol. 49, No. 7, August 28, 2001)
*Women aged 15 to 19 years old.
**Not available.

Percent of Births Attended by Midwives in 1999

National Percent = 7.7% of Live Births*

ALPHA ORDER

RANK ORDER

RANK	STATE	PERCENT	RANK	STATE	PERCENT
48	Alabama	2.0	1	New Mexico	27.2
2	Alaska	18.0	2	Alaska	18.0
14	Arizona	9.0	3	Vermont	17.9
45	Arkansas	2.2	4	Georgia	16.5
15	California	8.9	5	New Hampshire	15.4
12	Colorado	9.9	6	Oregon	15.2
19	Connecticut	8.5	7	Massachusetts	13.8
26	Delaware	6.1	8	Maine	12.6
9	Florida	12.0	9	Florida	12.0
4	Georgia	16.5	10	Rhode Island	11.7
40	Hawaii	3.7	11	New York	11.0
35	Idaho	4.4	12	Colorado	9.9
40	Illinois	3.7	12	Washington	9.9
43	Indiana	3.2	14	Arizona	9.0
40	Iowa	3.7	15	California	8.9
46	Kansas	2.1	16	Minnesota	8.8
37	Kentucky	4.1	16	Montana	8.8
46	Louisiana	2.1	18	West Virginia	8.7
8	Maine	12.6	19	Connecticut	8.5
23	Maryland	7.6	19	Utah	8.5
7	Massachusetts	13.8	21	Pennsylvania	7.9
23	Michigan	7.6	22	North Carolina	7.8
16	Minnesota	8.8	23	Maryland	7.6
49	Mississippi	1.7	23	Michigan	7.6
50	Missouri	1.3	25	Ohio	6.8
16	Montana	8.8	26	Delaware	6.1
39	Nebraska	3.9	26	Virginia	6.1
28	Nevada	6.0	28	Nevada	6.0
5	New Hampshire	15.4	29	New Jersey	5.6
29	New Jersey	5.6	30	Wisconsin	5.5
1	New Mexico	27.2	31	South Carolina	5.2
11	New York	11.0	32	North Dakota	5.0
22	North Carolina	7.8	33	Texas	4.8
32	North Dakota	5.0	34	South Dakota	4.7
25	Ohio	6.8	35	Idaho	4.4
37	Oklahoma	4.1	35	Tennessee	4.4
6	Oregon	15.2	37	Kentucky	4.1
21	Pennsylvania	7.9	37	Oklahoma	4.1
10	Rhode Island	11.7	39	Nebraska	3.9
31	South Carolina	5.2	40	Hawaii	3.7
34	South Dakota	4.7	40	Illinois	3.7
35	Tennessee	4.4	40	Iowa	3.7
33	Texas	4.8	43	Indiana	3.2
19	Utah	8.5	44	Wyoming	3.0
3	Vermont	17.9	45	Arkansas	2.2
26	Virginia	6.1	46	Kansas	2.1
12	Washington	9.9	46	Louisiana	2.1
18	West Virginia	8.7	48	Alabama	2.0
30	Wisconsin	5.5	49	Mississippi	1.7
44	Wyoming	3.0	50	Missouri	1.3

	District of Columbia	3.9

Source: U.S. Department of Health and Human Services, National Center for Health Statistics
unpublished data
*Final numbers. Includes certified nurse midwives and other midwives.

Reported Legal Abortions in 1997

National Total = 1,186,039 Abortions*

<table>
<tr><td colspan="4">ALPHA ORDER</td><td colspan="4">RANK ORDER</td></tr>
<tr><td>RANK</td><td>STATE</td><td>ABORTIONS</td><td>% of USA</td><td>RANK</td><td>STATE</td><td>ABORTIONS</td><td>% of USA</td></tr>
<tr><td>21</td><td>Alabama</td><td>13,063</td><td>1.1%</td><td>1</td><td>California</td><td>275,739</td><td>23.2%</td></tr>
<tr><td>46</td><td>Alaska</td><td>1,632</td><td>0.1%</td><td>2</td><td>New York</td><td>140,834</td><td>11.9%</td></tr>
<tr><td>23</td><td>Arizona</td><td>11,266</td><td>0.9%</td><td>3</td><td>Texas</td><td>84,680</td><td>7.1%</td></tr>
<tr><td>33</td><td>Arkansas</td><td>5,782</td><td>0.5%</td><td>4</td><td>Florida</td><td>81,692</td><td>6.9%</td></tr>
<tr><td>1</td><td>California</td><td>275,739</td><td>23.2%</td><td>5</td><td>Illinois</td><td>50,147</td><td>4.2%</td></tr>
<tr><td>29</td><td>Colorado</td><td>9,183</td><td>0.8%</td><td>6</td><td>Ohio</td><td>38,242</td><td>3.2%</td></tr>
<tr><td>18</td><td>Connecticut</td><td>13,802</td><td>1.2%</td><td>7</td><td>Pennsylvania</td><td>37,135</td><td>3.1%</td></tr>
<tr><td>36</td><td>Delaware</td><td>5,138</td><td>0.4%</td><td>8</td><td>Georgia</td><td>35,702</td><td>3.0%</td></tr>
<tr><td>4</td><td>Florida</td><td>81,692</td><td>6.9%</td><td>9</td><td>North Carolina</td><td>31,495</td><td>2.7%</td></tr>
<tr><td>8</td><td>Georgia</td><td>35,702</td><td>3.0%</td><td>10</td><td>New Jersey</td><td>30,654</td><td>2.6%</td></tr>
<tr><td>38</td><td>Hawaii</td><td>4,520</td><td>0.4%</td><td>11</td><td>Michigan</td><td>29,528</td><td>2.5%</td></tr>
<tr><td>49</td><td>Idaho</td><td>878</td><td>0.1%</td><td>12</td><td>Massachusetts</td><td>28,477</td><td>2.4%</td></tr>
<tr><td>5</td><td>Illinois</td><td>50,147</td><td>4.2%</td><td>13</td><td>Washington</td><td>26,932</td><td>2.3%</td></tr>
<tr><td>20</td><td>Indiana</td><td>13,208</td><td>1.1%</td><td>14</td><td>Virginia</td><td>26,089</td><td>2.2%</td></tr>
<tr><td>26</td><td>Iowa</td><td>10,022</td><td>0.8%</td><td>15</td><td>Tennessee</td><td>18,283</td><td>1.5%</td></tr>
<tr><td>24</td><td>Kansas</td><td>11,249</td><td>0.9%</td><td>16</td><td>Oregon</td><td>14,834</td><td>1.3%</td></tr>
<tr><td>30</td><td>Kentucky</td><td>7,033</td><td>0.6%</td><td>17</td><td>Minnesota</td><td>14,229</td><td>1.2%</td></tr>
<tr><td>22</td><td>Louisiana</td><td>11,739</td><td>1.0%</td><td>18</td><td>Connecticut</td><td>13,802</td><td>1.2%</td></tr>
<tr><td>43</td><td>Maine</td><td>2,545</td><td>0.2%</td><td>19</td><td>Wisconsin</td><td>13,218</td><td>1.1%</td></tr>
<tr><td>27</td><td>Maryland</td><td>9,869</td><td>0.8%</td><td>20</td><td>Indiana</td><td>13,208</td><td>1.1%</td></tr>
<tr><td>12</td><td>Massachusetts</td><td>28,477</td><td>2.4%</td><td>21</td><td>Alabama</td><td>13,063</td><td>1.1%</td></tr>
<tr><td>11</td><td>Michigan</td><td>29,528</td><td>2.5%</td><td>22</td><td>Louisiana</td><td>11,739</td><td>1.0%</td></tr>
<tr><td>17</td><td>Minnesota</td><td>14,229</td><td>1.2%</td><td>23</td><td>Arizona</td><td>11,266</td><td>0.9%</td></tr>
<tr><td>39</td><td>Mississippi</td><td>4,325</td><td>0.4%</td><td>24</td><td>Kansas</td><td>11,249</td><td>0.9%</td></tr>
<tr><td>25</td><td>Missouri</td><td>10,202</td><td>0.9%</td><td>25</td><td>Missouri</td><td>10,202</td><td>0.9%</td></tr>
<tr><td>41</td><td>Montana</td><td>2,809</td><td>0.2%</td><td>26</td><td>Iowa</td><td>10,022</td><td>0.8%</td></tr>
<tr><td>37</td><td>Nebraska</td><td>5,129</td><td>0.4%</td><td>27</td><td>Maryland</td><td>9,869</td><td>0.8%</td></tr>
<tr><td>31</td><td>Nevada</td><td>6,887</td><td>0.6%</td><td>28</td><td>South Carolina</td><td>9,212</td><td>0.8%</td></tr>
<tr><td>44</td><td>New Hampshire</td><td>2,069</td><td>0.2%</td><td>29</td><td>Colorado</td><td>9,183</td><td>0.8%</td></tr>
<tr><td>10</td><td>New Jersey</td><td>30,654</td><td>2.6%</td><td>30</td><td>Kentucky</td><td>7,033</td><td>0.6%</td></tr>
<tr><td>35</td><td>New Mexico</td><td>5,382</td><td>0.5%</td><td>31</td><td>Nevada</td><td>6,887</td><td>0.6%</td></tr>
<tr><td>2</td><td>New York</td><td>140,834</td><td>11.9%</td><td>32</td><td>Oklahoma</td><td>6,428</td><td>0.5%</td></tr>
<tr><td>9</td><td>North Carolina</td><td>31,495</td><td>2.7%</td><td>33</td><td>Arkansas</td><td>5,782</td><td>0.5%</td></tr>
<tr><td>47</td><td>North Dakota</td><td>1,226</td><td>0.1%</td><td>34</td><td>Rhode Island</td><td>5,478</td><td>0.5%</td></tr>
<tr><td>6</td><td>Ohio</td><td>38,242</td><td>3.2%</td><td>35</td><td>New Mexico</td><td>5,382</td><td>0.5%</td></tr>
<tr><td>32</td><td>Oklahoma</td><td>6,428</td><td>0.5%</td><td>36</td><td>Delaware</td><td>5,138</td><td>0.4%</td></tr>
<tr><td>16</td><td>Oregon</td><td>14,834</td><td>1.3%</td><td>37</td><td>Nebraska</td><td>5,129</td><td>0.4%</td></tr>
<tr><td>7</td><td>Pennsylvania</td><td>37,135</td><td>3.1%</td><td>38</td><td>Hawaii</td><td>4,520</td><td>0.4%</td></tr>
<tr><td>34</td><td>Rhode Island</td><td>5,478</td><td>0.5%</td><td>39</td><td>Mississippi</td><td>4,325</td><td>0.4%</td></tr>
<tr><td>28</td><td>South Carolina</td><td>9,212</td><td>0.8%</td><td>40</td><td>Utah</td><td>3,408</td><td>0.3%</td></tr>
<tr><td>48</td><td>South Dakota</td><td>919</td><td>0.1%</td><td>41</td><td>Montana</td><td>2,809</td><td>0.2%</td></tr>
<tr><td>15</td><td>Tennessee</td><td>18,283</td><td>1.5%</td><td>42</td><td>West Virginia</td><td>2,808</td><td>0.2%</td></tr>
<tr><td>3</td><td>Texas</td><td>84,680</td><td>7.1%</td><td>43</td><td>Maine</td><td>2,545</td><td>0.2%</td></tr>
<tr><td>40</td><td>Utah</td><td>3,408</td><td>0.3%</td><td>44</td><td>New Hampshire</td><td>2,069</td><td>0.2%</td></tr>
<tr><td>45</td><td>Vermont</td><td>1,955</td><td>0.2%</td><td>45</td><td>Vermont</td><td>1,955</td><td>0.2%</td></tr>
<tr><td>14</td><td>Virginia</td><td>26,089</td><td>2.2%</td><td>46</td><td>Alaska</td><td>1,632</td><td>0.1%</td></tr>
<tr><td>13</td><td>Washington</td><td>26,932</td><td>2.3%</td><td>47</td><td>North Dakota</td><td>1,226</td><td>0.1%</td></tr>
<tr><td>42</td><td>West Virginia</td><td>2,808</td><td>0.2%</td><td>48</td><td>South Dakota</td><td>919</td><td>0.1%</td></tr>
<tr><td>19</td><td>Wisconsin</td><td>13,218</td><td>1.1%</td><td>49</td><td>Idaho</td><td>878</td><td>0.1%</td></tr>
<tr><td>50</td><td>Wyoming</td><td>192</td><td>0.0%</td><td>50</td><td>Wyoming</td><td>192</td><td>0.0%</td></tr>
<tr><td></td><td></td><td></td><td></td><td></td><td>District of Columbia</td><td>8,771</td><td>0.7%</td></tr>
</table>

Source: U.S. Department of Health and Human Services, Centers for Disease Control and Prevention
  "Abortion Surveillance-United States, 1997" (Morbidity Mortality Weekly Report, Vol. 49, No. SS-11, 12/08/00)
*By state of occurrence.

Reported Legal Abortions per 1,000 Live Births in 1997

National Rate = 306 Abortions per 1,000 Live Births*

ALPHA ORDER

RANK	STATE	RATE
28	Alabama	214
34	Alaska	164
38	Arizona	149
36	Arkansas	159
2	California	525
35	Colorado	162
9	Connecticut	320
3	Delaware	501
5	Florida	425
10	Georgia	302
18	Hawaii	260
49	Idaho	47
15	Illinois	277
37	Indiana	158
16	Iowa	273
10	Kansas	302
45	Kentucky	132
32	Louisiana	178
31	Maine	186
41	Maryland	141
6	Massachusetts	354
25	Michigan	221
25	Minnesota	221
46	Mississippi	104
42	Missouri	138
19	Montana	259
27	Nebraska	220
21	Nevada	256
40	New Hampshire	145
17	New Jersey	271
29	New Mexico	200
1	New York	547
13	North Carolina	294
39	North Dakota	147
23	Ohio	252
44	Oklahoma	133
8	Oregon	339
20	Pennsylvania	257
4	Rhode Island	440
33	South Carolina	176
47	South Dakota	90
24	Tennessee	245
22	Texas	254
48	Utah	79
12	Vermont	296
14	Virginia	284
7	Washington	344
43	West Virginia	135
30	Wisconsin	199
50	Wyoming	30

RANK ORDER

RANK	STATE	RATE
1	New York	547
2	California	525
3	Delaware	501
4	Rhode Island	440
5	Florida	425
6	Massachusetts	354
7	Washington	344
8	Oregon	339
9	Connecticut	320
10	Georgia	302
10	Kansas	302
12	Vermont	296
13	North Carolina	294
14	Virginia	284
15	Illinois	277
16	Iowa	273
17	New Jersey	271
18	Hawaii	260
19	Montana	259
20	Pennsylvania	257
21	Nevada	256
22	Texas	254
23	Ohio	252
24	Tennessee	245
25	Michigan	221
25	Minnesota	221
27	Nebraska	220
28	Alabama	214
29	New Mexico	200
30	Wisconsin	199
31	Maine	186
32	Louisiana	178
33	South Carolina	176
34	Alaska	164
35	Colorado	162
36	Arkansas	159
37	Indiana	158
38	Arizona	149
39	North Dakota	147
40	New Hampshire	145
41	Maryland	141
42	Missouri	138
43	West Virginia	135
44	Oklahoma	133
45	Kentucky	132
46	Mississippi	104
47	South Dakota	90
48	Utah	79
49	Idaho	47
50	Wyoming	30
	District of Columbia**	NA

Source: U.S. Department of Health and Human Services, Centers for Disease Control and Prevention
    "Abortion Surveillance-United States, 1997" (Morbidity Mortality Weekly Report, Vol. 49, No. SS-11, 12/08/00)
*By state of occurrence.
**The District of Columbia's ratio was not listed but was noted as being greater than 1,000 abortions per 1,000 live births.

Reported Legal Abortions per 1,000 Women Ages 15 to 44 in 1997

National Rate = 20 Abortions per 1,000 Women Ages 15 to 44*

ALPHA ORDER

RANK	STATE	RATE
27	Alabama	13
30	Alaska	12
32	Arizona	11
32	Arkansas	11
1	California	38
36	Colorado	10
11	Connecticut	19
3	Delaware	30
4	Florida	27
8	Georgia	20
16	Hawaii	18
49	Idaho	3
11	Illinois	19
36	Indiana	10
18	Iowa	16
8	Kansas	20
42	Kentucky	8
30	Louisiana	12
38	Maine	9
42	Maryland	8
8	Massachusetts	20
27	Michigan	13
27	Minnesota	13
45	Mississippi	7
38	Missouri	9
20	Montana	15
24	Nebraska	14
11	Nevada	19
42	New Hampshire	8
17	New Jersey	17
24	New Mexico	14
2	New York	35
11	North Carolina	19
38	North Dakota	9
20	Ohio	15
38	Oklahoma	9
6	Oregon	21
24	Pennsylvania	14
5	Rhode Island	25
32	South Carolina	11
48	South Dakota	6
20	Tennessee	15
11	Texas	19
45	Utah	7
20	Vermont	15
18	Virginia	16
6	Washington	21
45	West Virginia	7
32	Wisconsin	11
50	Wyoming	2

RANK ORDER

RANK	STATE	RATE
1	California	38
2	New York	35
3	Delaware	30
4	Florida	27
5	Rhode Island	25
6	Oregon	21
6	Washington	21
8	Georgia	20
8	Kansas	20
8	Massachusetts	20
11	Connecticut	19
11	Illinois	19
11	Nevada	19
11	North Carolina	19
11	Texas	19
16	Hawaii	18
17	New Jersey	17
18	Iowa	16
18	Virginia	16
20	Montana	15
20	Ohio	15
20	Tennessee	15
20	Vermont	15
24	Nebraska	14
24	New Mexico	14
24	Pennsylvania	14
27	Alabama	13
27	Michigan	13
27	Minnesota	13
30	Alaska	12
30	Louisiana	12
32	Arizona	11
32	Arkansas	11
32	South Carolina	11
32	Wisconsin	11
36	Colorado	10
36	Indiana	10
38	Maine	9
38	Missouri	9
38	North Dakota	9
38	Oklahoma	9
42	Kentucky	8
42	Maryland	8
42	New Hampshire	8
45	Mississippi	7
45	Utah	7
45	West Virginia	7
48	South Dakota	6
49	Idaho	3
50	Wyoming	2
	District of Columbia	68

Source: U.S. Department of Health and Human Services, Centers for Disease Control and Prevention
    "Abortion Surveillance-United States, 1997" (Morbidity Mortality Weekly Report, Vol. 49, No. SS-11, 12/08/00)
*By state of occurrence.

Percent of Legal Abortions Obtained by Out-Of-State Residents in 1997

National Percent = 8.1% of Abortions*

ALPHA ORDER				RANK ORDER		
RANK	STATE	PERCENT		RANK	STATE	PERCENT
11	Alabama	15.0		1	Kansas	44.2
NA	Alaska**	NA		2	Delaware	34.5
41	Arizona	1.9		3	North Dakota	32.4
16	Arkansas	10.4		4	South Dakota	23.9
NA	California**	NA		5	Nebraska	22.0
20	Colorado	9.3		6	Kentucky	21.5
38	Connecticut	3.4		7	Rhode Island	18.9
2	Delaware	34.5		8	Tennessee	18.3
NA	Florida**	NA		9	Montana	17.3
18	Georgia	9.9		10	Vermont	17.1
42	Hawaii	0.4		11	Alabama	15.0
32	Idaho	4.3		12	Oregon	12.0
23	Illinois	7.8		13	West Virginia	11.7
33	Indiana	4.1		14	Nevada	11.3
NA	Iowa**	NA		15	North Carolina	11.2
1	Kansas	44.2		16	Arkansas	10.4
6	Kentucky	21.5		17	Missouri	10.1
NA	Louisiana**	NA		18	Georgia	9.9
39	Maine	3.2		19	Wyoming	9.4
35	Maryland	4.0		20	Colorado	9.3
26	Massachusetts	6.2		21	Minnesota	8.6
36	Michigan	3.9		22	Utah	8.0
21	Minnesota	8.6		23	Illinois	7.8
28	Mississippi	5.2		24	Ohio	6.6
17	Missouri	10.1		25	South Carolina	6.3
9	Montana	17.3		26	Massachusetts	6.2
5	Nebraska	22.0		27	Virginia	5.7
14	Nevada	11.3		28	Mississippi	5.2
NA	New Hampshire**	NA		29	New Mexico	5.1
40	New Jersey	2.4		30	Washington	4.6
29	New Mexico	5.1		31	Pennsylvania	4.5
NA	New York**	NA		32	Idaho	4.3
15	North Carolina	11.2		33	Indiana	4.1
3	North Dakota	32.4		33	Wisconsin	4.1
24	Ohio	6.6		35	Maryland	4.0
NA	Oklahoma**	NA		36	Michigan	3.9
12	Oregon	12.0		36	Texas	3.9
31	Pennsylvania	4.5		38	Connecticut	3.4
7	Rhode Island	18.9		39	Maine	3.2
25	South Carolina	6.3		40	New Jersey	2.4
4	South Dakota	23.9		41	Arizona	1.9
8	Tennessee	18.3		42	Hawaii	0.4
36	Texas	3.9		NA	Alaska**	NA
22	Utah	8.0		NA	California**	NA
10	Vermont	17.1		NA	Florida**	NA
27	Virginia	5.7		NA	Iowa**	NA
30	Washington	4.6		NA	Louisiana**	NA
13	West Virginia	11.7		NA	New Hampshire**	NA
33	Wisconsin	4.1		NA	New York**	NA
19	Wyoming	9.4		NA	Oklahoma**	NA
					District of Columbia	42.1

Source: U.S. Department of Health and Human Services, Centers for Disease Control and Prevention
   "Abortion Surveillance-United States, 1997" (Morbidity Mortality Weekly Report, Vol. 49, No. SS-11, 12/08/00)
By state of occurrence.
**Not reported.*

Percent of Reported Legal Abortions Obtained by White Women in 1997

Reporting States' Percent = 56.3% of Abortions*

ALPHA ORDER				RANK ORDER		
RANK	STATE	PERCENT		RANK	STATE	PERCENT
30	Alabama	51.6		1	Vermont	96.7
NA	Alaska**	NA		2	Idaho	93.3
12	Arizona	79.9		3	Maine	92.9
23	Arkansas	62.3		4	West Virginia	88.2
NA	California**	NA		5	North Dakota	88.1
16	Colorado	74.4		6	Wyoming	87.5
NA	Connecticut**	NA		7	Oregon	86.9
22	Delaware	63.0		8	New Mexico	86.3
NA	Florida**	NA		9	Utah	85.7
33	Georgia	42.9		10	South Dakota	85.6
38	Hawaii	27.0		11	Montana	83.1
2	Idaho	93.3		12	Arizona	79.9
NA	Illinois**	NA		13	Nevada	77.9
21	Indiana	64.5		14	Rhode Island	76.9
NA	Iowa**	NA		15	Kansas	75.4
15	Kansas	75.4		16	Colorado	74.4
17	Kentucky	73.9		17	Kentucky	73.9
32	Louisiana	45.3		18	Minnesota	73.3
3	Maine	92.9		19	Wisconsin	71.8
35	Maryland	34.6		20	Texas	71.1
NA	Massachusetts**	NA		21	Indiana	64.5
NA	Michigan**	NA		22	Delaware	63.0
18	Minnesota	73.3		23	Arkansas	62.3
36	Mississippi	32.8		24	Missouri	61.7
24	Missouri	61.7		25	Ohio	59.9
11	Montana	83.1		26	Pennsylvania	56.3
NA	Nebraska**	NA		27	Tennessee	56.0
13	Nevada	77.9		28	South Carolina	53.9
NA	New Hampshire**	NA		29	Virginia	53.2
37	New Jersey	32.5		30	Alabama	51.6
8	New Mexico	86.3		31	North Carolina	50.5
34	New York**	39.7		32	Louisiana	45.3
31	North Carolina	50.5		33	Georgia	42.9
5	North Dakota	88.1		34	New York**	39.7
25	Ohio	59.9		35	Maryland	34.6
NA	Oklahoma**	NA		36	Mississippi	32.8
7	Oregon	86.9		37	New Jersey	32.5
26	Pennsylvania	56.3		38	Hawaii	27.0
14	Rhode Island	76.9		NA	Alaska**	NA
28	South Carolina	53.9		NA	California**	NA
10	South Dakota	85.6		NA	Connecticut**	NA
27	Tennessee	56.0		NA	Florida**	NA
20	Texas	71.1		NA	Illinois**	NA
9	Utah	85.7		NA	Iowa**	NA
1	Vermont	96.7		NA	Massachusetts**	NA
29	Virginia	53.2		NA	Michigan**	NA
NA	Washington**	NA		NA	Nebraska**	NA
4	West Virginia	88.2		NA	New Hampshire**	NA
19	Wisconsin	71.8		NA	Oklahoma**	NA
6	Wyoming	87.5		NA	Washington**	NA
					District of Columbia	7.6

Source: U.S. Department of Health and Human Services, Centers for Disease Control and Prevention
   "Abortion Surveillance-United States, 1997" (Morbidity Mortality Weekly Report, Vol. 49, No. SS-11, 12/08/00)
*By state of occurrence. Includes those of Hispanic ethnicity. National percent is for reporting states only.
**Not reported. New York's number is for New York City only.

Percent of Reported Legal Abortions Obtained by Black Women in 1997

Reporting States' Percent = 34.6% of Abortions*

ALPHA ORDER

RANK	STATE	PERCENT
7	Alabama	46.0
NA	Alaska**	NA
28	Arizona	4.8
13	Arkansas	34.9
NA	California**	NA
26	Colorado	6.2
NA	Connecticut**	NA
15	Delaware	33.7
NA	Florida**	NA
3	Georgia	54.4
29	Hawaii	3.2
35	Idaho	1.1
NA	Illinois**	NA
17	Indiana	25.4
NA	Iowa**	NA
21	Kansas	18.7
20	Kentucky	21.5
4	Louisiana	52.5
34	Maine	1.4
2	Maryland	56.5
NA	Massachusetts**	NA
NA	Michigan**	NA
22	Minnesota	13.9
1	Mississippi	65.9
14	Missouri	33.8
37	Montana	0.3
NA	Nebraska**	NA
25	Nevada	8.0
NA	New Hampshire**	NA
6	New Jersey	47.3
31	New Mexico	2.7
5	New York	47.4
11	North Carolina	39.7
33	North Dakota	1.5
16	Ohio	32.4
NA	Oklahoma**	NA
27	Oregon	5.4
10	Pennsylvania	40.4
23	Rhode Island	13.1
8	South Carolina	43.7
29	South Dakota	3.2
9	Tennessee	41.7
19	Texas	21.7
32	Utah	1.7
35	Vermont	1.1
12	Virginia	39.3
NA	Washington**	NA
24	West Virginia	10.5
18	Wisconsin	22.6
38	Wyoming	0.0

RANK ORDER

RANK	STATE	PERCENT
1	Mississippi	65.9
2	Maryland	56.5
3	Georgia	54.4
4	Louisiana	52.5
5	New York	47.4
6	New Jersey	47.3
7	Alabama	46.0
8	South Carolina	43.7
9	Tennessee	41.7
10	Pennsylvania	40.4
11	North Carolina	39.7
12	Virginia	39.3
13	Arkansas	34.9
14	Missouri	33.8
15	Delaware	33.7
16	Ohio	32.4
17	Indiana	25.4
18	Wisconsin	22.6
19	Texas	21.7
20	Kentucky	21.5
21	Kansas	18.7
22	Minnesota	13.9
23	Rhode Island	13.1
24	West Virginia	10.5
25	Nevada	8.0
26	Colorado	6.2
27	Oregon	5.4
28	Arizona	4.8
29	Hawaii	3.2
29	South Dakota	3.2
31	New Mexico	2.7
32	Utah	1.7
33	North Dakota	1.5
34	Maine	1.4
35	Idaho	1.1
35	Vermont	1.1
37	Montana	0.3
38	Wyoming	0.0
NA	Alaska**	NA
NA	California**	NA
NA	Connecticut**	NA
NA	Florida**	NA
NA	Illinois**	NA
NA	Iowa**	NA
NA	Massachusetts**	NA
NA	Michigan**	NA
NA	Nebraska**	NA
NA	New Hampshire**	NA
NA	Oklahoma**	NA
NA	Washington**	NA

	District of Columbia	76.4

Source: U.S. Department of Health and Human Services, Centers for Disease Control and Prevention
   "Abortion Surveillance-United States, 1997" (Morbidity Mortality Weekly Report, Vol. 49, No. SS-11, 12/08/00)
*By state of occurrence. National percent is for reporting states only.
**Not reported. New York's number is for New York City only.

Percent of Reported Legal Abortions Obtained by Married Women in 1997

Reporting States' Percent = 18.5% of Abortions*

ALPHA ORDER

RANK ORDER

RANK	STATE	PERCENT		RANK	STATE	PERCENT
27	Alabama	17.2		1	Utah	35.0
NA	Alaska**	NA		2	Nevada	23.2
NA	Arizona**	NA		3	Oregon	22.1
19	Arkansas	18.2		4	South Dakota	21.9
NA	California**	NA		5	Vermont	21.7
13	Colorado	19.1		6	Missouri	20.6
NA	Connecticut**	NA		7	North Dakota	20.5
36	Delaware	15.7		8	North Carolina	20.3
NA	Florida**	NA		9	Texas	20.2
19	Georgia	18.2		10	Massachusetts	20.1
26	Hawaii	17.5		11	Kansas	19.8
15	Idaho	19.0		12	Tennessee	19.2
35	Illinois	16.3		13	Colorado	19.1
37	Indiana	14.1		13	New York**	19.1
NA	Iowa**	NA		15	Idaho	19.0
11	Kansas	19.8		15	Minnesota	19.0
28	Kentucky	17.1		17	Wyoming	18.8
NA	Louisiana**	NA		18	Maryland	18.3
22	Maine	17.9		19	Arkansas	18.2
18	Maryland	18.3		19	Georgia	18.2
10	Massachusetts	20.1		21	Rhode Island	18.1
34	Michigan	16.5		22	Maine	17.9
15	Minnesota	19.0		22	South Carolina	17.9
38	Mississippi	13.0		24	Montana	17.7
6	Missouri	20.6		24	Wisconsin	17.7
24	Montana	17.7		26	Hawaii	17.5
NA	Nebraska**	NA		27	Alabama	17.2
2	Nevada	23.2		28	Kentucky	17.1
NA	New Hampshire**	NA		28	New Jersey	17.1
28	New Jersey	17.1		30	New Mexico	16.9
30	New Mexico	16.9		31	Ohio	16.8
13	New York**	19.1		32	West Virginia	16.7
8	North Carolina	20.3		33	Pennsylvania	16.6
7	North Dakota	20.5		34	Michigan	16.5
31	Ohio	16.8		35	Illinois	16.3
NA	Oklahoma**	NA		36	Delaware	15.7
3	Oregon	22.1		37	Indiana	14.1
33	Pennsylvania	16.6		38	Mississippi	13.0
21	Rhode Island	18.1		NA	Alaska**	NA
22	South Carolina	17.9		NA	Arizona**	NA
4	South Dakota	21.9		NA	California**	NA
12	Tennessee	19.2		NA	Connecticut**	NA
9	Texas	20.2		NA	Florida**	NA
1	Utah	35.0		NA	Iowa**	NA
5	Vermont	21.7		NA	Louisiana**	NA
NA	Virginia**	NA		NA	Nebraska**	NA
NA	Washington**	NA		NA	New Hampshire**	NA
32	West Virginia	16.7		NA	Oklahoma**	NA
24	Wisconsin	17.7		NA	Virginia**	NA
17	Wyoming	18.8		NA	Washington**	NA
					District of Columbia**	NA

Source: U.S. Department of Health and Human Services, Centers for Disease Control and Prevention
     "Abortion Surveillance-United States, 1997" (Morbidity Mortality Weekly Report, Vol. 49, No. SS-11, 12/08/00)
*By state of occurrence. National percent is for reporting states only.
**Not reported. New York's percentage is for New York City only.

Percent of Reported Legal Abortions Obtained by Unmarried Women in 1997

Reporting States' Percent = 78.8% of Abortions*

ALPHA ORDER			RANK ORDER		
RANK	STATE	PERCENT	RANK	STATE	PERCENT
10	Alabama	82.0	1	Mississippi	86.9
NA	Alaska**	NA	2	Delaware	84.3
NA	Arizona**	NA	3	Pennsylvania	83.3
17	Arkansas	80.4	4	Michigan	83.0
NA	California**	NA	4	West Virginia	83.0
18	Colorado	80.2	6	New Jersey	82.6
NA	Connecticut**	NA	7	Hawaii	82.2
2	Delaware	84.3	8	New Mexico	82.1
NA	Florida**	NA	8	South Carolina	82.1
11	Georgia	81.8	10	Alabama	82.0
7	Hawaii	82.2	11	Georgia	81.8
14	Idaho	81.0	12	Kentucky	81.3
13	Illinois	81.1	13	Illinois	81.1
33	Indiana	73.1	14	Idaho	81.0
NA	Iowa**	NA	15	Tennessee	80.8
19	Kansas	80.1	16	Wyoming	80.7
12	Kentucky	81.3	17	Arkansas	80.4
NA	Louisiana**	NA	18	Colorado	80.2
29	Maine	76.2	19	Kansas	80.1
21	Maryland	79.6	20	Ohio	79.7
36	Massachusetts	72.1	21	Maryland	79.6
4	Michigan	83.0	22	Minnesota	79.1
22	Minnesota	79.1	23	North Dakota	79.0
1	Mississippi	86.9	24	New York**	78.2
25	Missouri	77.7	25	Missouri	77.7
30	Montana	75.8	25	South Dakota	77.7
NA	Nebraska**	NA	27	Texas	77.5
32	Nevada	74.5	27	Wisconsin	77.5
NA	New Hampshire**	NA	29	Maine	76.2
6	New Jersey	82.6	30	Montana	75.8
8	New Mexico	82.1	31	Oregon	74.8
24	New York**	78.2	32	Nevada	74.5
37	North Carolina	70.3	33	Indiana	73.1
23	North Dakota	79.0	33	Rhode Island	73.1
20	Ohio	79.7	35	Vermont	72.3
NA	Oklahoma**	NA	36	Massachusetts	72.1
31	Oregon	74.8	37	North Carolina	70.3
3	Pennsylvania	83.3	38	Utah	65.0
33	Rhode Island	73.1	NA	Alaska**	NA
8	South Carolina	82.1	NA	Arizona**	NA
25	South Dakota	77.7	NA	California**	NA
15	Tennessee	80.8	NA	Connecticut**	NA
27	Texas	77.5	NA	Florida**	NA
38	Utah	65.0	NA	Iowa**	NA
35	Vermont	72.3	NA	Louisiana**	NA
NA	Virginia**	NA	NA	Nebraska**	NA
NA	Washington**	NA	NA	New Hampshire**	NA
4	West Virginia	83.0	NA	Oklahoma**	NA
27	Wisconsin	77.5	NA	Virginia**	NA
16	Wyoming	80.7	NA	Washington**	NA
				District of Columbia**	NA

Source: U.S. Department of Health and Human Services, Centers for Disease Control and Prevention
    "Abortion Surveillance-United States, 1997" (Morbidity Mortality Weekly Report, Vol. 49, No. SS-11, 12/08/00)
*By state of occurrence. National percent is for reporting states only.
**Not reported. New York's percentage is for New York City only.

Reported Legal Abortions Obtained by Teenagers in 1997

Reporting States' Total = 150,531 Abortions Obtained by Teenagers*

ALPHA ORDER

RANK	STATE	ABORTIONS	% of USA
15	Alabama	2,832	1.9%
40	Alaska	349	0.2%
21	Arizona	2,248	1.5%
28	Arkansas	1,327	0.9%
NA	California**	NA	NA
22	Colorado	2,189	1.5%
14	Connecticut	3,038	2.0%
27	Delaware	1,334	0.9%
NA	Florida**	NA	NA
5	Georgia	7,043	4.7%
33	Hawaii	1,088	0.7%
43	Idaho	236	0.2%
NA	Illinois**	NA	NA
17	Indiana	2,759	1.8%
NA	Iowa**	NA	NA
18	Kansas	2,672	1.8%
26	Kentucky	1,569	1.0%
20	Louisiana	2,432	1.6%
38	Maine	632	0.4%
25	Maryland	1,912	1.3%
11	Massachusetts	4,849	3.2%
7	Michigan	6,026	4.0%
16	Minnesota	2,763	1.8%
34	Mississippi	957	0.6%
24	Missouri	1,985	1.3%
36	Montana	695	0.5%
31	Nebraska	1,106	0.7%
29	Nevada	1,248	0.8%
NA	New Hampshire**	NA	NA
9	New Jersey	5,207	3.5%
30	New Mexico	1,198	0.8%
1	New York	26,440	17.6%
6	North Carolina	6,332	4.2%
41	North Dakota	280	0.2%
3	Ohio	8,149	5.4%
NA	Oklahoma**	NA	NA
13	Oregon	3,335	2.2%
4	Pennsylvania	7,174	4.8%
32	Rhode Island	1,096	0.7%
23	South Carolina	2,056	1.4%
42	South Dakota	249	0.2%
12	Tennessee	3,732	2.5%
2	Texas	15,020	10.0%
35	Utah	732	0.5%
39	Vermont	461	0.3%
10	Virginia	5,031	3.3%
8	Washington	5,728	3.8%
37	West Virginia	691	0.5%
19	Wisconsin	2,666	1.8%
44	Wyoming	33	0.0%

RANK ORDER

RANK	STATE	ABORTIONS	% of USA
1	New York	26,440	17.6%
2	Texas	15,020	10.0%
3	Ohio	8,149	5.4%
4	Pennsylvania	7,174	4.8%
5	Georgia	7,043	4.7%
6	North Carolina	6,332	4.2%
7	Michigan	6,026	4.0%
8	Washington	5,728	3.8%
9	New Jersey	5,207	3.5%
10	Virginia	5,031	3.3%
11	Massachusetts	4,849	3.2%
12	Tennessee	3,732	2.5%
13	Oregon	3,335	2.2%
14	Connecticut	3,038	2.0%
15	Alabama	2,832	1.9%
16	Minnesota	2,763	1.8%
17	Indiana	2,759	1.8%
18	Kansas	2,672	1.8%
19	Wisconsin	2,666	1.8%
20	Louisiana	2,432	1.6%
21	Arizona	2,248	1.5%
22	Colorado	2,189	1.5%
23	South Carolina	2,056	1.4%
24	Missouri	1,985	1.3%
25	Maryland	1,912	1.3%
26	Kentucky	1,569	1.0%
27	Delaware	1,334	0.9%
28	Arkansas	1,327	0.9%
29	Nevada	1,248	0.8%
30	New Mexico	1,198	0.8%
31	Nebraska	1,106	0.7%
32	Rhode Island	1,096	0.7%
33	Hawaii	1,088	0.7%
34	Mississippi	957	0.6%
35	Utah	732	0.5%
36	Montana	695	0.5%
37	West Virginia	691	0.5%
38	Maine	632	0.4%
39	Vermont	461	0.3%
40	Alaska	349	0.2%
41	North Dakota	280	0.2%
42	South Dakota	249	0.2%
43	Idaho	236	0.2%
44	Wyoming	33	0.0%
NA	California**	NA	NA
NA	Florida**	NA	NA
NA	Illinois**	NA	NA
NA	Iowa**	NA	NA
NA	New Hampshire**	NA	NA
NA	Oklahoma**	NA	NA
	District of Columbia	1,632	1.1%

Source: U.S. Department of Health and Human Services, Centers for Disease Control and Prevention
   "Abortion Surveillance-United States, 1997" (Morbidity Mortality Weekly Report, Vol. 49, No. SS-11, 12/08/00)
*Nineteen years old and younger by state of occurrence. National total is for reporting states only.
**Not reported.

Percent of Reported Legal Abortions Obtained by Teenagers in 1997

Reporting States' Percent = 19.8% of Abortions*

ALPHA ORDER

RANK ORDER

RANK	STATE	PERCENT		RANK	STATE	PERCENT
19	Alabama	21.7		1	South Dakota	27.1
22	Alaska	21.4		2	Idaho	26.9
31	Arizona	20.0		3	Delaware	26.0
11	Arkansas	23.0		4	Maine	24.8
NA	California**	NA		5	Montana	24.7
8	Colorado	23.8		6	West Virginia	24.6
18	Connecticut	22.0		7	Hawaii	24.1
3	Delaware	26.0		8	Colorado	23.8
NA	Florida**	NA		8	Kansas	23.8
33	Georgia	19.7		10	Vermont	23.6
7	Hawaii	24.1		11	Arkansas	23.0
2	Idaho	26.9		12	North Dakota	22.8
NA	Illinois**	NA		13	Oregon	22.5
25	Indiana	20.9		14	Kentucky	22.3
NA	Iowa**	NA		14	New Mexico	22.3
8	Kansas	23.8		14	South Carolina	22.3
14	Kentucky	22.3		17	Mississippi	22.1
26	Louisiana	20.7		18	Connecticut	22.0
4	Maine	24.8		19	Alabama	21.7
35	Maryland	19.4		20	Nebraska	21.6
43	Massachusetts	17.0		21	Utah	21.5
27	Michigan	20.4		22	Alaska	21.4
35	Minnesota	19.4		23	Ohio	21.3
17	Mississippi	22.1		23	Washington	21.3
34	Missouri	19.5		25	Indiana	20.9
5	Montana	24.7		26	Louisiana	20.7
20	Nebraska	21.6		27	Michigan	20.4
40	Nevada	18.1		27	Tennessee	20.4
NA	New Hampshire**	NA		29	Wisconsin	20.2
43	New Jersey	17.0		30	North Carolina	20.1
14	New Mexico	22.3		31	Arizona	20.0
39	New York	18.8		31	Rhode Island	20.0
30	North Carolina	20.1		33	Georgia	19.7
12	North Dakota	22.8		34	Missouri	19.5
23	Ohio	21.3		35	Maryland	19.4
NA	Oklahoma**	NA		35	Minnesota	19.4
13	Oregon	22.5		37	Pennsylvania	19.3
37	Pennsylvania	19.3		37	Virginia	19.3
31	Rhode Island	20.0		39	New York	18.8
14	South Carolina	22.3		40	Nevada	18.1
1	South Dakota	27.1		41	Texas	17.7
27	Tennessee	20.4		42	Wyoming	17.2
41	Texas	17.7		43	Massachusetts	17.0
21	Utah	21.5		43	New Jersey	17.0
10	Vermont	23.6		NA	California**	NA
37	Virginia	19.3		NA	Florida**	NA
23	Washington	21.3		NA	Illinois**	NA
6	West Virginia	24.6		NA	Iowa**	NA
29	Wisconsin	20.2		NA	New Hampshire**	NA
42	Wyoming	17.2		NA	Oklahoma**	NA

District of Columbia   18.6

Source: Morgan Quitno Press using data from US Dept of Health & Human Serv's, Centers for Disease Control-Prevention
"Abortion Surveillance-United States, 1997" (Morbidity Mortality Weekly Report, Vol. 49, No. SS-11, 12/08/00)
*Nineteen and younger by state of occurrence. National percent is for reporting states only.
**Not reported.

Reported Legal Abortions Obtained by Teenagers 17 Years and Younger in 1997

Reporting States' Total = 61,341 Abortions*

ALPHA ORDER

RANK	STATE	ABORTIONS	% of USA
16	Alabama	1,135	1.9%
40	Alaska	144	0.2%
22	Arizona	885	1.4%
30	Arkansas	548	0.9%
NA	California**	NA	NA
20	Colorado	1,011	1.6%
14	Connecticut	1,340	2.2%
27	Delaware	609	1.0%
NA	Florida**	NA	NA
4	Georgia	3,032	4.9%
31	Hawaii	476	0.8%
43	Idaho	101	0.2%
NA	Illinois**	NA	NA
19	Indiana	1,024	1.7%
NA	Iowa**	NA	NA
15	Kansas	1,146	1.9%
26	Kentucky	634	1.0%
21	Louisiana	946	1.5%
37	Maine	290	0.5%
24	Maryland	793	1.3%
11	Massachusetts	1,925	3.1%
8	Michigan	2,372	3.9%
17	Minnesota	1,083	1.8%
33	Mississippi	380	0.6%
25	Missouri	782	1.3%
35	Montana	302	0.5%
32	Nebraska	461	0.8%
29	Nevada	552	0.9%
NA	New Hampshire**	NA	NA
9	New Jersey	2,023	3.3%
28	New Mexico	553	0.9%
1	New York	11,388	18.6%
7	North Carolina	2,433	4.0%
41	North Dakota	115	0.2%
3	Ohio	3,444	5.6%
NA	Oklahoma**	NA	NA
13	Oregon	1,412	2.3%
5	Pennsylvania	2,594	4.2%
34	Rhode Island	355	0.6%
23	South Carolina	871	1.4%
42	South Dakota	114	0.2%
12	Tennessee	1,513	2.5%
2	Texas	5,505	9.0%
38	Utah	269	0.4%
39	Vermont	186	0.3%
10	Virginia	1,995	3.3%
6	Washington	2,560	4.2%
36	West Virginia	294	0.5%
18	Wisconsin	1,071	1.7%
44	Wyoming	18	0.0%

RANK ORDER

RANK	STATE	ABORTIONS	% of USA
1	New York	11,388	18.6%
2	Texas	5,505	9.0%
3	Ohio	3,444	5.6%
4	Georgia	3,032	4.9%
5	Pennsylvania	2,594	4.2%
6	Washington	2,560	4.2%
7	North Carolina	2,433	4.0%
8	Michigan	2,372	3.9%
9	New Jersey	2,023	3.3%
10	Virginia	1,995	3.3%
11	Massachusetts	1,925	3.1%
12	Tennessee	1,513	2.5%
13	Oregon	1,412	2.3%
14	Connecticut	1,340	2.2%
15	Kansas	1,146	1.9%
16	Alabama	1,135	1.9%
17	Minnesota	1,083	1.8%
18	Wisconsin	1,071	1.7%
19	Indiana	1,024	1.7%
20	Colorado	1,011	1.6%
21	Louisiana	946	1.5%
22	Arizona	885	1.4%
23	South Carolina	871	1.4%
24	Maryland	793	1.3%
25	Missouri	782	1.3%
26	Kentucky	634	1.0%
27	Delaware	609	1.0%
28	New Mexico	553	0.9%
29	Nevada	552	0.9%
30	Arkansas	548	0.9%
31	Hawaii	476	0.8%
32	Nebraska	461	0.8%
33	Mississippi	380	0.6%
34	Rhode Island	355	0.6%
35	Montana	302	0.5%
36	West Virginia	294	0.5%
37	Maine	290	0.5%
38	Utah	269	0.4%
39	Vermont	186	0.3%
40	Alaska	144	0.2%
41	North Dakota	115	0.2%
42	South Dakota	114	0.2%
43	Idaho	101	0.2%
44	Wyoming	18	0.0%
NA	California**	NA	NA
NA	Florida**	NA	NA
NA	Illinois**	NA	NA
NA	Iowa**	NA	NA
NA	New Hampshire**	NA	NA
NA	Oklahoma**	NA	NA
	District of Columbia	657	1.1%

Source: Morgan Quitno Press using data from US Dept of Health & Human Serv's, Centers for Disease Control-Prevention "Abortion Surveillance-United States, 1997" (Morbidity Mortality Weekly Report, Vol. 49, No. SS-11, 12/08/00)
*By state of occurrence. National total is for reporting states only.
**Not reported.

Percent of Reported Legal Abortions Obtained
By Teenagers 17 Years and Younger in 1997
Reporting States' Percent = 8.1% of Abortions*

ALPHA ORDER			RANK ORDER		
RANK	STATE	PERCENT	RANK	STATE	PERCENT
24	Alabama	8.7	1	South Dakota	12.4
22	Alaska	8.8	2	Delaware	11.9
33	Arizona	7.9	3	Idaho	11.5
12	Arkansas	9.5	4	Maine	11.4
NA	California**	NA	5	Colorado	11.0
5	Colorado	11.0	6	Montana	10.8
11	Connecticut	9.7	7	Hawaii	10.5
2	Delaware	11.9	7	West Virginia	10.5
NA	Florida**	NA	9	New Mexico	10.3
25	Georgia	8.5	10	Kansas	10.2
7	Hawaii	10.5	11	Connecticut	9.7
3	Idaho	11.5	12	Arkansas	9.5
NA	Illinois**	NA	12	Oregon	9.5
35	Indiana	7.8	12	South Carolina	9.5
NA	Iowa**	NA	12	Vermont	9.5
10	Kansas	10.2	12	Washington	9.5
19	Kentucky	9.0	17	North Dakota	9.4
27	Louisiana	8.1	17	Wyoming	9.4
4	Maine	11.4	19	Kentucky	9.0
30	Maryland	8.0	19	Nebraska	9.0
41	Massachusetts	6.8	19	Ohio	9.0
30	Michigan	8.0	22	Alaska	8.8
38	Minnesota	7.6	22	Mississippi	8.8
22	Mississippi	8.8	24	Alabama	8.7
36	Missouri	7.7	25	Georgia	8.5
6	Montana	10.8	26	Tennessee	8.3
19	Nebraska	9.0	27	Louisiana	8.1
30	Nevada	8.0	27	New York	8.1
NA	New Hampshire**	NA	27	Wisconsin	8.1
42	New Jersey	6.6	30	Maryland	8.0
9	New Mexico	10.3	30	Michigan	8.0
27	New York	8.1	30	Nevada	8.0
36	North Carolina	7.7	33	Arizona	7.9
17	North Dakota	9.4	33	Utah	7.9
19	Ohio	9.0	35	Indiana	7.8
NA	Oklahoma**	NA	36	Missouri	7.7
12	Oregon	9.5	36	North Carolina	7.7
40	Pennsylvania	7.0	38	Minnesota	7.6
43	Rhode Island	6.5	38	Virginia	7.6
12	South Carolina	9.5	40	Pennsylvania	7.0
1	South Dakota	12.4	41	Massachusetts	6.8
26	Tennessee	8.3	42	New Jersey	6.6
43	Texas	6.5	43	Rhode Island	6.5
33	Utah	7.9	43	Texas	6.5
12	Vermont	9.5	NA	California**	NA
38	Virginia	7.6	NA	Florida**	NA
12	Washington	9.5	NA	Illinois**	NA
7	West Virginia	10.5	NA	Iowa**	NA
27	Wisconsin	8.1	NA	New Hampshire**	NA
17	Wyoming	9.4	NA	Oklahoma**	NA

District of Columbia 7.5

Source: Morgan Quitno Press using data from US Dept of Health & Human Serv's, Centers for Disease Control-Prevention
"Abortion Surveillance-United States, 1997" (Morbidity Mortality Weekly Report, Vol. 49, No. SS-11, 12/08/00)
*By state of occurrence. National percent is for reporting states only.
**Not reported.

Percent of Teenage Abortions Obtained
By Teenagers 17 Years and Younger in 1997
Reporting States' Percent = 40.7% of Teenage Abortions*

ALPHA ORDER

RANK ORDER

RANK	STATE	PERCENT		RANK	STATE	PERCENT
29	Alabama	40.1		1	Wyoming	54.5
22	Alaska	41.3		2	Colorado	46.2
33	Arizona	39.4		2	New Mexico	46.2
22	Arkansas	41.3		4	Maine	45.9
NA	California**	NA		5	South Dakota	45.8
2	Colorado	46.2		6	Delaware	45.7
9	Connecticut	44.1		7	Washington	44.7
6	Delaware	45.7		8	Nevada	44.2
NA	Florida**	NA		9	Connecticut	44.1
13	Georgia	43.0		10	Hawaii	43.8
10	Hawaii	43.8		11	Montana	43.5
15	Idaho	42.8		12	New York	43.1
NA	Illinois**	NA		13	Georgia	43.0
40	Indiana	37.1		14	Kansas	42.9
NA	Iowa**	NA		15	Idaho	42.8
14	Kansas	42.9		16	West Virginia	42.5
26	Kentucky	40.4		17	South Carolina	42.4
37	Louisiana	38.9		18	Ohio	42.3
4	Maine	45.9		18	Oregon	42.3
21	Maryland	41.5		20	Nebraska	41.7
30	Massachusetts	39.7		21	Maryland	41.5
33	Michigan	39.4		22	Alaska	41.3
36	Minnesota	39.2		22	Arkansas	41.3
30	Mississippi	39.7		24	North Dakota	41.1
33	Missouri	39.4		25	Tennessee	40.5
11	Montana	43.5		26	Kentucky	40.4
20	Nebraska	41.7		27	Vermont	40.3
8	Nevada	44.2		28	Wisconsin	40.2
NA	New Hampshire**	NA		29	Alabama	40.1
37	New Jersey	38.9		30	Massachusetts	39.7
2	New Mexico	46.2		30	Mississippi	39.7
12	New York	43.1		30	Virginia	39.7
39	North Carolina	38.4		33	Arizona	39.4
24	North Dakota	41.1		33	Michigan	39.4
18	Ohio	42.3		33	Missouri	39.4
NA	Oklahoma**	NA		36	Minnesota	39.2
18	Oregon	42.3		37	Louisiana	38.9
43	Pennsylvania	36.2		37	New Jersey	38.9
44	Rhode Island	32.4		39	North Carolina	38.4
17	South Carolina	42.4		40	Indiana	37.1
5	South Dakota	45.8		41	Texas	36.7
25	Tennessee	40.5		41	Utah	36.7
41	Texas	36.7		43	Pennsylvania	36.2
41	Utah	36.7		44	Rhode Island	32.4
27	Vermont	40.3		NA	California**	NA
30	Virginia	39.7		NA	Florida**	NA
7	Washington	44.7		NA	Illinois**	NA
16	West Virginia	42.5		NA	Iowa**	NA
28	Wisconsin	40.2		NA	New Hampshire**	NA
1	Wyoming	54.5		NA	Oklahoma**	NA

District of Columbia   40.3

Source: Morgan Quitno Press using data from US Dept of Health & Human Serv's, Centers for Disease Control-Prevention
"Abortion Surveillance-United States, 1997" (Morbidity Mortality Weekly Report, Vol. 49, No. SS-11, 12/08/00)
*By state of occurrence. National percent is for reporting states only.
**Not reported.

Reported Legal Abortions Performed at 12 Weeks or Less of Gestation in 1997

Reporting States' Total = 616,419 Abortions*

ALPHA ORDER

RANK	STATE	ABORTIONS	% of USA
16	Alabama	11,460	1.9%
NA	Alaska**	NA	NA
18	Arizona	9,618	1.6%
28	Arkansas	4,704	0.8%
NA	California**	NA	NA
24	Colorado	7,808	1.3%
14	Connecticut	12,482	2.0%
30	Delaware	4,493	0.7%
NA	Florida**	NA	NA
5	Georgia	29,515	4.8%
31	Hawaii	4,015	0.7%
40	Idaho	838	0.1%
NA	Illinois**	NA	NA
13	Indiana	12,518	2.0%
NA	Iowa**	NA	NA
23	Kansas	9,105	1.5%
26	Kentucky	5,741	0.9%
20	Louisiana	9,389	1.5%
34	Maine	2,511	0.4%
19	Maryland	9,412	1.5%
NA	Massachusetts**	NA	NA
6	Michigan	26,076	4.2%
15	Minnesota	12,399	2.0%
32	Mississippi	3,827	0.6%
21	Missouri	9,310	1.5%
35	Montana	2,485	0.4%
NA	Nebraska**	NA	NA
25	Nevada	6,041	1.0%
NA	New Hampshire**	NA	NA
9	New Jersey	23,673	3.8%
29	New Mexico	4,524	0.7%
1	New York	117,345	19.0%
7	North Carolina	25,495	4.1%
38	North Dakota	1,072	0.2%
4	Ohio	32,300	5.2%
NA	Oklahoma**	NA	NA
12	Oregon	13,028	2.1%
3	Pennsylvania	32,726	5.3%
27	Rhode Island	4,925	0.8%
22	South Carolina	9,123	1.5%
39	South Dakota	915	0.1%
11	Tennessee	17,317	2.8%
2	Texas	73,643	11.9%
33	Utah	3,088	0.5%
37	Vermont	1,870	0.3%
8	Virginia	24,974	4.1%
10	Washington	22,973	3.7%
36	West Virginia	2,384	0.4%
17	Wisconsin	11,113	1.8%
41	Wyoming	184	0.0%

RANK ORDER

RANK	STATE	ABORTIONS	% of USA
1	New York	117,345	19.0%
2	Texas	73,643	11.9%
3	Pennsylvania	32,726	5.3%
4	Ohio	32,300	5.2%
5	Georgia	29,515	4.8%
6	Michigan	26,076	4.2%
7	North Carolina	25,495	4.1%
8	Virginia	24,974	4.1%
9	New Jersey	23,673	3.8%
10	Washington	22,973	3.7%
11	Tennessee	17,317	2.8%
12	Oregon	13,028	2.1%
13	Indiana	12,518	2.0%
14	Connecticut	12,482	2.0%
15	Minnesota	12,399	2.0%
16	Alabama	11,460	1.9%
17	Wisconsin	11,113	1.8%
18	Arizona	9,618	1.6%
19	Maryland	9,412	1.5%
20	Louisiana	9,389	1.5%
21	Missouri	9,310	1.5%
22	South Carolina	9,123	1.5%
23	Kansas	9,105	1.5%
24	Colorado	7,808	1.3%
25	Nevada	6,041	1.0%
26	Kentucky	5,741	0.9%
27	Rhode Island	4,925	0.8%
28	Arkansas	4,704	0.8%
29	New Mexico	4,524	0.7%
30	Delaware	4,493	0.7%
31	Hawaii	4,015	0.7%
32	Mississippi	3,827	0.6%
33	Utah	3,088	0.5%
34	Maine	2,511	0.4%
35	Montana	2,485	0.4%
36	West Virginia	2,384	0.4%
37	Vermont	1,870	0.3%
38	North Dakota	1,072	0.2%
39	South Dakota	915	0.1%
40	Idaho	838	0.1%
41	Wyoming	184	0.0%
NA	Alaska**	NA	NA
NA	California**	NA	NA
NA	Florida**	NA	NA
NA	Illinois**	NA	NA
NA	Iowa**	NA	NA
NA	Massachusetts**	NA	NA
NA	Nebraska**	NA	NA
NA	New Hampshire**	NA	NA
NA	Oklahoma**	NA	NA
	District of Columbia**	NA	NA

Source: Morgan Quitno Press using data from US Dept of Health & Human Serv's, Centers for Disease Control-Prevention
"Abortion Surveillance-United States, 1997" (Morbidity Mortality Weekly Report, Vol. 49, No. SS-11, 12/08/00)
*By state of occurrence. National total is for reporting states only.
**Not reported.

Percent of Reported Legal Abortions Performed
At 12 Weeks or Less of Gestation in 1997
Reporting States' Percent = 86.2% of Abortions*

ALPHA ORDER

RANK	STATE	PERCENT
21	Alabama	87.7
NA	Alaska**	NA
28	Arizona	85.4
37	Arkansas	81.4
NA	California**	NA
30	Colorado	85.0
13	Connecticut	90.4
24	Delaware	87.4
NA	Florida**	NA
35	Georgia	82.7
15	Hawaii	88.8
7	Idaho	95.4
NA	Illinois**	NA
9	Indiana	94.8
NA	Iowa**	NA
38	Kansas	80.9
36	Kentucky	81.6
40	Louisiana	80.0
3	Maine	98.7
7	Maryland	95.4
NA	Massachusetts**	NA
18	Michigan	88.3
26	Minnesota	87.1
16	Mississippi	88.5
11	Missouri	91.3
16	Montana	88.5
NA	Nebraska**	NA
21	Nevada	87.7
NA	New Hampshire**	NA
41	New Jersey	77.2
33	New Mexico	84.1
34	New York	83.3
38	North Carolina	80.9
24	North Dakota	87.4
32	Ohio	84.5
NA	Oklahoma**	NA
20	Oregon	87.8
19	Pennsylvania	88.1
14	Rhode Island	89.9
2	South Carolina	99.0
1	South Dakota	99.6
10	Tennessee	94.7
27	Texas	87.0
12	Utah	90.6
5	Vermont	95.7
5	Virginia	95.7
29	Washington	85.3
31	West Virginia	84.9
21	Wisconsin	87.7
4	Wyoming	95.8

RANK ORDER

RANK	STATE	PERCENT
1	South Dakota	99.6
2	South Carolina	99.0
3	Maine	98.7
4	Wyoming	95.8
5	Vermont	95.7
5	Virginia	95.7
7	Idaho	95.4
7	Maryland	95.4
9	Indiana	94.8
10	Tennessee	94.7
11	Missouri	91.3
12	Utah	90.6
13	Connecticut	90.4
14	Rhode Island	89.9
15	Hawaii	88.8
16	Mississippi	88.5
16	Montana	88.5
18	Michigan	88.3
19	Pennsylvania	88.1
20	Oregon	87.8
21	Alabama	87.7
21	Nevada	87.7
21	Wisconsin	87.7
24	Delaware	87.4
24	North Dakota	87.4
26	Minnesota	87.1
27	Texas	87.0
28	Arizona	85.4
29	Washington	85.3
30	Colorado	85.0
31	West Virginia	84.9
32	Ohio	84.5
33	New Mexico	84.1
34	New York	83.3
35	Georgia	82.7
36	Kentucky	81.6
37	Arkansas	81.4
38	Kansas	80.9
38	North Carolina	80.9
40	Louisiana	80.0
41	New Jersey	77.2
NA	Alaska**	NA
NA	California**	NA
NA	Florida**	NA
NA	Illinois**	NA
NA	Iowa**	NA
NA	Massachusetts**	NA
NA	Nebraska**	NA
NA	New Hampshire**	NA
NA	Oklahoma**	NA
	District of Columbia**	NA

Source: Morgan Quitno Press using data from US Dept of Health & Human Serv's, Centers for Disease Control-Prevention
"Abortion Surveillance-United States, 1997" (Morbidity Mortality Weekly Report, Vol. 49, No. SS-11, 12/08/00)
*By state of occurrence. National percent is for reporting states only.
**Not reported.

Reported Legal Abortions Performed At or After 21 Weeks of Gestation in 1997

Reporting States' Total = 9,985 Abortions*

ALPHA ORDER

RANK	STATE	ABORTIONS	% of USA
19	Alabama	53	0.5%
NA	Alaska**	NA	NA
38	Arizona	0	0.0%
29	Arkansas	8	0.1%
NA	California**	NA	NA
13	Colorado	152	1.5%
30	Connecticut	4	0.0%
27	Delaware	10	0.1%
NA	Florida**	NA	NA
2	Georgia	1,376	13.8%
22	Hawaii	28	0.3%
30	Idaho	4	0.0%
NA	Illinois**	NA	NA
38	Indiana	0	0.0%
NA	Iowa**	NA	NA
4	Kansas	807	8.1%
15	Kentucky	129	1.3%
8	Louisiana	339	3.4%
34	Maine	1	0.0%
34	Maryland	1	0.0%
NA	Massachusetts**	NA	NA
11	Michigan	221	2.2%
16	Minnesota	102	1.0%
26	Mississippi	15	0.2%
21	Missouri	45	0.5%
20	Montana	47	0.5%
NA	Nebraska**	NA	NA
18	Nevada	69	0.7%
NA	New Hampshire**	NA	NA
5	New Jersey	660	6.6%
22	New Mexico	28	0.3%
1	New York	2,506	25.1%
12	North Carolina	217	2.2%
38	North Dakota	0	0.0%
6	Ohio	647	6.5%
NA	Oklahoma**	NA	NA
10	Oregon	266	2.7%
9	Pennsylvania	285	2.9%
28	Rhode Island	9	0.1%
22	South Carolina	28	0.3%
38	South Dakota	0	0.0%
25	Tennessee	19	0.2%
3	Texas	1,047	10.5%
32	Utah	3	0.0%
33	Vermont	2	0.0%
17	Virginia	96	1.0%
7	Washington	607	6.1%
34	West Virginia	1	0.0%
13	Wisconsin	152	1.5%
34	Wyoming	1	0.0%

RANK ORDER

RANK	STATE	ABORTIONS	% of USA
1	New York	2,506	25.1%
2	Georgia	1,376	13.8%
3	Texas	1,047	10.5%
4	Kansas	807	8.1%
5	New Jersey	660	6.6%
6	Ohio	647	6.5%
7	Washington	607	6.1%
8	Louisiana	339	3.4%
9	Pennsylvania	285	2.9%
10	Oregon	266	2.7%
11	Michigan	221	2.2%
12	North Carolina	217	2.2%
13	Colorado	152	1.5%
13	Wisconsin	152	1.5%
15	Kentucky	129	1.3%
16	Minnesota	102	1.0%
17	Virginia	96	1.0%
18	Nevada	69	0.7%
19	Alabama	53	0.5%
20	Montana	47	0.5%
21	Missouri	45	0.5%
22	Hawaii	28	0.3%
22	New Mexico	28	0.3%
22	South Carolina	28	0.3%
25	Tennessee	19	0.2%
26	Mississippi	15	0.2%
27	Delaware	10	0.1%
28	Rhode Island	9	0.1%
29	Arkansas	8	0.1%
30	Connecticut	4	0.0%
30	Idaho	4	0.0%
32	Utah	3	0.0%
33	Vermont	2	0.0%
34	Maine	1	0.0%
34	Maryland	1	0.0%
34	West Virginia	1	0.0%
34	Wyoming	1	0.0%
38	Arizona	0	0.0%
38	Indiana	0	0.0%
38	North Dakota	0	0.0%
38	South Dakota	0	0.0%
NA	Alaska**	NA	NA
NA	California**	NA	NA
NA	Florida**	NA	NA
NA	Illinois**	NA	NA
NA	Iowa**	NA	NA
NA	Massachusetts**	NA	NA
NA	Nebraska**	NA	NA
NA	New Hampshire**	NA	NA
NA	Oklahoma**	NA	NA
	District of Columbia**	NA	NA

Source: U.S. Department of Health and Human Services, Centers for Disease Control and Prevention
"Abortion Surveillance-United States, 1997" (Morbidity Mortality Weekly Report, Vol. 49, No. SS-11, 12/08/00)
*By state of occurrence. National total is for reporting states only.
**Not reported.

Percent of Reported Legal Abortions Performed At or After
21 Weeks of Gestation in 1997
Reporting States' Percent = 1.4% of Abortions*

ALPHA ORDER

RANK ORDER

RANK	STATE	PERCENT
23	Alabama	0.4
NA	Alaska**	NA
34	Arizona	0.0
30	Arkansas	0.1
NA	California**	NA
9	Colorado	1.7
34	Connecticut	0.0
28	Delaware	0.2
NA	Florida**	NA
2	Georgia	3.9
19	Hawaii	0.6
20	Idaho	0.5
NA	Illinois**	NA
34	Indiana	0.0
NA	Iowa**	NA
1	Kansas	7.2
6	Kentucky	1.8
3	Louisiana	2.9
34	Maine	0.0
34	Maryland	0.0
NA	Massachusetts**	NA
16	Michigan	0.7
16	Minnesota	0.7
26	Mississippi	0.3
23	Missouri	0.4
9	Montana	1.7
NA	Nebraska**	NA
14	Nevada	1.0
NA	New Hampshire**	NA
5	New Jersey	2.2
20	New Mexico	0.5
6	New York	1.8
16	North Carolina	0.7
34	North Dakota	0.0
9	Ohio	1.7
NA	Oklahoma**	NA
6	Oregon	1.8
15	Pennsylvania	0.8
28	Rhode Island	0.2
26	South Carolina	0.3
34	South Dakota	0.0
30	Tennessee	0.1
12	Texas	1.2
30	Utah	0.1
30	Vermont	0.1
23	Virginia	0.4
4	Washington	2.3
34	West Virginia	0.0
12	Wisconsin	1.2
20	Wyoming	0.5

RANK	STATE	PERCENT
1	Kansas	7.2
2	Georgia	3.9
3	Louisiana	2.9
4	Washington	2.3
5	New Jersey	2.2
6	Kentucky	1.8
6	New York	1.8
6	Oregon	1.8
9	Colorado	1.7
9	Montana	1.7
9	Ohio	1.7
12	Texas	1.2
12	Wisconsin	1.2
14	Nevada	1.0
15	Pennsylvania	0.8
16	Michigan	0.7
16	Minnesota	0.7
16	North Carolina	0.7
19	Hawaii	0.6
20	Idaho	0.5
20	New Mexico	0.5
20	Wyoming	0.5
23	Alabama	0.4
23	Missouri	0.4
23	Virginia	0.4
26	Mississippi	0.3
26	South Carolina	0.3
28	Delaware	0.2
28	Rhode Island	0.2
30	Arkansas	0.1
30	Tennessee	0.1
30	Utah	0.1
30	Vermont	0.1
34	Arizona	0.0
34	Connecticut	0.0
34	Indiana	0.0
34	Maine	0.0
34	Maryland	0.0
34	North Dakota	0.0
34	South Dakota	0.0
34	West Virginia	0.0
NA	Alaska**	NA
NA	California**	NA
NA	Florida**	NA
NA	Illinois**	NA
NA	Iowa**	NA
NA	Massachusetts**	NA
NA	Nebraska**	NA
NA	New Hampshire**	NA
NA	Oklahoma**	NA
	District of Columbia**	NA

Source: Morgan Quitno Press using data from US Dept of Health & Human Serv's, Centers for Disease Control-Prevention
"Abortion Surveillance-United States, 1997" (Morbidity Mortality Weekly Report, Vol. 49, No. SS-11, 12/08/00)
*By state of occurrence. National percent is for reporting states only.
**Not reported.

II. DEATHS

76   Deaths in 2000
77   Death Rate in 2000
78   Births to Deaths Ratio in 2000
79   Deaths in 1999
80   Death Rate in 1999
81   Age-Adjusted Death Rate in 1999
82   Death Rate in 1990
83   Death Rate in 1980
84   Infant Deaths in 2000
85   Infant Mortality Rate in 2000
86   Infant Deaths in 1999
87   Infant Mortality Rate in 1999
88   Infant Mortality Rate in 1990
89   Infant Mortality Rate in 1980
90   Percent Change in Infant Mortality Rate: 1990 to 1999
91   Percent Change in Infant Mortality Rate: 1980 to 1999
92   White Infant Deaths in 1999
93   White Infant Mortality Rate in 1999
94   Black Infant Deaths in 1999
95   Black Infant Mortality Rate in 1999
96   Percent Change in White Infant Mortality Rate: 1990 to 1999
97   Percent Change in Black Infant Mortality Rate: 1990 to 1999
98   Neonatal Deaths in 1999
99   Neonatal Death Rate in 1999
100 White Neonatal Deaths in 1999
101 White Neonatal Death Rate in 1999
102 Black Neonatal Deaths in 1999
103 Black Neonatal Death Rate in 1999
104 Deaths by AIDS Through 1999
105 Deaths by AIDS in 1999
106 Death Rate by AIDS in 1999
107 Age-Adjusted Death Rate by AIDS in 1999
108 Estimated Deaths by Cancer in 2002
109 Estimated Death Rate by Cancer in 2002
110 Age-Adjusted Death Rate by Cancer for Males in 1998
111 Age-Adjusted Death Rate by Cancer for Females in 1998
112 Estimated Deaths by Female Breast Cancer in 2002
113 Estimated Death Rate by Female Breast Cancer in 2002
114 Estimated Deaths by Colon and Rectum Cancer in 2002
115 Estimated Death Rate by Colon and Rectum Cancer in 2002
116 Estimated Deaths by Leukemia in 2002
117 Estimated Death Rate by Leukemia in 2002
118 Estimated Deaths by Liver Cancer in 2002
119 Estimated Death Rate by Liver Cancer in 2002
120 Estimated Deaths by Lung Cancer in 2002
121 Estimated Death Rate by Lung Cancer in 2002
122 Estimated Deaths by Non-Hodgkin's Lymphoma in 2002
123 Estimated Death Rate by Non-Hodgkin's Lymphoma in 2002
124 Estimated Deaths by Pancreatic Cancer in 2002
125 Estimated Death Rate by Pancreatic Cancer in 2002
126 Estimated Deaths by Prostate Cancer in 2002
127 Estimated Death Rate by Prostate Cancer in 2002
128 Estimated Deaths by Ovarian Cancer in 2002
129 Estimated Death Rate by Ovarian Cancer in 2002
130 Estimated Deaths by Brain Cancer in 2002
131 Estimated Death Rate by Brain Cancer in 2002
132 Deaths by Alzheimer's Disease in 1999
133 Death Rate by Alzheimer's Disease in 1999
134 Age-Adjusted Death Rate by Alzheimer's Disease in 1999
135 Deaths by Atherosclerosis in 1999
136 Death Rate by Atherosclerosis in 1999

II. DEATHS (Continued)

137 Age-Adjusted Death Rate by Atherosclerosis in 1999
138 Deaths by Cerebrovascular Diseases in 1999
139 Death Rate by Cerebrovascular Diseases in 1999
140 Age-Adjusted Death Rate by Cerebrovascular Diseases in 1999
141 Deaths by Chronic Liver Disease and Cirrhosis in 1999
142 Death Rate by Chronic Liver Disease and Cirrhosis in 1999
143 Age-Adjusted Death Rate by Chronic Liver Disease and Cirrhosis in 1999
144 Deaths by Chronic Lower Respiratory Diseases in 1999
145 Death Rate by Chronic Lower Respiratory Diseases in 1999
146 Age-Adjusted Death Rate by Chronic Lower Respiratory Diseases in 1999
147 Deaths by Diabetes Mellitus in 1999
148 Death Rate by Diabetes Mellitus in 1999
149 Age-Adjusted Death Rate by Diabetes Mellitus in 1999
150 Deaths by Diseases of the Heart in 1999
151 Death Rate by Diseases of the Heart in 1999
152 Age-Adjusted Death Rate by Diseases of the Heart in 1999
153 Deaths by Malignant Neoplasms in 1999
154 Death Rate by Malignant Neoplasms in 1999
155 Age-Adjusted Death Rate by Malignant Neoplasms in 1999
156 Deaths by Pneumonia and Influenza in 1999
157 Death Rate by Pneumonia and Influenza in 1999
158 Age-Adjusted Death Rate by Pneumonia and Influenza in 1999
159 Deaths by Tuberculosis in 1999
160 Death Rate by Tuberculosis in 1999
161 Age-Adjusted Death Rate by Tuberculosis in 1999
162 Deaths by Injury in 1999
163 Death Rate by Injury in 1999
164 Age-Adjusted Death Rate by Injury in 1999
165 Deaths by Accidents in 1999
166 Death Rate by Accidents in 1999
167 Age-Adjusted Death Rate by Accidents in 1999
168 Deaths by Motor Vehicle Accidents in 1999
169 Death Rate by Motor Vehicle Accidents in 1999
170 Age-Adjusted Death Rate by Motor Vehicle Accidents in 1999
171 Deaths by Homicide in 1999
172 Death Rate by Homicide in 1999
173 Age-Adjusted Death Rate by Homicide in 1999
174 Deaths by Suicide in 1999
175 Death Rate by Suicide in 1999
176 Age-Adjusted Death Rate by Suicide in 1999
177 Years Lost by Premature Death in 1999
178 Years Lost by Premature Death from Cancer in 1999
179 Years Lost by Premature Death from Heart Disease in 1999
180 Years Lost by Premature Death from Homicide in 1999
181 Years Lost by Premature Death from Suicide in 1999
182 Years Lost by Premature Death from Unintentional Injuries in 1999
183 Alcohol-Induced Deaths in 1999
184 Death Rate by Alcohol-Induced Deaths in 1999
185 Age-Adjusted Death Rate by Alcohol-Induced Deaths in 1999
186 Drug-Induced Deaths in 1999
187 Death Rate from Drug-Induced Deaths in 1999
188 Age-Adjusted Death Rate from Drug-Induced Deaths in 1999
189 Occupational Fatalities in 2000
190 Occupational Fatality Rate in 2000

Deaths in 2000

National Total = 2,404,598 Deaths*

ALPHA ORDER					RANK ORDER			
RANK	STATE	DEATHS	% of USA		RANK	STATE	DEATHS	% of USA
17	Alabama	45,075	1.9%		1	California	229,535	9.5%
49	Alaska	2,911	0.1%		2	Florida	164,401	6.8%
21	Arizona	40,524	1.7%		3	New York	158,137	6.6%
29	Arkansas	28,231	1.2%		4	Texas	148,554	6.2%
1	California	229,535	9.5%		5	Pennsylvania	130,814	5.4%
31	Colorado	27,335	1.1%		6	Illinois	106,712	4.4%
26	Connecticut	30,237	1.3%		7	Michigan	86,967	3.6%
45	Delaware	6,862	0.3%		8	New Jersey	75,681	3.1%
2	Florida	164,401	6.8%		9	North Carolina	71,995	3.0%
10	Georgia	63,980	2.7%		10	Georgia	63,980	2.7%
42	Hawaii	8,292	0.3%		11	Massachusetts	56,475	2.3%
41	Idaho	9,564	0.4%		12	Virginia	56,161	2.3%
6	Illinois	106,712	4.4%		13	Indiana	55,848	2.3%
13	Indiana	55,848	2.3%		14	Tennessee	55,318	2.3%
30	Iowa	28,082	1.2%		15	Missouri	54,880	2.3%
32	Kansas	24,720	1.0%		16	Wisconsin	46,519	1.9%
22	Kentucky	39,532	1.6%		17	Alabama	45,075	1.9%
20	Louisiana	41,150	1.7%		18	Washington	43,976	1.8%
37	Maine	12,377	0.5%		19	Maryland	43,779	1.8%
19	Maryland	43,779	1.8%		20	Louisiana	41,150	1.7%
11	Massachusetts	56,475	2.3%		21	Arizona	40,524	1.7%
7	Michigan	86,967	3.6%		22	Kentucky	39,532	1.6%
23	Minnesota	37,752	1.6%		23	Minnesota	37,752	1.6%
28	Mississippi	28,671	1.2%		24	South Carolina	36,948	1.5%
15	Missouri	54,880	2.3%		25	Oklahoma	35,265	1.5%
43	Montana	8,104	0.3%		26	Connecticut	30,237	1.3%
35	Nebraska	14,988	0.6%		27	Oregon	29,562	1.2%
34	Nevada	15,263	0.6%		28	Mississippi	28,671	1.2%
40	New Hampshire	9,703	0.4%		29	Arkansas	28,231	1.2%
8	New Jersey	75,681	3.1%		30	Iowa	28,082	1.2%
36	New Mexico	13,488	0.6%		31	Colorado	27,335	1.1%
3	New York	158,137	6.6%		32	Kansas	24,720	1.0%
9	North Carolina	71,995	3.0%		33	West Virginia	21,078	0.9%
46	North Dakota	5,860	0.2%		34	Nevada	15,263	0.6%
NA	Ohio**	NA	NA		35	Nebraska	14,988	0.6%
25	Oklahoma	35,265	1.5%		36	New Mexico	13,488	0.6%
27	Oregon	29,562	1.2%		37	Maine	12,377	0.5%
5	Pennsylvania	130,814	5.4%		38	Utah	12,370	0.5%
39	Rhode Island	10,030	0.4%		39	Rhode Island	10,030	0.4%
24	South Carolina	36,948	1.5%		40	New Hampshire	9,703	0.4%
44	South Dakota	7,024	0.3%		41	Idaho	9,564	0.4%
14	Tennessee	55,318	2.3%		42	Hawaii	8,292	0.3%
4	Texas	148,554	6.2%		43	Montana	8,104	0.3%
38	Utah	12,370	0.5%		44	South Dakota	7,024	0.3%
47	Vermont	5,142	0.2%		45	Delaware	6,862	0.3%
12	Virginia	56,161	2.3%		46	North Dakota	5,860	0.2%
18	Washington	43,976	1.8%		47	Vermont	5,142	0.2%
33	West Virginia	21,078	0.9%		48	Wyoming	3,918	0.2%
16	Wisconsin	46,519	1.9%		49	Alaska	2,911	0.1%
48	Wyoming	3,918	0.2%		NA	Ohio**	NA	NA
						District of Columbia	5,957	0.2%

Source: U.S. Department of Health and Human Services, National Center for Health Statistics
    "National Vital Statistics Reports" (Vol. 49, No. 12, October 9, 2001)
*Preliminary data by state of residence.
**Not available.

Death Rate in 2000

National Rate = 873.6 Deaths per 100,000 Population*

ALPHA ORDER

RANK ORDER

RANK	STATE	RATE		RANK	STATE	RATE
7	Alabama	1,027.3		1	West Virginia	1,169.5
49	Alaska	467.9		2	Arkansas	1,095.7
34	Arizona	830.0		3	Pennsylvania	1,091.5
2	Arkansas	1,095.7		4	Florida	1,072.3
46	California	682.5		5	Oklahoma	1,043.3
47	Colorado	660.8		6	Mississippi	1,028.7
22	Connecticut	917.0		7	Alabama	1,027.3
25	Delaware	900.2		8	Rhode Island	1,006.9
4	Florida	1,072.3		9	Tennessee	999.7
38	Georgia	805.5		10	Missouri	997.4
45	Hawaii	703.2		11	Kentucky	991.9
43	Idaho	751.1		12	Maine	983.4
30	Illinois	875.7		13	Iowa	976.0
17	Indiana	934.5		14	South Dakota	952.7
13	Iowa	976.0		15	South Carolina	941.5
20	Kansas	927.3		16	Louisiana	940.6
11	Kentucky	991.9		17	Indiana	934.5
16	Louisiana	940.6		18	North Dakota	931.2
12	Maine	983.4		19	North Carolina	929.3
33	Maryland	838.9		20	Kansas	927.3
24	Massachusetts	910.3		21	New Jersey	922.4
29	Michigan	876.8		22	Connecticut	917.0
40	Minnesota	782.0		23	Montana	912.7
6	Mississippi	1,028.7		24	Massachusetts	910.3
10	Missouri	997.4		25	Delaware	900.2
23	Montana	912.7		26	Nebraska	897.3
26	Nebraska	897.3		27	Oregon	884.8
36	Nevada	811.7		28	Wisconsin	878.5
39	New Hampshire	798.0		29	Michigan	876.8
21	New Jersey	922.4		30	Illinois	875.7
41	New Mexico	771.7		31	New York	865.2
31	New York	865.2		32	Vermont	860.1
19	North Carolina	929.3		33	Maryland	838.9
18	North Dakota	931.2		34	Arizona	830.0
NA	Ohio**	NA		35	Wyoming	814.7
5	Oklahoma	1,043.3		36	Nevada	811.7
27	Oregon	884.8		37	Virginia	805.7
3	Pennsylvania	1,091.5		38	Georgia	805.5
8	Rhode Island	1,006.9		39	New Hampshire	798.0
15	South Carolina	941.5		40	Minnesota	782.0
14	South Dakota	952.7		41	New Mexico	771.7
9	Tennessee	999.7		42	Washington	756.8
44	Texas	728.6		43	Idaho	751.1
48	Utah	571.5		44	Texas	728.6
32	Vermont	860.1		45	Hawaii	703.2
37	Virginia	805.7		46	California	682.5
42	Washington	756.8		47	Colorado	660.8
1	West Virginia	1,169.5		48	Utah	571.5
28	Wisconsin	878.5		49	Alaska	467.9
35	Wyoming	814.7		NA	Ohio**	NA
					District of Columbia	1,149.2

Source: U.S. Department of Health and Human Services, National Center for Health Statistics
   "National Vital Statistics Reports" (Vol. 49, No. 12, October 9, 2001)
*Preliminary data by state of residence. Not age-adjusted.
**Not available.

Births to Deaths Ratio in 2000

National Ratio = 1.69 Births for Every Death in 2000

ALPHA ORDER

RANK ORDER

RANK	STATE	RATIO
38	Alabama	1.40
2	Alaska	3.44
8	Arizona	2.10
41	Arkansas	1.35
5	California	2.32
4	Colorado	2.39
35	Connecticut	1.43
21	Delaware	1.61
46	Florida	1.24
9	Georgia	2.07
7	Hawaii	2.12
6	Idaho	2.13
15	Illinois	1.73
25	Indiana	1.56
40	Iowa	1.37
21	Kansas	1.61
36	Kentucky	1.42
18	Louisiana	1.65
48	Maine	1.10
16	Maryland	1.70
33	Massachusetts	1.45
24	Michigan	1.57
13	Minnesota	1.79
27	Mississippi	1.54
39	Missouri	1.39
41	Montana	1.35
19	Nebraska	1.64
10	Nevada	2.03
30	New Hampshire	1.51
28	New Jersey	1.52
11	New Mexico	2.02
20	New York	1.63
17	North Carolina	1.67
43	North Dakota	1.31
NA	Ohio**	NA
36	Oklahoma	1.42
26	Oregon	1.55
47	Pennsylvania	1.12
45	Rhode Island	1.25
28	South Carolina	1.52
32	South Dakota	1.47
34	Tennessee	1.44
3	Texas	2.47
1	Utah	3.83
44	Vermont	1.26
14	Virginia	1.76
12	Washington	1.84
49	West Virginia	0.99
31	Wisconsin	1.49
23	Wyoming	1.59

RANK	STATE	RATIO
1	Utah	3.83
2	Alaska	3.44
3	Texas	2.47
4	Colorado	2.39
5	California	2.32
6	Idaho	2.13
7	Hawaii	2.12
8	Arizona	2.10
9	Georgia	2.07
10	Nevada	2.03
11	New Mexico	2.02
12	Washington	1.84
13	Minnesota	1.79
14	Virginia	1.76
15	Illinois	1.73
16	Maryland	1.70
17	North Carolina	1.67
18	Louisiana	1.65
19	Nebraska	1.64
20	New York	1.63
21	Delaware	1.61
21	Kansas	1.61
23	Wyoming	1.59
24	Michigan	1.57
25	Indiana	1.56
26	Oregon	1.55
27	Mississippi	1.54
28	New Jersey	1.52
28	South Carolina	1.52
30	New Hampshire	1.51
31	Wisconsin	1.49
32	South Dakota	1.47
33	Massachusetts	1.45
34	Tennessee	1.44
35	Connecticut	1.43
36	Kentucky	1.42
36	Oklahoma	1.42
38	Alabama	1.40
39	Missouri	1.39
40	Iowa	1.37
41	Arkansas	1.35
41	Montana	1.35
43	North Dakota	1.31
44	Vermont	1.26
45	Rhode Island	1.25
46	Florida	1.24
47	Pennsylvania	1.12
48	Maine	1.10
49	West Virginia	0.99
NA	Ohio**	NA

District of Columbia	1.29

Source: Morgan Quitno Press using data from U.S. Dept. of Health & Human Services, National Center for Health Statistics
"National Vital Statistics Reports" (Vol. 49, No. 5, July 24, 2001)
*Preliminary data by state of residence.
**Not available.

Deaths in 1999

National Total = 2,391,399 Deaths*

ALPHA ORDER

RANK	STATE	DEATHS	% of USA
18	Alabama	44,806	1.9%
50	Alaska	2,708	0.1%
22	Arizona	40,050	1.7%
31	Arkansas	27,925	1.2%
1	California	229,380	9.6%
32	Colorado	27,114	1.1%
27	Connecticut	29,446	1.2%
46	Delaware	6,666	0.3%
2	Florida	163,224	6.8%
11	Georgia	62,028	2.6%
43	Hawaii	8,270	0.3%
41	Idaho	9,579	0.4%
7	Illinois	108,436	4.5%
15	Indiana	55,303	2.3%
29	Iowa	28,411	1.2%
33	Kansas	24,472	1.0%
23	Kentucky	39,321	1.6%
21	Louisiana	41,238	1.7%
38	Maine	12,261	0.5%
20	Maryland	43,089	1.8%
13	Massachusetts	55,840	2.3%
8	Michigan	87,232	3.6%
24	Minnesota	38,537	1.6%
30	Mississippi	28,185	1.2%
12	Missouri	55,931	2.3%
44	Montana	8,128	0.3%
35	Nebraska	15,579	0.7%
36	Nevada	15,082	0.6%
42	New Hampshire	9,537	0.4%
9	New Jersey	73,981	3.1%
37	New Mexico	13,676	0.6%
3	New York	159,927	6.7%
10	North Carolina	69,600	2.9%
47	North Dakota	6,103	0.3%
6	Ohio	108,517	4.5%
26	Oklahoma	34,700	1.5%
28	Oregon	29,422	1.2%
5	Pennsylvania	130,283	5.4%
40	Rhode Island	9,708	0.4%
25	South Carolina	36,053	1.5%
45	South Dakota	6,953	0.3%
16	Tennessee	53,765	2.2%
4	Texas	146,858	6.1%
39	Utah	12,058	0.5%
48	Vermont	4,993	0.2%
14	Virginia	55,320	2.3%
19	Washington	43,865	1.8%
34	West Virginia	21,049	0.9%
17	Wisconsin	46,672	2.0%
49	Wyoming	4,042	0.2%

RANK ORDER

RANK	STATE	DEATHS	% of USA
1	California	229,380	9.6%
2	Florida	163,224	6.8%
3	New York	159,927	6.7%
4	Texas	146,858	6.1%
5	Pennsylvania	130,283	5.4%
6	Ohio	108,517	4.5%
7	Illinois	108,436	4.5%
8	Michigan	87,232	3.6%
9	New Jersey	73,981	3.1%
10	North Carolina	69,600	2.9%
11	Georgia	62,028	2.6%
12	Missouri	55,931	2.3%
13	Massachusetts	55,840	2.3%
14	Virginia	55,320	2.3%
15	Indiana	55,303	2.3%
16	Tennessee	53,765	2.2%
17	Wisconsin	46,672	2.0%
18	Alabama	44,806	1.9%
19	Washington	43,865	1.8%
20	Maryland	43,089	1.8%
21	Louisiana	41,238	1.7%
22	Arizona	40,050	1.7%
23	Kentucky	39,321	1.6%
24	Minnesota	38,537	1.6%
25	South Carolina	36,053	1.5%
26	Oklahoma	34,700	1.5%
27	Connecticut	29,446	1.2%
28	Oregon	29,422	1.2%
29	Iowa	28,411	1.2%
30	Mississippi	28,185	1.2%
31	Arkansas	27,925	1.2%
32	Colorado	27,114	1.1%
33	Kansas	24,472	1.0%
34	West Virginia	21,049	0.9%
35	Nebraska	15,579	0.7%
36	Nevada	15,082	0.6%
37	New Mexico	13,676	0.6%
38	Maine	12,261	0.5%
39	Utah	12,058	0.5%
40	Rhode Island	9,708	0.4%
41	Idaho	9,579	0.4%
42	New Hampshire	9,537	0.4%
43	Hawaii	8,270	0.3%
44	Montana	8,128	0.3%
45	South Dakota	6,953	0.3%
46	Delaware	6,666	0.3%
47	North Dakota	6,103	0.3%
48	Vermont	4,993	0.2%
49	Wyoming	4,042	0.2%
50	Alaska	2,708	0.1%
	District of Columbia	6,076	0.3%

Source: U.S. Department of Health and Human Services, National Center for Health Statistics
    "National Vital Statistics Reports" (Vol. 49, No. 8, September 21, 2001)
*Final data by state of residence.

Death Rate in 1999

National Rate = 877.0 Deaths per 100,000 Population*

ALPHA ORDER

RANK	STATE	RATE
6	Alabama	1,025.3
50	Alaska	437.1
35	Arizona	838.2
2	Arkansas	1,094.5
47	California	692.0
48	Colorado	668.5
26	Connecticut	897.2
30	Delaware	884.6
4	Florida	1,080.1
40	Georgia	796.4
46	Hawaii	697.6
43	Idaho	765.3
27	Illinois	894.1
19	Indiana	930.6
10	Iowa	990.1
21	Kansas	922.1
9	Kentucky	992.7
17	Louisiana	943.2
13	Maine	978.5
37	Maryland	833.2
25	Massachusetts	904.3
31	Michigan	884.4
38	Minnesota	807.0
8	Mississippi	1,018.0
7	Missouri	1,022.8
22	Montana	920.7
18	Nebraska	935.1
36	Nevada	833.6
41	New Hampshire	794.0
24	New Jersey	908.5
42	New Mexico	786.0
32	New York	878.9
23	North Carolina	909.7
15	North Dakota	963.1
14	Ohio	964.0
5	Oklahoma	1,033.3
29	Oregon	887.2
3	Pennsylvania	1,086.2
12	Rhode Island	979.8
20	South Carolina	927.8
16	South Dakota	948.4
11	Tennessee	980.5
45	Texas	732.7
49	Utah	566.1
34	Vermont	840.9
39	Virginia	804.9
44	Washington	762.0
1	West Virginia	1,164.9
28	Wisconsin	888.9
33	Wyoming	842.8

RANK ORDER

RANK	STATE	RATE
1	West Virginia	1,164.9
2	Arkansas	1,094.5
3	Pennsylvania	1,086.2
4	Florida	1,080.1
5	Oklahoma	1,033.3
6	Alabama	1,025.3
7	Missouri	1,022.8
8	Mississippi	1,018.0
9	Kentucky	992.7
10	Iowa	990.1
11	Tennessee	980.5
12	Rhode Island	979.8
13	Maine	978.5
14	Ohio	964.0
15	North Dakota	963.1
16	South Dakota	948.4
17	Louisiana	943.2
18	Nebraska	935.1
19	Indiana	930.6
20	South Carolina	927.8
21	Kansas	922.1
22	Montana	920.7
23	North Carolina	909.7
24	New Jersey	908.5
25	Massachusetts	904.3
26	Connecticut	897.2
27	Illinois	894.1
28	Wisconsin	888.9
29	Oregon	887.2
30	Delaware	884.6
31	Michigan	884.4
32	New York	878.9
33	Wyoming	842.8
34	Vermont	840.9
35	Arizona	838.2
36	Nevada	833.6
37	Maryland	833.2
38	Minnesota	807.0
39	Virginia	804.9
40	Georgia	796.4
41	New Hampshire	794.0
42	New Mexico	786.0
43	Idaho	765.3
44	Washington	762.0
45	Texas	732.7
46	Hawaii	697.6
47	California	692.0
48	Colorado	668.5
49	Utah	566.1
50	Alaska	437.1

	District of Columbia	1,170.7

Source: U.S. Department of Health and Human Services, National Center for Health Statistics
    "National Vital Statistics Reports" (Vol. 49, No. 8, September 21, 2001)
*Final data by state of residence. Not age-adjusted.

Age-Adjusted Death Rate in 1999

National Rate = 881.9 Deaths per 100,000 Population*

ALPHA ORDER

RANK	STATE	RATE
3	Alabama	1,021.1
36	Alaska	834.4
29	Arizona	850.1
6	Arkansas	1,005.4
48	California	791.0
45	Colorado	801.2
46	Connecticut	792.3
21	Delaware	904.6
37	Florida	833.9
10	Georgia	983.9
50	Hawaii	680.3
38	Idaho	825.2
22	Illinois	903.1
14	Indiana	941.4
42	Iowa	815.3
28	Kansas	850.5
5	Kentucky	1,012.8
2	Louisiana	1,040.7
23	Maine	896.3
16	Maryland	911.2
40	Massachusetts	816.7
19	Michigan	906.9
47	Minnesota	792.2
1	Mississippi	1,064.9
12	Missouri	954.1
26	Montana	861.2
32	Nebraska	838.7
11	Nevada	967.1
35	New Hampshire	835.2
27	New Jersey	857.8
25	New Mexico	875.7
34	New York	836.0
13	North Carolina	943.6
44	North Dakota	802.6
15	Ohio	933.6
9	Oklahoma	985.0
31	Oregon	839.2
18	Pennsylvania	907.5
43	Rhode Island	812.8
8	South Carolina	996.0
39	South Dakota	820.2
7	Tennessee	1,001.9
24	Texas	892.2
49	Utah	787.1
30	Vermont	843.9
20	Virginia	905.9
41	Washington	816.1
4	West Virginia	1,013.3
33	Wisconsin	838.1
17	Wyoming	909.0

RANK ORDER

RANK	STATE	RATE
1	Mississippi	1,064.9
2	Louisiana	1,040.7
3	Alabama	1,021.1
4	West Virginia	1,013.3
5	Kentucky	1,012.8
6	Arkansas	1,005.4
7	Tennessee	1,001.9
8	South Carolina	996.0
9	Oklahoma	985.0
10	Georgia	983.9
11	Nevada	967.1
12	Missouri	954.1
13	North Carolina	943.6
14	Indiana	941.4
15	Ohio	933.6
16	Maryland	911.2
17	Wyoming	909.0
18	Pennsylvania	907.5
19	Michigan	906.9
20	Virginia	905.9
21	Delaware	904.6
22	Illinois	903.1
23	Maine	896.3
24	Texas	892.2
25	New Mexico	875.7
26	Montana	861.2
27	New Jersey	857.8
28	Kansas	850.5
29	Arizona	850.1
30	Vermont	843.9
31	Oregon	839.2
32	Nebraska	838.7
33	Wisconsin	838.1
34	New York	836.0
35	New Hampshire	835.2
36	Alaska	834.4
37	Florida	833.9
38	Idaho	825.2
39	South Dakota	820.2
40	Massachusetts	816.7
41	Washington	816.1
42	Iowa	815.3
43	Rhode Island	812.8
44	North Dakota	802.6
45	Colorado	801.2
46	Connecticut	792.3
47	Minnesota	792.2
48	California	791.0
49	Utah	787.1
50	Hawaii	680.3
	District of Columbia	1,082.7

Source: U.S. Department of Health and Human Services, National Center for Health Statistics
   "National Vital Statistics Reports" (Vol. 49, No. 8, September 21, 2001)
*Final data by state of residence. Age-adjusted rates eliminate the distorting effects of the aging of the population.
Rates based on the year 2000 standard population.

Death Rate in 1990

National Rate = 863 Deaths per 100,000 Population*

ALPHA ORDER

RANK	STATE	RATE
7	Alabama	974
50	Alaska	398
37	Arizona	784
2	Arkansas	1,048
44	California	719
47	Colorado	655
32	Connecticut	840
27	Delaware	864
3	Florida	1,038
35	Georgia	799
48	Hawaii	611
42	Idaho	740
19	Illinois	900
21	Indiana	894
8	Iowa	968
20	Kansas	899
11	Kentucky	951
22	Louisiana	890
18	Maine	905
34	Maryland	803
24	Massachusetts	884
31	Michigan	847
36	Minnesota	795
6	Mississippi	976
5	Missouri	984
29	Montana	859
14	Nebraska	936
38	Nevada	775
40	New Hampshire	765
16	New Jersey	910
46	New Mexico	701
13	New York	938
27	North Carolina	864
22	North Dakota	890
15	Ohio	911
9	Oklahoma	966
24	Oregon	884
4	Pennsylvania	1,026
10	Rhode Island	954
30	South Carolina	852
17	South Dakota	909
12	Tennessee	949
43	Texas	738
49	Utah	533
33	Vermont	817
38	Virginia	775
41	Washington	762
1	West Virginia	1,080
26	Wisconsin	874
45	Wyoming	706

RANK ORDER

RANK	STATE	RATE
1	West Virginia	1,080
2	Arkansas	1,048
3	Florida	1,038
4	Pennsylvania	1,026
5	Missouri	984
6	Mississippi	976
7	Alabama	974
8	Iowa	968
9	Oklahoma	966
10	Rhode Island	954
11	Kentucky	951
12	Tennessee	949
13	New York	938
14	Nebraska	936
15	Ohio	911
16	New Jersey	910
17	South Dakota	909
18	Maine	905
19	Illinois	900
20	Kansas	899
21	Indiana	894
22	Louisiana	890
22	North Dakota	890
24	Massachusetts	884
24	Oregon	884
26	Wisconsin	874
27	Delaware	864
27	North Carolina	864
29	Montana	859
30	South Carolina	852
31	Michigan	847
32	Connecticut	840
33	Vermont	817
34	Maryland	803
35	Georgia	799
36	Minnesota	795
37	Arizona	784
38	Nevada	775
38	Virginia	775
40	New Hampshire	765
41	Washington	762
42	Idaho	740
43	Texas	738
44	California	719
45	Wyoming	706
46	New Mexico	701
47	Colorado	655
48	Hawaii	611
49	Utah	533
50	Alaska	398
	District of Columbia	1,200

Source: U.S. Department of Health and Human Services, National Center for Health Statistics
    "Monthly Vital Statistics Report" (Vol. 41, No. 7(S), January 7, 1993)
*Final data by state of residence. Not age adjusted.

Death Rate in 1980

National Rate = 877 Deaths per 100,000 Population*

ALPHA ORDER				RANK ORDER		
RANK	STATE	RATE		RANK	STATE	RATE
18	Alabama	912		1	Florida	1,072
50	Alaska	425		2	Pennsylvania	1,041
40	Arizona	784		3	Missouri	1,008
4	Arkansas	994		4	Arkansas	994
39	California	786		5	West Virginia	987
47	Colorado	654		6	New York	984
23	Connecticut	877		6	Rhode Island	984
27	Delaware	847		8	Maine	960
1	Florida	1,072		9	Massachusetts	959
35	Georgia	809		10	South Dakota	947
49	Hawaii	515		11	Mississippi	937
44	Idaho	715		12	New Jersey	936
20	Illinois	899		13	Oklahoma	932
25	Indiana	862		14	Iowa	930
14	Iowa	930		14	Kansas	930
14	Kansas	930		16	Kentucky	922
16	Kentucky	922		17	Nebraska	920
28	Louisiana	846		18	Alabama	912
8	Maine	960		19	Ohio	911
36	Maryland	806		20	Illinois	899
9	Massachusetts	959		21	Vermont	895
34	Michigan	811		22	Tennessee	887
33	Minnesota	817		23	Connecticut	877
11	Mississippi	937		24	Wisconsin	867
3	Missouri	1,008		25	Indiana	862
28	Montana	846		26	North Dakota	856
17	Nebraska	920		27	Delaware	847
43	Nevada	735		28	Louisiana	846
30	New Hampshire	830		28	Montana	846
12	New Jersey	936		30	New Hampshire	830
45	New Mexico	696		31	Oregon	827
6	New York	984		32	North Carolina	823
32	North Carolina	823		33	Minnesota	817
26	North Dakota	856		34	Michigan	811
19	Ohio	911		35	Georgia	809
13	Oklahoma	932		36	Maryland	806
31	Oregon	827		37	South Carolina	805
2	Pennsylvania	1,041		38	Virginia	794
6	Rhode Island	984		39	California	786
37	South Carolina	805		40	Arizona	784
10	South Dakota	947		41	Washington	773
22	Tennessee	887		42	Texas	758
42	Texas	758		43	Nevada	735
48	Utah	554		44	Idaho	715
21	Vermont	895		45	New Mexico	696
38	Virginia	794		46	Wyoming	684
41	Washington	773		47	Colorado	654
5	West Virginia	987		48	Utah	554
24	Wisconsin	867		49	Hawaii	515
46	Wyoming	684		50	Alaska	425
					District of Columbia	1,109

Source: U.S. Department of Health and Human Services, National Center for Health Statistics
"Vital Statistics of the United States 1980" and "Monthly Vital Statistics Report"
*Final data by state of residence. Not age adjusted.

Infant Deaths in 2000

National Total = 27,200 Infant Deaths*

ALPHA ORDER

RANK	STATE	DEATHS	% of USA
18	Alabama	560	2.1%
47	Alaska	51	0.2%
19	Arizona	556	2.0%
29	Arkansas	279	1.0%
1	California	2,917	10.7%
24	Colorado	413	1.5%
33	Connecticut	242	0.9%
41	Delaware	117	0.4%
5	Florida	1,429	5.3%
10	Georgia	1,013	3.7%
40	Hawaii	121	0.4%
39	Idaho	150	0.6%
4	Illinois	1,578	5.8%
13	Indiana	656	2.4%
34	Iowa	216	0.8%
30	Kansas	278	1.0%
27	Kentucky	385	1.4%
15	Louisiana	624	2.3%
46	Maine	62	0.2%
16	Maryland	604	2.2%
23	Massachusetts	422	1.6%
7	Michigan	1,082	4.0%
25	Minnesota	401	1.5%
22	Mississippi	450	1.7%
17	Missouri	578	2.1%
44	Montana	68	0.3%
38	Nebraska	152	0.6%
35	Nevada	202	0.7%
45	New Hampshire	66	0.2%
11	New Jersey	780	2.9%
36	New Mexico	194	0.7%
3	New York	1,594	5.9%
8	North Carolina	1,056	3.9%
47	North Dakota	51	0.2%
6	Ohio	1,269	4.7%
26	Oklahoma	394	1.4%
31	Oregon	259	1.0%
9	Pennsylvania	1,030	3.8%
43	Rhode Island	85	0.3%
20	South Carolina	524	1.9%
42	South Dakota	96	0.4%
14	Tennessee	641	2.4%
2	Texas	2,195	8.1%
32	Utah	245	0.9%
50	Vermont	30	0.1%
12	Virginia	685	2.5%
28	Washington	380	1.4%
37	West Virginia	161	0.6%
21	Wisconsin	463	1.7%
49	Wyoming	38	0.1%

RANK ORDER

RANK	STATE	DEATHS	% of USA
1	California	2,917	10.7%
2	Texas	2,195	8.1%
3	New York	1,594	5.9%
4	Illinois	1,578	5.8%
5	Florida	1,429	5.3%
6	Ohio	1,269	4.7%
7	Michigan	1,082	4.0%
8	North Carolina	1,056	3.9%
9	Pennsylvania	1,030	3.8%
10	Georgia	1,013	3.7%
11	New Jersey	780	2.9%
12	Virginia	685	2.5%
13	Indiana	656	2.4%
14	Tennessee	641	2.4%
15	Louisiana	624	2.3%
16	Maryland	604	2.2%
17	Missouri	578	2.1%
18	Alabama	560	2.1%
19	Arizona	556	2.0%
20	South Carolina	524	1.9%
21	Wisconsin	463	1.7%
22	Mississippi	450	1.7%
23	Massachusetts	422	1.6%
24	Colorado	413	1.5%
25	Minnesota	401	1.5%
26	Oklahoma	394	1.4%
27	Kentucky	385	1.4%
28	Washington	380	1.4%
29	Arkansas	279	1.0%
30	Kansas	278	1.0%
31	Oregon	259	1.0%
32	Utah	245	0.9%
33	Connecticut	242	0.9%
34	Iowa	216	0.8%
35	Nevada	202	0.7%
36	New Mexico	194	0.7%
37	West Virginia	161	0.6%
38	Nebraska	152	0.6%
39	Idaho	150	0.6%
40	Hawaii	121	0.4%
41	Delaware	117	0.4%
42	South Dakota	96	0.4%
43	Rhode Island	85	0.3%
44	Montana	68	0.3%
45	New Hampshire	66	0.2%
46	Maine	62	0.2%
47	Alaska	51	0.2%
47	North Dakota	51	0.2%
49	Wyoming	38	0.1%
50	Vermont	30	0.1%
	District of Columbia	101	0.4%

Source: U.S. Department of Health and Human Services, National Center for Health Statistics
"National Vital Statistics Reports" (Vol. 49, No. 6, August 22, 2001)
For 12 months ending December 2000. Provisional data. Deaths under 1 year old by state of residence.

Infant Mortality Rate in 2000

National Rate = 6.7 Infant Deaths per 1,000 Live Births*

ALPHA ORDER

RANK	STATE	RATE
7	Alabama	9.0
46	Alaska	5.1
29	Arizona	6.8
19	Arkansas	7.5
42	California	5.6
32	Colorado	6.6
42	Connecticut	5.6
1	Delaware	10.8
20	Florida	7.2
13	Georgia	8.0
22	Hawaii	7.1
17	Idaho	7.6
8	Illinois	8.6
17	Indiana	7.6
41	Iowa	5.7
25	Kansas	7.0
25	Kentucky	7.0
4	Louisiana	9.3
50	Maine	4.5
9	Maryland	8.4
45	Massachusetts	5.2
12	Michigan	8.1
38	Minnesota	6.1
2	Mississippi	10.6
16	Missouri	7.7
35	Montana	6.2
34	Nebraska	6.3
27	Nevada	6.9
47	New Hampshire	4.7
29	New Jersey	6.8
20	New Mexico	7.2
35	New York	6.2
5	North Carolina	9.2
32	North Dakota	6.6
10	Ohio	8.2
13	Oklahoma	8.0
40	Oregon	5.8
22	Pennsylvania	7.1
27	Rhode Island	6.9
3	South Carolina	9.5
6	South Dakota	9.1
10	Tennessee	8.2
35	Texas	6.2
44	Utah	5.3
49	Vermont	4.6
22	Virginia	7.1
47	Washington	4.7
15	West Virginia	7.9
29	Wisconsin	6.8
38	Wyoming	6.1

RANK ORDER

RANK	STATE	RATE
1	Delaware	10.8
2	Mississippi	10.6
3	South Carolina	9.5
4	Louisiana	9.3
5	North Carolina	9.2
6	South Dakota	9.1
7	Alabama	9.0
8	Illinois	8.6
9	Maryland	8.4
10	Ohio	8.2
10	Tennessee	8.2
12	Michigan	8.1
13	Georgia	8.0
13	Oklahoma	8.0
15	West Virginia	7.9
16	Missouri	7.7
17	Idaho	7.6
17	Indiana	7.6
19	Arkansas	7.5
20	Florida	7.2
20	New Mexico	7.2
22	Hawaii	7.1
22	Pennsylvania	7.1
22	Virginia	7.1
25	Kansas	7.0
25	Kentucky	7.0
27	Nevada	6.9
27	Rhode Island	6.9
29	Arizona	6.8
29	New Jersey	6.8
29	Wisconsin	6.8
32	Colorado	6.6
32	North Dakota	6.6
34	Nebraska	6.3
35	Montana	6.2
35	New York	6.2
35	Texas	6.2
38	Minnesota	6.1
38	Wyoming	6.1
40	Oregon	5.8
41	Iowa	5.7
42	California	5.6
42	Connecticut	5.6
44	Utah	5.3
45	Massachusetts	5.2
46	Alaska	5.1
47	New Hampshire	4.7
47	Washington	4.7
49	Vermont	4.6
50	Maine	4.5

| | District of Columbia | 12.6 |

Source: U.S. Department of Health and Human Services, National Center for Health Statistics
"National Vital Statistics Reports" (Vol. 49, No. 6, August 22, 2001)
*For 12 months ending December 2000. Provisional data. Deaths under 1 year old by state of residence.

Infant Deaths in 1999

National Total = 27,937 Infant Deaths*

ALPHA ORDER				RANK ORDER			
RANK	STATE	DEATHS	% of USA	RANK	STATE	DEATHS	% of USA
15	Alabama	606	2.2%	1	California	2,800	10.0%
47	Alaska	57	0.2%	2	Texas	2,164	7.7%
20	Arizona	548	2.0%	3	New York	1,627	5.8%
29	Arkansas	292	1.0%	4	Illinois	1,550	5.5%
1	California	2,800	10.0%	5	Florida	1,452	5.2%
25	Colorado	416	1.5%	6	Ohio	1,244	4.5%
31	Connecticut	265	0.9%	7	Michigan	1,077	3.9%
43	Delaware	79	0.3%	8	Pennsylvania	1,058	3.8%
5	Florida	1,452	5.2%	9	Georgia	1,040	3.7%
9	Georgia	1,040	3.7%	10	North Carolina	1,038	3.7%
40	Hawaii	120	0.4%	11	New Jersey	766	2.7%
39	Idaho	134	0.5%	12	Virginia	693	2.5%
4	Illinois	1,550	5.5%	13	Indiana	686	2.5%
13	Indiana	686	2.5%	14	Louisiana	621	2.2%
34	Iowa	215	0.8%	15	Alabama	606	2.2%
30	Kansas	283	1.0%	16	Maryland	601	2.2%
26	Kentucky	411	1.5%	17	Tennessee	599	2.1%
14	Louisiana	621	2.2%	18	Missouri	585	2.1%
46	Maine	66	0.2%	19	South Carolina	563	2.0%
16	Maryland	601	2.2%	20	Arizona	548	2.0%
23	Massachusetts	417	1.5%	21	Wisconsin	459	1.6%
7	Michigan	1,077	3.9%	22	Mississippi	433	1.5%
27	Minnesota	408	1.5%	23	Massachusetts	417	1.5%
22	Mississippi	433	1.5%	23	Oklahoma	417	1.5%
18	Missouri	585	2.1%	25	Colorado	416	1.5%
44	Montana	72	0.3%	26	Kentucky	411	1.5%
37	Nebraska	163	0.6%	27	Minnesota	408	1.5%
35	Nevada	193	0.7%	28	Washington	400	1.4%
42	New Hampshire	82	0.3%	29	Arkansas	292	1.0%
11	New Jersey	766	2.7%	30	Kansas	283	1.0%
36	New Mexico	188	0.7%	31	Connecticut	265	0.9%
3	New York	1,627	5.8%	32	Oregon	261	0.9%
10	North Carolina	1,038	3.7%	33	Utah	224	0.8%
48	North Dakota	52	0.2%	34	Iowa	215	0.8%
6	Ohio	1,244	4.5%	35	Nevada	193	0.7%
23	Oklahoma	417	1.5%	36	New Mexico	188	0.7%
32	Oregon	261	0.9%	37	Nebraska	163	0.6%
8	Pennsylvania	1,058	3.8%	38	West Virginia	154	0.6%
45	Rhode Island	71	0.3%	39	Idaho	134	0.5%
19	South Carolina	563	2.0%	40	Hawaii	120	0.4%
41	South Dakota	94	0.3%	41	South Dakota	94	0.3%
17	Tennessee	599	2.1%	42	New Hampshire	82	0.3%
2	Texas	2,164	7.7%	43	Delaware	79	0.3%
33	Utah	224	0.8%	44	Montana	72	0.3%
50	Vermont	38	0.1%	45	Rhode Island	71	0.3%
12	Virginia	693	2.5%	46	Maine	66	0.2%
28	Washington	400	1.4%	47	Alaska	57	0.2%
38	West Virginia	154	0.6%	48	North Dakota	52	0.2%
21	Wisconsin	459	1.6%	49	Wyoming	42	0.2%
49	Wyoming	42	0.2%	50	Vermont	38	0.1%
					District of Columbia	113	0.4%

Source: U.S. Department of Health and Human Services, National Center for Health Statistics
"National Vital Statistics Reports" (Vol. 49, No. 8, September 21, 2001)
*Final data. Deaths under 1 year old by state of residence.

Infant Mortality Rate in 1999

National Rate = 7.1 Infant Deaths per 1,000 Live Births*

ALPHA ORDER

RANK ORDER

RANK	STATE	RATE		RANK	STATE	RATE
3	Alabama	9.8		1	South Carolina	10.2
43	Alaska	5.7		2	Mississippi	10.1
27	Arizona	6.8		3	Alabama	9.8
13	Arkansas	8.0		4	Louisiana	9.2
46	California	5.4		5	North Carolina	9.1
30	Colorado	6.7		6	South Dakota	8.9
39	Connecticut	6.1		7	Illinois	8.5
18	Delaware	7.4		7	Oklahoma	8.5
18	Florida	7.4		9	Maryland	8.4
10	Georgia	8.2		10	Georgia	8.2
24	Hawaii	7.0		10	Ohio	8.2
30	Idaho	6.7		12	Michigan	8.1
7	Illinois	8.5		13	Arkansas	8.0
13	Indiana	8.0		13	Indiana	8.0
43	Iowa	5.7		15	Missouri	7.8
21	Kansas	7.3		16	Tennessee	7.7
17	Kentucky	7.6		17	Kentucky	7.6
4	Louisiana	9.2		18	Delaware	7.4
49	Maine	4.8		18	Florida	7.4
9	Maryland	8.4		18	West Virginia	7.4
47	Massachusetts	5.2		21	Kansas	7.3
12	Michigan	8.1		21	Pennsylvania	7.3
37	Minnesota	6.2		21	Virginia	7.3
2	Mississippi	10.1		24	Hawaii	7.0
15	Missouri	7.8		25	New Mexico	6.9
30	Montana	6.7		25	Wyoming	6.9
27	Nebraska	6.8		27	Arizona	6.8
35	Nevada	6.6		27	Nebraska	6.8
40	New Hampshire	5.8		27	North Dakota	6.8
30	New Jersey	6.7		30	Colorado	6.7
25	New Mexico	6.9		30	Idaho	6.7
36	New York	6.4		30	Montana	6.7
5	North Carolina	9.1		30	New Jersey	6.7
27	North Dakota	6.8		30	Wisconsin	6.7
10	Ohio	8.2		35	Nevada	6.6
7	Oklahoma	8.5		36	New York	6.4
40	Oregon	5.8		37	Minnesota	6.2
21	Pennsylvania	7.3		37	Texas	6.2
43	Rhode Island	5.7		39	Connecticut	6.1
1	South Carolina	10.2		40	New Hampshire	5.8
6	South Dakota	8.9		40	Oregon	5.8
16	Tennessee	7.7		40	Vermont	5.8
37	Texas	6.2		43	Alaska	5.7
49	Utah	4.8		43	Iowa	5.7
40	Vermont	5.8		43	Rhode Island	5.7
21	Virginia	7.3		46	California	5.4
48	Washington	5.0		47	Massachusetts	5.2
18	West Virginia	7.4		48	Washington	5.0
30	Wisconsin	6.7		49	Maine	4.8
25	Wyoming	6.9		49	Utah	4.8
					District of Columbia	15.0

Source: U.S. Department of Health and Human Services, National Center for Health Statistics
"National Vital Statistics Reports" (Vol. 49, No. 8, September 21, 2001)
*Final data. Deaths under 1 year old by state of residence.

Infant Mortality Rate in 1990

National Rate = 9.2 Infant Deaths per 1,000 Live Births*

ALPHA ORDER				RANK ORDER		
RANK	**STATE**	**RATE**		**RANK**	**STATE**	**RATE**
5	Alabama	10.8		1	Georgia	12.4
9	Alaska	10.5		2	Mississippi	12.1
27	Arizona	8.8		3	South Carolina	11.7
22	Arkansas	9.2		4	Louisiana	11.1
41	California	7.9		5	Alabama	10.8
27	Colorado	8.8		5	Illinois	10.8
41	Connecticut	7.9		7	Michigan	10.7
12	Delaware	10.1		8	North Carolina	10.6
16	Florida	9.6		9	Alaska	10.5
1	Georgia	12.4		10	Tennessee	10.3
48	Hawaii	6.7		11	Virginia	10.2
29	Idaho	8.7		12	Delaware	10.1
5	Illinois	10.8		12	South Dakota	10.1
16	Indiana	9.6		14	West Virginia	9.9
37	Iowa	8.1		15	Ohio	9.8
32	Kansas	8.4		16	Florida	9.6
31	Kentucky	8.5		16	Indiana	9.6
4	Louisiana	11.1		16	Maryland	9.6
50	Maine	6.2		16	New York	9.6
16	Maryland	9.6		16	Pennsylvania	9.6
47	Massachusetts	7.0		21	Missouri	9.4
7	Michigan	10.7		22	Arkansas	9.2
45	Minnesota	7.3		22	Oklahoma	9.2
2	Mississippi	12.1		24	Montana	9.0
21	Missouri	9.4		24	New Jersey	9.0
24	Montana	9.0		24	New Mexico	9.0
34	Nebraska	8.3		27	Arizona	8.8
32	Nevada	8.4		27	Colorado	8.8
46	New Hampshire	7.1		29	Idaho	8.7
24	New Jersey	9.0		30	Wyoming	8.6
24	New Mexico	9.0		31	Kentucky	8.5
16	New York	9.6		32	Kansas	8.4
8	North Carolina	10.6		32	Nevada	8.4
40	North Dakota	8.0		34	Nebraska	8.3
15	Ohio	9.8		34	Oregon	8.3
22	Oklahoma	9.2		36	Wisconsin	8.2
34	Oregon	8.3		37	Iowa	8.1
16	Pennsylvania	9.6		37	Rhode Island	8.1
37	Rhode Island	8.1		37	Texas	8.1
3	South Carolina	11.7		40	North Dakota	8.0
12	South Dakota	10.1		41	California	7.9
10	Tennessee	10.3		41	Connecticut	7.9
37	Texas	8.1		43	Washington	7.8
44	Utah	7.5		44	Utah	7.5
49	Vermont	6.4		45	Minnesota	7.3
11	Virginia	10.2		46	New Hampshire	7.1
43	Washington	7.8		47	Massachusetts	7.0
14	West Virginia	9.9		48	Hawaii	6.7
36	Wisconsin	8.2		49	Vermont	6.4
30	Wyoming	8.6		50	Maine	6.2
					District of Columbia	20.7

Source: U.S. Department of Health and Human Services, National Center for Health Statistics
   "Monthly Vital Statistics Report" (Vol. 41, No. 7(S), January 7, 1993)
*Final data by state of residence. Infant deaths are those under 1 year old.

Infant Mortality Rate in 1980

National Rate = 12.6 Infant Deaths per 1,000 Live Births*

ALPHA ORDER				RANK ORDER		
RANK	STATE	RATE		RANK	STATE	RATE
3	Alabama	15.2		1	Mississippi	17.0
24	Alaska	12.3		2	South Carolina	15.6
21	Arizona	12.4		3	Alabama	15.2
17	Arkansas	12.7		4	Illinois	14.8
35	California	11.1		5	Florida	14.6
46	Colorado	10.1		6	Georgia	14.5
34	Connecticut	11.2		6	North Carolina	14.5
10	Delaware	13.9		8	Louisiana	14.3
5	Florida	14.6		9	Maryland	14.1
6	Georgia	14.5		10	Delaware	13.9
44	Hawaii	10.3		11	Virginia	13.6
38	Idaho	10.7		12	Tennessee	13.5
4	Illinois	14.8		13	Pennsylvania	13.2
28	Indiana	11.9		14	Kentucky	12.9
29	Iowa	11.8		15	Michigan	12.8
42	Kansas	10.4		15	Ohio	12.8
14	Kentucky	12.9		17	Arkansas	12.7
8	Louisiana	14.3		17	Oklahoma	12.7
50	Maine	9.2		19	New Jersey	12.5
9	Maryland	14.1		19	New York	12.5
41	Massachusetts	10.5		21	Arizona	12.4
15	Michigan	12.8		21	Missouri	12.4
47	Minnesota	10.0		21	Montana	12.4
1	Mississippi	17.0		24	Alaska	12.3
21	Missouri	12.4		25	Oregon	12.2
21	Montana	12.4		25	Texas	12.2
32	Nebraska	11.5		27	North Dakota	12.1
38	Nevada	10.7		28	Indiana	11.9
48	New Hampshire	9.9		29	Iowa	11.8
19	New Jersey	12.5		29	Washington	11.8
32	New Mexico	11.5		29	West Virginia	11.8
19	New York	12.5		32	Nebraska	11.5
6	North Carolina	14.5		32	New Mexico	11.5
27	North Dakota	12.1		34	Connecticut	11.2
15	Ohio	12.8		35	California	11.1
17	Oklahoma	12.7		36	Rhode Island	11.0
25	Oregon	12.2		37	South Dakota	10.9
13	Pennsylvania	13.2		38	Idaho	10.7
36	Rhode Island	11.0		38	Nevada	10.7
2	South Carolina	15.6		38	Vermont	10.7
37	South Dakota	10.9		41	Massachusetts	10.5
12	Tennessee	13.5		42	Kansas	10.4
25	Texas	12.2		42	Utah	10.4
42	Utah	10.4		44	Hawaii	10.3
38	Vermont	10.7		44	Wisconsin	10.3
11	Virginia	13.6		46	Colorado	10.1
29	Washington	11.8		47	Minnesota	10.0
29	West Virginia	11.8		48	New Hampshire	9.9
44	Wisconsin	10.3		49	Wyoming	9.8
49	Wyoming	9.8		50	Maine	9.2
					District of Columbia	25.0

Source: U.S. Department of Health and Human Services, National Center for Health Statistics
"Monthly Vital Statistics Report"
*Final data by state of residence. Deaths under 1 year old, exclusive of fetal deaths.

Percent Change in Infant Mortality Rate: 1990 to 1999

National Percent Change = 22.8% Decrease*

ALPHA ORDER

RANK	STATE	PERCENT CHANGE		RANK	STATE	PERCENT CHANGE
3	Alabama	(9.3)		1	Hawaii	4.5
50	Alaska	(45.7)		2	Oklahoma	(7.6)
26	Arizona	(22.7)		3	Alabama	(9.3)
9	Arkansas	(13.0)		4	Vermont	(9.4)
45	California	(31.6)		5	Kentucky	(10.6)
32	Colorado	(23.9)		6	South Dakota	(11.9)
27	Connecticut	(22.8)		7	Maryland	(12.5)
40	Delaware	(26.7)		8	South Carolina	(12.8)
28	Florida	(22.9)		9	Arkansas	(13.0)
47	Georgia	(33.9)		10	Kansas	(13.1)
1	Hawaii	4.5		11	North Carolina	(14.2)
29	Idaho	(23.0)		12	North Dakota	(15.0)
23	Illinois	(21.3)		13	Minnesota	(15.1)
16	Indiana	(16.7)		14	Ohio	(16.3)
42	Iowa	(29.6)		15	Mississippi	(16.5)
10	Kansas	(13.1)		16	Indiana	(16.7)
5	Kentucky	(10.6)		17	Missouri	(17.0)
18	Louisiana	(17.1)		18	Louisiana	(17.1)
25	Maine	(22.6)		19	Nebraska	(18.1)
7	Maryland	(12.5)		20	New Hampshire	(18.3)
39	Massachusetts	(25.7)		20	Wisconsin	(18.3)
34	Michigan	(24.3)		22	Wyoming	(19.8)
13	Minnesota	(15.1)		23	Illinois	(21.3)
15	Mississippi	(16.5)		24	Nevada	(21.4)
17	Missouri	(17.0)		25	Maine	(22.6)
37	Montana	(25.6)		26	Arizona	(22.7)
19	Nebraska	(18.1)		27	Connecticut	(22.8)
24	Nevada	(21.4)		28	Florida	(22.9)
20	New Hampshire	(18.3)		29	Idaho	(23.0)
37	New Jersey	(25.6)		30	New Mexico	(23.3)
30	New Mexico	(23.3)		31	Texas	(23.5)
46	New York	(33.3)		32	Colorado	(23.9)
11	North Carolina	(14.2)		33	Pennsylvania	(24.0)
12	North Dakota	(15.0)		34	Michigan	(24.3)
14	Ohio	(16.3)		35	Tennessee	(25.2)
2	Oklahoma	(7.6)		36	West Virginia	(25.3)
44	Oregon	(30.1)		37	Montana	(25.6)
33	Pennsylvania	(24.0)		37	New Jersey	(25.6)
42	Rhode Island	(29.6)		39	Massachusetts	(25.7)
8	South Carolina	(12.8)		40	Delaware	(26.7)
6	South Dakota	(11.9)		41	Virginia	(28.4)
35	Tennessee	(25.2)		42	Iowa	(29.6)
31	Texas	(23.5)		42	Rhode Island	(29.6)
49	Utah	(36.0)		44	Oregon	(30.1)
4	Vermont	(9.4)		45	California	(31.6)
41	Virginia	(28.4)		46	New York	(33.3)
48	Washington	(35.9)		47	Georgia	(33.9)
36	West Virginia	(25.3)		48	Washington	(35.9)
20	Wisconsin	(18.3)		49	Utah	(36.0)
22	Wyoming	(19.8)		50	Alaska	(45.7)

RANK ORDER

District of Columbia   (27.5)

Source: Morgan Quitno Press using data from US Dept of Health & Human Services, National Center for Health Statistics "Monthly Vital Statistics Report" (Vol. 41, No. 7(S), January 7, 1993) and "National Vital Statistics Reports" (Vol. 49, No. 8, September 21, 2001)

*By state of residence. Infant deaths are those under 1 year old.

Percent Change in Infant Mortality Rate: 1980 to 1999

National Percent Change = 43.7% Decrease*

ALPHA ORDER

RANK	STATE	PERCENT CHANGE
10	Alabama	(35.5)
48	Alaska	(53.7)
32	Arizona	(45.2)
14	Arkansas	(37.0)
45	California	(51.4)
7	Colorado	(33.7)
33	Connecticut	(45.5)
38	Delaware	(46.8)
43	Florida	(49.3)
29	Georgia	(43.4)
4	Hawaii	(32.0)
18	Idaho	(37.4)
27	Illinois	(42.6)
5	Indiana	(32.8)
46	Iowa	(51.7)
3	Kansas	(29.8)
25	Kentucky	(41.1)
11	Louisiana	(35.7)
39	Maine	(47.8)
22	Maryland	(40.4)
44	Massachusetts	(50.5)
13	Michigan	(36.7)
19	Minnesota	(38.0)
23	Mississippi	(40.6)
15	Missouri	(37.1)
35	Montana	(46.0)
24	Nebraska	(40.9)
20	Nevada	(38.3)
26	New Hampshire	(41.4)
37	New Jersey	(46.4)
21	New Mexico	(40.0)
41	New York	(48.8)
16	North Carolina	(37.2)
30	North Dakota	(43.8)
12	Ohio	(35.9)
6	Oklahoma	(33.1)
47	Oregon	(52.5)
31	Pennsylvania	(44.7)
40	Rhode Island	(48.2)
8	South Carolina	(34.6)
1	South Dakota	(18.3)
28	Tennessee	(43.0)
42	Texas	(49.2)
49	Utah	(53.8)
34	Vermont	(45.8)
36	Virginia	(46.3)
50	Washington	(57.6)
17	West Virginia	(37.3)
9	Wisconsin	(35.0)
2	Wyoming	(29.6)

RANK ORDER

RANK	STATE	PERCENT CHANGE
1	South Dakota	(18.3)
2	Wyoming	(29.6)
3	Kansas	(29.8)
4	Hawaii	(32.0)
5	Indiana	(32.8)
6	Oklahoma	(33.1)
7	Colorado	(33.7)
8	South Carolina	(34.6)
9	Wisconsin	(35.0)
10	Alabama	(35.5)
11	Louisiana	(35.7)
12	Ohio	(35.9)
13	Michigan	(36.7)
14	Arkansas	(37.0)
15	Missouri	(37.1)
16	North Carolina	(37.2)
17	West Virginia	(37.3)
18	Idaho	(37.4)
19	Minnesota	(38.0)
20	Nevada	(38.3)
21	New Mexico	(40.0)
22	Maryland	(40.4)
23	Mississippi	(40.6)
24	Nebraska	(40.9)
25	Kentucky	(41.1)
26	New Hampshire	(41.4)
27	Illinois	(42.6)
28	Tennessee	(43.0)
29	Georgia	(43.4)
30	North Dakota	(43.8)
31	Pennsylvania	(44.7)
32	Arizona	(45.2)
33	Connecticut	(45.5)
34	Vermont	(45.8)
35	Montana	(46.0)
36	Virginia	(46.3)
37	New Jersey	(46.4)
38	Delaware	(46.8)
39	Maine	(47.8)
40	Rhode Island	(48.2)
41	New York	(48.8)
42	Texas	(49.2)
43	Florida	(49.3)
44	Massachusetts	(50.5)
45	California	(51.4)
46	Iowa	(51.7)
47	Oregon	(52.5)
48	Alaska	(53.7)
49	Utah	(53.8)
50	Washington	(57.6)

District of Columbia (40.0)

Source: Morgan Quitno Press using data from US Dept of Health & Human Services, National Center for Health Statistics
"National Vital Statistics Reports" (Vol. 49, No. 8, September 21, 2001)
"Vital Statistics of the United States, 1980" (Vol. I-Natality, issued 1984) and unpublished data
*Final data by state of residence. Infant deaths are those occurring under 1 year, exclusive of fetal deaths.

White Infant Deaths in 1999

National Total = 18,067 Deaths*

ALPHA ORDER

RANK	STATE	DEATHS	% of USA
24	Alabama	288	1.6%
48	Alaska	31	0.2%
11	Arizona	442	2.4%
32	Arkansas	198	1.1%
1	California	2,106	11.7%
16	Colorado	359	2.0%
31	Connecticut	205	1.1%
49	Delaware	30	0.2%
6	Florida	825	4.6%
13	Georgia	435	2.4%
50	Hawaii	19	0.1%
39	Idaho	127	0.7%
4	Illinois	877	4.9%
10	Indiana	525	2.9%
33	Iowa	189	1.0%
27	Kansas	234	1.3%
17	Kentucky	347	1.9%
28	Louisiana	228	1.3%
42	Maine	62	0.3%
29	Maryland	226	1.3%
20	Massachusetts	329	1.8%
8	Michigan	630	3.5%
22	Minnesota	310	1.7%
34	Mississippi	153	0.8%
15	Missouri	366	2.0%
43	Montana	55	0.3%
38	Nebraska	128	0.7%
34	Nevada	153	0.8%
40	New Hampshire	78	0.4%
12	New Jersey	441	2.4%
36	New Mexico	148	0.8%
3	New York	1,009	5.6%
9	North Carolina	560	3.1%
45	North Dakota	39	0.2%
5	Ohio	846	4.7%
23	Oklahoma	308	1.7%
25	Oregon	237	1.3%
7	Pennsylvania	702	3.9%
44	Rhode Island	54	0.3%
26	South Carolina	235	1.3%
41	South Dakota	67	0.4%
18	Tennessee	342	1.9%
2	Texas	1,630	9.0%
30	Utah	212	1.2%
47	Vermont	38	0.2%
14	Virginia	387	2.1%
21	Washington	319	1.8%
37	West Virginia	145	0.8%
18	Wisconsin	342	1.9%
45	Wyoming	39	0.2%

RANK ORDER

RANK	STATE	DEATHS	% of USA
1	California	2,106	11.7%
2	Texas	1,630	9.0%
3	New York	1,009	5.6%
4	Illinois	877	4.9%
5	Ohio	846	4.7%
6	Florida	825	4.6%
7	Pennsylvania	702	3.9%
8	Michigan	630	3.5%
9	North Carolina	560	3.1%
10	Indiana	525	2.9%
11	Arizona	442	2.4%
12	New Jersey	441	2.4%
13	Georgia	435	2.4%
14	Virginia	387	2.1%
15	Missouri	366	2.0%
16	Colorado	359	2.0%
17	Kentucky	347	1.9%
18	Tennessee	342	1.9%
18	Wisconsin	342	1.9%
20	Massachusetts	329	1.8%
21	Washington	319	1.8%
22	Minnesota	310	1.7%
23	Oklahoma	308	1.7%
24	Alabama	288	1.6%
25	Oregon	237	1.3%
26	South Carolina	235	1.3%
27	Kansas	234	1.3%
28	Louisiana	228	1.3%
29	Maryland	226	1.3%
30	Utah	212	1.2%
31	Connecticut	205	1.1%
32	Arkansas	198	1.1%
33	Iowa	189	1.0%
34	Mississippi	153	0.8%
34	Nevada	153	0.8%
36	New Mexico	148	0.8%
37	West Virginia	145	0.8%
38	Nebraska	128	0.7%
39	Idaho	127	0.7%
40	New Hampshire	78	0.4%
41	South Dakota	67	0.4%
42	Maine	62	0.3%
43	Montana	55	0.3%
44	Rhode Island	54	0.3%
45	North Dakota	39	0.2%
45	Wyoming	39	0.2%
47	Vermont	38	0.2%
48	Alaska	31	0.2%
49	Delaware	30	0.2%
50	Hawaii	19	0.1%
	District of Columbia	12	0.1%

Source: U.S. Department of Health and Human Services, National Center for Health Statistics
"National Vital Statistics Reports" (Vol. 49, No. 8, September 21, 2001)
*Final data. Deaths of infants under 1 year old, exclusive of fetal deaths. Based on race of the mother.

White Infant Mortality Rate in 1999

National Rate = 5.8 White Infant Deaths per 1,000 White Live Births*

ALPHA ORDER			RANK ORDER		
RANK	STATE	RATE	RANK	STATE	RATE
7	Alabama	6.9	1	Oklahoma	8.0
46	Alaska	4.7	2	South Dakota	7.7
18	Arizona	6.2	3	West Virginia	7.3
5	Arkansas	7.0	4	Kentucky	7.1
42	California	5.0	5	Arkansas	7.0
16	Colorado	6.3	5	Indiana	7.0
29	Connecticut	5.7	7	Alabama	6.9
49	Delaware	3.9	7	North Carolina	6.9
33	Florida	5.6	9	Kansas	6.8
37	Georgia	5.4	9	Mississippi	6.8
NA	Hawaii**	NA	9	Wyoming	6.8
13	Idaho	6.6	12	South Carolina	6.7
16	Illinois	6.3	13	Idaho	6.6
5	Indiana	7.0	13	Ohio	6.6
39	Iowa	5.3	15	New Mexico	6.5
9	Kansas	6.8	16	Colorado	6.3
4	Kentucky	7.1	16	Illinois	6.3
21	Louisiana	5.9	18	Arizona	6.2
46	Maine	4.7	19	Nevada	6.1
41	Maryland	5.1	20	Michigan	6.0
44	Massachusetts	4.8	21	Louisiana	5.9
20	Michigan	6.0	21	Montana	5.9
37	Minnesota	5.4	21	Nebraska	5.9
9	Mississippi	6.8	21	Vermont	5.9
25	Missouri	5.8	25	Missouri	5.8
21	Montana	5.9	25	North Dakota	5.8
21	Nebraska	5.9	25	Pennsylvania	5.8
19	Nevada	6.1	25	Wisconsin	5.8
29	New Hampshire	5.7	29	Connecticut	5.7
40	New Jersey	5.2	29	New Hampshire	5.7
15	New Mexico	6.5	29	Oregon	5.7
35	New York	5.5	29	Tennessee	5.7
7	North Carolina	6.9	33	Florida	5.6
25	North Dakota	5.8	33	Virginia	5.6
13	Ohio	6.6	35	New York	5.5
1	Oklahoma	8.0	35	Texas	5.5
29	Oregon	5.7	37	Georgia	5.4
25	Pennsylvania	5.8	37	Minnesota	5.4
42	Rhode Island	5.0	39	Iowa	5.3
12	South Carolina	6.7	40	New Jersey	5.2
2	South Dakota	7.7	41	Maryland	5.1
29	Tennessee	5.7	42	California	5.0
35	Texas	5.5	42	Rhode Island	5.0
44	Utah	4.8	44	Massachusetts	4.8
21	Vermont	5.9	44	Utah	4.8
33	Virginia	5.6	46	Alaska	4.7
46	Washington	4.7	46	Maine	4.7
3	West Virginia	7.3	46	Washington	4.7
25	Wisconsin	5.8	49	Delaware	3.9
9	Wyoming	6.8	NA	Hawaii**	NA
				District of Columbia**	NA

Source: U.S. Department of Health and Human Services, National Center for Health Statistics
"National Vital Statistics Reports" (Vol. 49, No. 8, September 21, 2001)
*Final data. Deaths of infants under 1 year old, exclusive of fetal deaths. Based on race of the mother.
**Not available, fewer than 20 white infant deaths.

Black Infant Deaths in 1999

National Total = 8,822 Deaths*

ALPHA ORDER

RANK ORDER

RANK	STATE	DEATHS	% of USA
14	Alabama	316	3.6%
41	Alaska	4	0.0%
28	Arizona	52	0.6%
22	Arkansas	92	1.0%
6	California	457	5.2%
31	Colorado	47	0.5%
27	Connecticut	57	0.6%
30	Delaware	48	0.5%
2	Florida	611	6.9%
3	Georgia	583	6.6%
39	Hawaii	8	0.1%
42	Idaho	3	0.0%
1	Illinois	630	7.1%
20	Indiana	158	1.8%
34	Iowa	24	0.3%
32	Kansas	41	0.5%
25	Kentucky	63	0.7%
10	Louisiana	386	4.4%
42	Maine	3	0.0%
11	Maryland	355	4.0%
23	Massachusetts	80	0.9%
8	Michigan	430	4.9%
26	Minnesota	62	0.7%
17	Mississippi	275	3.1%
19	Missouri	213	2.4%
48	Montana	0	0.0%
34	Nebraska	24	0.3%
33	Nevada	29	0.3%
46	New Hampshire	1	0.0%
15	New Jersey	299	3.4%
37	New Mexico	11	0.1%
4	New York	568	6.4%
7	North Carolina	441	5.0%
48	North Dakota	0	0.0%
9	Ohio	388	4.4%
24	Oklahoma	72	0.8%
40	Oregon	6	0.1%
12	Pennsylvania	343	3.9%
36	Rhode Island	12	0.1%
13	South Carolina	322	3.6%
42	South Dakota	3	0.0%
18	Tennessee	251	2.8%
5	Texas	502	5.7%
45	Utah	2	0.0%
48	Vermont	0	0.0%
16	Virginia	288	3.3%
29	Washington	50	0.6%
38	West Virginia	9	0.1%
21	Wisconsin	104	1.2%
46	Wyoming	1	0.0%

RANK	STATE	DEATHS	% of USA
1	Illinois	630	7.1%
2	Florida	611	6.9%
3	Georgia	583	6.6%
4	New York	568	6.4%
5	Texas	502	5.7%
6	California	457	5.2%
7	North Carolina	441	5.0%
8	Michigan	430	4.9%
9	Ohio	388	4.4%
10	Louisiana	386	4.4%
11	Maryland	355	4.0%
12	Pennsylvania	343	3.9%
13	South Carolina	322	3.6%
14	Alabama	316	3.6%
15	New Jersey	299	3.4%
16	Virginia	288	3.3%
17	Mississippi	275	3.1%
18	Tennessee	251	2.8%
19	Missouri	213	2.4%
20	Indiana	158	1.8%
21	Wisconsin	104	1.2%
22	Arkansas	92	1.0%
23	Massachusetts	80	0.9%
24	Oklahoma	72	0.8%
25	Kentucky	63	0.7%
26	Minnesota	62	0.7%
27	Connecticut	57	0.6%
28	Arizona	52	0.6%
29	Washington	50	0.6%
30	Delaware	48	0.5%
31	Colorado	47	0.5%
32	Kansas	41	0.5%
33	Nevada	29	0.3%
34	Iowa	24	0.3%
34	Nebraska	24	0.3%
36	Rhode Island	12	0.1%
37	New Mexico	11	0.1%
38	West Virginia	9	0.1%
39	Hawaii	8	0.1%
40	Oregon	6	0.1%
41	Alaska	4	0.0%
42	Idaho	3	0.0%
42	Maine	3	0.0%
42	South Dakota	3	0.0%
45	Utah	2	0.0%
46	New Hampshire	1	0.0%
46	Wyoming	1	0.0%
48	Montana	0	0.0%
48	North Dakota	0	0.0%
48	Vermont	0	0.0%
	District of Columbia	98	1.1%

Source: U.S. Department of Health and Human Services, National Center for Health Statistics
    "National Vital Statistics Reports" (Vol. 49, No. 8, September 21, 2001)
*Final data. Deaths of infants under 1 year old, exclusive of fetal deaths. Based on race of the mother.

Black Infant Mortality Rate in 1999

National Rate = 14.6 Black Infant Deaths per 1,000 Black Live Births*

ALPHA ORDER

RANK	STATE	RATE
13	Alabama	16.0
NA	Alaska**	NA
2	Arizona	19.1
32	Arkansas	12.0
29	California	12.9
12	Colorado	16.2
33	Connecticut	10.6
6	Delaware	18.0
26	Florida	13.6
25	Georgia	13.8
NA	Hawaii**	NA
NA	Idaho**	NA
5	Illinois	18.4
9	Indiana	17.0
1	Iowa	20.6
21	Kansas	14.4
30	Kentucky	12.7
22	Louisiana	14.2
NA	Maine**	NA
20	Maryland	14.6
35	Massachusetts	9.8
7	Michigan	17.9
17	Minnesota	15.4
22	Mississippi	14.2
3	Missouri	18.9
NA	Montana**	NA
3	Nebraska	18.9
27	Nevada	13.2
NA	New Hampshire**	NA
24	New Jersey	14.1
NA	New Mexico**	NA
33	New York	10.6
16	North Carolina	15.5
NA	North Dakota**	NA
8	Ohio	17.6
15	Oklahoma	15.6
NA	Oregon**	NA
11	Pennsylvania	16.8
NA	Rhode Island**	NA
10	South Carolina	16.9
NA	South Dakota**	NA
18	Tennessee	15.2
31	Texas	12.5
NA	Utah**	NA
NA	Vermont**	NA
28	Virginia	13.0
19	Washington	15.0
NA	West Virginia**	NA
13	Wisconsin	16.0
NA	Wyoming**	NA

RANK ORDER

RANK	STATE	RATE
1	Iowa	20.6
2	Arizona	19.1
3	Missouri	18.9
3	Nebraska	18.9
5	Illinois	18.4
6	Delaware	18.0
7	Michigan	17.9
8	Ohio	17.6
9	Indiana	17.0
10	South Carolina	16.9
11	Pennsylvania	16.8
12	Colorado	16.2
13	Alabama	16.0
13	Wisconsin	16.0
15	Oklahoma	15.6
16	North Carolina	15.5
17	Minnesota	15.4
18	Tennessee	15.2
19	Washington	15.0
20	Maryland	14.6
21	Kansas	14.4
22	Louisiana	14.2
22	Mississippi	14.2
24	New Jersey	14.1
25	Georgia	13.8
26	Florida	13.6
27	Nevada	13.2
28	Virginia	13.0
29	California	12.9
30	Kentucky	12.7
31	Texas	12.5
32	Arkansas	12.0
33	Connecticut	10.6
33	New York	10.6
35	Massachusetts	9.8
NA	Alaska**	NA
NA	Hawaii**	NA
NA	Idaho**	NA
NA	Maine**	NA
NA	Montana**	NA
NA	New Hampshire**	NA
NA	New Mexico**	NA
NA	North Dakota**	NA
NA	Oregon**	NA
NA	Rhode Island**	NA
NA	South Dakota**	NA
NA	Utah**	NA
NA	Vermont**	NA
NA	West Virginia**	NA
NA	Wyoming**	NA

District of Columbia   19.0

Source: U.S. Department of Health and Human Services, National Center for Health Statistics
 "National Vital Statistics Reports" (Vol. 49, No. 8, September 21, 2001)
*Final data. Deaths of infants under 1 year old, exclusive of fetal deaths. Based on race of the mother.
**Not available, fewer than 20 black infant deaths.

Percent Change in White Infant Mortality Rate: 1990 to 1999

National Percent Change = 24.7% Decrease*

ALPHA ORDER

RANK	STATE	PERCENT CHANGE
8	Alabama	(16.9)
48	Alaska	(44.7)
28	Arizona	(24.4)
5	Arkansas	(12.5)
43	California	(34.2)
30	Colorado	(25.0)
6	Connecticut	(13.6)
49	Delaware	(46.6)
34	Florida	(26.3)
47	Georgia	(40.7)
NA	Hawaii**	NA
25	Idaho	(24.1)
11	Illinois	(18.2)
19	Indiana	(21.3)
42	Iowa	(32.1)
4	Kansas	(11.7)
3	Kentucky	(11.3)
12	Louisiana	(19.2)
27	Maine	(24.2)
20	Maryland	(21.5)
36	Massachusetts	(28.4)
25	Michigan	(24.1)
14	Minnesota	(19.4)
17	Mississippi	(20.0)
32	Missouri	(25.6)
41	Montana	(31.4)
10	Nebraska	(18.1)
29	Nevada	(24.7)
18	New Hampshire	(20.8)
23	New Jersey	(23.5)
40	New Mexico	(30.1)
37	New York	(28.6)
8	North Carolina	(16.9)
35	North Dakota	(26.6)
16	Ohio	(19.5)
7	Oklahoma	(14.9)
39	Oregon	(29.6)
32	Pennsylvania	(25.6)
46	Rhode Island	(39.8)
13	South Carolina	(19.3)
2	South Dakota	(10.5)
38	Tennessee	(28.8)
21	Texas	(22.5)
44	Utah	(35.1)
1	Vermont	(9.2)
31	Virginia	(25.3)
45	Washington	(38.2)
24	West Virginia	(24.0)
14	Wisconsin	(19.4)
22	Wyoming	(22.7)

RANK ORDER

RANK	STATE	PERCENT CHANGE
1	Vermont	(9.2)
2	South Dakota	(10.5)
3	Kentucky	(11.3)
4	Kansas	(11.7)
5	Arkansas	(12.5)
6	Connecticut	(13.6)
7	Oklahoma	(14.9)
8	Alabama	(16.9)
8	North Carolina	(16.9)
10	Nebraska	(18.1)
11	Illinois	(18.2)
12	Louisiana	(19.2)
13	South Carolina	(19.3)
14	Minnesota	(19.4)
14	Wisconsin	(19.4)
16	Ohio	(19.5)
17	Mississippi	(20.0)
18	New Hampshire	(20.8)
19	Indiana	(21.3)
20	Maryland	(21.5)
21	Texas	(22.5)
22	Wyoming	(22.7)
23	New Jersey	(23.5)
24	West Virginia	(24.0)
25	Idaho	(24.1)
25	Michigan	(24.1)
27	Maine	(24.2)
28	Arizona	(24.4)
29	Nevada	(24.7)
30	Colorado	(25.0)
31	Virginia	(25.3)
32	Missouri	(25.6)
32	Pennsylvania	(25.6)
34	Florida	(26.3)
35	North Dakota	(26.6)
36	Massachusetts	(28.4)
37	New York	(28.6)
38	Tennessee	(28.8)
39	Oregon	(29.6)
40	New Mexico	(30.1)
41	Montana	(31.4)
42	Iowa	(32.1)
43	California	(34.2)
44	Utah	(35.1)
45	Washington	(38.2)
46	Rhode Island	(39.8)
47	Georgia	(40.7)
48	Alaska	(44.7)
49	Delaware	(46.6)
NA	Hawaii**	NA
	District of Columbia**	NA

Source: Morgan Quitno Press using data from US Dept of Health & Human Services, National Center for Health Statistics
"National Vital Statistics Reports" (Vol. 49, No. 8, September 21, 2001) and "Vital Statistics of the United States"
*Final data. Deaths of infants under 1 year old, exclusive of fetal deaths. Based on race of the mother.
**Not available, fewer than 20 white infant deaths.

Percent Change in Black Infant Mortality Rate: 1990 to 1999

National Percent Change = 14.1% Decrease*

ALPHA ORDER

RANK	STATE	PERCENT CHANGE
9	Alabama	0.6
NA	Alaska**	NA
2	Arizona	14.4
23	Arkansas	(11.8)
18	California	(9.2)
11	Colorado	(1.8)
34	Connecticut	(33.8)
17	Delaware	(7.2)
29	Florida	(16.0)
32	Georgia	(23.3)
NA	Hawaii**	NA
NA	Idaho**	NA
27	Illinois	(14.4)
6	Indiana	6.3
2	Iowa	14.4
15	Kansas	(6.5)
16	Kentucky	(6.6)
26	Louisiana	(13.9)
NA	Maine**	NA
20	Maryland	(10.4)
14	Massachusetts	(5.8)
28	Michigan	(14.8)
31	Minnesota	(21.8)
23	Mississippi	(11.8)
5	Missouri	8.0
NA	Montana**	NA
4	Nebraska	12.5
7	Nevada	5.6
NA	New Hampshire**	NA
30	New Jersey	(18.5)
NA	New Mexico**	NA
35	New York	(38.7)
12	North Carolina	(3.1)
NA	North Dakota**	NA
13	Ohio	(3.8)
1	Oklahoma	18.2
NA	Oregon**	NA
21	Pennsylvania	(10.6)
NA	Rhode Island**	NA
10	South Carolina	(1.2)
NA	South Dakota**	NA
25	Tennessee	(13.1)
19	Texas	(10.1)
NA	Utah**	NA
NA	Vermont**	NA
33	Virginia	(30.9)
8	Washington	3.4
NA	West Virginia**	NA
22	Wisconsin	(11.6)
NA	Wyoming**	NA

RANK ORDER

RANK	STATE	PERCENT CHANGE
1	Oklahoma	18.2
2	Arizona	14.4
2	Iowa	14.4
4	Nebraska	12.5
5	Missouri	8.0
6	Indiana	6.3
7	Nevada	5.6
8	Washington	3.4
9	Alabama	0.6
10	South Carolina	(1.2)
11	Colorado	(1.8)
12	North Carolina	(3.1)
13	Ohio	(3.8)
14	Massachusetts	(5.8)
15	Kansas	(6.5)
16	Kentucky	(6.6)
17	Delaware	(7.2)
18	California	(9.2)
19	Texas	(10.1)
20	Maryland	(10.4)
21	Pennsylvania	(10.6)
22	Wisconsin	(11.6)
23	Arkansas	(11.8)
23	Mississippi	(11.8)
25	Tennessee	(13.1)
26	Louisiana	(13.9)
27	Illinois	(14.4)
28	Michigan	(14.8)
29	Florida	(16.0)
30	New Jersey	(18.5)
31	Minnesota	(21.8)
32	Georgia	(23.3)
33	Virginia	(30.9)
34	Connecticut	(33.8)
35	New York	(38.7)
NA	Alaska**	NA
NA	Hawaii**	NA
NA	Idaho**	NA
NA	Maine**	NA
NA	Montana**	NA
NA	New Hampshire**	NA
NA	New Mexico**	NA
NA	North Dakota**	NA
NA	Oregon**	NA
NA	Rhode Island**	NA
NA	South Dakota**	NA
NA	Utah**	NA
NA	Vermont**	NA
NA	West Virginia**	NA
NA	Wyoming**	NA

District of Columbia (22.1)

Source: Morgan Quitno Press using data from US Dept of Health & Human Services, National Center for Health Statistics
"National Vital Statistics Reports" (Vol. 49, No. 8, September 21, 2001) and "Vital Statistics of the United States"
*Final data. Deaths of infants under 1 year old, exclusive of fetal deaths. Based on race of the mother.
**Not available, fewer than 20 black infant deaths.

Neonatal Deaths in 1999

National Total = 18,728 Deaths*

ALPHA ORDER

RANK ORDER

RANK	STATE	DEATHS	% of USA		RANK	STATE	DEATHS	% of USA
19	Alabama	383	2.0%		1	California	1,852	9.9%
48	Alaska	26	0.1%		2	Texas	1,365	7.3%
20	Arizona	363	1.9%		3	New York	1,142	6.1%
32	Arkansas	168	0.9%		4	Illinois	1,083	5.8%
1	California	1,852	9.9%		5	Florida	967	5.2%
23	Colorado	268	1.4%		6	Ohio	845	4.5%
29	Connecticut	205	1.1%		7	North Carolina	767	4.1%
43	Delaware	55	0.3%		8	Pennsylvania	743	4.0%
5	Florida	967	5.2%		9	Michigan	734	3.9%
10	Georgia	699	3.7%		10	Georgia	699	3.7%
40	Hawaii	84	0.4%		11	New Jersey	555	3.0%
39	Idaho	92	0.5%		12	Virginia	483	2.6%
4	Illinois	1,083	5.8%		13	Indiana	452	2.4%
13	Indiana	452	2.4%		14	Maryland	420	2.2%
34	Iowa	128	0.7%		15	Louisiana	394	2.1%
30	Kansas	191	1.0%		16	South Carolina	392	2.1%
25	Kentucky	261	1.4%		17	Tennessee	389	2.1%
15	Louisiana	394	2.1%		18	Missouri	385	2.1%
45	Maine	51	0.3%		19	Alabama	383	2.0%
14	Maryland	420	2.2%		20	Arizona	363	1.9%
21	Massachusetts	332	1.8%		21	Massachusetts	332	1.8%
9	Michigan	734	3.9%		22	Wisconsin	294	1.6%
25	Minnesota	261	1.4%		23	Colorado	268	1.4%
24	Mississippi	265	1.4%		24	Mississippi	265	1.4%
18	Missouri	385	2.1%		25	Kentucky	261	1.4%
47	Montana	32	0.2%		25	Minnesota	261	1.4%
36	Nebraska	108	0.6%		27	Washington	256	1.4%
35	Nevada	114	0.6%		28	Oklahoma	243	1.3%
41	New Hampshire	60	0.3%		29	Connecticut	205	1.1%
11	New Jersey	555	3.0%		30	Kansas	191	1.0%
37	New Mexico	107	0.6%		30	Oregon	191	1.0%
3	New York	1,142	6.1%		32	Arkansas	168	0.9%
7	North Carolina	767	4.1%		33	Utah	148	0.8%
46	North Dakota	33	0.2%		34	Iowa	128	0.7%
6	Ohio	845	4.5%		35	Nevada	114	0.6%
28	Oklahoma	243	1.3%		36	Nebraska	108	0.6%
30	Oregon	191	1.0%		37	New Mexico	107	0.6%
8	Pennsylvania	743	4.0%		38	West Virginia	97	0.5%
44	Rhode Island	53	0.3%		39	Idaho	92	0.5%
16	South Carolina	392	2.1%		40	Hawaii	84	0.4%
42	South Dakota	57	0.3%		41	New Hampshire	60	0.3%
17	Tennessee	389	2.1%		42	South Dakota	57	0.3%
2	Texas	1,365	7.3%		43	Delaware	55	0.3%
33	Utah	148	0.8%		44	Rhode Island	53	0.3%
50	Vermont	22	0.1%		45	Maine	51	0.3%
12	Virginia	483	2.6%		46	North Dakota	33	0.2%
27	Washington	256	1.4%		47	Montana	32	0.2%
38	West Virginia	97	0.5%		48	Alaska	26	0.1%
22	Wisconsin	294	1.6%		49	Wyoming	25	0.1%
49	Wyoming	25	0.1%		50	Vermont	22	0.1%
						District of Columbia	88	0.5%

*Source: U.S. Department of Health and Human Services, National Center for Health Statistics
"National Vital Statistics Reports" (Vol. 49, No. 8, September 21, 2001)*
*Final data. Deaths of infants under 28 days, exclusive of fetal deaths.

Neonatal Death Rate in 1999

National Rate = 4.7 Deaths per 1,000 Live Births*

ALPHA ORDER			RANK ORDER		
RANK	STATE	RATE	RANK	STATE	RATE
3	Alabama	6.2	1	South Carolina	7.1
50	Alaska	2.6	2	North Carolina	6.7
28	Arizona	4.5	3	Alabama	6.2
26	Arkansas	4.6	3	Mississippi	6.2
44	California	3.6	5	Illinois	5.9
31	Colorado	4.3	5	Louisiana	5.9
24	Connecticut	4.7	7	Maryland	5.8
13	Delaware	5.2	8	Georgia	5.5
19	Florida	4.9	8	Michigan	5.5
8	Georgia	5.5	8	Ohio	5.5
19	Hawaii	4.9	11	South Dakota	5.4
26	Idaho	4.6	12	Indiana	5.3
5	Illinois	5.9	13	Delaware	5.2
12	Indiana	5.3	14	Missouri	5.1
45	Iowa	3.4	14	Pennsylvania	5.1
19	Kansas	4.9	14	Virginia	5.1
23	Kentucky	4.8	17	Oklahoma	5.0
5	Louisiana	5.9	17	Tennessee	5.0
43	Maine	3.7	19	Florida	4.9
7	Maryland	5.8	19	Hawaii	4.9
37	Massachusetts	4.1	19	Kansas	4.9
8	Michigan	5.5	19	New Jersey	4.9
39	Minnesota	4.0	23	Kentucky	4.8
3	Mississippi	6.2	24	Connecticut	4.7
14	Missouri	5.1	24	West Virginia	4.7
49	Montana	3.0	26	Arkansas	4.6
28	Nebraska	4.5	26	Idaho	4.6
40	Nevada	3.9	28	Arizona	4.5
31	New Hampshire	4.3	28	Nebraska	4.5
19	New Jersey	4.9	28	New York	4.5
40	New Mexico	3.9	31	Colorado	4.3
28	New York	4.5	31	New Hampshire	4.3
2	North Carolina	6.7	31	North Dakota	4.3
31	North Dakota	4.3	31	Rhode Island	4.3
8	Ohio	5.5	31	Wisconsin	4.3
17	Oklahoma	5.0	36	Oregon	4.2
36	Oregon	4.2	37	Massachusetts	4.1
14	Pennsylvania	5.1	37	Wyoming	4.1
31	Rhode Island	4.3	39	Minnesota	4.0
1	South Carolina	7.1	40	Nevada	3.9
11	South Dakota	5.4	40	New Mexico	3.9
17	Tennessee	5.0	40	Texas	3.9
40	Texas	3.9	43	Maine	3.7
47	Utah	3.2	44	California	3.6
45	Vermont	3.4	45	Iowa	3.4
14	Virginia	5.1	45	Vermont	3.4
47	Washington	3.2	47	Utah	3.2
24	West Virginia	4.7	47	Washington	3.2
31	Wisconsin	4.3	49	Montana	3.0
37	Wyoming	4.1	50	Alaska	2.6
				District of Columbia	11.7

Source: U.S. Department of Health and Human Services, National Center for Health Statistics
"National Vital Statistics Reports" (Vol. 49, No. 8, September 21, 2001)
*Final data. Deaths of infants under 28 days, exclusive of fetal deaths.

White Neonatal Deaths in 1999

National Total = 12,164 Deaths*

ALPHA ORDER

RANK	STATE	DEATHS	% of USA
24	Alabama	176	1.4%
50	Alaska	15	0.1%
12	Arizona	300	2.5%
32	Arkansas	120	1.0%
1	California	1,425	11.7%
17	Colorado	232	1.9%
27	Connecticut	159	1.3%
48	Delaware	20	0.2%
6	Florida	566	4.7%
13	Georgia	286	2.4%
49	Hawaii	16	0.1%
38	Idaho	86	0.7%
4	Illinois	623	5.1%
10	Indiana	349	2.9%
33	Iowa	113	0.9%
26	Kansas	161	1.3%
18	Kentucky	220	1.8%
30	Louisiana	143	1.2%
41	Maine	47	0.4%
28	Maryland	153	1.3%
14	Massachusetts	261	2.1%
8	Michigan	424	3.5%
22	Minnesota	203	1.7%
35	Mississippi	92	0.8%
16	Missouri	238	2.0%
45	Montana	23	0.2%
39	Nebraska	84	0.7%
34	Nevada	93	0.8%
40	New Hampshire	59	0.5%
11	New Jersey	329	2.7%
37	New Mexico	87	0.7%
3	New York	720	5.9%
9	North Carolina	413	3.4%
44	North Dakota	26	0.2%
5	Ohio	581	4.8%
23	Oklahoma	191	1.6%
25	Oregon	174	1.4%
7	Pennsylvania	496	4.1%
43	Rhode Island	42	0.3%
28	South Carolina	153	1.3%
42	South Dakota	44	0.4%
20	Tennessee	219	1.8%
2	Texas	1,036	8.5%
31	Utah	141	1.2%
46	Vermont	22	0.2%
15	Virginia	255	2.1%
21	Washington	206	1.7%
35	West Virginia	92	0.8%
18	Wisconsin	220	1.8%
46	Wyoming	22	0.2%

RANK ORDER

RANK	STATE	DEATHS	% of USA
1	California	1,425	11.7%
2	Texas	1,036	8.5%
3	New York	720	5.9%
4	Illinois	623	5.1%
5	Ohio	581	4.8%
6	Florida	566	4.7%
7	Pennsylvania	496	4.1%
8	Michigan	424	3.5%
9	North Carolina	413	3.4%
10	Indiana	349	2.9%
11	New Jersey	329	2.7%
12	Arizona	300	2.5%
13	Georgia	286	2.4%
14	Massachusetts	261	2.1%
15	Virginia	255	2.1%
16	Missouri	238	2.0%
17	Colorado	232	1.9%
18	Kentucky	220	1.8%
18	Wisconsin	220	1.8%
20	Tennessee	219	1.8%
21	Washington	206	1.7%
22	Minnesota	203	1.7%
23	Oklahoma	191	1.6%
24	Alabama	176	1.4%
25	Oregon	174	1.4%
26	Kansas	161	1.3%
27	Connecticut	159	1.3%
28	Maryland	153	1.3%
28	South Carolina	153	1.3%
30	Louisiana	143	1.2%
31	Utah	141	1.2%
32	Arkansas	120	1.0%
33	Iowa	113	0.9%
34	Nevada	93	0.8%
35	Mississippi	92	0.8%
35	West Virginia	92	0.8%
37	New Mexico	87	0.7%
38	Idaho	86	0.7%
39	Nebraska	84	0.7%
40	New Hampshire	59	0.5%
41	Maine	47	0.4%
42	South Dakota	44	0.4%
43	Rhode Island	42	0.3%
44	North Dakota	26	0.2%
45	Montana	23	0.2%
46	Vermont	22	0.2%
46	Wyoming	22	0.2%
48	Delaware	20	0.2%
49	Hawaii	16	0.1%
50	Alaska	15	0.1%
	District of Columbia	8	0.1%

Source: U.S. Department of Health and Human Services, National Center for Health Statistics
"National Vital Statistics Reports" (Vol. 49, No. 8, September 21, 2001)
*Final data. Deaths of infants under 28 days, exclusive of fetal deaths. Based on race of the mother.

White Neonatal Death Rate in 1999

National Rate = 3.9 White Neonatal Deaths per 1,000 White Live Births*

ALPHA ORDER				RANK ORDER		
RANK	**STATE**	**RATE**		**RANK**	**STATE**	**RATE**
14	Alabama	4.2		1	North Carolina	5.1
NA	Alaska**	NA		1	South Dakota	5.1
14	Arizona	4.2		3	Oklahoma	4.9
14	Arkansas	4.2		4	Kansas	4.7
41	California	3.4		5	Indiana	4.6
18	Colorado	4.1		5	West Virginia	4.6
10	Connecticut	4.4		7	Idaho	4.5
47	Delaware	2.6		7	Kentucky	4.5
22	Florida	3.9		7	Ohio	4.5
37	Georgia	3.5		10	Connecticut	4.4
NA	Hawaii**	NA		10	Illinois	4.4
7	Idaho	4.5		10	South Carolina	4.4
10	Illinois	4.4		13	New Hampshire	4.3
5	Indiana	4.6		14	Alabama	4.2
44	Iowa	3.2		14	Arizona	4.2
4	Kansas	4.7		14	Arkansas	4.2
7	Kentucky	4.5		14	Oregon	4.2
32	Louisiana	3.7		18	Colorado	4.1
37	Maine	3.5		18	Mississippi	4.1
41	Maryland	3.4		18	Pennsylvania	4.1
28	Massachusetts	3.8		21	Michigan	4.0
21	Michigan	4.0		22	Florida	3.9
37	Minnesota	3.5		22	Nebraska	3.9
18	Mississippi	4.1		22	New Jersey	3.9
28	Missouri	3.8		22	New York	3.9
48	Montana	2.5		22	North Dakota	3.9
22	Nebraska	3.9		22	Rhode Island	3.9
32	Nevada	3.7		28	Massachusetts	3.8
13	New Hampshire	4.3		28	Missouri	3.8
22	New Jersey	3.9		28	New Mexico	3.8
28	New Mexico	3.8		28	Wyoming	3.8
22	New York	3.9		32	Louisiana	3.7
1	North Carolina	5.1		32	Nevada	3.7
22	North Dakota	3.9		32	Virginia	3.7
7	Ohio	4.5		32	Wisconsin	3.7
3	Oklahoma	4.9		36	Tennessee	3.6
14	Oregon	4.2		37	Georgia	3.5
18	Pennsylvania	4.1		37	Maine	3.5
22	Rhode Island	3.9		37	Minnesota	3.5
10	South Carolina	4.4		37	Texas	3.5
1	South Dakota	5.1		41	California	3.4
36	Tennessee	3.6		41	Maryland	3.4
37	Texas	3.5		41	Vermont	3.4
44	Utah	3.2		44	Iowa	3.2
41	Vermont	3.4		44	Utah	3.2
32	Virginia	3.7		46	Washington	3.0
46	Washington	3.0		47	Delaware	2.6
5	West Virginia	4.6		48	Montana	2.5
32	Wisconsin	3.7		NA	Alaska**	NA
28	Wyoming	3.8		NA	Hawaii**	NA
					District of Columbia**	NA

Source: U.S. Department of Health and Human Services, National Center for Health Statistics
   "National Vital Statistics Reports" (Vol. 49, No. 8, September 21, 2001)
Final data. Deaths of infants under 28 days, exclusive of fetal deaths. Based on race of the mother.
**Not available. Fewer than 20 white neonatal deaths.*

Black Neonatal Deaths in 1999

National Total = 5,920 Deaths*

<table>
<tr><td colspan="4">ALPHA ORDER</td><td colspan="4">RANK ORDER</td></tr>
<tr><td>RANK</td><td>STATE</td><td>DEATHS</td><td>% of USA</td><td>RANK</td><td>STATE</td><td>DEATHS</td><td>% of USA</td></tr>
<tr><td>16</td><td>Alabama</td><td>205</td><td>3.5%</td><td>1</td><td>Illinois</td><td>430</td><td>7.3%</td></tr>
<tr><td>41</td><td>Alaska</td><td>3</td><td>0.1%</td><td>2</td><td>Georgia</td><td>400</td><td>6.8%</td></tr>
<tr><td>29</td><td>Arizona</td><td>31</td><td>0.5%</td><td>3</td><td>Florida</td><td>392</td><td>6.6%</td></tr>
<tr><td>23</td><td>Arkansas</td><td>46</td><td>0.8%</td><td>4</td><td>New York</td><td>386</td><td>6.5%</td></tr>
<tr><td>8</td><td>California</td><td>281</td><td>4.7%</td><td>5</td><td>North Carolina</td><td>326</td><td>5.5%</td></tr>
<tr><td>29</td><td>Colorado</td><td>31</td><td>0.5%</td><td>6</td><td>Texas</td><td>311</td><td>5.3%</td></tr>
<tr><td>24</td><td>Connecticut</td><td>45</td><td>0.8%</td><td>7</td><td>Michigan</td><td>299</td><td>5.1%</td></tr>
<tr><td>28</td><td>Delaware</td><td>35</td><td>0.6%</td><td>8</td><td>California</td><td>281</td><td>4.7%</td></tr>
<tr><td>3</td><td>Florida</td><td>392</td><td>6.6%</td><td>9</td><td>Ohio</td><td>261</td><td>4.4%</td></tr>
<tr><td>2</td><td>Georgia</td><td>400</td><td>6.8%</td><td>10</td><td>Maryland</td><td>253</td><td>4.3%</td></tr>
<tr><td>38</td><td>Hawaii</td><td>5</td><td>0.1%</td><td>11</td><td>Louisiana</td><td>248</td><td>4.2%</td></tr>
<tr><td>44</td><td>Idaho</td><td>2</td><td>0.0%</td><td>12</td><td>Pennsylvania</td><td>237</td><td>4.0%</td></tr>
<tr><td>1</td><td>Illinois</td><td>430</td><td>7.3%</td><td>13</td><td>South Carolina</td><td>235</td><td>4.0%</td></tr>
<tr><td>20</td><td>Indiana</td><td>100</td><td>1.7%</td><td>14</td><td>Virginia</td><td>213</td><td>3.6%</td></tr>
<tr><td>35</td><td>Iowa</td><td>14</td><td>0.2%</td><td>15</td><td>New Jersey</td><td>209</td><td>3.5%</td></tr>
<tr><td>32</td><td>Kansas</td><td>23</td><td>0.4%</td><td>16</td><td>Alabama</td><td>205</td><td>3.5%</td></tr>
<tr><td>25</td><td>Kentucky</td><td>40</td><td>0.7%</td><td>17</td><td>Mississippi</td><td>170</td><td>2.9%</td></tr>
<tr><td>11</td><td>Louisiana</td><td>248</td><td>4.2%</td><td>18</td><td>Tennessee</td><td>164</td><td>2.8%</td></tr>
<tr><td>41</td><td>Maine</td><td>3</td><td>0.1%</td><td>19</td><td>Missouri</td><td>145</td><td>2.4%</td></tr>
<tr><td>10</td><td>Maryland</td><td>253</td><td>4.3%</td><td>20</td><td>Indiana</td><td>100</td><td>1.7%</td></tr>
<tr><td>21</td><td>Massachusetts</td><td>66</td><td>1.1%</td><td>21</td><td>Massachusetts</td><td>66</td><td>1.1%</td></tr>
<tr><td>7</td><td>Michigan</td><td>299</td><td>5.1%</td><td>22</td><td>Wisconsin</td><td>65</td><td>1.1%</td></tr>
<tr><td>26</td><td>Minnesota</td><td>39</td><td>0.7%</td><td>23</td><td>Arkansas</td><td>46</td><td>0.8%</td></tr>
<tr><td>17</td><td>Mississippi</td><td>170</td><td>2.9%</td><td>24</td><td>Connecticut</td><td>45</td><td>0.8%</td></tr>
<tr><td>19</td><td>Missouri</td><td>145</td><td>2.4%</td><td>25</td><td>Kentucky</td><td>40</td><td>0.7%</td></tr>
<tr><td>46</td><td>Montana</td><td>0</td><td>0.0%</td><td>26</td><td>Minnesota</td><td>39</td><td>0.7%</td></tr>
<tr><td>33</td><td>Nebraska</td><td>15</td><td>0.3%</td><td>27</td><td>Oklahoma</td><td>38</td><td>0.6%</td></tr>
<tr><td>33</td><td>Nevada</td><td>15</td><td>0.3%</td><td>28</td><td>Delaware</td><td>35</td><td>0.6%</td></tr>
<tr><td>46</td><td>New Hampshire</td><td>0</td><td>0.0%</td><td>29</td><td>Arizona</td><td>31</td><td>0.5%</td></tr>
<tr><td>15</td><td>New Jersey</td><td>209</td><td>3.5%</td><td>29</td><td>Colorado</td><td>31</td><td>0.5%</td></tr>
<tr><td>36</td><td>New Mexico</td><td>9</td><td>0.2%</td><td>29</td><td>Washington</td><td>31</td><td>0.5%</td></tr>
<tr><td>4</td><td>New York</td><td>386</td><td>6.5%</td><td>32</td><td>Kansas</td><td>23</td><td>0.4%</td></tr>
<tr><td>5</td><td>North Carolina</td><td>326</td><td>5.5%</td><td>33</td><td>Nebraska</td><td>15</td><td>0.3%</td></tr>
<tr><td>46</td><td>North Dakota</td><td>0</td><td>0.0%</td><td>33</td><td>Nevada</td><td>15</td><td>0.3%</td></tr>
<tr><td>9</td><td>Ohio</td><td>261</td><td>4.4%</td><td>35</td><td>Iowa</td><td>14</td><td>0.2%</td></tr>
<tr><td>27</td><td>Oklahoma</td><td>38</td><td>0.6%</td><td>36</td><td>New Mexico</td><td>9</td><td>0.2%</td></tr>
<tr><td>40</td><td>Oregon</td><td>4</td><td>0.1%</td><td>36</td><td>Rhode Island</td><td>9</td><td>0.2%</td></tr>
<tr><td>12</td><td>Pennsylvania</td><td>237</td><td>4.0%</td><td>38</td><td>Hawaii</td><td>5</td><td>0.1%</td></tr>
<tr><td>36</td><td>Rhode Island</td><td>9</td><td>0.2%</td><td>38</td><td>West Virginia</td><td>5</td><td>0.1%</td></tr>
<tr><td>13</td><td>South Carolina</td><td>235</td><td>4.0%</td><td>40</td><td>Oregon</td><td>4</td><td>0.1%</td></tr>
<tr><td>41</td><td>South Dakota</td><td>3</td><td>0.1%</td><td>41</td><td>Alaska</td><td>3</td><td>0.1%</td></tr>
<tr><td>18</td><td>Tennessee</td><td>164</td><td>2.8%</td><td>41</td><td>Maine</td><td>3</td><td>0.1%</td></tr>
<tr><td>6</td><td>Texas</td><td>311</td><td>5.3%</td><td>41</td><td>South Dakota</td><td>3</td><td>0.1%</td></tr>
<tr><td>46</td><td>Utah</td><td>0</td><td>0.0%</td><td>44</td><td>Idaho</td><td>2</td><td>0.0%</td></tr>
<tr><td>46</td><td>Vermont</td><td>0</td><td>0.0%</td><td>45</td><td>Wyoming</td><td>1</td><td>0.0%</td></tr>
<tr><td>14</td><td>Virginia</td><td>213</td><td>3.6%</td><td>46</td><td>Montana</td><td>0</td><td>0.0%</td></tr>
<tr><td>29</td><td>Washington</td><td>31</td><td>0.5%</td><td>46</td><td>New Hampshire</td><td>0</td><td>0.0%</td></tr>
<tr><td>38</td><td>West Virginia</td><td>5</td><td>0.1%</td><td>46</td><td>North Dakota</td><td>0</td><td>0.0%</td></tr>
<tr><td>22</td><td>Wisconsin</td><td>65</td><td>1.1%</td><td>46</td><td>Utah</td><td>0</td><td>0.0%</td></tr>
<tr><td>45</td><td>Wyoming</td><td>1</td><td>0.0%</td><td>46</td><td>Vermont</td><td>0</td><td>0.0%</td></tr>
<tr><td></td><td></td><td></td><td></td><td></td><td>District of Columbia</td><td>77</td><td>1.3%</td></tr>
</table>

Source: U.S. Department of Health and Human Services, National Center for Health Statistics
  "National Vital Statistics Reports" (Vol. 49, No. 8, September 21, 2001)
*Final data. Deaths of infants under 28 days, exclusive of fetal deaths. Based on race of the mother.

Black Neonatal Death Rate in 1999

National Rate = 9.8 Black Neonatal Deaths per 1,000 Black Live Births*

ALPHA ORDER

RANK ORDER

RANK	STATE	RATE		RANK	STATE	RATE
12	Alabama	10.4		1	Delaware	13.1
NA	Alaska**	NA		2	Missouri	12.9
9	Arizona	11.4		3	Illinois	12.6
32	Arkansas	6.0		4	Michigan	12.4
29	California	7.9		5	South Carolina	12.3
11	Colorado	10.7		6	Ohio	11.8
24	Connecticut	8.4		7	Pennsylvania	11.6
1	Delaware	13.1		8	North Carolina	11.5
23	Florida	8.7		9	Arizona	11.4
19	Georgia	9.5		10	Indiana	10.8
NA	Hawaii**	NA		11	Colorado	10.7
NA	Idaho**	NA		12	Alabama	10.4
3	Illinois	12.6		12	Maryland	10.4
10	Indiana	10.8		14	Wisconsin	10.0
NA	Iowa**	NA		15	New Jersey	9.9
26	Kansas	8.1		15	Tennessee	9.9
28	Kentucky	8.0		17	Minnesota	9.7
21	Louisiana	9.1		18	Virginia	9.6
NA	Maine**	NA		19	Georgia	9.5
12	Maryland	10.4		20	Washington	9.3
26	Massachusetts	8.1		21	Louisiana	9.1
4	Michigan	12.4		22	Mississippi	8.8
17	Minnesota	9.7		23	Florida	8.7
22	Mississippi	8.8		24	Connecticut	8.4
2	Missouri	12.9		25	Oklahoma	8.2
NA	Montana**	NA		26	Kansas	8.1
NA	Nebraska**	NA		26	Massachusetts	8.1
NA	Nevada**	NA		28	Kentucky	8.0
NA	New Hampshire**	NA		29	California	7.9
15	New Jersey	9.9		30	Texas	7.8
NA	New Mexico**	NA		31	New York	7.2
31	New York	7.2		32	Arkansas	6.0
8	North Carolina	11.5		NA	Alaska**	NA
NA	North Dakota**	NA		NA	Hawaii**	NA
6	Ohio	11.8		NA	Idaho**	NA
25	Oklahoma	8.2		NA	Iowa**	NA
NA	Oregon**	NA		NA	Maine**	NA
7	Pennsylvania	11.6		NA	Montana**	NA
NA	Rhode Island**	NA		NA	Nebraska**	NA
5	South Carolina	12.3		NA	Nevada**	NA
NA	South Dakota**	NA		NA	New Hampshire**	NA
15	Tennessee	9.9		NA	New Mexico**	NA
30	Texas	7.8		NA	North Dakota**	NA
NA	Utah**	NA		NA	Oregon**	NA
NA	Vermont**	NA		NA	Rhode Island**	NA
18	Virginia	9.6		NA	South Dakota**	NA
20	Washington	9.3		NA	Utah**	NA
NA	West Virginia**	NA		NA	Vermont**	NA
14	Wisconsin	10.0		NA	West Virginia**	NA
NA	Wyoming**	NA		NA	Wyoming**	NA

District of Columbia   14.9

Source: U.S. Department of Health and Human Services, National Center for Health Statistics
"National Vital Statistics Reports" (Vol. 49, No. 8, September 21, 2001)
*Final data. Deaths of infants under 28 days, exclusive of fetal deaths. Based on race of the mother.
**Not available. Fewer than 20 black neonatal deaths.

Deaths by AIDS Through 1999

National Total = 338,831 Deaths*

ALPHA ORDER

RANK	STATE	DEATHS	% of USA
23	Alabama	2,925	0.9%
46	Alaska	189	0.1%
21	Arizona	3,429	1.0%
32	Arkansas	1,158	0.3%
2	California	55,430	16.4%
22	Colorado	3,290	1.0%
18	Connecticut	4,290	1.3%
36	Delaware	980	0.3%
3	Florida	32,876	9.7%
6	Georgia	12,180	3.6%
35	Hawaii	991	0.3%
44	Idaho	258	0.1%
7	Illinois	11,228	3.3%
24	Indiana	2,587	0.8%
39	Iowa	633	0.2%
33	Kansas	1,072	0.3%
31	Kentucky	1,401	0.4%
14	Louisiana	5,913	1.7%
42	Maine	510	0.2%
9	Maryland	8,996	2.7%
11	Massachusetts	6,737	2.0%
15	Michigan	5,722	1.7%
28	Minnesota	1,855	0.5%
26	Mississippi	2,051	0.6%
19	Missouri	3,694	1.1%
47	Montana	169	0.0%
40	Nebraska	523	0.2%
30	Nevada	1,547	0.5%
43	New Hampshire	353	0.1%
5	New Jersey	20,460	6.0%
34	New Mexico	994	0.3%
1	New York	65,437	19.3%
10	North Carolina	7,300	2.2%
50	North Dakota	66	0.0%
12	Ohio	6,121	1.8%
27	Oklahoma	1,908	0.6%
25	Oregon	2,171	0.6%
8	Pennsylvania	10,498	3.1%
37	Rhode Island	837	0.2%
17	South Carolina	4,330	1.3%
48	South Dakota	99	0.0%
20	Tennessee	3,538	1.0%
4	Texas	23,272	6.9%
38	Utah	656	0.2%
45	Vermont	199	0.1%
13	Virginia	5,925	1.7%
16	Washington	4,358	1.3%
41	West Virginia	521	0.2%
29	Wisconsin	1,727	0.5%
49	Wyoming	82	0.0%

RANK ORDER

RANK	STATE	DEATHS	% of USA
1	New York	65,437	19.3%
2	California	55,430	16.4%
3	Florida	32,876	9.7%
4	Texas	23,272	6.9%
5	New Jersey	20,460	6.0%
6	Georgia	12,180	3.6%
7	Illinois	11,228	3.3%
8	Pennsylvania	10,498	3.1%
9	Maryland	8,996	2.7%
10	North Carolina	7,300	2.2%
11	Massachusetts	6,737	2.0%
12	Ohio	6,121	1.8%
13	Virginia	5,925	1.7%
14	Louisiana	5,913	1.7%
15	Michigan	5,722	1.7%
16	Washington	4,358	1.3%
17	South Carolina	4,330	1.3%
18	Connecticut	4,290	1.3%
19	Missouri	3,694	1.1%
20	Tennessee	3,538	1.0%
21	Arizona	3,429	1.0%
22	Colorado	3,290	1.0%
23	Alabama	2,925	0.9%
24	Indiana	2,587	0.8%
25	Oregon	2,171	0.6%
26	Mississippi	2,051	0.6%
27	Oklahoma	1,908	0.6%
28	Minnesota	1,855	0.5%
29	Wisconsin	1,727	0.5%
30	Nevada	1,547	0.5%
31	Kentucky	1,401	0.4%
32	Arkansas	1,158	0.3%
33	Kansas	1,072	0.3%
34	New Mexico	994	0.3%
35	Hawaii	991	0.3%
36	Delaware	980	0.3%
37	Rhode Island	837	0.2%
38	Utah	656	0.2%
39	Iowa	633	0.2%
40	Nebraska	523	0.2%
41	West Virginia	521	0.2%
42	Maine	510	0.2%
43	New Hampshire	353	0.1%
44	Idaho	258	0.1%
45	Vermont	199	0.1%
46	Alaska	189	0.1%
47	Montana	169	0.0%
48	South Dakota	99	0.0%
49	Wyoming	82	0.0%
50	North Dakota	66	0.0%

District of Columbia   5,345   1.6%

Source: Morgan Quitno Press using data from US Dept of Health & Human Services, National Center for Health Statistics (http://wonder.cdc.gov/WONDER/) and "National Vital Statistics Reports" (Vol. 49, No. 8, September 21, 2001)
*Cumulative deaths through 1999. However, due to reporting delays, these totals should increase. AIDS is Acquired Immunodeficiency Syndrome. The definition of what AIDS is was expanded in 1985, 1987 and 1993.

Deaths by AIDS in 1999

National Total = 14,802 Deaths*

ALPHA ORDER

RANK	STATE	DEATHS	% of USA
19	Alabama	177	1.2%
43	Alaska	13	0.1%
21	Arizona	153	1.0%
31	Arkansas	67	0.5%
3	California	1,593	10.8%
26	Colorado	104	0.7%
18	Connecticut	203	1.4%
32	Delaware	65	0.4%
2	Florida	1,657	11.2%
6	Georgia	786	5.3%
36	Hawaii	29	0.2%
47	Idaho	5	0.0%
8	Illinois	548	3.7%
23	Indiana	111	0.7%
39	Iowa	21	0.1%
34	Kansas	43	0.3%
28	Kentucky	76	0.5%
11	Louisiana	373	2.5%
42	Maine	17	0.1%
7	Maryland	592	4.0%
15	Massachusetts	257	1.7%
17	Michigan	238	1.6%
30	Minnesota	72	0.5%
20	Mississippi	156	1.1%
22	Missouri	150	1.0%
46	Montana	6	0.0%
41	Nebraska	20	0.1%
25	Nevada	105	0.7%
44	New Hampshire	12	0.1%
5	New Jersey	913	6.2%
36	New Mexico	29	0.2%
1	New York	2,375	16.0%
10	North Carolina	466	3.1%
49	North Dakota	3	0.0%
16	Ohio	244	1.6%
27	Oklahoma	103	0.7%
29	Oregon	75	0.5%
9	Pennsylvania	498	3.4%
35	Rhode Island	35	0.2%
12	South Carolina	307	2.1%
47	South Dakota	5	0.0%
14	Tennessee	258	1.7%
4	Texas	1,072	7.2%
36	Utah	29	0.2%
44	Vermont	12	0.1%
13	Virginia	265	1.8%
24	Washington	110	0.7%
39	West Virginia	21	0.1%
32	Wisconsin	65	0.4%
50	Wyoming	2	0.0%

RANK ORDER

RANK	STATE	DEATHS	% of USA
1	New York	2,375	16.0%
2	Florida	1,657	11.2%
3	California	1,593	10.8%
4	Texas	1,072	7.2%
5	New Jersey	913	6.2%
6	Georgia	786	5.3%
7	Maryland	592	4.0%
8	Illinois	548	3.7%
9	Pennsylvania	498	3.4%
10	North Carolina	466	3.1%
11	Louisiana	373	2.5%
12	South Carolina	307	2.1%
13	Virginia	265	1.8%
14	Tennessee	258	1.7%
15	Massachusetts	257	1.7%
16	Ohio	244	1.6%
17	Michigan	238	1.6%
18	Connecticut	203	1.4%
19	Alabama	177	1.2%
20	Mississippi	156	1.1%
21	Arizona	153	1.0%
22	Missouri	150	1.0%
23	Indiana	111	0.7%
24	Washington	110	0.7%
25	Nevada	105	0.7%
26	Colorado	104	0.7%
27	Oklahoma	103	0.7%
28	Kentucky	76	0.5%
29	Oregon	75	0.5%
30	Minnesota	72	0.5%
31	Arkansas	67	0.5%
32	Delaware	65	0.4%
32	Wisconsin	65	0.4%
34	Kansas	43	0.3%
35	Rhode Island	35	0.2%
36	Hawaii	29	0.2%
36	New Mexico	29	0.2%
36	Utah	29	0.2%
39	Iowa	21	0.1%
39	West Virginia	21	0.1%
41	Nebraska	20	0.1%
42	Maine	17	0.1%
43	Alaska	13	0.1%
44	New Hampshire	12	0.1%
44	Vermont	12	0.1%
46	Montana	6	0.0%
47	Idaho	5	0.0%
47	South Dakota	5	0.0%
49	North Dakota	3	0.0%
50	Wyoming	2	0.0%
	District of Columbia	266	1.8%

Source: U.S. Department of Health and Human Services, National Center for Health Statistics
   "National Vital Statistics Reports" (Vol. 49, No. 8, September 21, 2001)
*AIDS is Acquired Immunodeficiency Syndrome. It is a specific group of diseases or conditions which are indicative
of severe immunosuppression related to infection with the Human Immunodeficiency Virus (HIV).

Death Rate by AIDS in 1999

National Rate = 5.4 Deaths per 100,000 Population*

ALPHA ORDER

RANK	STATE	RATE
19	Alabama	4.1
NA	Alaska**	NA
22	Arizona	3.2
25	Arkansas	2.6
14	California	4.8
25	Colorado	2.6
9	Connecticut	6.2
6	Delaware	8.6
4	Florida	11.0
5	Georgia	10.1
27	Hawaii	2.4
NA	Idaho**	NA
16	Illinois	4.5
31	Indiana	1.9
41	Iowa	0.7
35	Kansas	1.6
31	Kentucky	1.9
7	Louisiana	8.5
NA	Maine**	NA
2	Maryland	11.4
17	Massachusetts	4.2
27	Michigan	2.4
36	Minnesota	1.5
12	Mississippi	5.6
24	Missouri	2.7
NA	Montana**	NA
38	Nebraska	1.2
11	Nevada	5.8
NA	New Hampshire**	NA
3	New Jersey	11.2
34	New Mexico	1.7
1	New York	13.1
10	North Carolina	6.1
NA	North Dakota**	NA
30	Ohio	2.2
23	Oklahoma	3.1
29	Oregon	2.3
17	Pennsylvania	4.2
21	Rhode Island	3.5
8	South Carolina	7.9
NA	South Dakota**	NA
15	Tennessee	4.7
13	Texas	5.3
37	Utah	1.4
NA	Vermont**	NA
20	Virginia	3.9
31	Washington	1.9
38	West Virginia	1.2
38	Wisconsin	1.2
NA	Wyoming**	NA

RANK ORDER

RANK	STATE	RATE
1	New York	13.1
2	Maryland	11.4
3	New Jersey	11.2
4	Florida	11.0
5	Georgia	10.1
6	Delaware	8.6
7	Louisiana	8.5
8	South Carolina	7.9
9	Connecticut	6.2
10	North Carolina	6.1
11	Nevada	5.8
12	Mississippi	5.6
13	Texas	5.3
14	California	4.8
15	Tennessee	4.7
16	Illinois	4.5
17	Massachusetts	4.2
17	Pennsylvania	4.2
19	Alabama	4.1
20	Virginia	3.9
21	Rhode Island	3.5
22	Arizona	3.2
23	Oklahoma	3.1
24	Missouri	2.7
25	Arkansas	2.6
25	Colorado	2.6
27	Hawaii	2.4
27	Michigan	2.4
29	Oregon	2.3
30	Ohio	2.2
31	Indiana	1.9
31	Kentucky	1.9
31	Washington	1.9
34	New Mexico	1.7
35	Kansas	1.6
36	Minnesota	1.5
37	Utah	1.4
38	Nebraska	1.2
38	West Virginia	1.2
38	Wisconsin	1.2
41	Iowa	0.7
NA	Alaska**	NA
NA	Idaho**	NA
NA	Maine**	NA
NA	Montana**	NA
NA	New Hampshire**	NA
NA	North Dakota**	NA
NA	South Dakota**	NA
NA	Vermont**	NA
NA	Wyoming**	NA
	District of Columbia	51.3

Source: U.S. Department of Health and Human Services, National Center for Health Statistics
"National Vital Statistics Reports" (Vol. 49, No. 8, September 21, 2001)
*AIDS is Acquired Immunodeficiency Syndrome. It is a specific group of diseases or conditions which are indicative of severe immunosuppression related to infection with the Human Immunodeficiency Virus (HIV). Not age-adjusted.
**Insufficient data to determine a reliable rate.

Age-Adjusted Death Rate by AIDS in 1999

National Rate = 5.4 Deaths per 100,000 Population*

ALPHA ORDER

RANK	STATE	RATE
18	Alabama	4.0
NA	Alaska**	NA
22	Arizona	3.4
24	Arkansas	2.8
14	California	4.8
26	Colorado	2.5
9	Connecticut	6.1
7	Delaware	8.5
2	Florida	11.3
5	Georgia	9.8
27	Hawaii	2.4
NA	Idaho**	NA
16	Illinois	4.5
31	Indiana	1.9
41	Iowa	0.8
34	Kansas	1.7
31	Kentucky	1.9
6	Louisiana	8.9
NA	Maine**	NA
3	Maryland	10.8
18	Massachusetts	4.0
27	Michigan	2.4
37	Minnesota	1.5
11	Mississippi	5.9
24	Missouri	2.8
NA	Montana**	NA
38	Nebraska	1.3
12	Nevada	5.7
NA	New Hampshire**	NA
3	New Jersey	10.8
34	New Mexico	1.7
1	New York	12.8
10	North Carolina	6.0
NA	North Dakota**	NA
30	Ohio	2.2
23	Oklahoma	3.2
29	Oregon	2.3
17	Pennsylvania	4.1
21	Rhode Island	3.6
8	South Carolina	7.8
NA	South Dakota**	NA
15	Tennessee	4.6
13	Texas	5.4
34	Utah	1.7
NA	Vermont**	NA
20	Virginia	3.7
31	Washington	1.9
39	West Virginia	1.2
39	Wisconsin	1.2
NA	Wyoming**	NA

RANK ORDER

RANK	STATE	RATE
1	New York	12.8
2	Florida	11.3
3	Maryland	10.8
3	New Jersey	10.8
5	Georgia	9.8
6	Louisiana	8.9
7	Delaware	8.5
8	South Carolina	7.8
9	Connecticut	6.1
10	North Carolina	6.0
11	Mississippi	5.9
12	Nevada	5.7
13	Texas	5.4
14	California	4.8
15	Tennessee	4.6
16	Illinois	4.5
17	Pennsylvania	4.1
18	Alabama	4.0
18	Massachusetts	4.0
20	Virginia	3.7
21	Rhode Island	3.6
22	Arizona	3.4
23	Oklahoma	3.2
24	Arkansas	2.8
24	Missouri	2.8
26	Colorado	2.5
27	Hawaii	2.4
27	Michigan	2.4
29	Oregon	2.3
30	Ohio	2.2
31	Indiana	1.9
31	Kentucky	1.9
31	Washington	1.9
34	Kansas	1.7
34	New Mexico	1.7
34	Utah	1.7
37	Minnesota	1.5
38	Nebraska	1.3
39	West Virginia	1.2
39	Wisconsin	1.2
41	Iowa	0.8
NA	Alaska**	NA
NA	Idaho**	NA
NA	Maine**	NA
NA	Montana**	NA
NA	New Hampshire**	NA
NA	North Dakota**	NA
NA	South Dakota**	NA
NA	Vermont**	NA
NA	Wyoming**	NA

District of Columbia 47.1

Source: U.S. Department of Health and Human Services, National Center for Health Statistics
   "National Vital Statistics Reports" (Vol. 49, No. 8, September 21, 2001)
*AIDS is Acquired Immunodeficiency Syndrome. It is a specific group of diseases or conditions which are indicative of severe immunosuppression related to infection with the Human Immunodeficiency Virus (HIV). Age-adjusted rates based on the year 2000 standard population.
**Insufficient data to determine a reliable rate.

Estimated Deaths by Cancer in 2002

National Estimated Total = 555,500 Deaths

ALPHA ORDER				RANK ORDER			
RANK	STATE	DEATHS	% of USA	RANK	STATE	DEATHS	% of USA
20	Alabama	9,800	1.8%	1	California	51,800	9.3%
50	Alaska	700	0.1%	2	Florida	39,900	7.2%
21	Arizona	9,600	1.7%	3	New York	36,200	6.5%
31	Arkansas	6,200	1.1%	4	Texas	34,500	6.2%
1	California	51,800	9.3%	5	Pennsylvania	29,800	5.4%
30	Colorado	6,300	1.1%	6	Ohio	25,400	4.6%
28	Connecticut	7,000	1.3%	7	Illinois	24,800	4.5%
45	Delaware	1,800	0.3%	8	Michigan	19,800	3.6%
2	Florida	39,900	7.2%	9	New Jersey	17,800	3.2%
11	Georgia	13,700	2.5%	10	North Carolina	16,500	3.0%
43	Hawaii	2,000	0.4%	11	Georgia	13,700	2.5%
42	Idaho	2,300	0.4%	11	Massachusetts	13,700	2.5%
7	Illinois	24,800	4.5%	13	Virginia	13,500	2.4%
14	Indiana	13,000	2.3%	14	Indiana	13,000	2.3%
29	Iowa	6,400	1.2%	15	Tennessee	12,600	2.3%
33	Kansas	5,300	1.0%	16	Missouri	12,300	2.2%
23	Kentucky	9,100	1.6%	17	Washington	11,100	2.0%
22	Louisiana	9,500	1.7%	18	Wisconsin	11,000	2.0%
37	Maine	3,000	0.5%	19	Maryland	10,200	1.8%
19	Maryland	10,200	1.8%	20	Alabama	9,800	1.8%
11	Massachusetts	13,700	2.5%	21	Arizona	9,600	1.7%
8	Michigan	19,800	3.6%	22	Louisiana	9,500	1.7%
24	Minnesota	9,000	1.6%	23	Kentucky	9,100	1.6%
31	Mississippi	6,200	1.1%	24	Minnesota	9,000	1.6%
16	Missouri	12,300	2.2%	25	South Carolina	8,400	1.5%
44	Montana	1,900	0.3%	26	Oklahoma	7,300	1.3%
36	Nebraska	3,300	0.6%	26	Oregon	7,300	1.3%
35	Nevada	4,100	0.7%	28	Connecticut	7,000	1.3%
39	New Hampshire	2,500	0.5%	29	Iowa	6,400	1.2%
9	New Jersey	17,800	3.2%	30	Colorado	6,300	1.1%
37	New Mexico	3,000	0.5%	31	Arkansas	6,200	1.1%
3	New York	36,200	6.5%	31	Mississippi	6,200	1.1%
10	North Carolina	16,500	3.0%	33	Kansas	5,300	1.0%
47	North Dakota	1,300	0.2%	34	West Virginia	4,700	0.8%
6	Ohio	25,400	4.6%	35	Nevada	4,100	0.7%
26	Oklahoma	7,300	1.3%	36	Nebraska	3,300	0.6%
26	Oregon	7,300	1.3%	37	Maine	3,000	0.5%
5	Pennsylvania	29,800	5.4%	37	New Mexico	3,000	0.5%
41	Rhode Island	2,400	0.4%	39	New Hampshire	2,500	0.5%
25	South Carolina	8,400	1.5%	39	Utah	2,500	0.5%
46	South Dakota	1,600	0.3%	41	Rhode Island	2,400	0.4%
15	Tennessee	12,600	2.3%	42	Idaho	2,300	0.4%
4	Texas	34,500	6.2%	43	Hawaii	2,000	0.4%
39	Utah	2,500	0.5%	44	Montana	1,900	0.3%
47	Vermont	1,300	0.2%	45	Delaware	1,800	0.3%
13	Virginia	13,500	2.4%	46	South Dakota	1,600	0.3%
17	Washington	11,100	2.0%	47	North Dakota	1,300	0.2%
34	West Virginia	4,700	0.8%	47	Vermont	1,300	0.2%
18	Wisconsin	11,000	2.0%	49	Wyoming	1,000	0.2%
49	Wyoming	1,000	0.2%	50	Alaska	700	0.1%
					District of Columbia	1,200	0.2%

Source: American Cancer Society
"Cancer Facts & Figures 2002" (Copyright 2002, Reprinted with permission from the American Cancer Society)

Estimated Death Rate by Cancer in 2002

National Estimated Rate = 195.1 Deaths per 100,000 Population*

ALPHA ORDER

RANK	STATE	RATE
10	Alabama	219.5
49	Alaska	110.3
41	Arizona	180.9
5	Arkansas	230.3
47	California	150.1
48	Colorado	142.6
26	Connecticut	204.4
7	Delaware	226.1
2	Florida	243.3
44	Georgia	163.4
45	Hawaii	163.3
42	Idaho	174.1
30	Illinois	198.7
17	Indiana	212.6
12	Iowa	218.9
33	Kansas	196.7
8	Kentucky	223.8
16	Louisiana	212.7
4	Maine	233.2
37	Maryland	189.8
15	Massachusetts	214.8
32	Michigan	198.2
40	Minnesota	181.0
14	Mississippi	216.9
13	Missouri	218.5
22	Montana	210.1
35	Nebraska	192.6
34	Nevada	194.7
31	New Hampshire	198.5
23	New Jersey	209.8
43	New Mexico	164.0
36	New York	190.4
29	North Carolina	201.6
25	North Dakota	204.9
9	Ohio	223.3
20	Oklahoma	211.0
21	Oregon	210.2
3	Pennsylvania	242.5
6	Rhode Island	226.6
24	South Carolina	206.7
19	South Dakota	211.5
10	Tennessee	219.5
46	Texas	161.8
50	Utah	110.1
18	Vermont	212.0
38	Virginia	187.8
39	Washington	185.4
1	West Virginia	260.8
27	Wisconsin	203.6
28	Wyoming	202.3

RANK ORDER

RANK	STATE	RATE
1	West Virginia	260.8
2	Florida	243.3
3	Pennsylvania	242.5
4	Maine	233.2
5	Arkansas	230.3
6	Rhode Island	226.6
7	Delaware	226.1
8	Kentucky	223.8
9	Ohio	223.3
10	Alabama	219.5
10	Tennessee	219.5
12	Iowa	218.9
13	Missouri	218.5
14	Mississippi	216.9
15	Massachusetts	214.8
16	Louisiana	212.7
17	Indiana	212.6
18	Vermont	212.0
19	South Dakota	211.5
20	Oklahoma	211.0
21	Oregon	210.2
22	Montana	210.1
23	New Jersey	209.8
24	South Carolina	206.7
25	North Dakota	204.9
26	Connecticut	204.4
27	Wisconsin	203.6
28	Wyoming	202.3
29	North Carolina	201.6
30	Illinois	198.7
31	New Hampshire	198.5
32	Michigan	198.2
33	Kansas	196.7
34	Nevada	194.7
35	Nebraska	192.6
36	New York	190.4
37	Maryland	189.8
38	Virginia	187.8
39	Washington	185.4
40	Minnesota	181.0
41	Arizona	180.9
42	Idaho	174.1
43	New Mexico	164.0
44	Georgia	163.4
45	Hawaii	163.3
46	Texas	161.8
47	California	150.1
48	Colorado	142.6
49	Alaska	110.3
50	Utah	110.1
	District of Columbia	209.9

Source: Morgan Quitno Press using data from American Cancer Society
"Cancer Facts & Figures 2002" (Copyright 2002, Reprinted with permission from the American Cancer Society)
*Rates calculated using 2001 Census resident population estimates. Not age-adjusted.

Age-Adjusted Death Rate by Cancer for Males in 1998

National Rate = 206.0 Deaths per 100,000 Male Population*

ALPHA ORDER

RANK	STATE	RATE
4	Alabama	237.5
42	Alaska	185.7
44	Arizona	181.8
6	Arkansas	232.2
45	California	179.2
48	Colorado	169.3
32	Connecticut	193.8
7	Delaware	231.4
29	Florida	200.1
10	Georgia	227.8
49	Hawaii	157.5
46	Idaho	175.9
20	Illinois	214.1
16	Indiana	218.9
33	Iowa	193.4
35	Kansas	192.0
3	Kentucky	245.3
1	Louisiana	248.7
12	Maine	222.5
13	Maryland	222.1
23	Massachusetts	211.5
27	Michigan	207.1
41	Minnesota	186.9
2	Mississippi	247.4
18	Missouri	216.0
37	Montana	188.9
38	Nebraska	188.0
25	Nevada	209.6
21	New Hampshire	213.2
24	New Jersey	210.8
47	New Mexico	172.8
30	New York	199.1
11	North Carolina	226.1
40	North Dakota	187.1
17	Ohio	218.3
22	Oklahoma	211.7
34	Oregon	192.8
19	Pennsylvania	215.5
14	Rhode Island	221.9
8	South Carolina	229.5
36	South Dakota	190.8
5	Tennessee	237.0
26	Texas	207.8
50	Utah	143.7
28	Vermont	206.5
15	Virginia	220.2
39	Washington	187.2
9	West Virginia	229.4
31	Wisconsin	196.0
43	Wyoming	182.6

RANK ORDER

RANK	STATE	RATE
1	Louisiana	248.7
2	Mississippi	247.4
3	Kentucky	245.3
4	Alabama	237.5
5	Tennessee	237.0
6	Arkansas	232.2
7	Delaware	231.4
8	South Carolina	229.5
9	West Virginia	229.4
10	Georgia	227.8
11	North Carolina	226.1
12	Maine	222.5
13	Maryland	222.1
14	Rhode Island	221.9
15	Virginia	220.2
16	Indiana	218.9
17	Ohio	218.3
18	Missouri	216.0
19	Pennsylvania	215.5
20	Illinois	214.1
21	New Hampshire	213.2
22	Oklahoma	211.7
23	Massachusetts	211.5
24	New Jersey	210.8
25	Nevada	209.6
26	Texas	207.8
27	Michigan	207.1
28	Vermont	206.5
29	Florida	200.1
30	New York	199.1
31	Wisconsin	196.0
32	Connecticut	193.8
33	Iowa	193.4
34	Oregon	192.8
35	Kansas	192.0
36	South Dakota	190.8
37	Montana	188.9
38	Nebraska	188.0
39	Washington	187.2
40	North Dakota	187.1
41	Minnesota	186.9
42	Alaska	185.7
43	Wyoming	182.6
44	Arizona	181.8
45	California	179.2
46	Idaho	175.9
47	New Mexico	172.8
48	Colorado	169.3
49	Hawaii	157.5
50	Utah	143.7
	District of Columbia	268.2

Source: American Cancer Society
"Cancer Facts & Figures 2002" (Copyright 2002, Reprinted with permission from the American Cancer Society)
*For 1994 to 1998. Age-adjusted to the 1970 U.S. standard population.

Age-Adjusted Death Rate by Cancer for Females in 1998

National Rate = 138.6 Deaths per 100,000 Female Population*

ALPHA ORDER

RANK	STATE	RATE
25	Alabama	138.1
24	Alaska	138.4
42	Arizona	125.8
23	Arkansas	138.9
37	California	132.3
48	Colorado	118.5
26	Connecticut	137.9
1	Delaware	158.6
34	Florida	134.2
32	Georgia	136.0
49	Hawaii	105.2
46	Idaho	122.7
14	Illinois	144.0
13	Indiana	145.2
38	Iowa	130.6
40	Kansas	130.1
8	Kentucky	150.1
7	Louisiana	150.4
4	Maine	150.8
5	Maryland	150.6
12	Massachusetts	145.5
21	Michigan	141.1
39	Minnesota	130.4
26	Mississippi	137.9
17	Missouri	143.0
41	Montana	129.8
43	Nebraska	125.4
2	Nevada	153.2
3	New Hampshire	152.1
5	New Jersey	150.6
47	New Mexico	122.1
19	New York	141.4
33	North Carolina	135.1
45	North Dakota	124.5
11	Ohio	147.4
28	Oklahoma	137.6
21	Oregon	141.1
15	Pennsylvania	143.8
10	Rhode Island	147.5
30	South Carolina	137.0
44	South Dakota	125.0
18	Tennessee	142.8
36	Texas	133.1
50	Utah	102.3
16	Vermont	143.5
19	Virginia	141.4
28	Washington	137.6
8	West Virginia	150.1
35	Wisconsin	133.9
31	Wyoming	136.1

RANK ORDER

RANK	STATE	RATE
1	Delaware	158.6
2	Nevada	153.2
3	New Hampshire	152.1
4	Maine	150.8
5	Maryland	150.6
5	New Jersey	150.6
7	Louisiana	150.4
8	Kentucky	150.1
8	West Virginia	150.1
10	Rhode Island	147.5
11	Ohio	147.4
12	Massachusetts	145.5
13	Indiana	145.2
14	Illinois	144.0
15	Pennsylvania	143.8
16	Vermont	143.5
17	Missouri	143.0
18	Tennessee	142.8
19	New York	141.4
19	Virginia	141.4
21	Michigan	141.1
21	Oregon	141.1
23	Arkansas	138.9
24	Alaska	138.4
25	Alabama	138.1
26	Connecticut	137.9
26	Mississippi	137.9
28	Oklahoma	137.6
28	Washington	137.6
30	South Carolina	137.0
31	Wyoming	136.1
32	Georgia	136.0
33	North Carolina	135.1
34	Florida	134.2
35	Wisconsin	133.9
36	Texas	133.1
37	California	132.3
38	Iowa	130.6
39	Minnesota	130.4
40	Kansas	130.1
41	Montana	129.8
42	Arizona	125.8
43	Nebraska	125.4
44	South Dakota	125.0
45	North Dakota	124.5
46	Idaho	122.7
47	New Mexico	122.1
48	Colorado	118.5
49	Hawaii	105.2
50	Utah	102.3
	District of Columbia	165.2

Source: American Cancer Society
"Cancer Facts & Figures 2002" (Copyright 2002, Reprinted with permission from the American Cancer Society)
*For 1994 to 1998. Age-adjusted to the 1970 U.S. standard population.

Estimated Deaths by Female Breast Cancer in 2002

National Estimated Total = 40,000 Deaths

ALPHA ORDER

RANK ORDER

RANK	STATE	DEATHS	% of USA		RANK	STATE	DEATHS	% of USA
22	Alabama	600	1.5%		1	California	3,900	9.8%
43	Alaska	100	0.3%		2	New York	2,900	7.3%
19	Arizona	700	1.8%		3	Florida	2,600	6.5%
31	Arkansas	400	1.0%		3	Texas	2,600	6.5%
1	California	3,900	9.8%		5	Pennsylvania	2,200	5.5%
26	Colorado	500	1.3%		6	Illinois	1,900	4.8%
26	Connecticut	500	1.3%		6	Ohio	1,900	4.8%
43	Delaware	100	0.3%		8	Michigan	1,400	3.5%
3	Florida	2,600	6.5%		8	New Jersey	1,400	3.5%
11	Georgia	1,000	2.5%		10	North Carolina	1,200	3.0%
43	Hawaii	100	0.3%		11	Georgia	1,000	2.5%
36	Idaho	200	0.5%		11	Virginia	1,000	2.5%
6	Illinois	1,900	4.8%		13	Indiana	900	2.3%
13	Indiana	900	2.3%		13	Massachusetts	900	2.3%
26	Iowa	500	1.3%		13	Tennessee	900	2.3%
31	Kansas	400	1.0%		16	Maryland	800	2.0%
22	Kentucky	600	1.5%		16	Missouri	800	2.0%
19	Louisiana	700	1.8%		16	Wisconsin	800	2.0%
36	Maine	200	0.5%		19	Arizona	700	1.8%
16	Maryland	800	2.0%		19	Louisiana	700	1.8%
13	Massachusetts	900	2.3%		19	Washington	700	1.8%
8	Michigan	1,400	3.5%		22	Alabama	600	1.5%
22	Minnesota	600	1.5%		22	Kentucky	600	1.5%
31	Mississippi	400	1.0%		22	Minnesota	600	1.5%
16	Missouri	800	2.0%		22	South Carolina	600	1.5%
43	Montana	100	0.3%		26	Colorado	500	1.3%
36	Nebraska	200	0.5%		26	Connecticut	500	1.3%
34	Nevada	300	0.8%		26	Iowa	500	1.3%
36	New Hampshire	200	0.5%		26	Oklahoma	500	1.3%
8	New Jersey	1,400	3.5%		26	Oregon	500	1.3%
36	New Mexico	200	0.5%		31	Arkansas	400	1.0%
2	New York	2,900	7.3%		31	Kansas	400	1.0%
10	North Carolina	1,200	3.0%		31	Mississippi	400	1.0%
43	North Dakota	100	0.3%		34	Nevada	300	0.8%
6	Ohio	1,900	4.8%		34	West Virginia	300	0.8%
26	Oklahoma	500	1.3%		36	Idaho	200	0.5%
26	Oregon	500	1.3%		36	Maine	200	0.5%
5	Pennsylvania	2,200	5.5%		36	Nebraska	200	0.5%
36	Rhode Island	200	0.5%		36	New Hampshire	200	0.5%
22	South Carolina	600	1.5%		36	New Mexico	200	0.5%
43	South Dakota	100	0.3%		36	Rhode Island	200	0.5%
13	Tennessee	900	2.3%		36	Utah	200	0.5%
3	Texas	2,600	6.5%		43	Alaska	100	0.3%
36	Utah	200	0.5%		43	Delaware	100	0.3%
43	Vermont	100	0.3%		43	Hawaii	100	0.3%
11	Virginia	1,000	2.5%		43	Montana	100	0.3%
19	Washington	700	1.8%		43	North Dakota	100	0.3%
34	West Virginia	300	0.8%		43	South Dakota	100	0.3%
16	Wisconsin	800	2.0%		43	Vermont	100	0.3%
43	Wyoming	100	0.3%		43	Wyoming	100	0.3%
						District of Columbia	100	0.3%

Source: American Cancer Society
"Cancer Facts & Figures 2002" (Copyright 2002, Reprinted with permission from the American Cancer Society)

Estimated Death Rate by Female Breast Cancer in 2002

National Estimated Rate = 27.9 Deaths per 100,000 Female Population*

ALPHA ORDER

RANK	STATE	RATE
38	Alabama	26.1
5	Alaska	33.0
35	Arizona	27.2
22	Arkansas	29.2
46	California	22.9
44	Colorado	23.4
29	Connecticut	28.5
39	Delaware	24.8
10	Florida	31.8
42	Georgia	24.0
50	Hawaii	16.6
13	Idaho	31.0
18	Illinois	30.0
25	Indiana	29.1
4	Iowa	33.5
21	Kansas	29.4
27	Kentucky	29.0
17	Louisiana	30.4
15	Maine	30.6
22	Maryland	29.2
34	Massachusetts	27.4
33	Michigan	27.6
41	Minnesota	24.2
35	Mississippi	27.2
31	Missouri	27.8
47	Montana	22.1
45	Nebraska	23.0
15	Nevada	30.6
10	New Hampshire	31.8
7	New Jersey	32.3
48	New Mexico	21.6
19	New York	29.5
22	North Carolina	29.2
12	North Dakota	31.1
6	Ohio	32.5
29	Oklahoma	28.5
27	Oregon	29.0
3	Pennsylvania	34.6
2	Rhode Island	36.7
25	South Carolina	29.1
37	South Dakota	26.3
14	Tennessee	30.8
39	Texas	24.8
49	Utah	18.0
9	Vermont	32.2
32	Virginia	27.7
43	Washington	23.7
7	West Virginia	32.3
19	Wisconsin	29.5
1	Wyoming	40.7

RANK ORDER

RANK	STATE	RATE
1	Wyoming	40.7
2	Rhode Island	36.7
3	Pennsylvania	34.6
4	Iowa	33.5
5	Alaska	33.0
6	Ohio	32.5
7	New Jersey	32.3
7	West Virginia	32.3
9	Vermont	32.2
10	Florida	31.8
10	New Hampshire	31.8
12	North Dakota	31.1
13	Idaho	31.0
14	Tennessee	30.8
15	Maine	30.6
15	Nevada	30.6
17	Louisiana	30.4
18	Illinois	30.0
19	New York	29.5
19	Wisconsin	29.5
21	Kansas	29.4
22	Arkansas	29.2
22	Maryland	29.2
22	North Carolina	29.2
25	Indiana	29.1
25	South Carolina	29.1
27	Kentucky	29.0
27	Oregon	29.0
29	Connecticut	28.5
29	Oklahoma	28.5
31	Missouri	27.8
32	Virginia	27.7
33	Michigan	27.6
34	Massachusetts	27.4
35	Arizona	27.2
35	Mississippi	27.2
37	South Dakota	26.3
38	Alabama	26.1
39	Delaware	24.8
39	Texas	24.8
41	Minnesota	24.2
42	Georgia	24.0
43	Washington	23.7
44	Colorado	23.4
45	Nebraska	23.0
46	California	22.9
47	Montana	22.1
48	New Mexico	21.6
49	Utah	18.0
50	Hawaii	16.6

District of Columbia 33.0

Source: Morgan Quitno Press using data from American Cancer Society
"Cancer Facts & Figures 2002" (Copyright 2002, Reprinted with permission from the American Cancer Society)
Rates calculated using 2000 Census resident female population figures. Not age-adjusted.

Estimated Deaths by Colon and Rectum Cancer in 2002

National Estimated Total = 56,600 Deaths

ALPHA ORDER

RANK	STATE	DEATHS	% of USA
24	Alabama	800	1.4%
48	Alaska	100	0.2%
21	Arizona	900	1.6%
30	Arkansas	600	1.1%
1	California	4,900	8.7%
30	Colorado	600	1.1%
27	Connecticut	700	1.2%
42	Delaware	200	0.4%
2	Florida	4,000	7.1%
15	Georgia	1,200	2.1%
42	Hawaii	200	0.4%
42	Idaho	200	0.4%
7	Illinois	2,600	4.6%
12	Indiana	1,400	2.5%
24	Iowa	800	1.4%
33	Kansas	500	0.9%
21	Kentucky	900	1.6%
19	Louisiana	1,000	1.8%
37	Maine	300	0.5%
17	Maryland	1,100	1.9%
11	Massachusetts	1,500	2.7%
8	Michigan	2,000	3.5%
21	Minnesota	900	1.6%
30	Mississippi	600	1.1%
14	Missouri	1,300	2.3%
42	Montana	200	0.4%
36	Nebraska	400	0.7%
33	Nevada	500	0.9%
37	New Hampshire	300	0.5%
9	New Jersey	1,900	3.4%
37	New Mexico	300	0.5%
2	New York	4,000	7.1%
10	North Carolina	1,600	2.8%
48	North Dakota	100	0.2%
6	Ohio	2,700	4.8%
27	Oklahoma	700	1.2%
27	Oregon	700	1.2%
5	Pennsylvania	3,300	5.8%
37	Rhode Island	300	0.5%
24	South Carolina	800	1.4%
42	South Dakota	200	0.4%
15	Tennessee	1,200	2.1%
4	Texas	3,600	6.4%
37	Utah	300	0.5%
42	Vermont	200	0.4%
12	Virginia	1,400	2.5%
19	Washington	1,000	1.8%
33	West Virginia	500	0.9%
17	Wisconsin	1,100	1.9%
48	Wyoming	100	0.2%

RANK ORDER

RANK	STATE	DEATHS	% of USA
1	California	4,900	8.7%
2	Florida	4,000	7.1%
2	New York	4,000	7.1%
4	Texas	3,600	6.4%
5	Pennsylvania	3,300	5.8%
6	Ohio	2,700	4.8%
7	Illinois	2,600	4.6%
8	Michigan	2,000	3.5%
9	New Jersey	1,900	3.4%
10	North Carolina	1,600	2.8%
11	Massachusetts	1,500	2.7%
12	Indiana	1,400	2.5%
12	Virginia	1,400	2.5%
14	Missouri	1,300	2.3%
15	Georgia	1,200	2.1%
15	Tennessee	1,200	2.1%
17	Maryland	1,100	1.9%
17	Wisconsin	1,100	1.9%
19	Louisiana	1,000	1.8%
19	Washington	1,000	1.8%
21	Arizona	900	1.6%
21	Kentucky	900	1.6%
21	Minnesota	900	1.6%
24	Alabama	800	1.4%
24	Iowa	800	1.4%
24	South Carolina	800	1.4%
27	Connecticut	700	1.2%
27	Oklahoma	700	1.2%
27	Oregon	700	1.2%
30	Arkansas	600	1.1%
30	Colorado	600	1.1%
30	Mississippi	600	1.1%
33	Kansas	500	0.9%
33	Nevada	500	0.9%
33	West Virginia	500	0.9%
36	Nebraska	400	0.7%
37	Maine	300	0.5%
37	New Hampshire	300	0.5%
37	New Mexico	300	0.5%
37	Rhode Island	300	0.5%
37	Utah	300	0.5%
42	Delaware	200	0.4%
42	Hawaii	200	0.4%
42	Idaho	200	0.4%
42	Montana	200	0.4%
42	South Dakota	200	0.4%
42	Vermont	200	0.4%
48	Alaska	100	0.2%
48	North Dakota	100	0.2%
48	Wyoming	100	0.2%
	District of Columbia	100	0.2%

Source: American Cancer Society
"Cancer Facts & Figures 2002" (Copyright 2002, Reprinted with permission from the American Cancer Society)

Estimated Death Rate by Colon and Rectum Cancer in 2002

National Estimated Rate = 19.9 Deaths per 100,000 Population*

ALPHA ORDER

RANK	STATE	RATE
38	Alabama	17.9
44	Alaska	15.8
39	Arizona	17.0
19	Arkansas	22.3
48	California	14.2
49	Colorado	13.6
27	Connecticut	20.4
7	Delaware	25.1
8	Florida	24.4
47	Georgia	14.3
43	Hawaii	16.3
46	Idaho	15.1
25	Illinois	20.8
16	Indiana	22.9
4	Iowa	27.4
36	Kansas	18.6
20	Kentucky	22.1
17	Louisiana	22.4
13	Maine	23.3
26	Maryland	20.5
12	Massachusetts	23.5
32	Michigan	20.0
37	Minnesota	18.1
22	Mississippi	21.0
15	Missouri	23.1
20	Montana	22.1
13	Nebraska	23.3
10	Nevada	23.7
9	New Hampshire	23.8
17	New Jersey	22.4
42	New Mexico	16.4
22	New York	21.0
34	North Carolina	19.5
44	North Dakota	15.8
10	Ohio	23.7
29	Oklahoma	20.2
29	Oregon	20.2
5	Pennsylvania	26.9
2	Rhode Island	28.3
33	South Carolina	19.7
6	South Dakota	26.4
24	Tennessee	20.9
40	Texas	16.9
50	Utah	13.2
1	Vermont	32.6
34	Virginia	19.5
41	Washington	16.7
3	West Virginia	27.7
27	Wisconsin	20.4
29	Wyoming	20.2

RANK ORDER

RANK	STATE	RATE
1	Vermont	32.6
2	Rhode Island	28.3
3	West Virginia	27.7
4	Iowa	27.4
5	Pennsylvania	26.9
6	South Dakota	26.4
7	Delaware	25.1
8	Florida	24.4
9	New Hampshire	23.8
10	Nevada	23.7
10	Ohio	23.7
12	Massachusetts	23.5
13	Maine	23.3
13	Nebraska	23.3
15	Missouri	23.1
16	Indiana	22.9
17	Louisiana	22.4
17	New Jersey	22.4
19	Arkansas	22.3
20	Kentucky	22.1
20	Montana	22.1
22	Mississippi	21.0
22	New York	21.0
24	Tennessee	20.9
25	Illinois	20.8
26	Maryland	20.5
27	Connecticut	20.4
27	Wisconsin	20.4
29	Oklahoma	20.2
29	Oregon	20.2
29	Wyoming	20.2
32	Michigan	20.0
33	South Carolina	19.7
34	North Carolina	19.5
34	Virginia	19.5
36	Kansas	18.6
37	Minnesota	18.1
38	Alabama	17.9
39	Arizona	17.0
40	Texas	16.9
41	Washington	16.7
42	New Mexico	16.4
43	Hawaii	16.3
44	Alaska	15.8
44	North Dakota	15.8
46	Idaho	15.1
47	Georgia	14.3
48	California	14.2
49	Colorado	13.6
50	Utah	13.2
	District of Columbia	17.5

Source: Morgan Quitno Press using data from American Cancer Society
"Cancer Facts & Figures 2002" (Copyright 2002, Reprinted with permission from the American Cancer Society)
*Rates calculated using 2001 Census resident population estimates. Not age-adjusted.

Estimated Deaths by Leukemia in 2002

National Estimated Total = 21,700 Deaths

ALPHA ORDER

RANK	STATE	DEATHS	% of USA
19	Alabama	400	1.8%
NA	Alaska*	NA	NA
19	Arizona	400	1.8%
31	Arkansas	200	0.9%
1	California	2,100	9.7%
23	Colorado	300	1.4%
23	Connecticut	300	1.4%
36	Delaware	100	0.5%
2	Florida	1,600	7.4%
11	Georgia	500	2.3%
36	Hawaii	100	0.5%
36	Idaho	100	0.5%
6	Illinois	1,000	4.6%
11	Indiana	500	2.3%
23	Iowa	300	1.4%
31	Kansas	200	0.9%
23	Kentucky	300	1.4%
23	Louisiana	300	1.4%
36	Maine	100	0.5%
19	Maryland	400	1.8%
11	Massachusetts	500	2.3%
9	Michigan	700	3.2%
19	Minnesota	400	1.8%
31	Mississippi	200	0.9%
11	Missouri	500	2.3%
36	Montana	100	0.5%
31	Nebraska	200	0.9%
36	Nevada	100	0.5%
36	New Hampshire	100	0.5%
8	New Jersey	800	3.7%
36	New Mexico	100	0.5%
3	New York	1,400	6.5%
10	North Carolina	600	2.8%
36	North Dakota	100	0.5%
6	Ohio	1,000	4.6%
23	Oklahoma	300	1.4%
23	Oregon	300	1.4%
5	Pennsylvania	1,100	5.1%
36	Rhode Island	100	0.5%
23	South Carolina	300	1.4%
36	South Dakota	100	0.5%
11	Tennessee	500	2.3%
4	Texas	1,300	6.0%
36	Utah	100	0.5%
NA	Vermont*	NA	NA
11	Virginia	500	2.3%
11	Washington	500	2.3%
31	West Virginia	200	0.9%
11	Wisconsin	500	2.3%
NA	Wyoming*	NA	NA

RANK ORDER

RANK	STATE	DEATHS	% of USA
1	California	2,100	9.7%
2	Florida	1,600	7.4%
3	New York	1,400	6.5%
4	Texas	1,300	6.0%
5	Pennsylvania	1,100	5.1%
6	Illinois	1,000	4.6%
6	Ohio	1,000	4.6%
8	New Jersey	800	3.7%
9	Michigan	700	3.2%
10	North Carolina	600	2.8%
11	Georgia	500	2.3%
11	Indiana	500	2.3%
11	Massachusetts	500	2.3%
11	Missouri	500	2.3%
11	Tennessee	500	2.3%
11	Virginia	500	2.3%
11	Washington	500	2.3%
11	Wisconsin	500	2.3%
19	Alabama	400	1.8%
19	Arizona	400	1.8%
19	Maryland	400	1.8%
19	Minnesota	400	1.8%
23	Colorado	300	1.4%
23	Connecticut	300	1.4%
23	Iowa	300	1.4%
23	Kentucky	300	1.4%
23	Louisiana	300	1.4%
23	Oklahoma	300	1.4%
23	Oregon	300	1.4%
23	South Carolina	300	1.4%
31	Arkansas	200	0.9%
31	Kansas	200	0.9%
31	Mississippi	200	0.9%
31	Nebraska	200	0.9%
31	West Virginia	200	0.9%
36	Delaware	100	0.5%
36	Hawaii	100	0.5%
36	Idaho	100	0.5%
36	Maine	100	0.5%
36	Montana	100	0.5%
36	Nevada	100	0.5%
36	New Hampshire	100	0.5%
36	New Mexico	100	0.5%
36	North Dakota	100	0.5%
36	Rhode Island	100	0.5%
36	South Dakota	100	0.5%
36	Utah	100	0.5%
NA	Alaska*	NA	NA
NA	Vermont*	NA	NA
NA	Wyoming*	NA	NA
	District of Columbia*	NA	NA

Source: American Cancer Society
"Cancer Facts & Figures 2002" (Copyright 2002, Reprinted with permission from the American Cancer Society)
Fewer than 50 deaths.

Estimated Death Rate by Leukemia in 2002

National Estimated Rate = 7.6 Deaths per 100,000 Population*

ALPHA ORDER

RANK	STATE	RATE
12	Alabama	9.0
NA	Alaska**	NA
29	Arizona	7.5
30	Arkansas	7.4
42	California	6.1
40	Colorado	6.8
15	Connecticut	8.8
3	Delaware	12.6
8	Florida	9.8
44	Georgia	6.0
21	Hawaii	8.2
28	Idaho	7.6
23	Illinois	8.0
21	Indiana	8.2
7	Iowa	10.3
30	Kansas	7.4
30	Kentucky	7.4
41	Louisiana	6.7
26	Maine	7.8
30	Maryland	7.4
26	Massachusetts	7.8
37	Michigan	7.0
23	Minnesota	8.0
37	Mississippi	7.0
14	Missouri	8.9
5	Montana	11.1
4	Nebraska	11.7
46	Nevada	4.7
25	New Hampshire	7.9
9	New Jersey	9.4
45	New Mexico	5.5
30	New York	7.4
36	North Carolina	7.3
1	North Dakota	15.8
15	Ohio	8.8
17	Oklahoma	8.7
19	Oregon	8.6
12	Pennsylvania	9.0
9	Rhode Island	9.4
30	South Carolina	7.4
2	South Dakota	13.2
17	Tennessee	8.7
42	Texas	6.1
47	Utah	4.4
NA	Vermont**	NA
37	Virginia	7.0
20	Washington	8.4
5	West Virginia	11.1
11	Wisconsin	9.3
NA	Wyoming**	NA

RANK ORDER

RANK	STATE	RATE
1	North Dakota	15.8
2	South Dakota	13.2
3	Delaware	12.6
4	Nebraska	11.7
5	Montana	11.1
5	West Virginia	11.1
7	Iowa	10.3
8	Florida	9.8
9	New Jersey	9.4
9	Rhode Island	9.4
11	Wisconsin	9.3
12	Alabama	9.0
12	Pennsylvania	9.0
14	Missouri	8.9
15	Connecticut	8.8
15	Ohio	8.8
17	Oklahoma	8.7
17	Tennessee	8.7
19	Oregon	8.6
20	Washington	8.4
21	Hawaii	8.2
21	Indiana	8.2
23	Illinois	8.0
23	Minnesota	8.0
25	New Hampshire	7.9
26	Maine	7.8
26	Massachusetts	7.8
28	Idaho	7.6
29	Arizona	7.5
30	Arkansas	7.4
30	Kansas	7.4
30	Kentucky	7.4
30	Maryland	7.4
30	New York	7.4
30	South Carolina	7.4
36	North Carolina	7.3
37	Michigan	7.0
37	Mississippi	7.0
37	Virginia	7.0
40	Colorado	6.8
41	Louisiana	6.7
42	California	6.1
42	Texas	6.1
44	Georgia	6.0
45	New Mexico	5.5
46	Nevada	4.7
47	Utah	4.4
NA	Alaska**	NA
NA	Vermont**	NA
NA	Wyoming**	NA
	District of Columbia**	NA

Source: Morgan Quitno Press using data from American Cancer Society
"Cancer Facts & Figures 2002" (Copyright 2002, Reprinted with permission from the American Cancer Society)
*Rates calculated using 2001 Census resident population estimates. Not age-adjusted.
**Fewer than 50 deaths.

Estimated Deaths by Liver Cancer in 2002

National Estimated Total = 14,100 Deaths

ALPHA ORDER

RANK	STATE	DEATHS	% of USA
10	Alabama	300	2.1%
NA	Alaska*	NA	NA
20	Arizona	200	1.4%
20	Arkansas	200	1.4%
1	California	1,800	12.8%
30	Colorado	100	0.7%
20	Connecticut	200	1.4%
NA	Delaware*	NA	NA
3	Florida	1,000	7.1%
10	Georgia	300	2.1%
30	Hawaii	100	0.7%
NA	Idaho*	NA	NA
6	Illinois	600	4.3%
10	Indiana	300	2.1%
30	Iowa	100	0.7%
30	Kansas	100	0.7%
20	Kentucky	200	1.4%
10	Louisiana	300	2.1%
30	Maine	100	0.7%
20	Maryland	200	1.4%
10	Massachusetts	300	2.1%
7	Michigan	500	3.5%
20	Minnesota	200	1.4%
20	Mississippi	200	1.4%
10	Missouri	300	2.1%
NA	Montana*	NA	NA
30	Nebraska	100	0.7%
30	Nevada	100	0.7%
30	New Hampshire	100	0.7%
7	New Jersey	500	3.5%
30	New Mexico	100	0.7%
3	New York	1,000	7.1%
10	North Carolina	300	2.1%
NA	North Dakota*	NA	NA
7	Ohio	500	3.5%
20	Oklahoma	200	1.4%
30	Oregon	100	0.7%
5	Pennsylvania	700	5.0%
30	Rhode Island	100	0.7%
20	South Carolina	200	1.4%
NA	South Dakota*	NA	NA
10	Tennessee	300	2.1%
2	Texas	1,200	8.5%
30	Utah	100	0.7%
NA	Vermont*	NA	NA
10	Virginia	300	2.1%
10	Washington	300	2.1%
30	West Virginia	100	0.7%
20	Wisconsin	200	1.4%
NA	Wyoming*	NA	NA

RANK ORDER

RANK	STATE	DEATHS	% of USA
1	California	1,800	12.8%
2	Texas	1,200	8.5%
3	Florida	1,000	7.1%
3	New York	1,000	7.1%
5	Pennsylvania	700	5.0%
6	Illinois	600	4.3%
7	Michigan	500	3.5%
7	New Jersey	500	3.5%
7	Ohio	500	3.5%
10	Alabama	300	2.1%
10	Georgia	300	2.1%
10	Indiana	300	2.1%
10	Louisiana	300	2.1%
10	Massachusetts	300	2.1%
10	Missouri	300	2.1%
10	North Carolina	300	2.1%
10	Tennessee	300	2.1%
10	Virginia	300	2.1%
10	Washington	300	2.1%
20	Arizona	200	1.4%
20	Arkansas	200	1.4%
20	Connecticut	200	1.4%
20	Kentucky	200	1.4%
20	Maryland	200	1.4%
20	Minnesota	200	1.4%
20	Mississippi	200	1.4%
20	Oklahoma	200	1.4%
20	South Carolina	200	1.4%
20	Wisconsin	200	1.4%
30	Colorado	100	0.7%
30	Hawaii	100	0.7%
30	Iowa	100	0.7%
30	Kansas	100	0.7%
30	Maine	100	0.7%
30	Nebraska	100	0.7%
30	Nevada	100	0.7%
30	New Hampshire	100	0.7%
30	New Mexico	100	0.7%
30	Oregon	100	0.7%
30	Rhode Island	100	0.7%
30	Utah	100	0.7%
30	West Virginia	100	0.7%
NA	Alaska*	NA	NA
NA	Delaware*	NA	NA
NA	Idaho*	NA	NA
NA	Montana*	NA	NA
NA	North Dakota*	NA	NA
NA	South Dakota*	NA	NA
NA	Vermont*	NA	NA
NA	Wyoming*	NA	NA
	District of Columbia*	NA	NA

Source: American Cancer Society
   "Cancer Facts & Figures 2002" (Copyright 2002, Reprinted with permission from the American Cancer Society)
*Fewer than 50 deaths.

Estimated Death Rate by Liver Cancer in 2002

National Estimated Rate = 5.0 Deaths per 100,000 Population*

ALPHA ORDER				RANK ORDER		
RANK	STATE	RATE		RANK	STATE	RATE
7	Alabama	6.7		1	Rhode Island	9.4
NA	Alaska**	NA		2	Hawaii	8.2
34	Arizona	3.8		3	New Hampshire	7.9
5	Arkansas	7.4		4	Maine	7.8
20	California	5.2		5	Arkansas	7.4
42	Colorado	2.3		6	Mississippi	7.0
11	Connecticut	5.8		7	Alabama	6.7
NA	Delaware**	NA		7	Louisiana	6.7
9	Florida	6.1		9	Florida	6.1
39	Georgia	3.6		10	New Jersey	5.9
2	Hawaii	8.2		11	Connecticut	5.8
NA	Idaho**	NA		11	Nebraska	5.8
27	Illinois	4.8		11	Oklahoma	5.8
24	Indiana	4.9		14	Pennsylvania	5.7
40	Iowa	3.4		15	Texas	5.6
35	Kansas	3.7		16	New Mexico	5.5
24	Kentucky	4.9		16	West Virginia	5.5
7	Louisiana	6.7		18	Missouri	5.3
4	Maine	7.8		18	New York	5.3
35	Maryland	3.7		20	California	5.2
28	Massachusetts	4.7		20	Tennessee	5.2
22	Michigan	5.0		22	Michigan	5.0
33	Minnesota	4.0		22	Washington	5.0
6	Mississippi	7.0		24	Indiana	4.9
18	Missouri	5.3		24	Kentucky	4.9
NA	Montana**	NA		24	South Carolina	4.9
11	Nebraska	5.8		27	Illinois	4.8
28	Nevada	4.7		28	Massachusetts	4.7
3	New Hampshire	7.9		28	Nevada	4.7
10	New Jersey	5.9		30	Ohio	4.4
16	New Mexico	5.5		30	Utah	4.4
18	New York	5.3		32	Virginia	4.2
35	North Carolina	3.7		33	Minnesota	4.0
NA	North Dakota**	NA		34	Arizona	3.8
30	Ohio	4.4		35	Kansas	3.7
11	Oklahoma	5.8		35	Maryland	3.7
41	Oregon	2.9		35	North Carolina	3.7
14	Pennsylvania	5.7		35	Wisconsin	3.7
1	Rhode Island	9.4		39	Georgia	3.6
24	South Carolina	4.9		40	Iowa	3.4
NA	South Dakota**	NA		41	Oregon	2.9
20	Tennessee	5.2		42	Colorado	2.3
15	Texas	5.6		NA	Alaska**	NA
30	Utah	4.4		NA	Delaware**	NA
NA	Vermont**	NA		NA	Idaho**	NA
32	Virginia	4.2		NA	Montana**	NA
22	Washington	5.0		NA	North Dakota**	NA
16	West Virginia	5.5		NA	South Dakota**	NA
35	Wisconsin	3.7		NA	Vermont**	NA
NA	Wyoming**	NA		NA	Wyoming**	NA
					District of Columbia**	NA

Source: Morgan Quitno Press using data from American Cancer Society
    "Cancer Facts & Figures 2002" (Copyright 2002, Reprinted with permission from the American Cancer Society)
*Rates calculated using 2001 Census resident population estimates. Not age-adjusted.
**Fewer than 50 deaths.

Estimated Deaths by Lung Cancer in 2002

National Estimated Total = 154,900 Deaths

ALPHA ORDER

RANK	STATE	DEATHS	% of USA
19	Alabama	2,900	1.9%
49	Alaska	200	0.1%
22	Arizona	2,700	1.7%
27	Arkansas	2,000	1.3%
1	California	13,100	8.5%
32	Colorado	1,500	1.0%
30	Connecticut	1,800	1.2%
42	Delaware	500	0.3%
2	Florida	11,900	7.7%
11	Georgia	4,000	2.6%
42	Hawaii	500	0.3%
41	Idaho	600	0.4%
7	Illinois	6,700	4.3%
11	Indiana	4,000	2.6%
31	Iowa	1,700	1.1%
32	Kansas	1,500	1.0%
17	Kentucky	3,100	2.0%
22	Louisiana	2,700	1.7%
36	Maine	900	0.6%
19	Maryland	2,900	1.9%
16	Massachusetts	3,600	2.3%
8	Michigan	5,500	3.6%
25	Minnesota	2,300	1.5%
29	Mississippi	1,900	1.2%
14	Missouri	3,800	2.5%
42	Montana	500	0.3%
36	Nebraska	900	0.6%
35	Nevada	1,300	0.8%
38	New Hampshire	700	0.5%
10	New Jersey	4,500	2.9%
38	New Mexico	700	0.5%
4	New York	9,100	5.9%
9	North Carolina	5,000	3.2%
48	North Dakota	300	0.2%
6	Ohio	7,300	4.7%
25	Oklahoma	2,300	1.5%
27	Oregon	2,000	1.3%
5	Pennsylvania	8,000	5.2%
38	Rhode Island	700	0.5%
24	South Carolina	2,400	1.5%
45	South Dakota	400	0.3%
11	Tennessee	4,000	2.6%
3	Texas	9,900	6.4%
45	Utah	400	0.3%
45	Vermont	400	0.3%
14	Virginia	3,800	2.5%
17	Washington	3,100	2.0%
32	West Virginia	1,500	1.0%
21	Wisconsin	2,800	1.8%
49	Wyoming	200	0.1%

RANK ORDER

RANK	STATE	DEATHS	% of USA
1	California	13,100	8.5%
2	Florida	11,900	7.7%
3	Texas	9,900	6.4%
4	New York	9,100	5.9%
5	Pennsylvania	8,000	5.2%
6	Ohio	7,300	4.7%
7	Illinois	6,700	4.3%
8	Michigan	5,500	3.6%
9	North Carolina	5,000	3.2%
10	New Jersey	4,500	2.9%
11	Georgia	4,000	2.6%
11	Indiana	4,000	2.6%
11	Tennessee	4,000	2.6%
14	Missouri	3,800	2.5%
14	Virginia	3,800	2.5%
16	Massachusetts	3,600	2.3%
17	Kentucky	3,100	2.0%
17	Washington	3,100	2.0%
19	Alabama	2,900	1.9%
19	Maryland	2,900	1.9%
21	Wisconsin	2,800	1.8%
22	Arizona	2,700	1.7%
22	Louisiana	2,700	1.7%
24	South Carolina	2,400	1.5%
25	Minnesota	2,300	1.5%
25	Oklahoma	2,300	1.5%
27	Arkansas	2,000	1.3%
27	Oregon	2,000	1.3%
29	Mississippi	1,900	1.2%
30	Connecticut	1,800	1.2%
31	Iowa	1,700	1.1%
32	Colorado	1,500	1.0%
32	Kansas	1,500	1.0%
32	West Virginia	1,500	1.0%
35	Nevada	1,300	0.8%
36	Maine	900	0.6%
36	Nebraska	900	0.6%
38	New Hampshire	700	0.5%
38	New Mexico	700	0.5%
38	Rhode Island	700	0.5%
41	Idaho	600	0.4%
42	Delaware	500	0.3%
42	Hawaii	500	0.3%
42	Montana	500	0.3%
45	South Dakota	400	0.3%
45	Utah	400	0.3%
45	Vermont	400	0.3%
48	North Dakota	300	0.2%
49	Alaska	200	0.1%
49	Wyoming	200	0.1%
	District of Columbia	300	0.2%

Source: American Cancer Society
"Cancer Facts & Figures 2002" (Copyright 2002, Reprinted with permission from the American Cancer Society)

Estimated Death Rate by Lung Cancer in 2002

National Estimated Rate = 54.4 Deaths per 100,000 Population*

ALPHA ORDER

RANK	STATE	RATE
14	Alabama	65.0
49	Alaska	31.5
37	Arizona	50.9
3	Arkansas	74.3
47	California	38.0
48	Colorado	34.0
33	Connecticut	52.6
16	Delaware	62.8
4	Florida	72.6
39	Georgia	47.7
44	Hawaii	40.8
43	Idaho	45.4
29	Illinois	53.7
11	Indiana	65.4
21	Iowa	58.2
24	Kansas	55.7
2	Kentucky	76.3
19	Louisiana	60.5
5	Maine	69.9
28	Maryland	54.0
23	Massachusetts	56.4
27	Michigan	55.1
42	Minnesota	46.3
8	Mississippi	66.5
7	Missouri	67.5
26	Montana	55.3
34	Nebraska	52.5
17	Nevada	61.7
25	New Hampshire	55.6
30	New Jersey	53.0
46	New Mexico	38.3
38	New York	47.9
18	North Carolina	61.1
40	North Dakota	47.3
15	Ohio	64.2
8	Oklahoma	66.5
22	Oregon	57.6
13	Pennsylvania	65.1
10	Rhode Island	66.1
20	South Carolina	59.1
31	South Dakota	52.9
6	Tennessee	69.7
41	Texas	46.4
50	Utah	17.6
12	Vermont	65.2
31	Virginia	52.9
35	Washington	51.8
1	West Virginia	83.2
35	Wisconsin	51.8
45	Wyoming	40.5

RANK ORDER

RANK	STATE	RATE
1	West Virginia	83.2
2	Kentucky	76.3
3	Arkansas	74.3
4	Florida	72.6
5	Maine	69.9
6	Tennessee	69.7
7	Missouri	67.5
8	Mississippi	66.5
8	Oklahoma	66.5
10	Rhode Island	66.1
11	Indiana	65.4
12	Vermont	65.2
13	Pennsylvania	65.1
14	Alabama	65.0
15	Ohio	64.2
16	Delaware	62.8
17	Nevada	61.7
18	North Carolina	61.1
19	Louisiana	60.5
20	South Carolina	59.1
21	Iowa	58.2
22	Oregon	57.6
23	Massachusetts	56.4
24	Kansas	55.7
25	New Hampshire	55.6
26	Montana	55.3
27	Michigan	55.1
28	Maryland	54.0
29	Illinois	53.7
30	New Jersey	53.0
31	South Dakota	52.9
31	Virginia	52.9
33	Connecticut	52.6
34	Nebraska	52.5
35	Washington	51.8
35	Wisconsin	51.8
37	Arizona	50.9
38	New York	47.9
39	Georgia	47.7
40	North Dakota	47.3
41	Texas	46.4
42	Minnesota	46.3
43	Idaho	45.4
44	Hawaii	40.8
45	Wyoming	40.5
46	New Mexico	38.3
47	California	38.0
48	Colorado	34.0
49	Alaska	31.5
50	Utah	17.6
	District of Columbia	52.5

Source: Morgan Quitno Press using data from American Cancer Society
"Cancer Facts & Figures 2002" (Copyright 2002, Reprinted with permission from the American Cancer Society)
*Rates calculated using 2001 Census resident population estimates. Not age-adjusted.

Estimated Deaths by Non-Hodgkin's Lymphoma in 2002

National Estimated Total = 24,400 Deaths

ALPHA ORDER					RANK ORDER			
RANK	STATE	DEATHS	% of USA		RANK	STATE	DEATHS	% of USA
21	Alabama	400	1.6%		1	California	2,300	9.4%
NA	Alaska*	NA	NA		2	Florida	1,800	7.4%
15	Arizona	500	2.0%		3	New York	1,500	6.1%
25	Arkansas	300	1.2%		3	Texas	1,500	6.1%
1	California	2,300	9.4%		5	Pennsylvania	1,400	5.7%
25	Colorado	300	1.2%		6	Ohio	1,200	4.9%
25	Connecticut	300	1.2%		7	Illinois	1,100	4.5%
36	Delaware	100	0.4%		8	Michigan	900	3.7%
2	Florida	1,800	7.4%		9	New Jersey	800	3.3%
15	Georgia	500	2.0%		10	Indiana	600	2.5%
36	Hawaii	100	0.4%		10	Massachusetts	600	2.5%
36	Idaho	100	0.4%		10	North Carolina	600	2.5%
7	Illinois	1,100	4.5%		10	Virginia	600	2.5%
10	Indiana	600	2.5%		10	Wisconsin	600	2.5%
25	Iowa	300	1.2%		15	Arizona	500	2.0%
32	Kansas	200	0.8%		15	Georgia	500	2.0%
21	Kentucky	400	1.6%		15	Minnesota	500	2.0%
21	Louisiana	400	1.6%		15	Missouri	500	2.0%
36	Maine	100	0.4%		15	Tennessee	500	2.0%
21	Maryland	400	1.6%		15	Washington	500	2.0%
10	Massachusetts	600	2.5%		21	Alabama	400	1.6%
8	Michigan	900	3.7%		21	Kentucky	400	1.6%
15	Minnesota	500	2.0%		21	Louisiana	400	1.6%
32	Mississippi	200	0.8%		21	Maryland	400	1.6%
15	Missouri	500	2.0%		25	Arkansas	300	1.2%
36	Montana	100	0.4%		25	Colorado	300	1.2%
32	Nebraska	200	0.8%		25	Connecticut	300	1.2%
36	Nevada	100	0.4%		25	Iowa	300	1.2%
36	New Hampshire	100	0.4%		25	Oklahoma	300	1.2%
9	New Jersey	800	3.3%		25	Oregon	300	1.2%
36	New Mexico	100	0.4%		25	South Carolina	300	1.2%
3	New York	1,500	6.1%		32	Kansas	200	0.8%
10	North Carolina	600	2.5%		32	Mississippi	200	0.8%
36	North Dakota	100	0.4%		32	Nebraska	200	0.8%
6	Ohio	1,200	4.9%		32	West Virginia	200	0.8%
25	Oklahoma	300	1.2%		36	Delaware	100	0.4%
25	Oregon	300	1.2%		36	Hawaii	100	0.4%
5	Pennsylvania	1,400	5.7%		36	Idaho	100	0.4%
36	Rhode Island	100	0.4%		36	Maine	100	0.4%
25	South Carolina	300	1.2%		36	Montana	100	0.4%
36	South Dakota	100	0.4%		36	Nevada	100	0.4%
15	Tennessee	500	2.0%		36	New Hampshire	100	0.4%
3	Texas	1,500	6.1%		36	New Mexico	100	0.4%
36	Utah	100	0.4%		36	North Dakota	100	0.4%
36	Vermont	100	0.4%		36	Rhode Island	100	0.4%
10	Virginia	600	2.5%		36	South Dakota	100	0.4%
15	Washington	500	2.0%		36	Utah	100	0.4%
32	West Virginia	200	0.8%		36	Vermont	100	0.4%
10	Wisconsin	600	2.5%		NA	Alaska*	NA	NA
NA	Wyoming*	NA	NA		NA	Wyoming*	NA	NA
					District of Columbia*		NA	NA

Source: American Cancer Society
    "Cancer Facts & Figures 2002" (Copyright 2002, Reprinted with permission from the American Cancer Society)
*Fewer than 50 deaths.

122

Estimated Death Rate by Non-Hodgkin's Lymphoma in 2002

National Estimated Rate = 8.6 Deaths per 100,000 Population*

ALPHA ORDER

RANK	STATE	RATE
21	Alabama	9.0
NA	Alaska**	NA
17	Arizona	9.4
7	Arkansas	11.1
44	California	6.7
43	Colorado	6.8
25	Connecticut	8.8
4	Delaware	12.6
11	Florida	11.0
45	Georgia	6.0
32	Hawaii	8.2
36	Idaho	7.6
25	Illinois	8.8
15	Indiana	9.8
13	Iowa	10.3
37	Kansas	7.4
15	Kentucky	9.8
21	Louisiana	9.0
35	Maine	7.8
37	Maryland	7.4
17	Massachusetts	9.4
21	Michigan	9.0
14	Minnesota	10.1
41	Mississippi	7.0
24	Missouri	8.9
7	Montana	11.1
5	Nebraska	11.7
47	Nevada	4.7
33	New Hampshire	7.9
17	New Jersey	9.4
46	New Mexico	5.5
33	New York	7.9
40	North Carolina	7.3
2	North Dakota	15.8
12	Ohio	10.6
27	Oklahoma	8.7
29	Oregon	8.6
6	Pennsylvania	11.4
17	Rhode Island	9.4
37	South Carolina	7.4
3	South Dakota	13.2
27	Tennessee	8.7
41	Texas	7.0
48	Utah	4.4
1	Vermont	16.3
31	Virginia	8.3
30	Washington	8.4
7	West Virginia	11.1
7	Wisconsin	11.1
NA	Wyoming**	NA

RANK ORDER

RANK	STATE	RATE
1	Vermont	16.3
2	North Dakota	15.8
3	South Dakota	13.2
4	Delaware	12.6
5	Nebraska	11.7
6	Pennsylvania	11.4
7	Arkansas	11.1
7	Montana	11.1
7	West Virginia	11.1
7	Wisconsin	11.1
11	Florida	11.0
12	Ohio	10.6
13	Iowa	10.3
14	Minnesota	10.1
15	Indiana	9.8
15	Kentucky	9.8
17	Arizona	9.4
17	Massachusetts	9.4
17	New Jersey	9.4
17	Rhode Island	9.4
21	Alabama	9.0
21	Louisiana	9.0
21	Michigan	9.0
24	Missouri	8.9
25	Connecticut	8.8
25	Illinois	8.8
27	Oklahoma	8.7
27	Tennessee	8.7
29	Oregon	8.6
30	Washington	8.4
31	Virginia	8.3
32	Hawaii	8.2
33	New Hampshire	7.9
33	New York	7.9
35	Maine	7.8
36	Idaho	7.6
37	Kansas	7.4
37	Maryland	7.4
37	South Carolina	7.4
40	North Carolina	7.3
41	Mississippi	7.0
41	Texas	7.0
43	Colorado	6.8
44	California	6.7
45	Georgia	6.0
46	New Mexico	5.5
47	Nevada	4.7
48	Utah	4.4
NA	Alaska**	NA
NA	Wyoming**	NA
	District of Columbia**	NA

Source: Morgan Quitno Press using data from American Cancer Society
     "Cancer Facts & Figures 2002" (Copyright 2002, Reprinted with permission from the American Cancer Society)
*Rates calculated using 2001 Census resident population estimates. Not age-adjusted.
**Fewer than 50 deaths.

Estimated Deaths by Pancreatic Cancer in 2002

National Estimated Total = 29,700 Deaths

<table>
<tr><td colspan="4">ALPHA ORDER</td><td colspan="4">RANK ORDER</td></tr>
<tr><th>RANK</th><th>STATE</th><th>DEATHS</th><th>% of USA</th><th>RANK</th><th>STATE</th><th>DEATHS</th><th>% of USA</th></tr>
<tr><td>20</td><td>Alabama</td><td>500</td><td>1.7%</td><td>1</td><td>California</td><td>2,800</td><td>9.4%</td></tr>
<tr><td>NA</td><td>Alaska*</td><td>NA</td><td>NA</td><td>2</td><td>New York</td><td>2,200</td><td>7.4%</td></tr>
<tr><td>20</td><td>Arizona</td><td>500</td><td>1.7%</td><td>3</td><td>Florida</td><td>2,100</td><td>7.1%</td></tr>
<tr><td>29</td><td>Arkansas</td><td>300</td><td>1.0%</td><td>4</td><td>Texas</td><td>1,800</td><td>6.1%</td></tr>
<tr><td>1</td><td>California</td><td>2,800</td><td>9.4%</td><td>5</td><td>Pennsylvania</td><td>1,600</td><td>5.4%</td></tr>
<tr><td>25</td><td>Colorado</td><td>400</td><td>1.3%</td><td>6</td><td>Illinois</td><td>1,300</td><td>4.4%</td></tr>
<tr><td>25</td><td>Connecticut</td><td>400</td><td>1.3%</td><td>6</td><td>Ohio</td><td>1,300</td><td>4.4%</td></tr>
<tr><td>39</td><td>Delaware</td><td>100</td><td>0.3%</td><td>8</td><td>Michigan</td><td>1,100</td><td>3.7%</td></tr>
<tr><td>3</td><td>Florida</td><td>2,100</td><td>7.1%</td><td>9</td><td>New Jersey</td><td>1,000</td><td>3.4%</td></tr>
<tr><td>12</td><td>Georgia</td><td>700</td><td>2.4%</td><td>10</td><td>Massachusetts</td><td>800</td><td>2.7%</td></tr>
<tr><td>39</td><td>Hawaii</td><td>100</td><td>0.3%</td><td>10</td><td>North Carolina</td><td>800</td><td>2.7%</td></tr>
<tr><td>39</td><td>Idaho</td><td>100</td><td>0.3%</td><td>12</td><td>Georgia</td><td>700</td><td>2.4%</td></tr>
<tr><td>6</td><td>Illinois</td><td>1,300</td><td>4.4%</td><td>12</td><td>Virginia</td><td>700</td><td>2.4%</td></tr>
<tr><td>14</td><td>Indiana</td><td>600</td><td>2.0%</td><td>14</td><td>Indiana</td><td>600</td><td>2.0%</td></tr>
<tr><td>29</td><td>Iowa</td><td>300</td><td>1.0%</td><td>14</td><td>Maryland</td><td>600</td><td>2.0%</td></tr>
<tr><td>29</td><td>Kansas</td><td>300</td><td>1.0%</td><td>14</td><td>Missouri</td><td>600</td><td>2.0%</td></tr>
<tr><td>25</td><td>Kentucky</td><td>400</td><td>1.3%</td><td>14</td><td>Tennessee</td><td>600</td><td>2.0%</td></tr>
<tr><td>20</td><td>Louisiana</td><td>500</td><td>1.7%</td><td>14</td><td>Washington</td><td>600</td><td>2.0%</td></tr>
<tr><td>34</td><td>Maine</td><td>200</td><td>0.7%</td><td>14</td><td>Wisconsin</td><td>600</td><td>2.0%</td></tr>
<tr><td>14</td><td>Maryland</td><td>600</td><td>2.0%</td><td>20</td><td>Alabama</td><td>500</td><td>1.7%</td></tr>
<tr><td>10</td><td>Massachusetts</td><td>800</td><td>2.7%</td><td>20</td><td>Arizona</td><td>500</td><td>1.7%</td></tr>
<tr><td>8</td><td>Michigan</td><td>1,100</td><td>3.7%</td><td>20</td><td>Louisiana</td><td>500</td><td>1.7%</td></tr>
<tr><td>20</td><td>Minnesota</td><td>500</td><td>1.7%</td><td>20</td><td>Minnesota</td><td>500</td><td>1.7%</td></tr>
<tr><td>29</td><td>Mississippi</td><td>300</td><td>1.0%</td><td>20</td><td>South Carolina</td><td>500</td><td>1.7%</td></tr>
<tr><td>14</td><td>Missouri</td><td>600</td><td>2.0%</td><td>25</td><td>Colorado</td><td>400</td><td>1.3%</td></tr>
<tr><td>39</td><td>Montana</td><td>100</td><td>0.3%</td><td>25</td><td>Connecticut</td><td>400</td><td>1.3%</td></tr>
<tr><td>34</td><td>Nebraska</td><td>200</td><td>0.7%</td><td>25</td><td>Kentucky</td><td>400</td><td>1.3%</td></tr>
<tr><td>34</td><td>Nevada</td><td>200</td><td>0.7%</td><td>25</td><td>Oregon</td><td>400</td><td>1.3%</td></tr>
<tr><td>39</td><td>New Hampshire</td><td>100</td><td>0.3%</td><td>29</td><td>Arkansas</td><td>300</td><td>1.0%</td></tr>
<tr><td>9</td><td>New Jersey</td><td>1,000</td><td>3.4%</td><td>29</td><td>Iowa</td><td>300</td><td>1.0%</td></tr>
<tr><td>34</td><td>New Mexico</td><td>200</td><td>0.7%</td><td>29</td><td>Kansas</td><td>300</td><td>1.0%</td></tr>
<tr><td>2</td><td>New York</td><td>2,200</td><td>7.4%</td><td>29</td><td>Mississippi</td><td>300</td><td>1.0%</td></tr>
<tr><td>10</td><td>North Carolina</td><td>800</td><td>2.7%</td><td>29</td><td>Oklahoma</td><td>300</td><td>1.0%</td></tr>
<tr><td>39</td><td>North Dakota</td><td>100</td><td>0.3%</td><td>34</td><td>Maine</td><td>200</td><td>0.7%</td></tr>
<tr><td>6</td><td>Ohio</td><td>1,300</td><td>4.4%</td><td>34</td><td>Nebraska</td><td>200</td><td>0.7%</td></tr>
<tr><td>29</td><td>Oklahoma</td><td>300</td><td>1.0%</td><td>34</td><td>Nevada</td><td>200</td><td>0.7%</td></tr>
<tr><td>25</td><td>Oregon</td><td>400</td><td>1.3%</td><td>34</td><td>New Mexico</td><td>200</td><td>0.7%</td></tr>
<tr><td>5</td><td>Pennsylvania</td><td>1,600</td><td>5.4%</td><td>34</td><td>West Virginia</td><td>200</td><td>0.7%</td></tr>
<tr><td>39</td><td>Rhode Island</td><td>100</td><td>0.3%</td><td>39</td><td>Delaware</td><td>100</td><td>0.3%</td></tr>
<tr><td>20</td><td>South Carolina</td><td>500</td><td>1.7%</td><td>39</td><td>Hawaii</td><td>100</td><td>0.3%</td></tr>
<tr><td>39</td><td>South Dakota</td><td>100</td><td>0.3%</td><td>39</td><td>Idaho</td><td>100</td><td>0.3%</td></tr>
<tr><td>14</td><td>Tennessee</td><td>600</td><td>2.0%</td><td>39</td><td>Montana</td><td>100</td><td>0.3%</td></tr>
<tr><td>4</td><td>Texas</td><td>1,800</td><td>6.1%</td><td>39</td><td>New Hampshire</td><td>100</td><td>0.3%</td></tr>
<tr><td>39</td><td>Utah</td><td>100</td><td>0.3%</td><td>39</td><td>North Dakota</td><td>100</td><td>0.3%</td></tr>
<tr><td>39</td><td>Vermont</td><td>100</td><td>0.3%</td><td>39</td><td>Rhode Island</td><td>100</td><td>0.3%</td></tr>
<tr><td>12</td><td>Virginia</td><td>700</td><td>2.4%</td><td>39</td><td>South Dakota</td><td>100</td><td>0.3%</td></tr>
<tr><td>14</td><td>Washington</td><td>600</td><td>2.0%</td><td>39</td><td>Utah</td><td>100</td><td>0.3%</td></tr>
<tr><td>34</td><td>West Virginia</td><td>200</td><td>0.7%</td><td>39</td><td>Vermont</td><td>100</td><td>0.3%</td></tr>
<tr><td>14</td><td>Wisconsin</td><td>600</td><td>2.0%</td><td>NA</td><td>Alaska*</td><td>NA</td><td>NA</td></tr>
<tr><td>NA</td><td>Wyoming*</td><td>NA</td><td>NA</td><td>NA</td><td>Wyoming*</td><td>NA</td><td>NA</td></tr>
<tr><td></td><td></td><td></td><td></td><td></td><td>District of Columbia</td><td>100</td><td>0.3%</td></tr>
</table>

Source: American Cancer Society
"Cancer Facts & Figures 2002" (Copyright 2002, Reprinted with permission from the American Cancer Society)
*Fewer than 50 deaths.

Estimated Death Rate by Pancreatic Cancer in 2002

National Estimated Rate = 10.4 Deaths per 100,000 Population*

ALPHA ORDER

RANK	STATE	RATE
16	Alabama	11.2
NA	Alaska**	NA
38	Arizona	9.4
19	Arkansas	11.1
45	California	8.1
40	Colorado	9.1
11	Connecticut	11.7
7	Delaware	12.6
6	Florida	12.8
43	Georgia	8.3
44	Hawaii	8.2
47	Idaho	7.6
29	Illinois	10.4
33	Indiana	9.8
30	Iowa	10.3
19	Kansas	11.1
33	Kentucky	9.8
16	Louisiana	11.2
3	Maine	15.5
16	Maryland	11.2
8	Massachusetts	12.5
24	Michigan	11.0
31	Minnesota	10.1
27	Mississippi	10.5
26	Missouri	10.7
19	Montana	11.1
11	Nebraska	11.7
37	Nevada	9.5
46	New Hampshire	7.9
10	New Jersey	11.8
25	New Mexico	10.9
13	New York	11.6
33	North Carolina	9.8
2	North Dakota	15.8
15	Ohio	11.4
41	Oklahoma	8.7
14	Oregon	11.5
5	Pennsylvania	13.0
38	Rhode Island	9.4
9	South Carolina	12.3
4	South Dakota	13.2
27	Tennessee	10.5
42	Texas	8.4
48	Utah	4.4
1	Vermont	16.3
36	Virginia	9.7
32	Washington	10.0
19	West Virginia	11.1
19	Wisconsin	11.1
NA	Wyoming**	NA

RANK ORDER

RANK	STATE	RATE
1	Vermont	16.3
2	North Dakota	15.8
3	Maine	15.5
4	South Dakota	13.2
5	Pennsylvania	13.0
6	Florida	12.8
7	Delaware	12.6
8	Massachusetts	12.5
9	South Carolina	12.3
10	New Jersey	11.8
11	Connecticut	11.7
11	Nebraska	11.7
13	New York	11.6
14	Oregon	11.5
15	Ohio	11.4
16	Alabama	11.2
16	Louisiana	11.2
16	Maryland	11.2
19	Arkansas	11.1
19	Kansas	11.1
19	Montana	11.1
19	West Virginia	11.1
19	Wisconsin	11.1
24	Michigan	11.0
25	New Mexico	10.9
26	Missouri	10.7
27	Mississippi	10.5
27	Tennessee	10.5
29	Illinois	10.4
30	Iowa	10.3
31	Minnesota	10.1
32	Washington	10.0
33	Indiana	9.8
33	Kentucky	9.8
33	North Carolina	9.8
36	Virginia	9.7
37	Nevada	9.5
38	Arizona	9.4
38	Rhode Island	9.4
40	Colorado	9.1
41	Oklahoma	8.7
42	Texas	8.4
43	Georgia	8.3
44	Hawaii	8.2
45	California	8.1
46	New Hampshire	7.9
47	Idaho	7.6
48	Utah	4.4
NA	Alaska**	NA
NA	Wyoming**	NA
	District of Columbia	17.5

Source: Morgan Quitno Press using data from American Cancer Society
    "Cancer Facts & Figures 2002" (Copyright 2002, Reprinted with permission from the American Cancer Society)
*Rates calculated using 2001 Census resident population estimates. Not age-adjusted.
**Fewer than 50 deaths.

Estimated Deaths by Prostate Cancer in 2002

National Estimated Total = 30,200 Deaths

<table>
<tr><td colspan="4">ALPHA ORDER</td><td colspan="4">RANK ORDER</td></tr>
<tr><td>RANK</td><td>STATE</td><td>DEATHS</td><td>% of USA</td><td>RANK</td><td>STATE</td><td>DEATHS</td><td>% of USA</td></tr>
<tr><td>15</td><td>Alabama</td><td>600</td><td>2.0%</td><td>1</td><td>California</td><td>2,800</td><td>9.3%</td></tr>
<tr><td>NA</td><td>Alaska*</td><td>NA</td><td>NA</td><td>2</td><td>Florida</td><td>2,200</td><td>7.3%</td></tr>
<tr><td>19</td><td>Arizona</td><td>500</td><td>1.7%</td><td>3</td><td>New York</td><td>1,900</td><td>6.3%</td></tr>
<tr><td>26</td><td>Arkansas</td><td>400</td><td>1.3%</td><td>3</td><td>Texas</td><td>1,900</td><td>6.3%</td></tr>
<tr><td>1</td><td>California</td><td>2,800</td><td>9.3%</td><td>5</td><td>Pennsylvania</td><td>1,600</td><td>5.3%</td></tr>
<tr><td>26</td><td>Colorado</td><td>400</td><td>1.3%</td><td>6</td><td>Illinois</td><td>1,400</td><td>4.6%</td></tr>
<tr><td>26</td><td>Connecticut</td><td>400</td><td>1.3%</td><td>7</td><td>Ohio</td><td>1,300</td><td>4.3%</td></tr>
<tr><td>39</td><td>Delaware</td><td>100</td><td>0.3%</td><td>8</td><td>Michigan</td><td>1,100</td><td>3.6%</td></tr>
<tr><td>2</td><td>Florida</td><td>2,200</td><td>7.3%</td><td>9</td><td>New Jersey</td><td>900</td><td>3.0%</td></tr>
<tr><td>11</td><td>Georgia</td><td>800</td><td>2.6%</td><td>9</td><td>North Carolina</td><td>900</td><td>3.0%</td></tr>
<tr><td>39</td><td>Hawaii</td><td>100</td><td>0.3%</td><td>11</td><td>Georgia</td><td>800</td><td>2.6%</td></tr>
<tr><td>39</td><td>Idaho</td><td>100</td><td>0.3%</td><td>11</td><td>Virginia</td><td>800</td><td>2.6%</td></tr>
<tr><td>6</td><td>Illinois</td><td>1,400</td><td>4.6%</td><td>13</td><td>Indiana</td><td>700</td><td>2.3%</td></tr>
<tr><td>13</td><td>Indiana</td><td>700</td><td>2.3%</td><td>13</td><td>Massachusetts</td><td>700</td><td>2.3%</td></tr>
<tr><td>26</td><td>Iowa</td><td>400</td><td>1.3%</td><td>15</td><td>Alabama</td><td>600</td><td>2.0%</td></tr>
<tr><td>32</td><td>Kansas</td><td>300</td><td>1.0%</td><td>15</td><td>Missouri</td><td>600</td><td>2.0%</td></tr>
<tr><td>26</td><td>Kentucky</td><td>400</td><td>1.3%</td><td>15</td><td>Tennessee</td><td>600</td><td>2.0%</td></tr>
<tr><td>19</td><td>Louisiana</td><td>500</td><td>1.7%</td><td>15</td><td>Wisconsin</td><td>600</td><td>2.0%</td></tr>
<tr><td>39</td><td>Maine</td><td>100</td><td>0.3%</td><td>19</td><td>Arizona</td><td>500</td><td>1.7%</td></tr>
<tr><td>19</td><td>Maryland</td><td>500</td><td>1.7%</td><td>19</td><td>Louisiana</td><td>500</td><td>1.7%</td></tr>
<tr><td>13</td><td>Massachusetts</td><td>700</td><td>2.3%</td><td>19</td><td>Maryland</td><td>500</td><td>1.7%</td></tr>
<tr><td>8</td><td>Michigan</td><td>1,100</td><td>3.6%</td><td>19</td><td>Minnesota</td><td>500</td><td>1.7%</td></tr>
<tr><td>19</td><td>Minnesota</td><td>500</td><td>1.7%</td><td>19</td><td>Oregon</td><td>500</td><td>1.7%</td></tr>
<tr><td>26</td><td>Mississippi</td><td>400</td><td>1.3%</td><td>19</td><td>South Carolina</td><td>500</td><td>1.7%</td></tr>
<tr><td>15</td><td>Missouri</td><td>600</td><td>2.0%</td><td>19</td><td>Washington</td><td>500</td><td>1.7%</td></tr>
<tr><td>39</td><td>Montana</td><td>100</td><td>0.3%</td><td>26</td><td>Arkansas</td><td>400</td><td>1.3%</td></tr>
<tr><td>34</td><td>Nebraska</td><td>200</td><td>0.7%</td><td>26</td><td>Colorado</td><td>400</td><td>1.3%</td></tr>
<tr><td>34</td><td>Nevada</td><td>200</td><td>0.7%</td><td>26</td><td>Connecticut</td><td>400</td><td>1.3%</td></tr>
<tr><td>39</td><td>New Hampshire</td><td>100</td><td>0.3%</td><td>26</td><td>Iowa</td><td>400</td><td>1.3%</td></tr>
<tr><td>9</td><td>New Jersey</td><td>900</td><td>3.0%</td><td>26</td><td>Kentucky</td><td>400</td><td>1.3%</td></tr>
<tr><td>34</td><td>New Mexico</td><td>200</td><td>0.7%</td><td>26</td><td>Mississippi</td><td>400</td><td>1.3%</td></tr>
<tr><td>3</td><td>New York</td><td>1,900</td><td>6.3%</td><td>32</td><td>Kansas</td><td>300</td><td>1.0%</td></tr>
<tr><td>9</td><td>North Carolina</td><td>900</td><td>3.0%</td><td>32</td><td>Oklahoma</td><td>300</td><td>1.0%</td></tr>
<tr><td>39</td><td>North Dakota</td><td>100</td><td>0.3%</td><td>34</td><td>Nebraska</td><td>200</td><td>0.7%</td></tr>
<tr><td>7</td><td>Ohio</td><td>1,300</td><td>4.3%</td><td>34</td><td>Nevada</td><td>200</td><td>0.7%</td></tr>
<tr><td>32</td><td>Oklahoma</td><td>300</td><td>1.0%</td><td>34</td><td>New Mexico</td><td>200</td><td>0.7%</td></tr>
<tr><td>19</td><td>Oregon</td><td>500</td><td>1.7%</td><td>34</td><td>Utah</td><td>200</td><td>0.7%</td></tr>
<tr><td>5</td><td>Pennsylvania</td><td>1,600</td><td>5.3%</td><td>34</td><td>West Virginia</td><td>200</td><td>0.7%</td></tr>
<tr><td>39</td><td>Rhode Island</td><td>100</td><td>0.3%</td><td>39</td><td>Delaware</td><td>100</td><td>0.3%</td></tr>
<tr><td>19</td><td>South Carolina</td><td>500</td><td>1.7%</td><td>39</td><td>Hawaii</td><td>100</td><td>0.3%</td></tr>
<tr><td>39</td><td>South Dakota</td><td>100</td><td>0.3%</td><td>39</td><td>Idaho</td><td>100</td><td>0.3%</td></tr>
<tr><td>15</td><td>Tennessee</td><td>600</td><td>2.0%</td><td>39</td><td>Maine</td><td>100</td><td>0.3%</td></tr>
<tr><td>3</td><td>Texas</td><td>1,900</td><td>6.3%</td><td>39</td><td>Montana</td><td>100</td><td>0.3%</td></tr>
<tr><td>34</td><td>Utah</td><td>200</td><td>0.7%</td><td>39</td><td>New Hampshire</td><td>100</td><td>0.3%</td></tr>
<tr><td>39</td><td>Vermont</td><td>100</td><td>0.3%</td><td>39</td><td>North Dakota</td><td>100</td><td>0.3%</td></tr>
<tr><td>11</td><td>Virginia</td><td>800</td><td>2.6%</td><td>39</td><td>Rhode Island</td><td>100</td><td>0.3%</td></tr>
<tr><td>19</td><td>Washington</td><td>500</td><td>1.7%</td><td>39</td><td>South Dakota</td><td>100</td><td>0.3%</td></tr>
<tr><td>34</td><td>West Virginia</td><td>200</td><td>0.7%</td><td>39</td><td>Vermont</td><td>100</td><td>0.3%</td></tr>
<tr><td>15</td><td>Wisconsin</td><td>600</td><td>2.0%</td><td>39</td><td>Wyoming</td><td>100</td><td>0.3%</td></tr>
<tr><td>39</td><td>Wyoming</td><td>100</td><td>0.3%</td><td>NA</td><td>Alaska*</td><td>NA</td><td>NA</td></tr>
<tr><td></td><td></td><td></td><td></td><td></td><td>District of Columbia</td><td>100</td><td>0.3%</td></tr>
</table>

Source: American Cancer Society
  "Cancer Facts & Figures 2002" (Copyright 2002, Reprinted with permission from the American Cancer Society)
*Fewer than 50 deaths.

Estimated Death Rate by Prostate Cancer in 2002

National Estimated Rate = 21.9 Deaths per 100,000 Male Population*

ALPHA ORDER

RANK	STATE	RATE
8	Alabama	28.0
NA	Alaska**	NA
38	Arizona	19.5
4	Arkansas	30.7
45	California	16.6
40	Colorado	18.5
14	Connecticut	24.3
12	Delaware	26.3
7	Florida	28.2
35	Georgia	19.9
47	Hawaii	16.4
49	Idaho	15.4
19	Illinois	23.0
17	Indiana	23.5
9	Iowa	27.9
24	Kansas	22.6
34	Kentucky	20.2
18	Louisiana	23.1
48	Maine	16.1
38	Maryland	19.5
21	Massachusetts	22.9
24	Michigan	22.6
33	Minnesota	20.5
6	Mississippi	29.1
29	Missouri	22.1
28	Montana	22.2
15	Nebraska	23.7
37	Nevada	19.6
46	New Hampshire	16.5
30	New Jersey	22.0
27	New Mexico	22.4
32	New York	20.8
22	North Carolina	22.8
3	North Dakota	31.2
16	Ohio	23.6
43	Oklahoma	17.7
5	Oregon	29.5
10	Pennsylvania	27.0
35	Rhode Island	19.9
13	South Carolina	25.7
11	South Dakota	26.7
31	Tennessee	21.7
41	Texas	18.4
42	Utah	17.9
2	Vermont	33.5
19	Virginia	23.0
44	Washington	17.0
23	West Virginia	22.7
24	Wisconsin	22.6
1	Wyoming	40.3

RANK ORDER

RANK	STATE	RATE
1	Wyoming	40.3
2	Vermont	33.5
3	North Dakota	31.2
4	Arkansas	30.7
5	Oregon	29.5
6	Mississippi	29.1
7	Florida	28.2
8	Alabama	28.0
9	Iowa	27.9
10	Pennsylvania	27.0
11	South Dakota	26.7
12	Delaware	26.3
13	South Carolina	25.7
14	Connecticut	24.3
15	Nebraska	23.7
16	Ohio	23.6
17	Indiana	23.5
18	Louisiana	23.1
19	Illinois	23.0
19	Virginia	23.0
21	Massachusetts	22.9
22	North Carolina	22.8
23	West Virginia	22.7
24	Kansas	22.6
24	Michigan	22.6
24	Wisconsin	22.6
27	New Mexico	22.4
28	Montana	22.2
29	Missouri	22.1
30	New Jersey	22.0
31	Tennessee	21.7
32	New York	20.8
33	Minnesota	20.5
34	Kentucky	20.2
35	Georgia	19.9
35	Rhode Island	19.9
37	Nevada	19.6
38	Arizona	19.5
38	Maryland	19.5
40	Colorado	18.5
41	Texas	18.4
42	Utah	17.9
43	Oklahoma	17.7
44	Washington	17.0
45	California	16.6
46	New Hampshire	16.5
47	Hawaii	16.4
48	Maine	16.1
49	Idaho	15.4
NA	Alaska**	NA
	District of Columbia	37.1

Source: Morgan Quitno Press using data from American Cancer Society
   "Cancer Facts & Figures 2002" (Copyright 2002, Reprinted with permission from the American Cancer Society)
*Rates calculated using 2000 Census resident male population figures. Not age-adjusted.
**Fewer than 50 deaths.

Estimated Deaths by Ovarian Cancer in 2002

National Estimated Total = 13,900 Deaths

ALPHA ORDER

RANK	STATE	DEATHS	% of USA
19	Alabama	200	1.4%
NA	Alaska*	NA	NA
19	Arizona	200	1.4%
30	Arkansas	100	0.7%
1	California	1,400	10.1%
19	Colorado	200	1.4%
19	Connecticut	200	1.4%
NA	Delaware*	NA	NA
2	Florida	1,000	7.2%
10	Georgia	400	2.9%
NA	Hawaii*	NA	NA
30	Idaho	100	0.7%
6	Illinois	600	4.3%
12	Indiana	300	2.2%
19	Iowa	200	1.4%
30	Kansas	100	0.7%
19	Kentucky	200	1.4%
19	Louisiana	200	1.4%
30	Maine	100	0.7%
19	Maryland	200	1.4%
12	Massachusetts	300	2.2%
8	Michigan	500	3.6%
19	Minnesota	200	1.4%
30	Mississippi	100	0.7%
12	Missouri	300	2.2%
30	Montana	100	0.7%
30	Nebraska	100	0.7%
30	Nevada	100	0.7%
30	New Hampshire	100	0.7%
8	New Jersey	500	3.6%
30	New Mexico	100	0.7%
3	New York	900	6.5%
10	North Carolina	400	2.9%
NA	North Dakota*	NA	NA
6	Ohio	600	4.3%
30	Oklahoma	100	0.7%
19	Oregon	200	1.4%
5	Pennsylvania	700	5.0%
30	Rhode Island	100	0.7%
19	South Carolina	200	1.4%
30	South Dakota	100	0.7%
12	Tennessee	300	2.2%
4	Texas	800	5.8%
30	Utah	100	0.7%
NA	Vermont*	NA	NA
12	Virginia	300	2.2%
12	Washington	300	2.2%
30	West Virginia	100	0.7%
12	Wisconsin	300	2.2%
NA	Wyoming*	NA	NA

RANK ORDER

RANK	STATE	DEATHS	% of USA
1	California	1,400	10.1%
2	Florida	1,000	7.2%
3	New York	900	6.5%
4	Texas	800	5.8%
5	Pennsylvania	700	5.0%
6	Illinois	600	4.3%
6	Ohio	600	4.3%
8	Michigan	500	3.6%
8	New Jersey	500	3.6%
10	Georgia	400	2.9%
10	North Carolina	400	2.9%
12	Indiana	300	2.2%
12	Massachusetts	300	2.2%
12	Missouri	300	2.2%
12	Tennessee	300	2.2%
12	Virginia	300	2.2%
12	Washington	300	2.2%
12	Wisconsin	300	2.2%
19	Alabama	200	1.4%
19	Arizona	200	1.4%
19	Colorado	200	1.4%
19	Connecticut	200	1.4%
19	Iowa	200	1.4%
19	Kentucky	200	1.4%
19	Louisiana	200	1.4%
19	Maryland	200	1.4%
19	Minnesota	200	1.4%
19	Oregon	200	1.4%
19	South Carolina	200	1.4%
30	Arkansas	100	0.7%
30	Idaho	100	0.7%
30	Kansas	100	0.7%
30	Maine	100	0.7%
30	Mississippi	100	0.7%
30	Montana	100	0.7%
30	Nebraska	100	0.7%
30	Nevada	100	0.7%
30	New Hampshire	100	0.7%
30	New Mexico	100	0.7%
30	Oklahoma	100	0.7%
30	Rhode Island	100	0.7%
30	South Dakota	100	0.7%
30	Utah	100	0.7%
30	West Virginia	100	0.7%
NA	Alaska*	NA	NA
NA	Delaware*	NA	NA
NA	Hawaii*	NA	NA
NA	North Dakota*	NA	NA
NA	Vermont*	NA	NA
NA	Wyoming*	NA	NA
	District of Columbia*	NA	NA

Source: American Cancer Society
 "Cancer Facts & Figures 2002" (Copyright 2002, Reprinted with permission from the American Cancer Society)
*Fewer than 50 deaths.

Estimated Death Rate by Ovarian Cancer in 2002

National Estimated Rate = 9.7 Deaths per 100,000 Female Population*

ALPHA ORDER

RANK	STATE	RATE
33	Alabama	8.7
NA	Alaska**	NA
38	Arizona	7.8
41	Arkansas	7.3
36	California	8.2
29	Colorado	9.4
12	Connecticut	11.4
NA	Delaware**	NA
8	Florida	12.2
27	Georgia	9.6
NA	Hawaii**	NA
5	Idaho	15.5
28	Illinois	9.5
23	Indiana	9.7
7	Iowa	13.4
40	Kansas	7.4
23	Kentucky	9.7
33	Louisiana	8.7
6	Maine	15.3
41	Maryland	7.3
31	Massachusetts	9.1
22	Michigan	9.9
37	Minnesota	8.1
43	Mississippi	6.8
17	Missouri	10.4
2	Montana	22.1
10	Nebraska	11.5
20	Nevada	10.2
4	New Hampshire	15.9
10	New Jersey	11.5
15	New Mexico	10.8
30	New York	9.2
23	North Carolina	9.7
NA	North Dakota**	NA
18	Ohio	10.3
44	Oklahoma	5.7
9	Oregon	11.6
14	Pennsylvania	11.0
3	Rhode Island	18.4
23	South Carolina	9.7
1	South Dakota	26.3
18	Tennessee	10.3
39	Texas	7.6
32	Utah	9.0
NA	Vermont**	NA
35	Virginia	8.3
21	Washington	10.1
15	West Virginia	10.8
13	Wisconsin	11.1
NA	Wyoming**	NA

RANK ORDER

RANK	STATE	RATE
1	South Dakota	26.3
2	Montana	22.1
3	Rhode Island	18.4
4	New Hampshire	15.9
5	Idaho	15.5
6	Maine	15.3
7	Iowa	13.4
8	Florida	12.2
9	Oregon	11.6
10	Nebraska	11.5
10	New Jersey	11.5
12	Connecticut	11.4
13	Wisconsin	11.1
14	Pennsylvania	11.0
15	New Mexico	10.8
15	West Virginia	10.8
17	Missouri	10.4
18	Ohio	10.3
18	Tennessee	10.3
20	Nevada	10.2
21	Washington	10.1
22	Michigan	9.9
23	Indiana	9.7
23	Kentucky	9.7
23	North Carolina	9.7
23	South Carolina	9.7
27	Georgia	9.6
28	Illinois	9.5
29	Colorado	9.4
30	New York	9.2
31	Massachusetts	9.1
32	Utah	9.0
33	Alabama	8.7
33	Louisiana	8.7
35	Virginia	8.3
36	California	8.2
37	Minnesota	8.1
38	Arizona	7.8
39	Texas	7.6
40	Kansas	7.4
41	Arkansas	7.3
41	Maryland	7.3
43	Mississippi	6.8
44	Oklahoma	5.7
NA	Alaska**	NA
NA	Delaware**	NA
NA	Hawaii**	NA
NA	North Dakota**	NA
NA	Vermont**	NA
NA	Wyoming**	NA
	District of Columbia**	NA

Source: Morgan Quitno Press using data from American Cancer Society
   "Cancer Facts & Figures 2002" (Copyright 2002, Reprinted with permission from the American Cancer Society)
*Rates calculated using 2000 Census resident female population figures. Not age-adjusted.
**Fewer than 50 deaths.

Estimated Deaths by Brain Cancer in 2002

National Estimated Total = 13,100 Deaths

ALPHA ORDER

RANK	STATE	DEATHS	% of USA
19	Alabama	200	1.5%
NA	Alaska*	NA	NA
19	Arizona	200	1.5%
19	Arkansas	200	1.5%
1	California	1,500	11.5%
19	Colorado	200	1.5%
31	Connecticut	100	0.8%
NA	Delaware*	NA	NA
2	Florida	900	6.9%
11	Georgia	300	2.3%
NA	Hawaii*	NA	NA
31	Idaho	100	0.8%
7	Illinois	500	3.8%
11	Indiana	300	2.3%
19	Iowa	200	1.5%
31	Kansas	100	0.8%
19	Kentucky	200	1.5%
19	Louisiana	200	1.5%
31	Maine	100	0.8%
19	Maryland	200	1.5%
11	Massachusetts	300	2.3%
8	Michigan	400	3.1%
19	Minnesota	200	1.5%
19	Mississippi	200	1.5%
11	Missouri	300	2.3%
NA	Montana*	NA	NA
31	Nebraska	100	0.8%
31	Nevada	100	0.8%
31	New Hampshire	100	0.8%
8	New Jersey	400	3.1%
31	New Mexico	100	0.8%
4	New York	800	6.1%
8	North Carolina	400	3.1%
NA	North Dakota*	NA	NA
5	Ohio	600	4.6%
31	Oklahoma	100	0.8%
19	Oregon	200	1.5%
5	Pennsylvania	600	4.6%
31	Rhode Island	100	0.8%
19	South Carolina	200	1.5%
31	South Dakota	100	0.8%
11	Tennessee	300	2.3%
2	Texas	900	6.9%
31	Utah	100	0.8%
NA	Vermont*	NA	NA
11	Virginia	300	2.3%
11	Washington	300	2.3%
31	West Virginia	100	0.8%
11	Wisconsin	300	2.3%
NA	Wyoming*	NA	NA

RANK ORDER

RANK	STATE	DEATHS	% of USA
1	California	1,500	11.5%
2	Florida	900	6.9%
2	Texas	900	6.9%
4	New York	800	6.1%
5	Ohio	600	4.6%
5	Pennsylvania	600	4.6%
7	Illinois	500	3.8%
8	Michigan	400	3.1%
8	New Jersey	400	3.1%
8	North Carolina	400	3.1%
11	Georgia	300	2.3%
11	Indiana	300	2.3%
11	Massachusetts	300	2.3%
11	Missouri	300	2.3%
11	Tennessee	300	2.3%
11	Virginia	300	2.3%
11	Washington	300	2.3%
11	Wisconsin	300	2.3%
19	Alabama	200	1.5%
19	Arizona	200	1.5%
19	Arkansas	200	1.5%
19	Colorado	200	1.5%
19	Iowa	200	1.5%
19	Kentucky	200	1.5%
19	Louisiana	200	1.5%
19	Maryland	200	1.5%
19	Minnesota	200	1.5%
19	Mississippi	200	1.5%
19	Oregon	200	1.5%
19	South Carolina	200	1.5%
31	Connecticut	100	0.8%
31	Idaho	100	0.8%
31	Kansas	100	0.8%
31	Maine	100	0.8%
31	Nebraska	100	0.8%
31	Nevada	100	0.8%
31	New Hampshire	100	0.8%
31	New Mexico	100	0.8%
31	Oklahoma	100	0.8%
31	Rhode Island	100	0.8%
31	South Dakota	100	0.8%
31	Utah	100	0.8%
31	West Virginia	100	0.8%
NA	Alaska*	NA	NA
NA	Delaware*	NA	NA
NA	Hawaii*	NA	NA
NA	Montana*	NA	NA
NA	North Dakota*	NA	NA
NA	Vermont*	NA	NA
NA	Wyoming*	NA	NA
	District of Columbia*	NA	NA

Source: American Cancer Society
   "Cancer Facts & Figures 2002" (Copyright 2002, Reprinted with permission from the American Cancer Society)
*Fewer than 50 deaths.

Estimated Death Rate by Brain Cancer in 2002

National Estimated Rate = 4.6 Deaths per 100,000 Population*

ALPHA ORDER			RANK ORDER		
RANK	STATE	RATE	RANK	STATE	RATE
27	Alabama	4.5	1	South Dakota	13.2
NA	Alaska**	NA	2	Rhode Island	9.4
38	Arizona	3.8	3	New Hampshire	7.9
6	Arkansas	7.4	4	Maine	7.8
31	California	4.3	5	Idaho	7.6
27	Colorado	4.5	6	Arkansas	7.4
42	Connecticut	2.9	7	Mississippi	7.0
NA	Delaware**	NA	8	Iowa	6.8
12	Florida	5.5	9	Nebraska	5.8
41	Georgia	3.6	9	Oregon	5.8
NA	Hawaii**	NA	11	Wisconsin	5.6
5	Idaho	7.6	12	Florida	5.5
35	Illinois	4.0	12	New Mexico	5.5
19	Indiana	4.9	12	West Virginia	5.5
8	Iowa	6.8	15	Missouri	5.3
39	Kansas	3.7	15	Ohio	5.3
19	Kentucky	4.9	17	Tennessee	5.2
27	Louisiana	4.5	18	Washington	5.0
4	Maine	7.8	19	Indiana	4.9
39	Maryland	3.7	19	Kentucky	4.9
24	Massachusetts	4.7	19	North Carolina	4.9
35	Michigan	4.0	19	Pennsylvania	4.9
35	Minnesota	4.0	19	South Carolina	4.9
7	Mississippi	7.0	24	Massachusetts	4.7
15	Missouri	5.3	24	Nevada	4.7
NA	Montana**	NA	24	New Jersey	4.7
9	Nebraska	5.8	27	Alabama	4.5
24	Nevada	4.7	27	Colorado	4.5
3	New Hampshire	7.9	27	Louisiana	4.5
24	New Jersey	4.7	30	Utah	4.4
12	New Mexico	5.5	31	California	4.3
32	New York	4.2	32	New York	4.2
19	North Carolina	4.9	32	Texas	4.2
NA	North Dakota**	NA	32	Virginia	4.2
15	Ohio	5.3	35	Illinois	4.0
42	Oklahoma	2.9	35	Michigan	4.0
9	Oregon	5.8	35	Minnesota	4.0
19	Pennsylvania	4.9	38	Arizona	3.8
2	Rhode Island	9.4	39	Kansas	3.7
19	South Carolina	4.9	39	Maryland	3.7
1	South Dakota	13.2	41	Georgia	3.6
17	Tennessee	5.2	42	Connecticut	2.9
32	Texas	4.2	42	Oklahoma	2.9
30	Utah	4.4	NA	Alaska**	NA
NA	Vermont**	NA	NA	Delaware**	NA
32	Virginia	4.2	NA	Hawaii**	NA
18	Washington	5.0	NA	Montana**	NA
12	West Virginia	5.5	NA	North Dakota**	NA
11	Wisconsin	5.6	NA	Vermont**	NA
NA	Wyoming**	NA	NA	Wyoming**	NA
				District of Columbia**	NA

Source: Morgan Quitno Press using data from American Cancer Society
"Cancer Facts & Figures 2002" (Copyright 2002, Reprinted with permission from the American Cancer Society)
Rates calculated using 2001 Census resident population estimates. Not age-adjusted.
**Fewer than 50 deaths.*

Deaths by Alzheimer's Disease in 1999

National Total = 44,536 Deaths*

ALPHA ORDER

RANK	STATE	DEATHS	% of USA
22	Alabama	772	1.7%
50	Alaska	24	0.1%
17	Arizona	963	2.2%
32	Arkansas	434	1.0%
1	California	4,532	10.2%
23	Colorado	756	1.7%
31	Connecticut	449	1.0%
48	Delaware	107	0.2%
2	Florida	3,059	6.9%
15	Georgia	1,080	2.4%
47	Hawaii	109	0.2%
40	Idaho	243	0.5%
6	Illinois	1,908	4.3%
13	Indiana	1,106	2.5%
25	Iowa	706	1.6%
30	Kansas	511	1.1%
24	Kentucky	728	1.6%
27	Louisiana	683	1.5%
33	Maine	429	1.0%
28	Maryland	681	1.5%
11	Massachusetts	1,182	2.7%
9	Michigan	1,431	3.2%
14	Minnesota	1,083	2.4%
34	Mississippi	356	0.8%
20	Missouri	914	2.1%
42	Montana	205	0.5%
35	Nebraska	331	0.7%
43	Nevada	174	0.4%
37	New Hampshire	266	0.6%
16	New Jersey	1,041	2.3%
38	New Mexico	248	0.6%
10	New York	1,357	3.0%
8	North Carolina	1,456	3.3%
44	North Dakota	155	0.3%
5	Ohio	2,099	4.7%
29	Oklahoma	553	1.2%
21	Oregon	866	1.9%
4	Pennsylvania	2,192	4.9%
41	Rhode Island	219	0.5%
26	South Carolina	690	1.5%
44	South Dakota	155	0.3%
18	Tennessee	944	2.1%
3	Texas	2,833	6.4%
39	Utah	245	0.6%
46	Vermont	127	0.3%
19	Virginia	917	2.1%
7	Washington	1,577	3.5%
36	West Virginia	314	0.7%
12	Wisconsin	1,170	2.6%
49	Wyoming	103	0.2%

RANK ORDER

RANK	STATE	DEATHS	% of USA
1	California	4,532	10.2%
2	Florida	3,059	6.9%
3	Texas	2,833	6.4%
4	Pennsylvania	2,192	4.9%
5	Ohio	2,099	4.7%
6	Illinois	1,908	4.3%
7	Washington	1,577	3.5%
8	North Carolina	1,456	3.3%
9	Michigan	1,431	3.2%
10	New York	1,357	3.0%
11	Massachusetts	1,182	2.7%
12	Wisconsin	1,170	2.6%
13	Indiana	1,106	2.5%
14	Minnesota	1,083	2.4%
15	Georgia	1,080	2.4%
16	New Jersey	1,041	2.3%
17	Arizona	963	2.2%
18	Tennessee	944	2.1%
19	Virginia	917	2.1%
20	Missouri	914	2.1%
21	Oregon	866	1.9%
22	Alabama	772	1.7%
23	Colorado	756	1.7%
24	Kentucky	728	1.6%
25	Iowa	706	1.6%
26	South Carolina	690	1.5%
27	Louisiana	683	1.5%
28	Maryland	681	1.5%
29	Oklahoma	553	1.2%
30	Kansas	511	1.1%
31	Connecticut	449	1.0%
32	Arkansas	434	1.0%
33	Maine	429	1.0%
34	Mississippi	356	0.8%
35	Nebraska	331	0.7%
36	West Virginia	314	0.7%
37	New Hampshire	266	0.6%
38	New Mexico	248	0.6%
39	Utah	245	0.6%
40	Idaho	243	0.5%
41	Rhode Island	219	0.5%
42	Montana	205	0.5%
43	Nevada	174	0.4%
44	North Dakota	155	0.3%
44	South Dakota	155	0.3%
46	Vermont	127	0.3%
47	Hawaii	109	0.2%
48	Delaware	107	0.2%
49	Wyoming	103	0.2%
50	Alaska	24	0.1%
	District of Columbia	53	0.1%

Source: U.S. Department of Health and Human Services, National Center for Health Statistics
"National Vital Statistics Reports" (Vol. 49, No. 8, September 21, 2001)
Final data by state of residence. A degenerative disease of the brain cells producing loss of memory and general intellectual impairment. It usually affects people over age 65. As the disease progresses, a variety of symptoms may become apparent, including confusion, irritability, and restlessness, as well as disorientation and impaired judgment and concentration.

Death Rate by Alzheimer's Disease in 1999

National Rate = 16.3 Deaths per 100,000 Population*

ALPHA ORDER

RANK	STATE	RATE
27	Alabama	17.7
50	Alaska	3.9
14	Arizona	20.2
30	Arkansas	17.0
40	California	13.7
21	Colorado	18.6
40	Connecticut	13.7
37	Delaware	14.2
14	Florida	20.2
39	Georgia	13.9
48	Hawaii	9.2
17	Idaho	19.4
33	Illinois	15.7
21	Indiana	18.6
4	Iowa	24.6
18	Kansas	19.3
24	Kentucky	18.4
34	Louisiana	15.6
1	Maine	34.2
43	Maryland	13.2
19	Massachusetts	19.1
35	Michigan	14.5
7	Minnesota	22.7
44	Mississippi	12.9
31	Missouri	16.7
6	Montana	23.2
16	Nebraska	19.9
47	Nevada	9.6
9	New Hampshire	22.1
45	New Jersey	12.8
36	New Mexico	14.3
49	New York	7.5
20	North Carolina	19.0
5	North Dakota	24.5
21	Ohio	18.6
32	Oklahoma	16.5
3	Oregon	26.1
25	Pennsylvania	18.3
9	Rhode Island	22.1
26	South Carolina	17.8
13	South Dakota	21.1
29	Tennessee	17.2
38	Texas	14.1
46	Utah	11.5
12	Vermont	21.4
42	Virginia	13.3
2	Washington	27.4
28	West Virginia	17.4
8	Wisconsin	22.3
11	Wyoming	21.5

RANK ORDER

RANK	STATE	RATE
1	Maine	34.2
2	Washington	27.4
3	Oregon	26.1
4	Iowa	24.6
5	North Dakota	24.5
6	Montana	23.2
7	Minnesota	22.7
8	Wisconsin	22.3
9	New Hampshire	22.1
9	Rhode Island	22.1
11	Wyoming	21.5
12	Vermont	21.4
13	South Dakota	21.1
14	Arizona	20.2
14	Florida	20.2
16	Nebraska	19.9
17	Idaho	19.4
18	Kansas	19.3
19	Massachusetts	19.1
20	North Carolina	19.0
21	Colorado	18.6
21	Indiana	18.6
21	Ohio	18.6
24	Kentucky	18.4
25	Pennsylvania	18.3
26	South Carolina	17.8
27	Alabama	17.7
28	West Virginia	17.4
29	Tennessee	17.2
30	Arkansas	17.0
31	Missouri	16.7
32	Oklahoma	16.5
33	Illinois	15.7
34	Louisiana	15.6
35	Michigan	14.5
36	New Mexico	14.3
37	Delaware	14.2
38	Texas	14.1
39	Georgia	13.9
40	California	13.7
40	Connecticut	13.7
42	Virginia	13.3
43	Maryland	13.2
44	Mississippi	12.9
45	New Jersey	12.8
46	Utah	11.5
47	Nevada	9.6
48	Hawaii	9.2
49	New York	7.5
50	Alaska	3.9
	District of Columbia	10.2

Source: U.S. Department of Health and Human Services, National Center for Health Statistics
"National Vital Statistics Reports" (Vol. 49, No. 8, September 21, 2001)
*Final data by state of residence. A degenerative disease of the brain cells producing loss of memory and general intellectual impairment. It usually affects people over age 65. As the disease progresses, a variety of symptoms may become apparent, including confusion, irritability, and restlessness, as well as disorientation and impaired judgment and concentration. Not age-adjusted.

Age-Adjusted Death Rate by Alzheimer's Disease in 1999

National Rate = 16.5 Deaths per 100,000 Population*

ALPHA ORDER

RANK	STATE	RATE
24	Alabama	18.0
47	Alaska	11.8
9	Arizona	21.2
36	Arkansas	15.3
32	California	16.2
3	Colorado	24.4
48	Connecticut	11.4
36	Delaware	15.3
43	Florida	14.4
16	Georgia	19.1
49	Hawaii	9.3
9	Idaho	21.2
34	Illinois	15.7
17	Indiana	19.0
19	Iowa	18.4
27	Kansas	16.6
15	Kentucky	19.4
19	Louisiana	18.4
1	Maine	30.7
36	Maryland	15.3
29	Massachusetts	16.4
39	Michigan	15.1
7	Minnesota	21.3
44	Mississippi	13.7
40	Missouri	15.0
7	Montana	21.3
29	Nebraska	16.4
44	Nevada	13.7
6	New Hampshire	23.3
46	New Jersey	12.0
26	New Mexico	17.1
50	New York	7.0
13	North Carolina	20.7
22	North Dakota	18.2
23	Ohio	18.1
35	Oklahoma	15.5
5	Oregon	24.1
42	Pennsylvania	14.5
27	Rhode Island	16.6
11	South Carolina	21.1
29	South Dakota	16.4
21	Tennessee	18.3
18	Texas	18.6
25	Utah	17.2
11	Vermont	21.1
33	Virginia	16.1
2	Washington	29.7
40	West Virginia	15.0
14	Wisconsin	20.0
4	Wyoming	24.3

RANK ORDER

RANK	STATE	RATE
1	Maine	30.7
2	Washington	29.7
3	Colorado	24.4
4	Wyoming	24.3
5	Oregon	24.1
6	New Hampshire	23.3
7	Minnesota	21.3
7	Montana	21.3
9	Arizona	21.2
9	Idaho	21.2
11	South Carolina	21.1
11	Vermont	21.1
13	North Carolina	20.7
14	Wisconsin	20.0
15	Kentucky	19.4
16	Georgia	19.1
17	Indiana	19.0
18	Texas	18.6
19	Iowa	18.4
19	Louisiana	18.4
21	Tennessee	18.3
22	North Dakota	18.2
23	Ohio	18.1
24	Alabama	18.0
25	Utah	17.2
26	New Mexico	17.1
27	Kansas	16.6
27	Rhode Island	16.6
29	Massachusetts	16.4
29	Nebraska	16.4
29	South Dakota	16.4
32	California	16.2
33	Virginia	16.1
34	Illinois	15.7
35	Oklahoma	15.5
36	Arkansas	15.3
36	Delaware	15.3
36	Maryland	15.3
39	Michigan	15.1
40	Missouri	15.0
40	West Virginia	15.0
42	Pennsylvania	14.5
43	Florida	14.4
44	Mississippi	13.7
44	Nevada	13.7
46	New Jersey	12.0
47	Alaska	11.8
48	Connecticut	11.4
49	Hawaii	9.3
50	New York	7.0

District of Columbia 9.2

Source: U.S. Department of Health and Human Services, National Center for Health Statistics
"National Vital Statistics Reports" (Vol. 49, No. 8, September 21, 2001)
*Final data by state of residence. A degenerative disease of the brain cells producing loss of memory and general intellectual impairment. It usually affects people over age 65. As the disease progresses, a variety of symptoms may become apparent, including confusion, irritability, and restlessness, as well as disorientation and impaired judgment and concentration. Age-adjusted rates based on the year 2000 standard population.

Deaths by Atherosclerosis in 1999

National Total = 14,979 Deaths*

ALPHA ORDER

RANK	STATE	DEATHS	% of USA
25	Alabama	215	1.4%
49	Alaska	15	0.1%
21	Arizona	278	1.9%
33	Arkansas	156	1.0%
1	California	1,825	12.2%
9	Colorado	484	3.2%
30	Connecticut	170	1.1%
49	Delaware	15	0.1%
2	Florida	1,035	6.9%
11	Georgia	463	3.1%
45	Hawaii	32	0.2%
42	Idaho	46	0.3%
7	Illinois	611	4.1%
14	Indiana	404	2.7%
17	Iowa	326	2.2%
15	Kansas	345	2.3%
31	Kentucky	159	1.1%
24	Louisiana	219	1.5%
44	Maine	39	0.3%
28	Maryland	187	1.2%
19	Massachusetts	322	2.1%
8	Michigan	579	3.9%
26	Minnesota	209	1.4%
35	Mississippi	101	0.7%
20	Missouri	315	2.1%
41	Montana	51	0.3%
32	Nebraska	158	1.1%
40	Nevada	60	0.4%
38	New Hampshire	74	0.5%
12	New Jersey	439	2.9%
36	New Mexico	81	0.5%
5	New York	638	4.3%
13	North Carolina	423	2.8%
43	North Dakota	45	0.3%
6	Ohio	626	4.2%
10	Oklahoma	476	3.2%
27	Oregon	199	1.3%
4	Pennsylvania	641	4.3%
37	Rhode Island	77	0.5%
34	South Carolina	104	0.7%
45	South Dakota	32	0.2%
18	Tennessee	323	2.2%
3	Texas	838	5.6%
39	Utah	70	0.5%
47	Vermont	20	0.1%
22	Virginia	249	1.7%
15	Washington	345	2.3%
29	West Virginia	173	1.2%
23	Wisconsin	243	1.6%
48	Wyoming	18	0.1%

RANK ORDER

RANK	STATE	DEATHS	% of USA
1	California	1,825	12.2%
2	Florida	1,035	6.9%
3	Texas	838	5.6%
4	Pennsylvania	641	4.3%
5	New York	638	4.3%
6	Ohio	626	4.2%
7	Illinois	611	4.1%
8	Michigan	579	3.9%
9	Colorado	484	3.2%
10	Oklahoma	476	3.2%
11	Georgia	463	3.1%
12	New Jersey	439	2.9%
13	North Carolina	423	2.8%
14	Indiana	404	2.7%
15	Kansas	345	2.3%
15	Washington	345	2.3%
17	Iowa	326	2.2%
18	Tennessee	323	2.2%
19	Massachusetts	322	2.1%
20	Missouri	315	2.1%
21	Arizona	278	1.9%
22	Virginia	249	1.7%
23	Wisconsin	243	1.6%
24	Louisiana	219	1.5%
25	Alabama	215	1.4%
26	Minnesota	209	1.4%
27	Oregon	199	1.3%
28	Maryland	187	1.2%
29	West Virginia	173	1.2%
30	Connecticut	170	1.1%
31	Kentucky	159	1.1%
32	Nebraska	158	1.1%
33	Arkansas	156	1.0%
34	South Carolina	104	0.7%
35	Mississippi	101	0.7%
36	New Mexico	81	0.5%
37	Rhode Island	77	0.5%
38	New Hampshire	74	0.5%
39	Utah	70	0.5%
40	Nevada	60	0.4%
41	Montana	51	0.3%
42	Idaho	46	0.3%
43	North Dakota	45	0.3%
44	Maine	39	0.3%
45	Hawaii	32	0.2%
45	South Dakota	32	0.2%
47	Vermont	20	0.1%
48	Wyoming	18	0.1%
49	Alaska	15	0.1%
49	Delaware	15	0.1%
	District of Columbia	26	0.2%

Source: U.S. Department of Health and Human Services, National Center for Health Statistics
(http://wonder.cdc.gov/WONDER/)
Final data by state of residence. Atherosclerosis is a form of hardening of the arteries.

Death Rate by Atherosclerosis in 1999

National Rate = 5.5 Deaths per 100,000 Population*

ALPHA ORDER

RANK	STATE	RATE
30	Alabama	4.9
49	Alaska**	2.4
18	Arizona	5.8
12	Arkansas	6.1
22	California	5.5
3	Colorado	11.9
26	Connecticut	5.2
50	Delaware**	2.0
9	Florida	6.8
15	Georgia	5.9
47	Hawaii	2.7
38	Idaho	3.7
28	Illinois	5.0
9	Indiana	6.8
4	Iowa	11.4
2	Kansas	13.0
36	Kentucky	4.0
28	Louisiana	5.0
46	Maine	3.1
39	Maryland	3.6
26	Massachusetts	5.2
15	Michigan	5.9
33	Minnesota	4.4
39	Mississippi	3.6
18	Missouri	5.8
18	Montana	5.8
6	Nebraska	9.5
44	Nevada	3.3
11	New Hampshire	6.2
24	New Jersey	5.4
31	New Mexico	4.7
42	New York	3.5
22	North Carolina	5.5
8	North Dakota	7.1
21	Ohio	5.6
1	Oklahoma	14.2
13	Oregon	6.0
25	Pennsylvania	5.3
7	Rhode Island	7.8
47	South Carolina	2.7
33	South Dakota	4.4
15	Tennessee	5.9
35	Texas	4.2
44	Utah	3.3
43	Vermont	3.4
39	Virginia	3.6
13	Washington	6.0
5	West Virginia	9.6
32	Wisconsin	4.6
37	Wyoming**	3.8

RANK ORDER

RANK	STATE	RATE
1	Oklahoma	14.2
2	Kansas	13.0
3	Colorado	11.9
4	Iowa	11.4
5	West Virginia	9.6
6	Nebraska	9.5
7	Rhode Island	7.8
8	North Dakota	7.1
9	Florida	6.8
9	Indiana	6.8
11	New Hampshire	6.2
12	Arkansas	6.1
13	Oregon	6.0
13	Washington	6.0
15	Georgia	5.9
15	Michigan	5.9
15	Tennessee	5.9
18	Arizona	5.8
18	Missouri	5.8
18	Montana	5.8
21	Ohio	5.6
22	California	5.5
22	North Carolina	5.5
24	New Jersey	5.4
25	Pennsylvania	5.3
26	Connecticut	5.2
26	Massachusetts	5.2
28	Illinois	5.0
28	Louisiana	5.0
30	Alabama	4.9
31	New Mexico	4.7
32	Wisconsin	4.6
33	Minnesota	4.4
33	South Dakota	4.4
35	Texas	4.2
36	Kentucky	4.0
37	Wyoming**	3.8
38	Idaho	3.7
39	Maryland	3.6
39	Mississippi	3.6
39	Virginia	3.6
42	New York	3.5
43	Vermont	3.4
44	Nevada	3.3
44	Utah	3.3
46	Maine	3.1
47	Hawaii	2.7
47	South Carolina	2.7
49	Alaska**	2.4
50	Delaware**	2.0
	District of Columbia	5.0

Source: U.S. Department of Health and Human Services, National Center for Health Statistics
(http://wonder.cdc.gov/WONDER/)
*Final data by state of residence. Atherosclerosis is a form of hardening of the arteries. Not age-adjusted.
**Due to low numbers of deaths, rates for these states should be interpreted with caution.

Age-Adjusted Death Rate by Atherosclerosis in 1999

National Rate = 5.5 Deaths per 100,000 Population*

ALPHA ORDER

RANK	STATE	RATE
27	Alabama	5.0
31	Alaska**	4.7
13	Arizona	6.1
19	Arkansas	5.5
9	California	6.5
1	Colorado	15.5
34	Connecticut	4.3
50	Delaware**	2.0
29	Florida	4.9
6	Georgia	8.0
49	Hawaii	2.7
42	Idaho	4.0
27	Illinois	5.0
8	Indiana	6.9
4	Iowa	8.5
3	Kansas	11.1
37	Kentucky	4.2
16	Louisiana	5.9
48	Maine	2.8
37	Maryland	4.2
32	Massachusetts	4.5
13	Michigan	6.1
41	Minnesota	4.1
43	Mississippi	3.9
24	Missouri	5.2
23	Montana	5.3
7	Nebraska	7.7
32	Nevada	4.5
9	New Hampshire	6.5
25	New Jersey	5.1
19	New Mexico	5.5
46	New York	3.3
15	North Carolina	6.0
25	North Dakota	5.1
21	Ohio	5.4
2	Oklahoma	13.3
18	Oregon	5.6
34	Pennsylvania	4.3
16	Rhode Island	5.9
47	South Carolina	3.1
44	South Dakota	3.5
12	Tennessee	6.2
21	Texas	5.4
29	Utah	4.9
45	Vermont	3.4
34	Virginia	4.3
9	Washington	6.5
5	West Virginia	8.3
37	Wisconsin	4.2
37	Wyoming**	4.2

RANK ORDER

RANK	STATE	RATE
1	Colorado	15.5
2	Oklahoma	13.3
3	Kansas	11.1
4	Iowa	8.5
5	West Virginia	8.3
6	Georgia	8.0
7	Nebraska	7.7
8	Indiana	6.9
9	California	6.5
9	New Hampshire	6.5
9	Washington	6.5
12	Tennessee	6.2
13	Arizona	6.1
13	Michigan	6.1
15	North Carolina	6.0
16	Louisiana	5.9
16	Rhode Island	5.9
18	Oregon	5.6
19	Arkansas	5.5
19	New Mexico	5.5
21	Ohio	5.4
21	Texas	5.4
23	Montana	5.3
24	Missouri	5.2
25	New Jersey	5.1
25	North Dakota	5.1
27	Alabama	5.0
27	Illinois	5.0
29	Florida	4.9
29	Utah	4.9
31	Alaska**	4.7
32	Massachusetts	4.5
32	Nevada	4.5
34	Connecticut	4.3
34	Pennsylvania	4.3
34	Virginia	4.3
37	Kentucky	4.2
37	Maryland	4.2
37	Wisconsin	4.2
37	Wyoming**	4.2
41	Minnesota	4.1
42	Idaho	4.0
43	Mississippi	3.9
44	South Dakota	3.5
45	Vermont	3.4
46	New York	3.3
47	South Carolina	3.1
48	Maine	2.8
49	Hawaii	2.7
50	Delaware**	2.0
	District of Columbia	4.5

Source: U.S. Department of Health and Human Services, National Center for Health Statistics
(http://wonder.cdc.gov/WONDER/)
*Final data by state of residence. Atherosclerosis is a form of hardening of the arteries. Age-adjusted rates based on the year 2000 standard population.
**Due to low numbers of deaths, rates for these states should be interpreted with caution.

Deaths by Cerebrovascular Diseases in 1999

National Total = 167,366 Deaths*

<table>
<tr><td colspan="4">ALPHA ORDER</td><td colspan="4">RANK ORDER</td></tr>
<tr><td>RANK</td><td>STATE</td><td>DEATHS</td><td>% of USA</td><td>RANK</td><td>STATE</td><td>DEATHS</td><td>% of USA</td></tr>
<tr><td>19</td><td>Alabama</td><td>3,148</td><td>1.9%</td><td>1</td><td>California</td><td>17,962</td><td>10.7%</td></tr>
<tr><td>50</td><td>Alaska</td><td>171</td><td>0.1%</td><td>2</td><td>Florida</td><td>10,560</td><td>6.3%</td></tr>
<tr><td>26</td><td>Arizona</td><td>2,600</td><td>1.6%</td><td>3</td><td>Texas</td><td>10,414</td><td>6.2%</td></tr>
<tr><td>29</td><td>Arkansas</td><td>2,255</td><td>1.3%</td><td>4</td><td>Pennsylvania</td><td>8,600</td><td>5.1%</td></tr>
<tr><td>1</td><td>California</td><td>17,962</td><td>10.7%</td><td>5</td><td>New York</td><td>8,124</td><td>4.9%</td></tr>
<tr><td>33</td><td>Colorado</td><td>1,834</td><td>1.1%</td><td>6</td><td>Illinois</td><td>7,714</td><td>4.6%</td></tr>
<tr><td>30</td><td>Connecticut</td><td>1,933</td><td>1.2%</td><td>7</td><td>Ohio</td><td>7,235</td><td>4.3%</td></tr>
<tr><td>47</td><td>Delaware</td><td>365</td><td>0.2%</td><td>8</td><td>Michigan</td><td>6,041</td><td>3.6%</td></tr>
<tr><td>2</td><td>Florida</td><td>10,560</td><td>6.3%</td><td>9</td><td>North Carolina</td><td>5,626</td><td>3.4%</td></tr>
<tr><td>10</td><td>Georgia</td><td>4,416</td><td>2.6%</td><td>10</td><td>Georgia</td><td>4,416</td><td>2.6%</td></tr>
<tr><td>41</td><td>Hawaii</td><td>762</td><td>0.5%</td><td>11</td><td>New Jersey</td><td>4,122</td><td>2.5%</td></tr>
<tr><td>40</td><td>Idaho</td><td>771</td><td>0.5%</td><td>12</td><td>Virginia</td><td>4,110</td><td>2.5%</td></tr>
<tr><td>6</td><td>Illinois</td><td>7,714</td><td>4.6%</td><td>13</td><td>Tennessee</td><td>4,103</td><td>2.5%</td></tr>
<tr><td>14</td><td>Indiana</td><td>4,057</td><td>2.4%</td><td>14</td><td>Indiana</td><td>4,057</td><td>2.4%</td></tr>
<tr><td>28</td><td>Iowa</td><td>2,317</td><td>1.4%</td><td>15</td><td>Missouri</td><td>3,950</td><td>2.4%</td></tr>
<tr><td>32</td><td>Kansas</td><td>1,841</td><td>1.1%</td><td>16</td><td>Wisconsin</td><td>3,869</td><td>2.3%</td></tr>
<tr><td>24</td><td>Kentucky</td><td>2,710</td><td>1.6%</td><td>17</td><td>Washington</td><td>3,718</td><td>2.2%</td></tr>
<tr><td>25</td><td>Louisiana</td><td>2,684</td><td>1.6%</td><td>18</td><td>Massachusetts</td><td>3,548</td><td>2.1%</td></tr>
<tr><td>37</td><td>Maine</td><td>879</td><td>0.5%</td><td>19</td><td>Alabama</td><td>3,148</td><td>1.9%</td></tr>
<tr><td>22</td><td>Maryland</td><td>2,892</td><td>1.7%</td><td>20</td><td>Minnesota</td><td>2,997</td><td>1.8%</td></tr>
<tr><td>18</td><td>Massachusetts</td><td>3,548</td><td>2.1%</td><td>21</td><td>South Carolina</td><td>2,974</td><td>1.8%</td></tr>
<tr><td>8</td><td>Michigan</td><td>6,041</td><td>3.6%</td><td>22</td><td>Maryland</td><td>2,892</td><td>1.7%</td></tr>
<tr><td>20</td><td>Minnesota</td><td>2,997</td><td>1.8%</td><td>23</td><td>Oregon</td><td>2,799</td><td>1.7%</td></tr>
<tr><td>31</td><td>Mississippi</td><td>1,854</td><td>1.1%</td><td>24</td><td>Kentucky</td><td>2,710</td><td>1.6%</td></tr>
<tr><td>15</td><td>Missouri</td><td>3,950</td><td>2.4%</td><td>25</td><td>Louisiana</td><td>2,684</td><td>1.6%</td></tr>
<tr><td>44</td><td>Montana</td><td>595</td><td>0.4%</td><td>26</td><td>Arizona</td><td>2,600</td><td>1.6%</td></tr>
<tr><td>35</td><td>Nebraska</td><td>1,176</td><td>0.7%</td><td>27</td><td>Oklahoma</td><td>2,481</td><td>1.5%</td></tr>
<tr><td>36</td><td>Nevada</td><td>882</td><td>0.5%</td><td>28</td><td>Iowa</td><td>2,317</td><td>1.4%</td></tr>
<tr><td>42</td><td>New Hampshire</td><td>669</td><td>0.4%</td><td>29</td><td>Arkansas</td><td>2,255</td><td>1.3%</td></tr>
<tr><td>11</td><td>New Jersey</td><td>4,122</td><td>2.5%</td><td>30</td><td>Connecticut</td><td>1,933</td><td>1.2%</td></tr>
<tr><td>39</td><td>New Mexico</td><td>817</td><td>0.5%</td><td>31</td><td>Mississippi</td><td>1,854</td><td>1.1%</td></tr>
<tr><td>5</td><td>New York</td><td>8,124</td><td>4.9%</td><td>32</td><td>Kansas</td><td>1,841</td><td>1.1%</td></tr>
<tr><td>9</td><td>North Carolina</td><td>5,626</td><td>3.4%</td><td>33</td><td>Colorado</td><td>1,834</td><td>1.1%</td></tr>
<tr><td>46</td><td>North Dakota</td><td>513</td><td>0.3%</td><td>34</td><td>West Virginia</td><td>1,323</td><td>0.8%</td></tr>
<tr><td>7</td><td>Ohio</td><td>7,235</td><td>4.3%</td><td>35</td><td>Nebraska</td><td>1,176</td><td>0.7%</td></tr>
<tr><td>27</td><td>Oklahoma</td><td>2,481</td><td>1.5%</td><td>36</td><td>Nevada</td><td>882</td><td>0.5%</td></tr>
<tr><td>23</td><td>Oregon</td><td>2,799</td><td>1.7%</td><td>37</td><td>Maine</td><td>879</td><td>0.5%</td></tr>
<tr><td>4</td><td>Pennsylvania</td><td>8,600</td><td>5.1%</td><td>38</td><td>Utah</td><td>869</td><td>0.5%</td></tr>
<tr><td>43</td><td>Rhode Island</td><td>633</td><td>0.4%</td><td>39</td><td>New Mexico</td><td>817</td><td>0.5%</td></tr>
<tr><td>21</td><td>South Carolina</td><td>2,974</td><td>1.8%</td><td>40</td><td>Idaho</td><td>771</td><td>0.5%</td></tr>
<tr><td>45</td><td>South Dakota</td><td>547</td><td>0.3%</td><td>41</td><td>Hawaii</td><td>762</td><td>0.5%</td></tr>
<tr><td>13</td><td>Tennessee</td><td>4,103</td><td>2.5%</td><td>42</td><td>New Hampshire</td><td>669</td><td>0.4%</td></tr>
<tr><td>3</td><td>Texas</td><td>10,414</td><td>6.2%</td><td>43</td><td>Rhode Island</td><td>633</td><td>0.4%</td></tr>
<tr><td>38</td><td>Utah</td><td>869</td><td>0.5%</td><td>44</td><td>Montana</td><td>595</td><td>0.4%</td></tr>
<tr><td>48</td><td>Vermont</td><td>344</td><td>0.2%</td><td>45</td><td>South Dakota</td><td>547</td><td>0.3%</td></tr>
<tr><td>12</td><td>Virginia</td><td>4,110</td><td>2.5%</td><td>46</td><td>North Dakota</td><td>513</td><td>0.3%</td></tr>
<tr><td>17</td><td>Washington</td><td>3,718</td><td>2.2%</td><td>47</td><td>Delaware</td><td>365</td><td>0.2%</td></tr>
<tr><td>34</td><td>West Virginia</td><td>1,323</td><td>0.8%</td><td>48</td><td>Vermont</td><td>344</td><td>0.2%</td></tr>
<tr><td>16</td><td>Wisconsin</td><td>3,869</td><td>2.3%</td><td>49</td><td>Wyoming</td><td>265</td><td>0.2%</td></tr>
<tr><td>49</td><td>Wyoming</td><td>265</td><td>0.2%</td><td>50</td><td>Alaska</td><td>171</td><td>0.1%</td></tr>
<tr><td></td><td></td><td></td><td></td><td></td><td>District of Columbia</td><td>297</td><td>0.2%</td></tr>
</table>

Source: U.S. Department of Health and Human Services, National Center for Health Statistics
"National Vital Statistics Reports" (Vol. 49, No. 8, September 21, 2001)
*Final data by state of residence. Cerebrovascular diseases include stroke and other disorders of the blood vessels of the brain.

Death Rate by Cerebrovascular Diseases in 1999

National Rate = 61.4 Deaths per 100,000 Population*

ALPHA ORDER

RANK	STATE	RATE
13	Alabama	72.0
50	Alaska	27.6
40	Arizona	54.4
1	Arkansas	88.4
41	California	54.2
47	Colorado	45.2
33	Connecticut	58.9
45	Delaware	48.4
17	Florida	69.9
36	Georgia	56.7
24	Hawaii	64.3
29	Idaho	61.6
27	Illinois	63.6
20	Indiana	68.3
4	Iowa	80.7
18	Kansas	69.4
19	Kentucky	68.4
30	Louisiana	61.4
16	Maine	70.1
37	Maryland	55.9
35	Massachusetts	57.5
31	Michigan	61.2
28	Minnesota	62.8
22	Mississippi	67.0
12	Missouri	72.2
21	Montana	67.4
15	Nebraska	70.6
44	Nevada	48.7
38	New Hampshire	55.7
43	New Jersey	50.6
46	New Mexico	47.0
48	New York	44.6
10	North Carolina	73.5
3	North Dakota	81.0
24	Ohio	64.3
8	Oklahoma	73.9
2	Oregon	84.4
14	Pennsylvania	71.7
26	Rhode Island	63.9
5	South Carolina	76.5
7	South Dakota	74.6
6	Tennessee	74.8
42	Texas	52.0
49	Utah	40.8
34	Vermont	57.9
32	Virginia	59.8
23	Washington	64.6
11	West Virginia	73.2
9	Wisconsin	73.7
39	Wyoming	55.3

RANK ORDER

RANK	STATE	RATE
1	Arkansas	88.4
2	Oregon	84.4
3	North Dakota	81.0
4	Iowa	80.7
5	South Carolina	76.5
6	Tennessee	74.8
7	South Dakota	74.6
8	Oklahoma	73.9
9	Wisconsin	73.7
10	North Carolina	73.5
11	West Virginia	73.2
12	Missouri	72.2
13	Alabama	72.0
14	Pennsylvania	71.7
15	Nebraska	70.6
16	Maine	70.1
17	Florida	69.9
18	Kansas	69.4
19	Kentucky	68.4
20	Indiana	68.3
21	Montana	67.4
22	Mississippi	67.0
23	Washington	64.6
24	Hawaii	64.3
24	Ohio	64.3
26	Rhode Island	63.9
27	Illinois	63.6
28	Minnesota	62.8
29	Idaho	61.6
30	Louisiana	61.4
31	Michigan	61.2
32	Virginia	59.8
33	Connecticut	58.9
34	Vermont	57.9
35	Massachusetts	57.5
36	Georgia	56.7
37	Maryland	55.9
38	New Hampshire	55.7
39	Wyoming	55.3
40	Arizona	54.4
41	California	54.2
42	Texas	52.0
43	New Jersey	50.6
44	Nevada	48.7
45	Delaware	48.4
46	New Mexico	47.0
47	Colorado	45.2
48	New York	44.6
49	Utah	40.8
50	Alaska	27.6
	District of Columbia	57.2

Source: U.S. Department of Health and Human Services, National Center for Health Statistics
   "National Vital Statistics Reports" (Vol. 49, No. 8, September 21, 2001)
*Final data by state of residence. Cerebrovascular diseases include stroke and other disorders of the blood vessels of the brain. Not age-adjusted.

Age-Adjusted Death Rate by Cerebrovascular Diseases in 1999

National Rate = 61.8 Deaths per 100,000 Population*

ALPHA ORDER

RANK	STATE	RATE		RANK	STATE	RATE
7	Alabama	72.4		1	South Carolina	85.6
10	Alaska	70.7		2	Arkansas	80.0
42	Arizona	56.1		3	Oregon	78.6
2	Arkansas	80.0		4	North Carolina	78.1
24	California	63.2		5	Tennessee	78.0
41	Colorado	57.0		6	Georgia	73.6
47	Connecticut	50.1		7	Alabama	72.4
45	Delaware	50.4		8	Kentucky	71.0
44	Florida	51.5		9	Mississippi	70.8
6	Georgia	73.6		10	Alaska	70.7
24	Hawaii	63.2		11	Oklahoma	69.8
17	Idaho	67.2		11	Virginia	69.8
20	Illinois	63.9		11	Washington	69.8
15	Indiana	69.4		14	Louisiana	69.6
28	Iowa	62.7		15	Indiana	69.4
31	Kansas	61.7		16	Wisconsin	67.9
8	Kentucky	71.0		17	Idaho	67.2
14	Louisiana	69.6		18	Texas	66.2
21	Maine	63.4		19	Missouri	66.1
26	Maryland	63.1		20	Illinois	63.9
46	Massachusetts	50.3		21	Maine	63.4
23	Michigan	63.3		21	North Dakota	63.4
37	Minnesota	60.1		23	Michigan	63.3
9	Mississippi	70.8		24	California	63.2
19	Missouri	66.1		24	Hawaii	63.2
29	Montana	62.2		26	Maryland	63.1
35	Nebraska	60.6		26	West Virginia	63.1
33	Nevada	60.7		28	Iowa	62.7
38	New Hampshire	58.6		29	Montana	62.2
49	New Jersey	47.5		30	Ohio	62.1
43	New Mexico	54.5		31	Kansas	61.7
50	New York	42.1		31	Wyoming	61.7
4	North Carolina	78.1		33	Nevada	60.7
21	North Dakota	63.4		33	South Dakota	60.7
30	Ohio	62.1		35	Nebraska	60.6
11	Oklahoma	69.8		36	Utah	60.2
3	Oregon	78.6		37	Minnesota	60.1
39	Pennsylvania	58.0		38	New Hampshire	58.6
48	Rhode Island	49.9		39	Pennsylvania	58.0
1	South Carolina	85.6		40	Vermont	57.7
33	South Dakota	60.7		41	Colorado	57.0
5	Tennessee	78.0		42	Arizona	56.1
18	Texas	66.2		43	New Mexico	54.5
36	Utah	60.2		44	Florida	51.5
40	Vermont	57.7		45	Delaware	50.4
11	Virginia	69.8		46	Massachusetts	50.3
11	Washington	69.8		47	Connecticut	50.1
26	West Virginia	63.1		48	Rhode Island	49.9
16	Wisconsin	67.9		49	New Jersey	47.5
31	Wyoming	61.7		50	New York	42.1
					District of Columbia	52.2

Source: U.S. Department of Health and Human Services, National Center for Health Statistics
"National Vital Statistics Reports" (Vol. 49, No. 8, September 21, 2001)
*Final data by state of residence. Cerebrovascular diseases include stroke and other disorders of the blood vessels of the brain. Age-adjusted rates based on the year 2000 standard population.

Deaths by Chronic Liver Disease and Cirrhosis in 1999

National Total = 26,259 Deaths*

ALPHA ORDER

RANK ORDER

RANK	STATE	DEATHS	% of USA
21	Alabama	412	1.6%
50	Alaska	46	0.2%
11	Arizona	653	2.5%
33	Arkansas	218	0.8%
1	California	3,572	13.6%
24	Colorado	391	1.5%
29	Connecticut	301	1.1%
46	Delaware	68	0.3%
3	Florida	1,972	7.5%
12	Georgia	627	2.4%
45	Hawaii	70	0.3%
42	Idaho	88	0.3%
5	Illinois	1,095	4.2%
18	Indiana	444	1.7%
34	Iowa	209	0.8%
36	Kansas	188	0.7%
25	Kentucky	386	1.5%
23	Louisiana	392	1.5%
38	Maine	128	0.5%
17	Maryland	481	1.8%
13	Massachusetts	590	2.2%
6	Michigan	1,029	3.9%
27	Minnesota	313	1.2%
32	Mississippi	250	1.0%
19	Missouri	428	1.6%
41	Montana	91	0.3%
39	Nebraska	123	0.5%
31	Nevada	268	1.0%
43	New Hampshire	87	0.3%
9	New Jersey	791	3.0%
30	New Mexico	288	1.1%
4	New York	1,534	5.8%
10	North Carolina	731	2.8%
47	North Dakota	56	0.2%
8	Ohio	1,007	3.8%
26	Oklahoma	365	1.4%
28	Oregon	306	1.2%
7	Pennsylvania	1,024	3.9%
40	Rhode Island	119	0.5%
20	South Carolina	415	1.6%
44	South Dakota	82	0.3%
14	Tennessee	549	2.1%
2	Texas	2,104	8.0%
37	Utah	138	0.5%
48	Vermont	52	0.2%
16	Virginia	525	2.0%
15	Washington	532	2.0%
35	West Virginia	207	0.8%
22	Wisconsin	408	1.6%
49	Wyoming	49	0.2%

RANK	STATE	DEATHS	% of USA
1	California	3,572	13.6%
2	Texas	2,104	8.0%
3	Florida	1,972	7.5%
4	New York	1,534	5.8%
5	Illinois	1,095	4.2%
6	Michigan	1,029	3.9%
7	Pennsylvania	1,024	3.9%
8	Ohio	1,007	3.8%
9	New Jersey	791	3.0%
10	North Carolina	731	2.8%
11	Arizona	653	2.5%
12	Georgia	627	2.4%
13	Massachusetts	590	2.2%
14	Tennessee	549	2.1%
15	Washington	532	2.0%
16	Virginia	525	2.0%
17	Maryland	481	1.8%
18	Indiana	444	1.7%
19	Missouri	428	1.6%
20	South Carolina	415	1.6%
21	Alabama	412	1.6%
22	Wisconsin	408	1.6%
23	Louisiana	392	1.5%
24	Colorado	391	1.5%
25	Kentucky	386	1.5%
26	Oklahoma	365	1.4%
27	Minnesota	313	1.2%
28	Oregon	306	1.2%
29	Connecticut	301	1.1%
30	New Mexico	288	1.1%
31	Nevada	268	1.0%
32	Mississippi	250	1.0%
33	Arkansas	218	0.8%
34	Iowa	209	0.8%
35	West Virginia	207	0.8%
36	Kansas	188	0.7%
37	Utah	138	0.5%
38	Maine	128	0.5%
39	Nebraska	123	0.5%
40	Rhode Island	119	0.5%
41	Montana	91	0.3%
42	Idaho	88	0.3%
43	New Hampshire	87	0.3%
44	South Dakota	82	0.3%
45	Hawaii	70	0.3%
46	Delaware	68	0.3%
47	North Dakota	56	0.2%
48	Vermont	52	0.2%
49	Wyoming	49	0.2%
50	Alaska	46	0.2%
	District of Columbia	57	0.2%

Source: U.S. Department of Health and Human Services, National Center for Health Statistics
"National Vital Statistics Reports" (Vol. 49, No. 8, September 21, 2001)
*Final data by state of residence. Cirrhosis of the liver is characterized by the replacement of normal tissue with fibrous tissue and the loss of functional liver cells. It can result from alcohol abuse, nutritional deprivation, or infection especially by the hepatitis virus.

Death Rate by Chronic Liver Disease and Cirrhosis in 1999

National Rate = 9.6 Deaths per 100,000 Population*

ALPHA ORDER

RANK	STATE	RATE
22	Alabama	9.4
42	Alaska	7.4
3	Arizona	13.7
34	Arkansas	8.5
9	California	10.8
19	Colorado	9.6
24	Connecticut	9.2
27	Delaware	9.0
4	Florida	13.0
37	Georgia	8.1
50	Hawaii	5.9
47	Idaho	7.0
27	Illinois	9.0
41	Indiana	7.5
44	Iowa	7.3
46	Kansas	7.1
17	Kentucky	9.7
27	Louisiana	9.0
14	Maine	10.2
23	Maryland	9.3
19	Massachusetts	9.6
12	Michigan	10.4
48	Minnesota	6.6
27	Mississippi	9.0
38	Missouri	7.8
13	Montana	10.3
42	Nebraska	7.4
2	Nevada	14.8
45	New Hampshire	7.2
17	New Jersey	9.7
1	New Mexico	16.6
36	New York	8.4
19	North Carolina	9.6
32	North Dakota	8.8
31	Ohio	8.9
8	Oklahoma	10.9
24	Oregon	9.2
34	Pennsylvania	8.5
5	Rhode Island	12.0
10	South Carolina	10.7
7	South Dakota	11.2
16	Tennessee	10.0
11	Texas	10.5
49	Utah	6.5
32	Vermont	8.8
40	Virginia	7.6
24	Washington	9.2
6	West Virginia	11.5
38	Wisconsin	7.8
14	Wyoming	10.2

RANK ORDER

RANK	STATE	RATE
1	New Mexico	16.6
2	Nevada	14.8
3	Arizona	13.7
4	Florida	13.0
5	Rhode Island	12.0
6	West Virginia	11.5
7	South Dakota	11.2
8	Oklahoma	10.9
9	California	10.8
10	South Carolina	10.7
11	Texas	10.5
12	Michigan	10.4
13	Montana	10.3
14	Maine	10.2
14	Wyoming	10.2
16	Tennessee	10.0
17	Kentucky	9.7
17	New Jersey	9.7
19	Colorado	9.6
19	Massachusetts	9.6
19	North Carolina	9.6
22	Alabama	9.4
23	Maryland	9.3
24	Connecticut	9.2
24	Oregon	9.2
24	Washington	9.2
27	Delaware	9.0
27	Illinois	9.0
27	Louisiana	9.0
27	Mississippi	9.0
31	Ohio	8.9
32	North Dakota	8.8
32	Vermont	8.8
34	Arkansas	8.5
34	Pennsylvania	8.5
36	New York	8.4
37	Georgia	8.1
38	Missouri	7.8
38	Wisconsin	7.8
40	Virginia	7.6
41	Indiana	7.5
42	Alaska	7.4
42	Nebraska	7.4
44	Iowa	7.3
45	New Hampshire	7.2
46	Kansas	7.1
47	Idaho	7.0
48	Minnesota	6.6
49	Utah	6.5
50	Hawaii	5.9
	District of Columbia	11.0

Source: U.S. Department of Health and Human Services, National Center for Health Statistics
    "National Vital Statistics Reports" (Vol. 49, No. 8, September 21, 2001)
*Final data by state of residence. Cirrhosis of the liver is characterized by the replacement of normal tissue with fibrous tissue and the loss of functional liver cells. It can result from alcohol abuse, nutritional deprivation, or infection especially by the hepatitis virus. Not age-adjusted.

Age-Adjusted Death Rate by Chronic Liver Disease and Cirrhosis in 1999

National Rate = 9.7 Deaths per 100,000 Population*

ALPHA ORDER

RANK	STATE	RATE
26	Alabama	9.2
15	Alaska	9.8
3	Arizona	14.0
37	Arkansas	8.2
4	California	12.0
15	Colorado	9.8
32	Connecticut	8.7
29	Delaware	9.0
6	Florida	11.4
29	Georgia	9.0
50	Hawaii	5.5
44	Idaho	7.5
26	Illinois	9.2
44	Indiana	7.5
49	Iowa	6.7
47	Kansas	7.1
18	Kentucky	9.6
21	Louisiana	9.5
21	Maine	9.5
21	Maryland	9.5
26	Massachusetts	9.2
11	Michigan	10.6
48	Minnesota	6.8
21	Mississippi	9.5
41	Missouri	7.6
17	Montana	9.7
46	Nebraska	7.4
2	Nevada	15.0
41	New Hampshire	7.6
25	New Jersey	9.3
1	New Mexico	17.3
37	New York	8.2
18	North Carolina	9.6
32	North Dakota	8.7
32	Ohio	8.7
10	Oklahoma	10.7
31	Oregon	8.8
41	Pennsylvania	7.6
6	Rhode Island	11.4
9	South Carolina	10.8
6	South Dakota	11.4
14	Tennessee	9.9
5	Texas	11.8
32	Utah	8.7
36	Vermont	8.6
39	Virginia	8.0
18	Washington	9.6
13	West Virginia	10.0
40	Wisconsin	7.7
12	Wyoming	10.4

RANK ORDER

RANK	STATE	RATE
1	New Mexico	17.3
2	Nevada	15.0
3	Arizona	14.0
4	California	12.0
5	Texas	11.8
6	Florida	11.4
6	Rhode Island	11.4
6	South Dakota	11.4
9	South Carolina	10.8
10	Oklahoma	10.7
11	Michigan	10.6
12	Wyoming	10.4
13	West Virginia	10.0
14	Tennessee	9.9
15	Alaska	9.8
15	Colorado	9.8
17	Montana	9.7
18	Kentucky	9.6
18	North Carolina	9.6
18	Washington	9.6
21	Louisiana	9.5
21	Maine	9.5
21	Maryland	9.5
21	Mississippi	9.5
25	New Jersey	9.3
26	Alabama	9.2
26	Illinois	9.2
26	Massachusetts	9.2
29	Delaware	9.0
29	Georgia	9.0
31	Oregon	8.8
32	Connecticut	8.7
32	North Dakota	8.7
32	Ohio	8.7
32	Utah	8.7
36	Vermont	8.6
37	Arkansas	8.2
37	New York	8.2
39	Virginia	8.0
40	Wisconsin	7.7
41	Missouri	7.6
41	New Hampshire	7.6
41	Pennsylvania	7.6
44	Idaho	7.5
44	Indiana	7.5
46	Nebraska	7.4
47	Kansas	7.1
48	Minnesota	6.8
49	Iowa	6.7
50	Hawaii	5.5
	District of Columbia	10.3

Source: U.S. Department of Health and Human Services, National Center for Health Statistics
"National Vital Statistics Reports" (Vol. 49, No. 8, September 21, 2001)
*Final data by state of residence. Cirrhosis of the liver is characterized by the replacement of normal tissue with fibrous tissue and the loss of functional liver cells. It can result from alcohol abuse, nutritional deprivation, or infection especially by the hepatitis virus. Age-adjusted rates based on the year 2000 standard population.

Deaths by Chronic Lower Respiratory Diseases in 1999

National Total = 124,181 Deaths*

RANK	STATE	DEATHS	% of USA
21	Alabama	2,179	1.8%
50	Alaska	146	0.1%
18	Arizona	2,553	2.1%
32	Arkansas	1,358	1.1%
1	California	13,165	10.6%
24	Colorado	1,894	1.5%
30	Connecticut	1,435	1.2%
46	Delaware	327	0.3%
2	Florida	9,131	7.4%
12	Georgia	3,056	2.5%
48	Hawaii	290	0.2%
40	Idaho	568	0.5%
7	Illinois	5,155	4.2%
13	Indiana	3,053	2.5%
28	Iowa	1,643	1.3%
31	Kansas	1,386	1.1%
19	Kentucky	2,327	1.9%
29	Louisiana	1,610	1.3%
38	Maine	751	0.6%
23	Maryland	1,943	1.6%
14	Massachusetts	2,862	2.3%
8	Michigan	4,316	3.5%
22	Minnesota	1,994	1.6%
33	Mississippi	1,267	1.0%
11	Missouri	3,068	2.5%
41	Montana	566	0.5%
36	Nebraska	945	0.8%
35	Nevada	1,029	0.8%
39	New Hampshire	592	0.5%
10	New Jersey	3,130	2.5%
37	New Mexico	848	0.7%
4	New York	7,086	5.7%
9	North Carolina	3,591	2.9%
49	North Dakota	273	0.2%
6	Ohio	5,858	4.7%
27	Oklahoma	1,751	1.4%
25	Oregon	1,765	1.4%
5	Pennsylvania	6,141	4.9%
43	Rhode Island	495	0.4%
26	South Carolina	1,752	1.4%
45	South Dakota	335	0.3%
15	Tennessee	2,748	2.2%
3	Texas	7,518	6.1%
42	Utah	559	0.5%
47	Vermont	300	0.2%
17	Virginia	2,699	2.2%
16	Washington	2,713	2.2%
34	West Virginia	1,236	1.0%
20	Wisconsin	2,270	1.8%
44	Wyoming	338	0.3%

RANK	STATE	DEATHS	% of USA
1	California	13,165	10.6%
2	Florida	9,131	7.4%
3	Texas	7,518	6.1%
4	New York	7,086	5.7%
5	Pennsylvania	6,141	4.9%
6	Ohio	5,858	4.7%
7	Illinois	5,155	4.2%
8	Michigan	4,316	3.5%
9	North Carolina	3,591	2.9%
10	New Jersey	3,130	2.5%
11	Missouri	3,068	2.5%
12	Georgia	3,056	2.5%
13	Indiana	3,053	2.5%
14	Massachusetts	2,862	2.3%
15	Tennessee	2,748	2.2%
16	Washington	2,713	2.2%
17	Virginia	2,699	2.2%
18	Arizona	2,553	2.1%
19	Kentucky	2,327	1.9%
20	Wisconsin	2,270	1.8%
21	Alabama	2,179	1.8%
22	Minnesota	1,994	1.6%
23	Maryland	1,943	1.6%
24	Colorado	1,894	1.5%
25	Oregon	1,765	1.4%
26	South Carolina	1,752	1.4%
27	Oklahoma	1,751	1.4%
28	Iowa	1,643	1.3%
29	Louisiana	1,610	1.3%
30	Connecticut	1,435	1.2%
31	Kansas	1,386	1.1%
32	Arkansas	1,358	1.1%
33	Mississippi	1,267	1.0%
34	West Virginia	1,236	1.0%
35	Nevada	1,029	0.8%
36	Nebraska	945	0.8%
37	New Mexico	848	0.7%
38	Maine	751	0.6%
39	New Hampshire	592	0.5%
40	Idaho	568	0.5%
41	Montana	566	0.5%
42	Utah	559	0.5%
43	Rhode Island	495	0.4%
44	Wyoming	338	0.3%
45	South Dakota	335	0.3%
46	Delaware	327	0.3%
47	Vermont	300	0.2%
48	Hawaii	290	0.2%
49	North Dakota	273	0.2%
50	Alaska	146	0.1%
	District of Columbia	166	0.1%

Source: U.S. Department of Health and Human Services, National Center for Health Statistics
"National Vital Statistics Reports" (Vol. 49, No. 8, September 21, 2001)
*Final data by state of residence. Chronic lower respiratory diseases are diseases of the lungs including bronchitis, emphysema and asthma. Includes allied conditions.

Death Rate by Chronic Lower Respiratory Diseases in 1999

National Rate = 45.5 Deaths per 100,000 Population*

ALPHA ORDER

RANK	STATE	RATE
22	Alabama	49.9
50	Alaska	23.6
11	Arizona	53.4
12	Arkansas	53.2
40	California	39.7
27	Colorado	46.7
34	Connecticut	43.7
35	Delaware	43.4
4	Florida	60.4
42	Georgia	39.2
49	Hawaii	24.5
31	Idaho	45.4
38	Illinois	42.5
17	Indiana	51.4
7	Iowa	57.3
14	Kansas	52.2
6	Kentucky	58.8
47	Louisiana	36.8
5	Maine	59.9
45	Maryland	37.6
28	Massachusetts	46.3
33	Michigan	43.8
39	Minnesota	41.8
29	Mississippi	45.8
10	Missouri	56.1
3	Montana	64.1
9	Nebraska	56.7
8	Nevada	56.9
23	New Hampshire	49.3
44	New Jersey	38.4
24	New Mexico	48.7
43	New York	38.9
26	North Carolina	46.9
37	North Dakota	43.1
16	Ohio	52.0
15	Oklahoma	52.1
12	Oregon	53.2
18	Pennsylvania	51.2
21	Rhode Island	50.0
32	South Carolina	45.1
30	South Dakota	45.7
20	Tennessee	50.1
46	Texas	37.5
48	Utah	26.2
19	Vermont	50.5
41	Virginia	39.3
25	Washington	47.1
2	West Virginia	68.4
36	Wisconsin	43.2
1	Wyoming	70.5

RANK ORDER

RANK	STATE	RATE
1	Wyoming	70.5
2	West Virginia	68.4
3	Montana	64.1
4	Florida	60.4
5	Maine	59.9
6	Kentucky	58.8
7	Iowa	57.3
8	Nevada	56.9
9	Nebraska	56.7
10	Missouri	56.1
11	Arizona	53.4
12	Arkansas	53.2
12	Oregon	53.2
14	Kansas	52.2
15	Oklahoma	52.1
16	Ohio	52.0
17	Indiana	51.4
18	Pennsylvania	51.2
19	Vermont	50.5
20	Tennessee	50.1
21	Rhode Island	50.0
22	Alabama	49.9
23	New Hampshire	49.3
24	New Mexico	48.7
25	Washington	47.1
26	North Carolina	46.9
27	Colorado	46.7
28	Massachusetts	46.3
29	Mississippi	45.8
30	South Dakota	45.7
31	Idaho	45.4
32	South Carolina	45.1
33	Michigan	43.8
34	Connecticut	43.7
35	Delaware	43.4
36	Wisconsin	43.2
37	North Dakota	43.1
38	Illinois	42.5
39	Minnesota	41.8
40	California	39.7
41	Virginia	39.3
42	Georgia	39.2
43	New York	38.9
44	New Jersey	38.4
45	Maryland	37.6
46	Texas	37.5
47	Louisiana	36.8
48	Utah	26.2
49	Hawaii	24.5
50	Alaska	23.6
	District of Columbia	32.0

Source: U.S. Department of Health and Human Services, National Center for Health Statistics
    "National Vital Statistics Reports" (Vol. 49, No. 8, September 21, 2001)
*Final data by state of residence. Chronic lower respiratory diseases are diseases of the lungs including bronchitis, emphysema and asthma. Includes allied conditions. Not age-adjusted.

Age-Adjusted Death Rate by Chronic Lower Respiratory Diseases in 1999

National Rate = 45.8 Deaths per 100,000 Population*

ALPHA ORDER

RANK ORDER

RANK	STATE	RATE		RANK	STATE	RATE
23	Alabama	49.3		1	Wyoming	76.6
7	Alaska	55.7		2	Nevada	66.5
10	Arizona	53.3		3	Montana	60.0
26	Arkansas	48.2		4	Kentucky	59.7
31	California	46.0		5	West Virginia	58.1
6	Colorado	57.9		6	Colorado	57.9
45	Connecticut	38.0		7	Alaska	55.7
35	Delaware	43.9		8	New Mexico	55.0
34	Florida	44.0		9	Maine	54.6
19	Georgia	50.1		10	Arizona	53.3
50	Hawaii	23.6		11	Missouri	52.3
21	Idaho	49.7		12	New Hampshire	52.1
36	Illinois	43.2		13	Indiana	52.0
13	Indiana	52.0		14	Vermont	51.5
29	Iowa	47.5		15	Nebraska	51.3
24	Kansas	48.8		16	Washington	51.2
4	Kentucky	59.7		17	Tennessee	51.1
41	Louisiana	41.0		18	Oregon	50.4
9	Maine	54.6		19	Georgia	50.1
37	Maryland	41.7		20	Ohio	49.9
38	Massachusetts	41.6		21	Idaho	49.7
32	Michigan	44.8		22	Oklahoma	49.6
38	Minnesota	41.6		23	Alabama	49.3
27	Mississippi	48.1		24	Kansas	48.8
11	Missouri	52.3		25	North Carolina	48.4
3	Montana	60.0		26	Arkansas	48.2
15	Nebraska	51.3		27	Mississippi	48.1
2	Nevada	66.5		28	South Carolina	48.0
12	New Hampshire	52.1		29	Iowa	47.5
49	New Jersey	36.0		30	Texas	47.2
8	New Mexico	55.0		31	California	46.0
47	New York	37.0		32	Michigan	44.8
25	North Carolina	48.4		33	Virginia	44.6
48	North Dakota	36.2		34	Florida	44.0
20	Ohio	49.9		35	Delaware	43.9
22	Oklahoma	49.6		36	Illinois	43.2
18	Oregon	50.4		37	Maryland	41.7
38	Pennsylvania	41.6		38	Massachusetts	41.6
43	Rhode Island	40.6		38	Minnesota	41.6
28	South Carolina	48.0		38	Pennsylvania	41.6
44	South Dakota	39.3		41	Louisiana	41.0
17	Tennessee	51.1		42	Wisconsin	40.8
30	Texas	47.2		43	Rhode Island	40.6
46	Utah	37.8		44	South Dakota	39.3
14	Vermont	51.5		45	Connecticut	38.0
33	Virginia	44.6		46	Utah	37.8
16	Washington	51.2		47	New York	37.0
5	West Virginia	58.1		48	North Dakota	36.2
42	Wisconsin	40.8		49	New Jersey	36.0
1	Wyoming	76.6		50	Hawaii	23.6
					District of Columbia	29.3

Source: U.S. Department of Health and Human Services, National Center for Health Statistics
    "National Vital Statistics Reports" (Vol. 49, No. 8, September 21, 2001)
*Final data by state of residence. Chronic lower respiratory diseases are diseases of the lungs including bronchitis, emphysema and asthma. Includes allied conditions. Age-adjusted rates based on the year 2000 standard population.

Deaths by Diabetes Mellitus in 1999

National Total = 68,399 Deaths*

RANK	STATE	DEATHS	% of USA
19	Alabama	1,341	2.0%
50	Alaska	67	0.1%
25	Arizona	1,063	1.6%
29	Arkansas	691	1.0%
1	California	6,401	9.4%
33	Colorado	639	0.9%
29	Connecticut	691	1.0%
47	Delaware	179	0.3%
3	Florida	4,357	6.4%
15	Georgia	1,448	2.1%
44	Hawaii	211	0.3%
41	Idaho	267	0.4%
7	Illinois	3,004	4.4%
12	Indiana	1,591	2.3%
31	Iowa	684	1.0%
32	Kansas	650	1.0%
23	Kentucky	1,133	1.7%
11	Louisiana	1,687	2.5%
38	Maine	348	0.5%
17	Maryland	1,422	2.1%
18	Massachusetts	1,354	2.0%
8	Michigan	2,587	3.8%
22	Minnesota	1,249	1.8%
34	Mississippi	593	0.9%
13	Missouri	1,554	2.3%
42	Montana	244	0.4%
37	Nebraska	372	0.5%
40	Nevada	286	0.4%
39	New Hampshire	294	0.4%
9	New Jersey	2,436	3.6%
35	New Mexico	517	0.8%
4	New York	3,799	5.6%
10	North Carolina	2,050	3.0%
45	North Dakota	203	0.3%
6	Ohio	3,675	5.4%
26	Oklahoma	986	1.4%
27	Oregon	860	1.3%
5	Pennsylvania	3,742	5.5%
43	Rhode Island	236	0.3%
24	South Carolina	1,118	1.6%
46	South Dakota	196	0.3%
16	Tennessee	1,436	2.1%
2	Texas	4,931	7.2%
36	Utah	472	0.7%
47	Vermont	179	0.3%
14	Virginia	1,486	2.2%
20	Washington	1,307	1.9%
28	West Virginia	734	1.1%
21	Wisconsin	1,273	1.9%
49	Wyoming	135	0.2%

RANK	STATE	DEATHS	% of USA
1	California	6,401	9.4%
2	Texas	4,931	7.2%
3	Florida	4,357	6.4%
4	New York	3,799	5.6%
5	Pennsylvania	3,742	5.5%
6	Ohio	3,675	5.4%
7	Illinois	3,004	4.4%
8	Michigan	2,587	3.8%
9	New Jersey	2,436	3.6%
10	North Carolina	2,050	3.0%
11	Louisiana	1,687	2.5%
12	Indiana	1,591	2.3%
13	Missouri	1,554	2.3%
14	Virginia	1,486	2.2%
15	Georgia	1,448	2.1%
16	Tennessee	1,436	2.1%
17	Maryland	1,422	2.1%
18	Massachusetts	1,354	2.0%
19	Alabama	1,341	2.0%
20	Washington	1,307	1.9%
21	Wisconsin	1,273	1.9%
22	Minnesota	1,249	1.8%
23	Kentucky	1,133	1.7%
24	South Carolina	1,118	1.6%
25	Arizona	1,063	1.6%
26	Oklahoma	986	1.4%
27	Oregon	860	1.3%
28	West Virginia	734	1.1%
29	Arkansas	691	1.0%
29	Connecticut	691	1.0%
31	Iowa	684	1.0%
32	Kansas	650	1.0%
33	Colorado	639	0.9%
34	Mississippi	593	0.9%
35	New Mexico	517	0.8%
36	Utah	472	0.7%
37	Nebraska	372	0.5%
38	Maine	348	0.5%
39	New Hampshire	294	0.4%
40	Nevada	286	0.4%
41	Idaho	267	0.4%
42	Montana	244	0.4%
43	Rhode Island	236	0.3%
44	Hawaii	211	0.3%
45	North Dakota	203	0.3%
46	South Dakota	196	0.3%
47	Delaware	179	0.3%
47	Vermont	179	0.3%
49	Wyoming	135	0.2%
50	Alaska	67	0.1%
	District of Columbia	221	0.3%

Source: U.S. Department of Health and Human Services, National Center for Health Statistics
"National Vital Statistics Reports" (Vol. 49, No. 8, September 21, 2001)

*Final data by state of residence. A severe, chronic form of diabetes caused by insufficient production of insulin and resulting in abnormal metabolism of carbohydrates, fats, and proteins. The disease, which typically appears in childhood or adolescence, is characterized by increased sugar levels in the blood and urine, excessive thirst and frequent urination.

Death Rate by Diabetes Mellitus in 1999

National Rate = 25.1 Deaths per 100,000 Population*

ALPHA ORDER

RANK ORDER

RANK	STATE	RATE
6	Alabama	30.7
50	Alaska	10.8
37	Arizona	22.2
19	Arkansas	27.1
45	California	19.3
48	Colorado	15.8
43	Connecticut	21.1
32	Delaware	23.8
11	Florida	28.8
46	Georgia	18.6
47	Hawaii	17.8
42	Idaho	21.3
27	Illinois	24.8
20	Indiana	26.8
32	Iowa	23.8
29	Kansas	24.5
13	Kentucky	28.6
2	Louisiana	38.6
16	Maine	27.8
18	Maryland	27.5
39	Massachusetts	21.9
23	Michigan	26.2
23	Minnesota	26.2
41	Mississippi	21.4
14	Missouri	28.4
17	Montana	27.6
36	Nebraska	22.3
48	Nevada	15.8
29	New Hampshire	24.5
8	New Jersey	29.9
9	New Mexico	29.7
44	New York	20.9
20	North Carolina	26.8
4	North Dakota	32.0
3	Ohio	32.6
10	Oklahoma	29.4
26	Oregon	25.9
5	Pennsylvania	31.2
32	Rhode Island	23.8
11	South Carolina	28.8
22	South Dakota	26.7
23	Tennessee	26.2
28	Texas	24.6
37	Utah	22.2
7	Vermont	30.1
40	Virginia	21.6
35	Washington	22.7
1	West Virginia	40.6
31	Wisconsin	24.2
15	Wyoming	28.1

RANK	STATE	RATE
1	West Virginia	40.6
2	Louisiana	38.6
3	Ohio	32.6
4	North Dakota	32.0
5	Pennsylvania	31.2
6	Alabama	30.7
7	Vermont	30.1
8	New Jersey	29.9
9	New Mexico	29.7
10	Oklahoma	29.4
11	Florida	28.8
11	South Carolina	28.8
13	Kentucky	28.6
14	Missouri	28.4
15	Wyoming	28.1
16	Maine	27.8
17	Montana	27.6
18	Maryland	27.5
19	Arkansas	27.1
20	Indiana	26.8
20	North Carolina	26.8
22	South Dakota	26.7
23	Michigan	26.2
23	Minnesota	26.2
23	Tennessee	26.2
26	Oregon	25.9
27	Illinois	24.8
28	Texas	24.6
29	Kansas	24.5
29	New Hampshire	24.5
31	Wisconsin	24.2
32	Delaware	23.8
32	Iowa	23.8
32	Rhode Island	23.8
35	Washington	22.7
36	Nebraska	22.3
37	Arizona	22.2
37	Utah	22.2
39	Massachusetts	21.9
40	Virginia	21.6
41	Mississippi	21.4
42	Idaho	21.3
43	Connecticut	21.1
44	New York	20.9
45	California	19.3
46	Georgia	18.6
47	Hawaii	17.8
48	Colorado	15.8
48	Nevada	15.8
50	Alaska	10.8

District of Columbia — 42.6

Source: U.S. Department of Health and Human Services, National Center for Health Statistics
"National Vital Statistics Reports" (Vol. 49, No. 8, September 21, 2001)
*Final data by state of residence. A severe, chronic form of diabetes caused by insufficient production of insulin and resulting in abnormal metabolism of carbohydrates, fats, and proteins. The disease, which typically appears in childhood or adolescence, is characterized by increased sugar levels in the blood and urine, excessive thirst and frequent urination. Not age-adjusted.

Age-Adjusted Death Rate by Diabetes Mellitus in 1999

National Rate = 25.2 Deaths per 100,000 Population*

ALPHA ORDER

RANK	STATE	RATE
7	Alabama	30.4
32	Alaska	23.6
38	Arizona	22.4
27	Arkansas	24.9
40	California	22.2
47	Colorado	19.1
48	Connecticut	18.8
30	Delaware	24.2
41	Florida	22.1
34	Georgia	23.1
50	Hawaii	17.1
34	Idaho	23.1
26	Illinois	25.2
16	Indiana	27.1
45	Iowa	19.9
37	Kansas	23.0
12	Kentucky	29.0
1	Louisiana	42.5
25	Maine	25.4
10	Maryland	30.0
44	Massachusetts	20.0
18	Michigan	26.8
21	Minnesota	26.0
38	Mississippi	22.4
19	Missouri	26.6
22	Montana	25.9
42	Nebraska	20.5
49	Nevada	17.8
22	New Hampshire	25.9
13	New Jersey	28.2
3	New Mexico	32.7
45	New York	19.9
15	North Carolina	27.4
17	North Dakota	27.0
5	Ohio	31.5
14	Oklahoma	28.1
28	Oregon	24.6
22	Pennsylvania	25.9
43	Rhode Island	20.4
8	South Carolina	30.3
33	South Dakota	23.5
19	Tennessee	26.6
10	Texas	30.0
4	Utah	31.6
6	Vermont	30.7
31	Virginia	24.0
29	Washington	24.5
2	West Virginia	34.9
34	Wisconsin	23.1
9	Wyoming	30.2

RANK ORDER

RANK	STATE	RATE
1	Louisiana	42.5
2	West Virginia	34.9
3	New Mexico	32.7
4	Utah	31.6
5	Ohio	31.5
6	Vermont	30.7
7	Alabama	30.4
8	South Carolina	30.3
9	Wyoming	30.2
10	Maryland	30.0
10	Texas	30.0
12	Kentucky	29.0
13	New Jersey	28.2
14	Oklahoma	28.1
15	North Carolina	27.4
16	Indiana	27.1
17	North Dakota	27.0
18	Michigan	26.8
19	Missouri	26.6
19	Tennessee	26.6
21	Minnesota	26.0
22	Montana	25.9
22	New Hampshire	25.9
22	Pennsylvania	25.9
25	Maine	25.4
26	Illinois	25.2
27	Arkansas	24.9
28	Oregon	24.6
29	Washington	24.5
30	Delaware	24.2
31	Virginia	24.0
32	Alaska	23.6
33	South Dakota	23.5
34	Georgia	23.1
34	Idaho	23.1
34	Wisconsin	23.1
37	Kansas	23.0
38	Arizona	22.4
38	Mississippi	22.4
40	California	22.2
41	Florida	22.1
42	Nebraska	20.5
43	Rhode Island	20.4
44	Massachusetts	20.0
45	Iowa	19.9
45	New York	19.9
47	Colorado	19.1
48	Connecticut	18.8
49	Nevada	17.8
50	Hawaii	17.1
	District of Columbia	38.9

Source: U.S. Department of Health and Human Services, National Center for Health Statistics "National Vital Statistics Reports" (Vol. 49, No. 8, September 21, 2001)
Final data by state of residence. A severe, chronic form of diabetes caused by insufficient production of insulin and resulting in abnormal metabolism of carbohydrates, fats, and proteins. The disease, which typically appears in childhood or adolescence, is characterized by increased sugar levels in the blood and urine, excessive thirst and frequent urination. Age-adjusted rates based on the year 2000 standard population.

Deaths by Diseases of the Heart in 1999

National Total = 725,192 Deaths*

ALPHA ORDER				RANK ORDER			
RANK	STATE	DEATHS	% of USA	RANK	STATE	DEATHS	% of USA
18	Alabama	13,419	1.9%	1	California	71,930	9.9%
50	Alaska	563	0.1%	2	New York	58,987	8.1%
24	Arizona	10,800	1.5%	3	Florida	51,434	7.1%
30	Arkansas	8,315	1.1%	4	Texas	43,418	6.0%
1	California	71,930	9.9%	5	Pennsylvania	41,707	5.8%
34	Colorado	6,420	0.9%	6	Illinois	33,387	4.6%
28	Connecticut	9,127	1.3%	7	Ohio	33,192	4.6%
46	Delaware	2,011	0.3%	8	Michigan	27,693	3.8%
3	Florida	51,434	7.1%	9	New Jersey	23,493	3.2%
12	Georgia	17,597	2.4%	10	North Carolina	19,191	2.6%
43	Hawaii	2,410	0.3%	11	Missouri	17,974	2.5%
42	Idaho	2,532	0.3%	12	Georgia	17,597	2.4%
6	Illinois	33,387	4.6%	13	Indiana	16,661	2.3%
13	Indiana	16,661	2.3%	14	Tennessee	16,280	2.2%
29	Iowa	8,699	1.2%	15	Massachusetts	15,871	2.2%
32	Kansas	6,975	1.0%	16	Virginia	15,329	2.1%
19	Kentucky	12,098	1.7%	17	Wisconsin	13,827	1.9%
21	Louisiana	12,007	1.7%	18	Alabama	13,419	1.9%
38	Maine	3,418	0.5%	19	Kentucky	12,098	1.7%
20	Maryland	12,080	1.7%	20	Maryland	12,080	1.7%
15	Massachusetts	15,871	2.2%	21	Louisiana	12,007	1.7%
8	Michigan	27,693	3.8%	22	Washington	11,515	1.6%
26	Minnesota	9,533	1.3%	23	Oklahoma	11,263	1.6%
27	Mississippi	9,336	1.3%	24	Arizona	10,800	1.5%
11	Missouri	17,974	2.5%	25	South Carolina	9,981	1.4%
44	Montana	2,049	0.3%	26	Minnesota	9,533	1.3%
35	Nebraska	4,497	0.6%	27	Mississippi	9,336	1.3%
36	Nevada	4,231	0.6%	28	Connecticut	9,127	1.3%
41	New Hampshire	2,751	0.4%	29	Iowa	8,699	1.2%
9	New Jersey	23,493	3.2%	30	Arkansas	8,315	1.1%
37	New Mexico	3,452	0.5%	31	Oregon	7,263	1.0%
2	New York	58,987	8.1%	32	Kansas	6,975	1.0%
10	North Carolina	19,191	2.6%	33	West Virginia	6,822	0.9%
47	North Dakota	1,833	0.3%	34	Colorado	6,420	0.9%
7	Ohio	33,192	4.6%	35	Nebraska	4,497	0.6%
23	Oklahoma	11,263	1.6%	36	Nevada	4,231	0.6%
31	Oregon	7,263	1.0%	37	New Mexico	3,452	0.5%
5	Pennsylvania	41,707	5.8%	38	Maine	3,418	0.5%
39	Rhode Island	3,008	0.4%	39	Rhode Island	3,008	0.4%
25	South Carolina	9,981	1.4%	40	Utah	2,786	0.4%
45	South Dakota	2,024	0.3%	41	New Hampshire	2,751	0.4%
14	Tennessee	16,280	2.2%	42	Idaho	2,532	0.3%
4	Texas	43,418	6.0%	43	Hawaii	2,410	0.3%
40	Utah	2,786	0.4%	44	Montana	2,049	0.3%
48	Vermont	1,342	0.2%	45	South Dakota	2,024	0.3%
16	Virginia	15,329	2.1%	46	Delaware	2,011	0.3%
22	Washington	11,515	1.6%	47	North Dakota	1,833	0.3%
33	West Virginia	6,822	0.9%	48	Vermont	1,342	0.2%
17	Wisconsin	13,827	1.9%	49	Wyoming	1,009	0.1%
49	Wyoming	1,009	0.1%	50	Alaska	563	0.1%
					District of Columbia	1,652	0.2%

Source: U.S. Department of Health and Human Services, National Center for Health Statistics
   "National Vital Statistics Reports" (Vol. 49, No. 8, September 21, 2001)
*Final data by state of residence.

Death Rate by Diseases of the Heart in 1999

National Rate = 265.9 Deaths per 100,000 Population*

ALPHA ORDER

RANK	STATE	RATE
9	Alabama	307.1
50	Alaska	90.9
35	Arizona	226.0
7	Arkansas	325.9
40	California	217.0
48	Colorado	158.3
19	Connecticut	278.1
25	Delaware	266.9
3	Florida	340.4
37	Georgia	225.9
43	Hawaii	203.3
44	Idaho	202.3
21	Illinois	275.3
18	Indiana	280.4
12	Iowa	303.2
27	Kansas	262.8
10	Kentucky	305.4
22	Louisiana	274.6
23	Maine	272.8
32	Maryland	233.6
28	Massachusetts	257.0
17	Michigan	280.8
46	Minnesota	199.6
4	Mississippi	337.2
6	Missouri	328.7
33	Montana	232.1
24	Nebraska	269.9
31	Nevada	233.9
34	New Hampshire	229.0
16	New Jersey	288.5
47	New Mexico	198.4
8	New York	324.2
30	North Carolina	250.8
15	North Dakota	289.3
14	Ohio	294.9
5	Oklahoma	335.4
39	Oregon	219.0
2	Pennsylvania	347.7
11	Rhode Island	303.6
29	South Carolina	256.9
20	South Dakota	276.1
13	Tennessee	296.9
41	Texas	216.6
49	Utah	130.8
35	Vermont	226.0
38	Virginia	223.0
45	Washington	200.0
1	West Virginia	377.5
26	Wisconsin	263.3
42	Wyoming	210.4

RANK ORDER

RANK	STATE	RATE
1	West Virginia	377.5
2	Pennsylvania	347.7
3	Florida	340.4
4	Mississippi	337.2
5	Oklahoma	335.4
6	Missouri	328.7
7	Arkansas	325.9
8	New York	324.2
9	Alabama	307.1
10	Kentucky	305.4
11	Rhode Island	303.6
12	Iowa	303.2
13	Tennessee	296.9
14	Ohio	294.9
15	North Dakota	289.3
16	New Jersey	288.5
17	Michigan	280.8
18	Indiana	280.4
19	Connecticut	278.1
20	South Dakota	276.1
21	Illinois	275.3
22	Louisiana	274.6
23	Maine	272.8
24	Nebraska	269.9
25	Delaware	266.9
26	Wisconsin	263.3
27	Kansas	262.8
28	Massachusetts	257.0
29	South Carolina	256.9
30	North Carolina	250.8
31	Nevada	233.9
32	Maryland	233.6
33	Montana	232.1
34	New Hampshire	229.0
35	Arizona	226.0
35	Vermont	226.0
37	Georgia	225.9
38	Virginia	223.0
39	Oregon	219.0
40	California	217.0
41	Texas	216.6
42	Wyoming	210.4
43	Hawaii	203.3
44	Idaho	202.3
45	Washington	200.0
46	Minnesota	199.6
47	New Mexico	198.4
48	Colorado	158.3
49	Utah	130.8
50	Alaska	90.9
	District of Columbia	318.3

Source: U.S. Department of Health and Human Services, National Center for Health Statistics
   "National Vital Statistics Reports" (Vol. 49, No. 8, September 21, 2001)
*Final data by state of residence. Not age-adjusted.

Age-Adjusted Death Rate by Diseases of the Heart in 1999

National Rate = 267.8 Deaths per 100,000 Population*

ALPHA ORDER

RANK	STATE	RATE
6	Alabama	306.8
47	Alaska	196.1
38	Arizona	230.8
10	Arkansas	296.5
26	California	252.8
48	Colorado	195.3
32	Connecticut	240.7
19	Delaware	275.9
25	Florida	253.0
12	Georgia	288.0
46	Hawaii	198.8
42	Idaho	220.0
18	Illinois	277.8
15	Indiana	284.2
30	Iowa	242.9
33	Kansas	237.5
4	Kentucky	313.4
5	Louisiana	308.2
27	Maine	247.5
23	Maryland	259.9
39	Massachusetts	228.8
11	Michigan	289.1
49	Minnesota	194.1
1	Mississippi	354.9
9	Missouri	302.9
44	Montana	215.2
34	Nebraska	236.9
16	Nevada	281.8
31	New Hampshire	241.5
21	New Jersey	271.0
40	New Mexico	226.7
7	New York	305.6
22	North Carolina	262.7
35	North Dakota	235.6
13	Ohio	285.1
3	Oklahoma	317.4
45	Oregon	205.7
14	Pennsylvania	284.8
29	Rhode Island	243.6
17	South Carolina	280.1
36	South Dakota	231.6
8	Tennessee	305.5
20	Texas	271.5
50	Utah	190.5
41	Vermont	225.6
24	Virginia	255.5
43	Washington	215.6
2	West Virginia	325.4
28	Wisconsin	245.4
37	Wyoming	231.1

RANK ORDER

RANK	STATE	RATE
1	Mississippi	354.9
2	West Virginia	325.4
3	Oklahoma	317.4
4	Kentucky	313.4
5	Louisiana	308.2
6	Alabama	306.8
7	New York	305.6
8	Tennessee	305.5
9	Missouri	302.9
10	Arkansas	296.5
11	Michigan	289.1
12	Georgia	288.0
13	Ohio	285.1
14	Pennsylvania	284.8
15	Indiana	284.2
16	Nevada	281.8
17	South Carolina	280.1
18	Illinois	277.8
19	Delaware	275.9
20	Texas	271.5
21	New Jersey	271.0
22	North Carolina	262.7
23	Maryland	259.9
24	Virginia	255.5
25	Florida	253.0
26	California	252.8
27	Maine	247.5
28	Wisconsin	245.4
29	Rhode Island	243.6
30	Iowa	242.9
31	New Hampshire	241.5
32	Connecticut	240.7
33	Kansas	237.5
34	Nebraska	236.9
35	North Dakota	235.6
36	South Dakota	231.6
37	Wyoming	231.1
38	Arizona	230.8
39	Massachusetts	228.8
40	New Mexico	226.7
41	Vermont	225.6
42	Idaho	220.0
43	Washington	215.6
44	Montana	215.2
45	Oregon	205.7
46	Hawaii	198.8
47	Alaska	196.1
48	Colorado	195.3
49	Minnesota	194.1
50	Utah	190.5
	District of Columbia	289.9

Source: U.S. Department of Health and Human Services, National Center for Health Statistics
"National Vital Statistics Reports" (Vol. 49, No. 8, September 21, 2001)
*Final data by state of residence. Age-adjusted rates based on the year 2000 standard population.

Deaths by Malignant Neoplasms in 1999

National Total = 549,838 Deaths*

ALPHA ORDER

RANK	STATE	DEATHS	% of USA
20	Alabama	9,506	1.7%
50	Alaska	633	0.1%
22	Arizona	9,006	1.6%
31	Arkansas	6,137	1.1%
1	California	53,067	9.7%
32	Colorado	5,863	1.1%
27	Connecticut	7,054	1.3%
45	Delaware	1,737	0.3%
2	Florida	38,478	7.0%
13	Georgia	13,225	2.4%
43	Hawaii	1,916	0.3%
42	Idaho	2,162	0.4%
7	Illinois	25,024	4.6%
14	Indiana	12,898	2.3%
29	Iowa	6,346	1.2%
33	Kansas	5,334	1.0%
23	Kentucky	8,925	1.6%
21	Louisiana	9,412	1.7%
37	Maine	3,035	0.6%
19	Maryland	10,143	1.8%
11	Massachusetts	13,853	2.5%
8	Michigan	19,744	3.6%
24	Minnesota	8,892	1.6%
30	Mississippi	6,143	1.1%
15	Missouri	12,186	2.2%
44	Montana	1,854	0.3%
36	Nebraska	3,410	0.6%
35	Nevada	3,556	0.6%
40	New Hampshire	2,408	0.4%
9	New Jersey	18,178	3.3%
38	New Mexico	2,857	0.5%
3	New York	37,609	6.8%
10	North Carolina	15,815	2.9%
47	North Dakota	1,366	0.2%
6	Ohio	25,233	4.6%
26	Oklahoma	7,312	1.3%
28	Oregon	6,905	1.3%
5	Pennsylvania	30,312	5.5%
39	Rhode Island	2,463	0.4%
25	South Carolina	8,089	1.5%
46	South Dakota	1,632	0.3%
16	Tennessee	11,943	2.2%
4	Texas	32,755	6.0%
41	Utah	2,393	0.4%
48	Vermont	1,255	0.2%
12	Virginia	13,365	2.4%
18	Washington	10,653	1.9%
34	West Virginia	4,762	0.9%
17	Wisconsin	10,755	2.0%
49	Wyoming	899	0.2%

RANK ORDER

RANK	STATE	DEATHS	% of USA
1	California	53,067	9.7%
2	Florida	38,478	7.0%
3	New York	37,609	6.8%
4	Texas	32,755	6.0%
5	Pennsylvania	30,312	5.5%
6	Ohio	25,233	4.6%
7	Illinois	25,024	4.6%
8	Michigan	19,744	3.6%
9	New Jersey	18,178	3.3%
10	North Carolina	15,815	2.9%
11	Massachusetts	13,853	2.5%
12	Virginia	13,365	2.4%
13	Georgia	13,225	2.4%
14	Indiana	12,898	2.3%
15	Missouri	12,186	2.2%
16	Tennessee	11,943	2.2%
17	Wisconsin	10,755	2.0%
18	Washington	10,653	1.9%
19	Maryland	10,143	1.8%
20	Alabama	9,506	1.7%
21	Louisiana	9,412	1.7%
22	Arizona	9,006	1.6%
23	Kentucky	8,925	1.6%
24	Minnesota	8,892	1.6%
25	South Carolina	8,089	1.5%
26	Oklahoma	7,312	1.3%
27	Connecticut	7,054	1.3%
28	Oregon	6,905	1.3%
29	Iowa	6,346	1.2%
30	Mississippi	6,143	1.1%
31	Arkansas	6,137	1.1%
32	Colorado	5,863	1.1%
33	Kansas	5,334	1.0%
34	West Virginia	4,762	0.9%
35	Nevada	3,556	0.6%
36	Nebraska	3,410	0.6%
37	Maine	3,035	0.6%
38	New Mexico	2,857	0.5%
39	Rhode Island	2,463	0.4%
40	New Hampshire	2,408	0.4%
41	Utah	2,393	0.4%
42	Idaho	2,162	0.4%
43	Hawaii	1,916	0.3%
44	Montana	1,854	0.3%
45	Delaware	1,737	0.3%
46	South Dakota	1,632	0.3%
47	North Dakota	1,366	0.2%
48	Vermont	1,255	0.2%
49	Wyoming	899	0.2%
50	Alaska	633	0.1%
	District of Columbia	1,340	0.2%

Source: U.S. Department of Health and Human Services, National Center for Health Statistics
"National Vital Statistics Reports" (Vol. 49, No. 8, September 21, 2001)
*Final data by state of residence. Neoplasms are abnormal tissue, tumors. Includes many cancers.

Death Rate by Malignant Neoplasms in 1999

National Rate = 201.6 Deaths per 100,000 Population*

ALPHA ORDER

RANK ORDER

RANK	STATE	RATE		RANK	STATE	RATE
18	Alabama	217.5		1	West Virginia	263.5
50	Alaska	102.2		2	Florida	254.6
38	Arizona	188.5		3	Pennsylvania	252.7
6	Arkansas	240.5		4	Rhode Island	248.6
47	California	160.1		5	Maine	242.2
48	Colorado	144.5		6	Arkansas	240.5
22	Connecticut	214.9		7	Delaware	230.5
7	Delaware	230.5		8	Kentucky	225.3
2	Florida	254.6		9	Massachusetts	224.3
43	Georgia	169.8		10	Ohio	224.2
46	Hawaii	161.6		11	New Jersey	223.2
42	Idaho	172.7		12	Missouri	222.8
29	Illinois	206.3		13	South Dakota	222.6
19	Indiana	217.0		14	Mississippi	221.9
15	Iowa	221.2		15	Iowa	221.2
32	Kansas	201.0		16	Tennessee	217.8
8	Kentucky	225.3		17	Oklahoma	217.7
21	Louisiana	215.3		18	Alabama	217.5
5	Maine	242.2		19	Indiana	217.0
36	Maryland	196.1		20	North Dakota	215.6
9	Massachusetts	224.3		21	Louisiana	215.3
34	Michigan	200.2		22	Connecticut	214.9
40	Minnesota	186.2		23	Vermont	211.4
14	Mississippi	221.9		24	Montana	210.0
12	Missouri	222.8		25	Oregon	208.2
24	Montana	210.0		25	South Carolina	208.2
31	Nebraska	204.7		27	New York	206.7
35	Nevada	196.5		27	North Carolina	206.7
33	New Hampshire	200.5		29	Illinois	206.3
11	New Jersey	223.2		30	Wisconsin	204.8
44	New Mexico	164.2		31	Nebraska	204.7
27	New York	206.7		32	Kansas	201.0
27	North Carolina	206.7		33	New Hampshire	200.5
20	North Dakota	215.6		34	Michigan	200.2
10	Ohio	224.2		35	Nevada	196.5
17	Oklahoma	217.7		36	Maryland	196.1
25	Oregon	208.2		37	Virginia	194.5
3	Pennsylvania	252.7		38	Arizona	188.5
4	Rhode Island	248.6		39	Wyoming	187.4
25	South Carolina	208.2		40	Minnesota	186.2
13	South Dakota	222.6		41	Washington	185.1
16	Tennessee	217.8		42	Idaho	172.7
45	Texas	163.4		43	Georgia	169.8
49	Utah	112.4		44	New Mexico	164.2
23	Vermont	211.4		45	Texas	163.4
37	Virginia	194.5		46	Hawaii	161.6
41	Washington	185.1		47	California	160.1
1	West Virginia	263.5		48	Colorado	144.5
30	Wisconsin	204.8		49	Utah	112.4
39	Wyoming	187.4		50	Alaska	102.2
					District of Columbia	258.2

Source: U.S. Department of Health and Human Services, National Center for Health Statistics
"National Vital Statistics Reports" (Vol. 49, No. 8, September 21, 2001)
*Final data by state of residence. Neoplasms are abnormal tissue, tumors. Includes many cancers. Not age-adjusted.

Age-Adjusted Death Rate by Malignant Neoplasms in 1999

National Rate = 202.7 Deaths per 100,000 Population*

ALPHA ORDER

RANK ORDER

RANK	STATE	RATE	RANK	STATE	RATE
14	Alabama	213.5	1	Louisiana	233.9
44	Alaska	187.0	2	Mississippi	232.4
43	Arizona	188.0	3	Delaware	231.0
7	Arkansas	220.6	4	Kentucky	226.1
46	California	183.1	5	West Virginia	225.6
48	Colorado	169.8	6	Maine	223.2
37	Connecticut	194.5	7	Arkansas	220.6
3	Delaware	231.0	8	Indiana	219.1
35	Florida	196.2	9	Tennessee	218.6
26	Georgia	206.5	10	Ohio	216.2
50	Hawaii	154.7	11	South Carolina	216.1
45	Idaho	186.5	12	Nevada	214.8
22	Illinois	210.5	13	Rhode Island	214.0
8	Indiana	219.1	14	Alabama	213.5
40	Iowa	191.2	14	Virginia	213.5
38	Kansas	193.0	16	Vermont	213.1
4	Kentucky	226.1	17	Pennsylvania	212.7
1	Louisiana	233.9	18	Maryland	212.0
6	Maine	223.2	19	New Hampshire	211.3
18	Maryland	212.0	20	Missouri	210.7
24	Massachusetts	207.8	21	New Jersey	210.6
27	Michigan	204.1	22	Illinois	210.5
41	Minnesota	189.1	23	North Carolina	210.3
2	Mississippi	232.4	24	Massachusetts	207.8
20	Missouri	210.7	24	Oklahoma	207.8
35	Montana	196.2	26	Georgia	206.5
39	Nebraska	191.7	27	Michigan	204.1
12	Nevada	214.8	28	South Dakota	201.0
19	New Hampshire	211.3	29	Washington	199.0
21	New Jersey	210.6	30	Oregon	198.4
47	New Mexico	180.1	31	New York	197.8
31	New York	197.8	32	Wisconsin	197.7
23	North Carolina	210.3	33	Wyoming	197.5
42	North Dakota	188.4	34	Texas	196.8
10	Ohio	216.2	35	Florida	196.2
24	Oklahoma	207.8	35	Montana	196.2
30	Oregon	198.4	37	Connecticut	194.5
17	Pennsylvania	212.7	38	Kansas	193.0
13	Rhode Island	214.0	39	Nebraska	191.7
11	South Carolina	216.1	40	Iowa	191.2
28	South Dakota	201.0	41	Minnesota	189.1
9	Tennessee	218.6	42	North Dakota	188.4
34	Texas	196.8	43	Arizona	188.0
49	Utah	157.1	44	Alaska	187.0
16	Vermont	213.1	45	Idaho	186.5
14	Virginia	213.5	46	California	183.1
29	Washington	199.0	47	New Mexico	180.1
5	West Virginia	225.6	48	Colorado	169.8
32	Wisconsin	197.7	49	Utah	157.1
33	Wyoming	197.5	50	Hawaii	154.7
				District of Columbia	236.9

Source: U.S. Department of Health and Human Services, National Center for Health Statistics
  "National Vital Statistics Reports" (Vol. 49, No. 8, September 21, 2001)
*Final data by state of residence. Neoplasms are abnormal tissue, tumors. Includes many cancers. Age-adjusted rates based on the year 2000 standard population.

Deaths by Pneumonia and Influenza in 1999

National Total = 63,730 Deaths*

ALPHA ORDER

RANK	STATE	DEATHS	% of USA
20	Alabama	1,228	1.9%
50	Alaska	46	0.1%
18	Arizona	1,287	2.0%
31	Arkansas	741	1.2%
2	California	4,560	7.2%
29	Colorado	807	1.3%
27	Connecticut	885	1.4%
47	Delaware	155	0.2%
4	Florida	3,328	5.2%
13	Georgia	1,703	2.7%
44	Hawaii	229	0.4%
40	Idaho	289	0.5%
5	Illinois	3,121	4.9%
17	Indiana	1,362	2.1%
23	Iowa	1,082	1.7%
33	Kansas	676	1.1%
21	Kentucky	1,198	1.9%
25	Louisiana	1,008	1.6%
41	Maine	287	0.5%
22	Maryland	1,140	1.8%
10	Massachusetts	1,904	3.0%
8	Michigan	2,307	3.6%
24	Minnesota	1,077	1.7%
30	Mississippi	801	1.3%
12	Missouri	1,716	2.7%
43	Montana	252	0.4%
35	Nebraska	459	0.7%
38	Nevada	319	0.5%
45	New Hampshire	187	0.3%
9	New Jersey	2,075	3.3%
37	New Mexico	374	0.6%
1	New York	5,482	8.6%
11	North Carolina	1,891	3.0%
46	North Dakota	157	0.2%
7	Ohio	2,641	4.1%
26	Oklahoma	1,007	1.6%
32	Oregon	695	1.1%
6	Pennsylvania	3,116	4.9%
39	Rhode Island	300	0.5%
28	South Carolina	883	1.4%
42	South Dakota	264	0.4%
15	Tennessee	1,588	2.5%
3	Texas	3,534	5.5%
36	Utah	391	0.6%
48	Vermont	134	0.2%
14	Virginia	1,594	2.5%
19	Washington	1,259	2.0%
34	West Virginia	520	0.8%
16	Wisconsin	1,425	2.2%
49	Wyoming	130	0.2%

RANK ORDER

RANK	STATE	DEATHS	% of USA
1	New York	5,482	8.6%
2	California	4,560	7.2%
3	Texas	3,534	5.5%
4	Florida	3,328	5.2%
5	Illinois	3,121	4.9%
6	Pennsylvania	3,116	4.9%
7	Ohio	2,641	4.1%
8	Michigan	2,307	3.6%
9	New Jersey	2,075	3.3%
10	Massachusetts	1,904	3.0%
11	North Carolina	1,891	3.0%
12	Missouri	1,716	2.7%
13	Georgia	1,703	2.7%
14	Virginia	1,594	2.5%
15	Tennessee	1,588	2.5%
16	Wisconsin	1,425	2.2%
17	Indiana	1,362	2.1%
18	Arizona	1,287	2.0%
19	Washington	1,259	2.0%
20	Alabama	1,228	1.9%
21	Kentucky	1,198	1.9%
22	Maryland	1,140	1.8%
23	Iowa	1,082	1.7%
24	Minnesota	1,077	1.7%
25	Louisiana	1,008	1.6%
26	Oklahoma	1,007	1.6%
27	Connecticut	885	1.4%
28	South Carolina	883	1.4%
29	Colorado	807	1.3%
30	Mississippi	801	1.3%
31	Arkansas	741	1.2%
32	Oregon	695	1.1%
33	Kansas	676	1.1%
34	West Virginia	520	0.8%
35	Nebraska	459	0.7%
36	Utah	391	0.6%
37	New Mexico	374	0.6%
38	Nevada	319	0.5%
39	Rhode Island	300	0.5%
40	Idaho	289	0.5%
41	Maine	287	0.5%
42	South Dakota	264	0.4%
43	Montana	252	0.4%
44	Hawaii	229	0.4%
45	New Hampshire	187	0.3%
46	North Dakota	157	0.2%
47	Delaware	155	0.2%
48	Vermont	134	0.2%
49	Wyoming	130	0.2%
50	Alaska	46	0.1%
	District of Columbia	116	0.2%

Source: U.S. Department of Health and Human Services, National Center for Health Statistics
"National Vital Statistics Reports" (Vol. 49, No. 8, September 21, 2001)
*Final data by state of residence.

156

Death Rate by Pneumonia and Influenza in 1999

National Rate = 23.4 Deaths per 100,000 Population*

ALPHA ORDER

RANK	STATE	RATE
14	Alabama	28.1
50	Alaska	7.4
19	Arizona	26.9
9	Arkansas	29.0
49	California	13.8
43	Colorado	19.9
18	Connecticut	27.0
42	Delaware	20.6
36	Florida	22.0
38	Georgia	21.9
44	Hawaii	19.3
29	Idaho	23.1
21	Illinois	25.7
31	Indiana	22.9
1	Iowa	37.7
22	Kansas	25.5
6	Kentucky	30.2
29	Louisiana	23.1
31	Maine	22.9
36	Maryland	22.0
4	Massachusetts	30.8
27	Michigan	23.4
34	Minnesota	22.6
11	Mississippi	28.9
3	Missouri	31.4
13	Montana	28.5
15	Nebraska	27.6
46	Nevada	17.6
48	New Hampshire	15.6
22	New Jersey	25.5
40	New Mexico	21.5
7	New York	30.1
25	North Carolina	24.7
24	North Dakota	24.8
26	Ohio	23.5
8	Oklahoma	30.0
41	Oregon	21.0
20	Pennsylvania	26.0
5	Rhode Island	30.3
33	South Carolina	22.7
2	South Dakota	36.0
9	Tennessee	29.0
46	Texas	17.6
45	Utah	18.4
34	Vermont	22.6
28	Virginia	23.2
38	Washington	21.9
12	West Virginia	28.8
16	Wisconsin	27.1
16	Wyoming	27.1

RANK ORDER

RANK	STATE	RATE
1	Iowa	37.7
2	South Dakota	36.0
3	Missouri	31.4
4	Massachusetts	30.8
5	Rhode Island	30.3
6	Kentucky	30.2
7	New York	30.1
8	Oklahoma	30.0
9	Arkansas	29.0
9	Tennessee	29.0
11	Mississippi	28.9
12	West Virginia	28.8
13	Montana	28.5
14	Alabama	28.1
15	Nebraska	27.6
16	Wisconsin	27.1
16	Wyoming	27.1
18	Connecticut	27.0
19	Arizona	26.9
20	Pennsylvania	26.0
21	Illinois	25.7
22	Kansas	25.5
22	New Jersey	25.5
24	North Dakota	24.8
25	North Carolina	24.7
26	Ohio	23.5
27	Michigan	23.4
28	Virginia	23.2
29	Idaho	23.1
29	Louisiana	23.1
31	Indiana	22.9
31	Maine	22.9
33	South Carolina	22.7
34	Minnesota	22.6
34	Vermont	22.6
36	Florida	22.0
36	Maryland	22.0
38	Georgia	21.9
38	Washington	21.9
40	New Mexico	21.5
41	Oregon	21.0
42	Delaware	20.6
43	Colorado	19.9
44	Hawaii	19.3
45	Utah	18.4
46	Nevada	17.6
46	Texas	17.6
48	New Hampshire	15.6
49	California	13.8
50	Alaska	7.4

| | District of Columbia | 22.4 |

Source: U.S. Department of Health and Human Services, National Center for Health Statistics
   "National Vital Statistics Reports" (Vol. 49, No. 8, September 21, 2001)
*Final data by state of residence. Not age-adjusted.

Age-Adjusted Death Rate by Pneumonia and Influenza in 1999

National Rate = 23.6 Deaths per 100,000 Population*

ALPHA ORDER

RANK ORDER

RANK	STATE	RATE		RANK	STATE	RATE
7	Alabama	28.6		1	Kentucky	31.6
44	Alaska	19.7		2	Mississippi	30.5
12	Arizona	28.0		2	Wyoming	30.5
19	Arkansas	26.2		4	Tennessee	30.3
50	California	16.1		5	Georgia	28.8
23	Colorado	25.1		6	Iowa	28.7
35	Connecticut	22.7		7	Alabama	28.6
40	Delaware	21.7		8	Missouri	28.5
49	Florida	16.3		9	South Dakota	28.4
5	Georgia	28.8		10	New York	28.2
47	Hawaii	19.2		11	Oklahoma	28.1
22	Idaho	25.2		12	Arizona	28.0
21	Illinois	25.7		13	Virginia	27.5
31	Indiana	23.3		14	Utah	27.0
6	Iowa	28.7		15	Massachusetts	26.8
39	Kansas	22.2		16	Louisiana	26.6
1	Kentucky	31.6		17	North Carolina	26.5
16	Louisiana	26.6		18	Montana	26.4
43	Maine	20.6		19	Arkansas	26.2
23	Maryland	25.1		20	South Carolina	25.9
15	Massachusetts	26.8		21	Illinois	25.7
28	Michigan	24.2		22	Idaho	25.2
41	Minnesota	21.2		23	Colorado	25.1
2	Mississippi	30.5		23	Maryland	25.1
8	Missouri	28.5		23	New Mexico	25.1
18	Montana	26.4		26	West Virginia	25.0
33	Nebraska	23.1		27	Wisconsin	24.7
35	Nevada	22.7		28	Michigan	24.2
48	New Hampshire	16.4		29	New Jersey	23.9
29	New Jersey	23.9		30	Washington	23.6
23	New Mexico	25.1		31	Indiana	23.3
10	New York	28.2		32	Rhode Island	23.2
17	North Carolina	26.5		33	Nebraska	23.1
45	North Dakota	19.5		34	Ohio	22.8
34	Ohio	22.8		35	Connecticut	22.7
11	Oklahoma	28.1		35	Nevada	22.7
45	Oregon	19.5		37	Texas	22.5
42	Pennsylvania	21.1		38	Vermont	22.4
32	Rhode Island	23.2		39	Kansas	22.2
20	South Carolina	25.9		40	Delaware	21.7
9	South Dakota	28.4		41	Minnesota	21.2
4	Tennessee	30.3		42	Pennsylvania	21.1
37	Texas	22.5		43	Maine	20.6
14	Utah	27.0		44	Alaska	19.7
38	Vermont	22.4		45	North Dakota	19.5
13	Virginia	27.5		45	Oregon	19.5
30	Washington	23.6		47	Hawaii	19.2
26	West Virginia	25.0		48	New Hampshire	16.4
27	Wisconsin	24.7		49	Florida	16.3
2	Wyoming	30.5		50	California	16.1

District of Columbia 20.2

Source: U.S. Department of Health and Human Services, National Center for Health Statistics
   "National Vital Statistics Reports" (Vol. 49, No. 8, September 21, 2001)
*Final data by state of residence. Age-adjusted rates based on the year 2000 standard population.

Deaths by Tuberculosis in 1999

National Total = 930 Deaths*

ALPHA ORDER				RANK ORDER			
RANK	STATE	DEATHS	% of USA	RANK	STATE	DEATHS	% of USA
19	Alabama	16	1.7%	1	California	157	16.9%
40	Alaska	2	0.2%	2	Texas	91	9.8%
14	Arizona	21	2.3%	3	Florida	69	7.4%
24	Arkansas	12	1.3%	4	New York	61	6.6%
1	California	157	16.9%	5	Illinois	38	4.1%
28	Colorado	8	0.9%	6	Georgia	37	4.0%
32	Connecticut	5	0.5%	6	Pennsylvania	37	4.0%
40	Delaware	2	0.2%	8	Ohio	30	3.2%
3	Florida	69	7.4%	9	Michigan	27	2.9%
6	Georgia	37	4.0%	10	New Jersey	25	2.7%
33	Hawaii	4	0.4%	11	Louisiana	23	2.5%
33	Idaho	4	0.4%	11	North Carolina	23	2.5%
5	Illinois	38	4.1%	11	Tennessee	23	2.5%
23	Indiana	13	1.4%	14	Arizona	21	2.3%
37	Iowa	3	0.3%	15	Maryland	20	2.2%
33	Kansas	4	0.4%	15	Virginia	20	2.2%
20	Kentucky	15	1.6%	17	Missouri	19	2.0%
11	Louisiana	23	2.5%	18	South Carolina	17	1.8%
37	Maine	3	0.3%	19	Alabama	16	1.7%
15	Maryland	20	2.2%	20	Kentucky	15	1.6%
26	Massachusetts	9	1.0%	20	Mississippi	15	1.6%
9	Michigan	27	2.9%	20	Oklahoma	15	1.6%
30	Minnesota	6	0.6%	23	Indiana	13	1.4%
20	Mississippi	15	1.6%	24	Arkansas	12	1.3%
17	Missouri	19	2.0%	25	New Mexico	11	1.2%
40	Montana	2	0.2%	26	Massachusetts	9	1.0%
40	Nebraska	2	0.2%	26	Washington	9	1.0%
29	Nevada	7	0.8%	28	Colorado	8	0.9%
46	New Hampshire	1	0.1%	29	Nevada	7	0.8%
10	New Jersey	25	2.7%	30	Minnesota	6	0.6%
25	New Mexico	11	1.2%	30	Wisconsin	6	0.6%
4	New York	61	6.6%	32	Connecticut	5	0.5%
11	North Carolina	23	2.5%	33	Hawaii	4	0.4%
49	North Dakota	0	0.0%	33	Idaho	4	0.4%
8	Ohio	30	3.2%	33	Kansas	4	0.4%
20	Oklahoma	15	1.6%	33	Rhode Island	4	0.4%
40	Oregon	2	0.2%	37	Iowa	3	0.3%
6	Pennsylvania	37	4.0%	37	Maine	3	0.3%
33	Rhode Island	4	0.4%	37	South Dakota	3	0.3%
18	South Carolina	17	1.8%	40	Alaska	2	0.2%
37	South Dakota	3	0.3%	40	Delaware	2	0.2%
11	Tennessee	23	2.5%	40	Montana	2	0.2%
2	Texas	91	9.8%	40	Nebraska	2	0.2%
40	Utah	2	0.2%	40	Oregon	2	0.2%
46	Vermont	1	0.1%	40	Utah	2	0.2%
15	Virginia	20	2.2%	46	New Hampshire	1	0.1%
26	Washington	9	1.0%	46	Vermont	1	0.1%
46	West Virginia	1	0.1%	46	West Virginia	1	0.1%
30	Wisconsin	6	0.6%	49	North Dakota	0	0.0%
49	Wyoming	0	0.0%	49	Wyoming	0	0.0%
					District of Columbia	5	0.5%

Source: U.S. Department of Health and Human Services, National Center for Health Statistics
(http://wonder.cdc.gov/WONDER/)
*By state of residence.

Death Rate by Tuberculosis in 1999

National Rate = 0.3 Deaths per 100,000 Population*

ALPHA ORDER			RANK ORDER		
RANK	STATE	RATE	RANK	STATE	RATE
9	Alabama	0.4	1	New Mexico	0.6
19	Alaska	0.3	2	Arkansas	0.5
9	Arizona	0.4	2	California	0.5
2	Arkansas	0.5	2	Florida	0.5
2	California	0.5	2	Georgia	0.5
32	Colorado	0.2	2	Louisiana	0.5
32	Connecticut	0.2	2	Mississippi	0.5
19	Delaware	0.3	2	Texas	0.5
2	Florida	0.5	9	Alabama	0.4
2	Georgia	0.5	9	Arizona	0.4
19	Hawaii	0.3	9	Kentucky	0.4
19	Idaho	0.3	9	Maryland	0.4
19	Illinois	0.3	9	Nevada	0.4
32	Indiana	0.2	9	Oklahoma	0.4
40	Iowa	0.1	9	Rhode Island	0.4
32	Kansas	0.2	9	South Carolina	0.4
9	Kentucky	0.4	9	South Dakota	0.4
2	Louisiana	0.5	9	Tennessee	0.4
32	Maine	0.2	19	Alaska	0.3
9	Maryland	0.4	19	Delaware	0.3
40	Massachusetts	0.1	19	Hawaii	0.3
19	Michigan	0.3	19	Idaho	0.3
40	Minnesota	0.1	19	Illinois	0.3
2	Mississippi	0.5	19	Michigan	0.3
19	Missouri	0.3	19	Missouri	0.3
32	Montana	0.2	19	New Jersey	0.3
40	Nebraska	0.1	19	New York	0.3
9	Nevada	0.4	19	North Carolina	0.3
40	New Hampshire	0.1	19	Ohio	0.3
19	New Jersey	0.3	19	Pennsylvania	0.3
1	New Mexico	0.6	19	Virginia	0.3
19	New York	0.3	32	Colorado	0.2
19	North Carolina	0.3	32	Connecticut	0.2
49	North Dakota	0.0	32	Indiana	0.2
19	Ohio	0.3	32	Kansas	0.2
9	Oklahoma	0.4	32	Maine	0.2
40	Oregon	0.1	32	Montana	0.2
19	Pennsylvania	0.3	32	Vermont	0.2
9	Rhode Island	0.4	32	Washington	0.2
9	South Carolina	0.4	40	Iowa	0.1
9	South Dakota	0.4	40	Massachusetts	0.1
9	Tennessee	0.4	40	Minnesota	0.1
2	Texas	0.5	40	Nebraska	0.1
40	Utah	0.1	40	New Hampshire	0.1
32	Vermont	0.2	40	Oregon	0.1
19	Virginia	0.3	40	Utah	0.1
32	Washington	0.2	40	West Virginia	0.1
40	West Virginia	0.1	40	Wisconsin	0.1
40	Wisconsin	0.1	49	North Dakota	0.0
49	Wyoming	0.0	49	Wyoming	0.0
				District of Columbia	1.0

Source: U.S. Department of Health and Human Services, National Center for Health Statistics
(http://wonder.cdc.gov/WONDER/)
*By state of residence. Not age-adjusted. Due to low numbers of deaths, rates for all states should be interpreted with caution.

Age-Adjusted Death Rate by Tuberculosis in 1999

National Rate = 0.3 Deaths per 100,000 Population*

ALPHA ORDER

RANK	STATE	RATE
9	Alabama	0.4
9	Alaska	0.4
4	Arizona	0.5
9	Arkansas	0.4
4	California	0.5
32	Colorado	0.2
38	Connecticut	0.1
20	Delaware	0.3
9	Florida	0.4
4	Georgia	0.5
20	Hawaii	0.3
20	Idaho	0.3
20	Illinois	0.3
32	Indiana	0.2
38	Iowa	0.1
38	Kansas	0.1
9	Kentucky	0.4
2	Louisiana	0.6
32	Maine	0.2
9	Maryland	0.4
38	Massachusetts	0.1
20	Michigan	0.3
38	Minnesota	0.1
2	Mississippi	0.6
20	Missouri	0.3
32	Montana	0.2
38	Nebraska	0.1
9	Nevada	0.4
38	New Hampshire	0.1
20	New Jersey	0.3
1	New Mexico	0.7
20	New York	0.3
20	North Carolina	0.3
48	North Dakota	0.0
20	Ohio	0.3
9	Oklahoma	0.4
38	Oregon	0.1
20	Pennsylvania	0.3
9	Rhode Island	0.4
4	South Carolina	0.5
9	South Dakota	0.4
9	Tennessee	0.4
4	Texas	0.5
38	Utah	0.1
32	Vermont	0.2
20	Virginia	0.3
32	Washington	0.2
48	West Virginia	0.0
38	Wisconsin	0.1
48	Wyoming	0.0

RANK ORDER

RANK	STATE	RATE
1	New Mexico	0.7
2	Louisiana	0.6
2	Mississippi	0.6
4	Arizona	0.5
4	California	0.5
4	Georgia	0.5
4	South Carolina	0.5
4	Texas	0.5
9	Alabama	0.4
9	Alaska	0.4
9	Arkansas	0.4
9	Florida	0.4
9	Kentucky	0.4
9	Maryland	0.4
9	Nevada	0.4
9	Oklahoma	0.4
9	Rhode Island	0.4
9	South Dakota	0.4
9	Tennessee	0.4
20	Delaware	0.3
20	Hawaii	0.3
20	Idaho	0.3
20	Illinois	0.3
20	Michigan	0.3
20	Missouri	0.3
20	New Jersey	0.3
20	New York	0.3
20	North Carolina	0.3
20	Ohio	0.3
20	Pennsylvania	0.3
20	Virginia	0.3
32	Colorado	0.2
32	Indiana	0.2
32	Maine	0.2
32	Montana	0.2
32	Vermont	0.2
32	Washington	0.2
38	Connecticut	0.1
38	Iowa	0.1
38	Kansas	0.1
38	Massachusetts	0.1
38	Minnesota	0.1
38	Nebraska	0.1
38	New Hampshire	0.1
38	Oregon	0.1
38	Utah	0.1
38	Wisconsin	0.1
48	North Dakota	0.0
48	West Virginia	0.0
48	Wyoming	0.0
	District of Columbia	0.9

Source: U.S. Department of Health and Human Services, National Center for Health Statistics
    (http://wonder.cdc.gov/WONDER/)
*By state of residence. Due to low numbers of deaths, rates for all states should be interpreted with caution.
Age-adjusted rates based on the year 2000 standard population.

Deaths by Injury in 1999

National Total = 143,948 Deaths*

ALPHA ORDER

ALPHA ORDER

RANK	STATE	DEATHS	% of USA
16	Alabama	3,306	2.3%
45	Alaska	441	0.3%
13	Arizona	3,450	2.4%
29	Arkansas	1,802	1.3%
1	California	14,341	10.0%
25	Colorado	2,292	1.6%
34	Connecticut	1,428	1.0%
46	Delaware	377	0.3%
3	Florida	8,954	6.2%
10	Georgia	4,585	3.2%
44	Hawaii	467	0.3%
39	Idaho	809	0.6%
6	Illinois	6,168	4.3%
15	Indiana	3,323	2.3%
32	Iowa	1,481	1.0%
31	Kansas	1,562	1.1%
22	Kentucky	2,410	1.7%
18	Louisiana	2,942	2.0%
40	Maine	658	0.5%
26	Maryland	2,262	1.6%
28	Massachusetts	1,867	1.3%
8	Michigan	4,921	3.4%
23	Minnesota	2,348	1.6%
27	Mississippi	2,258	1.6%
12	Missouri	3,550	2.5%
41	Montana	656	0.5%
38	Nebraska	906	0.6%
35	Nevada	1,281	0.9%
42	New Hampshire	487	0.3%
17	New Jersey	3,088	2.1%
33	New Mexico	1,454	1.0%
4	New York	6,962	4.8%
9	North Carolina	4,825	3.4%
49	North Dakota	353	0.2%
7	Ohio	5,182	3.6%
24	Oklahoma	2,332	1.6%
30	Oregon	1,784	1.2%
5	Pennsylvania	6,537	4.5%
47	Rhode Island	375	0.3%
21	South Carolina	2,632	1.8%
43	South Dakota	477	0.3%
11	Tennessee	3,826	2.7%
2	Texas	10,551	7.3%
37	Utah	983	0.7%
50	Vermont	289	0.2%
14	Virginia	3,424	2.4%
19	Washington	2,920	2.0%
36	West Virginia	1,126	0.8%
20	Wisconsin	2,750	1.9%
48	Wyoming	369	0.3%

RANK ORDER

RANK	STATE	DEATHS	% of USA
1	California	14,341	10.0%
2	Texas	10,551	7.3%
3	Florida	8,954	6.2%
4	New York	6,962	4.8%
5	Pennsylvania	6,537	4.5%
6	Illinois	6,168	4.3%
7	Ohio	5,182	3.6%
8	Michigan	4,921	3.4%
9	North Carolina	4,825	3.4%
10	Georgia	4,585	3.2%
11	Tennessee	3,826	2.7%
12	Missouri	3,550	2.5%
13	Arizona	3,450	2.4%
14	Virginia	3,424	2.4%
15	Indiana	3,323	2.3%
16	Alabama	3,306	2.3%
17	New Jersey	3,088	2.1%
18	Louisiana	2,942	2.0%
19	Washington	2,920	2.0%
20	Wisconsin	2,750	1.9%
21	South Carolina	2,632	1.8%
22	Kentucky	2,410	1.7%
23	Minnesota	2,348	1.6%
24	Oklahoma	2,332	1.6%
25	Colorado	2,292	1.6%
26	Maryland	2,262	1.6%
27	Mississippi	2,258	1.6%
28	Massachusetts	1,867	1.3%
29	Arkansas	1,802	1.3%
30	Oregon	1,784	1.2%
31	Kansas	1,562	1.1%
32	Iowa	1,481	1.0%
33	New Mexico	1,454	1.0%
34	Connecticut	1,428	1.0%
35	Nevada	1,281	0.9%
36	West Virginia	1,126	0.8%
37	Utah	983	0.7%
38	Nebraska	906	0.6%
39	Idaho	809	0.6%
40	Maine	658	0.5%
41	Montana	656	0.5%
42	New Hampshire	487	0.3%
43	South Dakota	477	0.3%
44	Hawaii	467	0.3%
45	Alaska	441	0.3%
46	Delaware	377	0.3%
47	Rhode Island	375	0.3%
48	Wyoming	369	0.3%
49	North Dakota	353	0.2%
50	Vermont	289	0.2%
	District of Columbia	377	0.3%

Source: U.S. Department of Health and Human Services, National Center for Health Statistics
   (http://wonder.cdc.gov/WONDER/)
By state of residence. Injury as used here includes Accidents (including motor vehicle), Suicides, Homicides and "Other" undetermined.

Death Rate by Injury in 1999

National Rate = 52.8 Deaths per 100,000 Population*

ALPHA ORDER				RANK ORDER		
RANK	STATE	RATE		RANK	STATE	RATE
4	Alabama	75.7		1	New Mexico	83.6
7	Alaska	71.2		2	Mississippi	81.6
6	Arizona	72.2		3	Wyoming	76.9
9	Arkansas	70.6		4	Alabama	75.7
44	California	43.3		5	Montana	74.3
23	Colorado	56.5		6	Arizona	72.2
43	Connecticut	43.5		7	Alaska	71.2
35	Delaware	50.0		8	Nevada	70.8
20	Florida	59.3		9	Arkansas	70.6
21	Georgia	58.9		10	Tennessee	69.8
46	Hawaii	39.4		11	Oklahoma	69.4
16	Idaho	64.6		12	South Carolina	67.7
33	Illinois	50.9		13	Louisiana	67.3
24	Indiana	55.9		14	South Dakota	65.1
32	Iowa	51.6		15	Missouri	64.9
21	Kansas	58.9		16	Idaho	64.6
19	Kentucky	60.8		17	North Carolina	63.1
13	Louisiana	67.3		18	West Virginia	62.3
30	Maine	52.5		19	Kentucky	60.8
42	Maryland	43.7		20	Florida	59.3
50	Massachusetts	30.2		21	Georgia	58.9
36	Michigan	49.9		21	Kansas	58.9
38	Minnesota	49.2		23	Colorado	56.5
2	Mississippi	81.6		24	Indiana	55.9
15	Missouri	64.9		25	North Dakota	55.7
5	Montana	74.3		26	Pennsylvania	54.5
27	Nebraska	54.4		27	Nebraska	54.4
8	Nevada	70.8		28	Oregon	53.8
45	New Hampshire	40.5		29	Texas	52.6
48	New Jersey	37.9		30	Maine	52.5
1	New Mexico	83.6		31	Wisconsin	52.4
47	New York	38.3		32	Iowa	51.6
17	North Carolina	63.1		33	Illinois	50.9
25	North Dakota	55.7		34	Washington	50.7
41	Ohio	46.0		35	Delaware	50.0
11	Oklahoma	69.4		36	Michigan	49.9
28	Oregon	53.8		37	Virginia	49.8
26	Pennsylvania	54.5		38	Minnesota	49.2
49	Rhode Island	37.8		39	Vermont	48.7
12	South Carolina	67.7		40	Utah	46.2
14	South Dakota	65.1		41	Ohio	46.0
10	Tennessee	69.8		42	Maryland	43.7
29	Texas	52.6		43	Connecticut	43.5
40	Utah	46.2		44	California	43.3
39	Vermont	48.7		45	New Hampshire	40.5
37	Virginia	49.8		46	Hawaii	39.4
34	Washington	50.7		47	New York	38.3
18	West Virginia	62.3		48	New Jersey	37.9
31	Wisconsin	52.4		49	Rhode Island	37.8
3	Wyoming	76.9		50	Massachusetts	30.2
					District of Columbia	72.6

Source: U.S. Department of Health and Human Services, National Center for Health Statistics
(http://wonder.cdc.gov/WONDER/)
*By state of residence. Injury as used here includes Accidents (including motor vehicle), Suicides, Homicides and "Other" undetermined. Not age-adjusted.

Age-Adjusted Death Rate by Injury in 1999

National Rate = 52.7 Deaths per 100,000 Population*

ALPHA ORDER

RANK	STATE	RATE
5	Alabama	75.0
2	Alaska	83.5
6	Arizona	73.5
9	Arkansas	69.7
43	California	44.4
21	Colorado	59.3
44	Connecticut	42.1
36	Delaware	50.3
23	Florida	56.9
18	Georgia	61.9
46	Hawaii	39.2
14	Idaho	66.2
32	Illinois	51.0
24	Indiana	55.9
39	Iowa	48.1
22	Kansas	57.3
19	Kentucky	60.7
13	Louisiana	68.6
35	Maine	50.5
42	Maryland	44.7
50	Massachusetts	28.9
37	Michigan	50.1
38	Minnesota	48.3
3	Mississippi	82.3
15	Missouri	63.6
8	Montana	72.5
27	Nebraska	52.4
7	Nevada	73.4
45	New Hampshire	40.9
48	New Jersey	37.2
1	New Mexico	86.7
47	New York	37.6
15	North Carolina	63.6
28	North Dakota	52.3
41	Ohio	45.5
11	Oklahoma	69.0
26	Oregon	52.7
29	Pennsylvania	51.9
49	Rhode Island	35.5
12	South Carolina	68.7
17	South Dakota	63.0
10	Tennessee	69.6
25	Texas	55.2
30	Utah	51.4
39	Vermont	48.1
32	Virginia	51.0
31	Washington	51.1
20	West Virginia	59.7
32	Wisconsin	51.0
4	Wyoming	77.5

RANK ORDER

RANK	STATE	RATE
1	New Mexico	86.7
2	Alaska	83.5
3	Mississippi	82.3
4	Wyoming	77.5
5	Alabama	75.0
6	Arizona	73.5
7	Nevada	73.4
8	Montana	72.5
9	Arkansas	69.7
10	Tennessee	69.6
11	Oklahoma	69.0
12	South Carolina	68.7
13	Louisiana	68.6
14	Idaho	66.2
15	Missouri	63.6
15	North Carolina	63.6
17	South Dakota	63.0
18	Georgia	61.9
19	Kentucky	60.7
20	West Virginia	59.7
21	Colorado	59.3
22	Kansas	57.3
23	Florida	56.9
24	Indiana	55.9
25	Texas	55.2
26	Oregon	52.7
27	Nebraska	52.4
28	North Dakota	52.3
29	Pennsylvania	51.9
30	Utah	51.4
31	Washington	51.1
32	Illinois	51.0
32	Virginia	51.0
32	Wisconsin	51.0
35	Maine	50.5
36	Delaware	50.3
37	Michigan	50.1
38	Minnesota	48.3
39	Iowa	48.1
39	Vermont	48.1
41	Ohio	45.5
42	Maryland	44.7
43	California	44.4
44	Connecticut	42.1
45	New Hampshire	40.9
46	Hawaii	39.2
47	New York	37.6
48	New Jersey	37.2
49	Rhode Island	35.5
50	Massachusetts	28.9

	District of Columbia	71.3

Source: U.S. Department of Health and Human Services, National Center for Health Statistics (http://wonder.cdc.gov/WONDER/)

*By state of residence. Injury as used here includes Accidents (including motor vehicle), Suicides, Homicides and "Other" undetermined. Age-adjusted rates based on the year 2000 standard population.

Deaths by Accidents in 1999

National Total = 97,860 Deaths*

ALPHA ORDER

RANK	STATE	DEATHS	% of USA
13	Alabama	2,313	2.4%
44	Alaska	294	0.3%
16	Arizona	2,214	2.3%
29	Arkansas	1,287	1.3%
1	California	9,198	9.4%
26	Colorado	1,519	1.6%
33	Connecticut	1,034	1.1%
46	Delaware	267	0.3%
3	Florida	5,961	6.1%
10	Georgia	3,078	3.1%
45	Hawaii	293	0.3%
39	Idaho	597	0.6%
6	Illinois	4,125	4.2%
14	Indiana	2,309	2.4%
32	Iowa	1,123	1.1%
31	Kansas	1,126	1.2%
23	Kentucky	1,730	1.8%
19	Louisiana	1,940	2.0%
41	Maine	458	0.5%
28	Maryland	1,296	1.3%
27	Massachusetts	1,303	1.3%
9	Michigan	3,188	3.3%
22	Minnesota	1,772	1.8%
24	Mississippi	1,642	1.7%
12	Missouri	2,465	2.5%
40	Montana	461	0.5%
37	Nebraska	668	0.7%
36	Nevada	710	0.7%
43	New Hampshire	329	0.3%
15	New Jersey	2,227	2.3%
34	New Mexico	969	1.0%
4	New York	4,797	4.9%
8	North Carolina	3,290	3.4%
46	North Dakota	267	0.3%
7	Ohio	3,630	3.7%
25	Oklahoma	1,609	1.6%
30	Oregon	1,199	1.2%
5	Pennsylvania	4,614	4.7%
49	Rhode Island	243	0.2%
21	South Carolina	1,901	1.9%
42	South Dakota	351	0.4%
11	Tennessee	2,677	2.7%
2	Texas	7,227	7.4%
38	Utah	650	0.7%
50	Vermont	209	0.2%
16	Virginia	2,214	2.3%
20	Washington	1,914	2.0%
35	West Virginia	798	0.8%
18	Wisconsin	1,955	2.0%
48	Wyoming	258	0.3%

RANK ORDER

RANK	STATE	DEATHS	% of USA
1	California	9,198	9.4%
2	Texas	7,227	7.4%
3	Florida	5,961	6.1%
4	New York	4,797	4.9%
5	Pennsylvania	4,614	4.7%
6	Illinois	4,125	4.2%
7	Ohio	3,630	3.7%
8	North Carolina	3,290	3.4%
9	Michigan	3,188	3.3%
10	Georgia	3,078	3.1%
11	Tennessee	2,677	2.7%
12	Missouri	2,465	2.5%
13	Alabama	2,313	2.4%
14	Indiana	2,309	2.4%
15	New Jersey	2,227	2.3%
16	Arizona	2,214	2.3%
16	Virginia	2,214	2.3%
18	Wisconsin	1,955	2.0%
19	Louisiana	1,940	2.0%
20	Washington	1,914	2.0%
21	South Carolina	1,901	1.9%
22	Minnesota	1,772	1.8%
23	Kentucky	1,730	1.8%
24	Mississippi	1,642	1.7%
25	Oklahoma	1,609	1.6%
26	Colorado	1,519	1.6%
27	Massachusetts	1,303	1.3%
28	Maryland	1,296	1.3%
29	Arkansas	1,287	1.3%
30	Oregon	1,199	1.2%
31	Kansas	1,126	1.2%
32	Iowa	1,123	1.1%
33	Connecticut	1,034	1.1%
34	New Mexico	969	1.0%
35	West Virginia	798	0.8%
36	Nevada	710	0.7%
37	Nebraska	668	0.7%
38	Utah	650	0.7%
39	Idaho	597	0.6%
40	Montana	461	0.5%
41	Maine	458	0.5%
42	South Dakota	351	0.4%
43	New Hampshire	329	0.3%
44	Alaska	294	0.3%
45	Hawaii	293	0.3%
46	Delaware	267	0.3%
46	North Dakota	267	0.3%
48	Wyoming	258	0.3%
49	Rhode Island	243	0.2%
50	Vermont	209	0.2%
	District of Columbia	161	0.2%

Source: U.S. Department of Health and Human Services, National Center for Health Statistics
"National Vital Statistics Reports" (Vol. 49, No. 8, September 21, 2001)
*Final data by state of residence. Includes motor vehicle deaths, poisoning, falls, drowning and other accidents.

Death Rate by Accidents in 1999

National Rate = 35.9 Deaths per 100,000 Population*

ALPHA ORDER			RANK ORDER		
RANK	STATE	RATE	RANK	STATE	RATE
4	Alabama	52.9	1	Mississippi	59.3
12	Alaska	47.5	2	New Mexico	55.7
13	Arizona	46.3	3	Wyoming	53.8
6	Arkansas	50.4	4	Alabama	52.9
43	California	27.8	5	Montana	52.2
28	Colorado	37.4	6	Arkansas	50.4
41	Connecticut	31.5	7	South Carolina	48.9
34	Delaware	35.4	8	Tennessee	48.8
23	Florida	39.4	9	Oklahoma	47.9
22	Georgia	39.5	9	South Dakota	47.9
48	Hawaii	24.7	11	Idaho	47.7
11	Idaho	47.7	12	Alaska	47.5
36	Illinois	34.0	13	Arizona	46.3
26	Indiana	38.9	14	Missouri	45.1
25	Iowa	39.1	15	Louisiana	44.4
19	Kansas	42.4	16	West Virginia	44.2
17	Kentucky	43.7	17	Kentucky	43.7
15	Louisiana	44.4	18	North Carolina	43.0
31	Maine	36.6	19	Kansas	42.4
47	Maryland	25.1	20	North Dakota	42.1
50	Massachusetts	21.1	21	Nebraska	40.1
38	Michigan	32.3	22	Georgia	39.5
30	Minnesota	37.1	23	Florida	39.4
1	Mississippi	59.3	24	Nevada	39.2
14	Missouri	45.1	25	Iowa	39.1
5	Montana	52.2	26	Indiana	38.9
21	Nebraska	40.1	27	Pennsylvania	38.5
24	Nevada	39.2	28	Colorado	37.4
44	New Hampshire	27.4	29	Wisconsin	37.2
45	New Jersey	27.3	30	Minnesota	37.1
2	New Mexico	55.7	31	Maine	36.6
46	New York	26.4	32	Oregon	36.2
18	North Carolina	43.0	33	Texas	36.1
20	North Dakota	42.1	34	Delaware	35.4
39	Ohio	32.2	35	Vermont	35.2
9	Oklahoma	47.9	36	Illinois	34.0
32	Oregon	36.2	37	Washington	33.3
27	Pennsylvania	38.5	38	Michigan	32.3
49	Rhode Island	24.5	39	Ohio	32.2
7	South Carolina	48.9	39	Virginia	32.2
9	South Dakota	47.9	41	Connecticut	31.5
8	Tennessee	48.8	42	Utah	30.5
33	Texas	36.1	43	California	27.8
42	Utah	30.5	44	New Hampshire	27.4
35	Vermont	35.2	45	New Jersey	27.3
39	Virginia	32.2	46	New York	26.4
37	Washington	33.3	47	Maryland	25.1
16	West Virginia	44.2	48	Hawaii	24.7
29	Wisconsin	37.2	49	Rhode Island	24.5
3	Wyoming	53.8	50	Massachusetts	21.1
				District of Columbia	31.0

Source: U.S. Department of Health and Human Services, National Center for Health Statistics
   "National Vital Statistics Reports" (Vol. 49, No. 8, September 21, 2001)
*Final data by state of residence. Includes motor vehicle deaths, poisoning, falls, drowning and other accidents.
Not age-adjusted.

Age-Adjusted Death Rate by Accidents in 1999

National Rate = 35.9 Deaths per 100,000 Population*

ALPHA ORDER				RANK ORDER		
RANK	STATE	RATE		RANK	STATE	RATE
5	Alabama	52.6		1	Mississippi	60.0
3	Alaska	57.8		2	New Mexico	58.2
12	Arizona	47.1		3	Alaska	57.8
8	Arkansas	49.4		4	Wyoming	53.9
43	California	28.7		5	Alabama	52.6
22	Colorado	40.1		6	Montana	50.7
42	Connecticut	30.1		7	South Carolina	50.1
29	Delaware	36.1		8	Arkansas	49.4
27	Florida	37.3		9	Tennessee	49.0
18	Georgia	42.6		10	Idaho	48.7
48	Hawaii	24.5		11	Oklahoma	47.2
10	Idaho	48.7		12	Arizona	47.1
37	Illinois	34.1		13	South Dakota	45.7
24	Indiana	38.9		14	Louisiana	45.6
32	Iowa	35.8		15	Missouri	43.8
21	Kansas	40.9		16	Kentucky	43.7
16	Kentucky	43.7		17	North Carolina	43.6
14	Louisiana	45.6		18	Georgia	42.6
34	Maine	35.1		19	West Virginia	42.0
46	Maryland	26.1		20	Nevada	41.0
50	Massachusetts	19.9		21	Kansas	40.9
40	Michigan	32.6		22	Colorado	40.1
28	Minnesota	36.3		23	North Dakota	39.0
1	Mississippi	60.0		24	Indiana	38.9
15	Missouri	43.8		25	Texas	38.3
6	Montana	50.7		26	Nebraska	38.0
26	Nebraska	38.0		27	Florida	37.3
20	Nevada	41.0		28	Minnesota	36.3
44	New Hampshire	27.9		29	Delaware	36.1
45	New Jersey	26.7		30	Wisconsin	36.0
2	New Mexico	58.2		31	Pennsylvania	35.9
47	New York	25.8		32	Iowa	35.8
17	North Carolina	43.6		33	Oregon	35.3
23	North Dakota	39.0		34	Maine	35.1
41	Ohio	31.9		35	Vermont	34.8
11	Oklahoma	47.2		36	Utah	34.3
33	Oregon	35.3		37	Illinois	34.1
31	Pennsylvania	35.9		38	Virginia	33.6
49	Rhode Island	22.3		38	Washington	33.6
7	South Carolina	50.1		40	Michigan	32.6
13	South Dakota	45.7		41	Ohio	31.9
9	Tennessee	49.0		42	Connecticut	30.1
25	Texas	38.3		43	California	28.7
36	Utah	34.3		44	New Hampshire	27.9
35	Vermont	34.8		45	New Jersey	26.7
38	Virginia	33.6		46	Maryland	26.1
38	Washington	33.6		47	New York	25.8
19	West Virginia	42.0		48	Hawaii	24.5
30	Wisconsin	36.0		49	Rhode Island	22.3
4	Wyoming	53.9		50	Massachusetts	19.9
					District of Columbia	29.1

Source: U.S. Department of Health and Human Services, National Center for Health Statistics
    "National Vital Statistics Reports" (Vol. 49, No. 8, September 21, 2001)
*Final data by state of residence. Includes motor vehicle deaths, poisoning, falls, drowning and other accidents.
Age-adjusted rates based on the year 2000 standard population.

Deaths by Motor Vehicle Accidents in 1999

National Total = 42,401 Deaths*

<table>
<tr><th colspan="4">ALPHA ORDER</th><th colspan="4">RANK ORDER</th></tr>
<tr><th>RANK</th><th>STATE</th><th>DEATHS</th><th>% of USA</th><th>RANK</th><th>STATE</th><th>DEATHS</th><th>% of USA</th></tr>
<tr><td>12</td><td>Alabama</td><td>1,162</td><td>2.7%</td><td>1</td><td>Texas</td><td>3,669</td><td>8.7%</td></tr>
<tr><td>49</td><td>Alaska</td><td>87</td><td>0.2%</td><td>2</td><td>California</td><td>3,641</td><td>8.6%</td></tr>
<tr><td>18</td><td>Arizona</td><td>945</td><td>2.2%</td><td>3</td><td>Florida</td><td>2,872</td><td>6.8%</td></tr>
<tr><td>25</td><td>Arkansas</td><td>649</td><td>1.5%</td><td>4</td><td>New York</td><td>1,759</td><td>4.1%</td></tr>
<tr><td>2</td><td>California</td><td>3,641</td><td>8.6%</td><td>5</td><td>North Carolina</td><td>1,597</td><td>3.8%</td></tr>
<tr><td>27</td><td>Colorado</td><td>620</td><td>1.5%</td><td>6</td><td>Pennsylvania</td><td>1,580</td><td>3.7%</td></tr>
<tr><td>37</td><td>Connecticut</td><td>308</td><td>0.7%</td><td>7</td><td>Illinois</td><td>1,537</td><td>3.6%</td></tr>
<tr><td>46</td><td>Delaware</td><td>98</td><td>0.2%</td><td>8</td><td>Georgia</td><td>1,521</td><td>3.6%</td></tr>
<tr><td>3</td><td>Florida</td><td>2,872</td><td>6.8%</td><td>9</td><td>Ohio</td><td>1,427</td><td>3.4%</td></tr>
<tr><td>8</td><td>Georgia</td><td>1,521</td><td>3.6%</td><td>10</td><td>Michigan</td><td>1,411</td><td>3.3%</td></tr>
<tr><td>47</td><td>Hawaii</td><td>90</td><td>0.2%</td><td>11</td><td>Tennessee</td><td>1,322</td><td>3.1%</td></tr>
<tr><td>39</td><td>Idaho</td><td>278</td><td>0.7%</td><td>12</td><td>Alabama</td><td>1,162</td><td>2.7%</td></tr>
<tr><td>7</td><td>Illinois</td><td>1,537</td><td>3.6%</td><td>13</td><td>Missouri</td><td>1,061</td><td>2.5%</td></tr>
<tr><td>15</td><td>Indiana</td><td>988</td><td>2.3%</td><td>14</td><td>South Carolina</td><td>996</td><td>2.3%</td></tr>
<tr><td>30</td><td>Iowa</td><td>529</td><td>1.2%</td><td>15</td><td>Indiana</td><td>988</td><td>2.3%</td></tr>
<tr><td>29</td><td>Kansas</td><td>570</td><td>1.3%</td><td>16</td><td>Louisiana</td><td>976</td><td>2.3%</td></tr>
<tr><td>20</td><td>Kentucky</td><td>814</td><td>1.9%</td><td>17</td><td>Mississippi</td><td>956</td><td>2.3%</td></tr>
<tr><td>16</td><td>Louisiana</td><td>976</td><td>2.3%</td><td>18</td><td>Arizona</td><td>945</td><td>2.2%</td></tr>
<tr><td>41</td><td>Maine</td><td>199</td><td>0.5%</td><td>19</td><td>Virginia</td><td>897</td><td>2.1%</td></tr>
<tr><td>28</td><td>Maryland</td><td>609</td><td>1.4%</td><td>20</td><td>Kentucky</td><td>814</td><td>1.9%</td></tr>
<tr><td>31</td><td>Massachusetts</td><td>441</td><td>1.0%</td><td>21</td><td>Wisconsin</td><td>775</td><td>1.8%</td></tr>
<tr><td>10</td><td>Michigan</td><td>1,411</td><td>3.3%</td><td>22</td><td>Washington</td><td>732</td><td>1.7%</td></tr>
<tr><td>26</td><td>Minnesota</td><td>646</td><td>1.5%</td><td>23</td><td>New Jersey</td><td>727</td><td>1.7%</td></tr>
<tr><td>17</td><td>Mississippi</td><td>956</td><td>2.3%</td><td>24</td><td>Oklahoma</td><td>686</td><td>1.6%</td></tr>
<tr><td>13</td><td>Missouri</td><td>1,061</td><td>2.5%</td><td>25</td><td>Arkansas</td><td>649</td><td>1.5%</td></tr>
<tr><td>40</td><td>Montana</td><td>210</td><td>0.5%</td><td>26</td><td>Minnesota</td><td>646</td><td>1.5%</td></tr>
<tr><td>38</td><td>Nebraska</td><td>295</td><td>0.7%</td><td>27</td><td>Colorado</td><td>620</td><td>1.5%</td></tr>
<tr><td>36</td><td>Nevada</td><td>333</td><td>0.8%</td><td>28</td><td>Maryland</td><td>609</td><td>1.4%</td></tr>
<tr><td>45</td><td>New Hampshire</td><td>129</td><td>0.3%</td><td>29</td><td>Kansas</td><td>570</td><td>1.3%</td></tr>
<tr><td>23</td><td>New Jersey</td><td>727</td><td>1.7%</td><td>30</td><td>Iowa</td><td>529</td><td>1.2%</td></tr>
<tr><td>33</td><td>New Mexico</td><td>415</td><td>1.0%</td><td>31</td><td>Massachusetts</td><td>441</td><td>1.0%</td></tr>
<tr><td>4</td><td>New York</td><td>1,759</td><td>4.1%</td><td>32</td><td>Oregon</td><td>433</td><td>1.0%</td></tr>
<tr><td>5</td><td>North Carolina</td><td>1,597</td><td>3.8%</td><td>33</td><td>New Mexico</td><td>415</td><td>1.0%</td></tr>
<tr><td>44</td><td>North Dakota</td><td>134</td><td>0.3%</td><td>34</td><td>West Virginia</td><td>387</td><td>0.9%</td></tr>
<tr><td>9</td><td>Ohio</td><td>1,427</td><td>3.4%</td><td>35</td><td>Utah</td><td>364</td><td>0.9%</td></tr>
<tr><td>24</td><td>Oklahoma</td><td>686</td><td>1.6%</td><td>36</td><td>Nevada</td><td>333</td><td>0.8%</td></tr>
<tr><td>32</td><td>Oregon</td><td>433</td><td>1.0%</td><td>37</td><td>Connecticut</td><td>308</td><td>0.7%</td></tr>
<tr><td>6</td><td>Pennsylvania</td><td>1,580</td><td>3.7%</td><td>38</td><td>Nebraska</td><td>295</td><td>0.7%</td></tr>
<tr><td>48</td><td>Rhode Island</td><td>89</td><td>0.2%</td><td>39</td><td>Idaho</td><td>278</td><td>0.7%</td></tr>
<tr><td>14</td><td>South Carolina</td><td>996</td><td>2.3%</td><td>40</td><td>Montana</td><td>210</td><td>0.5%</td></tr>
<tr><td>42</td><td>South Dakota</td><td>174</td><td>0.4%</td><td>41</td><td>Maine</td><td>199</td><td>0.5%</td></tr>
<tr><td>11</td><td>Tennessee</td><td>1,322</td><td>3.1%</td><td>42</td><td>South Dakota</td><td>174</td><td>0.4%</td></tr>
<tr><td>1</td><td>Texas</td><td>3,669</td><td>8.7%</td><td>43</td><td>Wyoming</td><td>144</td><td>0.3%</td></tr>
<tr><td>35</td><td>Utah</td><td>364</td><td>0.9%</td><td>44</td><td>North Dakota</td><td>134</td><td>0.3%</td></tr>
<tr><td>50</td><td>Vermont</td><td>83</td><td>0.2%</td><td>45</td><td>New Hampshire</td><td>129</td><td>0.3%</td></tr>
<tr><td>19</td><td>Virginia</td><td>897</td><td>2.1%</td><td>46</td><td>Delaware</td><td>98</td><td>0.2%</td></tr>
<tr><td>22</td><td>Washington</td><td>732</td><td>1.7%</td><td>47</td><td>Hawaii</td><td>90</td><td>0.2%</td></tr>
<tr><td>34</td><td>West Virginia</td><td>387</td><td>0.9%</td><td>48</td><td>Rhode Island</td><td>89</td><td>0.2%</td></tr>
<tr><td>21</td><td>Wisconsin</td><td>775</td><td>1.8%</td><td>49</td><td>Alaska</td><td>87</td><td>0.2%</td></tr>
<tr><td>43</td><td>Wyoming</td><td>144</td><td>0.3%</td><td>50</td><td>Vermont</td><td>83</td><td>0.2%</td></tr>
<tr><td></td><td></td><td></td><td></td><td></td><td>District of Columbia</td><td>36</td><td>0.1%</td></tr>
</table>

Source: U.S. Department of Health and Human Services, National Center for Health Statistics
"National Vital Statistics Reports" (Vol. 49, No. 8, September 21, 2001)
*Final data by state of residence. These numbers are compiled from death certificates by the Centers for Disease Control and Prevention. They may differ from motor vehicle deaths collected by the U.S. Department of Transportation from other sources.

Death Rate by Motor Vehicle Accidents in 1999

National Rate = 15.5 Deaths per 100,000 Population*

ALPHA ORDER

RANK	STATE	RATE
3	Alabama	26.6
32	Alaska	14.0
18	Arizona	19.8
5	Arkansas	25.4
43	California	11.0
29	Colorado	15.3
46	Connecticut	9.4
38	Delaware	13.0
21	Florida	19.0
19	Georgia	19.5
49	Hawaii	7.6
11	Idaho	22.2
39	Illinois	12.7
27	Indiana	16.6
22	Iowa	18.4
12	Kansas	21.5
16	Kentucky	20.6
10	Louisiana	22.3
28	Maine	15.9
42	Maryland	11.8
50	Massachusetts	7.1
31	Michigan	14.3
34	Minnesota	13.5
1	Mississippi	34.5
20	Missouri	19.4
8	Montana	23.8
25	Nebraska	17.7
22	Nevada	18.4
44	New Hampshire	10.7
48	New Jersey	8.9
7	New Mexico	23.9
45	New York	9.7
15	North Carolina	20.9
14	North Dakota	21.1
39	Ohio	12.7
17	Oklahoma	20.4
36	Oregon	13.1
35	Pennsylvania	13.2
47	Rhode Island	9.0
4	South Carolina	25.6
9	South Dakota	23.7
6	Tennessee	24.1
24	Texas	18.3
26	Utah	17.1
32	Vermont	14.0
36	Virginia	13.1
39	Washington	12.7
13	West Virginia	21.4
30	Wisconsin	14.8
2	Wyoming	30.0

RANK ORDER

RANK	STATE	RATE
1	Mississippi	34.5
2	Wyoming	30.0
3	Alabama	26.6
4	South Carolina	25.6
5	Arkansas	25.4
6	Tennessee	24.1
7	New Mexico	23.9
8	Montana	23.8
9	South Dakota	23.7
10	Louisiana	22.3
11	Idaho	22.2
12	Kansas	21.5
13	West Virginia	21.4
14	North Dakota	21.1
15	North Carolina	20.9
16	Kentucky	20.6
17	Oklahoma	20.4
18	Arizona	19.8
19	Georgia	19.5
20	Missouri	19.4
21	Florida	19.0
22	Iowa	18.4
22	Nevada	18.4
24	Texas	18.3
25	Nebraska	17.7
26	Utah	17.1
27	Indiana	16.6
28	Maine	15.9
29	Colorado	15.3
30	Wisconsin	14.8
31	Michigan	14.3
32	Alaska	14.0
32	Vermont	14.0
34	Minnesota	13.5
35	Pennsylvania	13.2
36	Oregon	13.1
36	Virginia	13.1
38	Delaware	13.0
39	Illinois	12.7
39	Ohio	12.7
39	Washington	12.7
42	Maryland	11.8
43	California	11.0
44	New Hampshire	10.7
45	New York	9.7
46	Connecticut	9.4
47	Rhode Island	9.0
48	New Jersey	8.9
49	Hawaii	7.6
50	Massachusetts	7.1
	District of Columbia	6.9

Source: U.S. Department of Health and Human Services, National Center for Health Statistics
    "National Vital Statistics Reports" (Vol. 49, No. 8, September 21, 2001)
*Final data by state of residence. These numbers are compiled from death certificates by the Centers for Disease Control and Prevention. They may differ from motor vehicle deaths collected by the U.S. Department of Transportation from other sources. Not age-adjusted.

Age-Adjusted Death Rate by Motor Vehicle Accidents in 1999

National Rate = 15.5 Deaths per 100,000 Population*

ALPHA ORDER

RANK	STATE	RATE
3	Alabama	26.3
30	Alaska	15.4
18	Arizona	20.0
5	Arkansas	25.4
43	California	11.2
29	Colorado	15.5
46	Connecticut	9.5
36	Delaware	13.0
22	Florida	18.8
19	Georgia	19.8
49	Hawaii	7.6
11	Idaho	22.2
39	Illinois	12.7
27	Indiana	16.6
24	Iowa	18.0
12	Kansas	21.2
16	Kentucky	20.3
10	Louisiana	22.3
28	Maine	15.7
42	Maryland	12.0
50	Massachusetts	7.1
32	Michigan	14.3
34	Minnesota	13.5
1	Mississippi	34.5
20	Missouri	19.2
8	Montana	23.5
26	Nebraska	17.5
21	Nevada	18.9
44	New Hampshire	10.9
47	New Jersey	8.9
6	New Mexico	24.3
45	New York	9.6
14	North Carolina	20.9
15	North Dakota	20.4
41	Ohio	12.6
17	Oklahoma	20.2
38	Oregon	12.9
36	Pennsylvania	13.0
48	Rhode Island	8.8
4	South Carolina	25.5
8	South Dakota	23.5
7	Tennessee	24.0
23	Texas	18.7
25	Utah	17.7
33	Vermont	13.8
35	Virginia	13.1
39	Washington	12.7
13	West Virginia	21.0
31	Wisconsin	14.6
2	Wyoming	29.2

RANK ORDER

RANK	STATE	RATE
1	Mississippi	34.5
2	Wyoming	29.2
3	Alabama	26.3
4	South Carolina	25.5
5	Arkansas	25.4
6	New Mexico	24.3
7	Tennessee	24.0
8	Montana	23.5
8	South Dakota	23.5
10	Louisiana	22.3
11	Idaho	22.2
12	Kansas	21.2
13	West Virginia	21.0
14	North Carolina	20.9
15	North Dakota	20.4
16	Kentucky	20.3
17	Oklahoma	20.2
18	Arizona	20.0
19	Georgia	19.8
20	Missouri	19.2
21	Nevada	18.9
22	Florida	18.8
23	Texas	18.7
24	Iowa	18.0
25	Utah	17.7
26	Nebraska	17.5
27	Indiana	16.6
28	Maine	15.7
29	Colorado	15.5
30	Alaska	15.4
31	Wisconsin	14.6
32	Michigan	14.3
33	Vermont	13.8
34	Minnesota	13.5
35	Virginia	13.1
36	Delaware	13.0
36	Pennsylvania	13.0
38	Oregon	12.9
39	Illinois	12.7
39	Washington	12.7
41	Ohio	12.6
42	Maryland	12.0
43	California	11.2
44	New Hampshire	10.9
45	New York	9.6
46	Connecticut	9.5
47	New Jersey	8.9
48	Rhode Island	8.8
49	Hawaii	7.6
50	Massachusetts	7.1
	District of Columbia	6.9

Source: U.S. Department of Health and Human Services, National Center for Health Statistics
"National Vital Statistics Reports" (Vol. 49, No. 8, September 21, 2001)
*Final data by state of residence. These numbers are compiled from death certificates by the Centers for Disease Control and Prevention. They may differ from motor vehicle deaths collected by the U.S. Department of Transportation from other sources. Age-adjusted rates based on the year 2000 standard population.

Deaths by Homicide in 1999

National Total = 16,889 Homicides*

RANK	STATE	HOMICIDES	% of USA
14	Alabama	438	2.6%
38	Alaska	51	0.3%
12	Arizona	470	2.8%
27	Arkansas	179	1.1%
1	California	2,066	12.2%
25	Colorado	199	1.2%
33	Connecticut	120	0.7%
45	Delaware	24	0.1%
5	Florida	964	5.7%
9	Georgia	634	3.8%
40	Hawaii	38	0.2%
43	Idaho	31	0.2%
3	Illinois	1,023	6.1%
17	Indiana	386	2.3%
37	Iowa	53	0.3%
31	Kansas	137	0.8%
23	Kentucky	210	1.2%
11	Louisiana	484	2.9%
44	Maine	25	0.1%
10	Maryland	531	3.1%
32	Massachusetts	133	0.8%
6	Michigan	759	4.5%
30	Minnesota	139	0.8%
20	Mississippi	312	1.8%
18	Missouri	385	2.3%
42	Montana	33	0.2%
36	Nebraska	61	0.4%
28	Nevada	167	1.0%
47	New Hampshire	21	0.1%
21	New Jersey	298	1.8%
28	New Mexico	167	1.0%
4	New York	969	5.7%
7	North Carolina	651	3.9%
49	North Dakota	13	0.1%
13	Ohio	450	2.7%
22	Oklahoma	231	1.4%
34	Oregon	107	0.6%
8	Pennsylvania	639	3.8%
41	Rhode Island	36	0.2%
19	South Carolina	313	1.9%
46	South Dakota	23	0.1%
15	Tennessee	423	2.5%
2	Texas	1,319	7.8%
38	Utah	51	0.3%
48	Vermont	17	0.1%
16	Virginia	419	2.5%
26	Washington	190	1.1%
35	West Virginia	99	0.6%
24	Wisconsin	202	1.2%
49	Wyoming	13	0.1%

RANK	STATE	HOMICIDES	% of USA
1	California	2,066	12.2%
2	Texas	1,319	7.8%
3	Illinois	1,023	6.1%
4	New York	969	5.7%
5	Florida	964	5.7%
6	Michigan	759	4.5%
7	North Carolina	651	3.9%
8	Pennsylvania	639	3.8%
9	Georgia	634	3.8%
10	Maryland	531	3.1%
11	Louisiana	484	2.9%
12	Arizona	470	2.8%
13	Ohio	450	2.7%
14	Alabama	438	2.6%
15	Tennessee	423	2.5%
16	Virginia	419	2.5%
17	Indiana	386	2.3%
18	Missouri	385	2.3%
19	South Carolina	313	1.9%
20	Mississippi	312	1.8%
21	New Jersey	298	1.8%
22	Oklahoma	231	1.4%
23	Kentucky	210	1.2%
24	Wisconsin	202	1.2%
25	Colorado	199	1.2%
26	Washington	190	1.1%
27	Arkansas	179	1.1%
28	Nevada	167	1.0%
28	New Mexico	167	1.0%
30	Minnesota	139	0.8%
31	Kansas	137	0.8%
32	Massachusetts	133	0.8%
33	Connecticut	120	0.7%
34	Oregon	107	0.6%
35	West Virginia	99	0.6%
36	Nebraska	61	0.4%
37	Iowa	53	0.3%
38	Alaska	51	0.3%
38	Utah	51	0.3%
40	Hawaii	38	0.2%
41	Rhode Island	36	0.2%
42	Montana	33	0.2%
43	Idaho	31	0.2%
44	Maine	25	0.1%
45	Delaware	24	0.1%
46	South Dakota	23	0.1%
47	New Hampshire	21	0.1%
48	Vermont	17	0.1%
49	North Dakota	13	0.1%
49	Wyoming	13	0.1%
	District of Columbia	186	1.1%

Source: U.S. Department of Health and Human Services, National Center for Health Statistics
   "National Vital Statistics Reports" (Vol. 49, No. 8, September 21, 2001)
*By state of residence. Includes legal intervention. Homicide data shown here are collected by the Centers for Disease Control and Prevention based on death certificates and differ from murder data collected by the F.B.I. from other sources.

Death Rate by Homicide in 1999

National Rate = 6.2 Deaths per 100,000 Population*

ALPHA ORDER

RANK	STATE	RATE
4	Alabama	10.0
10	Alaska	8.2
5	Arizona	9.8
15	Arkansas	7.0
21	California	6.2
28	Colorado	4.9
31	Connecticut	3.7
37	Delaware	3.2
20	Florida	6.4
11	Georgia	8.1
37	Hawaii	3.2
42	Idaho	2.5
9	Illinois	8.4
19	Indiana	6.5
46	Iowa	1.8
27	Kansas	5.2
24	Kentucky	5.3
2	Louisiana	11.1
45	Maine	2.0
3	Maryland	10.3
44	Massachusetts	2.2
13	Michigan	7.7
41	Minnesota	2.9
1	Mississippi	11.3
15	Missouri	7.0
31	Montana	3.7
31	Nebraska	3.7
7	Nevada	9.2
47	New Hampshire	1.7
31	New Jersey	3.7
6	New Mexico	9.6
24	New York	5.3
8	North Carolina	8.5
NA	North Dakota**	NA
29	Ohio	4.0
17	Oklahoma	6.9
37	Oregon	3.2
24	Pennsylvania	5.3
35	Rhode Island	3.6
11	South Carolina	8.1
40	South Dakota	3.1
13	Tennessee	7.7
18	Texas	6.6
43	Utah	2.4
NA	Vermont**	NA
22	Virginia	6.1
36	Washington	3.3
23	West Virginia	5.5
30	Wisconsin	3.8
NA	Wyoming**	NA

RANK ORDER

RANK	STATE	RATE
1	Mississippi	11.3
2	Louisiana	11.1
3	Maryland	10.3
4	Alabama	10.0
5	Arizona	9.8
6	New Mexico	9.6
7	Nevada	9.2
8	North Carolina	8.5
9	Illinois	8.4
10	Alaska	8.2
11	Georgia	8.1
11	South Carolina	8.1
13	Michigan	7.7
13	Tennessee	7.7
15	Arkansas	7.0
15	Missouri	7.0
17	Oklahoma	6.9
18	Texas	6.6
19	Indiana	6.5
20	Florida	6.4
21	California	6.2
22	Virginia	6.1
23	West Virginia	5.5
24	Kentucky	5.3
24	New York	5.3
24	Pennsylvania	5.3
27	Kansas	5.2
28	Colorado	4.9
29	Ohio	4.0
30	Wisconsin	3.8
31	Connecticut	3.7
31	Montana	3.7
31	Nebraska	3.7
31	New Jersey	3.7
35	Rhode Island	3.6
36	Washington	3.3
37	Delaware	3.2
37	Hawaii	3.2
37	Oregon	3.2
40	South Dakota	3.1
41	Minnesota	2.9
42	Idaho	2.5
43	Utah	2.4
44	Massachusetts	2.2
45	Maine	2.0
46	Iowa	1.8
47	New Hampshire	1.7
NA	North Dakota**	NA
NA	Vermont**	NA
NA	Wyoming**	NA

	District of Columbia	35.8

Source: U.S. Department of Health and Human Services, National Center for Health Statistics
    "National Vital Statistics Reports" (Vol. 49, No. 8, September 21, 2001)
*By state of residence. Includes legal intervention. Homicide data shown here are collected by the Centers for Disease Control and Prevention based on death certificates and differ from murder data collected by the F.B.I. from other sources. Not age-adjusted.
**Insufficient data to determine a reliable rate.

Age-Adjusted Death Rate by Homicide in 1999

National Rate = 6.2 Deaths per 100,000 Population*

ALPHA ORDER

RANK	STATE	RATE
4	Alabama	9.9
8	Alaska	8.5
4	Arizona	9.9
15	Arkansas	7.1
21	California	6.1
28	Colorado	4.8
31	Connecticut	3.8
40	Delaware	3.1
18	Florida	6.7
12	Georgia	7.8
39	Hawaii	3.2
42	Idaho	2.4
9	Illinois	8.4
20	Indiana	6.4
46	Iowa	1.9
27	Kansas	5.1
26	Kentucky	5.2
2	Louisiana	10.9
45	Maine	2.0
3	Maryland	10.2
44	Massachusetts	2.2
13	Michigan	7.6
41	Minnesota	2.9
1	Mississippi	11.1
15	Missouri	7.1
30	Montana	3.9
35	Nebraska	3.6
7	Nevada	9.4
47	New Hampshire	1.7
33	New Jersey	3.7
6	New Mexico	9.6
25	New York	5.4
9	North Carolina	8.4
NA	North Dakota**	NA
29	Ohio	4.0
17	Oklahoma	6.9
36	Oregon	3.3
23	Pennsylvania	5.5
33	Rhode Island	3.7
11	South Carolina	7.9
36	South Dakota	3.3
13	Tennessee	7.6
19	Texas	6.5
42	Utah	2.4
NA	Vermont**	NA
22	Virginia	5.9
36	Washington	3.3
23	West Virginia	5.5
31	Wisconsin	3.8
NA	Wyoming**	NA

RANK ORDER

RANK	STATE	RATE
1	Mississippi	11.1
2	Louisiana	10.9
3	Maryland	10.2
4	Alabama	9.9
4	Arizona	9.9
6	New Mexico	9.6
7	Nevada	9.4
8	Alaska	8.5
9	Illinois	8.4
9	North Carolina	8.4
11	South Carolina	7.9
12	Georgia	7.8
13	Michigan	7.6
13	Tennessee	7.6
15	Arkansas	7.1
15	Missouri	7.1
17	Oklahoma	6.9
18	Florida	6.7
19	Texas	6.5
20	Indiana	6.4
21	California	6.1
22	Virginia	5.9
23	Pennsylvania	5.5
23	West Virginia	5.5
25	New York	5.4
26	Kentucky	5.2
27	Kansas	5.1
28	Colorado	4.8
29	Ohio	4.0
30	Montana	3.9
31	Connecticut	3.8
31	Wisconsin	3.8
33	New Jersey	3.7
33	Rhode Island	3.7
35	Nebraska	3.6
36	Oregon	3.3
36	South Dakota	3.3
36	Washington	3.3
39	Hawaii	3.2
40	Delaware	3.1
41	Minnesota	2.9
42	Idaho	2.4
42	Utah	2.4
44	Massachusetts	2.2
45	Maine	2.0
46	Iowa	1.9
47	New Hampshire	1.7
NA	North Dakota**	NA
NA	Vermont**	NA
NA	Wyoming**	NA
	District of Columbia	36.8

Source: U.S. Department of Health and Human Services, National Center for Health Statistics
   "National Vital Statistics Reports" (Vol. 49, No. 8, September 21, 2001)
*By state of residence. Includes legal intervention. Homicide data shown here are collected by the Centers for Disease Control and Prevention based on death certificates and differ from murder data collected by the F.B.I. from other sources. Age-adjusted rates based on the year 2000 standard population.
**Insufficient data to determine a reliable rate.

Deaths by Suicide in 1999

National Total = 29,199 Suicides*

ALPHA ORDER				RANK ORDER			
RANK	STATE	SUICIDES	% of USA	RANK	STATE	SUICIDES	% of USA
20	Alabama	555	1.9%	1	California	3,077	10.5%
46	Alaska	96	0.3%	2	Florida	2,029	6.9%
13	Arizona	766	2.6%	3	Texas	2,005	6.9%
30	Arkansas	336	1.2%	4	Pennsylvania	1,284	4.4%
1	California	3,077	10.5%	5	New York	1,196	4.1%
18	Colorado	574	2.0%	6	Ohio	1,102	3.8%
36	Connecticut	274	0.9%	7	Illinois	1,020	3.5%
48	Delaware	86	0.3%	8	Michigan	974	3.3%
2	Florida	2,029	6.9%	9	North Carolina	884	3.0%
10	Georgia	873	3.0%	10	Georgia	873	3.0%
43	Hawaii	136	0.5%	11	Washington	816	2.8%
38	Idaho	181	0.6%	12	Virginia	791	2.7%
7	Illinois	1,020	3.5%	13	Arizona	766	2.6%
16	Indiana	628	2.2%	14	Tennessee	726	2.5%
32	Iowa	305	1.0%	15	Missouri	700	2.4%
34	Kansas	299	1.0%	16	Indiana	628	2.2%
24	Kentucky	470	1.6%	17	Wisconsin	593	2.0%
21	Louisiana	518	1.8%	18	Colorado	574	2.0%
40	Maine	175	0.6%	19	New Jersey	563	1.9%
26	Maryland	435	1.5%	20	Alabama	555	1.9%
27	Massachusetts	431	1.5%	21	Louisiana	518	1.8%
8	Michigan	974	3.3%	22	Oklahoma	492	1.7%
25	Minnesota	437	1.5%	23	Oregon	478	1.6%
33	Mississippi	304	1.0%	24	Kentucky	470	1.6%
15	Missouri	700	2.4%	25	Minnesota	437	1.5%
41	Montana	162	0.6%	26	Maryland	435	1.5%
39	Nebraska	177	0.6%	27	Massachusetts	431	1.5%
29	Nevada	404	1.4%	28	South Carolina	418	1.4%
42	New Hampshire	137	0.5%	29	Nevada	404	1.4%
19	New Jersey	563	1.9%	30	Arkansas	336	1.2%
31	New Mexico	318	1.1%	31	New Mexico	318	1.1%
5	New York	1,196	4.1%	32	Iowa	305	1.0%
9	North Carolina	884	3.0%	33	Mississippi	304	1.0%
49	North Dakota	73	0.3%	34	Kansas	299	1.0%
6	Ohio	1,102	3.8%	35	Utah	282	1.0%
22	Oklahoma	492	1.7%	36	Connecticut	274	0.9%
23	Oregon	478	1.6%	37	West Virginia	229	0.8%
4	Pennsylvania	1,284	4.4%	38	Idaho	181	0.6%
46	Rhode Island	96	0.3%	39	Nebraska	177	0.6%
28	South Carolina	418	1.4%	40	Maine	175	0.6%
44	South Dakota	103	0.4%	41	Montana	162	0.6%
14	Tennessee	726	2.5%	42	New Hampshire	137	0.5%
3	Texas	2,005	6.9%	43	Hawaii	136	0.5%
35	Utah	282	1.0%	44	South Dakota	103	0.4%
50	Vermont	63	0.2%	45	Wyoming	98	0.3%
12	Virginia	791	2.7%	46	Alaska	96	0.3%
11	Washington	816	2.8%	46	Rhode Island	96	0.3%
37	West Virginia	229	0.8%	48	Delaware	86	0.3%
17	Wisconsin	593	2.0%	49	North Dakota	73	0.3%
45	Wyoming	98	0.3%	50	Vermont	63	0.2%
					District of Columbia	30	0.1%

*Source: U.S. Department of Health and Human Services, National Center for Health Statistics
"National Vital Statistics Reports" (Vol. 49, No. 8, September 21, 2001)
Final data by state of residence.

Death Rate by Suicide in 1999

National Rate = 10.7 Suicides per 100,000 Population*

<table>
<tr><td colspan="3">ALPHA ORDER</td><td colspan="3">RANK ORDER</td></tr>
<tr><th>RANK</th><th>STATE</th><th>RATE</th><th>RANK</th><th>STATE</th><th>RATE</th></tr>
<tr><td>19</td><td>Alabama</td><td>12.7</td><td>1</td><td>Nevada</td><td>22.3</td></tr>
<tr><td>6</td><td>Alaska</td><td>15.5</td><td>2</td><td>Wyoming</td><td>20.4</td></tr>
<tr><td>5</td><td>Arizona</td><td>16.0</td><td>3</td><td>Montana</td><td>18.4</td></tr>
<tr><td>15</td><td>Arkansas</td><td>13.2</td><td>4</td><td>New Mexico</td><td>18.3</td></tr>
<tr><td>43</td><td>California</td><td>9.3</td><td>5</td><td>Arizona</td><td>16.0</td></tr>
<tr><td>10</td><td>Colorado</td><td>14.2</td><td>6</td><td>Alaska</td><td>15.5</td></tr>
<tr><td>47</td><td>Connecticut</td><td>8.3</td><td>7</td><td>Oklahoma</td><td>14.7</td></tr>
<tr><td>27</td><td>Delaware</td><td>11.4</td><td>8</td><td>Idaho</td><td>14.5</td></tr>
<tr><td>14</td><td>Florida</td><td>13.4</td><td>9</td><td>Oregon</td><td>14.4</td></tr>
<tr><td>31</td><td>Georgia</td><td>11.2</td><td>10</td><td>Colorado</td><td>14.2</td></tr>
<tr><td>24</td><td>Hawaii</td><td>11.5</td><td>10</td><td>Washington</td><td>14.2</td></tr>
<tr><td>8</td><td>Idaho</td><td>14.5</td><td>12</td><td>Maine</td><td>14.0</td></tr>
<tr><td>45</td><td>Illinois</td><td>8.4</td><td>12</td><td>South Dakota</td><td>14.0</td></tr>
<tr><td>35</td><td>Indiana</td><td>10.6</td><td>14</td><td>Florida</td><td>13.4</td></tr>
<tr><td>35</td><td>Iowa</td><td>10.6</td><td>15</td><td>Arkansas</td><td>13.2</td></tr>
<tr><td>29</td><td>Kansas</td><td>11.3</td><td>15</td><td>Tennessee</td><td>13.2</td></tr>
<tr><td>21</td><td>Kentucky</td><td>11.9</td><td>15</td><td>Utah</td><td>13.2</td></tr>
<tr><td>22</td><td>Louisiana</td><td>11.8</td><td>18</td><td>Missouri</td><td>12.8</td></tr>
<tr><td>12</td><td>Maine</td><td>14.0</td><td>19</td><td>Alabama</td><td>12.7</td></tr>
<tr><td>45</td><td>Maryland</td><td>8.4</td><td>19</td><td>West Virginia</td><td>12.7</td></tr>
<tr><td>48</td><td>Massachusetts</td><td>7.0</td><td>21</td><td>Kentucky</td><td>11.9</td></tr>
<tr><td>40</td><td>Michigan</td><td>9.9</td><td>22</td><td>Louisiana</td><td>11.8</td></tr>
<tr><td>44</td><td>Minnesota</td><td>9.2</td><td>23</td><td>North Carolina</td><td>11.6</td></tr>
<tr><td>32</td><td>Mississippi</td><td>11.0</td><td>24</td><td>Hawaii</td><td>11.5</td></tr>
<tr><td>18</td><td>Missouri</td><td>12.8</td><td>24</td><td>North Dakota</td><td>11.5</td></tr>
<tr><td>3</td><td>Montana</td><td>18.4</td><td>24</td><td>Virginia</td><td>11.5</td></tr>
<tr><td>35</td><td>Nebraska</td><td>10.6</td><td>27</td><td>Delaware</td><td>11.4</td></tr>
<tr><td>1</td><td>Nevada</td><td>22.3</td><td>27</td><td>New Hampshire</td><td>11.4</td></tr>
<tr><td>27</td><td>New Hampshire</td><td>11.4</td><td>29</td><td>Kansas</td><td>11.3</td></tr>
<tr><td>49</td><td>New Jersey</td><td>6.9</td><td>29</td><td>Wisconsin</td><td>11.3</td></tr>
<tr><td>4</td><td>New Mexico</td><td>18.3</td><td>31</td><td>Georgia</td><td>11.2</td></tr>
<tr><td>50</td><td>New York</td><td>6.6</td><td>32</td><td>Mississippi</td><td>11.0</td></tr>
<tr><td>23</td><td>North Carolina</td><td>11.6</td><td>33</td><td>South Carolina</td><td>10.8</td></tr>
<tr><td>24</td><td>North Dakota</td><td>11.5</td><td>34</td><td>Pennsylvania</td><td>10.7</td></tr>
<tr><td>41</td><td>Ohio</td><td>9.8</td><td>35</td><td>Indiana</td><td>10.6</td></tr>
<tr><td>7</td><td>Oklahoma</td><td>14.7</td><td>35</td><td>Iowa</td><td>10.6</td></tr>
<tr><td>9</td><td>Oregon</td><td>14.4</td><td>35</td><td>Nebraska</td><td>10.6</td></tr>
<tr><td>34</td><td>Pennsylvania</td><td>10.7</td><td>35</td><td>Vermont</td><td>10.6</td></tr>
<tr><td>42</td><td>Rhode Island</td><td>9.7</td><td>39</td><td>Texas</td><td>10.0</td></tr>
<tr><td>33</td><td>South Carolina</td><td>10.8</td><td>40</td><td>Michigan</td><td>9.9</td></tr>
<tr><td>12</td><td>South Dakota</td><td>14.0</td><td>41</td><td>Ohio</td><td>9.8</td></tr>
<tr><td>15</td><td>Tennessee</td><td>13.2</td><td>42</td><td>Rhode Island</td><td>9.7</td></tr>
<tr><td>39</td><td>Texas</td><td>10.0</td><td>43</td><td>California</td><td>9.3</td></tr>
<tr><td>15</td><td>Utah</td><td>13.2</td><td>44</td><td>Minnesota</td><td>9.2</td></tr>
<tr><td>35</td><td>Vermont</td><td>10.6</td><td>45</td><td>Illinois</td><td>8.4</td></tr>
<tr><td>24</td><td>Virginia</td><td>11.5</td><td>45</td><td>Maryland</td><td>8.4</td></tr>
<tr><td>10</td><td>Washington</td><td>14.2</td><td>47</td><td>Connecticut</td><td>8.3</td></tr>
<tr><td>19</td><td>West Virginia</td><td>12.7</td><td>48</td><td>Massachusetts</td><td>7.0</td></tr>
<tr><td>29</td><td>Wisconsin</td><td>11.3</td><td>49</td><td>New Jersey</td><td>6.9</td></tr>
<tr><td>2</td><td>Wyoming</td><td>20.4</td><td>50</td><td>New York</td><td>6.6</td></tr>
<tr><td></td><td></td><td></td><td></td><td>District of Columbia</td><td>5.8</td></tr>
</table>

Source: U.S. Department of Health and Human Services, National Center for Health Statistics
"National Vital Statistics Reports" (Vol. 49, No. 8, September 21, 2001)
*Final data by state of residence. Not age-adjusted.

Age-Adjusted Death Rate by Suicide in 1999

National Rate = 10.7 Suicides per 100,000 Population*

ALPHA ORDER

RANK ORDER

RANK	STATE	RATE		RANK	STATE	RATE
19	Alabama	12.5		1	Nevada	23.0
5	Alaska	17.2		2	Wyoming	20.8
6	Arizona	16.5		3	New Mexico	18.8
15	Arkansas	13.2		4	Montana	18.0
42	California	9.6		5	Alaska	17.2
10	Colorado	14.3		6	Arizona	16.5
47	Connecticut	8.3		7	Idaho	15.0
29	Delaware	11.2		8	Oklahoma	14.9
17	Florida	12.9		9	Utah	14.7
23	Georgia	11.5		10	Colorado	14.3
23	Hawaii	11.5		11	Oregon	14.2
7	Idaho	15.0		11	Washington	14.2
45	Illinois	8.5		13	South Dakota	14.0
35	Indiana	10.6		14	Maine	13.4
37	Iowa	10.4		15	Arkansas	13.2
27	Kansas	11.3		16	Tennessee	13.0
22	Kentucky	11.7		17	Florida	12.9
21	Louisiana	12.1		18	Missouri	12.7
14	Maine	13.4		19	Alabama	12.5
46	Maryland	8.4		20	West Virginia	12.2
48	Massachusetts	6.8		21	Louisiana	12.1
40	Michigan	9.9		22	Kentucky	11.7
44	Minnesota	9.2		23	Georgia	11.5
29	Mississippi	11.2		23	Hawaii	11.5
18	Missouri	12.7		23	North Carolina	11.5
4	Montana	18.0		26	Virginia	11.4
33	Nebraska	10.8		27	Kansas	11.3
1	Nevada	23.0		27	New Hampshire	11.3
27	New Hampshire	11.3		29	Delaware	11.2
48	New Jersey	6.8		29	Mississippi	11.2
3	New Mexico	18.8		29	North Dakota	11.2
50	New York	6.5		29	Wisconsin	11.2
23	North Carolina	11.5		33	Nebraska	10.8
29	North Dakota	11.2		34	South Carolina	10.7
41	Ohio	9.7		35	Indiana	10.6
8	Oklahoma	14.9		36	Pennsylvania	10.5
11	Oregon	14.2		37	Iowa	10.4
36	Pennsylvania	10.5		37	Texas	10.4
42	Rhode Island	9.6		39	Vermont	10.3
34	South Carolina	10.7		40	Michigan	9.9
13	South Dakota	14.0		41	Ohio	9.7
16	Tennessee	13.0		42	California	9.6
37	Texas	10.4		42	Rhode Island	9.6
9	Utah	14.7		44	Minnesota	9.2
39	Vermont	10.3		45	Illinois	8.5
26	Virginia	11.4		46	Maryland	8.4
11	Washington	14.2		47	Connecticut	8.3
20	West Virginia	12.2		48	Massachusetts	6.8
29	Wisconsin	11.2		48	New Jersey	6.8
2	Wyoming	20.8		50	New York	6.5
					District of Columbia	5.4

Source: U.S. Department of Health and Human Services, National Center for Health Statistics
    "National Vital Statistics Reports" (Vol. 49, No. 8, September 21, 2001)
*Final data by state of residence. Age-adjusted rates based on the year 2000 standard population.

Years Lost by Premature Death in 1999

National Average = 7,734 Years Lost per 100,000 Population*

ALPHA ORDER

RANK	STATE	YEARS
3	Alabama	10,128
26	Alaska	7,690
17	Arizona	8,216
5	Arkansas	9,524
39	California	6,618
37	Colorado	6,686
42	Connecticut	6,525
21	Delaware	7,867
16	Florida	8,391
8	Georgia	9,028
47	Hawaii	6,215
34	Idaho	6,825
19	Illinois	8,011
18	Indiana	8,036
46	Iowa	6,343
30	Kansas	7,306
12	Kentucky	8,582
2	Louisiana	10,228
40	Maine	6,588
15	Maryland	8,397
49	Massachusetts	6,148
20	Michigan	8,010
50	Minnesota	5,985
1	Mississippi	11,083
14	Missouri	8,420
29	Montana	7,393
33	Nebraska	6,854
9	Nevada	8,970
48	New Hampshire	6,204
32	New Jersey	7,166
13	New Mexico	8,505
31	New York	7,223
10	North Carolina	8,844
41	North Dakota	6,562
24	Ohio	7,781
7	Oklahoma	9,181
35	Oregon	6,798
23	Pennsylvania	7,784
36	Rhode Island	6,750
4	South Carolina	9,915
25	South Dakota	7,777
6	Tennessee	9,346
27	Texas	7,669
43	Utah	6,503
44	Vermont	6,443
28	Virginia	7,417
45	Washington	6,401
11	West Virginia	8,750
38	Wisconsin	6,623
22	Wyoming	7,844

RANK ORDER

RANK	STATE	YEARS
1	Mississippi	11,083
2	Louisiana	10,228
3	Alabama	10,128
4	South Carolina	9,915
5	Arkansas	9,524
6	Tennessee	9,346
7	Oklahoma	9,181
8	Georgia	9,028
9	Nevada	8,970
10	North Carolina	8,844
11	West Virginia	8,750
12	Kentucky	8,582
13	New Mexico	8,505
14	Missouri	8,420
15	Maryland	8,397
16	Florida	8,391
17	Arizona	8,216
18	Indiana	8,036
19	Illinois	8,011
20	Michigan	8,010
21	Delaware	7,867
22	Wyoming	7,844
23	Pennsylvania	7,784
24	Ohio	7,781
25	South Dakota	7,777
26	Alaska	7,690
27	Texas	7,669
28	Virginia	7,417
29	Montana	7,393
30	Kansas	7,306
31	New York	7,223
32	New Jersey	7,166
33	Nebraska	6,854
34	Idaho	6,825
35	Oregon	6,798
36	Rhode Island	6,750
37	Colorado	6,686
38	Wisconsin	6,623
39	California	6,618
40	Maine	6,588
41	North Dakota	6,562
42	Connecticut	6,525
43	Utah	6,503
44	Vermont	6,443
45	Washington	6,401
46	Iowa	6,343
47	Hawaii	6,215
48	New Hampshire	6,204
49	Massachusetts	6,148
50	Minnesota	5,985
	District of Columbia	14,645

Source: U.S. Department of Health and Human Services, National Center for Health Statistics
    unpublished data
*Age-adjusted years of potential life lost due to death before age 75.

Years Lost by Premature Death from Cancer in 1999

National Average = 1,724 Years Lost per 100,000 Population*

ALPHA ORDER				RANK ORDER		
RANK	STATE	YEARS		RANK	STATE	YEARS
8	Alabama	1,892		1	Mississippi	2,144
47	Alaska	1,411		2	Louisiana	2,041
35	Arizona	1,606		3	West Virginia	2,002
7	Arkansas	1,965		4	South Carolina	1,994
42	California	1,546		5	Kentucky	1,969
50	Colorado	1,308		6	Tennessee	1,966
36	Connecticut	1,605		7	Arkansas	1,965
9	Delaware	1,886		8	Alabama	1,892
18	Florida	1,797		9	Delaware	1,886
17	Georgia	1,801		10	North Carolina	1,868
48	Hawaii	1,399		11	Rhode Island	1,853
43	Idaho	1,530		12	Ohio	1,847
25	Illinois	1,743		13	Maine	1,840
15	Indiana	1,821		14	Missouri	1,826
41	Iowa	1,550		15	Indiana	1,821
31	Kansas	1,657		16	Pennsylvania	1,817
5	Kentucky	1,969		17	Georgia	1,801
2	Louisiana	2,041		18	Florida	1,797
13	Maine	1,840		19	Oklahoma	1,793
21	Maryland	1,774		20	Virginia	1,789
30	Massachusetts	1,673		21	Maryland	1,774
26	Michigan	1,738		22	Vermont	1,757
40	Minnesota	1,553		23	New Hampshire	1,748
1	Mississippi	2,144		23	New Jersey	1,748
14	Missouri	1,826		25	Illinois	1,743
44	Montana	1,500		26	Michigan	1,738
38	Nebraska	1,577		27	Nevada	1,737
27	Nevada	1,737		28	New York	1,714
23	New Hampshire	1,748		29	South Dakota	1,702
23	New Jersey	1,748		30	Massachusetts	1,673
45	New Mexico	1,432		31	Kansas	1,657
28	New York	1,714		32	Texas	1,649
10	North Carolina	1,868		33	Wyoming	1,644
46	North Dakota	1,412		34	Wisconsin	1,621
12	Ohio	1,847		35	Arizona	1,606
19	Oklahoma	1,793		36	Connecticut	1,605
37	Oregon	1,580		37	Oregon	1,580
16	Pennsylvania	1,817		38	Nebraska	1,577
11	Rhode Island	1,853		39	Washington	1,570
4	South Carolina	1,994		40	Minnesota	1,553
29	South Dakota	1,702		41	Iowa	1,550
6	Tennessee	1,966		42	California	1,546
32	Texas	1,649		43	Idaho	1,530
49	Utah	1,325		44	Montana	1,500
22	Vermont	1,757		45	New Mexico	1,432
20	Virginia	1,789		46	North Dakota	1,412
39	Washington	1,570		47	Alaska	1,411
3	West Virginia	2,002		48	Hawaii	1,399
34	Wisconsin	1,621		49	Utah	1,325
33	Wyoming	1,644		50	Colorado	1,308
					District of Columbia	2,123

Source: U.S. Department of Health and Human Services, National Center for Health Statistics
    unpublished data
*Age-adjusted years of potential life lost due to death before age 75.

Years Lost by Premature Death from Heart Disease in 1999

National Average = 1,317 Years Lost per 100,000 Population*

ALPHA ORDER				RANK ORDER		
RANK	STATE	YEARS		RANK	STATE	YEARS
2	Alabama	1,848		1	Mississippi	2,173
45	Alaska	961		2	Alabama	1,848
27	Arizona	1,171		3	Louisiana	1,776
8	Arkansas	1,686		4	South Carolina	1,721
35	California	1,092		5	Tennessee	1,720
49	Colorado	859		6	Oklahoma	1,703
33	Connecticut	1,105		7	West Virginia	1,692
19	Delaware	1,369		8	Arkansas	1,686
23	Florida	1,293		9	Kentucky	1,629
10	Georgia	1,614		10	Georgia	1,614
25	Hawaii	1,185		11	Nevada	1,581
40	Idaho	1,002		12	Missouri	1,536
16	Illinois	1,450		13	Michigan	1,486
14	Indiana	1,461		14	Indiana	1,461
32	Iowa	1,114		15	North Carolina	1,457
36	Kansas	1,077		16	Illinois	1,450
9	Kentucky	1,629		17	Ohio	1,425
3	Louisiana	1,776		18	Pennsylvania	1,380
37	Maine	1,065		19	Delaware	1,369
20	Maryland	1,347		20	Maryland	1,347
39	Massachusetts	1,055		21	Texas	1,330
13	Michigan	1,486		22	Virginia	1,301
48	Minnesota	886		23	Florida	1,293
1	Mississippi	2,173		24	New York	1,279
12	Missouri	1,536		25	Hawaii	1,185
41	Montana	999		26	North Dakota	1,184
31	Nebraska	1,121		27	Arizona	1,171
11	Nevada	1,581		28	New Jersey	1,152
38	New Hampshire	1,059		29	Rhode Island	1,128
28	New Jersey	1,152		29	South Dakota	1,128
46	New Mexico	960		31	Nebraska	1,121
24	New York	1,279		32	Iowa	1,114
15	North Carolina	1,457		33	Connecticut	1,105
26	North Dakota	1,184		34	Wisconsin	1,102
17	Ohio	1,425		35	California	1,092
6	Oklahoma	1,703		36	Kansas	1,077
42	Oregon	998		37	Maine	1,065
18	Pennsylvania	1,380		38	New Hampshire	1,059
29	Rhode Island	1,128		39	Massachusetts	1,055
4	South Carolina	1,721		40	Idaho	1,002
29	South Dakota	1,128		41	Montana	999
5	Tennessee	1,720		42	Oregon	998
21	Texas	1,330		43	Vermont	997
50	Utah	759		44	Washington	965
43	Vermont	997		45	Alaska	961
22	Virginia	1,301		46	New Mexico	960
44	Washington	965		47	Wyoming	929
7	West Virginia	1,692		48	Minnesota	886
34	Wisconsin	1,102		49	Colorado	859
47	Wyoming	929		50	Utah	759
					District of Columbia	1,823

Source: U.S. Department of Health and Human Services, National Center for Health Statistics
       unpublished data
*Age-adjusted years of potential life lost due to death before age 75.

Years Lost by Premature Death from Homicide in 1999

National Average = 279 Years Lost per 100,000 Population*

ALPHA ORDER

RANK	STATE	YEARS
6	Alabama	421
10	Alaska	356
4	Arizona	438
16	Arkansas	308
21	California	276
25	Colorado	230
32	Connecticut	169
39	Delaware	134
18	Florida	300
12	Georgia	351
42	Hawaii	109
41	Idaho	115
7	Illinois	405
17	Indiana	304
46	Iowa	76
26	Kansas	226
28	Kentucky	218
2	Louisiana	486
45	Maine	91
1	Maryland	508
43	Massachusetts	105
13	Michigan	346
40	Minnesota	128
3	Mississippi	485
15	Missouri	331
35	Montana	162
34	Nebraska	164
8	Nevada	397
NA	New Hampshire**	NA
33	New Jersey	168
5	New Mexico	431
24	New York	246
9	North Carolina	373
NA	North Dakota**	NA
31	Ohio	173
19	Oklahoma	291
37	Oregon	153
22	Pennsylvania	265
30	Rhode Island	180
11	South Carolina	353
36	South Dakota	155
14	Tennessee	337
20	Texas	283
44	Utah	98
NA	Vermont**	NA
23	Virginia	258
38	Washington	148
27	West Virginia	223
29	Wisconsin	193
NA	Wyoming**	NA

RANK ORDER

RANK	STATE	YEARS
1	Maryland	508
2	Louisiana	486
3	Mississippi	485
4	Arizona	438
5	New Mexico	431
6	Alabama	421
7	Illinois	405
8	Nevada	397
9	North Carolina	373
10	Alaska	356
11	South Carolina	353
12	Georgia	351
13	Michigan	346
14	Tennessee	337
15	Missouri	331
16	Arkansas	308
17	Indiana	304
18	Florida	300
19	Oklahoma	291
20	Texas	283
21	California	276
22	Pennsylvania	265
23	Virginia	258
24	New York	246
25	Colorado	230
26	Kansas	226
27	West Virginia	223
28	Kentucky	218
29	Wisconsin	193
30	Rhode Island	180
31	Ohio	173
32	Connecticut	169
33	New Jersey	168
34	Nebraska	164
35	Montana	162
36	South Dakota	155
37	Oregon	153
38	Washington	148
39	Delaware	134
40	Minnesota	128
41	Idaho	115
42	Hawaii	109
43	Massachusetts	105
44	Utah	98
45	Maine	91
46	Iowa	76
NA	New Hampshire**	NA
NA	North Dakota**	NA
NA	Vermont**	NA
NA	Wyoming**	NA

District of Columbia   1,875

Source: U.S. Department of Health and Human Services, National Center for Health Statistics
unpublished data

*Age-adjusted years of potential life lost due to death before age 75.

**Data for states with fewer than 20 deaths from homicide for persons under 75 years of age are considered unreliable and are not shown.

Years Lost by Premature Death from Suicide in 1999

National Average = 343 Years Lost per 100,000 Population*

ALPHA ORDER				RANK ORDER		
RANK	STATE	YEARS		RANK	STATE	YEARS
19	Alabama	401		1	Wyoming	662
4	Alaska	584		2	Nevada	660
8	Arizona	501		3	New Mexico	642
12	Arkansas	448		4	Alaska	584
44	California	277		5	Montana	551
10	Colorado	467		6	Oklahoma	527
47	Connecticut	255		7	South Dakota	513
20	Delaware	400		8	Arizona	501
23	Florida	394		9	Utah	494
33	Georgia	353		10	Colorado	467
18	Hawaii	404		11	Idaho	455
11	Idaho	455		12	Arkansas	448
45	Illinois	275		13	Washington	445
31	Indiana	357		14	Oregon	433
34	Iowa	351		15	Tennessee	427
21	Kansas	399		16	Maine	426
30	Kentucky	376		16	Missouri	426
24	Louisiana	393		18	Hawaii	404
16	Maine	426		19	Alabama	401
46	Maryland	271		20	Delaware	400
48	Massachusetts	231		21	Kansas	399
38	Michigan	334		22	West Virginia	395
41	Minnesota	315		23	Florida	394
37	Mississippi	338		24	Louisiana	393
16	Missouri	426		24	North Dakota	393
5	Montana	551		26	New Hampshire	392
27	Nebraska	391		27	Nebraska	391
2	Nevada	660		28	North Carolina	388
26	New Hampshire	392		29	Wisconsin	378
49	New Jersey	215		30	Kentucky	376
3	New Mexico	642		31	Indiana	357
50	New York	209		32	Pennsylvania	354
28	North Carolina	388		33	Georgia	353
24	North Dakota	393		34	Iowa	351
42	Ohio	310		34	Virginia	351
6	Oklahoma	527		36	South Carolina	350
14	Oregon	433		37	Mississippi	338
32	Pennsylvania	354		38	Michigan	334
39	Rhode Island	330		39	Rhode Island	330
36	South Carolina	350		39	Texas	330
7	South Dakota	513		41	Minnesota	315
15	Tennessee	427		42	Ohio	310
39	Texas	330		43	Vermont	301
9	Utah	494		44	California	277
43	Vermont	301		45	Illinois	275
34	Virginia	351		46	Maryland	271
13	Washington	445		47	Connecticut	255
22	West Virginia	395		48	Massachusetts	231
29	Wisconsin	378		49	New Jersey	215
1	Wyoming	662		50	New York	209
					District of Columbia	186

*Source: U.S. Department of Health and Human Services, National Center for Health Statistics
   unpublished data*
Age-adjusted years of potential life lost due to death before age 75.

Years Lost by Premature Death from Unintentional Injuries in 1999

National Average = 1,048 Years Lost per 100,000 Population*

ALPHA ORDER

RANK	STATE	YEARS	RANK	STATE	YEARS
4	Alabama	1,651	1	Mississippi	1,912
3	Alaska	1,683	2	New Mexico	1,812
12	Arizona	1,435	3	Alaska	1,683
6	Arkansas	1,577	4	Alabama	1,651
41	California	864	5	Wyoming	1,644
26	Colorado	1,071	6	Arkansas	1,577
42	Connecticut	849	7	Montana	1,554
34	Delaware	969	8	South Carolina	1,500
19	Florida	1,236	9	Tennessee	1,490
21	Georgia	1,189	10	Louisiana	1,459
48	Hawaii	666	11	South Dakota	1,446
14	Idaho	1,385	12	Arizona	1,435
30	Illinois	1,000	13	Oklahoma	1,412
25	Indiana	1,124	14	Idaho	1,385
31	Iowa	990	15	Kentucky	1,295
23	Kansas	1,162	16	Nevada	1,284
15	Kentucky	1,295	17	West Virginia	1,280
10	Louisiana	1,459	18	North Carolina	1,255
29	Maine	1,003	19	Florida	1,236
45	Maryland	719	20	Missouri	1,228
50	Massachusetts	471	21	Georgia	1,189
37	Michigan	953	22	North Dakota	1,184
43	Minnesota	828	23	Kansas	1,162
1	Mississippi	1,912	24	Texas	1,150
20	Missouri	1,228	25	Indiana	1,124
7	Montana	1,554	26	Colorado	1,071
27	Nebraska	1,053	27	Nebraska	1,053
16	Nevada	1,284	28	Pennsylvania	1,041
44	New Hampshire	729	29	Maine	1,003
46	New Jersey	718	30	Illinois	1,000
2	New Mexico	1,812	31	Iowa	990
47	New York	713	32	Washington	989
18	North Carolina	1,255	33	Oregon	980
22	North Dakota	1,184	34	Delaware	969
39	Ohio	887	35	Utah	968
13	Oklahoma	1,412	36	Vermont	960
33	Oregon	980	37	Michigan	953
28	Pennsylvania	1,041	38	Wisconsin	949
49	Rhode Island	530	39	Ohio	887
8	South Carolina	1,500	40	Virginia	865
11	South Dakota	1,446	41	California	864
9	Tennessee	1,490	42	Connecticut	849
24	Texas	1,150	43	Minnesota	828
35	Utah	968	44	New Hampshire	729
36	Vermont	960	45	Maryland	719
40	Virginia	865	46	New Jersey	718
32	Washington	989	47	New York	713
17	West Virginia	1,280	48	Hawaii	666
38	Wisconsin	949	49	Rhode Island	530
5	Wyoming	1,644	50	Massachusetts	471

RANK ORDER

	District of Columbia	729

Source: U.S. Department of Health and Human Services, National Center for Health Statistics
    unpublished data

*Age-adjusted years of potential life lost due to death before age 75. Includes such subcategories as falls, drowning, fires/burns, poisonings and motor vehicle injuries.

Alcohol-Induced Deaths in 1999

National Total = 19,171 Deaths*

ALPHA ORDER

RANK ORDER

RANK	STATE	DEATHS	% of USA		RANK	STATE	DEATHS	% of USA
28	Alabama	242	1.3%		1	California	3,245	16.9%
39	Alaska	93	0.5%		2	Florida	1,266	6.6%
10	Arizona	466	2.4%		3	New York	1,220	6.4%
36	Arkansas	118	0.6%		4	Texas	1,163	6.1%
1	California	3,245	16.9%		5	North Carolina	670	3.5%
12	Colorado	462	2.4%		6	Illinois	636	3.3%
31	Connecticut	174	0.9%		7	Michigan	614	3.2%
46	Delaware	59	0.3%		8	Washington	557	2.9%
2	Florida	1,266	6.6%		9	Ohio	548	2.9%
11	Georgia	463	2.4%		10	Arizona	466	2.4%
49	Hawaii	37	0.2%		11	Georgia	463	2.4%
44	Idaho	74	0.4%		12	Colorado	462	2.4%
6	Illinois	636	3.3%		13	New Jersey	456	2.4%
24	Indiana	301	1.6%		14	Pennsylvania	450	2.3%
32	Iowa	150	0.8%		15	South Carolina	419	2.2%
34	Kansas	130	0.7%		16	Missouri	392	2.0%
30	Kentucky	230	1.2%		17	Tennessee	391	2.0%
26	Louisiana	291	1.5%		18	Massachusetts	351	1.8%
38	Maine	105	0.5%		19	Wisconsin	349	1.8%
21	Maryland	314	1.6%		20	Virginia	329	1.7%
18	Massachusetts	351	1.8%		21	Maryland	314	1.6%
7	Michigan	614	3.2%		22	Oregon	305	1.6%
23	Minnesota	302	1.6%		23	Minnesota	302	1.6%
32	Mississippi	150	0.8%		24	Indiana	301	1.6%
16	Missouri	392	2.0%		25	New Mexico	292	1.5%
43	Montana	75	0.4%		26	Louisiana	291	1.5%
40	Nebraska	90	0.5%		27	Nevada	250	1.3%
27	Nevada	250	1.3%		28	Alabama	242	1.3%
41	New Hampshire	89	0.5%		29	Oklahoma	240	1.3%
13	New Jersey	456	2.4%		30	Kentucky	230	1.2%
25	New Mexico	292	1.5%		31	Connecticut	174	0.9%
3	New York	1,220	6.4%		32	Iowa	150	0.8%
5	North Carolina	670	3.5%		32	Mississippi	150	0.8%
48	North Dakota	51	0.3%		34	Kansas	130	0.7%
9	Ohio	548	2.9%		35	Utah	127	0.7%
29	Oklahoma	240	1.3%		36	Arkansas	118	0.6%
22	Oregon	305	1.6%		37	West Virginia	116	0.6%
14	Pennsylvania	450	2.3%		38	Maine	105	0.5%
45	Rhode Island	69	0.4%		39	Alaska	93	0.5%
15	South Carolina	419	2.2%		40	Nebraska	90	0.5%
42	South Dakota	80	0.4%		41	New Hampshire	89	0.5%
17	Tennessee	391	2.0%		42	South Dakota	80	0.4%
4	Texas	1,163	6.1%		43	Montana	75	0.4%
35	Utah	127	0.7%		44	Idaho	74	0.4%
50	Vermont	36	0.2%		45	Rhode Island	69	0.4%
20	Virginia	329	1.7%		46	Delaware	59	0.3%
8	Washington	557	2.9%		47	Wyoming	57	0.3%
37	West Virginia	116	0.6%		48	North Dakota	51	0.3%
19	Wisconsin	349	1.8%		49	Hawaii	37	0.2%
47	Wyoming	57	0.3%		50	Vermont	36	0.2%
						District of Columbia	77	0.4%

Source: U.S. Department of Health and Human Services, National Center for Health Statistics
(http://wonder.cdc.gov/WONDER/)
*By state of residence. Includes excessive blood level of alcohol, accidental poisoning by alcohol and the
following alcohol-related causes: psychoses, dependence syndrome, polyneuropathy, cardiomyopathy, gastritis,
chronic liver disease and cirrhosis. Excludes accidents, homicides and other causes indirectly related to alcohol use.

Death Rate by Alcohol-Induced Deaths in 1999

National Rate = 7.0 Deaths per 100,000 Population*

ALPHA ORDER

RANK	STATE	RATE
38	Alabama	5.5
2	Alaska	15.0
8	Arizona	9.8
48	Arkansas	4.6
8	California	9.8
5	Colorado	11.4
41	Connecticut	5.3
17	Delaware	7.8
14	Florida	8.4
32	Georgia	5.9
50	Hawaii	3.1
32	Idaho	5.9
42	Illinois	5.2
44	Indiana	5.1
42	Iowa	5.2
45	Kansas	4.9
34	Kentucky	5.8
23	Louisiana	6.7
14	Maine	8.4
29	Maryland	6.1
36	Massachusetts	5.7
28	Michigan	6.2
27	Minnesota	6.3
39	Mississippi	5.4
19	Missouri	7.2
13	Montana	8.5
39	Nebraska	5.4
3	Nevada	13.8
18	New Hampshire	7.4
37	New Jersey	5.6
1	New Mexico	16.8
23	New York	6.7
12	North Carolina	8.8
16	North Dakota	8.0
45	Ohio	4.9
20	Oklahoma	7.1
11	Oregon	9.2
49	Pennsylvania	3.8
22	Rhode Island	7.0
7	South Carolina	10.8
6	South Dakota	10.9
20	Tennessee	7.1
34	Texas	5.8
31	Utah	6.0
29	Vermont	6.1
47	Virginia	4.8
10	Washington	9.7
26	West Virginia	6.4
25	Wisconsin	6.6
4	Wyoming	11.9

RANK ORDER

RANK	STATE	RATE
1	New Mexico	16.8
2	Alaska	15.0
3	Nevada	13.8
4	Wyoming	11.9
5	Colorado	11.4
6	South Dakota	10.9
7	South Carolina	10.8
8	Arizona	9.8
8	California	9.8
10	Washington	9.7
11	Oregon	9.2
12	North Carolina	8.8
13	Montana	8.5
14	Florida	8.4
14	Maine	8.4
16	North Dakota	8.0
17	Delaware	7.8
18	New Hampshire	7.4
19	Missouri	7.2
20	Oklahoma	7.1
20	Tennessee	7.1
22	Rhode Island	7.0
23	Louisiana	6.7
23	New York	6.7
25	Wisconsin	6.6
26	West Virginia	6.4
27	Minnesota	6.3
28	Michigan	6.2
29	Maryland	6.1
29	Vermont	6.1
31	Utah	6.0
32	Georgia	5.9
32	Idaho	5.9
34	Kentucky	5.8
34	Texas	5.8
36	Massachusetts	5.7
37	New Jersey	5.6
38	Alabama	5.5
39	Mississippi	5.4
39	Nebraska	5.4
41	Connecticut	5.3
42	Illinois	5.2
42	Iowa	5.2
44	Indiana	5.1
45	Kansas	4.9
45	Ohio	4.9
47	Virginia	4.8
48	Arkansas	4.6
49	Pennsylvania	3.8
50	Hawaii	3.1

District of Columbia		14.8

Source: U.S. Department of Health and Human Services, National Center for Health Statistics
       (http://wonder.cdc.gov/WONDER/)
*By state of residence. Includes excessive blood level of alcohol, accidental poisoning by alcohol and the
following alcohol-related causes: psychoses, dependence syndrome, polyneuropathy, cardiomyopathy, gastritis,
chronic liver disease and cirrhosis. Excludes accidents, homicides and other causes indirectly related to alcohol
use. Not age-adjusted.

184

Age-Adjusted Death Rate by Alcohol-Induced Deaths in 1999

National Rate = 7.1 Deaths per 100,000 Population*

ALPHA ORDER				RANK ORDER		
RANK	STATE	RATE		RANK	STATE	RATE
39	Alabama	5.4		1	New Mexico	17.4
2	Alaska	16.3		2	Alaska	16.3
9	Arizona	10.1		3	Nevada	13.8
48	Arkansas	4.6		4	Wyoming	11.7
7	California	10.7		5	Colorado	11.4
5	Colorado	11.4		5	South Dakota	11.4
42	Connecticut	5.2		7	California	10.7
17	Delaware	7.7		7	South Carolina	10.7
13	Florida	7.9		9	Arizona	10.1
28	Georgia	6.3		10	Washington	10.0
50	Hawaii	3.0		11	Oregon	8.8
31	Idaho	6.2		12	North Carolina	8.7
41	Illinois	5.3		13	Florida	7.9
43	Indiana	5.1		13	Maine	7.9
44	Iowa	5.0		13	Montana	7.9
44	Kansas	5.0		13	North Dakota	7.9
35	Kentucky	5.7		17	Delaware	7.7
23	Louisiana	6.9		17	Utah	7.7
13	Maine	7.9		19	New Hampshire	7.6
32	Maryland	6.1		20	Missouri	7.1
37	Massachusetts	5.6		20	Oklahoma	7.1
28	Michigan	6.3		22	Tennessee	7.0
27	Minnesota	6.5		23	Louisiana	6.9
35	Mississippi	5.7		23	Rhode Island	6.9
20	Missouri	7.1		25	New York	6.6
13	Montana	7.9		25	Wisconsin	6.6
38	Nebraska	5.5		27	Minnesota	6.5
3	Nevada	13.8		28	Georgia	6.3
19	New Hampshire	7.6		28	Michigan	6.3
39	New Jersey	5.4		28	Texas	6.3
1	New Mexico	17.4		31	Idaho	6.2
25	New York	6.6		32	Maryland	6.1
12	North Carolina	8.7		33	West Virginia	5.9
13	North Dakota	7.9		34	Vermont	5.8
46	Ohio	4.8		35	Kentucky	5.7
20	Oklahoma	7.1		35	Mississippi	5.7
11	Oregon	8.8		37	Massachusetts	5.6
49	Pennsylvania	3.5		38	Nebraska	5.5
23	Rhode Island	6.9		39	Alabama	5.4
7	South Carolina	10.7		39	New Jersey	5.4
5	South Dakota	11.4		41	Illinois	5.3
22	Tennessee	7.0		42	Connecticut	5.2
28	Texas	6.3		43	Indiana	5.1
17	Utah	7.7		44	Iowa	5.0
34	Vermont	5.8		44	Kansas	5.0
46	Virginia	4.8		46	Ohio	4.8
10	Washington	10.0		46	Virginia	4.8
33	West Virginia	5.9		48	Arkansas	4.6
25	Wisconsin	6.6		49	Pennsylvania	3.5
4	Wyoming	11.7		50	Hawaii	3.0
					District of Columbia	13.9

*Source: U.S. Department of Health and Human Services, National Center for Health Statistics
(http://wonder.cdc.gov/WONDER/)*

*By state of residence. Includes excessive blood level of alcohol, accidental poisoning by alcohol and the following alcohol-related causes: psychoses, dependence syndrome, polyneuropathy, cardiomyopathy, gastritis, chronic liver disease and cirrhosis. Excludes accidents, homicides and other causes indirectly related to alcohol use. Age-adjusted rates based on the year 2000 standard population.

Drug-Induced Deaths in 1999

National Total = 19,102 Deaths*

ALPHA ORDER

RANK	STATE	DEATHS	% of USA
29	Alabama	195	1.0%
43	Alaska	56	0.3%
11	Arizona	557	2.9%
33	Arkansas	121	0.6%
1	California	3,089	16.2%
16	Colorado	375	2.0%
19	Connecticut	330	1.7%
44	Delaware	54	0.3%
4	Florida	1,058	5.5%
18	Georgia	345	1.8%
36	Hawaii	83	0.4%
39	Idaho	66	0.3%
6	Illinois	872	4.6%
23	Indiana	249	1.3%
42	Iowa	59	0.3%
35	Kansas	99	0.5%
27	Kentucky	214	1.1%
24	Louisiana	245	1.3%
38	Maine	70	0.4%
9	Maryland	660	3.5%
13	Massachusetts	512	2.7%
8	Michigan	708	3.7%
32	Minnesota	167	0.9%
34	Mississippi	101	0.5%
21	Missouri	293	1.5%
45	Montana	48	0.3%
46	Nebraska	41	0.2%
26	Nevada	236	1.2%
40	New Hampshire	62	0.3%
7	New Jersey	757	4.0%
22	New Mexico	275	1.4%
3	New York	1,099	5.8%
14	North Carolina	401	2.1%
50	North Dakota	15	0.1%
12	Ohio	534	2.8%
30	Oklahoma	189	1.0%
20	Oregon	328	1.7%
5	Pennsylvania	1,048	5.5%
41	Rhode Island	61	0.3%
31	South Carolina	168	0.9%
49	South Dakota	20	0.1%
17	Tennessee	372	1.9%
2	Texas	1,250	6.5%
28	Utah	210	1.1%
47	Vermont	31	0.2%
15	Virginia	390	2.0%
10	Washington	596	3.1%
37	West Virginia	80	0.4%
25	Wisconsin	237	1.2%
48	Wyoming	21	0.1%

RANK ORDER

RANK	STATE	DEATHS	% of USA
1	California	3,089	16.2%
2	Texas	1,250	6.5%
3	New York	1,099	5.8%
4	Florida	1,058	5.5%
5	Pennsylvania	1,048	5.5%
6	Illinois	872	4.6%
7	New Jersey	757	4.0%
8	Michigan	708	3.7%
9	Maryland	660	3.5%
10	Washington	596	3.1%
11	Arizona	557	2.9%
12	Ohio	534	2.8%
13	Massachusetts	512	2.7%
14	North Carolina	401	2.1%
15	Virginia	390	2.0%
16	Colorado	375	2.0%
17	Tennessee	372	1.9%
18	Georgia	345	1.8%
19	Connecticut	330	1.7%
20	Oregon	328	1.7%
21	Missouri	293	1.5%
22	New Mexico	275	1.4%
23	Indiana	249	1.3%
24	Louisiana	245	1.3%
25	Wisconsin	237	1.2%
26	Nevada	236	1.2%
27	Kentucky	214	1.1%
28	Utah	210	1.1%
29	Alabama	195	1.0%
30	Oklahoma	189	1.0%
31	South Carolina	168	0.9%
32	Minnesota	167	0.9%
33	Arkansas	121	0.6%
34	Mississippi	101	0.5%
35	Kansas	99	0.5%
36	Hawaii	83	0.4%
37	West Virginia	80	0.4%
38	Maine	70	0.4%
39	Idaho	66	0.3%
40	New Hampshire	62	0.3%
41	Rhode Island	61	0.3%
42	Iowa	59	0.3%
43	Alaska	56	0.3%
44	Delaware	54	0.3%
45	Montana	48	0.3%
46	Nebraska	41	0.2%
47	Vermont	31	0.2%
48	Wyoming	21	0.1%
49	South Dakota	20	0.1%
50	North Dakota	15	0.1%
	District of Columbia	55	0.3%

Source: U.S. Department of Health and Human Services, National Center for Health Statistics
(http://wonder.cdc.gov/WONDER/)

*By state of residence. Includes drug psychoses, drug dependence, nondependent use excluding alcohol and tobacco, accidental poisoning or suicide by drugs, medicaments and biologicals. Excludes accidents, homicides and other causes indirectly related to drug use.

Death Rate from Drug-Induced Deaths in 1999

National Rate = 7.0 Deaths per 100,000 Population*

ALPHA ORDER

RANK	STATE	RATE
37	Alabama	4.5
12	Alaska	9.0
4	Arizona	11.7
35	Arkansas	4.7
9	California	9.3
11	Colorado	9.2
6	Connecticut	10.1
15	Delaware	7.2
18	Florida	7.0
39	Georgia	4.4
18	Hawaii	7.0
31	Idaho	5.3
15	Illinois	7.2
43	Indiana	4.2
50	Iowa	2.1
44	Kansas	3.7
28	Kentucky	5.4
25	Louisiana	5.6
25	Maine	5.6
3	Maryland	12.8
14	Massachusetts	8.3
15	Michigan	7.2
46	Minnesota	3.5
45	Mississippi	3.6
28	Missouri	5.4
28	Montana	5.4
48	Nebraska	2.5
2	Nevada	13.0
32	New Hampshire	5.2
9	New Jersey	9.3
1	New Mexico	15.8
23	New York	6.0
32	North Carolina	5.2
49	North Dakota**	2.4
35	Ohio	4.7
25	Oklahoma	5.6
7	Oregon	9.9
13	Pennsylvania	8.7
21	Rhode Island	6.2
42	South Carolina	4.3
47	South Dakota	2.7
20	Tennessee	6.8
21	Texas	6.2
7	Utah	9.9
32	Vermont	5.2
24	Virginia	5.7
5	Washington	10.4
39	West Virginia	4.4
37	Wisconsin	4.5
39	Wyoming	4.4

RANK ORDER

RANK	STATE	RATE
1	New Mexico	15.8
2	Nevada	13.0
3	Maryland	12.8
4	Arizona	11.7
5	Washington	10.4
6	Connecticut	10.1
7	Oregon	9.9
7	Utah	9.9
9	California	9.3
9	New Jersey	9.3
11	Colorado	9.2
12	Alaska	9.0
13	Pennsylvania	8.7
14	Massachusetts	8.3
15	Delaware	7.2
15	Illinois	7.2
15	Michigan	7.2
18	Florida	7.0
18	Hawaii	7.0
20	Tennessee	6.8
21	Rhode Island	6.2
21	Texas	6.2
23	New York	6.0
24	Virginia	5.7
25	Louisiana	5.6
25	Maine	5.6
25	Oklahoma	5.6
28	Kentucky	5.4
28	Missouri	5.4
28	Montana	5.4
31	Idaho	5.3
32	New Hampshire	5.2
32	North Carolina	5.2
32	Vermont	5.2
35	Arkansas	4.7
35	Ohio	4.7
37	Alabama	4.5
37	Wisconsin	4.5
39	Georgia	4.4
39	West Virginia	4.4
39	Wyoming	4.4
42	South Carolina	4.3
43	Indiana	4.2
44	Kansas	3.7
45	Mississippi	3.6
46	Minnesota	3.5
47	South Dakota	2.7
48	Nebraska	2.5
49	North Dakota**	2.4
50	Iowa	2.1
	District of Columbia	10.6

Source: U.S. Department of Health and Human Services, National Center for Health Statistics
(http://wonder.cdc.gov/WONDER/)

*By state of residence. Includes drug psychoses, drug dependence, nondependent use excluding alcohol and tobacco, accidental poisoning or suicide by drugs, medicaments and biologicals. Excludes accidents, homicides and other causes indirectly related to drug use. Not age-adjusted.

**Due to low numbers of deaths, rates for this state should be interpreted with caution.

Age-Adjusted Death Rate from Drug-Induced Deaths in 1999

National Rate = 7.0 Deaths per 100,000 Population*

ALPHA ORDER			RANK ORDER		
RANK	STATE	RATE	RANK	STATE	RATE
39	Alabama	4.4	1	New Mexico	16.2
9	Alaska	9.6	2	Nevada	13.0
3	Arizona	12.2	3	Arizona	12.2
35	Arkansas	4.9	4	Maryland	12.0
10	California	9.4	5	Utah	11.5
12	Colorado	9.0	6	Washington	10.2
7	Connecticut	9.9	7	Connecticut	9.9
18	Delaware	7.0	7	Oregon	9.9
15	Florida	7.2	9	Alaska	9.6
39	Georgia	4.4	10	California	9.4
19	Hawaii	6.9	11	New Jersey	9.1
27	Idaho	5.5	12	Colorado	9.0
15	Illinois	7.2	13	Pennsylvania	8.7
43	Indiana	4.2	14	Massachusetts	8.0
50	Iowa	2.1	15	Florida	7.2
44	Kansas	3.8	15	Illinois	7.2
31	Kentucky	5.3	17	Michigan	7.1
25	Louisiana	5.8	18	Delaware	7.0
29	Maine	5.4	19	Hawaii	6.9
4	Maryland	12.0	20	Tennessee	6.7
14	Massachusetts	8.0	21	Texas	6.4
17	Michigan	7.1	22	Rhode Island	6.1
46	Minnesota	3.5	23	New York	5.9
44	Mississippi	3.8	23	Oklahoma	5.9
29	Missouri	5.4	25	Louisiana	5.8
26	Montana	5.6	26	Montana	5.6
48	Nebraska	2.5	27	Idaho	5.5
2	Nevada	13.0	27	Virginia	5.5
33	New Hampshire	5.0	29	Maine	5.4
11	New Jersey	9.1	29	Missouri	5.4
1	New Mexico	16.2	31	Kentucky	5.3
23	New York	5.9	31	North Carolina	5.3
31	North Carolina	5.3	33	New Hampshire	5.0
49	North Dakota**	2.3	33	Vermont	5.0
36	Ohio	4.7	35	Arkansas	4.9
23	Oklahoma	5.9	36	Ohio	4.7
7	Oregon	9.9	37	Wisconsin	4.5
13	Pennsylvania	8.7	37	Wyoming	4.5
22	Rhode Island	6.1	39	Alabama	4.4
42	South Carolina	4.3	39	Georgia	4.4
47	South Dakota	2.8	39	West Virginia	4.4
20	Tennessee	6.7	42	South Carolina	4.3
21	Texas	6.4	43	Indiana	4.2
5	Utah	11.5	44	Kansas	3.8
33	Vermont	5.0	44	Mississippi	3.8
27	Virginia	5.5	46	Minnesota	3.5
6	Washington	10.2	47	South Dakota	2.8
39	West Virginia	4.4	48	Nebraska	2.5
37	Wisconsin	4.5	49	North Dakota**	2.3
37	Wyoming	4.5	50	Iowa	2.1
				District of Columbia	9.7

Source: U.S. Department of Health and Human Services, National Center for Health Statistics
(http://wonder.cdc.gov/WONDER/)
*By state of residence. Includes drug psychoses, drug dependence, nondependent use excluding alcohol and tobacco, accidental poisoning or suicide by drugs, medicaments and biologicals. Excludes accidents, homicides and other causes indirectly related to drug use. Age-adjusted rates based on the year 2000 standard population.
**Due to low numbers of deaths, rates for this state should be interpreted with caution.

Occupational Fatalities in 2000

National Total = 5,915 Deaths*

ALPHA ORDER

RANK	STATE	DEATHS	% of USA
24	Alabama	103	1.7%
35	Alaska	53	0.9%
18	Arizona	118	2.0%
23	Arkansas	106	1.8%
2	California	553	9.3%
19	Colorado	117	2.0%
34	Connecticut	55	0.9%
48	Delaware	13	0.2%
3	Florida	329	5.6%
9	Georgia	195	3.3%
46	Hawaii	20	0.3%
41	Idaho	35	0.6%
7	Illinois	205	3.5%
11	Indiana	159	2.7%
29	Iowa	71	1.2%
25	Kansas	85	1.4%
16	Kentucky	132	2.2%
15	Louisiana	143	2.4%
45	Maine	26	0.4%
26	Maryland	84	1.4%
31	Massachusetts	67	1.1%
12	Michigan	156	2.6%
30	Minnesota	68	1.1%
17	Mississippi	125	2.1%
13	Missouri	148	2.5%
39	Montana	42	0.7%
33	Nebraska	59	1.0%
37	Nevada	51	0.9%
48	New Hampshire	13	0.2%
20	New Jersey	115	1.9%
41	New Mexico	35	0.6%
5	New York	233	3.9%
4	North Carolina	234	4.0%
44	North Dakota	34	0.6%
6	Ohio	207	3.5%
27	Oklahoma	82	1.4%
36	Oregon	52	0.9%
8	Pennsylvania	199	3.4%
50	Rhode Island	7	0.1%
21	South Carolina	114	1.9%
41	South Dakota	35	0.6%
10	Tennessee	160	2.7%
1	Texas	572	9.7%
32	Utah	61	1.0%
47	Vermont	15	0.3%
13	Virginia	148	2.5%
28	Washington	75	1.3%
38	West Virginia	46	0.8%
22	Wisconsin	107	1.8%
40	Wyoming	36	0.6%

RANK ORDER

RANK	STATE	DEATHS	% of USA
1	Texas	572	9.7%
2	California	553	9.3%
3	Florida	329	5.6%
4	North Carolina	234	4.0%
5	New York	233	3.9%
6	Ohio	207	3.5%
7	Illinois	205	3.5%
8	Pennsylvania	199	3.4%
9	Georgia	195	3.3%
10	Tennessee	160	2.7%
11	Indiana	159	2.7%
12	Michigan	156	2.6%
13	Missouri	148	2.5%
13	Virginia	148	2.5%
15	Louisiana	143	2.4%
16	Kentucky	132	2.2%
17	Mississippi	125	2.1%
18	Arizona	118	2.0%
19	Colorado	117	2.0%
20	New Jersey	115	1.9%
21	South Carolina	114	1.9%
22	Wisconsin	107	1.8%
23	Arkansas	106	1.8%
24	Alabama	103	1.7%
25	Kansas	85	1.4%
26	Maryland	84	1.4%
27	Oklahoma	82	1.4%
28	Washington	75	1.3%
29	Iowa	71	1.2%
30	Minnesota	68	1.1%
31	Massachusetts	67	1.1%
32	Utah	61	1.0%
33	Nebraska	59	1.0%
34	Connecticut	55	0.9%
35	Alaska	53	0.9%
36	Oregon	52	0.9%
37	Nevada	51	0.9%
38	West Virginia	46	0.8%
39	Montana	42	0.7%
40	Wyoming	36	0.6%
41	Idaho	35	0.6%
41	New Mexico	35	0.6%
41	South Dakota	35	0.6%
44	North Dakota	34	0.6%
45	Maine	26	0.4%
46	Hawaii	20	0.3%
47	Vermont	15	0.3%
48	Delaware	13	0.2%
48	New Hampshire	13	0.2%
50	Rhode Island	7	0.1%
	District of Columbia	13	0.2%

Source: U.S. Department of Labor, Bureau of Labor Statistics
"National Census of Fatal Occupational Injuries, 2000" (press release, August 21, 2001)
*Includes four fatalities that occurred within the territorial boundaries of the United States but for which a state of incident could not be determined.

Occupational Fatality Rate in 2000

National Rate = 4.4 Deaths per 100,000 Workers*

ALPHA ORDER			RANK ORDER		
RANK	**STATE**	**RATE**	**RANK**	**STATE**	**RATE**
23	Alabama	5.1	1	Alaska	17.5
1	Alaska	17.5	2	Wyoming	13.8
23	Arizona	5.1	3	North Dakota	10.3
6	Arkansas	9.1	4	Mississippi	10.2
36	California	3.4	5	Montana	9.5
20	Colorado	5.3	6	Arkansas	9.1
39	Connecticut	3.3	7	South Dakota	8.9
40	Delaware	3.2	8	Louisiana	7.4
29	Florida	4.5	9	Kentucky	7.1
26	Georgia	4.9	10	Nebraska	6.6
35	Hawaii	3.5	11	Kansas	6.4
18	Idaho	5.4	12	North Carolina	6.2
36	Illinois	3.4	12	South Carolina	6.2
18	Indiana	5.4	14	Tennessee	5.9
27	Iowa	4.6	15	West Virginia	5.8
11	Kansas	6.4	16	Texas	5.7
9	Kentucky	7.1	16	Utah	5.7
8	Louisiana	7.4	18	Idaho	5.4
32	Maine	4.0	18	Indiana	5.4
42	Maryland	3.1	20	Colorado	5.3
48	Massachusetts	2.1	20	Nevada	5.3
40	Michigan	3.2	22	Missouri	5.2
47	Minnesota	2.5	23	Alabama	5.1
4	Mississippi	10.2	23	Arizona	5.1
22	Missouri	5.2	23	Oklahoma	5.1
5	Montana	9.5	26	Georgia	4.9
10	Nebraska	6.6	27	Iowa	4.6
20	Nevada	5.3	27	Vermont	4.6
49	New Hampshire	2.0	29	Florida	4.5
44	New Jersey	2.9	30	New Mexico	4.4
30	New Mexico	4.4	31	Virginia	4.2
45	New York	2.8	32	Maine	4.0
12	North Carolina	6.2	33	Ohio	3.7
3	North Dakota	10.3	33	Wisconsin	3.7
33	Ohio	3.7	35	Hawaii	3.5
23	Oklahoma	5.1	36	California	3.4
42	Oregon	3.1	36	Illinois	3.4
36	Pennsylvania	3.4	36	Pennsylvania	3.4
50	Rhode Island	1.5	39	Connecticut	3.3
12	South Carolina	6.2	40	Delaware	3.2
7	South Dakota	8.9	40	Michigan	3.2
14	Tennessee	5.9	42	Maryland	3.1
16	Texas	5.7	42	Oregon	3.1
16	Utah	5.7	44	New Jersey	2.9
27	Vermont	4.6	45	New York	2.8
31	Virginia	4.2	46	Washington	2.7
46	Washington	2.7	47	Minnesota	2.5
15	West Virginia	5.8	48	Massachusetts	2.1
33	Wisconsin	3.7	49	New Hampshire	2.0
2	Wyoming	13.8	50	Rhode Island	1.5
				District of Columbia	5.0

Source: Morgan Quitno Press using data from U.S. Department of Labor, Bureau of Labor Statistics
"National Census of Fatal Occupational Injuries, 2000" (press release, August 21, 2001)
*Based on employed civilian labor force. Does not include fatalities occurring outside the territorial boundaries of the United States.

III. FACILITIES

191   Community Hospitals in 2000
192   Rate of Community Hospitals in 2000
193   Community Hospitals per 1,000 Square Miles in 2000
194   Community Hospitals in Urban Areas in 2000
195   Percent of Community Hospitals in Urban Areas in 2000
196   Community Hospitals in Rural Areas in 2000
197   Percent of Community Hospitals in Rural Areas in 2000
198   Nongovernment Not-For-Profit Hospitals in 2000
199   Investor-Owned (For-Profit) Hospitals in 2000
200   State and Local Government-Owned Hospitals in 2000
201   Beds in Community Hospitals in 2000
202   Rate of Beds in Community Hospitals in 2000
203   Average Number of Beds per Community Hospital in 2000
204   Admissions to Community Hospitals in 2000
205   Inpatient Days in Community Hospitals in 2000
206   Average Daily Census in Community Hospitals in 2000
207   Average Stay in Community Hospitals in 2000
208   Occupancy Rate in Community Hospitals in 2000
209   Outpatient Visits to Community Hospitals in 2000
210   Emergency Outpatient Visits to Community Hospitals in 2000
211   Surgical Operations in Community Hospitals in 2000
212   Medicare and Medicaid Certified Facilities in 2002
213   Medicare and Medicaid Certified Hospitals in 2002
214   Beds in Medicare and Medicaid Certified Hospitals in 2002
215   Medicare and Medicaid Certified Children's Hospitals in 2002
216   Beds in Medicare and Medicaid Certified Children's Hospitals in 2002
217   Medicare and Medicaid Certified Rehabilitation Hospitals in 2002
218   Beds in Medicare and Medicaid Certified Rehabilitation Hospitals in 2002
219   Medicare and Medicaid Certified Psychiatric Hospitals in 2002
220   Beds in Medicare and Medicaid Certified Psychiatric Hospitals in 2002
221   Medicare and Medicaid Certified Community Mental Health Centers in 2002
222   Medicare and Medicaid Certified Outpatient Physical Therapy Facilities in 2002
223   Medicare and Medicaid Certified Rural Health Clinics in 2002
224   Medicare and Medicaid Certified Home Health Agencies in 2002
225   Medicare and Medicaid Certified Hospices in 2002
226   Hospice Patients in Residential Facilities in 2002
227   Medicare and Medicaid Certified Nursing Care Facilities in 2002
228   Beds in Medicare and Medicaid Certified Nursing Care Facilities in 2002
229   Rate of Beds in Medicare and Medicaid Certified Nursing Care Facilities in 2002
230   Nursing Home Occupancy Rate in 1999
231   Nursing Home Resident Rate in 1999
232   Nursing Home Population 85 Years Old and Older in 1999
233   Health Care Establishments in 1999
234   Offices and Clinics of Doctors of Medicine in 1997
235   Offices and Clinics of Dentists in 1997

Community Hospitals in 2000

National Total = 4,915 Hospitals*

ALPHA ORDER

RANK	STATE	HOSPITALS	% of USA
19	Alabama	108	2.2%
47	Alaska	18	0.4%
31	Arizona	61	1.2%
26	Arkansas	83	1.7%
2	California	389	7.9%
29	Colorado	69	1.4%
41	Connecticut	35	0.7%
50	Delaware	5	0.1%
5	Florida	202	4.1%
8	Georgia	151	3.1%
46	Hawaii	21	0.4%
37	Idaho	42	0.9%
6	Illinois	196	4.0%
18	Indiana	109	2.2%
16	Iowa	115	2.3%
11	Kansas	129	2.6%
21	Kentucky	105	2.1%
12	Louisiana	123	2.5%
40	Maine	37	0.8%
35	Maryland	49	1.0%
27	Massachusetts	80	1.6%
9	Michigan	146	3.0%
10	Minnesota	135	2.7%
22	Mississippi	95	1.9%
14	Missouri	119	2.4%
34	Montana	52	1.1%
24	Nebraska	85	1.7%
45	Nevada	22	0.4%
43	New Hampshire	28	0.6%
27	New Jersey	80	1.6%
41	New Mexico	35	0.7%
3	New York	215	4.4%
17	North Carolina	113	2.3%
37	North Dakota	42	0.9%
7	Ohio	163	3.3%
19	Oklahoma	108	2.2%
32	Oregon	59	1.2%
4	Pennsylvania	207	4.2%
49	Rhode Island	11	0.2%
30	South Carolina	63	1.3%
36	South Dakota	48	1.0%
13	Tennessee	121	2.5%
1	Texas	403	8.2%
37	Utah	42	0.9%
48	Vermont	14	0.3%
23	Virginia	88	1.8%
25	Washington	84	1.7%
33	West Virginia	57	1.2%
15	Wisconsin	118	2.4%
44	Wyoming	24	0.5%

RANK ORDER

RANK	STATE	HOSPITALS	% of USA
1	Texas	403	8.2%
2	California	389	7.9%
3	New York	215	4.4%
4	Pennsylvania	207	4.2%
5	Florida	202	4.1%
6	Illinois	196	4.0%
7	Ohio	163	3.3%
8	Georgia	151	3.1%
9	Michigan	146	3.0%
10	Minnesota	135	2.7%
11	Kansas	129	2.6%
12	Louisiana	123	2.5%
13	Tennessee	121	2.5%
14	Missouri	119	2.4%
15	Wisconsin	118	2.4%
16	Iowa	115	2.3%
17	North Carolina	113	2.3%
18	Indiana	109	2.2%
19	Alabama	108	2.2%
19	Oklahoma	108	2.2%
21	Kentucky	105	2.1%
22	Mississippi	95	1.9%
23	Virginia	88	1.8%
24	Nebraska	85	1.7%
25	Washington	84	1.7%
26	Arkansas	83	1.7%
27	Massachusetts	80	1.6%
27	New Jersey	80	1.6%
29	Colorado	69	1.4%
30	South Carolina	63	1.3%
31	Arizona	61	1.2%
32	Oregon	59	1.2%
33	West Virginia	57	1.2%
34	Montana	52	1.1%
35	Maryland	49	1.0%
36	South Dakota	48	1.0%
37	Idaho	42	0.9%
37	North Dakota	42	0.9%
37	Utah	42	0.9%
40	Maine	37	0.8%
41	Connecticut	35	0.7%
41	New Mexico	35	0.7%
43	New Hampshire	28	0.6%
44	Wyoming	24	0.5%
45	Nevada	22	0.4%
46	Hawaii	21	0.4%
47	Alaska	18	0.4%
48	Vermont	14	0.3%
49	Rhode Island	11	0.2%
50	Delaware	5	0.1%
	District of Columbia	11	0.2%

Source: American Hospital Association (Chicago, IL)
"Hospital Statistics" (2002 edition)
*Community hospitals are all nonfederal, short-term, general and special hospitals whose facilities and services are available to the public.

Rate of Community Hospitals in 2000

National Rate = 1.7 Community Hospitals per 100,000 Population*

ALPHA ORDER

RANK	STATE	RATE
18	Alabama	2.4
13	Alaska	2.9
41	Arizona	1.2
11	Arkansas	3.1
43	California	1.1
32	Colorado	1.6
46	Connecticut	1.0
50	Delaware	0.6
39	Florida	1.3
27	Georgia	1.8
29	Hawaii	1.7
9	Idaho	3.2
32	Illinois	1.6
27	Indiana	1.8
7	Iowa	3.9
6	Kansas	4.8
17	Kentucky	2.6
15	Louisiana	2.8
13	Maine	2.9
48	Maryland	0.9
39	Massachusetts	1.3
35	Michigan	1.5
16	Minnesota	2.7
8	Mississippi	3.3
22	Missouri	2.1
3	Montana	5.8
4	Nebraska	5.0
43	Nevada	1.1
19	New Hampshire	2.3
48	New Jersey	0.9
24	New Mexico	1.9
43	New York	1.1
36	North Carolina	1.4
1	North Dakota	6.6
36	Ohio	1.4
11	Oklahoma	3.1
29	Oregon	1.7
29	Pennsylvania	1.7
46	Rhode Island	1.0
32	South Carolina	1.6
2	South Dakota	6.4
22	Tennessee	2.1
24	Texas	1.9
24	Utah	1.9
19	Vermont	2.3
41	Virginia	1.2
36	Washington	1.4
9	West Virginia	3.2
21	Wisconsin	2.2
5	Wyoming	4.9

RANK ORDER

RANK	STATE	RATE
1	North Dakota	6.6
2	South Dakota	6.4
3	Montana	5.8
4	Nebraska	5.0
5	Wyoming	4.9
6	Kansas	4.8
7	Iowa	3.9
8	Mississippi	3.3
9	Idaho	3.2
9	West Virginia	3.2
11	Arkansas	3.1
11	Oklahoma	3.1
13	Alaska	2.9
13	Maine	2.9
15	Louisiana	2.8
16	Minnesota	2.7
17	Kentucky	2.6
18	Alabama	2.4
19	New Hampshire	2.3
19	Vermont	2.3
21	Wisconsin	2.2
22	Missouri	2.1
22	Tennessee	2.1
24	New Mexico	1.9
24	Texas	1.9
24	Utah	1.9
27	Georgia	1.8
27	Indiana	1.8
29	Hawaii	1.7
29	Oregon	1.7
29	Pennsylvania	1.7
32	Colorado	1.6
32	Illinois	1.6
32	South Carolina	1.6
35	Michigan	1.5
36	North Carolina	1.4
36	Ohio	1.4
36	Washington	1.4
39	Florida	1.3
39	Massachusetts	1.3
41	Arizona	1.2
41	Virginia	1.2
43	California	1.1
43	Nevada	1.1
43	New York	1.1
46	Connecticut	1.0
46	Rhode Island	1.0
48	Maryland	0.9
48	New Jersey	0.9
50	Delaware	0.6

District of Columbia — 1.9

Source: Morgan Quitno Press using data from American Hospital Association (Chicago, IL) "Hospital Statistics" (2002 edition)

*Community hospitals are all nonfederal, short-term, general and special hospitals whose facilities and services are available to the public.

Community Hospitals per 1,000 Square Miles in 2000

National Rate = 1.3 Community Hospitals*

<table>
<tr><td colspan="3">ALPHA ORDER</td><td colspan="3">RANK ORDER</td></tr>
<tr><td>RANK</td><td>STATE</td><td>RATE</td><td>RANK</td><td>STATE</td><td>RATE</td></tr>
<tr><td>20</td><td>Alabama</td><td>2.1</td><td>1</td><td>New Jersey</td><td>9.7</td></tr>
<tr><td>50</td><td>Alaska**</td><td>0.0</td><td>2</td><td>Rhode Island</td><td>8.9</td></tr>
<tr><td>43</td><td>Arizona</td><td>0.5</td><td>3</td><td>Massachusetts</td><td>8.7</td></tr>
<tr><td>29</td><td>Arkansas</td><td>1.6</td><td>4</td><td>Connecticut</td><td>6.3</td></tr>
<tr><td>18</td><td>California</td><td>2.4</td><td>5</td><td>Pennsylvania</td><td>4.5</td></tr>
<tr><td>39</td><td>Colorado</td><td>0.7</td><td>6</td><td>Maryland</td><td>4.0</td></tr>
<tr><td>4</td><td>Connecticut</td><td>6.3</td><td>6</td><td>New York</td><td>4.0</td></tr>
<tr><td>20</td><td>Delaware</td><td>2.1</td><td>8</td><td>Ohio</td><td>3.6</td></tr>
<tr><td>9</td><td>Florida</td><td>3.4</td><td>9</td><td>Florida</td><td>3.4</td></tr>
<tr><td>15</td><td>Georgia</td><td>2.6</td><td>9</td><td>Illinois</td><td>3.4</td></tr>
<tr><td>11</td><td>Hawaii</td><td>3.3</td><td>11</td><td>Hawaii</td><td>3.3</td></tr>
<tr><td>43</td><td>Idaho</td><td>0.5</td><td>12</td><td>Indiana</td><td>3.0</td></tr>
<tr><td>9</td><td>Illinois</td><td>3.4</td><td>12</td><td>New Hampshire</td><td>3.0</td></tr>
<tr><td>12</td><td>Indiana</td><td>3.0</td><td>14</td><td>Tennessee</td><td>2.9</td></tr>
<tr><td>24</td><td>Iowa</td><td>2.0</td><td>15</td><td>Georgia</td><td>2.6</td></tr>
<tr><td>29</td><td>Kansas</td><td>1.6</td><td>15</td><td>Kentucky</td><td>2.6</td></tr>
<tr><td>15</td><td>Kentucky</td><td>2.6</td><td>17</td><td>Louisiana</td><td>2.5</td></tr>
<tr><td>17</td><td>Louisiana</td><td>2.5</td><td>18</td><td>California</td><td>2.4</td></tr>
<tr><td>37</td><td>Maine</td><td>1.1</td><td>18</td><td>West Virginia</td><td>2.4</td></tr>
<tr><td>6</td><td>Maryland</td><td>4.0</td><td>20</td><td>Alabama</td><td>2.1</td></tr>
<tr><td>3</td><td>Massachusetts</td><td>8.7</td><td>20</td><td>Delaware</td><td>2.1</td></tr>
<tr><td>32</td><td>Michigan</td><td>1.5</td><td>20</td><td>North Carolina</td><td>2.1</td></tr>
<tr><td>29</td><td>Minnesota</td><td>1.6</td><td>20</td><td>Virginia</td><td>2.1</td></tr>
<tr><td>24</td><td>Mississippi</td><td>2.0</td><td>24</td><td>Iowa</td><td>2.0</td></tr>
<tr><td>28</td><td>Missouri</td><td>1.7</td><td>24</td><td>Mississippi</td><td>2.0</td></tr>
<tr><td>46</td><td>Montana</td><td>0.4</td><td>24</td><td>South Carolina</td><td>2.0</td></tr>
<tr><td>37</td><td>Nebraska</td><td>1.1</td><td>27</td><td>Wisconsin</td><td>1.8</td></tr>
<tr><td>48</td><td>Nevada</td><td>0.2</td><td>28</td><td>Missouri</td><td>1.7</td></tr>
<tr><td>12</td><td>New Hampshire</td><td>3.0</td><td>29</td><td>Arkansas</td><td>1.6</td></tr>
<tr><td>1</td><td>New Jersey</td><td>9.7</td><td>29</td><td>Kansas</td><td>1.6</td></tr>
<tr><td>47</td><td>New Mexico</td><td>0.3</td><td>29</td><td>Minnesota</td><td>1.6</td></tr>
<tr><td>6</td><td>New York</td><td>4.0</td><td>32</td><td>Michigan</td><td>1.5</td></tr>
<tr><td>20</td><td>North Carolina</td><td>2.1</td><td>32</td><td>Oklahoma</td><td>1.5</td></tr>
<tr><td>40</td><td>North Dakota</td><td>0.6</td><td>32</td><td>Texas</td><td>1.5</td></tr>
<tr><td>8</td><td>Ohio</td><td>3.6</td><td>32</td><td>Vermont</td><td>1.5</td></tr>
<tr><td>32</td><td>Oklahoma</td><td>1.5</td><td>36</td><td>Washington</td><td>1.2</td></tr>
<tr><td>40</td><td>Oregon</td><td>0.6</td><td>37</td><td>Maine</td><td>1.1</td></tr>
<tr><td>5</td><td>Pennsylvania</td><td>4.5</td><td>37</td><td>Nebraska</td><td>1.1</td></tr>
<tr><td>2</td><td>Rhode Island</td><td>8.9</td><td>39</td><td>Colorado</td><td>0.7</td></tr>
<tr><td>24</td><td>South Carolina</td><td>2.0</td><td>40</td><td>North Dakota</td><td>0.6</td></tr>
<tr><td>40</td><td>South Dakota</td><td>0.6</td><td>40</td><td>Oregon</td><td>0.6</td></tr>
<tr><td>14</td><td>Tennessee</td><td>2.9</td><td>40</td><td>South Dakota</td><td>0.6</td></tr>
<tr><td>32</td><td>Texas</td><td>1.5</td><td>43</td><td>Arizona</td><td>0.5</td></tr>
<tr><td>43</td><td>Utah</td><td>0.5</td><td>43</td><td>Idaho</td><td>0.5</td></tr>
<tr><td>32</td><td>Vermont</td><td>1.5</td><td>43</td><td>Utah</td><td>0.5</td></tr>
<tr><td>20</td><td>Virginia</td><td>2.1</td><td>46</td><td>Montana</td><td>0.4</td></tr>
<tr><td>36</td><td>Washington</td><td>1.2</td><td>47</td><td>New Mexico</td><td>0.3</td></tr>
<tr><td>18</td><td>West Virginia</td><td>2.4</td><td>48</td><td>Nevada</td><td>0.2</td></tr>
<tr><td>27</td><td>Wisconsin</td><td>1.8</td><td>48</td><td>Wyoming</td><td>0.2</td></tr>
<tr><td>48</td><td>Wyoming</td><td>0.2</td><td>50</td><td>Alaska**</td><td>0.0</td></tr>
<tr><td></td><td></td><td></td><td></td><td>District of Columbia***</td><td>NA</td></tr>
</table>

Source: Morgan Quitno Press using data from American Hospital Association (Chicago, IL)
"Hospital Statistics" (2002 edition)
*Based on 1990 Census land and water area figures. Community hospitals are nonfederal short-term general and other special hospitals, whose facilities and services are available to the public.
**Alaska has 18 community hospitals for its 615,230 square miles.
***The District of Columbia has 11 community hospitals for its 68 square miles.

Community Hospitals in Urban Areas in 2000

National Total = 2,740 Hospitals*

ALPHA ORDER				RANK ORDER			
RANK	STATE	HOSPITALS	% of USA	RANK	STATE	HOSPITALS	% of USA
16	Alabama	57	2.1%	1	California	348	12.7%
46	Alaska	3	0.1%	2	Texas	241	8.8%
20	Arizona	46	1.7%	3	New York	180	6.6%
29	Arkansas	28	1.0%	4	Florida	171	6.2%
1	California	348	12.7%	5	Pennsylvania	163	5.9%
27	Colorado	32	1.2%	6	Illinois	124	4.5%
28	Connecticut	29	1.1%	7	Ohio	111	4.1%
46	Delaware	3	0.1%	8	Michigan	88	3.2%
4	Florida	171	6.2%	9	New Jersey	80	2.9%
12	Georgia	67	2.4%	10	Louisiana	75	2.7%
39	Hawaii	12	0.4%	11	Massachusetts	69	2.5%
43	Idaho	7	0.3%	12	Georgia	67	2.4%
6	Illinois	124	4.5%	13	Indiana	64	2.3%
13	Indiana	64	2.3%	14	Missouri	61	2.2%
32	Iowa	21	0.8%	15	Tennessee	58	2.1%
31	Kansas	25	0.9%	16	Alabama	57	2.1%
26	Kentucky	33	1.2%	17	Wisconsin	56	2.0%
10	Louisiana	75	2.7%	18	Virginia	53	1.9%
42	Maine	8	0.3%	19	North Carolina	51	1.9%
23	Maryland	40	1.5%	20	Arizona	46	1.7%
11	Massachusetts	69	2.5%	21	Minnesota	45	1.6%
8	Michigan	88	3.2%	22	Washington	44	1.6%
21	Minnesota	45	1.6%	23	Maryland	40	1.5%
34	Mississippi	19	0.7%	23	Oklahoma	40	1.5%
14	Missouri	61	2.2%	25	South Carolina	35	1.3%
46	Montana	3	0.1%	26	Kentucky	33	1.2%
36	Nebraska	13	0.5%	27	Colorado	32	1.2%
36	Nevada	13	0.5%	28	Connecticut	29	1.1%
40	New Hampshire	10	0.4%	29	Arkansas	28	1.0%
9	New Jersey	80	2.9%	30	Oregon	27	1.0%
36	New Mexico	13	0.5%	31	Kansas	25	0.9%
3	New York	180	6.6%	32	Iowa	21	0.8%
19	North Carolina	51	1.9%	33	Utah	20	0.7%
44	North Dakota	6	0.2%	34	Mississippi	19	0.7%
7	Ohio	111	4.1%	35	West Virginia	18	0.7%
23	Oklahoma	40	1.5%	36	Nebraska	13	0.5%
30	Oregon	27	1.0%	36	Nevada	13	0.5%
5	Pennsylvania	163	5.9%	36	New Mexico	13	0.5%
40	Rhode Island	10	0.4%	39	Hawaii	12	0.4%
25	South Carolina	35	1.3%	40	New Hampshire	10	0.4%
45	South Dakota	5	0.2%	40	Rhode Island	10	0.4%
15	Tennessee	58	2.1%	42	Maine	8	0.3%
2	Texas	241	8.8%	43	Idaho	7	0.3%
33	Utah	20	0.7%	44	North Dakota	6	0.2%
49	Vermont	2	0.1%	45	South Dakota	5	0.2%
18	Virginia	53	1.9%	46	Alaska	3	0.1%
22	Washington	44	1.6%	46	Delaware	3	0.1%
35	West Virginia	18	0.7%	46	Montana	3	0.1%
17	Wisconsin	56	2.0%	49	Vermont	2	0.1%
49	Wyoming	2	0.1%	49	Wyoming	2	0.1%
					District of Columbia	11	0.4%

Source: American Hospital Association (Chicago, IL)
    "Hospital Statistics" (2002 edition)
*Community hospitals are all nonfederal, short-term, general and special hospitals whose facilities and services are available to the public. Urban is defined as any area inside a metropolitan statistical area as defined by the U.S. Office of Management and Budget.

Percent of Community Hospitals in Urban Areas in 2000

National Percent = 55.7% of Community Hospitals*

ALPHA ORDER

RANK	STATE	PERCENT
22	Alabama	52.8
43	Alaska	16.7
10	Arizona	75.4
35	Arkansas	33.7
3	California	89.5
28	Colorado	46.4
7	Connecticut	82.9
16	Delaware	60.0
5	Florida	84.7
31	Georgia	44.4
20	Hawaii	57.1
43	Idaho	16.7
12	Illinois	63.3
19	Indiana	58.7
42	Iowa	18.3
41	Kansas	19.4
38	Kentucky	31.4
13	Louisiana	61.0
39	Maine	21.6
8	Maryland	81.6
4	Massachusetts	86.3
14	Michigan	60.3
36	Minnesota	33.3
40	Mississippi	20.0
24	Missouri	51.3
50	Montana	5.8
45	Nebraska	15.3
18	Nevada	59.1
34	New Hampshire	35.7
1	New Jersey	100.0
32	New Mexico	37.1
6	New York	83.7
30	North Carolina	45.1
46	North Dakota	14.3
11	Ohio	68.1
33	Oklahoma	37.0
29	Oregon	45.8
9	Pennsylvania	78.7
2	Rhode Island	90.9
21	South Carolina	55.6
48	South Dakota	10.4
25	Tennessee	47.9
17	Texas	59.8
26	Utah	47.6
46	Vermont	14.3
15	Virginia	60.2
23	Washington	52.4
37	West Virginia	31.6
27	Wisconsin	47.5
49	Wyoming	8.3

RANK ORDER

RANK	STATE	PERCENT
1	New Jersey	100.0
2	Rhode Island	90.9
3	California	89.5
4	Massachusetts	86.3
5	Florida	84.7
6	New York	83.7
7	Connecticut	82.9
8	Maryland	81.6
9	Pennsylvania	78.7
10	Arizona	75.4
11	Ohio	68.1
12	Illinois	63.3
13	Louisiana	61.0
14	Michigan	60.3
15	Virginia	60.2
16	Delaware	60.0
17	Texas	59.8
18	Nevada	59.1
19	Indiana	58.7
20	Hawaii	57.1
21	South Carolina	55.6
22	Alabama	52.8
23	Washington	52.4
24	Missouri	51.3
25	Tennessee	47.9
26	Utah	47.6
27	Wisconsin	47.5
28	Colorado	46.4
29	Oregon	45.8
30	North Carolina	45.1
31	Georgia	44.4
32	New Mexico	37.1
33	Oklahoma	37.0
34	New Hampshire	35.7
35	Arkansas	33.7
36	Minnesota	33.3
37	West Virginia	31.6
38	Kentucky	31.4
39	Maine	21.6
40	Mississippi	20.0
41	Kansas	19.4
42	Iowa	18.3
43	Alaska	16.7
43	Idaho	16.7
45	Nebraska	15.3
46	North Dakota	14.3
46	Vermont	14.3
48	South Dakota	10.4
49	Wyoming	8.3
50	Montana	5.8

District of Columbia 100.0

Source: Morgan Quitno Press using data from American Hospital Association (Chicago, IL)
"Hospital Statistics" (2002 edition)
*Community hospitals are all nonfederal, short-term, general and special hospitals whose facilities and services are available to the public. Urban is defined as any area inside a metropolitan statistical area as defined by the U.S. Office of Management and Budget.

Community Hospitals in Rural Areas in 2000

National Total = 2,175 Hospitals*

ALPHA ORDER				RANK ORDER			
RANK	STATE	HOSPITALS	% of USA	RANK	STATE	HOSPITALS	% of USA
18	Alabama	51	2.3%	1	Texas	162	7.4%
40	Alaska	15	0.7%	2	Kansas	104	4.8%
40	Arizona	15	0.7%	3	Iowa	94	4.3%
16	Arkansas	55	2.5%	4	Minnesota	90	4.1%
24	California	41	1.9%	5	Georgia	84	3.9%
27	Colorado	37	1.7%	6	Mississippi	76	3.5%
47	Connecticut	6	0.3%	7	Illinois	72	3.3%
48	Delaware	2	0.1%	7	Kentucky	72	3.3%
33	Florida	31	1.4%	7	Nebraska	72	3.3%
5	Georgia	84	3.9%	10	Oklahoma	68	3.1%
44	Hawaii	9	0.4%	11	Tennessee	63	2.9%
29	Idaho	35	1.6%	12	North Carolina	62	2.9%
7	Illinois	72	3.3%	12	Wisconsin	62	2.9%
21	Indiana	45	2.1%	14	Michigan	58	2.7%
3	Iowa	94	4.3%	14	Missouri	58	2.7%
2	Kansas	104	4.8%	16	Arkansas	55	2.5%
7	Kentucky	72	3.3%	17	Ohio	52	2.4%
20	Louisiana	48	2.2%	18	Alabama	51	2.3%
34	Maine	29	1.3%	19	Montana	49	2.3%
44	Maryland	9	0.4%	20	Louisiana	48	2.2%
43	Massachusetts	11	0.5%	21	Indiana	45	2.1%
14	Michigan	58	2.7%	22	Pennsylvania	44	2.0%
4	Minnesota	90	4.1%	23	South Dakota	43	2.0%
6	Mississippi	76	3.5%	24	California	41	1.9%
14	Missouri	58	2.7%	25	Washington	40	1.8%
19	Montana	49	2.3%	26	West Virginia	39	1.8%
7	Nebraska	72	3.3%	27	Colorado	37	1.7%
44	Nevada	9	0.4%	28	North Dakota	36	1.7%
39	New Hampshire	18	0.8%	29	Idaho	35	1.6%
50	New Jersey	0	0.0%	29	New York	35	1.6%
36	New Mexico	22	1.0%	29	Virginia	35	1.6%
29	New York	35	1.6%	32	Oregon	32	1.5%
12	North Carolina	62	2.9%	33	Florida	31	1.4%
28	North Dakota	36	1.7%	34	Maine	29	1.3%
17	Ohio	52	2.4%	35	South Carolina	28	1.3%
10	Oklahoma	68	3.1%	36	New Mexico	22	1.0%
32	Oregon	32	1.5%	36	Utah	22	1.0%
22	Pennsylvania	44	2.0%	36	Wyoming	22	1.0%
49	Rhode Island	1	0.0%	39	New Hampshire	18	0.8%
35	South Carolina	28	1.3%	40	Alaska	15	0.7%
23	South Dakota	43	2.0%	40	Arizona	15	0.7%
11	Tennessee	63	2.9%	42	Vermont	12	0.6%
1	Texas	162	7.4%	43	Massachusetts	11	0.5%
36	Utah	22	1.0%	44	Hawaii	9	0.4%
42	Vermont	12	0.6%	44	Maryland	9	0.4%
29	Virginia	35	1.6%	44	Nevada	9	0.4%
25	Washington	40	1.8%	47	Connecticut	6	0.3%
26	West Virginia	39	1.8%	48	Delaware	2	0.1%
12	Wisconsin	62	2.9%	49	Rhode Island	1	0.0%
36	Wyoming	22	1.0%	50	New Jersey	0	0.0%
					District of Columbia	0	0.0%

Source: American Hospital Association (Chicago, IL)
    "Hospital Statistics" (2002 edition)
*Community hospitals are all nonfederal, short-term, general and special hospitals whose facilities and services are
available to the public. Rural is defined as any area outside a metropolitan statistical area as defined by the U.S.
Office of Management and Budget.

Percent of Community Hospitals in Rural Areas in 2000

National Percent = 44.3% of Community Hospitals*

ALPHA ORDER

RANK ORDER

RANK	STATE	PERCENT
29	Alabama	47.2
7	Alaska	83.3
41	Arizona	24.6
16	Arkansas	66.3
48	California	10.5
23	Colorado	53.6
44	Connecticut	17.1
35	Delaware	40.0
46	Florida	15.3
20	Georgia	55.6
31	Hawaii	42.9
7	Idaho	83.3
39	Illinois	36.7
32	Indiana	41.3
9	Iowa	81.7
10	Kansas	80.6
13	Kentucky	68.6
38	Louisiana	39.0
12	Maine	78.4
43	Maryland	18.4
47	Massachusetts	13.8
37	Michigan	39.7
15	Minnesota	66.7
11	Mississippi	80.0
27	Missouri	48.7
1	Montana	94.2
6	Nebraska	84.7
33	Nevada	40.9
17	New Hampshire	64.3
50	New Jersey	0.0
19	New Mexico	62.9
45	New York	16.3
21	North Carolina	54.9
4	North Dakota	85.7
40	Ohio	31.9
18	Oklahoma	63.0
22	Oregon	54.2
42	Pennsylvania	21.3
49	Rhode Island	9.1
30	South Carolina	44.4
3	South Dakota	89.6
26	Tennessee	52.1
34	Texas	40.2
25	Utah	52.4
4	Vermont	85.7
36	Virginia	39.8
28	Washington	47.6
14	West Virginia	68.4
24	Wisconsin	52.5
2	Wyoming	91.7

RANK	STATE	PERCENT
1	Montana	94.2
2	Wyoming	91.7
3	South Dakota	89.6
4	North Dakota	85.7
4	Vermont	85.7
6	Nebraska	84.7
7	Alaska	83.3
7	Idaho	83.3
9	Iowa	81.7
10	Kansas	80.6
11	Mississippi	80.0
12	Maine	78.4
13	Kentucky	68.6
14	West Virginia	68.4
15	Minnesota	66.7
16	Arkansas	66.3
17	New Hampshire	64.3
18	Oklahoma	63.0
19	New Mexico	62.9
20	Georgia	55.6
21	North Carolina	54.9
22	Oregon	54.2
23	Colorado	53.6
24	Wisconsin	52.5
25	Utah	52.4
26	Tennessee	52.1
27	Missouri	48.7
28	Washington	47.6
29	Alabama	47.2
30	South Carolina	44.4
31	Hawaii	42.9
32	Indiana	41.3
33	Nevada	40.9
34	Texas	40.2
35	Delaware	40.0
36	Virginia	39.8
37	Michigan	39.7
38	Louisiana	39.0
39	Illinois	36.7
40	Ohio	31.9
41	Arizona	24.6
42	Pennsylvania	21.3
43	Maryland	18.4
44	Connecticut	17.1
45	New York	16.3
46	Florida	15.3
47	Massachusetts	13.8
48	California	10.5
49	Rhode Island	9.1
50	New Jersey	0.0
	District of Columbia	0.0

Source: Morgan Quitno Press using data from American Hospital Association (Chicago, IL)
    "Hospital Statistics" (2002 edition)
*Community hospitals are all nonfederal, short-term, general and special hospitals whose facilities and services are available to the public. Rural is defined as any area outside a metropolitan statistical area as defined by the U.S. Office of Management and Budget.

Nongovernment Not-For-Profit Hospitals in 2000

National Total = 3,003 Hospitals*

<u>ALPHA ORDER</u>

RANK	STATE	HOSPITALS	% of USA
31	Alabama	39	1.3%
47	Alaska	10	0.3%
32	Arizona	37	1.2%
22	Arkansas	49	1.6%
1	California	224	7.5%
36	Colorado	32	1.1%
33	Connecticut	33	1.1%
49	Delaware	5	0.2%
10	Florida	88	2.9%
17	Georgia	62	2.1%
44	Hawaii	13	0.4%
45	Idaho	11	0.4%
4	Illinois	159	5.3%
21	Indiana	56	1.9%
19	Iowa	57	1.9%
18	Kansas	60	2.0%
12	Kentucky	72	2.4%
37	Louisiana	31	1.0%
33	Maine	33	1.1%
24	Maryland	47	1.6%
15	Massachusetts	70	2.3%
7	Michigan	124	4.1%
9	Minnesota	91	3.0%
38	Mississippi	26	0.9%
13	Missouri	71	2.4%
26	Montana	42	1.4%
25	Nebraska	43	1.4%
48	Nevada	7	0.2%
39	New Hampshire	24	0.8%
11	New Jersey	76	2.5%
41	New Mexico	20	0.7%
3	New York	183	6.1%
13	North Carolina	71	2.4%
30	North Dakota	40	1.3%
6	Ohio	137	4.6%
22	Oklahoma	49	1.6%
28	Oregon	41	1.4%
2	Pennsylvania	194	6.5%
45	Rhode Island	11	0.4%
41	South Carolina	20	0.7%
28	South Dakota	41	1.4%
19	Tennessee	57	1.9%
5	Texas	142	4.7%
40	Utah	22	0.7%
43	Vermont	14	0.5%
16	Virginia	66	2.2%
26	Washington	42	1.4%
33	West Virginia	33	1.1%
8	Wisconsin	115	3.8%
49	Wyoming	5	0.2%

<u>RANK ORDER</u>

RANK	STATE	HOSPITALS	% of USA
1	California	224	7.5%
2	Pennsylvania	194	6.5%
3	New York	183	6.1%
4	Illinois	159	5.3%
5	Texas	142	4.7%
6	Ohio	137	4.6%
7	Michigan	124	4.1%
8	Wisconsin	115	3.8%
9	Minnesota	91	3.0%
10	Florida	88	2.9%
11	New Jersey	76	2.5%
12	Kentucky	72	2.4%
13	Missouri	71	2.4%
13	North Carolina	71	2.4%
15	Massachusetts	70	2.3%
16	Virginia	66	2.2%
17	Georgia	62	2.1%
18	Kansas	60	2.0%
19	Iowa	57	1.9%
19	Tennessee	57	1.9%
21	Indiana	56	1.9%
22	Arkansas	49	1.6%
22	Oklahoma	49	1.6%
24	Maryland	47	1.6%
25	Nebraska	43	1.4%
26	Montana	42	1.4%
26	Washington	42	1.4%
28	Oregon	41	1.4%
28	South Dakota	41	1.4%
30	North Dakota	40	1.3%
31	Alabama	39	1.3%
32	Arizona	37	1.2%
33	Connecticut	33	1.1%
33	Maine	33	1.1%
33	West Virginia	33	1.1%
36	Colorado	32	1.1%
37	Louisiana	31	1.0%
38	Mississippi	26	0.9%
39	New Hampshire	24	0.8%
40	Utah	22	0.7%
41	New Mexico	20	0.7%
41	South Carolina	20	0.7%
43	Vermont	14	0.5%
44	Hawaii	13	0.4%
45	Idaho	11	0.4%
45	Rhode Island	11	0.4%
47	Alaska	10	0.3%
48	Nevada	7	0.2%
49	Delaware	5	0.2%
49	Wyoming	5	0.2%
	District of Columbia	8	0.3%

Source: American Hospital Association (Chicago, IL)
"Hospital Statistics" (2002 edition)
*Nongovernment not-for-profit hospitals are a subset of community hospitals.

Investor-Owned (For-Profit) Hospitals in 2000

National Total = 749 Hospitals*

ALPHA ORDER

RANK	STATE	HOSPITALS	% of USA
7	Alabama	29	3.9%
38	Alaska	1	0.1%
10	Arizona	19	2.5%
10	Arkansas	19	2.5%
3	California	94	12.6%
21	Colorado	9	1.2%
38	Connecticut	1	0.1%
44	Delaware	0	0.0%
2	Florida	95	12.7%
6	Georgia	33	4.4%
38	Hawaii	1	0.1%
31	Idaho	3	0.4%
21	Illinois	9	1.2%
17	Indiana	12	1.6%
44	Iowa	0	0.0%
25	Kansas	6	0.8%
12	Kentucky	18	2.4%
4	Louisiana	37	4.9%
38	Maine	1	0.1%
35	Maryland	2	0.3%
25	Massachusetts	6	0.8%
31	Michigan	3	0.4%
44	Minnesota	0	0.0%
8	Mississippi	24	3.2%
18	Missouri	11	1.5%
44	Montana	0	0.0%
38	Nebraska	1	0.1%
23	Nevada	8	1.1%
28	New Hampshire	4	0.5%
35	New Jersey	2	0.3%
25	New Mexico	6	0.8%
23	New York	8	1.1%
20	North Carolina	10	1.3%
35	North Dakota	2	0.3%
28	Ohio	4	0.5%
14	Oklahoma	14	1.9%
31	Oregon	3	0.4%
18	Pennsylvania	11	1.5%
44	Rhode Island	0	0.0%
9	South Carolina	20	2.7%
44	South Dakota	0	0.0%
4	Tennessee	37	4.9%
1	Texas	131	17.5%
16	Utah	13	1.7%
44	Vermont	0	0.0%
13	Virginia	17	2.3%
28	Washington	4	0.5%
14	West Virginia	14	1.9%
38	Wisconsin	1	0.1%
31	Wyoming	3	0.4%

RANK ORDER

RANK	STATE	HOSPITALS	% of USA
1	Texas	131	17.5%
2	Florida	95	12.7%
3	California	94	12.6%
4	Louisiana	37	4.9%
4	Tennessee	37	4.9%
6	Georgia	33	4.4%
7	Alabama	29	3.9%
8	Mississippi	24	3.2%
9	South Carolina	20	2.7%
10	Arizona	19	2.5%
10	Arkansas	19	2.5%
12	Kentucky	18	2.4%
13	Virginia	17	2.3%
14	Oklahoma	14	1.9%
14	West Virginia	14	1.9%
16	Utah	13	1.7%
17	Indiana	12	1.6%
18	Missouri	11	1.5%
18	Pennsylvania	11	1.5%
20	North Carolina	10	1.3%
21	Colorado	9	1.2%
21	Illinois	9	1.2%
23	Nevada	8	1.1%
23	New York	8	1.1%
25	Kansas	6	0.8%
25	Massachusetts	6	0.8%
25	New Mexico	6	0.8%
28	New Hampshire	4	0.5%
28	Ohio	4	0.5%
28	Washington	4	0.5%
31	Idaho	3	0.4%
31	Michigan	3	0.4%
31	Oregon	3	0.4%
31	Wyoming	3	0.4%
35	Maryland	2	0.3%
35	New Jersey	2	0.3%
35	North Dakota	2	0.3%
38	Alaska	1	0.1%
38	Connecticut	1	0.1%
38	Hawaii	1	0.1%
38	Maine	1	0.1%
38	Nebraska	1	0.1%
38	Wisconsin	1	0.1%
44	Delaware	0	0.0%
44	Iowa	0	0.0%
44	Minnesota	0	0.0%
44	Montana	0	0.0%
44	Rhode Island	0	0.0%
44	South Dakota	0	0.0%
44	Vermont	0	0.0%
	District of Columbia	3	0.4%

Source: American Hospital Association (Chicago, IL)
  "Hospital Statistics" (2002 edition)
*Investor-owned (for-profit) hospitals are a subset of community hospitals.

State and Local Government-Owned Hospitals in 2000

National Total = 1,163 Hospitals*

ALPHA ORDER					RANK ORDER			
RANK	STATE		HOSPITALS	% of USA	RANK	STATE		HOSPITALS	% of USA
12	Alabama	40	3.4%		1	Texas	130	11.2%
32	Alaska	7	0.6%		2	California	71	6.1%
37	Arizona	5	0.4%		3	Kansas	63	5.4%
26	Arkansas	15	1.3%		4	Iowa	58	5.0%
2	California	71	6.1%		5	Georgia	56	4.8%
16	Colorado	28	2.4%		6	Louisiana	55	4.7%
44	Connecticut	1	0.1%		7	Mississippi	45	3.9%
45	Delaware	0	0.0%		7	Oklahoma	45	3.9%
23	Florida	19	1.6%		9	Minnesota	44	3.8%
5	Georgia	56	4.8%		10	Indiana	41	3.5%
32	Hawaii	7	0.6%		10	Nebraska	41	3.5%
16	Idaho	28	2.4%		12	Alabama	40	3.4%
16	Illinois	28	2.4%		13	Washington	38	3.3%
10	Indiana	41	3.5%		14	Missouri	37	3.2%
4	Iowa	58	5.0%		15	North Carolina	32	2.8%
3	Kansas	63	5.4%		16	Colorado	28	2.4%
26	Kentucky	15	1.3%		16	Idaho	28	2.4%
6	Louisiana	55	4.7%		16	Illinois	28	2.4%
40	Maine	3	0.3%		19	Tennessee	27	2.3%
45	Maryland	0	0.0%		20	New York	24	2.1%
39	Massachusetts	4	0.3%		21	South Carolina	23	2.0%
23	Michigan	19	1.6%		22	Ohio	22	1.9%
9	Minnesota	44	3.8%		23	Florida	19	1.6%
7	Mississippi	45	3.9%		23	Michigan	19	1.6%
14	Missouri	37	3.2%		25	Wyoming	16	1.4%
29	Montana	10	0.9%		26	Arkansas	15	1.3%
10	Nebraska	41	3.5%		26	Kentucky	15	1.3%
32	Nevada	7	0.6%		26	Oregon	15	1.3%
45	New Hampshire	0	0.0%		29	Montana	10	0.9%
41	New Jersey	2	0.2%		29	West Virginia	10	0.9%
31	New Mexico	9	0.8%		31	New Mexico	9	0.8%
20	New York	24	2.1%		32	Alaska	7	0.6%
15	North Carolina	32	2.8%		32	Hawaii	7	0.6%
45	North Dakota	0	0.0%		32	Nevada	7	0.6%
22	Ohio	22	1.9%		32	South Dakota	7	0.6%
7	Oklahoma	45	3.9%		32	Utah	7	0.6%
26	Oregon	15	1.3%		37	Arizona	5	0.4%
41	Pennsylvania	2	0.2%		37	Virginia	5	0.4%
45	Rhode Island	0	0.0%		39	Massachusetts	4	0.3%
21	South Carolina	23	2.0%		40	Maine	3	0.3%
32	South Dakota	7	0.6%		41	New Jersey	2	0.2%
19	Tennessee	27	2.3%		41	Pennsylvania	2	0.2%
1	Texas	130	11.2%		41	Wisconsin	2	0.2%
32	Utah	7	0.6%		44	Connecticut	1	0.1%
45	Vermont	0	0.0%		45	Delaware	0	0.0%
37	Virginia	5	0.4%		45	Maryland	0	0.0%
13	Washington	38	3.3%		45	New Hampshire	0	0.0%
29	West Virginia	10	0.9%		45	North Dakota	0	0.0%
41	Wisconsin	2	0.2%		45	Rhode Island	0	0.0%
25	Wyoming	16	1.4%		45	Vermont	0	0.0%
						District of Columbia	0	0.0%

Source: American Hospital Association (Chicago, IL)
"Hospital Statistics" (2002 edition)
*State and local government-owned hospitals are a subset of community hospitals.

200

Beds in Community Hospitals in 2000

National Total = 823,560 Beds*

ALPHA ORDER					RANK ORDER			
RANK	STATE	BEDS	% of USA		RANK	STATE	BEDS	% of USA
19	Alabama	16,370	2.0%		1	California	72,707	8.8%
50	Alaska	1,417	0.2%		2	New York	66,434	8.1%
28	Arizona	10,864	1.3%		3	Texas	55,877	6.8%
30	Arkansas	9,784	1.2%		4	Florida	51,170	6.2%
1	California	72,707	8.8%		5	Pennsylvania	42,303	5.1%
31	Colorado	9,391	1.1%		6	Illinois	37,310	4.5%
34	Connecticut	7,719	0.9%		7	Ohio	33,849	4.1%
48	Delaware	1,839	0.2%		8	Michigan	26,074	3.2%
4	Florida	51,170	6.2%		9	New Jersey	25,307	3.1%
10	Georgia	23,875	2.9%		10	Georgia	23,875	2.9%
44	Hawaii	3,057	0.4%		11	North Carolina	23,081	2.8%
42	Idaho	3,485	0.4%		12	Tennessee	20,561	2.5%
6	Illinois	37,310	4.5%		13	Missouri	20,140	2.4%
14	Indiana	19,160	2.3%		14	Indiana	19,160	2.3%
23	Iowa	11,811	1.4%		15	Louisiana	17,544	2.1%
29	Kansas	10,821	1.3%		16	Virginia	16,869	2.0%
21	Kentucky	14,827	1.8%		17	Minnesota	16,705	2.0%
15	Louisiana	17,544	2.1%		18	Massachusetts	16,586	2.0%
41	Maine	3,700	0.4%		19	Alabama	16,370	2.0%
25	Maryland	11,192	1.4%		20	Wisconsin	15,329	1.9%
18	Massachusetts	16,586	2.0%		21	Kentucky	14,827	1.8%
8	Michigan	26,074	3.2%		22	Mississippi	13,598	1.7%
17	Minnesota	16,705	2.0%		23	Iowa	11,811	1.4%
22	Mississippi	13,598	1.7%		24	South Carolina	11,520	1.4%
13	Missouri	20,140	2.4%		25	Maryland	11,192	1.4%
38	Montana	4,255	0.5%		26	Washington	11,136	1.4%
32	Nebraska	8,161	1.0%		27	Oklahoma	11,112	1.3%
40	Nevada	3,810	0.5%		28	Arizona	10,864	1.3%
45	New Hampshire	2,865	0.3%		29	Kansas	10,821	1.3%
9	New Jersey	25,307	3.1%		30	Arkansas	9,784	1.2%
43	New Mexico	3,481	0.4%		31	Colorado	9,391	1.1%
2	New York	66,434	8.1%		32	Nebraska	8,161	1.0%
11	North Carolina	23,081	2.8%		33	West Virginia	7,966	1.0%
39	North Dakota	3,865	0.5%		34	Connecticut	7,719	0.9%
7	Ohio	33,849	4.1%		35	Oregon	6,631	0.8%
27	Oklahoma	11,112	1.3%		36	South Dakota	4,339	0.5%
35	Oregon	6,631	0.8%		37	Utah	4,330	0.5%
5	Pennsylvania	42,303	5.1%		38	Montana	4,255	0.5%
46	Rhode Island	2,400	0.3%		39	North Dakota	3,865	0.5%
24	South Carolina	11,520	1.4%		40	Nevada	3,810	0.5%
36	South Dakota	4,339	0.5%		41	Maine	3,700	0.4%
12	Tennessee	20,561	2.5%		42	Idaho	3,485	0.4%
3	Texas	55,877	6.8%		43	New Mexico	3,481	0.4%
37	Utah	4,330	0.5%		44	Hawaii	3,057	0.4%
49	Vermont	1,674	0.2%		45	New Hampshire	2,865	0.3%
16	Virginia	16,869	2.0%		46	Rhode Island	2,400	0.3%
26	Washington	11,136	1.4%		47	Wyoming	1,920	0.2%
33	West Virginia	7,966	1.0%		48	Delaware	1,839	0.2%
20	Wisconsin	15,329	1.9%		49	Vermont	1,674	0.2%
47	Wyoming	1,920	0.2%		50	Alaska	1,417	0.2%
						District of Columbia	3,339	0.4%

Source: American Hospital Association (Chicago, IL)
"Hospital Statistics" (2002 edition)
*All nonfederal short-term general and other special hospitals, whose facilities and services are available to the public. Includes beds in hospital and nursing home units.

Rate of Beds in Community Hospitals in 2000

National Rate = 292 Beds per 100,000 Population*

RANK	STATE	RATE		RANK	STATE	RATE
11	Alabama	368		1	North Dakota	603
40	Alaska	226		2	South Dakota	574
45	Arizona	210		3	Mississippi	477
13	Arkansas	365		3	Nebraska	477
43	California	214		5	Montana	471
42	Colorado	217		6	West Virginia	441
40	Connecticut	226		7	Iowa	403
37	Delaware	234		8	Kansas	402
20	Florida	319		9	Louisiana	392
25	Georgia	290		10	Wyoming	389
35	Hawaii	252		11	Alabama	368
31	Idaho	268		12	Kentucky	366
22	Illinois	300		13	Arkansas	365
21	Indiana	315		14	Tennessee	361
7	Iowa	403		15	Missouri	359
8	Kansas	402		16	New York	350
12	Kentucky	366		17	Pennsylvania	344
9	Louisiana	392		18	Minnesota	339
25	Maine	290		19	Oklahoma	322
44	Maryland	211		20	Florida	319
34	Massachusetts	261		21	Indiana	315
33	Michigan	262		22	Illinois	300
18	Minnesota	339		22	New Jersey	300
3	Mississippi	477		24	Ohio	298
15	Missouri	359		25	Georgia	290
5	Montana	471		25	Maine	290
3	Nebraska	477		27	North Carolina	286
49	Nevada	189		27	South Carolina	286
38	New Hampshire	231		29	Wisconsin	285
22	New Jersey	300		30	Vermont	275
48	New Mexico	191		31	Idaho	268
16	New York	350		32	Texas	267
27	North Carolina	286		33	Michigan	262
1	North Dakota	603		34	Massachusetts	261
24	Ohio	298		35	Hawaii	252
19	Oklahoma	322		36	Virginia	237
46	Oregon	193		37	Delaware	234
17	Pennsylvania	344		38	New Hampshire	231
39	Rhode Island	229		39	Rhode Island	229
27	South Carolina	286		40	Alaska	226
2	South Dakota	574		40	Connecticut	226
14	Tennessee	361		42	Colorado	217
32	Texas	267		43	California	214
46	Utah	193		44	Maryland	211
30	Vermont	275		45	Arizona	210
36	Virginia	237		46	Oregon	193
50	Washington	188		46	Utah	193
6	West Virginia	441		48	New Mexico	191
29	Wisconsin	285		49	Nevada	189
10	Wyoming	389		50	Washington	188
					District of Columbia	585

Source: Morgan Quitno Press using data from American Hospital Association (Chicago, IL)
"Hospital Statistics" (2002 edition)
*All nonfederal short-term general and other special hospitals, whose facilities and services are available to the public. Includes beds in hospital and nursing home units.

Average Number of Beds per Community Hospital in 2000

National Average = 168 Beds per Community Hospital*

ALPHA ORDER

RANK	STATE	BEDS
23	Alabama	152
50	Alaska	79
17	Arizona	178
35	Arkansas	118
14	California	187
30	Colorado	136
6	Connecticut	221
1	Delaware	368
4	Florida	253
22	Georgia	158
24	Hawaii	146
47	Idaho	83
13	Illinois	190
18	Indiana	176
37	Iowa	103
46	Kansas	84
27	Kentucky	141
25	Louisiana	143
41	Maine	100
5	Maryland	228
9	Massachusetts	207
16	Michigan	179
33	Minnesota	124
25	Mississippi	143
21	Missouri	169
48	Montana	82
43	Nebraska	96
19	Nevada	173
40	New Hampshire	102
2	New Jersey	316
42	New Mexico	99
3	New York	309
10	North Carolina	204
44	North Dakota	92
8	Ohio	208
37	Oklahoma	103
36	Oregon	112
10	Pennsylvania	204
7	Rhode Island	218
15	South Carolina	183
45	South Dakota	90
20	Tennessee	170
29	Texas	139
37	Utah	103
34	Vermont	120
12	Virginia	192
31	Washington	133
28	West Virginia	140
32	Wisconsin	130
49	Wyoming	80

RANK ORDER

RANK	STATE	BEDS
1	Delaware	368
2	New Jersey	316
3	New York	309
4	Florida	253
5	Maryland	228
6	Connecticut	221
7	Rhode Island	218
8	Ohio	208
9	Massachusetts	207
10	North Carolina	204
10	Pennsylvania	204
12	Virginia	192
13	Illinois	190
14	California	187
15	South Carolina	183
16	Michigan	179
17	Arizona	178
18	Indiana	176
19	Nevada	173
20	Tennessee	170
21	Missouri	169
22	Georgia	158
23	Alabama	152
24	Hawaii	146
25	Louisiana	143
25	Mississippi	143
27	Kentucky	141
28	West Virginia	140
29	Texas	139
30	Colorado	136
31	Washington	133
32	Wisconsin	130
33	Minnesota	124
34	Vermont	120
35	Arkansas	118
36	Oregon	112
37	Iowa	103
37	Oklahoma	103
37	Utah	103
40	New Hampshire	102
41	Maine	100
42	New Mexico	99
43	Nebraska	96
44	North Dakota	92
45	South Dakota	90
46	Kansas	84
47	Idaho	83
48	Montana	82
49	Wyoming	80
50	Alaska	79

District of Columbia   304

Source: Morgan Quitno Press using data from American Hospital Association (Chicago, IL)
        "Hospital Statistics" (2002 edition)
*All nonfederal short-term general and other special hospitals, whose facilities and services are available to the public. Includes beds in hospital and nursing home units.

Admissions to Community Hospitals in 2000

National Total = 33,089,467 Admissions*

ALPHA ORDER

RANK	STATE	ADMISSIONS	% of USA
17	Alabama	680,395	2.1%
50	Alaska	46,887	0.1%
23	Arizona	538,704	1.6%
29	Arkansas	368,287	1.1%
1	California	3,315,316	10.0%
28	Colorado	397,026	1.2%
31	Connecticut	348,780	1.1%
47	Delaware	83,318	0.3%
4	Florida	2,119,052	6.4%
11	Georgia	862,797	2.6%
43	Hawaii	99,937	0.3%
40	Idaho	123,187	0.4%
6	Illinois	1,530,800	4.6%
16	Indiana	699,511	2.1%
30	Iowa	359,682	1.1%
33	Kansas	310,256	0.9%
20	Kentucky	581,620	1.8%
18	Louisiana	654,323	2.0%
39	Maine	147,236	0.4%
19	Maryland	586,809	1.8%
13	Massachusetts	740,286	2.2%
8	Michigan	1,106,045	3.3%
21	Minnesota	570,672	1.7%
27	Mississippi	424,772	1.3%
12	Missouri	773,261	2.3%
44	Montana	99,273	0.3%
35	Nebraska	209,498	0.6%
36	Nevada	199,455	0.6%
42	New Hampshire	111,227	0.3%
9	New Jersey	1,073,619	3.2%
38	New Mexico	173,575	0.5%
2	New York	2,416,112	7.3%
10	North Carolina	970,742	2.9%
46	North Dakota	89,219	0.3%
7	Ohio	1,404,467	4.2%
26	Oklahoma	428,927	1.3%
32	Oregon	329,932	1.0%
5	Pennsylvania	1,796,081	5.4%
41	Rhode Island	119,070	0.4%
25	South Carolina	495,410	1.5%
45	South Dakota	98,508	0.3%
14	Tennessee	737,313	2.2%
3	Texas	2,366,652	7.2%
37	Utah	194,047	0.6%
48	Vermont	52,413	0.2%
15	Virginia	726,772	2.2%
24	Washington	504,836	1.5%
34	West Virginia	288,095	0.9%
22	Wisconsin	558,357	1.7%
49	Wyoming	47,852	0.1%

RANK ORDER

RANK	STATE	ADMISSIONS	% of USA
1	California	3,315,316	10.0%
2	New York	2,416,112	7.3%
3	Texas	2,366,652	7.2%
4	Florida	2,119,052	6.4%
5	Pennsylvania	1,796,081	5.4%
6	Illinois	1,530,800	4.6%
7	Ohio	1,404,467	4.2%
8	Michigan	1,106,045	3.3%
9	New Jersey	1,073,619	3.2%
10	North Carolina	970,742	2.9%
11	Georgia	862,797	2.6%
12	Missouri	773,261	2.3%
13	Massachusetts	740,286	2.2%
14	Tennessee	737,313	2.2%
15	Virginia	726,772	2.2%
16	Indiana	699,511	2.1%
17	Alabama	680,395	2.1%
18	Louisiana	654,323	2.0%
19	Maryland	586,809	1.8%
20	Kentucky	581,620	1.8%
21	Minnesota	570,672	1.7%
22	Wisconsin	558,357	1.7%
23	Arizona	538,704	1.6%
24	Washington	504,836	1.5%
25	South Carolina	495,410	1.5%
26	Oklahoma	428,927	1.3%
27	Mississippi	424,772	1.3%
28	Colorado	397,026	1.2%
29	Arkansas	368,287	1.1%
30	Iowa	359,682	1.1%
31	Connecticut	348,780	1.1%
32	Oregon	329,932	1.0%
33	Kansas	310,256	0.9%
34	West Virginia	288,095	0.9%
35	Nebraska	209,498	0.6%
36	Nevada	199,455	0.6%
37	Utah	194,047	0.6%
38	New Mexico	173,575	0.5%
39	Maine	147,236	0.4%
40	Idaho	123,187	0.4%
41	Rhode Island	119,070	0.4%
42	New Hampshire	111,227	0.3%
43	Hawaii	99,937	0.3%
44	Montana	99,273	0.3%
45	South Dakota	98,508	0.3%
46	North Dakota	89,219	0.3%
47	Delaware	83,318	0.3%
48	Vermont	52,413	0.2%
49	Wyoming	47,852	0.1%
50	Alaska	46,887	0.1%
	District of Columbia	129,056	0.4%

Source: American Hospital Association (Chicago, IL)
    "Hospital Statistics" (2002 edition)
*Admissions to all nonfederal short-term general and other special hospitals, whose facilities and services are available to the public. Includes admissions to hospital and nursing home units.

Inpatient Days in Community Hospitals in 2000

National Total = 192,420,368 Inpatient Days*

ALPHA ORDER

RANK	STATE	DAYS	% of USA
18	Alabama	3,585,804	1.9%
50	Alaska	293,707	0.2%
25	Arizona	2,501,003	1.3%
30	Arkansas	2,092,183	1.1%
2	California	17,481,600	9.1%
32	Colorado	1,986,526	1.0%
29	Connecticut	2,114,362	1.1%
47	Delaware	505,422	0.3%
4	Florida	11,345,469	5.9%
11	Georgia	5,479,389	2.8%
41	Hawaii	847,352	0.4%
44	Idaho	669,186	0.3%
6	Illinois	8,189,818	4.3%
17	Indiana	3,943,695	2.0%
26	Iowa	2,493,185	1.3%
31	Kansas	2,081,932	1.1%
20	Kentucky	3,333,314	1.7%
19	Louisiana	3,569,621	1.9%
40	Maine	867,352	0.5%
22	Maryland	2,993,513	1.6%
12	Massachusetts	4,289,840	2.2%
9	Michigan	6,176,230	3.2%
16	Minnesota	4,089,075	2.1%
23	Mississippi	2,929,248	1.5%
13	Missouri	4,269,800	2.2%
36	Montana	1,045,460	0.5%
34	Nebraska	1,760,490	0.9%
38	Nevada	984,845	0.5%
46	New Hampshire	611,919	0.3%
8	New Jersey	6,340,657	3.3%
43	New Mexico	731,708	0.4%
1	New York	19,074,063	9.9%
10	North Carolina	5,859,282	3.0%
42	North Dakota	841,256	0.4%
7	Ohio	7,556,261	3.9%
28	Oklahoma	2,280,050	1.2%
35	Oregon	1,435,545	0.7%
5	Pennsylvania	10,558,152	5.5%
45	Rhode Island	625,939	0.3%
24	South Carolina	2,916,386	1.5%
37	South Dakota	1,035,027	0.5%
14	Tennessee	4,225,812	2.2%
3	Texas	12,122,361	6.3%
39	Utah	886,846	0.5%
48	Vermont	407,915	0.2%
15	Virginia	4,161,981	2.2%
27	Washington	2,432,089	1.3%
33	West Virginia	1,772,580	0.9%
21	Wisconsin	3,331,095	1.7%
49	Wyoming	392,856	0.2%

RANK ORDER

RANK	STATE	DAYS	% of USA
1	New York	19,074,063	9.9%
2	California	17,481,600	9.1%
3	Texas	12,122,361	6.3%
4	Florida	11,345,469	5.9%
5	Pennsylvania	10,558,152	5.5%
6	Illinois	8,189,818	4.3%
7	Ohio	7,556,261	3.9%
8	New Jersey	6,340,657	3.3%
9	Michigan	6,176,230	3.2%
10	North Carolina	5,859,282	3.0%
11	Georgia	5,479,389	2.8%
12	Massachusetts	4,289,840	2.2%
13	Missouri	4,269,800	2.2%
14	Tennessee	4,225,812	2.2%
15	Virginia	4,161,981	2.2%
16	Minnesota	4,089,075	2.1%
17	Indiana	3,943,695	2.0%
18	Alabama	3,585,804	1.9%
19	Louisiana	3,569,621	1.9%
20	Kentucky	3,333,314	1.7%
21	Wisconsin	3,331,095	1.7%
22	Maryland	2,993,513	1.6%
23	Mississippi	2,929,248	1.5%
24	South Carolina	2,916,386	1.5%
25	Arizona	2,501,003	1.3%
26	Iowa	2,493,185	1.3%
27	Washington	2,432,089	1.3%
28	Oklahoma	2,280,050	1.2%
29	Connecticut	2,114,362	1.1%
30	Arkansas	2,092,183	1.1%
31	Kansas	2,081,932	1.1%
32	Colorado	1,986,526	1.0%
33	West Virginia	1,772,580	0.9%
34	Nebraska	1,760,490	0.9%
35	Oregon	1,435,545	0.7%
36	Montana	1,045,460	0.5%
37	South Dakota	1,035,027	0.5%
38	Nevada	984,845	0.5%
39	Utah	886,846	0.5%
40	Maine	867,352	0.5%
41	Hawaii	847,352	0.4%
42	North Dakota	841,256	0.4%
43	New Mexico	731,708	0.4%
44	Idaho	669,186	0.3%
45	Rhode Island	625,939	0.3%
46	New Hampshire	611,919	0.3%
47	Delaware	505,422	0.3%
48	Vermont	407,915	0.2%
49	Wyoming	392,856	0.2%
50	Alaska	293,707	0.2%
	District of Columbia	901,167	0.5%

Source: American Hospital Association (Chicago, IL)
  "Hospital Statistics" (2002 edition)
*Inpatient days in all nonfederal short-term general and other special hospitals, whose facilities and services are available to the public. Includes days in hospital and nursing home units.

Average Daily Census in Community Hospitals in 2000

National Average = 525,739 Inpatients*

ALPHA ORDER				RANK ORDER		
RANK	STATE	INPATIENTS		RANK	STATE	INPATIENTS
18	Alabama	9,797		1	New York	52,115
50	Alaska	802		2	California	47,764
25	Arizona	6,833		3	Texas	33,121
30	Arkansas	5,716		4	Florida	30,999
2	California	47,764		5	Pennsylvania	28,847
32	Colorado	5,428		6	Illinois	22,377
29	Connecticut	5,777		7	Ohio	20,646
47	Delaware	1,381		8	New Jersey	17,324
4	Florida	30,999		9	Michigan	16,875
11	Georgia	14,971		10	North Carolina	16,009
41	Hawaii	2,315		11	Georgia	14,971
44	Idaho	1,828		12	Massachusetts	11,721
6	Illinois	22,377		13	Missouri	11,666
17	Indiana	10,775		14	Tennessee	11,546
26	Iowa	6,812		15	Virginia	11,372
31	Kansas	5,688		16	Minnesota	11,172
20	Kentucky	9,107		17	Indiana	10,775
19	Louisiana	9,753		18	Alabama	9,797
40	Maine	2,370		19	Louisiana	9,753
22	Maryland	8,179		20	Kentucky	9,107
12	Massachusetts	11,721		21	Wisconsin	9,101
9	Michigan	16,875		22	Maryland	8,179
16	Minnesota	11,172		23	Mississippi	8,003
23	Mississippi	8,003		24	South Carolina	7,968
13	Missouri	11,666		25	Arizona	6,833
36	Montana	2,856		26	Iowa	6,812
34	Nebraska	4,810		27	Washington	6,645
38	Nevada	2,691		28	Oklahoma	6,230
46	New Hampshire	1,672		29	Connecticut	5,777
8	New Jersey	17,324		30	Arkansas	5,716
43	New Mexico	1,999		31	Kansas	5,688
1	New York	52,115		32	Colorado	5,428
10	North Carolina	16,009		33	West Virginia	4,843
42	North Dakota	2,299		34	Nebraska	4,810
7	Ohio	20,646		35	Oregon	3,922
28	Oklahoma	6,230		36	Montana	2,856
35	Oregon	3,922		37	South Dakota	2,828
5	Pennsylvania	28,847		38	Nevada	2,691
45	Rhode Island	1,710		39	Utah	2,423
24	South Carolina	7,968		40	Maine	2,370
37	South Dakota	2,828		41	Hawaii	2,315
14	Tennessee	11,546		42	North Dakota	2,299
3	Texas	33,121		43	New Mexico	1,999
39	Utah	2,423		44	Idaho	1,828
48	Vermont	1,115		45	Rhode Island	1,710
15	Virginia	11,372		46	New Hampshire	1,672
27	Washington	6,645		47	Delaware	1,381
33	West Virginia	4,843		48	Vermont	1,115
21	Wisconsin	9,101		49	Wyoming	1,073
49	Wyoming	1,073		50	Alaska	802
					District of Columbia	2,462

Source: Morgan Quitno Press using data from American Hospital Association (Chicago, IL)
"Hospital Statistics" (2002 edition)
*Average total of inpatients receiving care in all nonfederal short-term general and other special hospitals, whose facilities and services are available to the public. Excludes newborns.

Average Stay in Community Hospitals in 2000

National Average = 5.8 Days*

ALPHA ORDER

RANK	STATE	DAYS
38	Alabama	5.3
14	Alaska	6.3
47	Arizona	4.6
25	Arkansas	5.7
38	California	5.3
44	Colorado	5.0
16	Connecticut	6.1
16	Delaware	6.1
34	Florida	5.4
13	Georgia	6.4
4	Hawaii	8.5
34	Idaho	5.4
34	Illinois	5.4
29	Indiana	5.6
10	Iowa	6.9
12	Kansas	6.7
25	Kentucky	5.7
31	Louisiana	5.5
20	Maine	5.9
42	Maryland	5.1
24	Massachusetts	5.8
29	Michigan	5.6
9	Minnesota	7.2
10	Mississippi	6.9
31	Missouri	5.5
1	Montana	10.5
5	Nebraska	8.4
45	Nevada	4.9
31	New Hampshire	5.5
20	New Jersey	5.9
50	New Mexico	4.2
7	New York	7.9
18	North Carolina	6.0
3	North Dakota	9.4
34	Ohio	5.4
38	Oklahoma	5.3
49	Oregon	4.4
20	Pennsylvania	5.9
38	Rhode Island	5.3
20	South Carolina	5.9
1	South Dakota	10.5
25	Tennessee	5.7
42	Texas	5.1
47	Utah	4.6
8	Vermont	7.8
25	Virginia	5.7
46	Washington	4.8
15	West Virginia	6.2
18	Wisconsin	6.0
6	Wyoming	8.2

RANK ORDER

RANK	STATE	DAYS
1	Montana	10.5
1	South Dakota	10.5
3	North Dakota	9.4
4	Hawaii	8.5
5	Nebraska	8.4
6	Wyoming	8.2
7	New York	7.9
8	Vermont	7.8
9	Minnesota	7.2
10	Iowa	6.9
10	Mississippi	6.9
12	Kansas	6.7
13	Georgia	6.4
14	Alaska	6.3
15	West Virginia	6.2
16	Connecticut	6.1
16	Delaware	6.1
18	North Carolina	6.0
18	Wisconsin	6.0
20	Maine	5.9
20	New Jersey	5.9
20	Pennsylvania	5.9
20	South Carolina	5.9
24	Massachusetts	5.8
25	Arkansas	5.7
25	Kentucky	5.7
25	Tennessee	5.7
25	Virginia	5.7
29	Indiana	5.6
29	Michigan	5.6
31	Louisiana	5.5
31	Missouri	5.5
31	New Hampshire	5.5
34	Florida	5.4
34	Idaho	5.4
34	Illinois	5.4
34	Ohio	5.4
38	Alabama	5.3
38	California	5.3
38	Oklahoma	5.3
38	Rhode Island	5.3
42	Maryland	5.1
42	Texas	5.1
44	Colorado	5.0
45	Nevada	4.9
46	Washington	4.8
47	Arizona	4.6
47	Utah	4.6
49	Oregon	4.4
50	New Mexico	4.2
	District of Columbia	7.0

Source: American Hospital Association (Chicago, IL)
    "Hospital Statistics" (2002 edition)
*All nonfederal short-term general and other special hospitals, whose facilities and services are available to the public.

Occupancy Rate in Community Hospitals in 2000

National Rate = 63.8% of Community Hospital Beds Occupied*

ALPHA ORDER				RANK ORDER		
RANK	STATE	PERCENT		RANK	STATE	PERCENT
28	Alabama	59.8		1	New York	78.4
42	Alaska	56.6		2	Hawaii	75.7
21	Arizona	62.9		3	Delaware	75.1
36	Arkansas	58.4		4	Connecticut	74.8
17	California	65.7		5	Maryland	73.1
39	Colorado	57.8		6	Rhode Island	71.3
4	Connecticut	74.8		7	Massachusetts	70.7
3	Delaware	75.1		8	Nevada	70.6
26	Florida	60.6		9	North Carolina	69.4
22	Georgia	62.7		10	South Carolina	69.2
2	Hawaii	75.7		11	New Jersey	68.5
50	Idaho	52.5		12	Pennsylvania	68.2
27	Illinois	60.0		13	Virginia	67.4
43	Indiana	56.2		14	Montana	67.1
40	Iowa	57.7		15	Minnesota	66.9
49	Kansas	52.6		16	Vermont	66.6
23	Kentucky	61.4		17	California	65.7
48	Louisiana	55.6		18	South Dakota	65.2
20	Maine	64.1		19	Michigan	64.7
5	Maryland	73.1		20	Maine	64.1
7	Massachusetts	70.7		21	Arizona	62.9
19	Michigan	64.7		22	Georgia	62.7
15	Minnesota	66.9		23	Kentucky	61.4
34	Mississippi	58.9		24	Ohio	61.0
38	Missouri	57.9		25	West Virginia	60.8
14	Montana	67.1		26	Florida	60.6
34	Nebraska	58.9		27	Illinois	60.0
8	Nevada	70.6		28	Alabama	59.8
36	New Hampshire	58.4		29	Washington	59.7
11	New Jersey	68.5		30	North Dakota	59.5
41	New Mexico	57.4		31	Wisconsin	59.4
1	New York	78.4		32	Texas	59.3
9	North Carolina	69.4		33	Oregon	59.1
30	North Dakota	59.5		34	Mississippi	58.9
24	Ohio	61.0		34	Nebraska	58.9
45	Oklahoma	56.1		36	Arkansas	58.4
33	Oregon	59.1		36	New Hampshire	58.4
12	Pennsylvania	68.2		38	Missouri	57.9
6	Rhode Island	71.3		39	Colorado	57.8
10	South Carolina	69.2		40	Iowa	57.7
18	South Dakota	65.2		41	New Mexico	57.4
43	Tennessee	56.2		42	Alaska	56.6
32	Texas	59.3		43	Indiana	56.2
46	Utah	56.0		43	Tennessee	56.2
16	Vermont	66.6		45	Oklahoma	56.1
13	Virginia	67.4		46	Utah	56.0
29	Washington	59.7		47	Wyoming	55.9
25	West Virginia	60.8		48	Louisiana	55.6
31	Wisconsin	59.4		49	Kansas	52.6
47	Wyoming	55.9		50	Idaho	52.5

	District of Columbia	73.7

Source: Morgan Quitno Press using data from American Hospital Association (Chicago, IL)
"Hospital Statistics" (2002 edition)
*Average daily census compared to number of community hospital beds.

Outpatient Visits to Community Hospitals in 2000

National Total = 521,404,976 Visits*

<table>
<tr><td colspan="4">ALPHA ORDER</td><td colspan="4">RANK ORDER</td></tr>
<tr><th>RANK</th><th>STATE</th><th>VISITS</th><th>% of USA</th><th>RANK</th><th>STATE</th><th>VISITS</th><th>% of USA</th></tr>
<tr><td>22</td><td>Alabama</td><td>7,964,213</td><td>1.5%</td><td>1</td><td>New York</td><td>46,371,854</td><td>8.9%</td></tr>
<tr><td>48</td><td>Alaska</td><td>1,271,107</td><td>0.2%</td><td>2</td><td>California</td><td>44,944,427</td><td>8.6%</td></tr>
<tr><td>29</td><td>Arizona</td><td>5,300,106</td><td>1.0%</td><td>3</td><td>Pennsylvania</td><td>31,849,176</td><td>6.1%</td></tr>
<tr><td>34</td><td>Arkansas</td><td>4,407,079</td><td>0.8%</td><td>4</td><td>Texas</td><td>29,393,476</td><td>5.6%</td></tr>
<tr><td>2</td><td>California</td><td>44,944,427</td><td>8.6%</td><td>5</td><td>Ohio</td><td>26,857,304</td><td>5.2%</td></tr>
<tr><td>27</td><td>Colorado</td><td>6,712,721</td><td>1.3%</td><td>6</td><td>Illinois</td><td>25,099,563</td><td>4.8%</td></tr>
<tr><td>26</td><td>Connecticut</td><td>6,733,522</td><td>1.3%</td><td>7</td><td>Michigan</td><td>24,861,291</td><td>4.8%</td></tr>
<tr><td>47</td><td>Delaware</td><td>1,461,888</td><td>0.3%</td><td>8</td><td>Florida</td><td>21,793,588</td><td>4.2%</td></tr>
<tr><td>8</td><td>Florida</td><td>21,793,588</td><td>4.2%</td><td>9</td><td>Massachusetts</td><td>16,710,353</td><td>3.2%</td></tr>
<tr><td>14</td><td>Georgia</td><td>11,241,924</td><td>2.2%</td><td>10</td><td>New Jersey</td><td>16,307,273</td><td>3.1%</td></tr>
<tr><td>41</td><td>Hawaii</td><td>2,466,004</td><td>0.5%</td><td>11</td><td>Missouri</td><td>14,806,777</td><td>2.8%</td></tr>
<tr><td>43</td><td>Idaho</td><td>2,157,402</td><td>0.4%</td><td>12</td><td>Indiana</td><td>14,133,994</td><td>2.7%</td></tr>
<tr><td>6</td><td>Illinois</td><td>25,099,563</td><td>4.8%</td><td>13</td><td>North Carolina</td><td>12,378,653</td><td>2.4%</td></tr>
<tr><td>12</td><td>Indiana</td><td>14,133,994</td><td>2.7%</td><td>14</td><td>Georgia</td><td>11,241,924</td><td>2.2%</td></tr>
<tr><td>20</td><td>Iowa</td><td>9,156,991</td><td>1.8%</td><td>15</td><td>Wisconsin</td><td>10,854,252</td><td>2.1%</td></tr>
<tr><td>30</td><td>Kansas</td><td>5,255,273</td><td>1.0%</td><td>16</td><td>Tennessee</td><td>10,275,264</td><td>2.0%</td></tr>
<tr><td>21</td><td>Kentucky</td><td>8,696,720</td><td>1.7%</td><td>17</td><td>Louisiana</td><td>10,026,057</td><td>1.9%</td></tr>
<tr><td>17</td><td>Louisiana</td><td>10,026,057</td><td>1.9%</td><td>18</td><td>Washington</td><td>9,589,178</td><td>1.8%</td></tr>
<tr><td>37</td><td>Maine</td><td>3,247,494</td><td>0.6%</td><td>19</td><td>Virginia</td><td>9,543,474</td><td>1.8%</td></tr>
<tr><td>28</td><td>Maryland</td><td>6,017,622</td><td>1.2%</td><td>20</td><td>Iowa</td><td>9,156,991</td><td>1.8%</td></tr>
<tr><td>9</td><td>Massachusetts</td><td>16,710,353</td><td>3.2%</td><td>21</td><td>Kentucky</td><td>8,696,720</td><td>1.7%</td></tr>
<tr><td>7</td><td>Michigan</td><td>24,861,291</td><td>4.8%</td><td>22</td><td>Alabama</td><td>7,964,213</td><td>1.5%</td></tr>
<tr><td>24</td><td>Minnesota</td><td>7,335,612</td><td>1.4%</td><td>23</td><td>South Carolina</td><td>7,779,033</td><td>1.5%</td></tr>
<tr><td>35</td><td>Mississippi</td><td>3,707,797</td><td>0.7%</td><td>24</td><td>Minnesota</td><td>7,335,612</td><td>1.4%</td></tr>
<tr><td>11</td><td>Missouri</td><td>14,806,777</td><td>2.8%</td><td>25</td><td>Oregon</td><td>7,272,770</td><td>1.4%</td></tr>
<tr><td>40</td><td>Montana</td><td>2,648,576</td><td>0.5%</td><td>26</td><td>Connecticut</td><td>6,733,522</td><td>1.3%</td></tr>
<tr><td>36</td><td>Nebraska</td><td>3,405,399</td><td>0.7%</td><td>27</td><td>Colorado</td><td>6,712,721</td><td>1.3%</td></tr>
<tr><td>42</td><td>Nevada</td><td>2,192,118</td><td>0.4%</td><td>28</td><td>Maryland</td><td>6,017,622</td><td>1.2%</td></tr>
<tr><td>39</td><td>New Hampshire</td><td>2,763,353</td><td>0.5%</td><td>29</td><td>Arizona</td><td>5,300,106</td><td>1.0%</td></tr>
<tr><td>10</td><td>New Jersey</td><td>16,307,273</td><td>3.1%</td><td>30</td><td>Kansas</td><td>5,255,273</td><td>1.0%</td></tr>
<tr><td>38</td><td>New Mexico</td><td>3,100,634</td><td>0.6%</td><td>31</td><td>West Virginia</td><td>5,195,538</td><td>1.0%</td></tr>
<tr><td>1</td><td>New York</td><td>46,371,854</td><td>8.9%</td><td>32</td><td>Oklahoma</td><td>4,701,956</td><td>0.9%</td></tr>
<tr><td>13</td><td>North Carolina</td><td>12,378,653</td><td>2.4%</td><td>33</td><td>Utah</td><td>4,468,988</td><td>0.9%</td></tr>
<tr><td>46</td><td>North Dakota</td><td>1,694,969</td><td>0.3%</td><td>34</td><td>Arkansas</td><td>4,407,079</td><td>0.8%</td></tr>
<tr><td>5</td><td>Ohio</td><td>26,857,304</td><td>5.2%</td><td>35</td><td>Mississippi</td><td>3,707,797</td><td>0.7%</td></tr>
<tr><td>32</td><td>Oklahoma</td><td>4,701,956</td><td>0.9%</td><td>36</td><td>Nebraska</td><td>3,405,399</td><td>0.7%</td></tr>
<tr><td>25</td><td>Oregon</td><td>7,272,770</td><td>1.4%</td><td>37</td><td>Maine</td><td>3,247,494</td><td>0.6%</td></tr>
<tr><td>3</td><td>Pennsylvania</td><td>31,849,176</td><td>6.1%</td><td>38</td><td>New Mexico</td><td>3,100,634</td><td>0.6%</td></tr>
<tr><td>44</td><td>Rhode Island</td><td>2,080,945</td><td>0.4%</td><td>39</td><td>New Hampshire</td><td>2,763,353</td><td>0.5%</td></tr>
<tr><td>23</td><td>South Carolina</td><td>7,779,033</td><td>1.5%</td><td>40</td><td>Montana</td><td>2,648,576</td><td>0.5%</td></tr>
<tr><td>45</td><td>South Dakota</td><td>1,718,201</td><td>0.3%</td><td>41</td><td>Hawaii</td><td>2,466,004</td><td>0.5%</td></tr>
<tr><td>16</td><td>Tennessee</td><td>10,275,264</td><td>2.0%</td><td>42</td><td>Nevada</td><td>2,192,118</td><td>0.4%</td></tr>
<tr><td>4</td><td>Texas</td><td>29,393,476</td><td>5.6%</td><td>43</td><td>Idaho</td><td>2,157,402</td><td>0.4%</td></tr>
<tr><td>33</td><td>Utah</td><td>4,468,988</td><td>0.9%</td><td>44</td><td>Rhode Island</td><td>2,080,945</td><td>0.4%</td></tr>
<tr><td>49</td><td>Vermont</td><td>1,243,052</td><td>0.2%</td><td>45</td><td>South Dakota</td><td>1,718,201</td><td>0.3%</td></tr>
<tr><td>19</td><td>Virginia</td><td>9,543,474</td><td>1.8%</td><td>46</td><td>North Dakota</td><td>1,694,969</td><td>0.3%</td></tr>
<tr><td>18</td><td>Washington</td><td>9,589,178</td><td>1.8%</td><td>47</td><td>Delaware</td><td>1,461,888</td><td>0.3%</td></tr>
<tr><td>31</td><td>West Virginia</td><td>5,195,538</td><td>1.0%</td><td>48</td><td>Alaska</td><td>1,271,107</td><td>0.2%</td></tr>
<tr><td>15</td><td>Wisconsin</td><td>10,854,252</td><td>2.1%</td><td>49</td><td>Vermont</td><td>1,243,052</td><td>0.2%</td></tr>
<tr><td>50</td><td>Wyoming</td><td>878,608</td><td>0.2%</td><td>50</td><td>Wyoming</td><td>878,608</td><td>0.2%</td></tr>
<tr><td></td><td></td><td></td><td></td><td></td><td>District of Columbia</td><td>1,331,407</td><td>0.3%</td></tr>
</table>

Source: American Hospital Association (Chicago, IL)
    "Hospital Statistics" (2002 edition)
*All nonfederal short-term general and other special hospitals, whose facilities and services are available to the public. Includes emergency and other visits.

Emergency Outpatient Visits to Community Hospitals in 2000

National Total = 103,144,030 Visits*

ALPHA ORDER

RANK	STATE	VISITS	% of USA
18	Alabama	2,070,702	2.0%
50	Alaska	187,226	0.2%
24	Arizona	1,520,393	1.5%
29	Arkansas	1,170,079	1.1%
1	California	9,704,390	9.4%
27	Colorado	1,377,130	1.3%
28	Connecticut	1,323,999	1.3%
43	Delaware	286,231	0.3%
4	Florida	6,041,546	5.9%
9	Georgia	3,128,275	3.0%
45	Hawaii	253,452	0.2%
42	Idaho	409,030	0.4%
7	Illinois	4,497,815	4.4%
16	Indiana	2,187,447	2.1%
31	Iowa	1,050,606	1.0%
34	Kansas	889,390	0.9%
19	Kentucky	1,953,727	1.9%
17	Louisiana	2,143,846	2.1%
36	Maine	673,853	0.7%
23	Maryland	1,765,739	1.7%
12	Massachusetts	2,715,812	2.6%
8	Michigan	3,703,509	3.6%
26	Minnesota	1,454,970	1.4%
25	Mississippi	1,478,883	1.4%
15	Missouri	2,326,906	2.3%
44	Montana	270,905	0.3%
40	Nebraska	499,960	0.5%
37	Nevada	573,220	0.6%
39	New Hampshire	526,103	0.5%
11	New Jersey	2,853,236	2.8%
38	New Mexico	532,526	0.5%
3	New York	7,275,122	7.1%
10	North Carolina	2,983,548	2.9%
46	North Dakota	248,562	0.2%
5	Ohio	5,133,276	5.0%
30	Oklahoma	1,134,337	1.1%
32	Oregon	1,008,428	1.0%
6	Pennsylvania	4,727,149	4.6%
41	Rhode Island	440,098	0.4%
21	South Carolina	1,831,462	1.8%
49	South Dakota	196,054	0.2%
13	Tennessee	2,601,659	2.5%
2	Texas	7,375,580	7.2%
35	Utah	697,703	0.7%
47	Vermont	236,337	0.2%
14	Virginia	2,476,006	2.4%
20	Washington	1,932,238	1.9%
33	West Virginia	1,007,028	1.0%
22	Wisconsin	1,785,771	1.7%
48	Wyoming	198,691	0.2%

RANK ORDER

RANK	STATE	VISITS	% of USA
1	California	9,704,390	9.4%
2	Texas	7,375,580	7.2%
3	New York	7,275,122	7.1%
4	Florida	6,041,546	5.9%
5	Ohio	5,133,276	5.0%
6	Pennsylvania	4,727,149	4.6%
7	Illinois	4,497,815	4.4%
8	Michigan	3,703,509	3.6%
9	Georgia	3,128,275	3.0%
10	North Carolina	2,983,548	2.9%
11	New Jersey	2,853,236	2.8%
12	Massachusetts	2,715,812	2.6%
13	Tennessee	2,601,659	2.5%
14	Virginia	2,476,006	2.4%
15	Missouri	2,326,906	2.3%
16	Indiana	2,187,447	2.1%
17	Louisiana	2,143,846	2.1%
18	Alabama	2,070,702	2.0%
19	Kentucky	1,953,727	1.9%
20	Washington	1,932,238	1.9%
21	South Carolina	1,831,462	1.8%
22	Wisconsin	1,785,771	1.7%
23	Maryland	1,765,739	1.7%
24	Arizona	1,520,393	1.5%
25	Mississippi	1,478,883	1.4%
26	Minnesota	1,454,970	1.4%
27	Colorado	1,377,130	1.3%
28	Connecticut	1,323,999	1.3%
29	Arkansas	1,170,079	1.1%
30	Oklahoma	1,134,337	1.1%
31	Iowa	1,050,606	1.0%
32	Oregon	1,008,428	1.0%
33	West Virginia	1,007,028	1.0%
34	Kansas	889,390	0.9%
35	Utah	697,703	0.7%
36	Maine	673,853	0.7%
37	Nevada	573,220	0.6%
38	New Mexico	532,526	0.5%
39	New Hampshire	526,103	0.5%
40	Nebraska	499,960	0.5%
41	Rhode Island	440,098	0.4%
42	Idaho	409,030	0.4%
43	Delaware	286,231	0.3%
44	Montana	270,905	0.3%
45	Hawaii	253,452	0.2%
46	North Dakota	248,562	0.2%
47	Vermont	236,337	0.2%
48	Wyoming	198,691	0.2%
49	South Dakota	196,054	0.2%
50	Alaska	187,226	0.2%
	District of Columbia	284,075	0.3%

Source: American Hospital Association (Chicago, IL)
    "Hospital Statistics" (2002 edition)
All nonfederal short-term general and other special hospitals, whose facilities and services are available to the public.

Surgical Operations in Community Hospitals in 2000

National Total = 26,112,710 Surgical Operations*

ALPHA ORDER					RANK ORDER			
RANK	STATE	OPERATIONS	% of USA		RANK	STATE	OPERATIONS	% of USA
20	Alabama	486,164	1.9%		1	California	2,216,132	8.5%
48	Alaska	49,874	0.2%		2	New York	1,985,866	7.6%
26	Arizona	373,080	1.4%		3	Texas	1,760,843	6.7%
32	Arkansas	265,891	1.0%		4	Pennsylvania	1,532,805	5.9%
1	California	2,216,132	8.5%		5	Florida	1,431,022	5.5%
27	Colorado	345,026	1.3%		6	Ohio	1,199,906	4.6%
29	Connecticut	294,070	1.1%		7	Illinois	1,096,055	4.2%
43	Delaware	78,850	0.3%		8	Michigan	985,062	3.8%
5	Florida	1,431,022	5.5%		9	New Jersey	726,032	2.8%
10	Georgia	717,476	2.7%		10	Georgia	717,476	2.7%
45	Hawaii	75,162	0.3%		11	North Carolina	713,742	2.7%
42	Idaho	91,441	0.4%		12	Massachusetts	676,193	2.6%
7	Illinois	1,096,055	4.2%		13	Virginia	646,407	2.5%
15	Indiana	604,396	2.3%		14	Tennessee	641,122	2.5%
25	Iowa	395,612	1.5%		15	Indiana	604,396	2.3%
34	Kansas	246,720	0.9%		16	Missouri	588,765	2.3%
18	Kentucky	519,859	2.0%		17	Wisconsin	527,770	2.0%
21	Louisiana	458,089	1.8%		18	Kentucky	519,859	2.0%
38	Maine	153,200	0.6%		19	Maryland	513,772	2.0%
19	Maryland	513,772	2.0%		20	Alabama	486,164	1.9%
12	Massachusetts	676,193	2.6%		21	Louisiana	458,089	1.8%
8	Michigan	985,062	3.8%		22	Minnesota	428,273	1.6%
22	Minnesota	428,273	1.6%		23	South Carolina	427,034	1.6%
33	Mississippi	263,297	1.0%		24	Washington	424,517	1.6%
16	Missouri	588,765	2.3%		25	Iowa	395,612	1.5%
46	Montana	69,511	0.3%		26	Arizona	373,080	1.4%
35	Nebraska	191,780	0.7%		27	Colorado	345,026	1.3%
37	Nevada	156,930	0.6%		28	Oklahoma	300,273	1.1%
41	New Hampshire	102,402	0.4%		29	Connecticut	294,070	1.1%
9	New Jersey	726,032	2.8%		30	Oregon	273,905	1.0%
40	New Mexico	129,480	0.5%		31	West Virginia	267,191	1.0%
2	New York	1,985,866	7.6%		32	Arkansas	265,891	1.0%
11	North Carolina	713,742	2.7%		33	Mississippi	263,297	1.0%
47	North Dakota	68,816	0.3%		34	Kansas	246,720	0.9%
6	Ohio	1,199,906	4.6%		35	Nebraska	191,780	0.7%
28	Oklahoma	300,273	1.1%		36	Utah	184,159	0.7%
30	Oregon	273,905	1.0%		37	Nevada	156,930	0.6%
4	Pennsylvania	1,532,805	5.9%		38	Maine	153,200	0.6%
39	Rhode Island	129,629	0.5%		39	Rhode Island	129,629	0.5%
23	South Carolina	427,034	1.6%		40	New Mexico	129,480	0.5%
44	South Dakota	76,635	0.3%		41	New Hampshire	102,402	0.4%
14	Tennessee	641,122	2.5%		42	Idaho	91,441	0.4%
3	Texas	1,760,843	6.7%		43	Delaware	78,850	0.3%
36	Utah	184,159	0.7%		44	South Dakota	76,635	0.3%
49	Vermont	49,416	0.2%		45	Hawaii	75,162	0.3%
13	Virginia	646,407	2.5%		46	Montana	69,511	0.3%
24	Washington	424,517	1.6%		47	North Dakota	68,816	0.3%
31	West Virginia	267,191	1.0%		48	Alaska	49,874	0.2%
17	Wisconsin	527,770	2.0%		49	Vermont	49,416	0.2%
50	Wyoming	39,877	0.2%		50	Wyoming	39,877	0.2%
						District of Columbia	133,181	0.5%

Source: American Hospital Association (Chicago, IL)
"Hospital Statistics" (2002 edition)
*Includes inpatient and outpatient surgeries.

Medicare and Medicaid Certified Facilities in 2002

National Total = 230,241 Facilities*

ALPHA ORDER				RANK ORDER			
RANK	STATE	FACILITIES	% of USA	RANK	STATE	FACILITIES	% of USA
19	Alabama	3,973	1.7%	1	California	22,306	9.7%
49	Alaska	531	0.2%	2	Texas	18,476	8.0%
27	Arizona	3,273	1.4%	3	Florida	14,148	6.1%
31	Arkansas	2,710	1.2%	4	New York	12,154	5.3%
1	California	22,306	9.7%	5	Ohio	11,051	4.8%
30	Colorado	2,969	1.3%	6	Illinois	9,925	4.3%
29	Connecticut	3,182	1.4%	7	Pennsylvania	9,618	4.2%
47	Delaware	727	0.3%	8	Michigan	7,497	3.3%
3	Florida	14,148	6.1%	9	Georgia	7,175	3.1%
9	Georgia	7,175	3.1%	10	North Carolina	6,762	2.9%
45	Hawaii	929	0.4%	11	Indiana	6,157	2.7%
40	Idaho	1,073	0.5%	12	New Jersey	5,892	2.6%
6	Illinois	9,925	4.3%	13	Missouri	5,670	2.5%
11	Indiana	6,157	2.7%	14	Louisiana	5,182	2.3%
26	Iowa	3,544	1.5%	15	Virginia	5,116	2.2%
28	Kansas	3,206	1.4%	16	Tennessee	5,099	2.2%
25	Kentucky	3,599	1.6%	17	Massachusetts	4,595	2.0%
14	Louisiana	5,182	2.3%	18	Maryland	4,190	1.8%
38	Maine	1,328	0.6%	19	Alabama	3,973	1.7%
18	Maryland	4,190	1.8%	20	Wisconsin	3,829	1.7%
17	Massachusetts	4,595	2.0%	21	Washington	3,733	1.6%
8	Michigan	7,497	3.3%	22	Oklahoma	3,709	1.6%
24	Minnesota	3,629	1.6%	23	South Carolina	3,676	1.6%
32	Mississippi	2,664	1.2%	24	Minnesota	3,629	1.6%
13	Missouri	5,670	2.5%	25	Kentucky	3,599	1.6%
43	Montana	948	0.4%	26	Iowa	3,544	1.5%
35	Nebraska	1,877	0.8%	27	Arizona	3,273	1.4%
39	Nevada	1,199	0.5%	28	Kansas	3,206	1.4%
41	New Hampshire	1,065	0.5%	29	Connecticut	3,182	1.4%
12	New Jersey	5,892	2.6%	30	Colorado	2,969	1.3%
36	New Mexico	1,524	0.7%	31	Arkansas	2,710	1.2%
4	New York	12,154	5.3%	32	Mississippi	2,664	1.2%
10	North Carolina	6,762	2.9%	33	Oregon	2,440	1.1%
46	North Dakota	844	0.4%	34	West Virginia	2,069	0.9%
5	Ohio	11,051	4.8%	35	Nebraska	1,877	0.8%
22	Oklahoma	3,709	1.6%	36	New Mexico	1,524	0.7%
33	Oregon	2,440	1.1%	37	Utah	1,337	0.6%
7	Pennsylvania	9,618	4.2%	38	Maine	1,328	0.6%
44	Rhode Island	945	0.4%	39	Nevada	1,199	0.5%
23	South Carolina	3,676	1.6%	40	Idaho	1,073	0.5%
42	South Dakota	959	0.4%	41	New Hampshire	1,065	0.5%
16	Tennessee	5,099	2.2%	42	South Dakota	959	0.4%
2	Texas	18,476	8.0%	43	Montana	948	0.4%
37	Utah	1,337	0.6%	44	Rhode Island	945	0.4%
48	Vermont	541	0.2%	45	Hawaii	929	0.4%
15	Virginia	5,116	2.2%	46	North Dakota	844	0.4%
21	Washington	3,733	1.6%	47	Delaware	727	0.3%
34	West Virginia	2,069	0.9%	48	Vermont	541	0.2%
20	Wisconsin	3,829	1.7%	49	Alaska	531	0.2%
50	Wyoming	511	0.2%	50	Wyoming	511	0.2%
					District of Columbia	685	0.3%

Source: U.S. Department of Health and Human Services, Centers for Medicare and Medicaid Services OSCAR Report 10 (February 21, 2002)

*Certified by CMS to participate in the Medicare/Medicaid programs. All provider groups including hospitals, home health agencies, rural health centers, community mental health centers, nursing facilities, outpatient physical therapy facilities, hospices and laboratories. National total does not include 1,305 certified facilities in U.S. territories.

Medicare and Medicaid Certified Hospitals in 2002

National Total = 5,959 Hospitals*

<table>
<tr><td colspan="4">ALPHA ORDER</td><td colspan="4">RANK ORDER</td></tr>
<tr><td>RANK</td><td>STATE</td><td>HOSPITALS</td><td>% of USA</td><td>RANK</td><td>STATE</td><td>HOSPITALS</td><td>% of USA</td></tr>
<tr><td>19</td><td>Alabama</td><td>123</td><td>2.1%</td><td>1</td><td>Texas</td><td>481</td><td>8.1%</td></tr>
<tr><td>47</td><td>Alaska</td><td>24</td><td>0.4%</td><td>2</td><td>California</td><td>450</td><td>7.6%</td></tr>
<tr><td>29</td><td>Arizona</td><td>83</td><td>1.4%</td><td>3</td><td>New York</td><td>261</td><td>4.4%</td></tr>
<tr><td>26</td><td>Arkansas</td><td>105</td><td>1.8%</td><td>4</td><td>Pennsylvania</td><td>254</td><td>4.3%</td></tr>
<tr><td>2</td><td>California</td><td>450</td><td>7.6%</td><td>5</td><td>Florida</td><td>232</td><td>3.9%</td></tr>
<tr><td>29</td><td>Colorado</td><td>83</td><td>1.4%</td><td>6</td><td>Illinois</td><td>217</td><td>3.6%</td></tr>
<tr><td>41</td><td>Connecticut</td><td>46</td><td>0.8%</td><td>7</td><td>Ohio</td><td>207</td><td>3.5%</td></tr>
<tr><td>50</td><td>Delaware</td><td>11</td><td>0.2%</td><td>8</td><td>Louisiana</td><td>188</td><td>3.2%</td></tr>
<tr><td>5</td><td>Florida</td><td>232</td><td>3.9%</td><td>9</td><td>Georgia</td><td>178</td><td>3.0%</td></tr>
<tr><td>9</td><td>Georgia</td><td>178</td><td>3.0%</td><td>10</td><td>Michigan</td><td>174</td><td>2.9%</td></tr>
<tr><td>46</td><td>Hawaii</td><td>27</td><td>0.5%</td><td>11</td><td>Indiana</td><td>150</td><td>2.5%</td></tr>
<tr><td>40</td><td>Idaho</td><td>47</td><td>0.8%</td><td>11</td><td>Minnesota</td><td>150</td><td>2.5%</td></tr>
<tr><td>6</td><td>Illinois</td><td>217</td><td>3.6%</td><td>13</td><td>Kansas</td><td>149</td><td>2.5%</td></tr>
<tr><td>11</td><td>Indiana</td><td>150</td><td>2.5%</td><td>14</td><td>Tennessee</td><td>148</td><td>2.5%</td></tr>
<tr><td>20</td><td>Iowa</td><td>120</td><td>2.0%</td><td>15</td><td>Oklahoma</td><td>143</td><td>2.4%</td></tr>
<tr><td>13</td><td>Kansas</td><td>149</td><td>2.5%</td><td>16</td><td>Wisconsin</td><td>142</td><td>2.4%</td></tr>
<tr><td>23</td><td>Kentucky</td><td>115</td><td>1.9%</td><td>17</td><td>Missouri</td><td>138</td><td>2.3%</td></tr>
<tr><td>8</td><td>Louisiana</td><td>188</td><td>3.2%</td><td>18</td><td>North Carolina</td><td>133</td><td>2.2%</td></tr>
<tr><td>43</td><td>Maine</td><td>41</td><td>0.7%</td><td>19</td><td>Alabama</td><td>123</td><td>2.1%</td></tr>
<tr><td>32</td><td>Maryland</td><td>67</td><td>1.1%</td><td>20</td><td>Iowa</td><td>120</td><td>2.0%</td></tr>
<tr><td>22</td><td>Massachusetts</td><td>118</td><td>2.0%</td><td>20</td><td>Virginia</td><td>120</td><td>2.0%</td></tr>
<tr><td>10</td><td>Michigan</td><td>174</td><td>2.9%</td><td>22</td><td>Massachusetts</td><td>118</td><td>2.0%</td></tr>
<tr><td>11</td><td>Minnesota</td><td>150</td><td>2.5%</td><td>23</td><td>Kentucky</td><td>115</td><td>1.9%</td></tr>
<tr><td>24</td><td>Mississippi</td><td>107</td><td>1.8%</td><td>24</td><td>Mississippi</td><td>107</td><td>1.8%</td></tr>
<tr><td>17</td><td>Missouri</td><td>138</td><td>2.3%</td><td>24</td><td>New Jersey</td><td>107</td><td>1.8%</td></tr>
<tr><td>35</td><td>Montana</td><td>62</td><td>1.0%</td><td>26</td><td>Arkansas</td><td>105</td><td>1.8%</td></tr>
<tr><td>28</td><td>Nebraska</td><td>95</td><td>1.6%</td><td>27</td><td>Washington</td><td>99</td><td>1.7%</td></tr>
<tr><td>42</td><td>Nevada</td><td>42</td><td>0.7%</td><td>28</td><td>Nebraska</td><td>95</td><td>1.6%</td></tr>
<tr><td>44</td><td>New Hampshire</td><td>30</td><td>0.5%</td><td>29</td><td>Arizona</td><td>83</td><td>1.4%</td></tr>
<tr><td>24</td><td>New Jersey</td><td>107</td><td>1.8%</td><td>29</td><td>Colorado</td><td>83</td><td>1.4%</td></tr>
<tr><td>37</td><td>New Mexico</td><td>52</td><td>0.9%</td><td>31</td><td>South Carolina</td><td>75</td><td>1.3%</td></tr>
<tr><td>3</td><td>New York</td><td>261</td><td>4.4%</td><td>32</td><td>Maryland</td><td>67</td><td>1.1%</td></tr>
<tr><td>18</td><td>North Carolina</td><td>133</td><td>2.2%</td><td>33</td><td>South Dakota</td><td>65</td><td>1.1%</td></tr>
<tr><td>38</td><td>North Dakota</td><td>51</td><td>0.9%</td><td>33</td><td>West Virginia</td><td>65</td><td>1.1%</td></tr>
<tr><td>7</td><td>Ohio</td><td>207</td><td>3.5%</td><td>35</td><td>Montana</td><td>62</td><td>1.0%</td></tr>
<tr><td>15</td><td>Oklahoma</td><td>143</td><td>2.4%</td><td>35</td><td>Oregon</td><td>62</td><td>1.0%</td></tr>
<tr><td>35</td><td>Oregon</td><td>62</td><td>1.0%</td><td>37</td><td>New Mexico</td><td>52</td><td>0.9%</td></tr>
<tr><td>4</td><td>Pennsylvania</td><td>254</td><td>4.3%</td><td>38</td><td>North Dakota</td><td>51</td><td>0.9%</td></tr>
<tr><td>49</td><td>Rhode Island</td><td>15</td><td>0.3%</td><td>39</td><td>Utah</td><td>48</td><td>0.8%</td></tr>
<tr><td>31</td><td>South Carolina</td><td>75</td><td>1.3%</td><td>40</td><td>Idaho</td><td>47</td><td>0.8%</td></tr>
<tr><td>33</td><td>South Dakota</td><td>65</td><td>1.1%</td><td>41</td><td>Connecticut</td><td>46</td><td>0.8%</td></tr>
<tr><td>14</td><td>Tennessee</td><td>148</td><td>2.5%</td><td>42</td><td>Nevada</td><td>42</td><td>0.7%</td></tr>
<tr><td>1</td><td>Texas</td><td>481</td><td>8.1%</td><td>43</td><td>Maine</td><td>41</td><td>0.7%</td></tr>
<tr><td>39</td><td>Utah</td><td>48</td><td>0.8%</td><td>44</td><td>New Hampshire</td><td>30</td><td>0.5%</td></tr>
<tr><td>48</td><td>Vermont</td><td>16</td><td>0.3%</td><td>45</td><td>Wyoming</td><td>28</td><td>0.5%</td></tr>
<tr><td>20</td><td>Virginia</td><td>120</td><td>2.0%</td><td>46</td><td>Hawaii</td><td>27</td><td>0.5%</td></tr>
<tr><td>27</td><td>Washington</td><td>99</td><td>1.7%</td><td>47</td><td>Alaska</td><td>24</td><td>0.4%</td></tr>
<tr><td>33</td><td>West Virginia</td><td>65</td><td>1.1%</td><td>48</td><td>Vermont</td><td>16</td><td>0.3%</td></tr>
<tr><td>16</td><td>Wisconsin</td><td>142</td><td>2.4%</td><td>49</td><td>Rhode Island</td><td>15</td><td>0.3%</td></tr>
<tr><td>45</td><td>Wyoming</td><td>28</td><td>0.5%</td><td>50</td><td>Delaware</td><td>11</td><td>0.2%</td></tr>
<tr><td></td><td></td><td></td><td></td><td></td><td>District of Columbia</td><td>15</td><td>0.3%</td></tr>
</table>

Source: U.S. Department of Health and Human Services, Centers for Medicare and Medicaid Services
OSCAR Database (February 21, 2002)
*Certified by CMS to participate in the Medicare/Medicaid programs. Excludes licensed facilities that do not accept federal funding and facilities managed by the Department of Veterans Affairs. National total does not include 64 certified hospitals in U.S. territories.

Beds in Medicare and Medicaid Certified Hospitals in 2002

National Total = 956,437 Beds*

ALPHA ORDER

RANK ORDER

RANK	STATE	BEDS	% of USA	RANK	STATE	BEDS	% of USA
17	Alabama	20,382	2.1%	1	California	82,397	8.6%
50	Alaska	1,527	0.2%	2	New York	80,894	8.5%
27	Arizona	11,983	1.3%	3	Texas	57,409	6.0%
32	Arkansas	10,779	1.1%	4	Florida	52,644	5.5%
1	California	82,397	8.6%	5	Illinois	48,376	5.1%
29	Colorado	11,385	1.2%	6	Ohio	47,890	5.0%
31	Connecticut	10,795	1.1%	7	Pennsylvania	44,109	4.6%
47	Delaware	2,326	0.2%	8	New Jersey	31,790	3.3%
4	Florida	52,644	5.5%	9	Michigan	31,034	3.2%
11	Georgia	25,932	2.7%	10	North Carolina	26,372	2.8%
46	Hawaii	2,747	0.3%	11	Georgia	25,932	2.7%
45	Idaho	2,851	0.3%	12	Tennessee	24,971	2.6%
5	Illinois	48,376	5.1%	13	Missouri	24,909	2.6%
16	Indiana	21,101	2.2%	14	Virginia	22,450	2.3%
28	Iowa	11,905	1.2%	15	Louisiana	22,288	2.3%
30	Kansas	11,357	1.2%	16	Indiana	21,101	2.2%
20	Kentucky	17,414	1.8%	17	Alabama	20,382	2.1%
15	Louisiana	22,288	2.3%	18	Massachusetts	20,079	2.1%
39	Maine	4,124	0.4%	19	Wisconsin	19,746	2.1%
22	Maryland	16,620	1.7%	20	Kentucky	17,414	1.8%
18	Massachusetts	20,079	2.1%	21	Minnesota	17,180	1.8%
9	Michigan	31,034	3.2%	22	Maryland	16,620	1.7%
21	Minnesota	17,180	1.8%	23	Oklahoma	14,534	1.5%
25	Mississippi	12,915	1.4%	24	Washington	13,815	1.4%
13	Missouri	24,909	2.6%	25	Mississippi	12,915	1.4%
44	Montana	2,913	0.3%	26	South Carolina	12,485	1.3%
35	Nebraska	7,042	0.7%	27	Arizona	11,983	1.3%
37	Nevada	4,998	0.5%	28	Iowa	11,905	1.2%
41	New Hampshire	3,366	0.4%	29	Colorado	11,385	1.2%
8	New Jersey	31,790	3.3%	30	Kansas	11,357	1.2%
38	New Mexico	4,978	0.5%	31	Connecticut	10,795	1.1%
2	New York	80,894	8.5%	32	Arkansas	10,779	1.1%
10	North Carolina	26,372	2.8%	33	West Virginia	9,522	1.0%
43	North Dakota	3,290	0.3%	34	Oregon	7,951	0.8%
6	Ohio	47,890	5.0%	35	Nebraska	7,042	0.7%
23	Oklahoma	14,534	1.5%	36	Utah	5,288	0.6%
34	Oregon	7,951	0.8%	37	Nevada	4,998	0.5%
7	Pennsylvania	44,109	4.6%	38	New Mexico	4,978	0.5%
40	Rhode Island	3,903	0.4%	39	Maine	4,124	0.4%
26	South Carolina	12,485	1.3%	40	Rhode Island	3,903	0.4%
42	South Dakota	3,349	0.4%	41	New Hampshire	3,366	0.4%
12	Tennessee	24,971	2.6%	42	South Dakota	3,349	0.4%
3	Texas	57,409	6.0%	43	North Dakota	3,290	0.3%
36	Utah	5,288	0.6%	44	Montana	2,913	0.3%
48	Vermont	2,061	0.2%	45	Idaho	2,851	0.3%
14	Virginia	22,450	2.3%	46	Hawaii	2,747	0.3%
24	Washington	13,815	1.4%	47	Delaware	2,326	0.2%
33	West Virginia	9,522	1.0%	48	Vermont	2,061	0.2%
19	Wisconsin	19,746	2.1%	49	Wyoming	1,545	0.2%
49	Wyoming	1,545	0.2%	50	Alaska	1,527	0.2%
					District of Columbia	4,716	0.5%

Source: U.S. Department of Health and Human Services, Centers for Medicare and Medicaid Services OSCAR Database (February 21, 2002)

*Beds in hospitals certified by CMS to participate in the Medicare/Medicaid programs. Excludes licensed facilities that do not accept federal funding and facilities managed by the Department of Veterans Affairs. National total does not include 11,126 beds in U.S. territories.

Medicare and Medicaid Certified Children's Hospitals in 2002

National Total = 75 Hospitals*

ALPHA ORDER				RANK ORDER			
RANK	STATE	HOSPITALS	% of USA	RANK	STATE	HOSPITALS	% of USA
18	Alabama	1	1.3%	1	California	10	13.3%
33	Alaska	0	0.0%	2	Ohio	8	10.7%
18	Arizona	1	1.3%	2	Texas	8	10.7%
18	Arkansas	1	1.3%	4	Pennsylvania	5	6.7%
1	California	10	13.3%	5	Minnesota	3	4.0%
18	Colorado	1	1.3%	5	Virginia	3	4.0%
18	Connecticut	1	1.3%	7	Florida	2	2.7%
18	Delaware	1	1.3%	7	Georgia	2	2.7%
7	Florida	2	2.7%	7	Illinois	2	2.7%
7	Georgia	2	2.7%	7	Maryland	2	2.7%
18	Hawaii	1	1.3%	7	Massachusetts	2	2.7%
33	Idaho	0	0.0%	7	Missouri	2	2.7%
7	Illinois	2	2.7%	7	Nebraska	2	2.7%
18	Indiana	1	1.3%	7	New York	2	2.7%
33	Iowa	0	0.0%	7	Tennessee	2	2.7%
18	Kansas	1	1.3%	7	Washington	2	2.7%
33	Kentucky	0	0.0%	7	Wisconsin	2	2.7%
18	Louisiana	1	1.3%	18	Alabama	1	1.3%
33	Maine	0	0.0%	18	Arizona	1	1.3%
7	Maryland	2	2.7%	18	Arkansas	1	1.3%
7	Massachusetts	2	2.7%	18	Colorado	1	1.3%
18	Michigan	1	1.3%	18	Connecticut	1	1.3%
5	Minnesota	3	4.0%	18	Delaware	1	1.3%
33	Mississippi	0	0.0%	18	Hawaii	1	1.3%
7	Missouri	2	2.7%	18	Indiana	1	1.3%
33	Montana	0	0.0%	18	Kansas	1	1.3%
7	Nebraska	2	2.7%	18	Louisiana	1	1.3%
33	Nevada	0	0.0%	18	Michigan	1	1.3%
33	New Hampshire	0	0.0%	18	New Jersey	1	1.3%
18	New Jersey	1	1.3%	18	New Mexico	1	1.3%
18	New Mexico	1	1.3%	18	Oklahoma	1	1.3%
7	New York	2	2.7%	18	Utah	1	1.3%
33	North Carolina	0	0.0%	33	Alaska	0	0.0%
33	North Dakota	0	0.0%	33	Idaho	0	0.0%
2	Ohio	8	10.7%	33	Iowa	0	0.0%
18	Oklahoma	1	1.3%	33	Kentucky	0	0.0%
33	Oregon	0	0.0%	33	Maine	0	0.0%
4	Pennsylvania	5	6.7%	33	Mississippi	0	0.0%
33	Rhode Island	0	0.0%	33	Montana	0	0.0%
33	South Carolina	0	0.0%	33	Nevada	0	0.0%
33	South Dakota	0	0.0%	33	New Hampshire	0	0.0%
7	Tennessee	2	2.7%	33	North Carolina	0	0.0%
2	Texas	8	10.7%	33	North Dakota	0	0.0%
18	Utah	1	1.3%	33	Oregon	0	0.0%
33	Vermont	0	0.0%	33	Rhode Island	0	0.0%
5	Virginia	3	4.0%	33	South Carolina	0	0.0%
7	Washington	2	2.7%	33	South Dakota	0	0.0%
33	West Virginia	0	0.0%	33	Vermont	0	0.0%
7	Wisconsin	2	2.7%	33	West Virginia	0	0.0%
33	Wyoming	0	0.0%	33	Wyoming	0	0.0%
					District of Columbia	1	1.3%

Source: U.S. Department of Health and Human Services, Centers for Medicare and Medicaid Services
      OSCAR Report 10 (February 21, 2002)
*Certified by CMS to participate in the Medicare/Medicaid programs. National total does not include one facility in
U.S. territories. Excludes licensed facilities that do not accept federal funding and facilities managed by the
Department of Veterans Affairs.

Beds in Medicare and Medicaid Certified Children's Hospitals in 2002

National Total = 11,487 Beds*

RANK	STATE	BEDS	% of USA	RANK	STATE	BEDS	% of USA
	ALPHA ORDER				**RANK ORDER**		
19	Alabama	225	2.0%	1	Ohio	1,809	15.7%
33	Alaska	0	0.0%	2	California	1,500	13.1%
32	Arizona	15	0.1%	3	Texas	1,277	11.1%
13	Arkansas	280	2.4%	4	Pennsylvania	641	5.6%
2	California	1,500	13.1%	5	Massachusetts	425	3.7%
15	Colorado	253	2.2%	6	New York	405	3.5%
25	Connecticut	97	0.8%	7	Missouri	402	3.5%
25	Delaware	97	0.8%	8	Georgia	400	3.5%
9	Florida	376	3.3%	9	Florida	376	3.3%
8	Georgia	400	3.5%	10	Illinois	351	3.1%
20	Hawaii	201	1.7%	11	Minnesota	329	2.9%
33	Idaho	0	0.0%	12	Virginia	286	2.5%
10	Illinois	351	3.1%	13	Arkansas	280	2.4%
31	Indiana	20	0.2%	14	Washington	276	2.4%
33	Iowa	0	0.0%	15	Colorado	253	2.2%
29	Kansas	34	0.3%	16	Wisconsin	246	2.1%
33	Kentucky	0	0.0%	17	Utah	232	2.0%
21	Louisiana	188	1.6%	18	Michigan	228	2.0%
33	Maine	0	0.0%	19	Alabama	225	2.0%
23	Maryland	165	1.4%	20	Hawaii	201	1.7%
5	Massachusetts	425	3.7%	21	Louisiana	188	1.6%
18	Michigan	228	2.0%	22	Tennessee	175	1.5%
11	Minnesota	329	2.9%	23	Maryland	165	1.4%
33	Mississippi	0	0.0%	24	Nebraska	150	1.3%
7	Missouri	402	3.5%	25	Connecticut	97	0.8%
33	Montana	0	0.0%	25	Delaware	97	0.8%
24	Nebraska	150	1.3%	27	New Jersey	73	0.6%
33	Nevada	0	0.0%	28	Oklahoma	60	0.5%
33	New Hampshire	0	0.0%	29	Kansas	34	0.3%
27	New Jersey	73	0.6%	30	New Mexico	28	0.2%
30	New Mexico	28	0.2%	31	Indiana	20	0.2%
6	New York	405	3.5%	32	Arizona	15	0.1%
33	North Carolina	0	0.0%	33	Alaska	0	0.0%
33	North Dakota	0	0.0%	33	Idaho	0	0.0%
1	Ohio	1,809	15.7%	33	Iowa	0	0.0%
28	Oklahoma	60	0.5%	33	Kentucky	0	0.0%
33	Oregon	0	0.0%	33	Maine	0	0.0%
4	Pennsylvania	641	5.6%	33	Mississippi	0	0.0%
33	Rhode Island	0	0.0%	33	Montana	0	0.0%
33	South Carolina	0	0.0%	33	Nevada	0	0.0%
33	South Dakota	0	0.0%	33	New Hampshire	0	0.0%
22	Tennessee	175	1.5%	33	North Carolina	0	0.0%
3	Texas	1,277	11.1%	33	North Dakota	0	0.0%
17	Utah	232	2.0%	33	Oregon	0	0.0%
33	Vermont	0	0.0%	33	Rhode Island	0	0.0%
12	Virginia	286	2.5%	33	South Carolina	0	0.0%
14	Washington	276	2.4%	33	South Dakota	0	0.0%
33	West Virginia	0	0.0%	33	Vermont	0	0.0%
16	Wisconsin	246	2.1%	33	West Virginia	0	0.0%
33	Wyoming	0	0.0%	33	Wyoming	0	0.0%
					District of Columbia	243	2.1%

Source: U.S. Department of Health and Human Services, Centers for Medicare and Medicaid Services
   OSCAR Database (February 21, 2002)
*Beds in hospitals certified by CMS to participate in the Medicare/Medicaid programs. Excludes licensed facilities
that do not accept federal funding and facilities managed by the Department of Veterans Affairs. National total
does not include 215 beds in U.S. territories.

Medicare and Medicaid Certified Rehabilitation Hospitals in 2002

National Total = 217 Hospitals*

<table>
<tr><td colspan="4">ALPHA ORDER</td><td colspan="4">RANK ORDER</td></tr>
<tr><td>RANK</td><td>STATE</td><td>HOSPITALS</td><td>% of USA</td><td>RANK</td><td>STATE</td><td>HOSPITALS</td><td>% of USA</td></tr>
<tr><td>8</td><td>Alabama</td><td>6</td><td>2.8%</td><td>1</td><td>Texas</td><td>31</td><td>14.3%</td></tr>
<tr><td>43</td><td>Alaska</td><td>0</td><td>0.0%</td><td>2</td><td>Louisiana</td><td>28</td><td>12.9%</td></tr>
<tr><td>22</td><td>Arizona</td><td>3</td><td>1.4%</td><td>3</td><td>Pennsylvania</td><td>18</td><td>8.3%</td></tr>
<tr><td>8</td><td>Arkansas</td><td>6</td><td>2.8%</td><td>4</td><td>Florida</td><td>13</td><td>6.0%</td></tr>
<tr><td>5</td><td>California</td><td>9</td><td>4.1%</td><td>5</td><td>California</td><td>9</td><td>4.1%</td></tr>
<tr><td>27</td><td>Colorado</td><td>2</td><td>0.9%</td><td>6</td><td>Massachusetts</td><td>7</td><td>3.2%</td></tr>
<tr><td>31</td><td>Connecticut</td><td>1</td><td>0.5%</td><td>6</td><td>New Jersey</td><td>7</td><td>3.2%</td></tr>
<tr><td>31</td><td>Delaware</td><td>1</td><td>0.5%</td><td>8</td><td>Alabama</td><td>6</td><td>2.8%</td></tr>
<tr><td>4</td><td>Florida</td><td>13</td><td>6.0%</td><td>8</td><td>Arkansas</td><td>6</td><td>2.8%</td></tr>
<tr><td>27</td><td>Georgia</td><td>2</td><td>0.9%</td><td>8</td><td>Kentucky</td><td>6</td><td>2.8%</td></tr>
<tr><td>31</td><td>Hawaii</td><td>1</td><td>0.5%</td><td>8</td><td>West Virginia</td><td>6</td><td>2.8%</td></tr>
<tr><td>31</td><td>Idaho</td><td>1</td><td>0.5%</td><td>12</td><td>Indiana</td><td>5</td><td>2.3%</td></tr>
<tr><td>22</td><td>Illinois</td><td>3</td><td>1.4%</td><td>12</td><td>Michigan</td><td>5</td><td>2.3%</td></tr>
<tr><td>12</td><td>Indiana</td><td>5</td><td>2.3%</td><td>12</td><td>Tennessee</td><td>5</td><td>2.3%</td></tr>
<tr><td>43</td><td>Iowa</td><td>0</td><td>0.0%</td><td>12</td><td>Virginia</td><td>5</td><td>2.3%</td></tr>
<tr><td>16</td><td>Kansas</td><td>4</td><td>1.8%</td><td>16</td><td>Kansas</td><td>4</td><td>1.8%</td></tr>
<tr><td>8</td><td>Kentucky</td><td>6</td><td>2.8%</td><td>16</td><td>Missouri</td><td>4</td><td>1.8%</td></tr>
<tr><td>2</td><td>Louisiana</td><td>28</td><td>12.9%</td><td>16</td><td>Nevada</td><td>4</td><td>1.8%</td></tr>
<tr><td>31</td><td>Maine</td><td>1</td><td>0.5%</td><td>16</td><td>New Mexico</td><td>4</td><td>1.8%</td></tr>
<tr><td>22</td><td>Maryland</td><td>3</td><td>1.4%</td><td>16</td><td>New York</td><td>4</td><td>1.8%</td></tr>
<tr><td>6</td><td>Massachusetts</td><td>7</td><td>3.2%</td><td>16</td><td>South Carolina</td><td>4</td><td>1.8%</td></tr>
<tr><td>12</td><td>Michigan</td><td>5</td><td>2.3%</td><td>22</td><td>Arizona</td><td>3</td><td>1.4%</td></tr>
<tr><td>31</td><td>Minnesota</td><td>1</td><td>0.5%</td><td>22</td><td>Illinois</td><td>3</td><td>1.4%</td></tr>
<tr><td>31</td><td>Mississippi</td><td>1</td><td>0.5%</td><td>22</td><td>Maryland</td><td>3</td><td>1.4%</td></tr>
<tr><td>16</td><td>Missouri</td><td>4</td><td>1.8%</td><td>22</td><td>Ohio</td><td>3</td><td>1.4%</td></tr>
<tr><td>43</td><td>Montana</td><td>0</td><td>0.0%</td><td>22</td><td>Oklahoma</td><td>3</td><td>1.4%</td></tr>
<tr><td>31</td><td>Nebraska</td><td>1</td><td>0.5%</td><td>27</td><td>Colorado</td><td>2</td><td>0.9%</td></tr>
<tr><td>16</td><td>Nevada</td><td>4</td><td>1.8%</td><td>27</td><td>Georgia</td><td>2</td><td>0.9%</td></tr>
<tr><td>27</td><td>New Hampshire</td><td>2</td><td>0.9%</td><td>27</td><td>New Hampshire</td><td>2</td><td>0.9%</td></tr>
<tr><td>6</td><td>New Jersey</td><td>7</td><td>3.2%</td><td>27</td><td>North Carolina</td><td>2</td><td>0.9%</td></tr>
<tr><td>16</td><td>New Mexico</td><td>4</td><td>1.8%</td><td>31</td><td>Connecticut</td><td>1</td><td>0.5%</td></tr>
<tr><td>16</td><td>New York</td><td>4</td><td>1.8%</td><td>31</td><td>Delaware</td><td>1</td><td>0.5%</td></tr>
<tr><td>27</td><td>North Carolina</td><td>2</td><td>0.9%</td><td>31</td><td>Hawaii</td><td>1</td><td>0.5%</td></tr>
<tr><td>43</td><td>North Dakota</td><td>0</td><td>0.0%</td><td>31</td><td>Idaho</td><td>1</td><td>0.5%</td></tr>
<tr><td>22</td><td>Ohio</td><td>3</td><td>1.4%</td><td>31</td><td>Maine</td><td>1</td><td>0.5%</td></tr>
<tr><td>22</td><td>Oklahoma</td><td>3</td><td>1.4%</td><td>31</td><td>Minnesota</td><td>1</td><td>0.5%</td></tr>
<tr><td>43</td><td>Oregon</td><td>0</td><td>0.0%</td><td>31</td><td>Mississippi</td><td>1</td><td>0.5%</td></tr>
<tr><td>3</td><td>Pennsylvania</td><td>18</td><td>8.3%</td><td>31</td><td>Nebraska</td><td>1</td><td>0.5%</td></tr>
<tr><td>31</td><td>Rhode Island</td><td>1</td><td>0.5%</td><td>31</td><td>Rhode Island</td><td>1</td><td>0.5%</td></tr>
<tr><td>16</td><td>South Carolina</td><td>4</td><td>1.8%</td><td>31</td><td>Utah</td><td>1</td><td>0.5%</td></tr>
<tr><td>43</td><td>South Dakota</td><td>0</td><td>0.0%</td><td>31</td><td>Washington</td><td>1</td><td>0.5%</td></tr>
<tr><td>12</td><td>Tennessee</td><td>5</td><td>2.3%</td><td>31</td><td>Wisconsin</td><td>1</td><td>0.5%</td></tr>
<tr><td>1</td><td>Texas</td><td>31</td><td>14.3%</td><td>43</td><td>Alaska</td><td>0</td><td>0.0%</td></tr>
<tr><td>31</td><td>Utah</td><td>1</td><td>0.5%</td><td>43</td><td>Iowa</td><td>0</td><td>0.0%</td></tr>
<tr><td>43</td><td>Vermont</td><td>0</td><td>0.0%</td><td>43</td><td>Montana</td><td>0</td><td>0.0%</td></tr>
<tr><td>12</td><td>Virginia</td><td>5</td><td>2.3%</td><td>43</td><td>North Dakota</td><td>0</td><td>0.0%</td></tr>
<tr><td>31</td><td>Washington</td><td>1</td><td>0.5%</td><td>43</td><td>Oregon</td><td>0</td><td>0.0%</td></tr>
<tr><td>8</td><td>West Virginia</td><td>6</td><td>2.8%</td><td>43</td><td>South Dakota</td><td>0</td><td>0.0%</td></tr>
<tr><td>31</td><td>Wisconsin</td><td>1</td><td>0.5%</td><td>43</td><td>Vermont</td><td>0</td><td>0.0%</td></tr>
<tr><td>43</td><td>Wyoming</td><td>0</td><td>0.0%</td><td>43</td><td>Wyoming</td><td>0</td><td>0.0%</td></tr>
<tr><td></td><td></td><td></td><td></td><td></td><td>District of Columbia</td><td>1</td><td>0.5%</td></tr>
</table>

Source: U.S. Department of Health and Human Services, Centers for Medicare and Medicaid Services
    OSCAR Database (February 21, 2002)
*Certified by CMS to participate in the Medicare/Medicaid programs. Excludes licensed facilities that do not accept federal funding and facilities managed by the Department of Veterans Affairs. National total does not include one certified hospital in U.S. territories.

Beds in Medicare and Medicaid Certified Rehabilitation Hospitals in 2002

National Total = 13,779 Beds*

ALPHA ORDER

RANK	STATE	BEDS	% of USA
12	Alabama	336	2.4%
43	Alaska	0	0.0%
26	Arizona	165	1.2%
8	Arkansas	452	3.3%
7	California	529	3.8%
22	Colorado	202	1.5%
38	Connecticut	60	0.4%
38	Delaware	60	0.4%
3	Florida	858	6.2%
31	Georgia	108	0.8%
33	Hawaii	100	0.7%
41	Idaho	59	0.4%
10	Illinois	371	2.7%
11	Indiana	349	2.5%
43	Iowa	0	0.0%
18	Kansas	257	1.9%
15	Kentucky	306	2.2%
6	Louisiana	651	4.7%
33	Maine	100	0.7%
30	Maryland	121	0.9%
4	Massachusetts	739	5.4%
14	Michigan	315	2.3%
42	Minnesota	15	0.1%
29	Mississippi	124	0.9%
17	Missouri	260	1.9%
43	Montana	0	0.0%
38	Nebraska	60	0.4%
23	Nevada	197	1.4%
27	New Hampshire	152	1.1%
5	New Jersey	666	4.8%
28	New Mexico	149	1.1%
9	New York	428	3.1%
21	North Carolina	233	1.7%
43	North Dakota	0	0.0%
24	Ohio	170	1.2%
25	Oklahoma	167	1.2%
43	Oregon	0	0.0%
2	Pennsylvania	1,658	12.0%
35	Rhode Island	82	0.6%
20	South Carolina	239	1.7%
43	South Dakota	0	0.0%
13	Tennessee	330	2.4%
1	Texas	1,765	12.8%
37	Utah	76	0.6%
43	Vermont	0	0.0%
16	Virginia	281	2.0%
32	Washington	102	0.7%
19	West Virginia	246	1.8%
36	Wisconsin	81	0.6%
43	Wyoming	0	0.0%

RANK ORDER

RANK	STATE	BEDS	% of USA
1	Texas	1,765	12.8%
2	Pennsylvania	1,658	12.0%
3	Florida	858	6.2%
4	Massachusetts	739	5.4%
5	New Jersey	666	4.8%
6	Louisiana	651	4.7%
7	California	529	3.8%
8	Arkansas	452	3.3%
9	New York	428	3.1%
10	Illinois	371	2.7%
11	Indiana	349	2.5%
12	Alabama	336	2.4%
13	Tennessee	330	2.4%
14	Michigan	315	2.3%
15	Kentucky	306	2.2%
16	Virginia	281	2.0%
17	Missouri	260	1.9%
18	Kansas	257	1.9%
19	West Virginia	246	1.8%
20	South Carolina	239	1.7%
21	North Carolina	233	1.7%
22	Colorado	202	1.5%
23	Nevada	197	1.4%
24	Ohio	170	1.2%
25	Oklahoma	167	1.2%
26	Arizona	165	1.2%
27	New Hampshire	152	1.1%
28	New Mexico	149	1.1%
29	Mississippi	124	0.9%
30	Maryland	121	0.9%
31	Georgia	108	0.8%
32	Washington	102	0.7%
33	Hawaii	100	0.7%
33	Maine	100	0.7%
35	Rhode Island	82	0.6%
36	Wisconsin	81	0.6%
37	Utah	76	0.6%
38	Connecticut	60	0.4%
38	Delaware	60	0.4%
38	Nebraska	60	0.4%
41	Idaho	59	0.4%
42	Minnesota	15	0.1%
43	Alaska	0	0.0%
43	Iowa	0	0.0%
43	Montana	0	0.0%
43	North Dakota	0	0.0%
43	Oregon	0	0.0%
43	South Dakota	0	0.0%
43	Vermont	0	0.0%
43	Wyoming	0	0.0%
	District of Columbia	160	1.2%

Source: U.S. Department of Health and Human Services, Centers for Medicare and Medicaid Services OSCAR Database (February 21, 2002)

Beds in hospitals certified by CMS to participate in the Medicare/Medicaid programs. Excludes licensed facilities that do not accept federal funding and facilities managed by the Department of Veterans Affairs. National total does not include 30 beds in U.S. territories.

Medicare and Medicaid Certified Psychiatric Hospitals in 2002

National Total = 487 Psychiatric Hospitals*

ALPHA ORDER					RANK ORDER			
RANK	STATE		HOSPITALS	% of USA	RANK	STATE	HOSPITALS	% of USA
23	Alabama		9	1.8%	1	California	34	7.0%
43	Alaska		2	0.4%	2	New York	33	6.8%
25	Arizona		7	1.4%	3	Texas	30	6.2%
19	Arkansas		10	2.1%	4	Pennsylvania	24	4.9%
1	California		34	7.0%	5	Florida	23	4.7%
28	Colorado		6	1.2%	6	Indiana	19	3.9%
24	Connecticut		8	1.6%	7	Massachusetts	18	3.7%
37	Delaware		3	0.6%	8	Illinois	17	3.5%
5	Florida		23	4.7%	9	New Jersey	16	3.3%
13	Georgia		14	2.9%	9	Virginia	16	3.3%
49	Hawaii		1	0.2%	11	Louisiana	15	3.1%
31	Idaho		4	0.8%	11	Ohio	15	3.1%
8	Illinois		17	3.5%	13	Georgia	14	2.9%
6	Indiana		19	3.9%	13	Missouri	14	2.9%
31	Iowa		4	0.8%	15	Wisconsin	13	2.7%
31	Kansas		4	0.8%	16	Kentucky	11	2.3%
16	Kentucky		11	2.3%	16	North Carolina	11	2.3%
11	Louisiana		15	3.1%	16	Tennessee	11	2.3%
31	Maine		4	0.8%	19	Arkansas	10	2.1%
19	Maryland		10	2.1%	19	Maryland	10	2.1%
7	Massachusetts		18	3.7%	19	Michigan	10	2.1%
19	Michigan		10	2.1%	19	Oklahoma	10	2.1%
25	Minnesota		7	1.4%	23	Alabama	9	1.8%
37	Mississippi		3	0.6%	24	Connecticut	8	1.6%
13	Missouri		14	2.9%	25	Arizona	7	1.4%
43	Montana		2	0.4%	25	Minnesota	7	1.4%
29	Nebraska		5	1.0%	25	South Carolina	7	1.4%
31	Nevada		4	0.8%	28	Colorado	6	1.2%
43	New Hampshire		2	0.4%	29	Nebraska	5	1.0%
9	New Jersey		16	3.3%	29	Washington	5	1.0%
37	New Mexico		3	0.6%	31	Idaho	4	0.8%
2	New York		33	6.8%	31	Iowa	4	0.8%
16	North Carolina		11	2.3%	31	Kansas	4	0.8%
37	North Dakota		3	0.6%	31	Maine	4	0.8%
11	Ohio		15	3.1%	31	Nevada	4	0.8%
19	Oklahoma		10	2.1%	31	West Virginia	4	0.8%
37	Oregon		3	0.6%	37	Delaware	3	0.6%
4	Pennsylvania		24	4.9%	37	Mississippi	3	0.6%
43	Rhode Island		2	0.4%	37	New Mexico	3	0.6%
25	South Carolina		7	1.4%	37	North Dakota	3	0.6%
49	South Dakota		1	0.2%	37	Oregon	3	0.6%
16	Tennessee		11	2.3%	37	Utah	3	0.6%
3	Texas		30	6.2%	43	Alaska	2	0.4%
37	Utah		3	0.6%	43	Montana	2	0.4%
43	Vermont		2	0.4%	43	New Hampshire	2	0.4%
9	Virginia		16	3.3%	43	Rhode Island	2	0.4%
29	Washington		5	1.0%	43	Vermont	2	0.4%
31	West Virginia		4	0.8%	43	Wyoming	2	0.4%
15	Wisconsin		13	2.7%	49	Hawaii	1	0.2%
43	Wyoming		2	0.4%	49	South Dakota	1	0.2%
						District of Columbia	3	0.6%

Source: U.S. Department of Health and Human Services, Centers for Medicare and Medicaid Services
OSCAR Database (February 21, 2002)

*Certified by CMS to participate in the Medicare/Medicaid programs. Excludes licensed facilities that do not accept federal funding and facilities managed by the Department of Veterans Affairs. National total does not include four certified psychiatric hospitals in U.S. territories.

Beds in Medicare and Medicaid Certified Psychiatric Hospitals in 2002

National Total = 64,998 Beds*

ALPHA ORDER					RANK ORDER			
RANK	STATE	BEDS	% of USA		RANK	STATE	BEDS	% of USA
29	Alabama	693	1.1%		1	New York	11,982	18.4%
44	Alaska	188	0.3%		2	Pennsylvania	5,119	7.9%
28	Arizona	734	1.1%		3	New Jersey	3,018	4.6%
25	Arkansas	863	1.3%		4	North Carolina	2,857	4.4%
6	California	2,449	3.8%		5	Maryland	2,640	4.1%
26	Colorado	833	1.3%		6	California	2,449	3.8%
21	Connecticut	1,175	1.8%		7	Texas	2,413	3.7%
40	Delaware	242	0.4%		8	Michigan	2,025	3.1%
11	Florida	1,695	2.6%		9	Georgia	1,855	2.9%
9	Georgia	1,855	2.9%		10	Illinois	1,730	2.7%
49	Hawaii	88	0.1%		11	Florida	1,695	2.6%
48	Idaho	105	0.2%		12	Virginia	1,528	2.4%
10	Illinois	1,730	2.7%		13	Massachusetts	1,522	2.3%
18	Indiana	1,296	2.0%		14	Ohio	1,512	2.3%
37	Iowa	300	0.5%		15	Wisconsin	1,511	2.3%
31	Kansas	561	0.9%		16	Louisiana	1,451	2.2%
19	Kentucky	1,263	1.9%		17	Minnesota	1,368	2.1%
16	Louisiana	1,451	2.2%		18	Indiana	1,296	2.0%
34	Maine	364	0.6%		19	Kentucky	1,263	1.9%
5	Maryland	2,640	4.1%		20	Tennessee	1,205	1.9%
13	Massachusetts	1,522	2.3%		21	Connecticut	1,175	1.8%
8	Michigan	2,025	3.1%		22	Washington	1,142	1.8%
17	Minnesota	1,368	2.1%		23	Missouri	1,006	1.5%
42	Mississippi	223	0.3%		24	Nebraska	905	1.4%
23	Missouri	1,006	1.5%		25	Arkansas	863	1.3%
45	Montana	182	0.3%		26	Colorado	833	1.3%
24	Nebraska	905	1.4%		27	South Carolina	807	1.2%
35	Nevada	331	0.5%		28	Arizona	734	1.1%
36	New Hampshire	323	0.5%		29	Alabama	693	1.1%
3	New Jersey	3,018	4.6%		30	Oklahoma	641	1.0%
39	New Mexico	245	0.4%		31	Kansas	561	0.9%
1	New York	11,982	18.4%		32	West Virginia	485	0.7%
4	North Carolina	2,857	4.4%		33	Utah	473	0.7%
41	North Dakota	229	0.4%		34	Maine	364	0.6%
14	Ohio	1,512	2.3%		35	Nevada	331	0.5%
30	Oklahoma	641	1.0%		36	New Hampshire	323	0.5%
38	Oregon	296	0.5%		37	Iowa	300	0.5%
2	Pennsylvania	5,119	7.9%		38	Oregon	296	0.5%
46	Rhode Island	165	0.3%		39	New Mexico	245	0.4%
27	South Carolina	807	1.2%		40	Delaware	242	0.4%
47	South Dakota	133	0.2%		41	North Dakota	229	0.4%
20	Tennessee	1,205	1.9%		42	Mississippi	223	0.3%
7	Texas	2,413	3.7%		43	Vermont	205	0.3%
33	Utah	473	0.7%		44	Alaska	188	0.3%
43	Vermont	205	0.3%		45	Montana	182	0.3%
12	Virginia	1,528	2.4%		46	Rhode Island	165	0.3%
22	Washington	1,142	1.8%		47	South Dakota	133	0.2%
32	West Virginia	485	0.7%		48	Idaho	105	0.2%
15	Wisconsin	1,511	2.3%		49	Hawaii	88	0.1%
50	Wyoming	68	0.1%		50	Wyoming	68	0.1%
						District of Columbia	554	0.9%

Source: U.S. Department of Health and Human Services, Centers for Medicare and Medicaid Services
OSCAR Database (February 21, 2002)
*Beds in hospitals certified by CMS to participate in the Medicare/Medicaid programs. Excludes licensed facilities that do not accept federal funding and facilities managed by the Department of Veterans Affairs. National total does not include 903 beds in U.S. territories.

Medicare and Medicaid Certified Community Mental Health Centers in 2002

National Total = 674 Centers*

ALPHA ORDER

RANK	STATE	CENTERS	% of USA
2	Alabama	80	11.9%
43	Alaska	0	0.0%
32	Arizona	3	0.4%
17	Arkansas	14	2.1%
9	California	21	3.1%
17	Colorado	14	2.1%
31	Connecticut	4	0.6%
43	Delaware	0	0.0%
1	Florida	97	14.4%
23	Georgia	9	1.3%
43	Hawaii	0	0.0%
43	Idaho	0	0.0%
14	Illinois	16	2.4%
22	Indiana	11	1.6%
26	Iowa	7	1.0%
13	Kansas	17	2.5%
19	Kentucky	13	1.9%
5	Louisiana	34	5.0%
32	Maine	3	0.4%
28	Maryland	6	0.9%
15	Massachusetts	15	2.2%
23	Michigan	9	1.3%
19	Minnesota	13	1.9%
29	Mississippi	5	0.7%
11	Missouri	19	2.8%
38	Montana	2	0.3%
42	Nebraska	1	0.1%
38	Nevada	2	0.3%
38	New Hampshire	2	0.3%
4	New Jersey	38	5.6%
15	New Mexico	15	2.2%
26	New York	7	1.0%
8	North Carolina	22	3.3%
43	North Dakota	0	0.0%
7	Ohio	23	3.4%
25	Oklahoma	8	1.2%
21	Oregon	12	1.8%
12	Pennsylvania	18	2.7%
43	Rhode Island	0	0.0%
32	South Carolina	3	0.4%
38	South Dakota	2	0.3%
9	Tennessee	21	3.1%
3	Texas	46	6.8%
32	Utah	3	0.4%
43	Vermont	0	0.0%
29	Virginia	5	0.7%
6	Washington	28	4.2%
32	West Virginia	3	0.4%
43	Wisconsin	0	0.0%
32	Wyoming	3	0.4%

RANK ORDER

RANK	STATE	CENTERS	% of USA
1	Florida	97	14.4%
2	Alabama	80	11.9%
3	Texas	46	6.8%
4	New Jersey	38	5.6%
5	Louisiana	34	5.0%
6	Washington	28	4.2%
7	Ohio	23	3.4%
8	North Carolina	22	3.3%
9	California	21	3.1%
9	Tennessee	21	3.1%
11	Missouri	19	2.8%
12	Pennsylvania	18	2.7%
13	Kansas	17	2.5%
14	Illinois	16	2.4%
15	Massachusetts	15	2.2%
15	New Mexico	15	2.2%
17	Arkansas	14	2.1%
17	Colorado	14	2.1%
19	Kentucky	13	1.9%
19	Minnesota	13	1.9%
21	Oregon	12	1.8%
22	Indiana	11	1.6%
23	Georgia	9	1.3%
23	Michigan	9	1.3%
25	Oklahoma	8	1.2%
26	Iowa	7	1.0%
26	New York	7	1.0%
28	Maryland	6	0.9%
29	Mississippi	5	0.7%
29	Virginia	5	0.7%
31	Connecticut	4	0.6%
32	Arizona	3	0.4%
32	Maine	3	0.4%
32	South Carolina	3	0.4%
32	Utah	3	0.4%
32	West Virginia	3	0.4%
32	Wyoming	3	0.4%
38	Montana	2	0.3%
38	Nevada	2	0.3%
38	New Hampshire	2	0.3%
38	South Dakota	2	0.3%
42	Nebraska	1	0.1%
43	Alaska	0	0.0%
43	Delaware	0	0.0%
43	Hawaii	0	0.0%
43	Idaho	0	0.0%
43	North Dakota	0	0.0%
43	Rhode Island	0	0.0%
43	Vermont	0	0.0%
43	Wisconsin	0	0.0%
	District of Columbia	0	0.0%

Source: U.S. Department of Health and Human Services, Centers for Medicare and Medicaid Services
    OSCAR Report 10 (February 21, 2002)
*Certified by CMS to participate in the Medicare/Medicaid programs. Excludes licensed facilities that do not accept federal funding and facilities managed by the Department of Veterans Affairs. National total does not include nine certified mental health centers in U.S. territories.

Medicare and Medicaid Certified Outpatient Physical Therapy Facilities in 2002

National Total = 2,854 Facilities*

ALPHA ORDER

RANK	STATE	FACILITIES	% of USA
33	Alabama	21	0.7%
37	Alaska	17	0.6%
29	Arizona	30	1.1%
28	Arkansas	32	1.1%
3	California	219	7.7%
18	Colorado	53	1.9%
25	Connecticut	37	1.3%
34	Delaware	19	0.7%
1	Florida	250	8.8%
7	Georgia	127	4.4%
39	Hawaii	11	0.4%
39	Idaho	11	0.4%
12	Illinois	86	3.0%
17	Indiana	54	1.9%
24	Iowa	40	1.4%
31	Kansas	24	0.8%
13	Kentucky	65	2.3%
18	Louisiana	53	1.9%
32	Maine	23	0.8%
11	Maryland	89	3.1%
38	Massachusetts	16	0.6%
2	Michigan	222	7.8%
20	Minnesota	52	1.8%
21	Mississippi	46	1.6%
14	Missouri	60	2.1%
41	Montana	10	0.4%
43	Nebraska	9	0.3%
35	Nevada	18	0.6%
41	New Hampshire	10	0.4%
9	New Jersey	103	3.6%
27	New Mexico	33	1.2%
30	New York	27	0.9%
23	North Carolina	44	1.5%
46	North Dakota	5	0.2%
5	Ohio	136	4.8%
22	Oklahoma	45	1.6%
35	Oregon	18	0.6%
5	Pennsylvania	136	4.8%
49	Rhode Island	4	0.1%
16	South Carolina	55	1.9%
46	South Dakota	5	0.2%
10	Tennessee	96	3.4%
4	Texas	207	7.3%
43	Utah	9	0.3%
50	Vermont	2	0.1%
8	Virginia	118	4.1%
26	Washington	35	1.2%
45	West Virginia	7	0.2%
15	Wisconsin	58	2.0%
46	Wyoming	5	0.2%

RANK ORDER

RANK	STATE	FACILITIES	% of USA
1	Florida	250	8.8%
2	Michigan	222	7.8%
3	California	219	7.7%
4	Texas	207	7.3%
5	Ohio	136	4.8%
5	Pennsylvania	136	4.8%
7	Georgia	127	4.4%
8	Virginia	118	4.1%
9	New Jersey	103	3.6%
10	Tennessee	96	3.4%
11	Maryland	89	3.1%
12	Illinois	86	3.0%
13	Kentucky	65	2.3%
14	Missouri	60	2.1%
15	Wisconsin	58	2.0%
16	South Carolina	55	1.9%
17	Indiana	54	1.9%
18	Colorado	53	1.9%
18	Louisiana	53	1.9%
20	Minnesota	52	1.8%
21	Mississippi	46	1.6%
22	Oklahoma	45	1.6%
23	North Carolina	44	1.5%
24	Iowa	40	1.4%
25	Connecticut	37	1.3%
26	Washington	35	1.2%
27	New Mexico	33	1.2%
28	Arkansas	32	1.1%
29	Arizona	30	1.1%
30	New York	27	0.9%
31	Kansas	24	0.8%
32	Maine	23	0.8%
33	Alabama	21	0.7%
34	Delaware	19	0.7%
35	Nevada	18	0.6%
35	Oregon	18	0.6%
37	Alaska	17	0.6%
38	Massachusetts	16	0.6%
39	Hawaii	11	0.4%
39	Idaho	11	0.4%
41	Montana	10	0.4%
41	New Hampshire	10	0.4%
43	Nebraska	9	0.3%
43	Utah	9	0.3%
45	West Virginia	7	0.2%
46	North Dakota	5	0.2%
46	South Dakota	5	0.2%
46	Wyoming	5	0.2%
49	Rhode Island	4	0.1%
50	Vermont	2	0.1%
	District of Columbia	2	0.1%

*Source: U.S. Department of Health and Human Services, Centers for Medicare and Medicaid Services
OSCAR Report 10 (February 21, 2002)*
Certified by CMS to participate in the Medicare/Medicaid programs. Excludes licensed facilities that do not accept federal funding and facilities managed by the Department of Veterans Affairs. National total does not include two certified outpatient physical therapy facilities in U.S. territories.

Medicare and Medicaid Certified Rural Health Clinics in 2002

National Total = 3,298 Rural Health Clinics*

ALPHA ORDER

RANK	STATE	CLINICS	% of USA
23	Alabama	54	1.6%
41	Alaska	7	0.2%
41	Arizona	7	0.2%
14	Arkansas	77	2.3%
2	California	230	7.0%
29	Colorado	45	1.4%
45	Connecticut	0	0.0%
45	Delaware	0	0.0%
7	Florida	141	4.3%
11	Georgia	114	3.5%
45	Hawaii	0	0.0%
30	Idaho	37	1.1%
3	Illinois	194	5.9%
24	Indiana	51	1.5%
8	Iowa	130	3.9%
5	Kansas	155	4.7%
13	Kentucky	84	2.5%
24	Louisiana	51	1.5%
24	Maine	51	1.5%
45	Maryland	0	0.0%
45	Massachusetts	0	0.0%
5	Michigan	155	4.7%
19	Minnesota	61	1.8%
9	Mississippi	129	3.9%
4	Missouri	179	5.4%
31	Montana	36	1.1%
16	Nebraska	74	2.2%
43	Nevada	3	0.1%
35	New Hampshire	20	0.6%
45	New Jersey	0	0.0%
39	New Mexico	11	0.3%
40	New York	9	0.3%
10	North Carolina	117	3.5%
17	North Dakota	73	2.2%
37	Ohio	16	0.5%
27	Oklahoma	50	1.5%
33	Oregon	31	0.9%
28	Pennsylvania	49	1.5%
44	Rhode Island	1	0.0%
12	South Carolina	93	2.8%
22	South Dakota	57	1.7%
32	Tennessee	32	1.0%
1	Texas	358	10.9%
38	Utah	15	0.5%
34	Vermont	21	0.6%
21	Virginia	60	1.8%
15	Washington	76	2.3%
18	West Virginia	65	2.0%
19	Wisconsin	61	1.8%
36	Wyoming	18	0.5%

RANK ORDER

RANK	STATE	CLINICS	% of USA
1	Texas	358	10.9%
2	California	230	7.0%
3	Illinois	194	5.9%
4	Missouri	179	5.4%
5	Kansas	155	4.7%
5	Michigan	155	4.7%
7	Florida	141	4.3%
8	Iowa	130	3.9%
9	Mississippi	129	3.9%
10	North Carolina	117	3.5%
11	Georgia	114	3.5%
12	South Carolina	93	2.8%
13	Kentucky	84	2.5%
14	Arkansas	77	2.3%
15	Washington	76	2.3%
16	Nebraska	74	2.2%
17	North Dakota	73	2.2%
18	West Virginia	65	2.0%
19	Minnesota	61	1.8%
19	Wisconsin	61	1.8%
21	Virginia	60	1.8%
22	South Dakota	57	1.7%
23	Alabama	54	1.6%
24	Indiana	51	1.5%
24	Louisiana	51	1.5%
24	Maine	51	1.5%
27	Oklahoma	50	1.5%
28	Pennsylvania	49	1.5%
29	Colorado	45	1.4%
30	Idaho	37	1.1%
31	Montana	36	1.1%
32	Tennessee	32	1.0%
33	Oregon	31	0.9%
34	Vermont	21	0.6%
35	New Hampshire	20	0.6%
36	Wyoming	18	0.5%
37	Ohio	16	0.5%
38	Utah	15	0.5%
39	New Mexico	11	0.3%
40	New York	9	0.3%
41	Alaska	7	0.2%
41	Arizona	7	0.2%
43	Nevada	3	0.1%
44	Rhode Island	1	0.0%
45	Connecticut	0	0.0%
45	Delaware	0	0.0%
45	Hawaii	0	0.0%
45	Maryland	0	0.0%
45	Massachusetts	0	0.0%
45	New Jersey	0	0.0%
	District of Columbia	0	0.0%

Source: U.S. Department of Health and Human Services, Centers for Medicare and Medicaid Services
     OSCAR Report 10 (February 21, 2002)
*Certified by CMS to participate in the Medicare/Medicaid programs. Excludes licensed facilities that do not accept federal funding and facilities managed by the Department of Veterans Affairs. There are no certified rural health centers in U.S. territories.

Medicare and Medicaid Certified Home Health Agencies in 2002

National Total = 6,843 Home Health Agencies*

ALPHA ORDER

RANK	STATE	AGENCIES	% of USA
19	Alabama	140	2.0%
48	Alaska	16	0.2%
31	Arizona	63	0.9%
13	Arkansas	179	2.6%
2	California	534	7.8%
21	Colorado	129	1.9%
26	Connecticut	83	1.2%
47	Delaware	17	0.2%
4	Florida	322	4.7%
25	Georgia	94	1.4%
49	Hawaii	14	0.2%
37	Idaho	50	0.7%
6	Illinois	279	4.1%
16	Indiana	158	2.3%
12	Iowa	180	2.6%
20	Kansas	134	2.0%
24	Kentucky	110	1.6%
7	Louisiana	239	3.5%
43	Maine	36	0.5%
35	Maryland	53	0.8%
22	Massachusetts	125	1.8%
10	Michigan	196	2.9%
8	Minnesota	230	3.4%
32	Mississippi	61	0.9%
14	Missouri	167	2.4%
38	Montana	49	0.7%
29	Nebraska	67	1.0%
41	Nevada	37	0.5%
44	New Hampshire	35	0.5%
35	New Jersey	53	0.8%
30	New Mexico	65	0.9%
9	New York	207	3.0%
15	North Carolina	166	2.4%
45	North Dakota	31	0.5%
3	Ohio	334	4.9%
11	Oklahoma	189	2.8%
32	Oregon	61	0.9%
5	Pennsylvania	288	4.2%
46	Rhode Island	23	0.3%
27	South Carolina	72	1.1%
39	South Dakota	45	0.7%
18	Tennessee	142	2.1%
1	Texas	853	12.5%
40	Utah	42	0.6%
50	Vermont	13	0.2%
17	Virginia	156	2.3%
32	Washington	61	0.9%
28	West Virginia	68	1.0%
22	Wisconsin	125	1.8%
41	Wyoming	37	0.5%

RANK ORDER

RANK	STATE	AGENCIES	% of USA
1	Texas	853	12.5%
2	California	534	7.8%
3	Ohio	334	4.9%
4	Florida	322	4.7%
5	Pennsylvania	288	4.2%
6	Illinois	279	4.1%
7	Louisiana	239	3.5%
8	Minnesota	230	3.4%
9	New York	207	3.0%
10	Michigan	196	2.9%
11	Oklahoma	189	2.8%
12	Iowa	180	2.6%
13	Arkansas	179	2.6%
14	Missouri	167	2.4%
15	North Carolina	166	2.4%
16	Indiana	158	2.3%
17	Virginia	156	2.3%
18	Tennessee	142	2.1%
19	Alabama	140	2.0%
20	Kansas	134	2.0%
21	Colorado	129	1.9%
22	Massachusetts	125	1.8%
22	Wisconsin	125	1.8%
24	Kentucky	110	1.6%
25	Georgia	94	1.4%
26	Connecticut	83	1.2%
27	South Carolina	72	1.1%
28	West Virginia	68	1.0%
29	Nebraska	67	1.0%
30	New Mexico	65	0.9%
31	Arizona	63	0.9%
32	Mississippi	61	0.9%
32	Oregon	61	0.9%
32	Washington	61	0.9%
35	Maryland	53	0.8%
35	New Jersey	53	0.8%
37	Idaho	50	0.7%
38	Montana	49	0.7%
39	South Dakota	45	0.7%
40	Utah	42	0.6%
41	Nevada	37	0.5%
41	Wyoming	37	0.5%
43	Maine	36	0.5%
44	New Hampshire	35	0.5%
45	North Dakota	31	0.5%
46	Rhode Island	23	0.3%
47	Delaware	17	0.2%
48	Alaska	16	0.2%
49	Hawaii	14	0.2%
50	Vermont	13	0.2%
	District of Columbia	15	0.2%

Source: U.S. Department of Health and Human Services, Centers for Medicare and Medicaid Services OSCAR Database (February 21, 2002)

Certified by CMS to participate in the Medicare/Medicaid programs. Excludes agencies that do not accept federal funding. National total does not include 50 certified home health agencies in U.S. territories. A home health agency provides health services to individuals in their homes for the purpose of promoting, maintaining or restoring health or maximizing the level of independence, while minimizing the effects of disability and illness.

Medicare and Medicaid Certified Hospices in 2002

National Total = 2,250 Hospices*

ALPHA ORDER

RANK	STATE	HOSPICES	% of USA
9	Alabama	76	3.4%
50	Alaska	2	0.1%
25	Arizona	38	1.7%
20	Arkansas	46	2.0%
1	California	157	7.0%
29	Colorado	35	1.6%
34	Connecticut	26	1.2%
49	Delaware	5	0.2%
23	Florida	40	1.8%
7	Georgia	81	3.6%
47	Hawaii	7	0.3%
36	Idaho	24	1.1%
5	Illinois	85	3.8%
13	Indiana	60	2.7%
13	Iowa	60	2.7%
27	Kansas	37	1.6%
34	Kentucky	26	1.2%
21	Louisiana	44	2.0%
42	Maine	17	0.8%
30	Maryland	30	1.3%
25	Massachusetts	38	1.7%
6	Michigan	84	3.7%
12	Minnesota	63	2.8%
19	Mississippi	48	2.1%
11	Missouri	66	2.9%
37	Montana	22	1.0%
33	Nebraska	28	1.2%
45	Nevada	9	0.4%
38	New Hampshire	19	0.8%
23	New Jersey	40	1.8%
30	New Mexico	30	1.3%
16	New York	52	2.3%
10	North Carolina	73	3.2%
44	North Dakota	14	0.6%
4	Ohio	90	4.0%
8	Oklahoma	77	3.4%
22	Oregon	42	1.9%
3	Pennsylvania	115	5.1%
47	Rhode Island	7	0.3%
28	South Carolina	36	1.6%
43	South Dakota	15	0.7%
18	Tennessee	50	2.2%
2	Texas	131	5.8%
38	Utah	19	0.8%
45	Vermont	9	0.4%
16	Virginia	52	2.3%
30	Washington	30	1.3%
38	West Virginia	19	0.8%
15	Wisconsin	55	2.4%
41	Wyoming	18	0.8%

RANK ORDER

RANK	STATE	HOSPICES	% of USA
1	California	157	7.0%
2	Texas	131	5.8%
3	Pennsylvania	115	5.1%
4	Ohio	90	4.0%
5	Illinois	85	3.8%
6	Michigan	84	3.7%
7	Georgia	81	3.6%
8	Oklahoma	77	3.4%
9	Alabama	76	3.4%
10	North Carolina	73	3.2%
11	Missouri	66	2.9%
12	Minnesota	63	2.8%
13	Indiana	60	2.7%
13	Iowa	60	2.7%
15	Wisconsin	55	2.4%
16	New York	52	2.3%
16	Virginia	52	2.3%
18	Tennessee	50	2.2%
19	Mississippi	48	2.1%
20	Arkansas	46	2.0%
21	Louisiana	44	2.0%
22	Oregon	42	1.9%
23	Florida	40	1.8%
23	New Jersey	40	1.8%
25	Arizona	38	1.7%
25	Massachusetts	38	1.7%
27	Kansas	37	1.6%
28	South Carolina	36	1.6%
29	Colorado	35	1.6%
30	Maryland	30	1.3%
30	New Mexico	30	1.3%
30	Washington	30	1.3%
33	Nebraska	28	1.2%
34	Connecticut	26	1.2%
34	Kentucky	26	1.2%
36	Idaho	24	1.1%
37	Montana	22	1.0%
38	New Hampshire	19	0.8%
38	Utah	19	0.8%
38	West Virginia	19	0.8%
41	Wyoming	18	0.8%
42	Maine	17	0.8%
43	South Dakota	15	0.7%
44	North Dakota	14	0.6%
45	Nevada	9	0.4%
45	Vermont	9	0.4%
47	Hawaii	7	0.3%
47	Rhode Island	7	0.3%
49	Delaware	5	0.2%
50	Alaska	2	0.1%
	District of Columbia	3	0.1%

*Source: U.S. Department of Health and Human Services, Centers for Medicare and Medicaid Services
OSCAR Report 10 (February 21, 2002)*

*Certified by CMS to participate in the Medicare/Medicaid programs. Excludes licensed facilities that do not accept federal funding and facilities managed by the Department of Veterans Affairs. National total does not include 33 certified hospices in U.S. territories. An hospice provides specialized services for terminally ill people and their families.

Hospice Patients in Residential Facilities in 2002

National Total = 24,250 Patients*

ALPHA ORDER RANK	STATE	PATIENTS	% of USA		RANK ORDER RANK	STATE	PATIENTS	% of USA
29	Alabama	165	0.7%		1	Pennsylvania	4,273	17.6%
49	Alaska	0	0.0%		2	Florida	2,911	12.0%
20	Arizona	343	1.4%		3	Texas	2,288	9.4%
32	Arkansas	117	0.5%		4	Michigan	1,302	5.4%
7	California	957	3.9%		5	Oklahoma	1,250	5.2%
23	Colorado	295	1.2%		6	Ohio	1,239	5.1%
31	Connecticut	144	0.6%		7	California	957	3.9%
45	Delaware	7	0.0%		8	Indiana	925	3.8%
2	Florida	2,911	12.0%		9	Illinois	825	3.4%
12	Georgia	623	2.6%		10	Kentucky	689	2.8%
48	Hawaii	3	0.0%		11	Missouri	625	2.6%
44	Idaho	17	0.1%		12	Georgia	623	2.6%
9	Illinois	825	3.4%		13	New York	529	2.2%
8	Indiana	925	3.8%		14	Washington	463	1.9%
22	Iowa	296	1.2%		15	Kansas	394	1.6%
15	Kansas	394	1.6%		16	Minnesota	370	1.5%
10	Kentucky	689	2.8%		17	Massachusetts	365	1.5%
33	Louisiana	89	0.4%		18	Wisconsin	361	1.5%
38	Maine	46	0.2%		19	Oregon	360	1.5%
30	Maryland	163	0.7%		20	Arizona	343	1.4%
17	Massachusetts	365	1.5%		21	North Carolina	329	1.4%
4	Michigan	1,302	5.4%		22	Iowa	296	1.2%
16	Minnesota	370	1.5%		23	Colorado	295	1.2%
35	Mississippi	58	0.2%		24	New Jersey	259	1.1%
11	Missouri	625	2.6%		25	Nebraska	205	0.8%
41	Montana	30	0.1%		26	South Carolina	204	0.8%
25	Nebraska	205	0.8%		27	Tennessee	187	0.8%
37	Nevada	50	0.2%		28	Utah	167	0.7%
39	New Hampshire	38	0.2%		29	Alabama	165	0.7%
24	New Jersey	259	1.1%		30	Maryland	163	0.7%
34	New Mexico	86	0.4%		31	Connecticut	144	0.6%
13	New York	529	2.2%		32	Arkansas	117	0.5%
21	North Carolina	329	1.4%		33	Louisiana	89	0.4%
36	North Dakota	52	0.2%		34	New Mexico	86	0.4%
6	Ohio	1,239	5.1%		35	Mississippi	58	0.2%
5	Oklahoma	1,250	5.2%		36	North Dakota	52	0.2%
19	Oregon	360	1.5%		37	Nevada	50	0.2%
1	Pennsylvania	4,273	17.6%		38	Maine	46	0.2%
49	Rhode Island	0	0.0%		39	New Hampshire	38	0.2%
26	South Carolina	204	0.8%		40	Vermont	37	0.2%
47	South Dakota	4	0.0%		41	Montana	30	0.1%
27	Tennessee	187	0.8%		41	Virginia	30	0.1%
3	Texas	2,288	9.4%		43	West Virginia	28	0.1%
28	Utah	167	0.7%		44	Idaho	17	0.1%
40	Vermont	37	0.2%		45	Delaware	7	0.0%
41	Virginia	30	0.1%		46	Wyoming	6	0.0%
14	Washington	463	1.9%		47	South Dakota	4	0.0%
43	West Virginia	28	0.1%		48	Hawaii	3	0.0%
18	Wisconsin	361	1.5%		49	Alaska	0	0.0%
46	Wyoming	6	0.0%		49	Rhode Island	0	0.0%
						District of Columbia	46	0.2%

Source: U.S. Department of Health and Human Services, Centers for Medicare and Medicaid Services
   OSCAR Database (February 21, 2002)

*Patients in facilities certified by CMS to participate in the Medicare/Medicaid programs. Excludes licensed facilities that do not accept federal funding and facilities managed by the Department of Veterans Affairs. National total does not include seven patients in U.S. territories. An hospice provides specialized services for terminally ill people and their families.

Medicare and Medicaid Certified Nursing Care Facilities in 2002

National Total = 14,743 Nursing Care Facilities*

ALPHA ORDER

RANK	STATE	FACILITIES	% of USA
27	Alabama	223	1.5%
50	Alaska	15	0.1%
33	Arizona	139	0.9%
29	Arkansas	193	1.3%
1	California	1,247	8.5%
28	Colorado	201	1.4%
23	Connecticut	245	1.7%
48	Delaware	37	0.3%
5	Florida	718	4.9%
16	Georgia	329	2.2%
47	Hawaii	41	0.3%
41	Idaho	81	0.5%
7	Illinois	656	4.4%
8	Indiana	498	3.4%
17	Iowa	312	2.1%
20	Kansas	257	1.7%
18	Kentucky	303	2.1%
22	Louisiana	249	1.7%
34	Maine	122	0.8%
24	Maryland	237	1.6%
9	Massachusetts	488	3.3%
13	Michigan	389	2.6%
12	Minnesota	406	2.8%
32	Mississippi	148	1.0%
10	Missouri	458	3.1%
37	Montana	101	0.7%
31	Nebraska	171	1.2%
45	Nevada	44	0.3%
44	New Hampshire	67	0.5%
15	New Jersey	361	2.4%
43	New Mexico	70	0.5%
6	New York	665	4.5%
11	North Carolina	409	2.8%
40	North Dakota	86	0.6%
3	Ohio	901	6.1%
26	Oklahoma	231	1.6%
35	Oregon	121	0.8%
4	Pennsylvania	744	5.0%
38	Rhode Island	97	0.7%
30	South Carolina	177	1.2%
39	South Dakota	89	0.6%
19	Tennessee	285	1.9%
2	Texas	983	6.7%
41	Utah	81	0.5%
46	Vermont	43	0.3%
24	Virginia	237	1.6%
20	Washington	257	1.7%
36	West Virginia	116	0.8%
14	Wisconsin	362	2.5%
49	Wyoming	33	0.2%

RANK ORDER

RANK	STATE	FACILITIES	% of USA
1	California	1,247	8.5%
2	Texas	983	6.7%
3	Ohio	901	6.1%
4	Pennsylvania	744	5.0%
5	Florida	718	4.9%
6	New York	665	4.5%
7	Illinois	656	4.4%
8	Indiana	498	3.4%
9	Massachusetts	488	3.3%
10	Missouri	458	3.1%
11	North Carolina	409	2.8%
12	Minnesota	406	2.8%
13	Michigan	389	2.6%
14	Wisconsin	362	2.5%
15	New Jersey	361	2.4%
16	Georgia	329	2.2%
17	Iowa	312	2.1%
18	Kentucky	303	2.1%
19	Tennessee	285	1.9%
20	Kansas	257	1.7%
20	Washington	257	1.7%
22	Louisiana	249	1.7%
23	Connecticut	245	1.7%
24	Maryland	237	1.6%
24	Virginia	237	1.6%
26	Oklahoma	231	1.6%
27	Alabama	223	1.5%
28	Colorado	201	1.4%
29	Arkansas	193	1.3%
30	South Carolina	177	1.2%
31	Nebraska	171	1.2%
32	Mississippi	148	1.0%
33	Arizona	139	0.9%
34	Maine	122	0.8%
35	Oregon	121	0.8%
36	West Virginia	116	0.8%
37	Montana	101	0.7%
38	Rhode Island	97	0.7%
39	South Dakota	89	0.6%
40	North Dakota	86	0.6%
41	Idaho	81	0.5%
41	Utah	81	0.5%
43	New Mexico	70	0.5%
44	New Hampshire	67	0.5%
45	Nevada	44	0.3%
46	Vermont	43	0.3%
47	Hawaii	41	0.3%
48	Delaware	37	0.3%
49	Wyoming	33	0.2%
50	Alaska	15	0.1%
	District of Columbia	20	0.1%

Source: U.S. Department of Health and Human Services, Centers for Medicare and Medicaid Services
    OSCAR Report 10 (February 21, 2002)
*Certified by CMS to participate in the Medicare/Medicaid programs. Excludes licensed facilities that do not accept federal funding and facilities managed by the Department of Veterans Affairs. National total does not include nine certified nursing facilities in U.S. territories.

Beds in Medicare and Medicaid Certified Nursing Care Facilities in 2002

National Total = 1,520,276 Beds*

ALPHA ORDER

RANK	STATE	BEDS	% of USA
22	Alabama	24,816	1.6%
50	Alaska	744	0.0%
31	Arizona	15,462	1.0%
27	Arkansas	18,523	1.2%
2	California	110,372	7.3%
29	Colorado	16,968	1.1%
18	Connecticut	29,968	2.0%
46	Delaware	3,766	0.2%
7	Florida	78,347	5.2%
16	Georgia	36,228	2.4%
47	Hawaii	3,664	0.2%
44	Idaho	5,952	0.4%
6	Illinois	78,936	5.2%
10	Indiana	47,682	3.1%
25	Iowa	22,732	1.5%
28	Kansas	17,888	1.2%
23	Kentucky	24,077	1.6%
19	Louisiana	27,973	1.8%
37	Maine	7,763	0.5%
20	Maryland	27,856	1.8%
8	Massachusetts	52,150	3.4%
12	Michigan	43,239	2.8%
15	Minnesota	38,280	2.5%
33	Mississippi	12,570	0.8%
11	Missouri	43,766	2.9%
38	Montana	7,259	0.5%
32	Nebraska	13,180	0.9%
45	Nevada	4,646	0.3%
41	New Hampshire	6,494	0.4%
9	New Jersey	48,092	3.2%
42	New Mexico	6,395	0.4%
1	New York	120,558	7.9%
14	North Carolina	40,300	2.7%
40	North Dakota	6,571	0.4%
5	Ohio	85,543	5.6%
26	Oklahoma	20,419	1.3%
34	Oregon	11,060	0.7%
4	Pennsylvania	89,112	5.9%
35	Rhode Island	9,848	0.6%
30	South Carolina	16,749	1.1%
43	South Dakota	6,166	0.4%
17	Tennessee	31,100	2.0%
3	Texas	91,969	6.0%
39	Utah	6,798	0.4%
48	Vermont	3,559	0.2%
21	Virginia	26,642	1.8%
24	Washington	23,180	1.5%
36	West Virginia	9,065	0.6%
13	Wisconsin	40,383	2.7%
49	Wyoming	2,808	0.2%

RANK ORDER

RANK	STATE	BEDS	% of USA
1	New York	120,558	7.9%
2	California	110,372	7.3%
3	Texas	91,969	6.0%
4	Pennsylvania	89,112	5.9%
5	Ohio	85,543	5.6%
6	Illinois	78,936	5.2%
7	Florida	78,347	5.2%
8	Massachusetts	52,150	3.4%
9	New Jersey	48,092	3.2%
10	Indiana	47,682	3.1%
11	Missouri	43,766	2.9%
12	Michigan	43,239	2.8%
13	Wisconsin	40,383	2.7%
14	North Carolina	40,300	2.7%
15	Minnesota	38,280	2.5%
16	Georgia	36,228	2.4%
17	Tennessee	31,100	2.0%
18	Connecticut	29,968	2.0%
19	Louisiana	27,973	1.8%
20	Maryland	27,856	1.8%
21	Virginia	26,642	1.8%
22	Alabama	24,816	1.6%
23	Kentucky	24,077	1.6%
24	Washington	23,180	1.5%
25	Iowa	22,732	1.5%
26	Oklahoma	20,419	1.3%
27	Arkansas	18,523	1.2%
28	Kansas	17,888	1.2%
29	Colorado	16,968	1.1%
30	South Carolina	16,749	1.1%
31	Arizona	15,462	1.0%
32	Nebraska	13,180	0.9%
33	Mississippi	12,570	0.8%
34	Oregon	11,060	0.7%
35	Rhode Island	9,848	0.6%
36	West Virginia	9,065	0.6%
37	Maine	7,763	0.5%
38	Montana	7,259	0.5%
39	Utah	6,798	0.4%
40	North Dakota	6,571	0.4%
41	New Hampshire	6,494	0.4%
42	New Mexico	6,395	0.4%
43	South Dakota	6,166	0.4%
44	Idaho	5,952	0.4%
45	Nevada	4,646	0.3%
46	Delaware	3,766	0.2%
47	Hawaii	3,664	0.2%
48	Vermont	3,559	0.2%
49	Wyoming	2,808	0.2%
50	Alaska	744	0.0%
	District of Columbia	2,658	0.2%

Source: U.S. Department of Health and Human Services, Centers for Medicare and Medicaid Services
    OSCAR Database (February 21, 2002)

Beds in nursing care facilities certified by CMS to participate in the Medicare/Medicaid programs. National total does not include 160 beds in U.S. territories.

Rate of Beds in Medicare and Medicaid Certified Nursing Care Facilities in 2002

National Rate = 359 Beds per 1,000 Population 85 Years and Older*

ALPHA ORDER

RANK	STATE	RATE
25	Alabama	369
42	Alaska	282
48	Arizona	226
17	Arkansas	398
46	California	259
31	Colorado	352
6	Connecticut	466
26	Delaware	357
47	Florida	236
15	Georgia	412
49	Hawaii	209
36	Idaho	330
16	Illinois	411
1	Indiana	521
32	Iowa	349
33	Kansas	346
14	Kentucky	413
3	Louisiana	477
34	Maine	333
13	Maryland	416
7	Massachusetts	447
39	Michigan	304
7	Minnesota	447
40	Mississippi	293
10	Missouri	444
4	Montana	473
18	Nebraska	388
45	Nevada	273
28	New Hampshire	356
30	New Jersey	354
44	New Mexico	274
19	New York	387
22	North Carolina	382
9	North Dakota	446
2	Ohio	484
26	Oklahoma	357
50	Oregon	193
24	Pennsylvania	375
5	Rhode Island	471
34	South Carolina	333
21	South Dakota	383
22	Tennessee	382
19	Texas	387
37	Utah	313
28	Vermont	356
38	Virginia	305
43	Washington	276
41	West Virginia	285
11	Wisconsin	422
12	Wyoming	417

RANK ORDER

RANK	STATE	RATE
1	Indiana	521
2	Ohio	484
3	Louisiana	477
4	Montana	473
5	Rhode Island	471
6	Connecticut	466
7	Massachusetts	447
7	Minnesota	447
9	North Dakota	446
10	Missouri	444
11	Wisconsin	422
12	Wyoming	417
13	Maryland	416
14	Kentucky	413
15	Georgia	412
16	Illinois	411
17	Arkansas	398
18	Nebraska	388
19	New York	387
19	Texas	387
21	South Dakota	383
22	North Carolina	382
22	Tennessee	382
24	Pennsylvania	375
25	Alabama	369
26	Delaware	357
26	Oklahoma	357
28	New Hampshire	356
28	Vermont	356
30	New Jersey	354
31	Colorado	352
32	Iowa	349
33	Kansas	346
34	Maine	333
34	South Carolina	333
36	Idaho	330
37	Utah	313
38	Virginia	305
39	Michigan	304
40	Mississippi	293
41	West Virginia	285
42	Alaska	282
43	Washington	276
44	New Mexico	274
45	Nevada	273
46	California	259
47	Florida	236
48	Arizona	226
49	Hawaii	209
50	Oregon	193
	District of Columbia	296

Source: U.S. Department of Health and Human Services, Centers for Medicare and Medicaid Services
OSCAR Database (February 21, 2002)
*Beds in nursing care facilities certified by CMS to participate in the Medicare/Medicaid programs. National rate does not include beds or population in U.S. territories. Calculated using 2000 Census population count.

Nursing Home Occupancy Rate in 1999

National Rate = 82.7% of Beds in Nursing Homes Occupied

ALPHA ORDER

RANK ORDER

RANK	STATE	RATE		RANK	STATE	RATE
3	Alabama	92.5		1	New York	94.8
41	Alaska	76.4		2	Mississippi	93.7
41	Arizona	76.4		3	Alabama	92.5
38	Arkansas	77.3		4	Hawaii	92.2
32	California	81.3		4	North Dakota	92.2
27	Colorado	82.8		6	Vermont	91.8
9	Connecticut	91.5		7	New Hampshire	91.6
45	Delaware	74.0		7	South Dakota	91.6
28	Florida	82.6		9	Connecticut	91.5
10	Georgia	91.1		10	Georgia	91.1
4	Hawaii	92.2		11	Tennessee	90.4
44	Idaho	74.7		12	North Carolina	90.1
43	Illinois	76.3		13	Kentucky	90.0
49	Indiana	69.5		13	Virginia	90.0
35	Iowa	79.3		15	Minnesota	89.8
31	Kansas	81.4		15	West Virginia	89.8
13	Kentucky	90.0		17	Maine	89.7
37	Louisiana	78.7		17	New Jersey	89.7
17	Maine	89.7		19	Pennsylvania	88.7
29	Maryland	82.1		19	Rhode Island	88.7
21	Massachusetts	88.6		21	Massachusetts	88.6
25	Michigan	84.3		22	New Mexico	88.3
15	Minnesota	89.8		23	South Carolina	86.5
2	Mississippi	93.7		24	Wisconsin	85.5
46	Missouri	71.7		25	Michigan	84.3
34	Montana	79.8		26	Nebraska	83.3
26	Nebraska	83.3		27	Colorado	82.8
48	Nevada	70.7		28	Florida	82.6
7	New Hampshire	91.6		29	Maryland	82.1
17	New Jersey	89.7		30	Wyoming	81.9
22	New Mexico	88.3		31	Kansas	81.4
1	New York	94.8		32	California	81.3
12	North Carolina	90.1		32	Washington	81.3
4	North Dakota	92.2		34	Montana	79.8
36	Ohio	78.9		35	Iowa	79.3
47	Oklahoma	71.0		36	Ohio	78.9
40	Oregon	76.8		37	Louisiana	78.7
19	Pennsylvania	88.7		38	Arkansas	77.3
19	Rhode Island	88.7		39	Utah	77.2
23	South Carolina	86.5		40	Oregon	76.8
7	South Dakota	91.6		41	Alaska	76.4
11	Tennessee	90.4		41	Arizona	76.4
50	Texas	67.8		43	Illinois	76.3
39	Utah	77.2		44	Idaho	74.7
6	Vermont	91.8		45	Delaware	74.0
13	Virginia	90.0		46	Missouri	71.7
32	Washington	81.3		47	Oklahoma	71.0
15	West Virginia	89.8		48	Nevada	70.7
24	Wisconsin	85.5		49	Indiana	69.5
30	Wyoming	81.9		50	Texas	67.8
					District of Columbia	93.3

Source: U.S. Department of Health and Human Services, Centers for Medicare and Medicaid Services
   "Health, United States, 2001"

Nursing Home Resident Rate in 1999

National Rate = 358.0 Residents per 1,000 Population Age 85 and Older*

ALPHA ORDER

RANK	STATE	RATE
30	Alabama	358.7
43	Alaska	260.6
48	Arizona	208.7
9	Arkansas	444.1
45	California	254.9
32	Colorado	352.3
4	Connecticut	468.9
26	Delaware	370.6
47	Florida	214.3
18	Georgia	424.5
49	Hawaii	205.6
42	Idaho	261.4
12	Illinois	440.5
2	Indiana	479.2
6	Iowa	461.2
14	Kansas	438.7
23	Kentucky	398.3
1	Louisiana	550.5
35	Maine	339.4
25	Maryland	372.4
11	Massachusetts	440.7
40	Michigan	298.6
3	Minnesota	474.6
24	Mississippi	389.7
20	Missouri	402.2
22	Montana	399.5
10	Nebraska	440.8
46	Nevada	224.5
19	New Hampshire	405.1
34	New Jersey	344.1
39	New Mexico	299.3
29	New York	362.5
33	North Carolina	350.0
13	North Dakota	440.3
5	Ohio	468.8
16	Oklahoma	429.8
50	Oregon	187.9
27	Pennsylvania	367.5
15	Rhode Island	436.3
36	South Carolina	330.9
7	South Dakota	457.5
8	Tennessee	450.0
28	Texas	365.7
41	Utah	267.6
31	Vermont	356.4
37	Virginia	323.2
44	Washington	258.6
38	West Virginia	315.7
17	Wisconsin	427.3
21	Wyoming	400.5

RANK ORDER

RANK	STATE	RATE
1	Louisiana	550.5
2	Indiana	479.2
3	Minnesota	474.6
4	Connecticut	468.9
5	Ohio	468.8
6	Iowa	461.2
7	South Dakota	457.5
8	Tennessee	450.0
9	Arkansas	444.1
10	Nebraska	440.8
11	Massachusetts	440.7
12	Illinois	440.5
13	North Dakota	440.3
14	Kansas	438.7
15	Rhode Island	436.3
16	Oklahoma	429.8
17	Wisconsin	427.3
18	Georgia	424.5
19	New Hampshire	405.1
20	Missouri	402.2
21	Wyoming	400.5
22	Montana	399.5
23	Kentucky	398.3
24	Mississippi	389.7
25	Maryland	372.4
26	Delaware	370.6
27	Pennsylvania	367.5
28	Texas	365.7
29	New York	362.5
30	Alabama	358.7
31	Vermont	356.4
32	Colorado	352.3
33	North Carolina	350.0
34	New Jersey	344.1
35	Maine	339.4
36	South Carolina	330.9
37	Virginia	323.2
38	West Virginia	315.7
39	New Mexico	299.3
40	Michigan	298.6
41	Utah	267.6
42	Idaho	261.4
43	Alaska	260.6
44	Washington	258.6
45	California	254.9
46	Nevada	224.5
47	Florida	214.3
48	Arizona	208.7
49	Hawaii	205.6
50	Oregon	187.9
	District of Columbia	311.4

Source: U.S. Department of Health and Human Services, Centers for Medicare and Medicaid Services
        "Health, United States, 2001"
*Number of nursing home residents (all ages) per 1,000 resident population 85 years of age and over.

Nursing Home Population 85 Years Old and Older in 1999

National Total = 1,495,000*

ALPHA ORDER | | | | | RANK ORDER | | | |

RANK	STATE	POPULATION	% of USA		RANK	STATE	POPULATION	% of USA
24	Alabama	23,000	1.5%		1	New York	112,000	7.5%
50	Alaska	1,000	0.1%		2	California	108,000	7.2%
33	Arizona	14,000	0.9%		3	Illinois	85,000	5.7%
28	Arkansas	20,000	1.3%		3	Pennsylvania	85,000	5.7%
2	California	108,000	7.2%		3	Texas	85,000	5.7%
29	Colorado	17,000	1.1%		6	Ohio	83,000	5.6%
19	Connecticut	30,000	2.0%		7	Florida	69,000	4.6%
45	Delaware	4,000	0.3%		8	Massachusetts	51,000	3.4%
7	Florida	69,000	4.6%		9	New Jersey	46,000	3.1%
16	Georgia	36,000	2.4%		10	Indiana	43,000	2.9%
45	Hawaii	4,000	0.3%		10	Michigan	43,000	2.9%
44	Idaho	5,000	0.3%		12	Minnesota	40,000	2.7%
3	Illinois	85,000	5.7%		12	Wisconsin	40,000	2.7%
10	Indiana	43,000	2.9%		14	Missouri	39,000	2.6%
19	Iowa	30,000	2.0%		15	North Carolina	37,000	2.5%
24	Kansas	23,000	1.5%		16	Georgia	36,000	2.4%
24	Kentucky	23,000	1.5%		16	Tennessee	36,000	2.4%
18	Louisiana	31,000	2.1%		18	Louisiana	31,000	2.1%
37	Maine	8,000	0.5%		19	Connecticut	30,000	2.0%
22	Maryland	25,000	1.7%		19	Iowa	30,000	2.0%
8	Massachusetts	51,000	3.4%		21	Virginia	27,000	1.8%
10	Michigan	43,000	2.9%		22	Maryland	25,000	1.7%
12	Minnesota	40,000	2.7%		22	Oklahoma	25,000	1.7%
30	Mississippi	16,000	1.1%		24	Alabama	23,000	1.5%
14	Missouri	39,000	2.6%		24	Kansas	23,000	1.5%
40	Montana	6,000	0.4%		24	Kentucky	23,000	1.5%
31	Nebraska	15,000	1.0%		27	Washington	21,000	1.4%
45	Nevada	4,000	0.3%		28	Arkansas	20,000	1.3%
38	New Hampshire	7,000	0.5%		29	Colorado	17,000	1.1%
9	New Jersey	46,000	3.1%		30	Mississippi	16,000	1.1%
40	New Mexico	6,000	0.4%		31	Nebraska	15,000	1.0%
1	New York	112,000	7.5%		31	South Carolina	15,000	1.0%
15	North Carolina	37,000	2.5%		33	Arizona	14,000	0.9%
40	North Dakota	6,000	0.4%		34	Oregon	11,000	0.7%
6	Ohio	83,000	5.6%		35	West Virginia	10,000	0.7%
22	Oklahoma	25,000	1.7%		36	Rhode Island	9,000	0.6%
34	Oregon	11,000	0.7%		37	Maine	8,000	0.5%
3	Pennsylvania	85,000	5.7%		38	New Hampshire	7,000	0.5%
36	Rhode Island	9,000	0.6%		38	South Dakota	7,000	0.5%
31	South Carolina	15,000	1.0%		40	Montana	6,000	0.4%
38	South Dakota	7,000	0.5%		40	New Mexico	6,000	0.4%
16	Tennessee	36,000	2.4%		40	North Dakota	6,000	0.4%
3	Texas	85,000	5.7%		40	Utah	6,000	0.4%
40	Utah	6,000	0.4%		44	Idaho	5,000	0.3%
48	Vermont	3,000	0.2%		45	Delaware	4,000	0.3%
21	Virginia	27,000	1.8%		45	Hawaii	4,000	0.3%
27	Washington	21,000	1.4%		45	Nevada	4,000	0.3%
35	West Virginia	10,000	0.7%		48	Vermont	3,000	0.2%
12	Wisconsin	40,000	2.7%		48	Wyoming	3,000	0.2%
48	Wyoming	3,000	0.2%		50	Alaska	1,000	0.1%
						District of Columbia	3,000	0.2%

Source: MQ Press using data from U.S. Dept of Health & Human Services, Centers for Medicare and Medicaid Services
"Health, United States, 2001"
*Estimated using nursing home resident rate and population 85 years old and older.

Health Care Establishments in 1999

National Total = 524,252 Establishments*

ALPHA ORDER					RANK ORDER			
RANK	STATE	ESTABLISH'S	% of USA		RANK	STATE	ESTABLISH'S	% of USA
27	Alabama	6,761	1.3%		1	California	67,155	12.8%
48	Alaska	1,228	0.2%		2	New York	37,999	7.2%
20	Arizona	9,076	1.7%		3	Texas	36,032	6.9%
32	Arkansas	4,569	0.9%		4	Florida	34,372	6.6%
1	California	67,155	12.8%		5	Pennsylvania	25,733	4.9%
21	Colorado	8,558	1.6%		6	Illinois	21,310	4.1%
24	Connecticut	7,379	1.4%		7	Ohio	20,750	4.0%
46	Delaware	1,392	0.3%		8	Michigan	18,935	3.6%
4	Florida	34,372	6.6%		9	New Jersey	18,633	3.6%
10	Georgia	13,006	2.5%		10	Georgia	13,006	2.5%
40	Hawaii	2,479	0.5%		11	Massachusetts	12,788	2.4%
41	Idaho	2,462	0.5%		12	North Carolina	12,098	2.3%
6	Illinois	21,310	4.1%		13	Washington	11,529	2.2%
16	Indiana	9,996	1.9%		14	Virginia	11,422	2.2%
30	Iowa	5,299	1.0%		15	Maryland	10,707	2.0%
31	Kansas	4,918	0.9%		16	Indiana	9,996	1.9%
26	Kentucky	6,776	1.3%		17	Missouri	9,849	1.9%
23	Louisiana	7,997	1.5%		18	Tennessee	9,836	1.9%
39	Maine	2,841	0.5%		19	Wisconsin	9,261	1.8%
15	Maryland	10,707	2.0%		20	Arizona	9,076	1.7%
11	Massachusetts	12,788	2.4%		21	Colorado	8,558	1.6%
8	Michigan	18,935	3.6%		22	Minnesota	8,301	1.6%
22	Minnesota	8,301	1.6%		23	Louisiana	7,997	1.5%
34	Mississippi	3,809	0.7%		24	Connecticut	7,379	1.4%
17	Missouri	9,849	1.9%		25	Oregon	7,315	1.4%
44	Montana	1,948	0.4%		26	Kentucky	6,776	1.3%
38	Nebraska	2,875	0.5%		27	Alabama	6,761	1.3%
36	Nevada	3,327	0.6%		28	Oklahoma	6,561	1.3%
42	New Hampshire	2,281	0.4%		29	South Carolina	5,890	1.1%
9	New Jersey	18,633	3.6%		30	Iowa	5,299	1.0%
37	New Mexico	2,953	0.6%		31	Kansas	4,918	0.9%
2	New York	37,999	7.2%		32	Arkansas	4,569	0.9%
12	North Carolina	12,098	2.3%		33	Utah	3,868	0.7%
49	North Dakota	1,066	0.2%		34	Mississippi	3,809	0.7%
7	Ohio	20,750	4.0%		35	West Virginia	3,534	0.7%
28	Oklahoma	6,561	1.3%		36	Nevada	3,327	0.6%
25	Oregon	7,315	1.4%		37	New Mexico	2,953	0.6%
5	Pennsylvania	25,733	4.9%		38	Nebraska	2,875	0.5%
43	Rhode Island	2,188	0.4%		39	Maine	2,841	0.5%
29	South Carolina	5,890	1.1%		40	Hawaii	2,479	0.5%
45	South Dakota	1,401	0.3%		41	Idaho	2,462	0.5%
18	Tennessee	9,836	1.9%		42	New Hampshire	2,281	0.4%
3	Texas	36,032	6.9%		43	Rhode Island	2,188	0.4%
33	Utah	3,868	0.7%		44	Montana	1,948	0.4%
47	Vermont	1,304	0.2%		45	South Dakota	1,401	0.3%
14	Virginia	11,422	2.2%		46	Delaware	1,392	0.3%
13	Washington	11,529	2.2%		47	Vermont	1,304	0.2%
35	West Virginia	3,534	0.7%		48	Alaska	1,228	0.2%
19	Wisconsin	9,261	1.8%		49	North Dakota	1,066	0.2%
50	Wyoming	1,022	0.2%		50	Wyoming	1,022	0.2%
						District of Columbia	1,463	0.3%

Source: U.S. Bureau of the Census
   "County Business Patterns 1999 (NAICS)" (http://tier2.census.gov/cbp_naics/index.html)
*Includes establishments exempt from as well as subject to the federal income tax. Includes those establishments within the North American Industry Classification System (NAICS) classifications 621 (ambulatory health care services), 622 (hospitals) and 623 (nursing and residential care facilities).

Offices and Clinics of Doctors of Medicine in 1997

National Total = 185,094 Establishments*

ALPHA ORDER

RANK	STATE	ESTABLISH'S	% of USA
21	Alabama	2,694	1.5%
47	Alaska	356	0.2%
17	Arizona	3,269	1.8%
29	Arkansas	1,645	0.9%
1	California	24,079	13.0%
23	Colorado	2,586	1.4%
22	Connecticut	2,661	1.4%
45	Delaware	572	0.3%
4	Florida	13,784	7.4%
10	Georgia	5,081	2.7%
37	Hawaii	1,022	0.6%
42	Idaho	752	0.4%
8	Illinois	7,440	4.0%
16	Indiana	3,387	1.8%
34	Iowa	1,283	0.7%
32	Kansas	1,368	0.7%
24	Kentucky	2,474	1.3%
20	Louisiana	3,051	1.6%
39	Maine	838	0.5%
11	Maryland	4,343	2.3%
14	Massachusetts	3,844	2.1%
9	Michigan	6,234	3.4%
36	Minnesota	1,217	0.7%
30	Mississippi	1,520	0.8%
18	Missouri	3,160	1.7%
44	Montana	586	0.3%
40	Nebraska	774	0.4%
33	Nevada	1,335	0.7%
43	New Hampshire	656	0.4%
6	New Jersey	7,644	4.1%
38	New Mexico	941	0.5%
2	New York	15,137	8.2%
13	North Carolina	3,858	2.1%
50	North Dakota	191	0.1%
7	Ohio	7,573	4.1%
27	Oklahoma	2,189	1.2%
28	Oregon	2,040	1.1%
5	Pennsylvania	9,078	4.9%
41	Rhode Island	764	0.4%
25	South Carolina	2,216	1.2%
49	South Dakota	332	0.2%
15	Tennessee	3,620	2.0%
3	Texas	14,041	7.6%
35	Utah	1,219	0.7%
46	Vermont	360	0.2%
12	Virginia	4,277	2.3%
19	Washington	3,058	1.7%
31	West Virginia	1,415	0.8%
26	Wisconsin	2,198	1.2%
48	Wyoming	345	0.2%

RANK ORDER

RANK	STATE	ESTABLISH'S	% of USA
1	California	24,079	13.0%
2	New York	15,137	8.2%
3	Texas	14,041	7.6%
4	Florida	13,784	7.4%
5	Pennsylvania	9,078	4.9%
6	New Jersey	7,644	4.1%
7	Ohio	7,573	4.1%
8	Illinois	7,440	4.0%
9	Michigan	6,234	3.4%
10	Georgia	5,081	2.7%
11	Maryland	4,343	2.3%
12	Virginia	4,277	2.3%
13	North Carolina	3,858	2.1%
14	Massachusetts	3,844	2.1%
15	Tennessee	3,620	2.0%
16	Indiana	3,387	1.8%
17	Arizona	3,269	1.8%
18	Missouri	3,160	1.7%
19	Washington	3,058	1.7%
20	Louisiana	3,051	1.6%
21	Alabama	2,694	1.5%
22	Connecticut	2,661	1.4%
23	Colorado	2,586	1.4%
24	Kentucky	2,474	1.3%
25	South Carolina	2,216	1.2%
26	Wisconsin	2,198	1.2%
27	Oklahoma	2,189	1.2%
28	Oregon	2,040	1.1%
29	Arkansas	1,645	0.9%
30	Mississippi	1,520	0.8%
31	West Virginia	1,415	0.8%
32	Kansas	1,368	0.7%
33	Nevada	1,335	0.7%
34	Iowa	1,283	0.7%
35	Utah	1,219	0.7%
36	Minnesota	1,217	0.7%
37	Hawaii	1,022	0.6%
38	New Mexico	941	0.5%
39	Maine	838	0.5%
40	Nebraska	774	0.4%
41	Rhode Island	764	0.4%
42	Idaho	752	0.4%
43	New Hampshire	656	0.4%
44	Montana	586	0.3%
45	Delaware	572	0.3%
46	Vermont	360	0.2%
47	Alaska	356	0.2%
48	Wyoming	345	0.2%
49	South Dakota	332	0.2%
50	North Dakota	191	0.1%
	District of Columbia	587	0.3%

Source: U.S. Bureau of the Census
"1997 Economic Census, Health Care and Social Assistance" (EC97562A, October 1999)
*Includes only establishments subject to the federal income tax.

Offices and Clinics of Dentists in 1997

National Total = 114,178 Establishments*

ALPHA ORDER					RANK ORDER			
RANK	STATE	ESTABLISH'S	% of USA		RANK	STATE	ESTABLISH'S	% of USA
27	Alabama	1,356	1.2%		1	California	16,269	14.2%
45	Alaska	292	0.3%		2	New York	8,694	7.6%
24	Arizona	1,641	1.4%		3	Texas	6,691	5.9%
33	Arkansas	898	0.8%		4	Florida	6,182	5.4%
1	California	16,269	14.2%		5	Pennsylvania	5,433	4.8%
20	Colorado	2,042	1.8%		6	Illinois	5,383	4.7%
22	Connecticut	1,774	1.6%		7	Ohio	4,519	4.0%
49	Delaware	218	0.2%		8	Michigan	4,352	3.8%
4	Florida	6,182	5.4%		9	New Jersey	4,272	3.7%
13	Georgia	2,547	2.3%		10	Massachusetts	2,929	2.6%
36	Hawaii	657	0.6%		11	Washington	2,827	2.5%
41	Idaho	502	0.4%		12	Virginia	2,645	2.3%
6	Illinois	5,383	4.7%		13	Georgia	2,574	2.3%
16	Indiana	2,208	1.9%		14	Maryland	2,371	2.1%
30	Iowa	1,113	1.0%		15	North Carolina	2,323	2.0%
32	Kansas	1,012	0.9%		16	Indiana	2,208	1.9%
26	Kentucky	1,516	1.3%		17	Wisconsin	2,203	1.9%
25	Louisiana	1,541	1.3%		18	Missouri	2,052	1.8%
42	Maine	462	0.4%		19	Tennessee	2,050	1.8%
14	Maryland	2,371	2.1%		20	Colorado	2,042	1.8%
10	Massachusetts	2,929	2.6%		21	Minnesota	2,002	1.8%
8	Michigan	4,352	3.8%		22	Connecticut	1,774	1.6%
21	Minnesota	2,002	1.8%		23	Oregon	1,680	1.5%
34	Mississippi	780	0.7%		24	Arizona	1,641	1.4%
18	Missouri	2,052	1.8%		25	Louisiana	1,541	1.3%
43	Montana	419	0.4%		26	Kentucky	1,516	1.3%
35	Nebraska	754	0.7%		27	Alabama	1,356	1.2%
38	Nevada	575	0.5%		28	Oklahoma	1,268	1.1%
40	New Hampshire	533	0.5%		29	South Carolina	1,216	1.1%
9	New Jersey	4,272	3.7%		30	Iowa	1,113	1.0%
39	New Mexico	557	0.5%		31	Utah	1,088	1.0%
2	New York	8,694	7.6%		32	Kansas	1,012	0.9%
15	North Carolina	2,323	2.0%		33	Arkansas	898	0.8%
48	North Dakota	246	0.2%		34	Mississippi	780	0.7%
7	Ohio	4,519	4.0%		35	Nebraska	754	0.7%
28	Oklahoma	1,268	1.1%		36	Hawaii	657	0.6%
23	Oregon	1,680	1.5%		37	West Virginia	588	0.5%
5	Pennsylvania	5,433	4.8%		38	Nevada	575	0.5%
44	Rhode Island	410	0.4%		39	New Mexico	557	0.5%
29	South Carolina	1,216	1.1%		40	New Hampshire	533	0.5%
46	South Dakota	267	0.2%		41	Idaho	502	0.4%
19	Tennessee	2,050	1.8%		42	Maine	462	0.4%
3	Texas	6,691	5.9%		43	Montana	419	0.4%
31	Utah	1,088	1.0%		44	Rhode Island	410	0.4%
47	Vermont	256	0.2%		45	Alaska	292	0.3%
12	Virginia	2,645	2.3%		46	South Dakota	267	0.2%
11	Washington	2,827	2.5%		47	Vermont	256	0.2%
37	West Virginia	588	0.5%		48	North Dakota	246	0.2%
17	Wisconsin	2,203	1.9%		49	Delaware	218	0.2%
50	Wyoming	209	0.2%		50	Wyoming	209	0.2%
						District of Columbia	329	0.3%

Source: U.S. Bureau of the Census
   "1997 Economic Census, Health Care and Social Assistance" (EC97562A, October 1999)
*Includes only establishments subject to the federal income tax.

IV. FINANCE

236   Persons Not Covered by Health Insurance in 2000
237   Percent of Population Not Covered by Health Insurance in 2000
238   Persons Covered by Health Insurance in 2000
239   Percent of Population Covered by Health Insurance in 2000
240   Persons Not Covered by Health Insurance in 1996
241   Percent of Population Not Covered by Health Insurance in 1996
242   Change in Number of Persons Uninsured: 1996 to 2000
243   Percent Change in Number of Uninsured: 1996 to 2000
244   Change in Percent of Population Uninsured: 1996 to 2000
245   Percent of Children Not Covered by Health Insurance in 2000
246   State Children's Health Insurance Program Enrollment in 2001
247   Percent Change in State Children's Health Insurance Program Enrollment: 2000 to 2001
248   Percent of Children Enrolled in State Children's Health Insurance Program in 2001
249   Percent of Population Covered by Private Health Insurance in 2000
250   Percent of Population Covered by Employment-Based Private Health Insurance in 2000
251   Percent of Population Covered by Government Health Insurance in 2000
252   Percent of Population Covered by Military Health Insurance in 2000
253   Health Maintenance Organizations (HMOs) in 2001
254   Enrollees in Health Maintenance Organizations (HMOs) in 2001
255   Percent Change in Enrollees in Health Maintenance Organizations (HMOs): 2000 to 2001
256   Percent of Population Enrolled in Health Maintenance Organizations (HMOs) in 2001
257   Percent of Insured Population Enrolled in Health Maintenance Organizations (HMOs) in 2001
258   Medicare Enrollees in 2000
259   Medicare Benefit Payments in 2000
260   Medicare Payments per Enrollee in 2000
261   Percent of Population Enrolled in Medicare in 2000
262   Medicare Managed Care Enrollees in 2001
263   Percent of Medicare Enrollees in Managed Care Programs in 2001
264   Percent of Medicare Benefits Paid Through Managed Care in 2000
265   Percent of Medicare Benefits Paid Through Fee for Service Plans in 2000
266   Medicare Physicians in 1999
267   Percent of Physicians Participating in Medicare in 1999
268   Medicaid Enrollment in 2000
269   Percent of Population Enrolled in Medicaid in 2000
270   Percent of Children Covered by Medicaid in 2000
271   Medicaid Enrollment in 1999
272   Medicaid Expenditures in 1999
273   Percent Change in Medicaid Expenditures: 1997 to 1999
274   Medicaid Expenditures per Enrollee in 1999
275   Percent Change in Expenditures per Medicaid Enrollee: 1997 to 1999
276   Medicaid Managed Care Enrollment in 2000
277   Percent of Medicaid Enrollees in Managed Care in 2000
278   Federal Medicaid Matching Fund Rate for 2002
279   Personal Health Care Expenditures in 1998
280   Health Care Expenditures as a Percent of Gross State Product in 1998
281   Percent Change in Personal Health Care Expenditures: 1990 to 1998
282   Average Annual Change in Expenditures for Personal Health Care: 1990 to 1998
283   Per Capita Personal Health Care Expenditures in 1998
284   Percent Change in Per Capita Expenditures for Personal Health Care: 1990 to 1998
285   Average Annual Change in Per Capita Expenditures for Personal Health Care: 1990 to 1998
286   Per Capita Medicare Expenditures for Personal Health Care in 1998
287   Per Capita Medicaid Expenditures for Personal Health Care in 1998
288   Expenditures for Hospital Care in 1998
289   Percent of Total Personal Health Care Expenditures Spent on Hospital Care in 1998
290   Percent Change in Expenditures for Hospital Care: 1990 to 1998
291   Average Annual Change in Expenditures for Hospital Care: 1990 to 1998
292   Per Capita Expenditures for Hospital Care in 1998
293   Percent Change in Per Capita Expenditures for Hospital Care: 1990 to 1998
294   Average Annual Change in Per Capita Expenditures for Hospital Care: 1990 to 1998
295   Per Capita Medicare Expenditures for Hospital Care in 1998
296   Per Capita Medicaid Expenditures for Hospital Care in 1998
297   Expenditures for Physician and Other Professional Services in 1998

IV. FINANCE (Continued)

298 Percent of Total Personal Health Care Expenditures Spent on Physician and Other Professional Services in 1998
299 Percent Change in Expenditures for Physician and Other Professional Services: 1990 to 1998
300 Average Annual Change in Expenditures for Physician and Other Professional Services: 1990 to 1998
301 Per Capita Expenditures for Physician and Other Professional Services in 1998
302 Percent Change in Per Capita Expenditures for Physician and Other Professional Services: 1990 to 1998
303 Average Annual Change in Per Capita Expenditures for Physician Services: 1990 to 1998
304 Per Capita Medicare Expenditures for Physician Services in 1998
305 Per Capita Medicaid Expenditures for Physician Services in 1998
306 Expenditures for Prescription Drugs in 1998
307 Percent of Total Personal Health Care Expenditures Spent on Prescription Drugs in 1998
308 Percent Change in Expenditures for Prescription Drugs: 1990 to 1998
309 Average Annual Change in Expenditures for Prescription Drugs: 1990 to 1998
310 Per Capita Expenditures for Prescription Drugs in 1998
311 Percent Change in Per Capita Expenditures for Prescription Drugs: 1990 to 1998
312 Average Annual Change in Per Capita Expenditures for Prescription Drugs: 1990 to 1998
313 Expenditures for Dental Services in 1998
314 Percent of Total Personal Health Care Expenditures Spent on Dental Services in 1998
315 Average Annual Change in Expenditures for Dental Services: 1990 to 1998
316 Per Capita Expenditures for Dental Services in 1998
317 Per Capita Medicaid Expenditures for Dental Services in 1998
318 Expenditures for Other Personal Health Care Services in 1998
319 Percent of Total Personal Health Care Expenditures Spent on Other Personal Health Care Services in 1998
320 Average Annual Change in Expenditures for Other Personal Health Care Services: 1990 to 1998
321 Per Capita Expenditures for Other Personal Health Care Services in 1998
322 Expenditures for Home Health Care in 1998
323 Percent of Total Personal Health Care Expenditures Spent on Home Health Care in 1998
324 Average Annual Change in Expenditures for Home Health Care: 1990 to 1998
325 Per Capita Expenditures for Home Health Care in 1998
326 Per Capita Medicare Expenditures for Home Health Care in 1998
327 Per Capita Medicaid Expenditures for Home Health Care in 1998
328 Expenditures for Over-the-Counter Drugs and Other Medical Non-Durables in 1998
329 Percent of Total Personal Health Care Expenditures Spent on Over-the-Counter Drugs and Other Medical Non-Durables in 1998
330 Average Annual Change in Expenditures for Over-the-Counter Drugs and Other Medical Non-Durables: 1990 to 1998
331 Per Capita Expenditures for Over-the-Counter Drugs and Other Medical Non-Durables in 1998
332 Expenditures for Vision Products and Other Medical Durables in 1998
333 Percent of Total Personal Health Care Expenditures Spent on Vision Products and Other Medical Durables in 1998
334 Average Annual Change in Expenditures for Vision Products and Other Medical Durables: 1990 to 1998
335 Per Capita Expenditures for Vision Products and Other Medical Durables in 1998
336 Expenditures for Nursing Home Care in 1998
337 Percent of Total Personal Health Care Expenditures Spent on Nursing Home Care in 1998
338 Average Annual Change in Expenditures for Nursing Home Care: 1990 to 1998
339 Per Capita Expenditures for Nursing Home Care in 1998
340 Per Capita Medicare Expenditures for Nursing Home Care in 1998
341 Per Capita Medicaid Expenditures for Nursing Home Care in 1998
342 Estimated State Funds from the Tobacco Settlement Through 2025
343 State Government Expenditures for Health Programs in 1999
344 Per Capita State Government Expenditures for Health Programs in 1999
345 State Government Expenditures for Hospitals in 1999
346 Per Capita State Government Expenditures for Hospitals in 1999
347 Payroll of Health Care Establishments in 1999
348 Average Pay per Health Care Establishment Employee in 1999
349 Receipts per Health Service Establishment in 1997
350 Receipts per Hospital in 1997
351 Receipts per Office or Clinic of Doctors of Medicine in 1997
352 Receipts per Office or Clinic of Dentists in 1997

Persons Not Covered by Health Insurance in 2000

National Total = 38,683,000 Uninsured

ALPHA ORDER

RANK	STATE	UNINSURED	% of USA
18	Alabama	600,000	1.6%
42	Alaska	125,000	0.3%
14	Arizona	793,000	2.0%
30	Arkansas	364,000	0.9%
1	California	6,281,000	16.2%
22	Colorado	563,000	1.5%
35	Connecticut	263,000	0.7%
45	Delaware	82,000	0.2%
4	Florida	2,620,000	6.8%
7	Georgia	1,135,000	2.9%
43	Hawaii	117,000	0.3%
38	Idaho	196,000	0.5%
5	Illinois	1,659,000	4.3%
16	Indiana	701,000	1.8%
37	Iowa	248,000	0.6%
33	Kansas	301,000	0.8%
23	Kentucky	513,000	1.3%
13	Louisiana	810,000	2.1%
41	Maine	145,000	0.4%
24	Maryland	501,000	1.3%
19	Massachusetts	595,000	1.5%
9	Michigan	982,000	2.5%
27	Minnesota	430,000	1.1%
30	Mississippi	364,000	0.9%
20	Missouri	586,000	1.5%
40	Montana	162,000	0.4%
39	Nebraska	164,000	0.4%
32	Nevada	311,000	0.8%
44	New Hampshire	85,000	0.2%
8	New Jersey	1,049,000	2.7%
28	New Mexico	427,000	1.1%
3	New York	2,802,000	7.2%
10	North Carolina	980,000	2.5%
48	North Dakota	69,000	0.2%
6	Ohio	1,255,000	3.2%
17	Oklahoma	636,000	1.6%
25	Oregon	465,000	1.2%
11	Pennsylvania	905,000	2.3%
50	Rhode Island	55,000	0.1%
26	South Carolina	448,000	1.2%
45	South Dakota	82,000	0.2%
21	Tennessee	577,000	1.5%
2	Texas	4,425,000	11.4%
34	Utah	296,000	0.8%
49	Vermont	67,000	0.2%
12	Virginia	886,000	2.3%
15	Washington	780,000	2.0%
36	West Virginia	254,000	0.7%
29	Wisconsin	386,000	1.0%
47	Wyoming	70,000	0.2%

RANK ORDER

RANK	STATE	UNINSURED	% of USA
1	California	6,281,000	16.2%
2	Texas	4,425,000	11.4%
3	New York	2,802,000	7.2%
4	Florida	2,620,000	6.8%
5	Illinois	1,659,000	4.3%
6	Ohio	1,255,000	3.2%
7	Georgia	1,135,000	2.9%
8	New Jersey	1,049,000	2.7%
9	Michigan	982,000	2.5%
10	North Carolina	980,000	2.5%
11	Pennsylvania	905,000	2.3%
12	Virginia	886,000	2.3%
13	Louisiana	810,000	2.1%
14	Arizona	793,000	2.0%
15	Washington	780,000	2.0%
16	Indiana	701,000	1.8%
17	Oklahoma	636,000	1.6%
18	Alabama	600,000	1.6%
19	Massachusetts	595,000	1.5%
20	Missouri	586,000	1.5%
21	Tennessee	577,000	1.5%
22	Colorado	563,000	1.5%
23	Kentucky	513,000	1.3%
24	Maryland	501,000	1.3%
25	Oregon	465,000	1.2%
26	South Carolina	448,000	1.2%
27	Minnesota	430,000	1.1%
28	New Mexico	427,000	1.1%
29	Wisconsin	386,000	1.0%
30	Arkansas	364,000	0.9%
30	Mississippi	364,000	0.9%
32	Nevada	311,000	0.8%
33	Kansas	301,000	0.8%
34	Utah	296,000	0.8%
35	Connecticut	263,000	0.7%
36	West Virginia	254,000	0.7%
37	Iowa	248,000	0.6%
38	Idaho	196,000	0.5%
39	Nebraska	164,000	0.4%
40	Montana	162,000	0.4%
41	Maine	145,000	0.4%
42	Alaska	125,000	0.3%
43	Hawaii	117,000	0.3%
44	New Hampshire	85,000	0.2%
45	Delaware	82,000	0.2%
45	South Dakota	82,000	0.2%
47	Wyoming	70,000	0.2%
48	North Dakota	69,000	0.2%
49	Vermont	67,000	0.2%
50	Rhode Island	55,000	0.1%
	District of Columbia	73,000	0.2%

Source: U.S. Bureau of the Census
"Health Insurance Coverage Status by State for All People: 2000"
(http://ferret.bls.census.gov/macro/032001/health/h06_000.htm)

Percent of Population Not Covered by Health Insurance in 2000

National Percent = 14.0% of Population

ALPHA ORDER

RANK	STATE	PERCENT
18	Alabama	13.5
3	Alaska	19.3
9	Arizona	16.1
16	Arkansas	13.9
7	California	18.1
21	Colorado	13.3
46	Connecticut	7.9
37	Delaware	10.4
8	Florida	17.3
13	Georgia	14.6
39	Hawaii	10.1
10	Idaho	15.6
18	Illinois	13.5
28	Indiana	12.1
45	Iowa	8.7
31	Kansas	11.5
25	Kentucky	12.9
5	Louisiana	19.1
31	Maine	11.5
42	Maryland	9.8
43	Massachusetts	9.5
40	Michigan	9.9
44	Minnesota	9.0
23	Mississippi	13.1
36	Missouri	10.6
6	Montana	18.5
40	Nebraska	9.9
10	Nevada	15.6
49	New Hampshire	6.8
27	New Jersey	12.6
1	New Mexico	23.8
12	New York	15.2
24	North Carolina	13.0
33	North Dakota	11.3
34	Ohio	10.9
3	Oklahoma	19.3
17	Oregon	13.7
47	Pennsylvania	7.6
50	Rhode Island	5.9
29	South Carolina	11.9
30	South Dakota	11.8
38	Tennessee	10.3
2	Texas	21.5
20	Utah	13.4
35	Vermont	10.7
26	Virginia	12.7
21	Washington	13.3
15	West Virginia	14.3
48	Wisconsin	7.1
14	Wyoming	14.4

RANK ORDER

RANK	STATE	PERCENT
1	New Mexico	23.8
2	Texas	21.5
3	Alaska	19.3
3	Oklahoma	19.3
5	Louisiana	19.1
6	Montana	18.5
7	California	18.1
8	Florida	17.3
9	Arizona	16.1
10	Idaho	15.6
10	Nevada	15.6
12	New York	15.2
13	Georgia	14.6
14	Wyoming	14.4
15	West Virginia	14.3
16	Arkansas	13.9
17	Oregon	13.7
18	Alabama	13.5
18	Illinois	13.5
20	Utah	13.4
21	Colorado	13.3
21	Washington	13.3
23	Mississippi	13.1
24	North Carolina	13.0
25	Kentucky	12.9
26	Virginia	12.7
27	New Jersey	12.6
28	Indiana	12.1
29	South Carolina	11.9
30	South Dakota	11.8
31	Kansas	11.5
31	Maine	11.5
33	North Dakota	11.3
34	Ohio	10.9
35	Vermont	10.7
36	Missouri	10.6
37	Delaware	10.4
38	Tennessee	10.3
39	Hawaii	10.1
40	Michigan	9.9
40	Nebraska	9.9
42	Maryland	9.8
43	Massachusetts	9.5
44	Minnesota	9.0
45	Iowa	8.7
46	Connecticut	7.9
47	Pennsylvania	7.6
48	Wisconsin	7.1
49	New Hampshire	6.8
50	Rhode Island	5.9
	District of Columbia	14.4

Source: U.S. Bureau of the Census
"Health Insurance Coverage Status by State for All People: 2000"
(http://ferret.bls.census.gov/macro/032001/health/h06_000.htm)

Persons Covered by Health Insurance in 2000

National Total = 237,857,000 Insured

ALPHA ORDER

RANK	STATE	INSURED	% of USA
22	Alabama	3,851,000	1.6%
49	Alaska	522,000	0.2%
21	Arizona	4,124,000	1.7%
33	Arkansas	2,261,000	1.0%
1	California	28,454,000	12.0%
23	Colorado	3,665,000	1.5%
27	Connecticut	3,056,000	1.3%
45	Delaware	705,000	0.3%
4	Florida	12,537,000	5.3%
10	Georgia	6,638,000	2.8%
42	Hawaii	1,039,000	0.4%
41	Idaho	1,061,000	0.4%
6	Illinois	10,627,000	4.5%
14	Indiana	5,117,000	2.2%
30	Iowa	2,615,000	1.1%
32	Kansas	2,306,000	1.0%
24	Kentucky	3,462,000	1.5%
25	Louisiana	3,423,000	1.4%
40	Maine	1,121,000	0.5%
19	Maryland	4,618,000	1.9%
13	Massachusetts	5,661,000	2.4%
8	Michigan	8,964,000	3.8%
20	Minnesota	4,354,000	1.8%
31	Mississippi	2,425,000	1.0%
18	Missouri	4,930,000	2.1%
44	Montana	714,000	0.3%
37	Nebraska	1,494,000	0.6%
35	Nevada	1,680,000	0.7%
39	New Hampshire	1,155,000	0.5%
9	New Jersey	7,257,000	3.1%
38	New Mexico	1,366,000	0.6%
3	New York	15,608,000	6.6%
11	North Carolina	6,541,000	2.7%
48	North Dakota	538,000	0.2%
7	Ohio	10,284,000	4.3%
29	Oklahoma	2,651,000	1.1%
28	Oregon	2,935,000	1.2%
5	Pennsylvania	11,063,000	4.7%
43	Rhode Island	881,000	0.4%
26	South Carolina	3,321,000	1.4%
46	South Dakota	615,000	0.3%
17	Tennessee	5,003,000	2.1%
2	Texas	16,167,000	6.8%
34	Utah	1,913,000	0.8%
47	Vermont	564,000	0.2%
12	Virginia	6,091,000	2.6%
15	Washington	5,075,000	2.1%
36	West Virginia	1,524,000	0.6%
16	Wisconsin	5,032,000	2.1%
50	Wyoming	418,000	0.2%

RANK ORDER

RANK	STATE	INSURED	% of USA
1	California	28,454,000	12.0%
2	Texas	16,167,000	6.8%
3	New York	15,608,000	6.6%
4	Florida	12,537,000	5.3%
5	Pennsylvania	11,063,000	4.7%
6	Illinois	10,627,000	4.5%
7	Ohio	10,284,000	4.3%
8	Michigan	8,964,000	3.8%
9	New Jersey	7,257,000	3.1%
10	Georgia	6,638,000	2.8%
11	North Carolina	6,541,000	2.7%
12	Virginia	6,091,000	2.6%
13	Massachusetts	5,661,000	2.4%
14	Indiana	5,117,000	2.2%
15	Washington	5,075,000	2.1%
16	Wisconsin	5,032,000	2.1%
17	Tennessee	5,003,000	2.1%
18	Missouri	4,930,000	2.1%
19	Maryland	4,618,000	1.9%
20	Minnesota	4,354,000	1.8%
21	Arizona	4,124,000	1.7%
22	Alabama	3,851,000	1.6%
23	Colorado	3,665,000	1.5%
24	Kentucky	3,462,000	1.5%
25	Louisiana	3,423,000	1.4%
26	South Carolina	3,321,000	1.4%
27	Connecticut	3,056,000	1.3%
28	Oregon	2,935,000	1.2%
29	Oklahoma	2,651,000	1.1%
30	Iowa	2,615,000	1.1%
31	Mississippi	2,425,000	1.0%
32	Kansas	2,306,000	1.0%
33	Arkansas	2,261,000	1.0%
34	Utah	1,913,000	0.8%
35	Nevada	1,680,000	0.7%
36	West Virginia	1,524,000	0.6%
37	Nebraska	1,494,000	0.6%
38	New Mexico	1,366,000	0.6%
39	New Hampshire	1,155,000	0.5%
40	Maine	1,121,000	0.5%
41	Idaho	1,061,000	0.4%
42	Hawaii	1,039,000	0.4%
43	Rhode Island	881,000	0.4%
44	Montana	714,000	0.3%
45	Delaware	705,000	0.3%
46	South Dakota	615,000	0.3%
47	Vermont	564,000	0.2%
48	North Dakota	538,000	0.2%
49	Alaska	522,000	0.2%
50	Wyoming	418,000	0.2%
	District of Columbia	434,000	0.2%

Source: U.S. Bureau of the Census
"Health Insurance Coverage Status by State for All People: 2000"
(http://ferret.bls.census.gov/macro/032001/health/h06_000.htm)

Percent of Population Covered by Health Insurance in 2000

National Percent = 86.0% of Population

ALPHA ORDER

RANK	STATE	PERCENT
32	Alabama	86.5
47	Alaska	80.7
42	Arizona	83.9
35	Arkansas	86.1
44	California	81.9
29	Colorado	86.7
5	Connecticut	92.1
14	Delaware	89.6
43	Florida	82.7
38	Georgia	85.4
12	Hawaii	89.9
40	Idaho	84.4
32	Illinois	86.5
23	Indiana	87.9
6	Iowa	91.3
19	Kansas	88.5
26	Kentucky	87.1
46	Louisiana	80.9
19	Maine	88.5
9	Maryland	90.2
8	Massachusetts	90.5
10	Michigan	90.1
7	Minnesota	91.0
28	Mississippi	86.9
15	Missouri	89.4
45	Montana	81.5
10	Nebraska	90.1
40	Nevada	84.4
2	New Hampshire	93.2
24	New Jersey	87.4
50	New Mexico	76.2
39	New York	84.8
27	North Carolina	87.0
18	North Dakota	88.7
17	Ohio	89.1
47	Oklahoma	80.7
34	Oregon	86.3
4	Pennsylvania	92.4
1	Rhode Island	94.1
22	South Carolina	88.1
21	South Dakota	88.2
13	Tennessee	89.7
49	Texas	78.5
31	Utah	86.6
16	Vermont	89.3
25	Virginia	87.3
29	Washington	86.7
36	West Virginia	85.7
3	Wisconsin	92.9
37	Wyoming	85.6

RANK ORDER

RANK	STATE	PERCENT
1	Rhode Island	94.1
2	New Hampshire	93.2
3	Wisconsin	92.9
4	Pennsylvania	92.4
5	Connecticut	92.1
6	Iowa	91.3
7	Minnesota	91.0
8	Massachusetts	90.5
9	Maryland	90.2
10	Michigan	90.1
10	Nebraska	90.1
12	Hawaii	89.9
13	Tennessee	89.7
14	Delaware	89.6
15	Missouri	89.4
16	Vermont	89.3
17	Ohio	89.1
18	North Dakota	88.7
19	Kansas	88.5
19	Maine	88.5
21	South Dakota	88.2
22	South Carolina	88.1
23	Indiana	87.9
24	New Jersey	87.4
25	Virginia	87.3
26	Kentucky	87.1
27	North Carolina	87.0
28	Mississippi	86.9
29	Colorado	86.7
29	Washington	86.7
31	Utah	86.6
32	Alabama	86.5
32	Illinois	86.5
34	Oregon	86.3
35	Arkansas	86.1
36	West Virginia	85.7
37	Wyoming	85.6
38	Georgia	85.4
39	New York	84.8
40	Idaho	84.4
40	Nevada	84.4
42	Arizona	83.9
43	Florida	82.7
44	California	81.9
45	Montana	81.5
46	Louisiana	80.9
47	Alaska	80.7
47	Oklahoma	80.7
49	Texas	78.5
50	New Mexico	76.2
	District of Columbia	85.6

Source: U.S. Bureau of the Census
"Health Insurance Coverage Status by State for All People: 2000"
(http://ferret.bls.census.gov/macro/032001/health/h06_000.htm)

Persons Not Covered by Health Insurance in 1996

National Total = 41,716,000 Uninsured

ALPHA ORDER

RANK	STATE	UNINSURED	% of USA
26	Alabama	550,000	1.3%
46	Alaska	89,000	0.2%
10	Arizona	1,159,000	2.8%
25	Arkansas	566,000	1.4%
1	California	6,514,000	15.6%
19	Colorado	644,000	1.5%
32	Connecticut	368,000	0.9%
44	Delaware	98,000	0.2%
4	Florida	2,722,000	6.5%
6	Georgia	1,319,000	3.2%
43	Hawaii	101,000	0.2%
38	Idaho	196,000	0.5%
5	Illinois	1,337,000	3.2%
22	Indiana	600,000	1.4%
33	Iowa	335,000	0.8%
34	Kansas	292,000	0.7%
21	Kentucky	601,000	1.4%
12	Louisiana	890,000	2.1%
40	Maine	146,000	0.3%
23	Maryland	581,000	1.4%
16	Massachusetts	766,000	1.8%
13	Michigan	857,000	2.1%
29	Minnesota	480,000	1.2%
27	Mississippi	518,000	1.2%
18	Missouri	700,000	1.7%
41	Montana	124,000	0.3%
39	Nebraska	190,000	0.5%
36	Nevada	255,000	0.6%
42	New Hampshire	109,000	0.3%
7	New Jersey	1,317,000	3.2%
31	New Mexico	412,000	1.0%
3	New York	3,132,000	7.5%
9	North Carolina	1,160,000	2.8%
50	North Dakota	62,000	0.1%
8	Ohio	1,292,000	3.1%
24	Oklahoma	570,000	1.4%
28	Oregon	496,000	1.2%
11	Pennsylvania	1,133,000	2.7%
45	Rhode Island	93,000	0.2%
20	South Carolina	634,000	1.5%
47	South Dakota	67,000	0.2%
14	Tennessee	841,000	2.0%
2	Texas	4,680,000	11.2%
37	Utah	240,000	0.6%
49	Vermont	65,000	0.2%
15	Virginia	811,000	1.9%
17	Washington	761,000	1.8%
35	West Virginia	261,000	0.6%
30	Wisconsin	438,000	1.0%
48	Wyoming	66,000	0.2%

RANK ORDER

RANK	STATE	UNINSURED	% of USA
1	California	6,514,000	15.6%
2	Texas	4,680,000	11.2%
3	New York	3,132,000	7.5%
4	Florida	2,722,000	6.5%
5	Illinois	1,337,000	3.2%
6	Georgia	1,319,000	3.2%
7	New Jersey	1,317,000	3.2%
8	Ohio	1,292,000	3.1%
9	North Carolina	1,160,000	2.8%
10	Arizona	1,159,000	2.8%
11	Pennsylvania	1,133,000	2.7%
12	Louisiana	890,000	2.1%
13	Michigan	857,000	2.1%
14	Tennessee	841,000	2.0%
15	Virginia	811,000	1.9%
16	Massachusetts	766,000	1.8%
17	Washington	761,000	1.8%
18	Missouri	700,000	1.7%
19	Colorado	644,000	1.5%
20	South Carolina	634,000	1.5%
21	Kentucky	601,000	1.4%
22	Indiana	600,000	1.4%
23	Maryland	581,000	1.4%
24	Oklahoma	570,000	1.4%
25	Arkansas	566,000	1.4%
26	Alabama	550,000	1.3%
27	Mississippi	518,000	1.2%
28	Oregon	496,000	1.2%
29	Minnesota	480,000	1.2%
30	Wisconsin	438,000	1.0%
31	New Mexico	412,000	1.0%
32	Connecticut	368,000	0.9%
33	Iowa	335,000	0.8%
34	Kansas	292,000	0.7%
35	West Virginia	261,000	0.6%
36	Nevada	255,000	0.6%
37	Utah	240,000	0.6%
38	Idaho	196,000	0.5%
39	Nebraska	190,000	0.5%
40	Maine	146,000	0.3%
41	Montana	124,000	0.3%
42	New Hampshire	109,000	0.3%
43	Hawaii	101,000	0.2%
44	Delaware	98,000	0.2%
45	Rhode Island	93,000	0.2%
46	Alaska	89,000	0.2%
47	South Dakota	67,000	0.2%
48	Wyoming	66,000	0.2%
49	Vermont	65,000	0.2%
50	North Dakota	62,000	0.1%
	District of Columbia	80,000	0.2%

Source: U.S. Bureau of the Census
"Health Insurance Coverage: 1996" (http://www.census.gov/hhes/hlthins/cover96/c96tabf.html)

Percent of Population Not Covered by Health Insurance in 1996

National Percent = 15.6% of Population

ALPHA ORDER			RANK ORDER		
RANK	STATE	PERCENT	RANK	STATE	PERCENT
28	Alabama	12.9	1	Texas	24.3
23	Alaska	13.5	2	Arizona	24.1
2	Arizona	24.1	3	New Mexico	22.3
4	Arkansas	21.7	4	Arkansas	21.7
6	California	20.1	5	Louisiana	20.9
14	Colorado	16.6	6	California	20.1
40	Connecticut	11.0	7	Florida	18.9
26	Delaware	13.4	8	Mississippi	18.5
7	Florida	18.9	9	Georgia	17.8
9	Georgia	17.8	10	South Carolina	17.1
49	Hawaii	8.6	11	New York	17.0
15	Idaho	16.5	11	Oklahoma	17.0
38	Illinois	11.3	13	New Jersey	16.7
41	Indiana	10.6	14	Colorado	16.6
33	Iowa	11.6	15	Idaho	16.5
35	Kansas	11.4	16	North Carolina	16.0
18	Kentucky	15.4	17	Nevada	15.6
5	Louisiana	20.9	18	Kentucky	15.4
31	Maine	12.1	19	Oregon	15.3
35	Maryland	11.4	20	Tennessee	15.2
30	Massachusetts	12.4	21	West Virginia	14.9
48	Michigan	8.9	22	Montana	13.6
42	Minnesota	10.2	23	Alaska	13.5
8	Mississippi	18.5	23	Washington	13.5
27	Missouri	13.2	23	Wyoming	13.5
22	Montana	13.6	26	Delaware	13.4
35	Nebraska	11.4	27	Missouri	13.2
17	Nevada	15.6	28	Alabama	12.9
45	New Hampshire	9.5	29	Virginia	12.5
13	New Jersey	16.7	30	Massachusetts	12.4
3	New Mexico	22.3	31	Maine	12.1
11	New York	17.0	32	Utah	12.0
16	North Carolina	16.0	33	Iowa	11.6
44	North Dakota	9.8	34	Ohio	11.5
34	Ohio	11.5	35	Kansas	11.4
11	Oklahoma	17.0	35	Maryland	11.4
19	Oregon	15.3	35	Nebraska	11.4
45	Pennsylvania	9.5	38	Illinois	11.3
43	Rhode Island	9.9	39	Vermont	11.1
10	South Carolina	17.1	40	Connecticut	11.0
45	South Dakota	9.5	41	Indiana	10.6
20	Tennessee	15.2	42	Minnesota	10.2
1	Texas	24.3	43	Rhode Island	9.9
32	Utah	12.0	44	North Dakota	9.8
39	Vermont	11.1	45	New Hampshire	9.5
29	Virginia	12.5	45	Pennsylvania	9.5
23	Washington	13.5	45	South Dakota	9.5
21	West Virginia	14.9	48	Michigan	8.9
50	Wisconsin	8.4	49	Hawaii	8.6
23	Wyoming	13.5	50	Wisconsin	8.4
				District of Columbia	14.8

Source: U.S. Bureau of the Census
   "Health Insurance Coverage: 1996" (http://www.census.gov/hhes/hlthins/cover96/c96tabf.html)

Change in Number of Persons Uninsured: 1996 to 2000

National Change = 3,033,000 Decrease

ALPHA ORDER

RANK	STATE	CHANGE
8	Alabama	50,000
10	Alaska	36,000
50	Arizona	(366,000)
43	Arkansas	(202,000)
45	California	(233,000)
32	Colorado	(81,000)
36	Connecticut	(105,000)
22	Delaware	(16,000)
35	Florida	(102,000)
41	Georgia	(184,000)
12	Hawaii	16,000
19	Idaho	0
1	Illinois	322,000
3	Indiana	101,000
33	Iowa	(87,000)
15	Kansas	9,000
34	Kentucky	(88,000)
30	Louisiana	(80,000)
20	Maine	(1,000)
30	Maryland	(80,000)
39	Massachusetts	(171,000)
2	Michigan	125,000
28	Minnesota	(50,000)
38	Mississippi	(154,000)
37	Missouri	(114,000)
9	Montana	38,000
24	Nebraska	(26,000)
6	Nevada	56,000
23	New Hampshire	(24,000)
48	New Jersey	(268,000)
13	New Mexico	15,000
49	New York	(330,000)
40	North Carolina	(180,000)
16	North Dakota	7,000
26	Ohio	(37,000)
5	Oklahoma	66,000
25	Oregon	(31,000)
44	Pennsylvania	(228,000)
27	Rhode Island	(38,000)
42	South Carolina	(186,000)
13	South Dakota	15,000
47	Tennessee	(264,000)
46	Texas	(255,000)
6	Utah	56,000
18	Vermont	2,000
4	Virginia	75,000
11	Washington	19,000
21	West Virginia	(7,000)
29	Wisconsin	(52,000)
17	Wyoming	4,000

RANK ORDER

RANK	STATE	CHANGE
1	Illinois	322,000
2	Michigan	125,000
3	Indiana	101,000
4	Virginia	75,000
5	Oklahoma	66,000
6	Nevada	56,000
6	Utah	56,000
8	Alabama	50,000
9	Montana	38,000
10	Alaska	36,000
11	Washington	19,000
12	Hawaii	16,000
13	New Mexico	15,000
13	South Dakota	15,000
15	Kansas	9,000
16	North Dakota	7,000
17	Wyoming	4,000
18	Vermont	2,000
19	Idaho	0
20	Maine	(1,000)
21	West Virginia	(7,000)
22	Delaware	(16,000)
23	New Hampshire	(24,000)
24	Nebraska	(26,000)
25	Oregon	(31,000)
26	Ohio	(37,000)
27	Rhode Island	(38,000)
28	Minnesota	(50,000)
29	Wisconsin	(52,000)
30	Louisiana	(80,000)
30	Maryland	(80,000)
32	Colorado	(81,000)
33	Iowa	(87,000)
34	Kentucky	(88,000)
35	Florida	(102,000)
36	Connecticut	(105,000)
37	Missouri	(114,000)
38	Mississippi	(154,000)
39	Massachusetts	(171,000)
40	North Carolina	(180,000)
41	Georgia	(184,000)
42	South Carolina	(186,000)
43	Arkansas	(202,000)
44	Pennsylvania	(228,000)
45	California	(233,000)
46	Texas	(255,000)
47	Tennessee	(264,000)
48	New Jersey	(268,000)
49	New York	(330,000)
50	Arizona	(366,000)

| | District of Columbia | (7,000) |

Source: Morgan Quitno Press using data from U.S. Bureau of the Census
"Health Insurance Coverage: 1996" (http://www.census.gov/hhes/hlthins/cover96/c96tabf.html) and
"Health Insurance Coverage Status by State for All People: 2000"
(http://ferret.bls.census.gov/macro/032001/health/h06_000.htm)

Percent Change in Number of Uninsured: 1996 to 2000

National Percent Change = 7.3% Decrease

ALPHA ORDER

RANK	STATE	PERCENT CHANGE
13	Alabama	9.1
1	Alaska	40.4
48	Arizona	(31.6)
49	Arkansas	(35.7)
23	California	(3.6)
31	Colorado	(12.6)
44	Connecticut	(28.5)
37	Delaware	(16.3)
24	Florida	(3.7)
34	Georgia	(13.9)
8	Hawaii	15.8
19	Idaho	0.0
3	Illinois	24.1
7	Indiana	16.8
43	Iowa	(26.0)
16	Kansas	3.1
35	Kentucky	(14.6)
27	Louisiana	(9.0)
20	Maine	(0.7)
33	Maryland	(13.8)
42	Massachusetts	(22.3)
9	Michigan	14.6
28	Minnesota	(10.4)
46	Mississippi	(29.7)
37	Missouri	(16.3)
2	Montana	30.6
32	Nebraska	(13.7)
6	Nevada	22.0
41	New Hampshire	(22.0)
40	New Jersey	(20.3)
15	New Mexico	3.6
29	New York	(10.5)
36	North Carolina	(15.5)
11	North Dakota	11.3
22	Ohio	(2.9)
10	Oklahoma	11.6
26	Oregon	(6.3)
39	Pennsylvania	(20.1)
50	Rhode Island	(40.9)
45	South Carolina	(29.3)
5	South Dakota	22.4
47	Tennessee	(31.4)
25	Texas	(5.4)
4	Utah	23.3
16	Vermont	3.1
12	Virginia	9.2
18	Washington	2.5
21	West Virginia	(2.7)
30	Wisconsin	(11.9)
14	Wyoming	6.1

RANK ORDER

RANK	STATE	PERCENT CHANGE
1	Alaska	40.4
2	Montana	30.6
3	Illinois	24.1
4	Utah	23.3
5	South Dakota	22.4
6	Nevada	22.0
7	Indiana	16.8
8	Hawaii	15.8
9	Michigan	14.6
10	Oklahoma	11.6
11	North Dakota	11.3
12	Virginia	9.2
13	Alabama	9.1
14	Wyoming	6.1
15	New Mexico	3.6
16	Kansas	3.1
16	Vermont	3.1
18	Washington	2.5
19	Idaho	0.0
20	Maine	(0.7)
21	West Virginia	(2.7)
22	Ohio	(2.9)
23	California	(3.6)
24	Florida	(3.7)
25	Texas	(5.4)
26	Oregon	(6.3)
27	Louisiana	(9.0)
28	Minnesota	(10.4)
29	New York	(10.5)
30	Wisconsin	(11.9)
31	Colorado	(12.6)
32	Nebraska	(13.7)
33	Maryland	(13.8)
34	Georgia	(13.9)
35	Kentucky	(14.6)
36	North Carolina	(15.5)
37	Delaware	(16.3)
37	Missouri	(16.3)
39	Pennsylvania	(20.1)
40	New Jersey	(20.3)
41	New Hampshire	(22.0)
42	Massachusetts	(22.3)
43	Iowa	(26.0)
44	Connecticut	(28.5)
45	South Carolina	(29.3)
46	Mississippi	(29.7)
47	Tennessee	(31.4)
48	Arizona	(31.6)
49	Arkansas	(35.7)
50	Rhode Island	(40.9)

District of Columbia — (8.8)

Source: Morgan Quitno Press using data from U.S. Bureau of the Census
  "Health Insurance Coverage: 1996" (http://www.census.gov/hhes/hlthins/cover96/c96tabf.html) and
  "Health Insurance Coverage Status by State for All People: 2000"
  (http://ferret.bls.census.gov/macro/032001/health/h06_000.htm)

Change in Percent of Population Uninsured: 1996 to 2000

National Percent Change = 10.3% Decrease

ALPHA ORDER

RANK	STATE	PERCENT CHANGE
13	Alabama	4.7
1	Alaska	43.0
48	Arizona	(33.2)
49	Arkansas	(35.9)
25	California	(10.0)
37	Colorado	(19.9)
43	Connecticut	(28.2)
39	Delaware	(22.4)
23	Florida	(8.5)
34	Georgia	(18.0)
5	Hawaii	17.4
22	Idaho	(5.5)
4	Illinois	19.5
7	Indiana	14.2
42	Iowa	(25.0)
15	Kansas	0.9
33	Kentucky	(16.2)
24	Louisiana	(8.6)
20	Maine	(5.0)
31	Maryland	(14.0)
40	Massachusetts	(23.4)
10	Michigan	11.2
29	Minnesota	(11.8)
45	Mississippi	(29.2)
36	Missouri	(19.7)
2	Montana	36.0
30	Nebraska	(13.2)
16	Nevada	0.0
44	New Hampshire	(28.4)
41	New Jersey	(24.6)
11	New Mexico	6.7
27	New York	(10.6)
35	North Carolina	(18.8)
6	North Dakota	15.3
21	Ohio	(5.2)
8	Oklahoma	13.5
26	Oregon	(10.5)
38	Pennsylvania	(20.0)
50	Rhode Island	(40.4)
46	South Carolina	(30.4)
3	South Dakota	24.2
47	Tennessee	(32.2)
28	Texas	(11.5)
9	Utah	11.7
18	Vermont	(3.6)
14	Virginia	1.6
17	Washington	(1.5)
19	West Virginia	(4.0)
32	Wisconsin	(15.5)
11	Wyoming	6.7

RANK ORDER

RANK	STATE	PERCENT CHANGE
1	Alaska	43.0
2	Montana	36.0
3	South Dakota	24.2
4	Illinois	19.5
5	Hawaii	17.4
6	North Dakota	15.3
7	Indiana	14.2
8	Oklahoma	13.5
9	Utah	11.7
10	Michigan	11.2
11	New Mexico	6.7
11	Wyoming	6.7
13	Alabama	4.7
14	Virginia	1.6
15	Kansas	0.9
16	Nevada	0.0
17	Washington	(1.5)
18	Vermont	(3.6)
19	West Virginia	(4.0)
20	Maine	(5.0)
21	Ohio	(5.2)
22	Idaho	(5.5)
23	Florida	(8.5)
24	Louisiana	(8.6)
25	California	(10.0)
26	Oregon	(10.5)
27	New York	(10.6)
28	Texas	(11.5)
29	Minnesota	(11.8)
30	Nebraska	(13.2)
31	Maryland	(14.0)
32	Wisconsin	(15.5)
33	Kentucky	(16.2)
34	Georgia	(18.0)
35	North Carolina	(18.8)
36	Missouri	(19.7)
37	Colorado	(19.9)
38	Pennsylvania	(20.0)
39	Delaware	(22.4)
40	Massachusetts	(23.4)
41	New Jersey	(24.6)
42	Iowa	(25.0)
43	Connecticut	(28.2)
44	New Hampshire	(28.4)
45	Mississippi	(29.2)
46	South Carolina	(30.4)
47	Tennessee	(32.2)
48	Arizona	(33.2)
49	Arkansas	(35.9)
50	Rhode Island	(40.4)

District of Columbia (2.7)

Source: Morgan Quitno Press using data from U.S. Bureau of the Census
"Health Insurance Coverage: 1996" (http://www.census.gov/hhes/hlthins/cover96/c96tabf.html) and
"Health Insurance Coverage Status by State for All People: 2000"
(http://ferret.bls.census.gov/macro/032001/health/h06_000.htm)

Percent of Children Not Covered by Health Insurance in 2000

National Percent = 11.6% of Children*

ALPHA ORDER

RANK	STATE	PERCENT
32	Alabama	8.5
4	Alaska	17.7
14	Arizona	12.8
18	Arkansas	11.6
8	California	15.4
12	Colorado	13.7
49	Connecticut	2.6
42	Delaware	7.2
6	Florida	16.5
36	Georgia	8.1
35	Hawaii	8.3
10	Idaho	14.7
21	Illinois	10.8
11	Indiana	13.9
45	Iowa	6.2
20	Kansas	11.3
40	Kentucky	7.7
7	Louisiana	15.7
38	Maine	7.8
41	Maryland	7.4
38	Massachusetts	7.8
44	Michigan	6.7
27	Minnesota	9.3
29	Mississippi	9.2
32	Missouri	8.5
3	Montana	18.7
30	Nebraska	8.8
9	Nevada	14.9
43	New Hampshire	7.0
27	New Jersey	9.3
2	New Mexico	20.2
22	New York	10.5
23	North Carolina	10.1
16	North Dakota	11.9
26	Ohio	9.5
5	Oklahoma	16.8
13	Oregon	12.9
46	Pennsylvania	4.9
50	Rhode Island	2.5
31	South Carolina	8.6
18	South Dakota	11.6
47	Tennessee	4.7
1	Texas	21.5
23	Utah	10.1
32	Vermont	8.5
17	Virginia	11.7
36	Washington	8.1
25	West Virginia	9.8
48	Wisconsin	3.7
15	Wyoming	12.5

RANK ORDER

RANK	STATE	PERCENT
1	Texas	21.5
2	New Mexico	20.2
3	Montana	18.7
4	Alaska	17.7
5	Oklahoma	16.8
6	Florida	16.5
7	Louisiana	15.7
8	California	15.4
9	Nevada	14.9
10	Idaho	14.7
11	Indiana	13.9
12	Colorado	13.7
13	Oregon	12.9
14	Arizona	12.8
15	Wyoming	12.5
16	North Dakota	11.9
17	Virginia	11.7
18	Arkansas	11.6
18	South Dakota	11.6
20	Kansas	11.3
21	Illinois	10.8
22	New York	10.5
23	North Carolina	10.1
23	Utah	10.1
25	West Virginia	9.8
26	Ohio	9.5
27	Minnesota	9.3
27	New Jersey	9.3
29	Mississippi	9.2
30	Nebraska	8.8
31	South Carolina	8.6
32	Alabama	8.5
32	Missouri	8.5
32	Vermont	8.5
35	Hawaii	8.3
36	Georgia	8.1
36	Washington	8.1
38	Maine	7.8
38	Massachusetts	7.8
40	Kentucky	7.7
41	Maryland	7.4
42	Delaware	7.2
43	New Hampshire	7.0
44	Michigan	6.7
45	Iowa	6.2
46	Pennsylvania	4.9
47	Tennessee	4.7
48	Wisconsin	3.7
49	Connecticut	2.6
50	Rhode Island	2.5
	District of Columbia	9.9

Source: U.S. Bureau of the Census
   "Health Insurance Historical Table 5" (http://www.census.gov/hhes/hlthins/historic/hihistt5.html)
*Children under 18 years old.

State Children's Health Insurance Program Enrollment in 2001

National Total = 4,601,098 Children*

ALPHA ORDER

RANK	STATE	CHILDREN	% of USA
18	Alabama	68,179	1.5%
33	Alaska	21,831	0.5%
13	Arizona	86,863	1.9%
49	Arkansas	2,884	0.1%
2	California	693,048	15.1%
24	Colorado	45,773	1.0%
34	Connecticut	18,720	0.4%
45	Delaware	5,567	0.1%
4	Florida	298,705	6.5%
5	Georgia	182,762	4.0%
43	Hawaii	7,137	0.2%
38	Idaho	13,276	0.3%
14	Illinois	83,510	1.8%
22	Indiana	56,986	1.2%
32	Iowa	23,270	0.5%
28	Kansas	34,241	0.7%
19	Kentucky	66,796	1.5%
17	Louisiana	69,579	1.5%
31	Maine	27,003	0.6%
8	Maryland	109,983	2.4%
10	Massachusetts	105,072	2.3%
15	Michigan	76,181	1.7%
50	Minnesota	49	0.0%
23	Mississippi	52,436	1.1%
9	Missouri	106,594	2.3%
37	Montana	13,518	0.3%
36	Nebraska	13,933	0.3%
30	Nevada	28,026	0.6%
44	New Hampshire	5,982	0.1%
11	New Jersey	99,847	2.2%
39	New Mexico	10,347	0.2%
1	New York	872,949	19.0%
12	North Carolina	98,650	2.1%
47	North Dakota	3,404	0.1%
6	Ohio	158,265	3.4%
26	Oklahoma	38,858	0.8%
25	Oregon	41,468	0.9%
7	Pennsylvania	141,163	3.1%
35	Rhode Island	17,398	0.4%
20	South Carolina	66,183	1.4%
40	South Dakota	8,937	0.2%
41	Tennessee	8,615	0.2%
3	Texas	500,950	10.9%
27	Utah	34,655	0.8%
48	Vermont	2,996	0.1%
16	Virginia	73,102	1.6%
42	Washington	7,621	0.2%
29	West Virginia	33,144	0.7%
21	Wisconsin	57,183	1.2%
46	Wyoming	4,652	0.1%

RANK ORDER

RANK	STATE	CHILDREN	% of USA
1	New York	872,949	19.0%
2	California	693,048	15.1%
3	Texas	500,950	10.9%
4	Florida	298,705	6.5%
5	Georgia	182,762	4.0%
6	Ohio	158,265	3.4%
7	Pennsylvania	141,163	3.1%
8	Maryland	109,983	2.4%
9	Missouri	106,594	2.3%
10	Massachusetts	105,072	2.3%
11	New Jersey	99,847	2.2%
12	North Carolina	98,650	2.1%
13	Arizona	86,863	1.9%
14	Illinois	83,510	1.8%
15	Michigan	76,181	1.7%
16	Virginia	73,102	1.6%
17	Louisiana	69,579	1.5%
18	Alabama	68,179	1.5%
19	Kentucky	66,796	1.5%
20	South Carolina	66,183	1.4%
21	Wisconsin	57,183	1.2%
22	Indiana	56,986	1.2%
23	Mississippi	52,436	1.1%
24	Colorado	45,773	1.0%
25	Oregon	41,468	0.9%
26	Oklahoma	38,858	0.8%
27	Utah	34,655	0.8%
28	Kansas	34,241	0.7%
29	West Virginia	33,144	0.7%
30	Nevada	28,026	0.6%
31	Maine	27,003	0.6%
32	Iowa	23,270	0.5%
33	Alaska	21,831	0.5%
34	Connecticut	18,720	0.4%
35	Rhode Island	17,398	0.4%
36	Nebraska	13,933	0.3%
37	Montana	13,518	0.3%
38	Idaho	13,276	0.3%
39	New Mexico	10,347	0.2%
40	South Dakota	8,937	0.2%
41	Tennessee	8,615	0.2%
42	Washington	7,621	0.2%
43	Hawaii	7,137	0.2%
44	New Hampshire	5,982	0.1%
45	Delaware	5,567	0.1%
46	Wyoming	4,652	0.1%
47	North Dakota	3,404	0.1%
48	Vermont	2,996	0.1%
49	Arkansas	2,884	0.1%
50	Minnesota	49	0.0%
	District of Columbia	2,807	0.1%

Source: U.S. Department of Health and Human Services, Centers for Medicare and Medicaid Services "Children's Health Insurance Program" (http://www.hcfa.gov/init/children.htm)

*For fiscal year 2001. The State Children's Health Insurance Program (SCHIP) was created in 1997 to help states expand health insurance to children whose families earn too much to qualify for Medicaid, yet not enough to afford private health insurance.

Percent Change in State Children's Health Insurance
Program Enrollment: 2000 to 2001
National Percent Change = 38% Increase*

ALPHA ORDER

RANK	STATE	PERCENT CHANGE
29	Alabama	30
11	Alaska	63
20	Arizona	43
14	Arkansas	52
18	California	45
27	Colorado	31
45	Connecticut	0
32	Delaware	24
27	Florida	31
14	Georgia	52
2	Hawaii	216
44	Idaho	7
25	Illinois	34
31	Indiana	28
39	Iowa	17
29	Kansas	30
35	Kentucky	20
23	Louisiana	39
36	Maine	19
37	Maryland	18
47	Massachusetts	(7)
5	Michigan	105
6	Minnesota	104
4	Mississippi	156
19	Missouri	44
11	Montana	63
33	Nebraska	22
9	Nevada	76
22	New Hampshire	40
41	New Jersey	12
10	New Mexico	69
40	New York	13
46	North Carolina	(5)
26	North Dakota	32
21	Ohio	42
49	Oklahoma	(33)
41	Oregon	12
37	Pennsylvania	18
17	Rhode Island	51
43	South Carolina	11
14	South Dakota	52
50	Tennessee	(42)
1	Texas	284
24	Utah	37
48	Vermont	(27)
7	Virginia	94
3	Washington	191
13	West Virginia	53
34	Wisconsin	21
8	Wyoming	83

RANK ORDER

RANK	STATE	PERCENT CHANGE
1	Texas	284
2	Hawaii	216
3	Washington	191
4	Mississippi	156
5	Michigan	105
6	Minnesota	104
7	Virginia	94
8	Wyoming	83
9	Nevada	76
10	New Mexico	69
11	Alaska	63
11	Montana	63
13	West Virginia	53
14	Arkansas	52
14	Georgia	52
14	South Dakota	52
17	Rhode Island	51
18	California	45
19	Missouri	44
20	Arizona	43
21	Ohio	42
22	New Hampshire	40
23	Louisiana	39
24	Utah	37
25	Illinois	34
26	North Dakota	32
27	Colorado	31
27	Florida	31
29	Alabama	30
29	Kansas	30
31	Indiana	28
32	Delaware	24
33	Nebraska	22
34	Wisconsin	21
35	Kentucky	20
36	Maine	19
37	Maryland	18
37	Pennsylvania	18
39	Iowa	17
40	New York	13
41	New Jersey	12
41	Oregon	12
43	South Carolina	11
44	Idaho	7
45	Connecticut	0
46	North Carolina	(5)
47	Massachusetts	(7)
48	Vermont	(27)
49	Oklahoma	(33)
50	Tennessee	(42)

	District of Columbia	24

Source: U.S. Department of Health and Human Services, Centers for Medicare and Medicaid Services
   "Children's Health Insurance Program" (http://www.hcfa.gov/init/children.htm)
*For fiscal year 2001. The State Children's Health Insurance Program (SCHIP) was created in 1997 to help states expand health insurance to children whose families earn too much to qualify for Medicaid, yet not enough to afford private health insurance.

Percent of Children Enrolled in State Children's
Health Insurance Program in 2001
National Percent = 6.4% of Children 17 Years Old and Younger*

ALPHA ORDER

RANK	STATE	PERCENT
17	Alabama	6.1
2	Alaska	11.4
16	Arizona	6.4
49	Arkansas	0.4
9	California	7.5
30	Colorado	4.2
42	Connecticut	2.2
38	Delaware	2.9
6	Florida	8.2
5	Georgia	8.4
41	Hawaii	2.4
33	Idaho	3.6
40	Illinois	2.6
33	Indiana	3.6
36	Iowa	3.2
24	Kansas	4.8
14	Kentucky	6.7
19	Louisiana	5.7
3	Maine	9.0
8	Maryland	8.1
11	Massachusetts	7.0
38	Michigan	2.9
50	Minnesota	0.0
13	Mississippi	6.8
9	Missouri	7.5
18	Montana	5.9
37	Nebraska	3.1
20	Nevada	5.5
46	New Hampshire	1.9
24	New Jersey	4.8
44	New Mexico	2.0
1	New York	18.6
22	North Carolina	5.0
43	North Dakota	2.1
20	Ohio	5.5
28	Oklahoma	4.4
23	Oregon	4.9
24	Pennsylvania	4.8
11	Rhode Island	7.0
15	South Carolina	6.6
28	South Dakota	4.4
47	Tennessee	0.6
4	Texas	8.5
24	Utah	4.8
44	Vermont	2.0
30	Virginia	4.2
48	Washington	0.5
6	West Virginia	8.2
30	Wisconsin	4.2
33	Wyoming	3.6

RANK ORDER

RANK	STATE	PERCENT
1	New York	18.6
2	Alaska	11.4
3	Maine	9.0
4	Texas	8.5
5	Georgia	8.4
6	Florida	8.2
6	West Virginia	8.2
8	Maryland	8.1
9	California	7.5
9	Missouri	7.5
11	Massachusetts	7.0
11	Rhode Island	7.0
13	Mississippi	6.8
14	Kentucky	6.7
15	South Carolina	6.6
16	Arizona	6.4
17	Alabama	6.1
18	Montana	5.9
19	Louisiana	5.7
20	Nevada	5.5
20	Ohio	5.5
22	North Carolina	5.0
23	Oregon	4.9
24	Kansas	4.8
24	New Jersey	4.8
24	Pennsylvania	4.8
24	Utah	4.8
28	Oklahoma	4.4
28	South Dakota	4.4
30	Colorado	4.2
30	Virginia	4.2
30	Wisconsin	4.2
33	Idaho	3.6
33	Indiana	3.6
33	Wyoming	3.6
36	Iowa	3.2
37	Nebraska	3.1
38	Delaware	2.9
38	Michigan	2.9
40	Illinois	2.6
41	Hawaii	2.4
42	Connecticut	2.2
43	North Dakota	2.1
44	New Mexico	2.0
44	Vermont	2.0
46	New Hampshire	1.9
47	Tennessee	0.6
48	Washington	0.5
49	Arkansas	0.4
50	Minnesota	0.0
	District of Columbia	2.4

Source: MQ Press using data from U.S. Dept of Health & Human Services, Centers for Medicare and Medicaid Services
"Children's Health Insurance Program" (http://www.hcfa.gov/init/children.htm)
*For fiscal year 2001. The State Children's Health Insurance Program (SCHIP) was created in 1997 to help states expand health insurance to children whose families earn too much to qualify for Medicaid, yet not enough to afford private health insurance. Calculated using 2000 Census population counts.

Percent of Population Covered by Private Health Insurance in 2000

National Percent = 72.4% of Population

ALPHA ORDER				RANK ORDER		
RANK	STATE	PERCENT		RANK	STATE	PERCENT
35	Alabama	70.5		1	Iowa	84.6
47	Alaska	62.7		2	Minnesota	82.5
41	Arizona	67.7		3	Connecticut	82.4
43	Arkansas	66.5		4	Maryland	82.0
46	California	65.1		4	Wisconsin	82.0
20	Colorado	76.3		6	New Hampshire	81.9
3	Connecticut	82.4		7	Pennsylvania	81.7
21	Delaware	75.7		8	Rhode Island	79.4
42	Florida	66.7		9	Michigan	79.1
30	Georgia	73.0		10	South Dakota	78.9
15	Hawaii	77.7		11	Indiana	78.8
28	Idaho	73.5		12	Ohio	78.7
22	Illinois	75.0		13	Missouri	78.4
11	Indiana	78.8		14	North Dakota	78.1
1	Iowa	84.6		15	Hawaii	77.7
18	Kansas	76.9		16	Utah	77.5
32	Kentucky	72.2		17	New Jersey	77.3
47	Louisiana	62.7		18	Kansas	76.9
23	Maine	74.6		19	Nebraska	76.6
4	Maryland	82.0		20	Colorado	76.3
25	Massachusetts	74.3		21	Delaware	75.7
9	Michigan	79.1		22	Illinois	75.0
2	Minnesota	82.5		23	Maine	74.6
38	Mississippi	69.1		23	Washington	74.6
13	Missouri	78.4		25	Massachusetts	74.3
44	Montana	66.1		26	Virginia	74.2
19	Nebraska	76.6		27	North Carolina	73.7
34	Nevada	71.4		28	Idaho	73.5
6	New Hampshire	81.9		28	Oregon	73.5
17	New Jersey	77.3		30	Georgia	73.0
50	New Mexico	56.4		31	South Carolina	72.3
39	New York	68.3		32	Kentucky	72.2
27	North Carolina	73.7		33	Wyoming	72.1
14	North Dakota	78.1		34	Nevada	71.4
12	Ohio	78.7		35	Alabama	70.5
49	Oklahoma	62.6		36	Vermont	70.4
28	Oregon	73.5		37	Tennessee	70.3
7	Pennsylvania	81.7		38	Mississippi	69.1
8	Rhode Island	79.4		39	New York	68.3
31	South Carolina	72.3		40	West Virginia	67.9
10	South Dakota	78.9		41	Arizona	67.7
37	Tennessee	70.3		42	Florida	66.7
45	Texas	65.7		43	Arkansas	66.5
16	Utah	77.5		44	Montana	66.1
36	Vermont	70.4		45	Texas	65.7
26	Virginia	74.2		46	California	65.1
23	Washington	74.6		47	Alaska	62.7
40	West Virginia	67.9		47	Louisiana	62.7
4	Wisconsin	82.0		49	Oklahoma	62.6
33	Wyoming	72.1		50	New Mexico	56.4
				District of Columbia		68.0

Source: U.S. Bureau of the Census
"Health Insurance Historical Table 4" (http://www.census.gov/hhes/hlthins/historic/hihistt4.html)

Percent of Population Covered by Employment-Based
Private Health Insurance in 2000
National Percent = 64.1% of Population

ALPHA ORDER

RANK	STATE	PERCENT
32	Alabama	62.2
43	Alaska	57.9
40	Arizona	59.2
45	Arkansas	56.6
44	California	57.3
18	Colorado	67.3
3	Connecticut	73.0
13	Delaware	69.2
46	Florida	56.5
22	Georgia	66.1
14	Hawaii	68.4
34	Idaho	61.6
19	Illinois	66.5
14	Indiana	68.4
4	Iowa	72.5
28	Kansas	63.2
19	Kentucky	66.5
47	Louisiana	54.8
23	Maine	65.9
1	Maryland	75.6
21	Massachusetts	66.4
4	Michigan	72.5
8	Minnesota	71.4
41	Mississippi	59.0
16	Missouri	67.5
48	Montana	52.5
39	Nebraska	60.7
27	Nevada	63.9
6	New Hampshire	72.2
11	New Jersey	70.7
50	New Mexico	50.8
33	New York	61.8
24	North Carolina	65.8
37	North Dakota	60.8
8	Ohio	71.4
49	Oklahoma	52.4
28	Oregon	63.2
7	Pennsylvania	71.6
12	Rhode Island	69.7
25	South Carolina	64.9
35	South Dakota	61.2
31	Tennessee	63.0
42	Texas	58.5
10	Utah	71.0
30	Vermont	63.1
16	Virginia	67.5
25	Washington	64.9
36	West Virginia	61.1
2	Wisconsin	74.3
37	Wyoming	60.8

RANK ORDER

RANK	STATE	PERCENT
1	Maryland	75.6
2	Wisconsin	74.3
3	Connecticut	73.0
4	Iowa	72.5
4	Michigan	72.5
6	New Hampshire	72.2
7	Pennsylvania	71.6
8	Minnesota	71.4
8	Ohio	71.4
10	Utah	71.0
11	New Jersey	70.7
12	Rhode Island	69.7
13	Delaware	69.2
14	Hawaii	68.4
14	Indiana	68.4
16	Missouri	67.5
16	Virginia	67.5
18	Colorado	67.3
19	Illinois	66.5
19	Kentucky	66.5
21	Massachusetts	66.4
22	Georgia	66.1
23	Maine	65.9
24	North Carolina	65.8
25	South Carolina	64.9
25	Washington	64.9
27	Nevada	63.9
28	Kansas	63.2
28	Oregon	63.2
30	Vermont	63.1
31	Tennessee	63.0
32	Alabama	62.2
33	New York	61.8
34	Idaho	61.6
35	South Dakota	61.2
36	West Virginia	61.1
37	North Dakota	60.8
37	Wyoming	60.8
39	Nebraska	60.7
40	Arizona	59.2
41	Mississippi	59.0
42	Texas	58.5
43	Alaska	57.9
44	California	57.3
45	Arkansas	56.6
46	Florida	56.5
47	Louisiana	54.8
48	Montana	52.5
49	Oklahoma	52.4
50	New Mexico	50.8
	District of Columbia	60.7

Source: U.S. Bureau of the Census
"Health Insurance Historical Table 4" (http://www.census.gov/hhes/hlthins/historic/hihistt4.html)

Percent of Population Covered by Government Health Insurance in 2000

National Percent = 26.7% of Population*

ALPHA ORDER

RANK	STATE	PERCENT
16	Alabama	29.4
7	Alaska	32.9
27	Arizona	27.3
1	Arkansas	36.4
26	California	27.4
40	Colorado	24.2
33	Connecticut	25.2
31	Delaware	25.8
9	Florida	31.8
38	Georgia	24.4
17	Hawaii	29.3
24	Idaho	28.0
48	Illinois	21.7
41	Indiana	24.1
45	Iowa	23.4
15	Kansas	29.7
17	Kentucky	29.3
10	Louisiana	30.9
21	Maine	28.5
46	Maryland	23.3
19	Massachusetts	28.8
42	Michigan	23.9
49	Minnesota	20.5
2	Mississippi	35.5
43	Missouri	23.7
10	Montana	30.9
20	Nebraska	28.7
37	Nevada	24.6
33	New Hampshire	25.2
39	New Jersey	24.3
8	New Mexico	32.1
13	New York	30.0
24	North Carolina	28.0
27	North Dakota	27.3
47	Ohio	22.5
6	Oklahoma	33.5
29	Oregon	26.6
35	Pennsylvania	25.1
14	Rhode Island	29.9
12	South Carolina	30.1
22	South Dakota	28.2
4	Tennessee	34.8
44	Texas	23.6
50	Utah	20.1
5	Vermont	34.1
32	Virginia	25.4
30	Washington	26.2
3	West Virginia	35.0
36	Wisconsin	24.7
22	Wyoming	28.2

RANK ORDER

RANK	STATE	PERCENT
1	Arkansas	36.4
2	Mississippi	35.5
3	West Virginia	35.0
4	Tennessee	34.8
5	Vermont	34.1
6	Oklahoma	33.5
7	Alaska	32.9
8	New Mexico	32.1
9	Florida	31.8
10	Louisiana	30.9
10	Montana	30.9
12	South Carolina	30.1
13	New York	30.0
14	Rhode Island	29.9
15	Kansas	29.7
16	Alabama	29.4
17	Hawaii	29.3
17	Kentucky	29.3
19	Massachusetts	28.8
20	Nebraska	28.7
21	Maine	28.5
22	South Dakota	28.2
22	Wyoming	28.2
24	Idaho	28.0
24	North Carolina	28.0
26	California	27.4
27	Arizona	27.3
27	North Dakota	27.3
29	Oregon	26.6
30	Washington	26.2
31	Delaware	25.8
32	Virginia	25.4
33	Connecticut	25.2
33	New Hampshire	25.2
35	Pennsylvania	25.1
36	Wisconsin	24.7
37	Nevada	24.6
38	Georgia	24.4
39	New Jersey	24.3
40	Colorado	24.2
41	Indiana	24.1
42	Michigan	23.9
43	Missouri	23.7
44	Texas	23.6
45	Iowa	23.4
46	Maryland	23.3
47	Ohio	22.5
48	Illinois	21.7
49	Minnesota	20.5
50	Utah	20.1

District of Columbia — 29.0

Source: Morgan Quitno Press using data from U.S. Bureau of the Census
"Health Insurance Historical Table 4" (http://www.census.gov/hhes/hlthins/historic/hihistt4.html)
*Includes Medicaid, Medicare and Military health care.

Percent of Population Covered by Military Health Insurance in 2000

National Percent = 3.0% of Population*

ALPHA ORDER

RANK	STATE	PERCENT		RANK	STATE	PERCENT
28	Alabama	3.2		1	Alaska	12.9
1	Alaska	12.9		2	Virginia	7.8
18	Arizona	4.4		3	Kansas	7.5
10	Arkansas	5.3		4	Nebraska	7.1
31	California	2.9		4	Oklahoma	7.1
6	Colorado	5.9		6	Colorado	5.9
46	Connecticut	1.3		6	Wyoming	5.9
34	Delaware	2.2		8	Hawaii	5.6
30	Florida	3.1		9	Kentucky	5.4
16	Georgia	4.5		10	Arkansas	5.3
8	Hawaii	5.6		10	North Dakota	5.3
15	Idaho	4.6		12	Mississippi	5.1
46	Illinois	1.3		13	Montana	4.8
34	Indiana	2.2		14	North Carolina	4.7
36	Iowa	2.0		15	Idaho	4.6
3	Kansas	7.5		16	Georgia	4.5
9	Kentucky	5.4		16	Maine	4.5
18	Louisiana	4.4		18	Arizona	4.4
16	Maine	4.5		18	Louisiana	4.4
24	Maryland	3.4		20	New Mexico	4.3
50	Massachusetts	0.8		20	South Dakota	4.3
49	Michigan	0.9		22	Washington	4.1
46	Minnesota	1.3		23	South Carolina	3.7
12	Mississippi	5.1		24	Maryland	3.4
42	Missouri	1.6		24	Nevada	3.4
13	Montana	4.8		26	New Hampshire	3.3
4	Nebraska	7.1		26	Tennessee	3.3
24	Nevada	3.4		28	Alabama	3.2
26	New Hampshire	3.3		28	Texas	3.2
41	New Jersey	1.7		30	Florida	3.1
20	New Mexico	4.3		31	California	2.9
43	New York	1.5		32	Utah	2.7
14	North Carolina	4.7		33	West Virginia	2.6
10	North Dakota	5.3		34	Delaware	2.2
44	Ohio	1.4		34	Indiana	2.2
4	Oklahoma	7.1		36	Iowa	2.0
36	Oregon	2.0		36	Oregon	2.0
40	Pennsylvania	1.8		36	Vermont	2.0
44	Rhode Island	1.4		39	Wisconsin	1.9
23	South Carolina	3.7		40	Pennsylvania	1.8
20	South Dakota	4.3		41	New Jersey	1.7
26	Tennessee	3.3		42	Missouri	1.6
28	Texas	3.2		43	New York	1.5
32	Utah	2.7		44	Ohio	1.4
36	Vermont	2.0		44	Rhode Island	1.4
2	Virginia	7.8		46	Connecticut	1.3
22	Washington	4.1		46	Illinois	1.3
33	West Virginia	2.6		46	Minnesota	1.3
39	Wisconsin	1.9		49	Michigan	0.9
6	Wyoming	5.9		50	Massachusetts	0.8
					District of Columbia	2.0

Source: U.S. Bureau of the Census
   "Health Insurance Historical Table 4" (http://www.census.gov/hhes/hlthins/historic/hihistt4.html)
Includes CHAMPUS (Comprehensive Health and Medical Plan for Uniformed Services)/Tricare, Veterans and military health care.

Health Maintenance Organizations (HMOs) in 2001

National Total = 538 HMOs*

ALPHA ORDER

RANK	STATE	HMOs	% of USA
29	Alabama	5	0.9%
50	Alaska	0	0.0%
19	Arizona	10	1.9%
35	Arkansas	4	0.7%
2	California	33	6.1%
14	Colorado	13	2.4%
23	Connecticut	9	1.7%
35	Delaware	4	0.7%
3	Florida	32	5.9%
17	Georgia	11	2.0%
27	Hawaii	6	1.1%
41	Idaho	3	0.6%
9	Illinois	19	3.5%
14	Indiana	13	2.4%
41	Iowa	3	0.6%
25	Kansas	8	1.5%
29	Kentucky	5	0.9%
16	Louisiana	12	2.2%
35	Maine	4	0.7%
19	Maryland	10	1.9%
19	Massachusetts	10	1.9%
6	Michigan	25	4.6%
23	Minnesota	9	1.7%
41	Mississippi	3	0.6%
7	Missouri	20	3.7%
41	Montana	3	0.6%
29	Nebraska	5	0.9%
27	Nevada	6	1.1%
35	New Hampshire	4	0.7%
13	New Jersey	14	2.6%
35	New Mexico	4	0.7%
4	New York	31	5.8%
12	North Carolina	16	3.0%
46	North Dakota	2	0.4%
4	Ohio	31	5.8%
19	Oklahoma	10	1.9%
29	Oregon	5	0.9%
7	Pennsylvania	20	3.7%
41	Rhode Island	3	0.6%
29	South Carolina	5	0.9%
35	South Dakota	4	0.7%
11	Tennessee	17	3.2%
1	Texas	36	6.7%
26	Utah	7	1.3%
48	Vermont	1	0.2%
17	Virginia	11	2.0%
29	Washington	5	0.9%
46	West Virginia	2	0.4%
9	Wisconsin	19	3.5%
48	Wyoming	1	0.2%

RANK ORDER

RANK	STATE	HMOs	% of USA
1	Texas	36	6.7%
2	California	33	6.1%
3	Florida	32	5.9%
4	New York	31	5.8%
4	Ohio	31	5.8%
6	Michigan	25	4.6%
7	Missouri	20	3.7%
7	Pennsylvania	20	3.7%
9	Illinois	19	3.5%
9	Wisconsin	19	3.5%
11	Tennessee	17	3.2%
12	North Carolina	16	3.0%
13	New Jersey	14	2.6%
14	Colorado	13	2.4%
14	Indiana	13	2.4%
16	Louisiana	12	2.2%
17	Georgia	11	2.0%
17	Virginia	11	2.0%
19	Arizona	10	1.9%
19	Maryland	10	1.9%
19	Massachusetts	10	1.9%
19	Oklahoma	10	1.9%
23	Connecticut	9	1.7%
23	Minnesota	9	1.7%
25	Kansas	8	1.5%
26	Utah	7	1.3%
27	Hawaii	6	1.1%
27	Nevada	6	1.1%
29	Alabama	5	0.9%
29	Kentucky	5	0.9%
29	Nebraska	5	0.9%
29	Oregon	5	0.9%
29	South Carolina	5	0.9%
29	Washington	5	0.9%
35	Arkansas	4	0.7%
35	Delaware	4	0.7%
35	Maine	4	0.7%
35	New Hampshire	4	0.7%
35	New Mexico	4	0.7%
35	South Dakota	4	0.7%
41	Idaho	3	0.6%
41	Iowa	3	0.6%
41	Mississippi	3	0.6%
41	Montana	3	0.6%
41	Rhode Island	3	0.6%
46	North Dakota	2	0.4%
46	West Virginia	2	0.4%
48	Vermont	1	0.2%
48	Wyoming	1	0.2%
50	Alaska	0	0.0%
	District of Columbia	5	0.9%

Source: InterStudy Publications (Minneapolis, MN)

  "HMO Industry Report 11.2" (Press Release, October 31, 2001)

As of January 1, 2001. Total does not include one HMO in Guam and two in Puerto Rico. Health plans are allocated to states based upon their primary service areas. This means each plan is counted once. However, many plans serve more than one state.

Enrollees in Health Maintenance Organizations (HMOs) in 2001

National Total = 78,445,862 Enrollees*

ALPHA ORDER

RANK	STATE	ENROLLEES	% of USA
37	Alabama	288,480	0.4%
50	Alaska	0	0.0%
14	Arizona	1,660,995	2.1%
38	Arkansas	281,474	0.4%
1	California	18,073,792	23.0%
16	Colorado	1,565,812	2.0%
18	Connecticut	1,353,193	1.7%
41	Delaware	178,372	0.2%
3	Florida	4,757,158	6.1%
20	Georgia	1,304,253	1.7%
33	Hawaii	385,708	0.5%
45	Idaho	55,441	0.1%
10	Illinois	2,386,850	3.0%
26	Indiana	712,088	0.9%
40	Iowa	190,737	0.2%
31	Kansas	432,460	0.6%
21	Kentucky	1,228,308	1.6%
27	Louisiana	695,583	0.9%
36	Maine	356,014	0.5%
11	Maryland**	2,031,606	2.6%
6	Massachusetts	2,813,636	3.6%
8	Michigan	2,652,755	3.4%
17	Minnesota	1,385,078	1.8%
47	Mississippi	25,245	0.0%
13	Missouri	1,732,949	2.2%
44	Montana	69,800	0.1%
42	Nebraska	169,969	0.2%
32	Nevada	408,188	0.5%
29	New Hampshire	485,060	0.6%
7	New Jersey	2,664,436	3.4%
28	New Mexico	506,852	0.6%
2	New York	6,637,057	8.5%
19	North Carolina	1,311,292	1.7%
49	North Dakota	8,172	0.0%
9	Ohio	2,651,868	3.4%
30	Oklahoma	479,592	0.6%
22	Oregon	1,213,892	1.5%
4	Pennsylvania	4,099,592	5.2%
35	Rhode Island	366,695	0.5%
34	South Carolina	382,882	0.5%
43	South Dakota	73,032	0.1%
12	Tennessee	1,879,542	2.4%
5	Texas	3,655,939	4.7%
25	Utah	793,002	1.0%
46	Vermont	25,696	0.0%
23	Virginia**	1,144,030	1.5%
24	Washington	900,520	1.1%
39	West Virginia**	197,274	0.3%
15	Wisconsin	1,587,555	2.0%
48	Wyoming	8,600	0.0%

RANK ORDER

RANK	STATE	ENROLLEES	% of USA
1	California	18,073,792	23.0%
2	New York	6,637,057	8.5%
3	Florida	4,757,158	6.1%
4	Pennsylvania	4,099,592	5.2%
5	Texas	3,655,939	4.7%
6	Massachusetts	2,813,636	3.6%
7	New Jersey	2,664,436	3.4%
8	Michigan	2,652,755	3.4%
9	Ohio	2,651,868	3.4%
10	Illinois	2,386,850	3.0%
11	Maryland**	2,031,606	2.6%
12	Tennessee	1,879,542	2.4%
13	Missouri	1,732,949	2.2%
14	Arizona	1,660,995	2.1%
15	Wisconsin	1,587,555	2.0%
16	Colorado	1,565,812	2.0%
17	Minnesota	1,385,078	1.8%
18	Connecticut	1,353,193	1.7%
19	North Carolina	1,311,292	1.7%
20	Georgia	1,304,253	1.7%
21	Kentucky	1,228,308	1.6%
22	Oregon	1,213,892	1.5%
23	Virginia**	1,144,030	1.5%
24	Washington	900,520	1.1%
25	Utah	793,002	1.0%
26	Indiana	712,088	0.9%
27	Louisiana	695,583	0.9%
28	New Mexico	506,852	0.6%
29	New Hampshire	485,060	0.6%
30	Oklahoma	479,592	0.6%
31	Kansas	432,460	0.6%
32	Nevada	408,188	0.5%
33	Hawaii	385,708	0.5%
34	South Carolina	382,882	0.5%
35	Rhode Island	366,695	0.5%
36	Maine	356,014	0.5%
37	Alabama	288,480	0.4%
38	Arkansas	281,474	0.4%
39	West Virginia**	197,274	0.3%
40	Iowa	190,737	0.2%
41	Delaware	178,372	0.2%
42	Nebraska	169,969	0.2%
43	South Dakota	73,032	0.1%
44	Montana	69,800	0.1%
45	Idaho	55,441	0.1%
46	Vermont	25,696	0.0%
47	Mississippi	25,245	0.0%
48	Wyoming	8,600	0.0%
49	North Dakota	8,172	0.0%
50	Alaska	0	0.0%
	District of Columbia	177,338	0.2%

Source: InterStudy Publications (Minneapolis, MN)
"HMO Industry Report 11.2" (Press Release, October 31, 2001)
*As of January 1, 2001. Total does not include 1,089,057 enrollees in U.S. territories.
**Maryland, Virginia and West Virginia include partial enrollment from five HMOs serving the Washington, DC metropolitan area.

Percent Change in Enrollees in Health Maintenance Organizations (HMOs): 2000 to 2001
National Percent Change = 1.4% Decrease*

RANK	STATE	PERCENT CHANGE
38	Alabama	(8.4)
NA	Alaska**	NA
5	Arizona	14.4
10	Arkansas	6.2
14	California	3.4
25	Colorado	(2.3)
37	Connecticut	(7.6)
8	Delaware	8.0
20	Florida	0.2
29	Georgia	(3.6)
7	Hawaii	8.9
48	Idaho	(34.5)
32	Illinois	(4.5)
28	Indiana	(3.3)
36	Iowa	(7.2)
39	Kansas	(9.2)
23	Kentucky	(1.5)
35	Louisiana	(6.5)
3	Maine	27.5
43	Maryland	(10.5)
45	Massachusetts	(13.6)
19	Michigan	0.6
24	Minnesota	(1.6)
46	Mississippi	(17.1)
42	Missouri	(10.0)
6	Montana	13.5
39	Nebraska	(9.2)
31	Nevada	(4.0)
4	New Hampshire	19.7
11	New Jersey	5.7
47	New Mexico	(22.8)
16	New York	1.9
30	North Carolina	(3.9)
49	North Dakota	(48.4)
34	Ohio	(6.3)
26	Oklahoma	(2.5)
44	Oregon	(10.9)
18	Pennsylvania	0.9
27	Rhode Island	(2.8)
21	South Carolina	(0.7)
1	South Dakota	48.1
13	Tennessee	4.0
22	Texas	(1.3)
12	Utah	5.5
33	Vermont	(6.0)
41	Virginia	(9.9)
15	Washington	3.2
9	West Virginia	6.6
17	Wisconsin	1.4
2	Wyoming	29.8

RANK	STATE	PERCENT CHANGE
1	South Dakota	48.1
2	Wyoming	29.8
3	Maine	27.5
4	New Hampshire	19.7
5	Arizona	14.4
6	Montana	13.5
7	Hawaii	8.9
8	Delaware	8.0
9	West Virginia	6.6
10	Arkansas	6.2
11	New Jersey	5.7
12	Utah	5.5
13	Tennessee	4.0
14	California	3.4
15	Washington	3.2
16	New York	1.9
17	Wisconsin	1.4
18	Pennsylvania	0.9
19	Michigan	0.6
20	Florida	0.2
21	South Carolina	(0.7)
22	Texas	(1.3)
23	Kentucky	(1.5)
24	Minnesota	(1.6)
25	Colorado	(2.3)
26	Oklahoma	(2.5)
27	Rhode Island	(2.8)
28	Indiana	(3.3)
29	Georgia	(3.6)
30	North Carolina	(3.9)
31	Nevada	(4.0)
32	Illinois	(4.5)
33	Vermont	(6.0)
34	Ohio	(6.3)
35	Louisiana	(6.5)
36	Iowa	(7.2)
37	Connecticut	(7.6)
38	Alabama	(8.4)
39	Kansas	(9.2)
39	Nebraska	(9.2)
41	Virginia	(9.9)
42	Missouri	(10.0)
43	Maryland	(10.5)
44	Oregon	(10.9)
45	Massachusetts	(13.6)
46	Mississippi	(17.1)
47	New Mexico	(22.8)
48	Idaho	(34.5)
49	North Dakota	(48.4)
NA	Alaska**	NA

District of Columbia	(2.8)

Source: InterStudy Publications (Minneapolis, MN)
   "HMO Industry Report 11.2" (Press Release, October 31, 2001)
*As of January 1, 2001. National rate does not include enrollees in U.S. territories.
**Not applicable.

Percent of Population Enrolled in Health Maintenance Organizations (HMOs) in 2001
National Percent = 27.5% Enrolled in HMOs*

ALPHA ORDER

RANK ORDER

RANK	STATE	PERCENT
43	Alabama	6.5
50	Alaska	0.0
15	Arizona	31.3
38	Arkansas	10.5
1	California	52.4
6	Colorado	35.4
3	Connecticut	39.5
25	Delaware	22.4
19	Florida	29.0
32	Georgia	15.6
13	Hawaii	31.5
45	Idaho	4.2
27	Illinois	19.1
36	Indiana	11.6
43	Iowa	6.5
29	Kansas	16.0
17	Kentucky	30.2
32	Louisiana	15.6
21	Maine	27.7
5	Maryland	37.8
2	Massachusetts	44.1
23	Michigan	26.6
20	Minnesota	27.9
49	Mississippi	0.9
16	Missouri	30.8
42	Montana	7.7
39	Nebraska	9.9
26	Nevada	19.4
4	New Hampshire	38.5
14	New Jersey	31.4
21	New Mexico	27.7
8	New York	34.9
29	North Carolina	16.0
48	North Dakota	1.3
24	Ohio	23.3
35	Oklahoma	13.9
7	Oregon	35.0
11	Pennsylvania	33.4
10	Rhode Island	34.6
41	South Carolina	9.4
40	South Dakota	9.7
12	Tennessee	32.7
28	Texas	17.1
8	Utah	34.9
45	Vermont	4.2
31	Virginia	15.9
34	Washington	15.0
37	West Virginia	10.9
18	Wisconsin	29.4
47	Wyoming	1.7

RANK	STATE	PERCENT
1	California	52.4
2	Massachusetts	44.1
3	Connecticut	39.5
4	New Hampshire	38.5
5	Maryland	37.8
6	Colorado	35.4
7	Oregon	35.0
8	New York	34.9
8	Utah	34.9
10	Rhode Island	34.6
11	Pennsylvania	33.4
12	Tennessee	32.7
13	Hawaii	31.5
14	New Jersey	31.4
15	Arizona	31.3
16	Missouri	30.8
17	Kentucky	30.2
18	Wisconsin	29.4
19	Florida	29.0
20	Minnesota	27.9
21	Maine	27.7
21	New Mexico	27.7
23	Michigan	26.6
24	Ohio	23.3
25	Delaware	22.4
26	Nevada	19.4
27	Illinois	19.1
28	Texas	17.1
29	Kansas	16.0
29	North Carolina	16.0
31	Virginia	15.9
32	Georgia	15.6
32	Louisiana	15.6
34	Washington	15.0
35	Oklahoma	13.9
36	Indiana	11.6
37	West Virginia	10.9
38	Arkansas	10.5
39	Nebraska	9.9
40	South Dakota	9.7
41	South Carolina	9.4
42	Montana	7.7
43	Alabama	6.5
43	Iowa	6.5
45	Idaho	4.2
45	Vermont	4.2
47	Wyoming	1.7
48	North Dakota	1.3
49	Mississippi	0.9
50	Alaska	0.0

| | District of Columbia | 31.0 |

Source: Morgan Quitno Press using data from InterStudy Publications (Minneapolis, MN)
"HMO Industry Report 11.2" (Press Release, October 31, 2001)
*As of January 1, 2001. National percent does not include enrollees or population in U.S. territories.

Percent of Insured Population Enrolled in
Health Maintenance Organizations (HMOs) in 2001
National Percent = 33.4% of Insured are Enrolled in HMOs*

ALPHA ORDER

RANK	STATE	PERCENT
43	Alabama	7.5
50	Alaska	0.0
11	Arizona	40.3
38	Arkansas	12.4
1	California	63.5
5	Colorado	42.7
3	Connecticut	44.3
25	Delaware	25.3
12	Florida	37.9
31	Georgia	19.6
14	Hawaii	37.1
45	Idaho	5.2
28	Illinois	22.5
36	Indiana	13.9
44	Iowa	7.3
32	Kansas	18.8
18	Kentucky	35.5
29	Louisiana	20.3
20	Maine	31.8
4	Maryland	44.0
2	Massachusetts	49.7
23	Michigan	29.6
20	Minnesota	31.8
49	Mississippi	1.0
19	Missouri	35.2
42	Montana	9.8
41	Nebraska	11.4
26	Nevada	24.3
7	New Hampshire	42.0
17	New Jersey	36.7
14	New Mexico	37.1
6	New York	42.5
30	North Carolina	20.0
48	North Dakota	1.5
24	Ohio	25.8
34	Oklahoma	18.1
10	Oregon	41.4
14	Pennsylvania	37.1
8	Rhode Island	41.6
40	South Carolina	11.5
39	South Dakota	11.9
13	Tennessee	37.6
27	Texas	22.6
9	Utah	41.5
46	Vermont	4.6
32	Virginia	18.8
35	Washington	17.7
37	West Virginia	12.9
22	Wisconsin	31.5
47	Wyoming	2.1

RANK ORDER

RANK	STATE	PERCENT
1	California	63.5
2	Massachusetts	49.7
3	Connecticut	44.3
4	Maryland	44.0
5	Colorado	42.7
6	New York	42.5
7	New Hampshire	42.0
8	Rhode Island	41.6
9	Utah	41.5
10	Oregon	41.4
11	Arizona	40.3
12	Florida	37.9
13	Tennessee	37.6
14	Hawaii	37.1
14	New Mexico	37.1
14	Pennsylvania	37.1
17	New Jersey	36.7
18	Kentucky	35.5
19	Missouri	35.2
20	Maine	31.8
20	Minnesota	31.8
22	Wisconsin	31.5
23	Michigan	29.6
24	Ohio	25.8
25	Delaware	25.3
26	Nevada	24.3
27	Texas	22.6
28	Illinois	22.5
29	Louisiana	20.3
30	North Carolina	20.0
31	Georgia	19.6
32	Kansas	18.8
32	Virginia	18.8
34	Oklahoma	18.1
35	Washington	17.7
36	Indiana	13.9
37	West Virginia	12.9
38	Arkansas	12.4
39	South Dakota	11.9
40	South Carolina	11.5
41	Nebraska	11.4
42	Montana	9.8
43	Alabama	7.5
44	Iowa	7.3
45	Idaho	5.2
46	Vermont	4.6
47	Wyoming	2.1
48	North Dakota	1.5
49	Mississippi	1.0
50	Alaska	0.0
	District of Columbia	40.9

Source: Morgan Quitno Press using data from InterStudy Publications (Minneapolis, MN)
"HMO Industry Report 11.2" (Press Release, October 31, 2001)
*As of January 1, 2001. Calculated using estimated number of insured as of 2000 from the U.S. Census Bureau.

Medicare Enrollees in 2000

National Total = 39,140,386 Enrollees*

RANK	STATE	ENROLLEES	% of USA
19	Alabama	676,569	1.7%
50	Alaska	40,062	0.1%
20	Arizona	658,193	1.7%
31	Arkansas	435,880	1.1%
1	California	3,837,080	9.8%
30	Colorado	458,380	1.2%
26	Connecticut	511,611	1.3%
46	Delaware	109,575	0.3%
2	Florida	2,770,576	7.1%
12	Georgia	897,503	2.3%
42	Hawaii	161,787	0.4%
43	Idaho	161,362	0.4%
7	Illinois	1,628,744	4.2%
15	Indiana	844,835	2.2%
29	Iowa	475,854	1.2%
33	Kansas	389,103	1.0%
23	Kentucky	615,436	1.6%
24	Louisiana	597,485	1.5%
38	Maine	213,210	0.5%
22	Maryland	634,527	1.6%
11	Massachusetts	954,180	2.4%
8	Michigan	1,389,107	3.5%
21	Minnesota	648,272	1.7%
32	Mississippi	413,900	1.1%
14	Missouri	854,472	2.2%
44	Montana	135,415	0.3%
35	Nebraska	252,231	0.6%
37	Nevada	228,631	0.6%
41	New Hampshire	166,751	0.4%
9	New Jersey	1,194,539	3.1%
36	New Mexico	229,124	0.6%
3	New York	2,694,015	6.9%
10	North Carolina	1,111,273	2.8%
47	North Dakota	103,066	0.3%
6	Ohio	1,692,072	4.3%
27	Oklahoma	503,506	1.3%
28	Oregon	483,898	1.2%
5	Pennsylvania	2,088,116	5.3%
40	Rhode Island	170,331	0.4%
25	South Carolina	555,082	1.4%
45	South Dakota	118,979	0.3%
16	Tennessee	815,231	2.1%
4	Texas	2,223,175	5.7%
39	Utah	201,217	0.5%
48	Vermont	87,644	0.2%
13	Virginia	875,799	2.2%
18	Washington	725,018	1.9%
34	West Virginia	335,529	0.9%
17	Wisconsin	777,273	2.0%
49	Wyoming	64,448	0.2%

RANK	STATE	ENROLLEES	% of USA
1	California	3,837,080	9.8%
2	Florida	2,770,576	7.1%
3	New York	2,694,015	6.9%
4	Texas	2,223,175	5.7%
5	Pennsylvania	2,088,116	5.3%
6	Ohio	1,692,072	4.3%
7	Illinois	1,628,744	4.2%
8	Michigan	1,389,107	3.5%
9	New Jersey	1,194,539	3.1%
10	North Carolina	1,111,273	2.8%
11	Massachusetts	954,180	2.4%
12	Georgia	897,503	2.3%
13	Virginia	875,799	2.2%
14	Missouri	854,472	2.2%
15	Indiana	844,835	2.2%
16	Tennessee	815,231	2.1%
17	Wisconsin	777,273	2.0%
18	Washington	725,018	1.9%
19	Alabama	676,569	1.7%
20	Arizona	658,193	1.7%
21	Minnesota	648,272	1.7%
22	Maryland	634,527	1.6%
23	Kentucky	615,436	1.6%
24	Louisiana	597,485	1.5%
25	South Carolina	555,082	1.4%
26	Connecticut	511,611	1.3%
27	Oklahoma	503,506	1.3%
28	Oregon	483,898	1.2%
29	Iowa	475,854	1.2%
30	Colorado	458,380	1.2%
31	Arkansas	435,880	1.1%
32	Mississippi	413,900	1.1%
33	Kansas	389,103	1.0%
34	West Virginia	335,529	0.9%
35	Nebraska	252,231	0.6%
36	New Mexico	229,124	0.6%
37	Nevada	228,631	0.6%
38	Maine	213,210	0.5%
39	Utah	201,217	0.5%
40	Rhode Island	170,331	0.4%
41	New Hampshire	166,751	0.4%
42	Hawaii	161,787	0.4%
43	Idaho	161,362	0.4%
44	Montana	135,415	0.3%
45	South Dakota	118,979	0.3%
46	Delaware	109,575	0.3%
47	North Dakota	103,066	0.3%
48	Vermont	87,644	0.2%
49	Wyoming	64,448	0.2%
50	Alaska	40,062	0.1%
	District of Columbia	75,619	0.2%

*Source: U.S. Department of Health and Human Services, Centers for Medicare and Medicaid Services
"Medicare Estimated Benefit Payments by State" (http://www.hcfa.gov/stats/BENEPAY/bnpay00i.htm)
For fiscal year 2000. Includes aged and disabled enrollees. Total includes 525,000 enrollees in Puerto Rico and 329,701 enrollees in "other outlying areas."

Medicare Benefit Payments in 2000

National Total = $214,867,632,778*

ALPHA ORDER

RANK	STATE	BENEFITS	% of USA
19	Alabama	$3,884,939,060	1.8%
50	Alaska	188,624,044	0.1%
25	Arizona	2,937,976,231	1.4%
30	Arkansas	2,082,749,809	1.0%
1	California	23,620,610,542	11.0%
27	Colorado	2,337,864,957	1.1%
21	Connecticut	3,291,179,250	1.5%
47	Delaware	429,519,966	0.2%
2	Florida	19,220,607,977	8.9%
16	Georgia	4,110,655,928	1.9%
43	Hawaii	621,680,722	0.3%
41	Idaho	638,754,898	0.3%
7	Illinois	7,308,734,402	3.4%
13	Indiana	4,720,330,295	2.2%
34	Iowa	1,452,928,371	0.7%
31	Kansas	1,914,899,957	0.9%
22	Kentucky	3,153,190,792	1.5%
14	Louisiana	4,383,213,203	2.0%
40	Maine	793,162,952	0.4%
18	Maryland	3,998,320,142	1.9%
11	Massachusetts	5,465,762,999	2.5%
9	Michigan	6,269,417,011	2.9%
23	Minnesota	3,108,986,231	1.4%
28	Mississippi	2,247,917,430	1.0%
15	Missouri	4,273,990,871	2.0%
44	Montana	574,604,919	0.3%
35	Nebraska	1,224,833,404	0.6%
37	Nevada	1,069,328,044	0.5%
42	New Hampshire	628,752,777	0.3%
8	New Jersey	6,766,868,340	3.1%
39	New Mexico	853,675,941	0.4%
3	New York	18,653,025,253	8.7%
10	North Carolina	5,942,006,657	2.8%
46	North Dakota	500,700,180	0.2%
6	Ohio	9,310,104,645	4.3%
29	Oklahoma	2,137,385,847	1.0%
32	Oregon	1,852,665,125	0.9%
5	Pennsylvania	13,256,553,960	6.2%
36	Rhode Island	1,075,101,330	0.5%
24	South Carolina	2,946,661,184	1.4%
45	South Dakota	563,935,015	0.3%
12	Tennessee	4,906,775,721	2.3%
4	Texas	14,537,817,250	6.8%
38	Utah	917,794,670	0.4%
48	Vermont	314,536,271	0.1%
17	Virginia	4,037,966,718	1.9%
26	Washington	2,842,834,283	1.3%
33	West Virginia	1,655,615,997	0.8%
20	Wisconsin	3,497,823,831	1.6%
49	Wyoming	247,350,405	0.1%

RANK ORDER

RANK	STATE	BENEFITS	% of USA
1	California	$23,620,610,542	11.0%
2	Florida	19,220,607,977	8.9%
3	New York	18,653,025,253	8.7%
4	Texas	14,537,817,250	6.8%
5	Pennsylvania	13,256,553,960	6.2%
6	Ohio	9,310,104,645	4.3%
7	Illinois	7,308,734,402	3.4%
8	New Jersey	6,766,868,340	3.1%
9	Michigan	6,269,417,011	2.9%
10	North Carolina	5,942,006,657	2.8%
11	Massachusetts	5,465,762,999	2.5%
12	Tennessee	4,906,775,721	2.3%
13	Indiana	4,720,330,295	2.2%
14	Louisiana	4,383,213,203	2.0%
15	Missouri	4,273,990,871	2.0%
16	Georgia	4,110,655,928	1.9%
17	Virginia	4,037,966,718	1.9%
18	Maryland	3,998,320,142	1.9%
19	Alabama	3,884,939,060	1.8%
20	Wisconsin	3,497,823,831	1.6%
21	Connecticut	3,291,179,250	1.5%
22	Kentucky	3,153,190,792	1.5%
23	Minnesota	3,108,986,231	1.4%
24	South Carolina	2,946,661,184	1.4%
25	Arizona	2,937,976,231	1.4%
26	Washington	2,842,834,283	1.3%
27	Colorado	2,337,864,957	1.1%
28	Mississippi	2,247,917,430	1.0%
29	Oklahoma	2,137,385,847	1.0%
30	Arkansas	2,082,749,809	1.0%
31	Kansas	1,914,899,957	0.9%
32	Oregon	1,852,665,125	0.9%
33	West Virginia	1,655,615,997	0.8%
34	Iowa	1,452,928,371	0.7%
35	Nebraska	1,224,833,404	0.6%
36	Rhode Island	1,075,101,330	0.5%
37	Nevada	1,069,328,044	0.5%
38	Utah	917,794,670	0.4%
39	New Mexico	853,675,941	0.4%
40	Maine	793,162,952	0.4%
41	Idaho	638,754,898	0.3%
42	New Hampshire	628,752,777	0.3%
43	Hawaii	621,680,722	0.3%
44	Montana	574,604,919	0.3%
45	South Dakota	563,935,015	0.3%
46	North Dakota	500,700,180	0.2%
47	Delaware	429,519,966	0.2%
48	Vermont	314,536,271	0.1%
49	Wyoming	247,350,405	0.1%
50	Alaska	188,624,044	0.1%
	District of Columbia	784,390,711	0.4%

Source: U.S. Department of Health and Human Services, Centers for Medicare and Medicaid Services
   "Medicare Estimated Benefit Payments by State" (http://www.hcfa.gov/stats/BENEPAY/bnpay00i.htm)
*For fiscal year 2000. Includes payments to aged and disabled enrollees. Total includes $1,223,663,232 in
payments to enrollees in Puerto Rico and $88,843,026 to enrollees in "other outlying areas."

Medicare Payments per Enrollee in 2000

National Rate = $5,490*

ALPHA ORDER				RANK ORDER		
RANK	STATE	PER ENROLLEE		RANK	STATE	PER ENROLLEE
11	Alabama	$5,742		1	Louisiana	$7,336
29	Alaska	4,708		2	Florida	6,937
37	Arizona	4,464		3	New York	6,924
27	Arkansas	4,778		4	Texas	6,539
9	California	6,156		5	Connecticut	6,433
20	Colorado	5,100		6	Pennsylvania	6,349
5	Connecticut	6,433		7	Rhode Island	6,312
42	Delaware	3,920		8	Maryland	6,301
2	Florida	6,937		9	California	6,156
32	Georgia	4,580		10	Tennessee	6,019
43	Hawaii	3,843		11	Alabama	5,742
40	Idaho	3,959		12	Massachusetts	5,728
36	Illinois	4,487		13	New Jersey	5,665
14	Indiana	5,587		14	Indiana	5,587
50	Iowa	3,053		15	Ohio	5,502
23	Kansas	4,921		16	Mississippi	5,431
19	Kentucky	5,124		17	North Carolina	5,347
1	Louisiana	7,336		18	South Carolina	5,309
48	Maine	3,720		19	Kentucky	5,124
8	Maryland	6,301		20	Colorado	5,100
12	Massachusetts	5,728		21	Missouri	5,002
34	Michigan	4,513		22	West Virginia	4,934
26	Minnesota	4,796		23	Kansas	4,921
16	Mississippi	5,431		24	North Dakota	4,858
21	Missouri	5,002		25	Nebraska	4,856
39	Montana	4,243		26	Minnesota	4,796
25	Nebraska	4,856		27	Arkansas	4,778
30	Nevada	4,677		28	South Dakota	4,740
46	New Hampshire	3,771		29	Alaska	4,708
13	New Jersey	5,665		30	Nevada	4,677
47	New Mexico	3,726		31	Virginia	4,611
3	New York	6,924		32	Georgia	4,580
17	North Carolina	5,347		33	Utah	4,561
24	North Dakota	4,858		34	Michigan	4,513
15	Ohio	5,502		35	Wisconsin	4,500
38	Oklahoma	4,245		36	Illinois	4,487
45	Oregon	3,829		37	Arizona	4,464
6	Pennsylvania	6,349		38	Oklahoma	4,245
7	Rhode Island	6,312		39	Montana	4,243
18	South Carolina	5,309		40	Idaho	3,959
28	South Dakota	4,740		41	Washington	3,921
10	Tennessee	6,019		42	Delaware	3,920
4	Texas	6,539		43	Hawaii	3,843
33	Utah	4,561		44	Wyoming	3,838
49	Vermont	3,589		45	Oregon	3,829
31	Virginia	4,611		46	New Hampshire	3,771
41	Washington	3,921		47	New Mexico	3,726
22	West Virginia	4,934		48	Maine	3,720
35	Wisconsin	4,500		49	Vermont	3,589
44	Wyoming	3,838		50	Iowa	3,053
					District of Columbia	10,373

Source: U.S. Department of Health and Human Services, Centers for Medicare and Medicaid Services
"Medicare Estimated Benefit Payments by State" (http://www.hcfa.gov/stats/BENEPAY/bnpay00i.htm)
*For fiscal year 2000. Includes aged and disabled enrollees. National rate includes payments to enrollees in Puerto Rico and in "other outlying areas."

Percent of Population Enrolled in Medicare in 2000

National Percent = 13.6% of Population*

ALPHA ORDER				RANK ORDER		
RANK	STATE	PERCENT		RANK	STATE	PERCENT
10	Alabama	15.2		1	West Virginia	18.6
50	Alaska	6.4		2	Florida	17.3
38	Arizona	12.7		3	Pennsylvania	17.0
5	Arkansas	16.3		4	Maine	16.7
44	California	11.3		5	Arkansas	16.3
47	Colorado	10.6		5	Iowa	16.3
13	Connecticut	15.0		7	Rhode Island	16.2
28	Delaware	13.9		8	North Dakota	16.1
2	Florida	17.3		9	South Dakota	15.7
46	Georgia	10.9		10	Alabama	15.2
34	Hawaii	13.3		10	Kentucky	15.2
40	Idaho	12.4		10	Missouri	15.2
35	Illinois	13.1		13	Connecticut	15.0
28	Indiana	13.9		13	Massachusetts	15.0
5	Iowa	16.3		13	Montana	15.0
19	Kansas	14.5		16	Ohio	14.9
10	Kentucky	15.2		17	Nebraska	14.7
32	Louisiana	13.4		18	Oklahoma	14.6
4	Maine	16.7		19	Kansas	14.5
43	Maryland	11.9		19	Mississippi	14.5
13	Massachusetts	15.0		19	Wisconsin	14.5
27	Michigan	14.0		22	Vermont	14.4
35	Minnesota	13.1		23	Tennessee	14.3
19	Mississippi	14.5		24	New Jersey	14.2
10	Missouri	15.2		24	New York	14.2
13	Montana	15.0		26	Oregon	14.1
17	Nebraska	14.7		27	Michigan	14.0
44	Nevada	11.3		28	Delaware	13.9
32	New Hampshire	13.4		28	Indiana	13.9
24	New Jersey	14.2		30	North Carolina	13.8
39	New Mexico	12.6		30	South Carolina	13.8
24	New York	14.2		32	Louisiana	13.4
30	North Carolina	13.8		32	New Hampshire	13.4
8	North Dakota	16.1		34	Hawaii	13.3
16	Ohio	14.9		35	Illinois	13.1
18	Oklahoma	14.6		35	Minnesota	13.1
26	Oregon	14.1		37	Wyoming	13.0
3	Pennsylvania	17.0		38	Arizona	12.7
7	Rhode Island	16.2		39	New Mexico	12.6
30	South Carolina	13.8		40	Idaho	12.4
9	South Dakota	15.7		41	Virginia	12.3
23	Tennessee	14.3		41	Washington	12.3
47	Texas	10.6		43	Maryland	11.9
49	Utah	9.0		44	California	11.3
22	Vermont	14.4		44	Nevada	11.3
41	Virginia	12.3		46	Georgia	10.9
41	Washington	12.3		47	Colorado	10.6
1	West Virginia	18.6		47	Texas	10.6
19	Wisconsin	14.5		49	Utah	9.0
37	Wyoming	13.0		50	Alaska	6.4
					District of Columbia	13.2

Source: MQ Press using data from U.S. Dept of Health & Human Services, Centers for Medicare and Medicaid Services
"Medicare Estimated Benefit Payments by State" (http://www.hcfa.gov/stats/BENEPAY/bnpay00i.htm)
*For fiscal year 2000. Includes aged and disabled enrollees. National rate includes only residents of the 50 states and the District of Columbia.

Medicare Managed Care Enrollees in 2001

National Total = 6,059,675 Enrollees*

ALPHA ORDER

RANK ORDER

RANK	STATE	ENROLLEES	% of USA
22	Alabama	50,136	0.8%
44	Alaska	0	0.0%
7	Arizona	230,952	3.8%
32	Arkansas	15,676	0.3%
1	California	1,518,110	25.1%
12	Colorado	147,511	2.4%
19	Connecticut	71,965	1.2%
42	Delaware	880	0.0%
2	Florida	645,293	10.6%
27	Georgia	36,819	0.6%
20	Hawaii	58,334	1.0%
33	Idaho	12,923	0.2%
13	Illinois	147,064	2.4%
30	Indiana	19,824	0.3%
37	Iowa	7,192	0.1%
36	Kansas	9,048	0.1%
34	Kentucky	12,650	0.2%
17	Louisiana	80,622	1.3%
44	Maine	0	0.0%
29	Maryland	33,822	0.6%
8	Massachusetts	221,013	3.6%
18	Michigan	72,678	1.2%
15	Minnesota	82,923	1.4%
38	Mississippi	4,869	0.1%
10	Missouri	159,146	2.6%
44	Montana	0	0.0%
35	Nebraska	9,690	0.2%
16	Nevada	82,628	1.4%
41	New Hampshire	1,004	0.0%
14	New Jersey	145,168	2.4%
28	New Mexico	33,950	0.6%
4	New York	475,073	7.8%
23	North Carolina	48,027	0.8%
43	North Dakota	657	0.0%
5	Ohio	260,938	4.3%
24	Oklahoma	47,873	0.8%
9	Oregon	182,870	3.0%
3	Pennsylvania	511,854	8.4%
21	Rhode Island	58,095	1.0%
44	South Carolina	0	0.0%
40	South Dakota	1,272	0.0%
25	Tennessee	41,227	0.7%
6	Texas	250,419	4.1%
31	Utah	18,234	0.3%
44	Vermont	0	0.0%
39	Virginia	3,120	0.1%
11	Washington	153,389	2.5%
44	West Virginia	0	0.0%
26	Wisconsin	38,975	0.6%
44	Wyoming	0	0.0%

RANK	STATE	ENROLLEES	% of USA
1	California	1,518,110	25.1%
2	Florida	645,293	10.6%
3	Pennsylvania	511,854	8.4%
4	New York	475,073	7.8%
5	Ohio	260,938	4.3%
6	Texas	250,419	4.1%
7	Arizona	230,952	3.8%
8	Massachusetts	221,013	3.6%
9	Oregon	182,870	3.0%
10	Missouri	159,146	2.6%
11	Washington	153,389	2.5%
12	Colorado	147,511	2.4%
13	Illinois	147,064	2.4%
14	New Jersey	145,168	2.4%
15	Minnesota	82,923	1.4%
16	Nevada	82,628	1.4%
17	Louisiana	80,622	1.3%
18	Michigan	72,678	1.2%
19	Connecticut	71,965	1.2%
20	Hawaii	58,334	1.0%
21	Rhode Island	58,095	1.0%
22	Alabama	50,136	0.8%
23	North Carolina	48,027	0.8%
24	Oklahoma	47,873	0.8%
25	Tennessee	41,227	0.7%
26	Wisconsin	38,975	0.6%
27	Georgia	36,819	0.6%
28	New Mexico	33,950	0.6%
29	Maryland	33,822	0.6%
30	Indiana	19,824	0.3%
31	Utah	18,234	0.3%
32	Arkansas	15,676	0.3%
33	Idaho	12,923	0.2%
34	Kentucky	12,650	0.2%
35	Nebraska	9,690	0.2%
36	Kansas	9,048	0.1%
37	Iowa	7,192	0.1%
38	Mississippi	4,869	0.1%
39	Virginia	3,120	0.1%
40	South Dakota	1,272	0.0%
41	New Hampshire	1,004	0.0%
42	Delaware	880	0.0%
43	North Dakota	657	0.0%
44	Alaska	0	0.0%
44	Maine	0	0.0%
44	Montana	0	0.0%
44	South Carolina	0	0.0%
44	Vermont	0	0.0%
44	West Virginia	0	0.0%
44	Wyoming	0	0.0%
	District of Columbia	1,158	0.0%

Source: U.S. Department of Health and Human Services, Centers for Medicare and Medicaid Services
   "Medicare Managed Care Contract Report" (December 1, 2001, http://www.hcfa.gov/stats/mmcc1201.txt)
*As of December 1st. Includes TEFRA, Cost, and Health Care Prepayment Plans (HCPP) and other demo plans.
National total includes 54,604 enrollees in the United Mine Workers' plan not shown separately by state.

Percent of Medicare Enrollees in Managed Care Programs in 2001

National Percent = 16% of Medicare Enrollees*

ALPHA ORDER

RANK	STATE	PERCENT
25	Alabama	7
43	Alaska	0
5	Arizona	35
30	Arkansas	4
1	California	41
7	Colorado	33
16	Connecticut	14
38	Delaware	1
9	Florida	23
30	Georgia	4
3	Hawaii	37
24	Idaho	8
21	Illinois	10
34	Indiana	2
34	Iowa	2
34	Kansas	2
34	Kentucky	2
16	Louisiana	14
43	Maine	0
26	Maryland	5
9	Massachusetts	23
26	Michigan	5
18	Minnesota	13
38	Mississippi	1
12	Missouri	18
43	Montana	0
30	Nebraska	4
3	Nevada	37
38	New Hampshire	1
19	New Jersey	12
14	New Mexico	15
12	New York	18
30	North Carolina	4
38	North Dakota	1
14	Ohio	15
21	Oklahoma	10
2	Oregon	38
8	Pennsylvania	25
6	Rhode Island	34
43	South Carolina	0
38	South Dakota	1
26	Tennessee	5
20	Texas	11
23	Utah	9
43	Vermont	0
43	Virginia	0
11	Washington	22
43	West Virginia	0
26	Wisconsin	5
43	Wyoming	0

RANK ORDER

RANK	STATE	PERCENT
1	California	41
2	Oregon	38
3	Hawaii	37
3	Nevada	37
5	Arizona	35
6	Rhode Island	34
7	Colorado	33
8	Pennsylvania	25
9	Florida	23
9	Massachusetts	23
11	Washington	22
12	Missouri	18
12	New York	18
14	New Mexico	15
14	Ohio	15
16	Connecticut	14
16	Louisiana	14
18	Minnesota	13
19	New Jersey	12
20	Texas	11
21	Illinois	10
21	Oklahoma	10
23	Utah	9
24	Idaho	8
25	Alabama	7
26	Maryland	5
26	Michigan	5
26	Tennessee	5
26	Wisconsin	5
30	Arkansas	4
30	Georgia	4
30	Nebraska	4
30	North Carolina	4
34	Indiana	2
34	Iowa	2
34	Kansas	2
34	Kentucky	2
38	Delaware	1
38	Mississippi	1
38	New Hampshire	1
38	North Dakota	1
38	South Dakota	1
43	Alaska	0
43	Maine	0
43	Montana	0
43	South Carolina	0
43	Vermont	0
43	Virginia	0
43	West Virginia	0
43	Wyoming	0
	District of Columbia	2

Source: U.S. Department of Health and Human Services, Centers for Medicare and Medicaid Services
    "Medicare Managed Care Contract Report" (December 1, 2001, http://www.hcfa.gov/stats/mmcc1201.txt)
*As of December 1st. Includes TEFRA, Cost, and Health Care Prepayment Plans (HCPP) and other demo plans.
National figure includes enrollees in the United Mine Workers' plan not shown separately by state.

Percent of Medicare Benefits Paid Through Managed Care in 2000

National Percent = 18.5% of Payments*

RANK	STATE	PERCENT
25	Alabama	8.4
48	Alaska	0.0
1	Arizona	48.6
33	Arkansas	4.0
3	California	42.3
7	Colorado	33.7
14	Connecticut	18.1
29	Delaware	4.7
9	Florida	26.9
24	Georgia	8.5
4	Hawaii	42.0
28	Idaho	5.6
21	Illinois	13.5
26	Indiana	8.2
41	Iowa	0.8
37	Kansas	2.5
36	Kentucky	2.7
16	Louisiana	15.9
42	Maine	0.7
17	Maryland	15.2
12	Massachusetts	25.8
27	Michigan	7.5
22	Minnesota	10.8
45	Mississippi	0.4
13	Missouri	20.6
44	Montana	0.6
29	Nebraska	4.7
5	Nevada	41.0
34	New Hampshire	3.9
18	New Jersey	14.8
10	New Mexico	26.8
15	New York	16.5
35	North Carolina	3.5
46	North Dakota	0.2
20	Ohio	14.1
23	Oklahoma	10.2
2	Oregon	44.4
11	Pennsylvania	26.4
6	Rhode Island	34.7
48	South Carolina	0.0
47	South Dakota	0.1
31	Tennessee	4.6
19	Texas	14.3
40	Utah	2.0
42	Vermont	0.7
38	Virginia	2.2
8	Washington	29.0
38	West Virginia	2.2
32	Wisconsin	4.5
48	Wyoming	0.0

RANK	STATE	PERCENT
1	Arizona	48.6
2	Oregon	44.4
3	California	42.3
4	Hawaii	42.0
5	Nevada	41.0
6	Rhode Island	34.7
7	Colorado	33.7
8	Washington	29.0
9	Florida	26.9
10	New Mexico	26.8
11	Pennsylvania	26.4
12	Massachusetts	25.8
13	Missouri	20.6
14	Connecticut	18.1
15	New York	16.5
16	Louisiana	15.9
17	Maryland	15.2
18	New Jersey	14.8
19	Texas	14.3
20	Ohio	14.1
21	Illinois	13.5
22	Minnesota	10.8
23	Oklahoma	10.2
24	Georgia	8.5
25	Alabama	8.4
26	Indiana	8.2
27	Michigan	7.5
28	Idaho	5.6
29	Delaware	4.7
29	Nebraska	4.7
31	Tennessee	4.6
32	Wisconsin	4.5
33	Arkansas	4.0
34	New Hampshire	3.9
35	North Carolina	3.5
36	Kentucky	2.7
37	Kansas	2.5
38	Virginia	2.2
38	West Virginia	2.2
40	Utah	2.0
41	Iowa	0.8
42	Maine	0.7
42	Vermont	0.7
44	Montana	0.6
45	Mississippi	0.4
46	North Dakota	0.2
47	South Dakota	0.1
48	Alaska	0.0
48	South Carolina	0.0
48	Wyoming	0.0
	District of Columbia	17.0

Source: MQ Press using data from U.S. Dept of Health & Human Services, Centers for Medicare and Medicaid Services "Medicare Estimated Benefit Payments by State" (http://www.hcfa.gov/stats/BENEPAY/bnpay00i.htm)
For fiscal year 2000 by state of plan. National rate includes payments to enrollees in Puerto Rico and in "other outlying areas."

Percent of Medicare Benefits Paid Through Fee for Service Plans in 2000

National Percent = 81.5% of Payments*

<table>
<tr><th colspan="3">ALPHA ORDER</th><th colspan="3">RANK ORDER</th></tr>
<tr><th>RANK</th><th>STATE</th><th>PERCENT</th><th>RANK</th><th>STATE</th><th>PERCENT</th></tr>
<tr><td>26</td><td>Alabama</td><td>91.6</td><td>1</td><td>Alaska</td><td>100.0</td></tr>
<tr><td>1</td><td>Alaska</td><td>100.0</td><td>1</td><td>South Carolina</td><td>100.0</td></tr>
<tr><td>50</td><td>Arizona</td><td>51.4</td><td>1</td><td>Wyoming</td><td>100.0</td></tr>
<tr><td>18</td><td>Arkansas</td><td>96.0</td><td>4</td><td>South Dakota</td><td>99.9</td></tr>
<tr><td>48</td><td>California</td><td>57.7</td><td>5</td><td>North Dakota</td><td>99.8</td></tr>
<tr><td>44</td><td>Colorado</td><td>66.3</td><td>6</td><td>Mississippi</td><td>99.6</td></tr>
<tr><td>37</td><td>Connecticut</td><td>81.9</td><td>7</td><td>Montana</td><td>99.4</td></tr>
<tr><td>21</td><td>Delaware</td><td>95.3</td><td>8</td><td>Maine</td><td>99.3</td></tr>
<tr><td>42</td><td>Florida</td><td>73.1</td><td>8</td><td>Vermont</td><td>99.3</td></tr>
<tr><td>27</td><td>Georgia</td><td>91.5</td><td>10</td><td>Iowa</td><td>99.2</td></tr>
<tr><td>47</td><td>Hawaii</td><td>58.0</td><td>11</td><td>Utah</td><td>98.0</td></tr>
<tr><td>23</td><td>Idaho</td><td>94.4</td><td>12</td><td>Virginia</td><td>97.8</td></tr>
<tr><td>30</td><td>Illinois</td><td>86.5</td><td>12</td><td>West Virginia</td><td>97.8</td></tr>
<tr><td>25</td><td>Indiana</td><td>91.8</td><td>14</td><td>Kansas</td><td>97.5</td></tr>
<tr><td>10</td><td>Iowa</td><td>99.2</td><td>15</td><td>Kentucky</td><td>97.3</td></tr>
<tr><td>14</td><td>Kansas</td><td>97.5</td><td>16</td><td>North Carolina</td><td>96.5</td></tr>
<tr><td>15</td><td>Kentucky</td><td>97.3</td><td>17</td><td>New Hampshire</td><td>96.1</td></tr>
<tr><td>35</td><td>Louisiana</td><td>84.1</td><td>18</td><td>Arkansas</td><td>96.0</td></tr>
<tr><td>8</td><td>Maine</td><td>99.3</td><td>19</td><td>Wisconsin</td><td>95.5</td></tr>
<tr><td>34</td><td>Maryland</td><td>84.8</td><td>20</td><td>Tennessee</td><td>95.4</td></tr>
<tr><td>39</td><td>Massachusetts</td><td>74.2</td><td>21</td><td>Delaware</td><td>95.3</td></tr>
<tr><td>24</td><td>Michigan</td><td>92.5</td><td>21</td><td>Nebraska</td><td>95.3</td></tr>
<tr><td>29</td><td>Minnesota</td><td>89.2</td><td>23</td><td>Idaho</td><td>94.4</td></tr>
<tr><td>6</td><td>Mississippi</td><td>99.6</td><td>24</td><td>Michigan</td><td>92.5</td></tr>
<tr><td>38</td><td>Missouri</td><td>79.4</td><td>25</td><td>Indiana</td><td>91.8</td></tr>
<tr><td>7</td><td>Montana</td><td>99.4</td><td>26</td><td>Alabama</td><td>91.6</td></tr>
<tr><td>21</td><td>Nebraska</td><td>95.3</td><td>27</td><td>Georgia</td><td>91.5</td></tr>
<tr><td>46</td><td>Nevada</td><td>59.0</td><td>28</td><td>Oklahoma</td><td>89.8</td></tr>
<tr><td>17</td><td>New Hampshire</td><td>96.1</td><td>29</td><td>Minnesota</td><td>89.2</td></tr>
<tr><td>33</td><td>New Jersey</td><td>85.2</td><td>30</td><td>Illinois</td><td>86.5</td></tr>
<tr><td>41</td><td>New Mexico</td><td>73.2</td><td>31</td><td>Ohio</td><td>85.9</td></tr>
<tr><td>36</td><td>New York</td><td>83.5</td><td>32</td><td>Texas</td><td>85.7</td></tr>
<tr><td>16</td><td>North Carolina</td><td>96.5</td><td>33</td><td>New Jersey</td><td>85.2</td></tr>
<tr><td>5</td><td>North Dakota</td><td>99.8</td><td>34</td><td>Maryland</td><td>84.8</td></tr>
<tr><td>31</td><td>Ohio</td><td>85.9</td><td>35</td><td>Louisiana</td><td>84.1</td></tr>
<tr><td>28</td><td>Oklahoma</td><td>89.8</td><td>36</td><td>New York</td><td>83.5</td></tr>
<tr><td>49</td><td>Oregon</td><td>55.6</td><td>37</td><td>Connecticut</td><td>81.9</td></tr>
<tr><td>40</td><td>Pennsylvania</td><td>73.6</td><td>38</td><td>Missouri</td><td>79.4</td></tr>
<tr><td>45</td><td>Rhode Island</td><td>65.3</td><td>39</td><td>Massachusetts</td><td>74.2</td></tr>
<tr><td>1</td><td>South Carolina</td><td>100.0</td><td>40</td><td>Pennsylvania</td><td>73.6</td></tr>
<tr><td>4</td><td>South Dakota</td><td>99.9</td><td>41</td><td>New Mexico</td><td>73.2</td></tr>
<tr><td>20</td><td>Tennessee</td><td>95.4</td><td>42</td><td>Florida</td><td>73.1</td></tr>
<tr><td>32</td><td>Texas</td><td>85.7</td><td>43</td><td>Washington</td><td>71.0</td></tr>
<tr><td>11</td><td>Utah</td><td>98.0</td><td>44</td><td>Colorado</td><td>66.3</td></tr>
<tr><td>8</td><td>Vermont</td><td>99.3</td><td>45</td><td>Rhode Island</td><td>65.3</td></tr>
<tr><td>12</td><td>Virginia</td><td>97.8</td><td>46</td><td>Nevada</td><td>59.0</td></tr>
<tr><td>43</td><td>Washington</td><td>71.0</td><td>47</td><td>Hawaii</td><td>58.0</td></tr>
<tr><td>12</td><td>West Virginia</td><td>97.8</td><td>48</td><td>California</td><td>57.7</td></tr>
<tr><td>19</td><td>Wisconsin</td><td>95.5</td><td>49</td><td>Oregon</td><td>55.6</td></tr>
<tr><td>1</td><td>Wyoming</td><td>100.0</td><td>50</td><td>Arizona</td><td>51.4</td></tr>
<tr><td></td><td></td><td></td><td></td><td>District of Columbia</td><td>83.0</td></tr>
</table>

Source: MQ Press using data from U.S. Dept of Health & Human Services, Centers for Medicare and Medicaid Services
"Medicare Estimated Benefit Payments by State" (http://www.hcfa.gov/stats/BENEPAY/bnpay00i.htm)
*For fiscal year 2000 by state of provider. National rate includes payments to enrollees in Puerto Rico and in "other outlying areas."

Medicare Physicians in 1999

National Total = 830,372 Physicians*

ALPHA ORDER

RANK	STATE	PHYSICIANS	% of USA
26	Alabama	9,629	1.2%
49	Alaska	1,481	0.2%
24	Arizona	11,587	1.4%
31	Arkansas	6,972	0.8%
1	California	98,515	11.9%
22	Colorado	13,131	1.6%
23	Connecticut	12,279	1.5%
45	Delaware	2,440	0.3%
5	Florida	43,006	5.2%
12	Georgia	19,217	2.3%
40	Hawaii**	4,011	0.5%
27	Idaho	8,769	1.1%
44	Illinois	2,549	0.3%
7	Indiana	32,663	3.9%
18	Iowa	15,726	1.9%
32	Kansas	6,591	0.8%
29	Kentucky	8,620	1.0%
21	Louisiana	13,533	1.6%
9	Maine	28,566	3.4%
11	Maryland	19,364	2.3%
36	Massachusetts	4,646	0.6%
8	Michigan	29,112	3.5%
19	Minnesota	15,552	1.9%
17	Mississippi	16,560	2.0%
33	Missouri	5,414	0.7%
43	Montana	2,611	0.3%
13	Nebraska	18,405	2.2%
46	Nevada	2,311	0.3%
38	New Hampshire	4,234	0.5%
37	New Jersey	4,355	0.5%
10	New Mexico	28,374	3.4%
39	New York	4,197	0.5%
41	North Carolina	3,575	0.4%
2	North Dakota	73,216	8.8%
6	Ohio	32,841	4.0%
30	Oklahoma	7,570	0.9%
25	Oregon	9,934	1.2%
3	Pennsylvania	52,530	6.3%
42	Rhode Island	3,485	0.4%
28	South Carolina	8,682	1.0%
47	South Dakota	2,227	0.3%
20	Tennessee	15,149	1.8%
4	Texas	51,304	6.2%
34	Utah	5,001	0.6%
14	Vermont	17,312	2.1%
48	Virginia	2,226	0.3%
15	Washington	17,218	2.1%
16	West Virginia	16,627	2.0%
35	Wisconsin	4,948	0.6%
50	Wyoming	1,277	0.2%

RANK ORDER

RANK	STATE	PHYSICIANS	% of USA
1	California	98,515	11.9%
2	North Dakota	73,216	8.8%
3	Pennsylvania	52,530	6.3%
4	Texas	51,304	6.2%
5	Florida	43,006	5.2%
6	Ohio	32,841	4.0%
7	Indiana	32,663	3.9%
8	Michigan	29,112	3.5%
9	Maine	28,566	3.4%
10	New Mexico	28,374	3.4%
11	Maryland	19,364	2.3%
12	Georgia	19,217	2.3%
13	Nebraska	18,405	2.2%
14	Vermont	17,312	2.1%
15	Washington	17,218	2.1%
16	West Virginia	16,627	2.0%
17	Mississippi	16,560	2.0%
18	Iowa	15,726	1.9%
19	Minnesota	15,552	1.9%
20	Tennessee	15,149	1.8%
21	Louisiana	13,533	1.6%
22	Colorado	13,131	1.6%
23	Connecticut	12,279	1.5%
24	Arizona	11,587	1.4%
25	Oregon	9,934	1.2%
26	Alabama	9,629	1.2%
27	Idaho	8,769	1.1%
28	South Carolina	8,682	1.0%
29	Kentucky	8,620	1.0%
30	Oklahoma	7,570	0.9%
31	Arkansas	6,972	0.8%
32	Kansas	6,591	0.8%
33	Missouri	5,414	0.7%
34	Utah	5,001	0.6%
35	Wisconsin	4,948	0.6%
36	Massachusetts	4,646	0.6%
37	New Jersey	4,355	0.5%
38	New Hampshire	4,234	0.5%
39	New York	4,197	0.5%
40	Hawaii**	4,011	0.5%
41	North Carolina	3,575	0.4%
42	Rhode Island	3,485	0.4%
43	Montana	2,611	0.3%
44	Illinois	2,549	0.3%
45	Delaware	2,440	0.3%
46	Nevada	2,311	0.3%
47	South Dakota	2,227	0.3%
48	Virginia	2,226	0.3%
49	Alaska	1,481	0.2%
50	Wyoming	1,277	0.2%
	District of Columbia	4,449	0.5%

Source: U.S. Department of Health and Human Services, Centers for Medicare and Medicaid Services
   "Medicare Physician Registry" (July 1999)
Medicare Part B. "Physicians" include MD, DO, DDM, DDS, DPM, OD and CH. National total includes 6,376 physicians in Puerto Rico and the Virgin Islands.
**Physicians for Guam are included in Hawaii's total.*

Percent of Physicians Participating in Medicare in 1999

National Percent = 84.6% of Physicians Participate in Medicare*

ALPHA ORDER

RANK ORDER

RANK	STATE	PERCENT		RANK	STATE	PERCENT
2	Alabama	94.5		1	Kansas	94.7
41	Alaska	81.4		2	Alabama	94.5
21	Arizona	89.7		3	North Dakota	94.3
39	Arkansas	83.1		4	Utah	94.1
42	California	81.0		5	Massachusetts	94.0
33	Colorado	84.6		6	Maine	93.8
25	Connecticut	88.7		7	Nevada	93.3
35	Delaware	84.1		8	Ohio	93.2
46	Florida	77.6		9	Nebraska	92.4
37	Georgia	83.3		10	Kentucky	92.3
31	Hawaii	85.6		11	New Hampshire	92.2
47	Idaho	75.6		12	West Virginia	92.1
34	Illinois	84.2		13	Vermont	91.8
44	Indiana	79.0		14	Maryland	91.7
16	Iowa	91.1		14	Washington	91.7
1	Kansas	94.7		16	Iowa	91.1
10	Kentucky	92.3		17	Tennessee	90.9
49	Louisiana	73.5		18	South Carolina	90.0
6	Maine	93.8		19	Oklahoma	89.9
14	Maryland	91.7		20	Oregon	89.8
5	Massachusetts	94.0		21	Arizona	89.7
27	Michigan	87.7		22	Wisconsin	89.4
45	Minnesota	78.1		23	New Mexico	89.3
40	Mississippi	82.6		24	Missouri	89.2
24	Missouri	89.2		25	Connecticut	88.7
32	Montana	84.7		26	North Carolina	88.3
9	Nebraska	92.4		27	Michigan	87.7
7	Nevada	93.3		28	Virginia	87.2
11	New Hampshire	92.2		29	Wyoming	86.4
43	New Jersey	80.1		30	South Dakota	85.7
23	New Mexico	89.3		31	Hawaii	85.6
48	New York	75.3		32	Montana	84.7
26	North Carolina	88.3		33	Colorado	84.6
3	North Dakota	94.3		34	Illinois	84.2
8	Ohio	93.2		35	Delaware	84.1
19	Oklahoma	89.9		36	Pennsylvania	83.5
20	Oregon	89.8		37	Georgia	83.3
36	Pennsylvania	83.5		37	Texas	83.3
50	Rhode Island	71.7		39	Arkansas	83.1
18	South Carolina	90.0		40	Mississippi	82.6
30	South Dakota	85.7		41	Alaska	81.4
17	Tennessee	90.9		42	California	81.0
37	Texas	83.3		43	New Jersey	80.1
4	Utah	94.1		44	Indiana	79.0
13	Vermont	91.8		45	Minnesota	78.1
28	Virginia	87.2		46	Florida	77.6
14	Washington	91.7		47	Idaho	75.6
12	West Virginia	92.1		48	New York	75.3
22	Wisconsin	89.4		49	Louisiana	73.5
29	Wyoming	86.4		50	Rhode Island	71.7

District of Columbia   81.0

Source: U.S. Department of Health and Human Services, Centers for Medicare and Medicaid Services
"1999 Data Compendium" (July 1999)
*Medicare Part B. Physicians include MD's, DO's, limited license practitioners and non-physician practitioners.

Medicaid Enrollment in 2000

National Total = 34,471,373 Enrollees*

ALPHA ORDER

RANK ORDER

RANK	STATE	ENROLLEES	% of USA
17	Alabama	614,359	1.8%
45	Alaska	80,528	0.2%
22	Arizona	501,024	1.5%
28	Arkansas	423,342	1.2%
1	California	5,087,202	14.8%
32	Colorado	263,515	0.8%
30	Connecticut	321,706	0.9%
44	Delaware	99,128	0.3%
4	Florida	1,812,434	5.3%
12	Georgia	863,862	2.5%
39	Hawaii	152,507	0.4%
41	Idaho	122,018	0.4%
5	Illinois	1,423,907	4.1%
19	Indiana	585,783	1.7%
34	Iowa	220,525	0.6%
35	Kansas	196,331	0.6%
18	Kentucky	602,994	1.7%
15	Louisiana	724,135	2.1%
37	Maine	171,980	0.5%
24	Maryland	477,373	1.4%
11	Massachusetts	886,220	2.6%
9	Michigan	1,085,479	3.1%
26	Minnesota	449,700	1.3%
21	Mississippi	547,496	1.6%
13	Missouri	832,600	2.4%
48	Montana	70,685	0.2%
36	Nebraska	188,536	0.5%
43	Nevada	117,410	0.3%
46	New Hampshire	78,309	0.2%
16	New Jersey	645,812	1.9%
31	New Mexico	320,273	0.9%
2	New York	2,751,830	8.0%
10	North Carolina	904,974	2.6%
49	North Dakota	42,727	0.1%
8	Ohio	1,207,846	3.5%
27	Oklahoma	427,055	1.2%
29	Oregon	380,501	1.1%
7	Pennsylvania	1,315,585	3.8%
38	Rhode Island	153,549	0.4%
20	South Carolina	570,929	1.7%
47	South Dakota	76,517	0.2%
6	Tennessee	1,362,799	4.0%
3	Texas	1,923,799	5.6%
40	Utah	133,760	0.4%
42	Vermont	119,438	0.3%
25	Virginia	461,381	1.3%
14	Washington	781,549	2.3%
33	West Virginia	261,000	0.8%
23	Wisconsin	491,924	1.4%
50	Wyoming	38,109	0.1%

RANK	STATE	ENROLLEES	% of USA
1	California	5,087,202	14.8%
2	New York	2,751,830	8.0%
3	Texas	1,923,799	5.6%
4	Florida	1,812,434	5.3%
5	Illinois	1,423,907	4.1%
6	Tennessee	1,362,799	4.0%
7	Pennsylvania	1,315,585	3.8%
8	Ohio	1,207,846	3.5%
9	Michigan	1,085,479	3.1%
10	North Carolina	904,974	2.6%
11	Massachusetts	886,220	2.6%
12	Georgia	863,862	2.5%
13	Missouri	832,600	2.4%
14	Washington	781,549	2.3%
15	Louisiana	724,135	2.1%
16	New Jersey	645,812	1.9%
17	Alabama	614,359	1.8%
18	Kentucky	602,994	1.7%
19	Indiana	585,783	1.7%
20	South Carolina	570,929	1.7%
21	Mississippi	547,496	1.6%
22	Arizona	501,024	1.5%
23	Wisconsin	491,924	1.4%
24	Maryland	477,373	1.4%
25	Virginia	461,381	1.3%
26	Minnesota	449,700	1.3%
27	Oklahoma	427,055	1.2%
28	Arkansas	423,342	1.2%
29	Oregon	380,501	1.1%
30	Connecticut	321,706	0.9%
31	New Mexico	320,273	0.9%
32	Colorado	263,515	0.8%
33	West Virginia	261,000	0.8%
34	Iowa	220,525	0.6%
35	Kansas	196,331	0.6%
36	Nebraska	188,536	0.5%
37	Maine	171,980	0.5%
38	Rhode Island	153,549	0.4%
39	Hawaii	152,507	0.4%
40	Utah	133,760	0.4%
41	Idaho	122,018	0.4%
42	Vermont	119,438	0.3%
43	Nevada	117,410	0.3%
44	Delaware	99,128	0.3%
45	Alaska	80,528	0.2%
46	New Hampshire	78,309	0.2%
47	South Dakota	76,517	0.2%
48	Montana	70,685	0.2%
49	North Dakota	42,727	0.1%
50	Wyoming	38,109	0.1%
	District of Columbia	121,871	0.4%

Source: U.S. Department of Health and Human Services, Centers for Medicare and Medicaid Services "Medicaid Managed Care State Enrollment" (http://www.hcfa.gov/medicaid/omcpr00.pdf)
As of December 31, 2000. National total includes 977,057 Medicaid enrollees in Puerto Rico and the Virgin Islands

Percent of Population Enrolled in Medicaid in 2000

National Percent = 11.9% of Population*

ALPHA ORDER

RANK ORDER

RANK	STATE	PERCENT	RANK	STATE	PERCENT
15	Alabama	13.8	1	Tennessee	23.9
18	Alaska	12.8	2	Vermont	19.6
32	Arizona	9.7	3	Mississippi	19.2
6	Arkansas	15.8	4	New Mexico	17.6
7	California	15.0	5	Louisiana	16.2
48	Colorado	6.1	6	Arkansas	15.8
34	Connecticut	9.4	7	California	15.0
19	Delaware	12.6	8	Kentucky	14.9
23	Florida	11.3	8	Missouri	14.9
30	Georgia	10.5	10	Rhode Island	14.6
19	Hawaii	12.6	11	New York	14.5
34	Idaho	9.4	12	West Virginia	14.4
22	Illinois	11.4	13	South Carolina	14.2
33	Indiana	9.6	14	Massachusetts	13.9
43	Iowa	7.5	15	Alabama	13.8
44	Kansas	7.3	16	Maine	13.5
8	Kentucky	14.9	17	Washington	13.2
5	Louisiana	16.2	18	Alaska	12.8
16	Maine	13.5	19	Delaware	12.6
39	Maryland	9.0	19	Hawaii	12.6
14	Massachusetts	13.9	21	Oklahoma	12.4
27	Michigan	10.9	22	Illinois	11.4
38	Minnesota	9.1	23	Florida	11.3
3	Mississippi	19.2	24	North Carolina	11.2
8	Missouri	14.9	25	Oregon	11.1
40	Montana	7.8	26	Nebraska	11.0
26	Nebraska	11.0	27	Michigan	10.9
50	Nevada	5.8	28	Pennsylvania	10.7
47	New Hampshire	6.3	29	Ohio	10.6
41	New Jersey	7.7	30	Georgia	10.5
4	New Mexico	17.6	31	South Dakota	10.1
11	New York	14.5	32	Arizona	9.7
24	North Carolina	11.2	33	Indiana	9.6
45	North Dakota	6.7	34	Connecticut	9.4
29	Ohio	10.6	34	Idaho	9.4
21	Oklahoma	12.4	36	Texas	9.2
25	Oregon	11.1	36	Wisconsin	9.2
28	Pennsylvania	10.7	38	Minnesota	9.1
10	Rhode Island	14.6	39	Maryland	9.0
13	South Carolina	14.2	40	Montana	7.8
31	South Dakota	10.1	41	New Jersey	7.7
1	Tennessee	23.9	41	Wyoming	7.7
36	Texas	9.2	43	Iowa	7.5
49	Utah	6.0	44	Kansas	7.3
2	Vermont	19.6	45	North Dakota	6.7
46	Virginia	6.5	46	Virginia	6.5
17	Washington	13.2	47	New Hampshire	6.3
12	West Virginia	14.4	48	Colorado	6.1
36	Wisconsin	9.2	49	Utah	6.0
41	Wyoming	7.7	50	Nevada	5.8

District of Columbia 21.3

Source: MQ Press using data from U.S. Dept of Health & Human Services, Centers for Medicare and Medicaid Services
"Medicaid Managed Care State Enrollment" (http://www.hcfa.gov/medicaid/omcpr00.pdf)
*As of December 31, 2000. National percent does not include recipients or population in U.S. territories.

Percent of Children Covered by Medicaid in 2000

National Percent = 20.3% of Children*

ALPHA ORDER

RANK	STATE	PERCENT
9	Alabama	25.0
9	Alaska	25.0
16	Arizona	23.6
11	Arkansas	24.8
11	California	24.8
47	Colorado	11.1
45	Connecticut	13.3
18	Delaware	21.7
20	Florida	20.7
39	Georgia	16.6
22	Hawaii	20.5
21	Idaho	20.6
26	Illinois	18.5
44	Indiana	13.5
49	Iowa	10.2
46	Kansas	11.6
25	Kentucky	19.3
6	Louisiana	28.3
28	Maine	18.4
48	Maryland	10.9
7	Massachusetts	27.1
19	Michigan	21.1
42	Minnesota	14.1
4	Mississippi	30.1
24	Missouri	19.5
15	Montana	23.9
33	Nebraska	17.8
37	Nevada	17.2
26	New Hampshire	18.5
41	New Jersey	16.2
2	New Mexico	32.3
8	New York	26.5
23	North Carolina	19.6
30	North Dakota	18.0
34	Ohio	17.7
13	Oklahoma	24.7
31	Oregon	17.9
35	Pennsylvania	17.6
28	Rhode Island	18.4
17	South Carolina	21.8
43	South Dakota	14.0
3	Tennessee	30.6
36	Texas	17.5
38	Utah	17.1
1	Vermont	40.2
50	Virginia	7.8
13	Washington	24.7
5	West Virginia	29.2
39	Wisconsin	16.6
31	Wyoming	17.9

RANK ORDER

RANK	STATE	PERCENT
1	Vermont	40.2
2	New Mexico	32.3
3	Tennessee	30.6
4	Mississippi	30.1
5	West Virginia	29.2
6	Louisiana	28.3
7	Massachusetts	27.1
8	New York	26.5
9	Alabama	25.0
9	Alaska	25.0
11	Arkansas	24.8
11	California	24.8
13	Oklahoma	24.7
13	Washington	24.7
15	Montana	23.9
16	Arizona	23.6
17	South Carolina	21.8
18	Delaware	21.7
19	Michigan	21.1
20	Florida	20.7
21	Idaho	20.6
22	Hawaii	20.5
23	North Carolina	19.6
24	Missouri	19.5
25	Kentucky	19.3
26	Illinois	18.5
26	New Hampshire	18.5
28	Maine	18.4
28	Rhode Island	18.4
30	North Dakota	18.0
31	Oregon	17.9
31	Wyoming	17.9
33	Nebraska	17.8
34	Ohio	17.7
35	Pennsylvania	17.6
36	Texas	17.5
37	Nevada	17.2
38	Utah	17.1
39	Georgia	16.6
39	Wisconsin	16.6
41	New Jersey	16.2
42	Minnesota	14.1
43	South Dakota	14.0
44	Indiana	13.5
45	Connecticut	13.3
46	Kansas	11.6
47	Colorado	11.1
48	Maryland	10.9
49	Iowa	10.2
50	Virginia	7.8
	District of Columbia	29.5

Source: U.S. Bureau of the Census
   "Health Insurance Historical Table 5" (http://www.census.gov/hhes/hlthins/historic/hihistt5.html)
*Children under 18 years old.

Medicaid Enrollment in 1999

National Total = 42,061,552 Enrollees*

ALPHA ORDER

RANK	STATE	ENROLLEES	% of USA
21	Alabama	649,501	1.5%
45	Alaska	99,177	0.2%
22	Arizona	644,376	1.5%
29	Arkansas	483,257	1.1%
1	California	6,216,756	14.8%
33	Colorado	352,475	0.8%
30	Connecticut	409,554	1.0%
43	Delaware	113,253	0.3%
4	Florida	2,116,270	5.0%
10	Georgia	1,236,782	2.9%
37	Hawaii	203,159	0.5%
47	Idaho	93,983	0.2%
6	Illinois	1,698,504	4.0%
19	Indiana	668,491	1.6%
34	Iowa	313,328	0.7%
35	Kansas	260,382	0.6%
20	Kentucky	663,856	1.6%
16	Louisiana	774,796	1.8%
39	Maine	200,129	0.5%
23	Maryland	628,454	1.5%
12	Massachusetts	1,049,262	2.5%
9	Michigan	1,335,050	3.2%
24	Minnesota	585,449	1.4%
26	Mississippi	544,553	1.3%
14	Missouri	877,354	2.1%
46	Montana	95,942	0.2%
36	Nebraska	222,654	0.5%
41	Nevada	143,000	0.3%
44	New Hampshire	105,483	0.3%
15	New Jersey	843,793	2.0%
32	New Mexico	369,861	0.9%
2	New York	3,326,637	7.9%
11	North Carolina	1,205,499	2.9%
49	North Dakota	61,883	0.1%
8	Ohio	1,389,740	3.3%
28	Oklahoma	524,766	1.2%
27	Oregon	544,427	1.3%
5	Pennsylvania	1,772,839	4.2%
40	Rhode Island	154,535	0.4%
17	South Carolina	724,555	1.7%
48	South Dakota	91,979	0.2%
7	Tennessee	1,532,638	3.6%
3	Texas	2,676,056	6.4%
38	Utah	202,028	0.5%
42	Vermont	140,286	0.3%
18	Virginia	699,005	1.7%
13	Washington	895,148	2.1%
31	West Virginia	377,490	0.9%
25	Wisconsin	563,104	1.3%
50	Wyoming	51,835	0.1%

RANK ORDER

RANK	STATE	ENROLLEES	% of USA
1	California	6,216,756	14.8%
2	New York	3,326,637	7.9%
3	Texas	2,676,056	6.4%
4	Florida	2,116,270	5.0%
5	Pennsylvania	1,772,839	4.2%
6	Illinois	1,698,504	4.0%
7	Tennessee	1,532,638	3.6%
8	Ohio	1,389,740	3.3%
9	Michigan	1,335,050	3.2%
10	Georgia	1,236,782	2.9%
11	North Carolina	1,205,499	2.9%
12	Massachusetts	1,049,262	2.5%
13	Washington	895,148	2.1%
14	Missouri	877,354	2.1%
15	New Jersey	843,793	2.0%
16	Louisiana	774,796	1.8%
17	South Carolina	724,555	1.7%
18	Virginia	699,005	1.7%
19	Indiana	668,491	1.6%
20	Kentucky	663,856	1.6%
21	Alabama	649,501	1.5%
22	Arizona	644,376	1.5%
23	Maryland	628,454	1.5%
24	Minnesota	585,449	1.4%
25	Wisconsin	563,104	1.3%
26	Mississippi	544,553	1.3%
27	Oregon	544,427	1.3%
28	Oklahoma	524,766	1.2%
29	Arkansas	483,257	1.1%
30	Connecticut	409,554	1.0%
31	West Virginia	377,490	0.9%
32	New Mexico	369,861	0.9%
33	Colorado	352,475	0.8%
34	Iowa	313,328	0.7%
35	Kansas	260,382	0.6%
36	Nebraska	222,654	0.5%
37	Hawaii	203,159	0.5%
38	Utah	202,028	0.5%
39	Maine	200,129	0.5%
40	Rhode Island	154,535	0.4%
41	Nevada	143,000	0.3%
42	Vermont	140,286	0.3%
43	Delaware	113,253	0.3%
44	New Hampshire	105,483	0.3%
45	Alaska	99,177	0.2%
46	Montana	95,942	0.2%
47	Idaho	93,983	0.2%
48	South Dakota	91,979	0.2%
49	North Dakota	61,883	0.1%
50	Wyoming	51,835	0.1%
	District of Columbia	144,785	0.3%

Source: U.S. Department of Health and Human Services, Centers for Medicare and Medicaid Services
"Medicaid Recipients by Basis of Eligibility and by State: FY 1999" (HCFA-2082)
*For fiscal year 1999. National total includes 983,433 enrollees for U.S. territories.

Medicaid Expenditures in 1999

National Total = $180,948,767,296*

ALPHA ORDER

RANK	STATE	EXPENDITURES	% of USA
25	Alabama	$2,438,540,244	1.3%
46	Alaska	410,996,599	0.2%
26	Arizona	2,007,954,429	1.1%
31	Arkansas	1,460,724,048	0.8%
2	California	20,278,496,844	11.2%
28	Colorado	1,833,259,417	1.0%
19	Connecticut	2,975,667,138	1.6%
45	Delaware	456,731,853	0.3%
6	Florida	6,759,561,228	3.7%
13	Georgia	3,673,705,109	2.0%
41	Hawaii	586,224,188	0.3%
43	Idaho	514,711,236	0.3%
7	Illinois	6,447,404,285	3.6%
18	Indiana	3,017,190,702	1.7%
32	Iowa	1,397,271,906	0.8%
34	Kansas	1,222,928,982	0.7%
22	Kentucky	2,697,336,889	1.5%
16	Louisiana	3,282,146,476	1.8%
35	Maine	1,151,792,201	0.6%
20	Maryland	2,931,170,173	1.6%
9	Massachusetts	5,815,111,956	3.2%
8	Michigan	6,254,125,425	3.5%
17	Minnesota	3,079,902,394	1.7%
29	Mississippi	1,805,174,518	1.0%
14	Missouri	3,636,191,199	2.0%
47	Montana	385,697,755	0.2%
38	Nebraska	986,802,078	0.5%
42	Nevada	541,969,257	0.3%
39	New Hampshire	778,239,711	0.4%
10	New Jersey	5,775,479,739	3.2%
36	New Mexico	1,104,758,114	0.6%
1	New York	28,739,869,524	15.9%
11	North Carolina	4,885,503,195	2.7%
49	North Dakota	338,703,928	0.2%
5	Ohio	6,910,484,446	3.8%
30	Oklahoma	1,478,639,476	0.8%
27	Oregon	1,949,066,404	1.1%
4	Pennsylvania	9,627,196,439	5.3%
37	Rhode Island	1,049,349,806	0.6%
24	South Carolina	2,474,493,301	1.4%
48	South Dakota	376,117,181	0.2%
12	Tennessee	4,178,613,010	2.3%
3	Texas	10,398,353,951	5.7%
40	Utah	741,946,415	0.4%
44	Vermont	469,021,440	0.3%
23	Virginia	2,477,370,906	1.4%
15	Washington	3,529,717,373	2.0%
33	West Virginia	1,353,004,076	0.7%
21	Wisconsin	2,757,366,839	1.5%
50	Wyoming	200,684,719	0.1%

RANK ORDER

RANK	STATE	EXPENDITURES	% of USA
1	New York	$28,739,869,524	15.9%
2	California	20,278,496,844	11.2%
3	Texas	10,398,353,951	5.7%
4	Pennsylvania	9,627,196,439	5.3%
5	Ohio	6,910,484,446	3.8%
6	Florida	6,759,561,228	3.7%
7	Illinois	6,447,404,285	3.6%
8	Michigan	6,254,125,425	3.5%
9	Massachusetts	5,815,111,956	3.2%
10	New Jersey	5,775,479,739	3.2%
11	North Carolina	4,885,503,195	2.7%
12	Tennessee	4,178,613,010	2.3%
13	Georgia	3,673,705,109	2.0%
14	Missouri	3,636,191,199	2.0%
15	Washington	3,529,717,373	2.0%
16	Louisiana	3,282,146,476	1.8%
17	Minnesota	3,079,902,394	1.7%
18	Indiana	3,017,190,702	1.7%
19	Connecticut	2,975,667,138	1.6%
20	Maryland	2,931,170,173	1.6%
21	Wisconsin	2,757,366,839	1.5%
22	Kentucky	2,697,336,889	1.5%
23	Virginia	2,477,370,906	1.4%
24	South Carolina	2,474,493,301	1.4%
25	Alabama	2,438,540,244	1.3%
26	Arizona	2,007,954,429	1.1%
27	Oregon	1,949,066,404	1.1%
28	Colorado	1,833,259,417	1.0%
29	Mississippi	1,805,174,518	1.0%
30	Oklahoma	1,478,639,476	0.8%
31	Arkansas	1,460,724,048	0.8%
32	Iowa	1,397,271,906	0.8%
33	West Virginia	1,353,004,076	0.7%
34	Kansas	1,222,928,982	0.7%
35	Maine	1,151,792,201	0.6%
36	New Mexico	1,104,758,114	0.6%
37	Rhode Island	1,049,349,806	0.6%
38	Nebraska	986,802,078	0.5%
39	New Hampshire	778,239,711	0.4%
40	Utah	741,946,415	0.4%
41	Hawaii	586,224,188	0.3%
42	Nevada	541,969,257	0.3%
43	Idaho	514,711,236	0.3%
44	Vermont	469,021,440	0.3%
45	Delaware	456,731,853	0.3%
46	Alaska	410,996,599	0.2%
47	Montana	385,697,755	0.2%
48	South Dakota	376,117,181	0.2%
49	North Dakota	338,703,928	0.2%
50	Wyoming	200,684,719	0.1%
	District of Columbia	917,918,277	0.5%

Source: U.S. Department of Health and Human Services, Centers for Medicare and Medicaid Services
"Medicaid Financial Statistics Tables (HCFA-64 Report)"
For fiscal year 1999. National total includes $388,080,497 in expenditures in U.S. territories.

Percent Change in Medicaid Expenditures: 1997 to 1999

National Percent Change = 12.7% Increase*

ALPHA ORDER

RANK	STATE	PERCENT CHANGE
26	Alabama	10.8
21	Alaska	12.9
16	Arizona	15.4
25	Arkansas	11.2
4	California	24.9
9	Colorado	20.3
47	Connecticut	1.5
24	Delaware	11.6
43	Florida	4.8
45	Georgia	2.5
50	Hawaii	(6.8)
6	Idaho	21.6
48	Illinois	(0.9)
8	Indiana	21.0
28	Iowa	10.7
11	Kansas	18.9
42	Kentucky	4.9
34	Louisiana	7.4
39	Maine	5.6
31	Maryland	8.3
39	Massachusetts	5.6
22	Michigan	12.5
23	Minnesota	12.1
38	Mississippi	6.0
15	Missouri	15.7
49	Montana	(1.6)
1	Nebraska	34.9
26	Nevada	10.8
37	New Hampshire	6.3
41	New Jersey	5.4
14	New Mexico	16.8
13	New York	17.2
33	North Carolina	7.8
46	North Dakota	2.0
35	Ohio	7.3
5	Oklahoma	23.6
3	Oregon	26.2
10	Pennsylvania	19.2
18	Rhode Island	14.4
17	South Carolina	15.0
19	South Dakota	13.4
6	Tennessee	21.6
31	Texas	8.3
12	Utah	18.4
2	Vermont	30.8
30	Virginia	8.9
29	Washington	10.4
20	West Virginia	13.3
36	Wisconsin	7.1
44	Wyoming	3.3

RANK ORDER

RANK	STATE	PERCENT CHANGE
1	Nebraska	34.9
2	Vermont	30.8
3	Oregon	26.2
4	California	24.9
5	Oklahoma	23.6
6	Idaho	21.6
6	Tennessee	21.6
8	Indiana	21.0
9	Colorado	20.3
10	Pennsylvania	19.2
11	Kansas	18.9
12	Utah	18.4
13	New York	17.2
14	New Mexico	16.8
15	Missouri	15.7
16	Arizona	15.4
17	South Carolina	15.0
18	Rhode Island	14.4
19	South Dakota	13.4
20	West Virginia	13.3
21	Alaska	12.9
22	Michigan	12.5
23	Minnesota	12.1
24	Delaware	11.6
25	Arkansas	11.2
26	Alabama	10.8
26	Nevada	10.8
28	Iowa	10.7
29	Washington	10.4
30	Virginia	8.9
31	Maryland	8.3
31	Texas	8.3
33	North Carolina	7.8
34	Louisiana	7.4
35	Ohio	7.3
36	Wisconsin	7.1
37	New Hampshire	6.3
38	Mississippi	6.0
39	Maine	5.6
39	Massachusetts	5.6
41	New Jersey	5.4
42	Kentucky	4.9
43	Florida	4.8
44	Wyoming	3.3
45	Georgia	2.5
46	North Dakota	2.0
47	Connecticut	1.5
48	Illinois	(0.9)
49	Montana	(1.6)
50	Hawaii	(6.8)

District of Columbia — 15.3

Source: MQ Press using data from U.S. Dept of Health & Human Services, Centers for Medicare and Medicaid Services
   "Medicaid Financial Statistics Tables (HCFA-64 Report)"
*For fiscal years 1999 and 1997. National figure includes expenditures in U.S. territories.

Medicaid Expenditures per Enrollee in 1999

National Rate = $4,302 per Enrollee*

ALPHA ORDER

RANK	STATE	PER ENROLLEE
34	Alabama	$3,754
22	Alaska	4,144
44	Arizona	3,116
45	Arkansas	3,023
42	California	3,262
12	Colorado	5,201
3	Connecticut	7,266
27	Delaware	4,033
43	Florida	3,194
47	Georgia	2,970
48	Hawaii	2,886
8	Idaho	5,477
32	Illinois	3,796
18	Indiana	4,513
19	Iowa	4,459
15	Kansas	4,697
25	Kentucky	4,063
21	Louisiana	4,236
6	Maine	5,755
17	Maryland	4,664
7	Massachusetts	5,542
16	Michigan	4,685
11	Minnesota	5,261
41	Mississippi	3,315
22	Missouri	4,144
28	Montana	4,020
20	Nebraska	4,432
33	Nevada	3,790
2	New Hampshire	7,378
4	New Jersey	6,845
46	New Mexico	2,987
1	New York	8,639
26	North Carolina	4,053
9	North Dakota	5,473
13	Ohio	4,973
49	Oklahoma	2,818
37	Oregon	3,580
10	Pennsylvania	5,430
5	Rhode Island	6,790
39	South Carolina	3,415
24	South Dakota	4,089
50	Tennessee	2,726
30	Texas	3,886
35	Utah	3,672
40	Vermont	3,343
38	Virginia	3,544
29	Washington	3,943
36	West Virginia	3,584
14	Wisconsin	4,897
31	Wyoming	3,872

RANK ORDER

RANK	STATE	PER ENROLLEE
1	New York	$8,639
2	New Hampshire	7,378
3	Connecticut	7,266
4	New Jersey	6,845
5	Rhode Island	6,790
6	Maine	5,755
7	Massachusetts	5,542
8	Idaho	5,477
9	North Dakota	5,473
10	Pennsylvania	5,430
11	Minnesota	5,261
12	Colorado	5,201
13	Ohio	4,973
14	Wisconsin	4,897
15	Kansas	4,697
16	Michigan	4,685
17	Maryland	4,664
18	Indiana	4,513
19	Iowa	4,459
20	Nebraska	4,432
21	Louisiana	4,236
22	Alaska	4,144
22	Missouri	4,144
24	South Dakota	4,089
25	Kentucky	4,063
26	North Carolina	4,053
27	Delaware	4,033
28	Montana	4,020
29	Washington	3,943
30	Texas	3,886
31	Wyoming	3,872
32	Illinois	3,796
33	Nevada	3,790
34	Alabama	3,754
35	Utah	3,672
36	West Virginia	3,584
37	Oregon	3,580
38	Virginia	3,544
39	South Carolina	3,415
40	Vermont	3,343
41	Mississippi	3,315
42	California	3,262
43	Florida	3,194
44	Arizona	3,116
45	Arkansas	3,023
46	New Mexico	2,987
47	Georgia	2,970
48	Hawaii	2,886
49	Oklahoma	2,818
50	Tennessee	2,726
	District of Columbia	6,340

Source: MQ Press using data from U.S. Dept of Health & Human Services, Centers for Medicare and Medicaid Services
"Medicaid Financial Statistics Tables (HCFA-64 Report)"
*For fiscal year 1999. National figure includes expenditures and enrollees in U.S. territories.

Percent Change in Expenditures per Medicaid Enrollee: 1997 to 1999

National Percent Change = 6.5% Decrease*

ALPHA ORDER			RANK ORDER		
RANK	STATE	PERCENT CHANGE	RANK	STATE	PERCENT CHANGE
27	Alabama	(6.9)	1	Idaho	48.9
35	Alaska	(16.9)	2	Nebraska	23.2
22	Arizona	(3.2)	2	Oregon	23.2
33	Arkansas	(14.8)	4	Tennessee	12.4
20	California	(2.5)	5	New York	11.0
32	Colorado	(14.2)	6	West Virginia	7.8
NA	Connecticut**	NA	7	Ohio	7.7
36	Delaware	(17.3)	8	Kansas	6.3
40	Florida	(20.9)	9	Kentucky	5.0
16	Georgia	0.1	10	Iowa	3.7
25	Hawaii	(5.4)	11	Louisiana	3.5
1	Idaho	48.9	12	Texas	2.7
39	Illinois	(18.3)	13	Vermont	1.9
26	Indiana	(6.8)	14	New Mexico	1.2
10	Iowa	3.7	15	North Dakota	0.8
8	Kansas	6.3	16	Georgia	0.1
9	Kentucky	5.0	17	North Carolina	(0.4)
11	Louisiana	3.5	18	Mississippi	(1.8)
30	Maine	(11.7)	19	Montana	(2.0)
47	Maryland	(30.7)	20	California	(2.5)
44	Massachusetts	(27.2)	21	Wyoming	(2.6)
24	Michigan	(4.6)	22	Arizona	(3.2)
46	Minnesota	(28.9)	23	New Hampshire	(4.0)
18	Mississippi	(1.8)	24	Michigan	(4.6)
45	Missouri	(28.7)	25	Hawaii	(5.4)
19	Montana	(2.0)	26	Indiana	(6.8)
2	Nebraska	23.2	27	Alabama	(6.9)
38	Nevada	(18.2)	28	South Dakota	(7.0)
23	New Hampshire	(4.0)	29	Virginia	(7.2)
49	New Jersey	(32.8)	30	Maine	(11.7)
14	New Mexico	1.2	31	Rhode Island	(13.6)
5	New York	11.0	32	Colorado	(14.2)
17	North Carolina	(0.4)	33	Arkansas	(14.8)
15	North Dakota	0.8	34	Utah	(15.2)
7	Ohio	7.7	35	Alaska	(16.9)
43	Oklahoma	(25.6)	36	Delaware	(17.3)
2	Oregon	23.2	37	South Carolina	(17.5)
48	Pennsylvania	(31.1)	38	Nevada	(18.2)
31	Rhode Island	(13.6)	39	Illinois	(18.3)
37	South Carolina	(17.5)	40	Florida	(20.9)
28	South Dakota	(7.0)	41	Washington	(22.3)
4	Tennessee	12.4	42	Wisconsin	(25.4)
12	Texas	2.7	43	Oklahoma	(25.6)
34	Utah	(15.2)	44	Massachusetts	(27.2)
13	Vermont	1.9	45	Missouri	(28.7)
29	Virginia	(7.2)	46	Minnesota	(28.9)
41	Washington	(22.3)	47	Maryland	(30.7)
6	West Virginia	7.8	48	Pennsylvania	(31.1)
42	Wisconsin	(25.4)	49	New Jersey	(32.8)
21	Wyoming	(2.6)	NA	Connecticut**	NA

District of Columbia   1.9

Source: MQ Press using data from U.S. Dept of Health & Human Services, Centers for Medicare and Medicaid Services
  "Medicaid Financial Statistics Tables (HCFA-64 Report)"
*For fiscal years 1999 and 1997. National figure includes expenditures and enrollees in U.S. territories.
**Not available.

Medicaid Managed Care Enrollment in 2000

National Total = 19,553,382 Enrollees*

ALPHA ORDER

RANK	STATE	ENROLLEES	% of USA
19	Alabama	337,979	1.7%
49	Alaska	0	0.0%
13	Arizona	438,512	2.2%
23	Arkansas	267,470	1.4%
1	California	2,611,101	13.4%
27	Colorado	232,419	1.2%
28	Connecticut	232,213	1.2%
39	Delaware	79,364	0.4%
3	Florida	1,115,391	5.7%
6	Georgia	834,697	4.3%
34	Hawaii	119,576	0.6%
46	Idaho	34,961	0.2%
32	Illinois	137,225	0.7%
14	Indiana	407,034	2.1%
30	Iowa	189,198	1.0%
36	Kansas	113,693	0.6%
12	Kentucky	479,499	2.5%
42	Louisiana	52,174	0.3%
38	Maine	85,098	0.4%
15	Maryland	400,765	2.0%
11	Massachusetts	597,777	3.1%
4	Michigan	1,085,479	5.6%
22	Minnesota	279,057	1.4%
26	Mississippi	235,152	1.2%
17	Missouri	339,799	1.7%
43	Montana	43,383	0.2%
31	Nebraska	144,421	0.7%
44	Nevada	38,705	0.2%
48	New Hampshire	5,079	0.0%
16	New Jersey	394,330	2.0%
29	New Mexico	208,587	1.1%
8	New York	694,014	3.5%
9	North Carolina	634,292	3.2%
47	North Dakota	23,114	0.1%
24	Ohio	251,115	1.3%
21	Oklahoma	291,656	1.5%
18	Oregon	339,753	1.7%
5	Pennsylvania	1,005,502	5.1%
37	Rhode Island	106,554	0.5%
45	South Carolina	34,987	0.2%
41	South Dakota	58,134	0.3%
2	Tennessee	1,362,799	7.0%
10	Texas	608,774	3.1%
33	Utah	121,000	0.6%
40	Vermont	63,329	0.3%
20	Virginia	293,695	1.5%
7	Washington	781,549	4.0%
35	West Virginia	114,327	0.6%
25	Wisconsin	245,685	1.3%
49	Wyoming	0	0.0%

RANK ORDER

RANK	STATE	ENROLLEES	% of USA
1	California	2,611,101	13.4%
2	Tennessee	1,362,799	7.0%
3	Florida	1,115,391	5.7%
4	Michigan	1,085,479	5.6%
5	Pennsylvania	1,005,502	5.1%
6	Georgia	834,697	4.3%
7	Washington	781,549	4.0%
8	New York	694,014	3.5%
9	North Carolina	634,292	3.2%
10	Texas	608,774	3.1%
11	Massachusetts	597,777	3.1%
12	Kentucky	479,499	2.5%
13	Arizona	438,512	2.2%
14	Indiana	407,034	2.1%
15	Maryland	400,765	2.0%
16	New Jersey	394,330	2.0%
17	Missouri	339,799	1.7%
18	Oregon	339,753	1.7%
19	Alabama	337,979	1.7%
20	Virginia	293,695	1.5%
21	Oklahoma	291,656	1.5%
22	Minnesota	279,057	1.4%
23	Arkansas	267,470	1.4%
24	Ohio	251,115	1.3%
25	Wisconsin	245,685	1.3%
26	Mississippi	235,152	1.2%
27	Colorado	232,419	1.2%
28	Connecticut	232,213	1.2%
29	New Mexico	208,587	1.1%
30	Iowa	189,198	1.0%
31	Nebraska	144,421	0.7%
32	Illinois	137,225	0.7%
33	Utah	121,000	0.6%
34	Hawaii	119,576	0.6%
35	West Virginia	114,327	0.6%
36	Kansas	113,693	0.6%
37	Rhode Island	106,554	0.5%
38	Maine	85,098	0.4%
39	Delaware	79,364	0.4%
40	Vermont	63,329	0.3%
41	South Dakota	58,134	0.3%
42	Louisiana	52,174	0.3%
43	Montana	43,383	0.2%
44	Nevada	38,705	0.2%
45	South Carolina	34,987	0.2%
46	Idaho	34,961	0.2%
47	North Dakota	23,114	0.1%
48	New Hampshire	5,079	0.0%
49	Alaska	0	0.0%
49	Wyoming	0	0.0%
	District of Columbia	78,940	0.4%

Source: U.S. Department of Health and Human Services, Centers for Medicare and Medicaid Services
"Medicaid Managed Care State Enrollment" (http://www.hcfa.gov/medicaid/omcpr00.pdf)
*As of December 31, 2000. Enrollment in state health care reform programs that expand eligibility beyond traditional Medicaid standards. National total includes 904,025 Medicaid managed care enrollees in Puerto Rico.

Percent of Medicaid Enrollees in Managed Care in 2000

National Percent = 56.7% of Medicaid Enrollees*

ALPHA ORDER

RANK	STATE	PERCENT
31	Alabama	55.0
49	Alaska	0.0
8	Arizona	87.5
25	Arkansas	63.2
34	California	51.3
7	Colorado	88.2
17	Connecticut	72.2
11	Delaware	80.1
27	Florida	61.5
4	Georgia	96.6
13	Hawaii	78.4
42	Idaho	28.7
45	Illinois	9.6
19	Indiana	69.5
9	Iowa	85.8
30	Kansas	57.9
12	Kentucky	79.5
46	Louisiana	7.2
36	Maine	49.5
10	Maryland	84.0
22	Massachusetts	67.5
1	Michigan	100.0
26	Minnesota	62.1
38	Mississippi	43.0
39	Missouri	40.8
28	Montana	61.4
14	Nebraska	76.6
40	Nevada	33.0
47	New Hampshire	6.5
29	New Jersey	61.1
23	New Mexico	65.1
43	New York	25.2
18	North Carolina	70.1
32	North Dakota	54.1
44	Ohio	20.8
21	Oklahoma	68.3
6	Oregon	89.3
15	Pennsylvania	76.4
20	Rhode Island	69.4
48	South Carolina	6.1
16	South Dakota	76.0
1	Tennessee	100.0
41	Texas	31.6
5	Utah	90.5
33	Vermont	53.0
24	Virginia	63.7
1	Washington	100.0
37	West Virginia	43.8
35	Wisconsin	49.9
49	Wyoming	0.0

RANK ORDER

RANK	STATE	PERCENT
1	Michigan	100.0
1	Tennessee	100.0
1	Washington	100.0
4	Georgia	96.6
5	Utah	90.5
6	Oregon	89.3
7	Colorado	88.2
8	Arizona	87.5
9	Iowa	85.8
10	Maryland	84.0
11	Delaware	80.1
12	Kentucky	79.5
13	Hawaii	78.4
14	Nebraska	76.6
15	Pennsylvania	76.4
16	South Dakota	76.0
17	Connecticut	72.2
18	North Carolina	70.1
19	Indiana	69.5
20	Rhode Island	69.4
21	Oklahoma	68.3
22	Massachusetts	67.5
23	New Mexico	65.1
24	Virginia	63.7
25	Arkansas	63.2
26	Minnesota	62.1
27	Florida	61.5
28	Montana	61.4
29	New Jersey	61.1
30	Kansas	57.9
31	Alabama	55.0
32	North Dakota	54.1
33	Vermont	53.0
34	California	51.3
35	Wisconsin	49.9
36	Maine	49.5
37	West Virginia	43.8
38	Mississippi	43.0
39	Missouri	40.8
40	Nevada	33.0
41	Texas	31.6
42	Idaho	28.7
43	New York	25.2
44	Ohio	20.8
45	Illinois	9.6
46	Louisiana	7.2
47	New Hampshire	6.5
48	South Carolina	6.1
49	Alaska	0.0
49	Wyoming	0.0
	District of Columbia	64.8

Source: U.S. Department of Health and Human Services, Centers for Medicare and Medicaid Services
  "Medicaid Managed Care State Enrollment" (http://www.hcfa.gov/medicaid/omcpr00.pdf)
*As of December 31, 2000. Enrollment in state health care reform programs that expand eligibility beyond traditional Medicaid standards. National percent includes Medicaid enrollees in Puerto Rico and the Virgin Islands.

Federal Medicaid Matching Fund Rate for 2002

National Average = 72.31% of States' Funds Matched by Federal Government*

ALPHA ORDER				RANK ORDER		
RANK	STATE	RATE		RANK	STATE	RATE
7	Alabama	79.32		1	Mississippi	83.26
35	Alaska	67.11		2	West Virginia	82.69
16	Arizona	75.49		3	New Mexico	81.13
5	Arkansas	80.85		4	Montana	80.98
38	California	65.98		5	Arkansas	80.85
40	Colorado	65.00		6	Idaho	79.71
40	Connecticut	65.00		7	Alabama	79.32
40	Delaware	65.00		8	Oklahoma	79.30
31	Florida	69.50		9	Louisiana	79.21
28	Georgia	71.30		10	Utah	79.00
33	Hawaii	69.44		11	Kentucky	78.96
6	Idaho	79.71		12	North Dakota	78.91
40	Illinois	65.00		13	South Carolina	78.54
20	Indiana	73.43		14	Maine	76.61
19	Iowa	74.00		15	South Dakota	76.15
24	Kansas	72.14		16	Arizona	75.49
11	Kentucky	78.96		17	Tennessee	74.55
9	Louisiana	79.21		18	Vermont	74.14
14	Maine	76.61		19	Iowa	74.00
40	Maryland	65.00		20	Indiana	73.43
40	Massachusetts	65.00		21	Wyoming	73.38
32	Michigan	69.45		22	North Carolina	73.02
40	Minnesota	65.00		23	Missouri	72.74
1	Mississippi	83.26		24	Kansas	72.14
23	Missouri	72.74		25	Texas	72.12
4	Montana	80.98		26	Nebraska	71.69
26	Nebraska	71.69		27	Oregon	71.44
40	Nevada	65.00		28	Georgia	71.30
40	New Hampshire	65.00		29	Ohio	71.15
40	New Jersey	65.00		30	Wisconsin	71.00
3	New Mexico	81.13		31	Florida	69.50
40	New York	65.00		32	Michigan	69.45
22	North Carolina	73.02		33	Hawaii	69.44
12	North Dakota	78.91		34	Pennsylvania	68.26
29	Ohio	71.15		35	Alaska	67.11
8	Oklahoma	79.30		36	Rhode Island	66.72
27	Oregon	71.44		37	Virginia	66.02
34	Pennsylvania	68.26		38	California	65.98
36	Rhode Island	66.72		39	Washington	65.26
13	South Carolina	78.54		40	Colorado	65.00
15	South Dakota	76.15		40	Connecticut	65.00
17	Tennessee	74.55		40	Delaware	65.00
25	Texas	72.12		40	Illinois	65.00
10	Utah	79.00		40	Maryland	65.00
18	Vermont	74.14		40	Massachusetts	65.00
37	Virginia	66.02		40	Minnesota	65.00
39	Washington	65.26		40	Nevada	65.00
2	West Virginia	82.69		40	New Hampshire	65.00
30	Wisconsin	71.00		40	New Jersey	65.00
21	Wyoming	73.38		40	New York	65.00
					District of Columbia	79.00

Source: U.S. Department of Health and Human Services, Centers for Medicare and Medicaid Services
"Enhanced Federal Medical Assistance Percentages" (Federal Register, 2/23/00)
*For fiscal year 2002. These are "enhanced" matching rates established by the Children's Health Insurance
Program, signed into law in August 1997. Sixty-five percent is the minimum. National average is a simple average of
the 51 individual rates and is not weighted for population or funds.

Personal Health Care Expenditures in 1998

National Total = $1,016,383,000,000*

ALPHA ORDER

RANK	STATE	EXPENDITURES	% of USA
22	Alabama	$16,056,000,000	1.6%
48	Alaska	2,299,000,000	0.2%
24	Arizona	14,782,000,000	1.5%
33	Arkansas	8,463,000,000	0.8%
1	California	110,057,000,000	10.8%
26	Colorado	13,669,000,000	1.3%
23	Connecticut	15,221,000,000	1.5%
44	Delaware	3,106,000,000	0.3%
4	Florida	59,724,000,000	5.9%
12	Georgia	27,219,000,000	2.7%
40	Hawaii	4,658,000,000	0.5%
43	Idaho	3,397,000,000	0.3%
6	Illinois	44,305,000,000	4.4%
15	Indiana	21,259,000,000	2.1%
30	Iowa	10,198,000,000	1.0%
31	Kansas	9,394,000,000	0.9%
25	Kentucky	14,414,000,000	1.4%
21	Louisiana	16,500,000,000	1.6%
39	Maine	4,925,000,000	0.5%
19	Maryland	19,646,000,000	1.9%
10	Massachusetts	30,039,000,000	3.0%
8	Michigan	35,647,000,000	3.5%
17	Minnesota	20,313,000,000	2.0%
32	Mississippi	8,882,000,000	0.9%
16	Missouri	20,911,000,000	2.1%
46	Montana	2,838,000,000	0.3%
35	Nebraska	6,095,000,000	0.6%
37	Nevada	5,606,000,000	0.6%
40	New Hampshire	4,658,000,000	0.5%
9	New Jersey	32,695,000,000	3.2%
38	New Mexico	5,344,000,000	0.5%
2	New York	85,785,000,000	8.4%
11	North Carolina	27,327,000,000	2.7%
47	North Dakota	2,680,000,000	0.3%
7	Ohio	42,581,000,000	4.2%
28	Oklahoma	10,988,000,000	1.1%
29	Oregon	10,840,000,000	1.1%
5	Pennsylvania	51,322,000,000	5.0%
42	Rhode Island	4,515,000,000	0.4%
27	South Carolina	13,204,000,000	1.3%
45	South Dakota	2,842,000,000	0.3%
14	Tennessee	22,021,000,000	2.2%
3	Texas	67,750,000,000	6.7%
36	Utah	5,944,000,000	0.6%
49	Vermont	2,066,000,000	0.2%
13	Virginia	22,261,000,000	2.2%
20	Washington	19,292,000,000	1.9%
34	West Virginia	7,037,000,000	0.7%
18	Wisconsin	19,945,000,000	2.0%
50	Wyoming	1,407,000,000	0.1%

RANK ORDER

RANK	STATE	EXPENDITURES	% of USA
1	California	$110,057,000,000	10.8%
2	New York	85,785,000,000	8.4%
3	Texas	67,750,000,000	6.7%
4	Florida	59,724,000,000	5.9%
5	Pennsylvania	51,322,000,000	5.0%
6	Illinois	44,305,000,000	4.4%
7	Ohio	42,581,000,000	4.2%
8	Michigan	35,647,000,000	3.5%
9	New Jersey	32,695,000,000	3.2%
10	Massachusetts	30,039,000,000	3.0%
11	North Carolina	27,327,000,000	2.7%
12	Georgia	27,219,000,000	2.7%
13	Virginia	22,261,000,000	2.2%
14	Tennessee	22,021,000,000	2.2%
15	Indiana	21,259,000,000	2.1%
16	Missouri	20,911,000,000	2.1%
17	Minnesota	20,313,000,000	2.0%
18	Wisconsin	19,945,000,000	2.0%
19	Maryland	19,646,000,000	1.9%
20	Washington	19,292,000,000	1.9%
21	Louisiana	16,500,000,000	1.6%
22	Alabama	16,056,000,000	1.6%
23	Connecticut	15,221,000,000	1.5%
24	Arizona	14,782,000,000	1.5%
25	Kentucky	14,414,000,000	1.4%
26	Colorado	13,669,000,000	1.3%
27	South Carolina	13,204,000,000	1.3%
28	Oklahoma	10,988,000,000	1.1%
29	Oregon	10,840,000,000	1.1%
30	Iowa	10,198,000,000	1.0%
31	Kansas	9,394,000,000	0.9%
32	Mississippi	8,882,000,000	0.9%
33	Arkansas	8,463,000,000	0.8%
34	West Virginia	7,037,000,000	0.7%
35	Nebraska	6,095,000,000	0.6%
36	Utah	5,944,000,000	0.6%
37	Nevada	5,606,000,000	0.6%
38	New Mexico	5,344,000,000	0.5%
39	Maine	4,925,000,000	0.5%
40	Hawaii	4,658,000,000	0.5%
40	New Hampshire	4,658,000,000	0.5%
42	Rhode Island	4,515,000,000	0.4%
43	Idaho	3,397,000,000	0.3%
44	Delaware	3,106,000,000	0.3%
45	South Dakota	2,842,000,000	0.3%
46	Montana	2,838,000,000	0.3%
47	North Dakota	2,680,000,000	0.3%
48	Alaska	2,299,000,000	0.2%
49	Vermont	2,066,000,000	0.2%
50	Wyoming	1,407,000,000	0.1%
	District of Columbia	4,258,000,000	0.4%

Source: U.S. Department of Health and Human Services, Centers for Medicare and Medicaid Services
"State Health Care Expenditures" (http://www.hcfa.gov/stats/nhe-oact/stateestimates/)
*By state of provider. Includes hospital care, physician services, dental services, home health care, drugs, vision products, nursing home care and other personal health care services and products.

Health Care Expenditures as a Percent of Gross State Product in 1998

National Percent = 11.6% of Total Gross State Product*

ALPHA ORDER				RANK ORDER		
RANK	STATE	PERCENT		RANK	STATE	PERCENT
5	Alabama	14.6		1	West Virginia	17.6
47	Alaska	9.5		2	North Dakota	15.6
34	Arizona	11.0		3	Maine	15.2
11	Arkansas	13.7		4	Rhode Island	14.8
44	California	9.8		5	Alabama	14.6
45	Colorado	9.6		6	Florida	14.3
36	Connecticut	10.7		6	Mississippi	14.3
48	Delaware	9.2		6	Montana	14.3
6	Florida	14.3		9	Pennsylvania	14.1
36	Georgia	10.7		10	Tennessee	13.8
30	Hawaii	11.7		11	Arkansas	13.7
34	Idaho	11.0		12	Kentucky	13.5
39	Illinois	10.4		12	Oklahoma	13.5
23	Indiana	12.2		14	South Dakota	13.4
25	Iowa	12.1		15	South Carolina	13.2
23	Kansas	12.2		16	Louisiana	12.8
12	Kentucky	13.5		16	Missouri	12.8
16	Louisiana	12.8		18	Vermont	12.7
3	Maine	15.2		19	Minnesota	12.6
28	Maryland	11.9		19	Wisconsin	12.6
21	Massachusetts	12.5		21	Massachusetts	12.5
25	Michigan	12.1		21	Ohio	12.5
19	Minnesota	12.6		23	Indiana	12.2
6	Mississippi	14.3		23	Kansas	12.2
16	Missouri	12.8		25	Iowa	12.1
6	Montana	14.3		25	Michigan	12.1
29	Nebraska	11.8		25	New York	12.1
49	Nevada	8.9		28	Maryland	11.9
32	New Hampshire	11.3		29	Nebraska	11.8
41	New Jersey	10.2		30	Hawaii	11.7
33	New Mexico	11.2		31	North Carolina	11.6
25	New York	12.1		32	New Hampshire	11.3
31	North Carolina	11.6		33	New Mexico	11.2
2	North Dakota	15.6		34	Arizona	11.0
21	Ohio	12.5		34	Idaho	11.0
12	Oklahoma	13.5		36	Connecticut	10.7
40	Oregon	10.3		36	Georgia	10.7
9	Pennsylvania	14.1		38	Texas	10.5
4	Rhode Island	14.8		39	Illinois	10.4
15	South Carolina	13.2		40	Oregon	10.3
14	South Dakota	13.4		41	New Jersey	10.2
10	Tennessee	13.8		42	Utah	10.0
38	Texas	10.5		42	Washington	10.0
42	Utah	10.0		44	California	9.8
18	Vermont	12.7		45	Colorado	9.6
45	Virginia	9.6		45	Virginia	9.6
42	Washington	10.0		47	Alaska	9.5
1	West Virginia	17.6		48	Delaware	9.2
19	Wisconsin	12.6		49	Nevada	8.9
50	Wyoming	8.0		50	Wyoming	8.0
					District of Columbia	7.9

Source: MQ Press using data from U.S. Dept of Health & Human Services, Centers for Medicare and Medicaid Services
"State Health Care Expenditures" (http://www.hcfa.gov/stats/nhe-oact/stateestimates/)
*By state of provider. Includes hospital care, physician services, dental services, home health care, drugs, vision products, nursing home care and other personal health care services and products.

Percent Change in Personal Health Care Expenditures: 1990 to 1998

National Percent Change = 66.0% Increase*

ALPHA ORDER				RANK ORDER		
RANK	STATE	PERCENT CHANGE		RANK	STATE	PERCENT CHANGE
21	Alabama	75.2		1	Idaho	100.2
30	Alaska	70.7		2	Nevada	99.8
26	Arizona	72.6		3	North Carolina	98.8
28	Arkansas	71.8		4	South Carolina	94.0
50	California	48.0		5	Mississippi	87.8
19	Colorado	76.6		5	South Dakota	87.8
49	Connecticut	52.0		7	Kentucky	84.3
14	Delaware	79.7		8	Utah	83.9
37	Florida	66.9		9	New Mexico	83.2
16	Georgia	77.9		10	Maine	82.7
31	Hawaii	69.7		11	New Hampshire	82.1
1	Idaho	100.2		12	Tennessee	80.3
44	Illinois	60.4		13	Texas	79.8
35	Indiana	67.5		14	Delaware	79.7
33	Iowa	68.1		15	West Virginia	79.1
32	Kansas	69.6		16	Georgia	77.9
7	Kentucky	84.3		17	Wyoming	77.4
39	Louisiana	65.4		18	Minnesota	77.2
10	Maine	82.7		19	Colorado	76.6
36	Maryland	67.1		20	Vermont	76.3
47	Massachusetts	57.9		21	Alabama	75.2
43	Michigan	61.1		22	Montana	74.3
18	Minnesota	77.2		22	Wisconsin	74.3
5	Mississippi	87.8		24	Oregon	73.5
40	Missouri	64.8		25	Oklahoma	72.8
22	Montana	74.3		26	Arizona	72.6
26	Nebraska	72.6		26	Nebraska	72.6
2	Nevada	99.8		28	Arkansas	71.8
11	New Hampshire	82.1		29	Washington	71.1
42	New Jersey	62.1		30	Alaska	70.7
9	New Mexico	83.2		31	Hawaii	69.7
45	New York	59.1		32	Kansas	69.6
3	North Carolina	98.8		33	Iowa	68.1
41	North Dakota	63.5		34	Virginia	68.0
46	Ohio	58.3		35	Indiana	67.5
25	Oklahoma	72.8		36	Maryland	67.1
24	Oregon	73.5		37	Florida	66.9
48	Pennsylvania	57.3		38	Rhode Island	65.5
38	Rhode Island	65.5		39	Louisiana	65.4
4	South Carolina	94.0		40	Missouri	64.8
5	South Dakota	87.8		41	North Dakota	63.5
12	Tennessee	80.3		42	New Jersey	62.1
13	Texas	79.8		43	Michigan	61.1
8	Utah	83.9		44	Illinois	60.4
20	Vermont	76.3		45	New York	59.1
34	Virginia	68.0		46	Ohio	58.3
29	Washington	71.1		47	Massachusetts	57.9
15	West Virginia	79.1		48	Pennsylvania	57.3
22	Wisconsin	74.3		49	Connecticut	52.0
17	Wyoming	77.4		50	California	48.0
					District of Columbia	19.5

Source: MQ Press using data from U.S. Dept of Health & Human Services, Centers for Medicare and Medicaid Services
"State Health Care Expenditures" (http://www.hcfa.gov/stats/nhe-oact/stateestimates/)
*By state of provider. Includes hospital care, physician services, dental services, home health care, drugs, vision products, nursing home care and other personal health care services and products.

Average Annual Change in Expenditures for
Personal Health Care: 1990 to 1998
National Percent Change = 13.9% Average Annual Increase*

ALPHA ORDER

RANK ORDER

RANK	STATE	PERCENT CHANGE	RANK	STATE	PERCENT CHANGE
19	Alabama	14.3	1	Florida	17.6
22	Alaska	14.1	1	New Hampshire	17.6
3	Arizona	17.0	3	Arizona	17.0
26	Arkansas	13.8	4	Georgia	16.4
26	California	13.8	4	Nevada	16.4
22	Colorado	14.1	6	North Carolina	16.0
8	Connecticut	15.6	7	South Carolina	15.8
12	Delaware	15.1	8	Connecticut	15.6
1	Florida	17.6	8	New Mexico	15.6
4	Georgia	16.4	10	New Jersey	15.3
15	Hawaii	14.6	11	Utah	15.2
33	Idaho	13.3	12	Delaware	15.1
48	Illinois	11.4	13	Virginia	15.0
30	Indiana	13.6	14	Tennessee	14.7
50	Iowa	11.2	15	Hawaii	14.6
45	Kansas	11.8	15	Texas	14.6
22	Kentucky	14.1	15	Vermont	14.6
28	Louisiana	13.7	18	Washington	14.5
19	Maine	14.3	19	Alabama	14.3
21	Maryland	14.2	19	Maine	14.3
22	Massachusetts	14.1	21	Maryland	14.2
49	Michigan	11.3	22	Alaska	14.1
33	Minnesota	13.3	22	Colorado	14.1
35	Mississippi	13.1	22	Kentucky	14.1
38	Missouri	12.9	22	Massachusetts	14.1
39	Montana	12.8	26	Arkansas	13.8
46	Nebraska	11.7	26	California	13.8
4	Nevada	16.4	28	Louisiana	13.7
1	New Hampshire	17.6	28	Rhode Island	13.7
10	New Jersey	15.3	30	Indiana	13.6
8	New Mexico	15.6	30	Pennsylvania	13.6
32	New York	13.4	32	New York	13.4
6	North Carolina	16.0	33	Idaho	13.3
40	North Dakota	12.7	33	Minnesota	13.3
36	Ohio	13.0	35	Mississippi	13.1
44	Oklahoma	11.9	36	Ohio	13.0
36	Oregon	13.0	36	Oregon	13.0
30	Pennsylvania	13.6	38	Missouri	12.9
28	Rhode Island	13.7	39	Montana	12.8
7	South Carolina	15.8	40	North Dakota	12.7
40	South Dakota	12.7	40	South Dakota	12.7
14	Tennessee	14.7	42	Wisconsin	12.6
15	Texas	14.6	43	West Virginia	12.0
11	Utah	15.2	44	Oklahoma	11.9
15	Vermont	14.6	45	Kansas	11.8
13	Virginia	15.0	46	Nebraska	11.7
18	Washington	14.5	46	Wyoming	11.7
43	West Virginia	12.0	48	Illinois	11.4
42	Wisconsin	12.6	49	Michigan	11.3
46	Wyoming	11.7	50	Iowa	11.2

| | | | | District of Columbia | 12.5 |

Source: U.S. Department of Health and Human Services, Centers for Medicare and Medicaid Services
"State Health Care Expenditures" (http://www.hcfa.gov/stats/nhe-oact/stateestimates/)
*By state of provider. Includes hospital care, physician services, dental services, home health care, drugs, vision products, nursing home care and other personal health care services and products.

Per Capita Personal Health Care Expenditures in 1998

National Per Capita = $3,761*

ALPHA ORDER			RANK ORDER		
RANK	STATE	PER CAPITA	RANK	STATE	PER CAPITA
23	Alabama	$3,690	1	Massachusetts	$4,889
22	Alaska	3,737	2	New York	4,724
46	Arizona	3,167	3	Connecticut	4,651
39	Arkansas	3,334	4	Rhode Island	4,571
38	California	3,367	5	Minnesota	4,298
34	Colorado	3,444	6	Pennsylvania	4,276
3	Connecticut	4,651	7	North Dakota	4,202
8	Delaware	4,174	8	Delaware	4,174
11	Florida	4,006	9	Tennessee	4,053
30	Georgia	3,564	10	New Jersey	4,039
14	Hawaii	3,913	11	Florida	4,006
50	Idaho	2,760	12	Maine	3,948
24	Illinois	3,671	13	New Hampshire	3,928
29	Indiana	3,599	14	Hawaii	3,913
30	Iowa	3,564	15	South Dakota	3,889
32	Kansas	3,560	16	West Virginia	3,884
26	Kentucky	3,664	17	Missouri	3,846
21	Louisiana	3,782	18	Maryland	3,830
12	Maine	3,948	19	Wisconsin	3,819
18	Maryland	3,830	20	Ohio	3,789
1	Massachusetts	4,889	21	Louisiana	3,782
27	Michigan	3,630	22	Alaska	3,737
5	Minnesota	4,298	23	Alabama	3,690
43	Mississippi	3,228	24	Illinois	3,671
17	Missouri	3,846	25	Nebraska	3,670
44	Montana	3,227	26	Kentucky	3,664
25	Nebraska	3,670	27	Michigan	3,630
45	Nevada	3,215	28	North Carolina	3,621
13	New Hampshire	3,928	29	Indiana	3,599
10	New Jersey	4,039	30	Georgia	3,564
47	New Mexico	3,083	30	Iowa	3,564
2	New York	4,724	32	Kansas	3,560
28	North Carolina	3,621	33	Vermont	3,498
7	North Dakota	4,202	34	Colorado	3,444
20	Ohio	3,789	35	South Carolina	3,439
41	Oklahoma	3,290	36	Texas	3,437
40	Oregon	3,303	37	Washington	3,392
6	Pennsylvania	4,276	38	California	3,367
4	Rhode Island	4,571	39	Arkansas	3,334
35	South Carolina	3,439	40	Oregon	3,303
15	South Dakota	3,889	41	Oklahoma	3,290
9	Tennessee	4,053	42	Virginia	3,279
36	Texas	3,437	43	Mississippi	3,228
49	Utah	2,830	44	Montana	3,227
33	Vermont	3,498	45	Nevada	3,215
42	Virginia	3,279	46	Arizona	3,167
37	Washington	3,392	47	New Mexico	3,083
16	West Virginia	3,884	48	Wyoming	2,931
19	Wisconsin	3,819	49	Utah	2,830
48	Wyoming	2,931	50	Idaho	2,760
				District of Columbia	8,166

Source: MQ Press using data from U.S. Dept of Health & Human Services, Centers for Medicare and Medicaid Services "State Health Care Expenditures" (http://www.hcfa.gov/stats/nhe-oact/stateestimates/)
*By state of provider. Per capita calculated using resident population. These figures may be skewed due to residents crossing state borders for care. Includes hospital care, physician services, dental services, home health care, drugs, vision products, nursing home care and other personal health care services and products.

Percent Change in Per Capita Expenditures for
Personal Health Care: 1990 to 1998
National Percent Change = 53.3% Increase*

ALPHA ORDER

RANK ORDER

RANK	STATE	PERCENT CHANGE	RANK	STATE	PERCENT CHANGE
18	Alabama	63.1	1	Maine	80.4
37	Alaska	53.5	2	South Dakota	79.1
49	Arizona	36.1	3	West Virginia	77.2
24	Arkansas	59.4	4	South Carolina	76.8
50	California	35.6	5	Mississippi	75.9
46	Colorado	47.0	6	North Carolina	75.4
39	Connecticut	52.8	7	Kentucky	73.0
21	Delaware	61.6	8	New Hampshire	70.7
47	Florida	45.7	9	Vermont	68.5
42	Georgia	51.5	10	Rhode Island	68.4
26	Hawaii	58.6	11	Wyoming	67.6
12	Idaho	64.6	12	Idaho	64.6
41	Illinois	52.1	13	Minnesota	64.5
29	Indiana	57.5	14	Nebraska	64.3
17	Iowa	63.3	15	Wisconsin	63.6
24	Kansas	59.4	16	North Dakota	63.4
7	Kentucky	73.0	17	Iowa	63.3
23	Louisiana	60.0	18	Alabama	63.1
1	Maine	80.4	19	Oklahoma	62.9
30	Maryland	56.3	20	Tennessee	62.3
35	Massachusetts	54.7	21	Delaware	61.6
40	Michigan	52.7	22	New Mexico	60.7
13	Minnesota	64.5	23	Louisiana	60.0
5	Mississippi	75.9	24	Arkansas	59.4
33	Missouri	55.4	24	Kansas	59.4
26	Montana	58.6	26	Hawaii	58.6
14	Nebraska	64.3	26	Montana	58.6
48	Nevada	39.6	28	New York	57.7
8	New Hampshire	70.7	29	Indiana	57.5
34	New Jersey	55.3	30	Maryland	56.3
22	New Mexico	60.7	31	Pennsylvania	55.9
28	New York	57.7	32	Texas	55.5
6	North Carolina	75.4	33	Missouri	55.4
16	North Dakota	63.4	34	New Jersey	55.3
38	Ohio	53.0	35	Massachusetts	54.7
19	Oklahoma	62.9	36	Virginia	53.7
44	Oregon	51.2	37	Alaska	53.5
31	Pennsylvania	55.9	38	Ohio	53.0
10	Rhode Island	68.4	39	Connecticut	52.8
4	South Carolina	76.8	40	Michigan	52.7
2	South Dakota	79.1	41	Illinois	52.1
20	Tennessee	62.3	42	Georgia	51.5
32	Texas	55.5	43	Utah	51.4
43	Utah	51.4	44	Oregon	51.2
9	Vermont	68.5	45	Washington	47.4
36	Virginia	53.7	46	Colorado	47.0
45	Washington	47.4	47	Florida	45.7
3	West Virginia	77.2	48	Nevada	39.6
15	Wisconsin	63.6	49	Arizona	36.1
11	Wyoming	67.6	50	California	35.6
				District of Columbia	38.4

Source: MQ Press using data from U.S. Dept of Health & Human Services, Centers for Medicare and Medicaid Services
"State Health Care Expenditures" (http://www.hcfa.gov/stats/nhe-oact/stateestimates/)
*By state of provider. Per capita calculated using resident population. These figures may be skewed due to
residents crossing state borders for care. Includes hospital care, physician services, dental services, home health
care, drugs, vision products, nursing home care and other personal health care services and products.

Average Annual Change in Per Capita Expenditures
For Personal Health Care: 1990 to 1998
National Percent Change = 5.5% Average Annual Increase*

ALPHA ORDER				RANK ORDER		
RANK	STATE	PERCENT CHANGE		RANK	STATE	PERCENT CHANGE
15	Alabama	6.3		1	Maine	7.7
36	Alaska	5.5		2	South Dakota	7.6
49	Arizona	3.9		3	South Carolina	7.4
23	Arkansas	6.0		3	West Virginia	7.4
49	California	3.9		5	Mississippi	7.3
46	Colorado	4.9		5	North Carolina	7.3
39	Connecticut	5.4		7	Kentucky	7.1
20	Delaware	6.2		8	New Hampshire	6.9
47	Florida	4.8		9	Rhode Island	6.7
42	Georgia	5.3		9	Vermont	6.7
26	Hawaii	5.9		9	Wyoming	6.7
12	Idaho	6.4		12	Idaho	6.4
39	Illinois	5.4		12	Minnesota	6.4
29	Indiana	5.8		12	Nebraska	6.4
15	Iowa	6.3		15	Alabama	6.3
23	Kansas	6.0		15	Iowa	6.3
7	Kentucky	7.1		15	North Dakota	6.3
23	Louisiana	6.0		15	Oklahoma	6.3
1	Maine	7.7		15	Wisconsin	6.3
30	Maryland	5.7		20	Delaware	6.2
35	Massachusetts	5.6		20	Tennessee	6.2
39	Michigan	5.4		22	New Mexico	6.1
12	Minnesota	6.4		23	Arkansas	6.0
5	Mississippi	7.3		23	Kansas	6.0
30	Missouri	5.7		23	Louisiana	6.0
26	Montana	5.9		26	Hawaii	5.9
12	Nebraska	6.4		26	Montana	5.9
48	Nevada	4.3		26	New York	5.9
8	New Hampshire	6.9		29	Indiana	5.8
30	New Jersey	5.7		30	Maryland	5.7
22	New Mexico	6.1		30	Missouri	5.7
26	New York	5.9		30	New Jersey	5.7
5	North Carolina	7.3		30	Pennsylvania	5.7
15	North Dakota	6.3		30	Texas	5.7
36	Ohio	5.5		35	Massachusetts	5.6
15	Oklahoma	6.3		36	Alaska	5.5
42	Oregon	5.3		36	Ohio	5.5
30	Pennsylvania	5.7		36	Virginia	5.5
9	Rhode Island	6.7		39	Connecticut	5.4
3	South Carolina	7.4		39	Illinois	5.4
2	South Dakota	7.6		39	Michigan	5.4
20	Tennessee	6.2		42	Georgia	5.3
30	Texas	5.7		42	Oregon	5.3
42	Utah	5.3		42	Utah	5.3
9	Vermont	6.7		45	Washington	5.0
36	Virginia	5.5		46	Colorado	4.9
45	Washington	5.0		47	Florida	4.8
3	West Virginia	7.4		48	Nevada	4.3
15	Wisconsin	6.3		49	Arizona	3.9
9	Wyoming	6.7		49	California	3.9
					District of Columbia	4.1

Source: MQ Press using data from U.S. Dept of Health & Human Services, Centers for Medicare and Medicaid Services
"State Health Care Expenditures" (http://www.hcfa.gov/stats/nhe-oact/stateestimates/)
*By state of provider. Per capita calculated using resident population. These figures may be skewed due to
residents crossing state borders for care. Includes hospital care, physician services, dental services, home health
care, drugs, vision products, nursing home care and other personal health care services and products.

Per Capita Medicare Expenditures for Personal Health Care in 1998

National Per Capita = $775*

ALPHA ORDER

RANK ORDER

RANK	STATE	PER CAPITA		RANK	STATE	PER CAPITA
12	Alabama	$817		1	Florida	$1,138
50	Alaska	289		2	Pennsylvania	1,077
28	Arizona	679		3	Massachusetts	1,047
17	Arkansas	777		4	Rhode Island	1,040
24	California	705		5	Louisiana	1,009
44	Colorado	553		6	Connecticut	937
6	Connecticut	937		7	New York	926
33	Delaware	638		8	Missouri	864
1	Florida	1,138		9	Tennessee	848
36	Georgia	605		10	West Virginia	846
48	Hawaii	426		11	New Jersey	832
46	Idaho	467		12	Alabama	817
25	Illinois	692		13	Mississippi	812
23	Indiana	718		14	Michigan	789
34	Iowa	626		15	Ohio	784
31	Kansas	658		16	Oklahoma	781
21	Kentucky	735		17	Arkansas	777
5	Louisiana	1,009		18	Maryland	750
19	Maine	741		19	Maine	741
18	Maryland	750		20	North Dakota	738
3	Massachusetts	1,047		21	Kentucky	735
14	Michigan	789		22	Texas	732
40	Minnesota	586		23	Indiana	718
13	Mississippi	812		24	California	705
8	Missouri	864		25	Illinois	692
37	Montana	595		26	Nevada	690
32	Nebraska	650		27	North Carolina	688
26	Nevada	690		28	Arizona	679
39	New Hampshire	589		29	South Dakota	673
11	New Jersey	832		30	South Carolina	662
45	New Mexico	515		31	Kansas	658
7	New York	926		32	Nebraska	650
27	North Carolina	688		33	Delaware	638
20	North Dakota	738		34	Iowa	626
15	Ohio	784		35	Wisconsin	611
16	Oklahoma	781		36	Georgia	605
38	Oregon	593		37	Montana	595
2	Pennsylvania	1,077		38	Oregon	593
4	Rhode Island	1,040		39	New Hampshire	589
30	South Carolina	662		40	Minnesota	586
29	South Dakota	673		41	Vermont	567
9	Tennessee	848		42	Virginia	565
22	Texas	732		43	Washington	562
49	Utah	410		44	Colorado	553
41	Vermont	567		45	New Mexico	515
42	Virginia	565		46	Idaho	467
43	Washington	562		47	Wyoming	433
10	West Virginia	846		48	Hawaii	426
35	Wisconsin	611		49	Utah	410
47	Wyoming	433		50	Alaska	289
					District of Columbia	1,552

Source: MQ Press using data from U.S. Dept of Health & Human Services, Centers for Medicare and Medicaid Services "State Health Care Expenditures" (http://www.hcfa.gov/stats/nhe-oact/stateestimates/)
*By state of provider. Per capita calculated using resident population. These figures may be skewed due to residents crossing state borders for care. Includes hospital care, physician services, dental services, home health care, drugs, vision products, nursing home care and other personal health care services and products.

Per Capita Medicaid Expenditures for Personal Health Care in 1998

National Per Capita = $589*

<table>
<tr><td colspan="3">ALPHA ORDER</td><td colspan="3">RANK ORDER</td></tr>
<tr><td>RANK</td><td>STATE</td><td>PER CAPITA</td><td>RANK</td><td>STATE</td><td>PER CAPITA</td></tr>
<tr><td>35</td><td>Alabama</td><td>$474</td><td>1</td><td>New York</td><td>$1,486</td></tr>
<tr><td>18</td><td>Alaska</td><td>582</td><td>2</td><td>Rhode Island</td><td>973</td></tr>
<tr><td>46</td><td>Arizona</td><td>371</td><td>3</td><td>Massachusetts</td><td>928</td></tr>
<tr><td>23</td><td>Arkansas</td><td>548</td><td>4</td><td>Maine</td><td>849</td></tr>
<tr><td>37</td><td>California</td><td>436</td><td>5</td><td>Connecticut</td><td>816</td></tr>
<tr><td>45</td><td>Colorado</td><td>379</td><td>6</td><td>Louisiana</td><td>717</td></tr>
<tr><td>5</td><td>Connecticut</td><td>816</td><td>7</td><td>West Virginia</td><td>700</td></tr>
<tr><td>29</td><td>Delaware</td><td>531</td><td>8</td><td>Pennsylvania</td><td>680</td></tr>
<tr><td>41</td><td>Florida</td><td>421</td><td>9</td><td>Tennessee</td><td>660</td></tr>
<tr><td>38</td><td>Georgia</td><td>428</td><td>10</td><td>Vermont</td><td>657</td></tr>
<tr><td>28</td><td>Hawaii</td><td>535</td><td>11</td><td>Kentucky</td><td>627</td></tr>
<tr><td>47</td><td>Idaho</td><td>367</td><td>12</td><td>Minnesota</td><td>614</td></tr>
<tr><td>21</td><td>Illinois</td><td>560</td><td>13</td><td>North Carolina</td><td>599</td></tr>
<tr><td>39</td><td>Indiana</td><td>426</td><td>14</td><td>New Hampshire</td><td>598</td></tr>
<tr><td>19</td><td>Iowa</td><td>579</td><td>15</td><td>New Jersey</td><td>590</td></tr>
<tr><td>44</td><td>Kansas</td><td>400</td><td>16</td><td>South Carolina</td><td>587</td></tr>
<tr><td>11</td><td>Kentucky</td><td>627</td><td>17</td><td>Ohio</td><td>585</td></tr>
<tr><td>6</td><td>Louisiana</td><td>717</td><td>18</td><td>Alaska</td><td>582</td></tr>
<tr><td>4</td><td>Maine</td><td>849</td><td>19</td><td>Iowa</td><td>579</td></tr>
<tr><td>34</td><td>Maryland</td><td>490</td><td>20</td><td>New Mexico</td><td>568</td></tr>
<tr><td>3</td><td>Massachusetts</td><td>928</td><td>21</td><td>Illinois</td><td>560</td></tr>
<tr><td>25</td><td>Michigan</td><td>546</td><td>22</td><td>Mississippi</td><td>550</td></tr>
<tr><td>12</td><td>Minnesota</td><td>614</td><td>23</td><td>Arkansas</td><td>548</td></tr>
<tr><td>22</td><td>Mississippi</td><td>550</td><td>23</td><td>Washington</td><td>548</td></tr>
<tr><td>26</td><td>Missouri</td><td>540</td><td>25</td><td>Michigan</td><td>546</td></tr>
<tr><td>36</td><td>Montana</td><td>458</td><td>26</td><td>Missouri</td><td>540</td></tr>
<tr><td>30</td><td>Nebraska</td><td>523</td><td>27</td><td>North Dakota</td><td>538</td></tr>
<tr><td>50</td><td>Nevada</td><td>286</td><td>28</td><td>Hawaii</td><td>535</td></tr>
<tr><td>14</td><td>New Hampshire</td><td>598</td><td>29</td><td>Delaware</td><td>531</td></tr>
<tr><td>15</td><td>New Jersey</td><td>590</td><td>30</td><td>Nebraska</td><td>523</td></tr>
<tr><td>20</td><td>New Mexico</td><td>568</td><td>31</td><td>Wisconsin</td><td>516</td></tr>
<tr><td>1</td><td>New York</td><td>1,486</td><td>32</td><td>Oregon</td><td>510</td></tr>
<tr><td>13</td><td>North Carolina</td><td>599</td><td>33</td><td>South Dakota</td><td>494</td></tr>
<tr><td>27</td><td>North Dakota</td><td>538</td><td>34</td><td>Maryland</td><td>490</td></tr>
<tr><td>17</td><td>Ohio</td><td>585</td><td>35</td><td>Alabama</td><td>474</td></tr>
<tr><td>43</td><td>Oklahoma</td><td>401</td><td>36</td><td>Montana</td><td>458</td></tr>
<tr><td>32</td><td>Oregon</td><td>510</td><td>37</td><td>California</td><td>436</td></tr>
<tr><td>8</td><td>Pennsylvania</td><td>680</td><td>38</td><td>Georgia</td><td>428</td></tr>
<tr><td>2</td><td>Rhode Island</td><td>973</td><td>39</td><td>Indiana</td><td>426</td></tr>
<tr><td>16</td><td>South Carolina</td><td>587</td><td>39</td><td>Texas</td><td>426</td></tr>
<tr><td>33</td><td>South Dakota</td><td>494</td><td>41</td><td>Florida</td><td>421</td></tr>
<tr><td>9</td><td>Tennessee</td><td>660</td><td>42</td><td>Wyoming</td><td>419</td></tr>
<tr><td>39</td><td>Texas</td><td>426</td><td>43</td><td>Oklahoma</td><td>401</td></tr>
<tr><td>49</td><td>Utah</td><td>322</td><td>44</td><td>Kansas</td><td>400</td></tr>
<tr><td>10</td><td>Vermont</td><td>657</td><td>45</td><td>Colorado</td><td>379</td></tr>
<tr><td>48</td><td>Virginia</td><td>325</td><td>46</td><td>Arizona</td><td>371</td></tr>
<tr><td>23</td><td>Washington</td><td>548</td><td>47</td><td>Idaho</td><td>367</td></tr>
<tr><td>7</td><td>West Virginia</td><td>700</td><td>48</td><td>Virginia</td><td>325</td></tr>
<tr><td>31</td><td>Wisconsin</td><td>516</td><td>49</td><td>Utah</td><td>322</td></tr>
<tr><td>42</td><td>Wyoming</td><td>419</td><td>50</td><td>Nevada</td><td>286</td></tr>
<tr><td></td><td></td><td></td><td></td><td>District of Columbia</td><td>1,365</td></tr>
</table>

Source: MQ Press using data from U.S. Dept of Health & Human Services, Centers for Medicare and Medicaid Services
"State Health Care Expenditures" (http://www.hcfa.gov/stats/nhe-oact/stateestimates/)
*By state of provider. Per capita calculated using resident population. These figures may be skewed due to residents crossing state borders for care. Includes hospital care, physician services, dental services, home health care, drugs, vision products, nursing home care and other personal health care services and products.

Expenditures for Hospital Care in 1998

National Total = $380,050,000,000*

ALPHA ORDER					RANK ORDER			
RANK	STATE	EXPENDITURES	% of USA		RANK	STATE	EXPENDITURES	% of USA
20	Alabama	$6,618,000,000	1.7%		1	California	$34,948,000,000	9.2%
48	Alaska	986,000,000	0.3%		2	New York	32,636,000,000	8.6%
25	Arizona	4,977,000,000	1.3%		3	Texas	25,322,000,000	6.7%
33	Arkansas	3,324,000,000	0.9%		4	Pennsylvania	20,213,000,000	5.3%
1	California	34,948,000,000	9.2%		5	Florida	19,742,000,000	5.2%
26	Colorado	4,850,000,000	1.3%		6	Illinois	17,996,000,000	4.7%
27	Connecticut	4,686,000,000	1.2%		7	Ohio	16,763,000,000	4.4%
47	Delaware	1,166,000,000	0.3%		8	Michigan	14,641,000,000	3.9%
5	Florida	19,742,000,000	5.2%		9	Massachusetts	11,305,000,000	3.0%
12	Georgia	10,396,000,000	2.7%		10	New Jersey	11,191,000,000	2.9%
40	Hawaii	1,775,000,000	0.5%		11	North Carolina	10,987,000,000	2.9%
45	Idaho	1,236,000,000	0.3%		12	Georgia	10,396,000,000	2.7%
6	Illinois	17,996,000,000	4.7%		13	Missouri	8,828,000,000	2.3%
15	Indiana	8,515,000,000	2.2%		14	Virginia	8,689,000,000	2.3%
29	Iowa	4,084,000,000	1.1%		15	Indiana	8,515,000,000	2.2%
31	Kansas	3,580,000,000	0.9%		16	Tennessee	8,276,000,000	2.2%
23	Kentucky	5,731,000,000	1.5%		17	Maryland	7,313,000,000	1.9%
19	Louisiana	7,139,000,000	1.9%		18	Wisconsin	7,252,000,000	1.9%
39	Maine	1,846,000,000	0.5%		19	Louisiana	7,139,000,000	1.9%
17	Maryland	7,313,000,000	1.9%		20	Alabama	6,618,000,000	1.7%
9	Massachusetts	11,305,000,000	3.0%		21	Minnesota	6,540,000,000	1.7%
8	Michigan	14,641,000,000	3.9%		22	Washington	6,362,000,000	1.7%
21	Minnesota	6,540,000,000	1.7%		23	Kentucky	5,731,000,000	1.5%
30	Mississippi	3,848,000,000	1.0%		24	South Carolina	5,597,000,000	1.5%
13	Missouri	8,828,000,000	2.3%		25	Arizona	4,977,000,000	1.3%
46	Montana	1,224,000,000	0.3%		26	Colorado	4,850,000,000	1.3%
35	Nebraska	2,597,000,000	0.7%		27	Connecticut	4,686,000,000	1.2%
38	Nevada	1,865,000,000	0.5%		28	Oklahoma	4,218,000,000	1.1%
42	New Hampshire	1,559,000,000	0.4%		29	Iowa	4,084,000,000	1.1%
10	New Jersey	11,191,000,000	2.9%		30	Mississippi	3,848,000,000	1.0%
36	New Mexico	2,317,000,000	0.6%		31	Kansas	3,580,000,000	0.9%
2	New York	32,636,000,000	8.6%		32	Oregon	3,545,000,000	0.9%
11	North Carolina	10,987,000,000	2.9%		33	Arkansas	3,324,000,000	0.9%
43	North Dakota	1,282,000,000	0.3%		34	West Virginia	2,955,000,000	0.8%
7	Ohio	16,763,000,000	4.4%		35	Nebraska	2,597,000,000	0.7%
28	Oklahoma	4,218,000,000	1.1%		36	New Mexico	2,317,000,000	0.6%
32	Oregon	3,545,000,000	0.9%		37	Utah	2,290,000,000	0.6%
4	Pennsylvania	20,213,000,000	5.3%		38	Nevada	1,865,000,000	0.5%
41	Rhode Island	1,702,000,000	0.4%		39	Maine	1,846,000,000	0.5%
24	South Carolina	5,597,000,000	1.5%		40	Hawaii	1,775,000,000	0.5%
44	South Dakota	1,257,000,000	0.3%		41	Rhode Island	1,702,000,000	0.4%
16	Tennessee	8,276,000,000	2.2%		42	New Hampshire	1,559,000,000	0.4%
3	Texas	25,322,000,000	6.7%		43	North Dakota	1,282,000,000	0.3%
37	Utah	2,290,000,000	0.6%		44	South Dakota	1,257,000,000	0.3%
49	Vermont	712,000,000	0.2%		45	Idaho	1,236,000,000	0.3%
14	Virginia	8,689,000,000	2.3%		46	Montana	1,224,000,000	0.3%
22	Washington	6,362,000,000	1.7%		47	Delaware	1,166,000,000	0.3%
34	West Virginia	2,955,000,000	0.8%		48	Alaska	986,000,000	0.3%
18	Wisconsin	7,252,000,000	1.9%		49	Vermont	712,000,000	0.2%
50	Wyoming	582,000,000	0.2%		50	Wyoming	582,000,000	0.2%
						District of Columbia	2,585,000,000	0.7%

Source: U.S. Department of Health and Human Services, Centers for Medicare and Medicaid Services
    "State Health Care Expenditures" (http://www.hcfa.gov/stats/nhe-oact/stateestimates/)
By state of provider.

Percent of Total Personal Health Care Expenditures
Spent on Hospital Care in 1998
National Percent = 37.4%*

ALPHA ORDER

RANK ORDER

RANK	STATE	PERCENT	RANK	STATE	PERCENT
13	Alabama	41.2	1	North Dakota	47.8
7	Alaska	42.9	2	South Dakota	44.2
42	Arizona	33.7	3	New Mexico	43.4
22	Arkansas	39.3	4	Louisiana	43.3
49	California	31.8	4	Mississippi	43.3
39	Colorado	35.5	6	Montana	43.1
50	Connecticut	30.8	7	Alaska	42.9
33	Delaware	37.5	8	Nebraska	42.6
45	Florida	33.1	9	South Carolina	42.4
26	Georgia	38.2	10	Missouri	42.2
27	Hawaii	38.1	11	West Virginia	42.0
37	Idaho	36.4	12	Wyoming	41.4
15	Illinois	40.6	13	Alabama	41.2
17	Indiana	40.1	14	Michigan	41.1
18	Iowa	40.0	15	Illinois	40.6
27	Kansas	38.1	16	North Carolina	40.2
19	Kentucky	39.8	17	Indiana	40.1
4	Louisiana	43.3	18	Iowa	40.0
33	Maine	37.5	19	Kentucky	39.8
36	Maryland	37.2	20	Ohio	39.4
31	Massachusetts	37.6	20	Pennsylvania	39.4
14	Michigan	41.1	22	Arkansas	39.3
48	Minnesota	32.2	23	Virginia	39.0
4	Mississippi	43.3	24	Utah	38.5
10	Missouri	42.2	25	Oklahoma	38.4
6	Montana	43.1	26	Georgia	38.2
8	Nebraska	42.6	27	Hawaii	38.1
44	Nevada	33.3	27	Kansas	38.1
43	New Hampshire	33.5	29	New York	38.0
41	New Jersey	34.2	30	Rhode Island	37.7
3	New Mexico	43.4	31	Massachusetts	37.6
29	New York	38.0	31	Tennessee	37.6
16	North Carolina	40.2	33	Delaware	37.5
1	North Dakota	47.8	33	Maine	37.5
20	Ohio	39.4	35	Texas	37.4
25	Oklahoma	38.4	36	Maryland	37.2
47	Oregon	32.7	37	Idaho	36.4
20	Pennsylvania	39.4	37	Wisconsin	36.4
30	Rhode Island	37.7	39	Colorado	35.5
9	South Carolina	42.4	40	Vermont	34.5
2	South Dakota	44.2	41	New Jersey	34.2
31	Tennessee	37.6	42	Arizona	33.7
35	Texas	37.4	43	New Hampshire	33.5
24	Utah	38.5	44	Nevada	33.3
40	Vermont	34.5	45	Florida	33.1
23	Virginia	39.0	46	Washington	33.0
46	Washington	33.0	47	Oregon	32.7
11	West Virginia	42.0	48	Minnesota	32.2
37	Wisconsin	36.4	49	California	31.8
12	Wyoming	41.4	50	Connecticut	30.8
				District of Columbia	60.7

Source: MQ Press using data from U.S. Dept of Health & Human Services, Centers for Medicare and Medicaid Services "State Health Care Expenditures" (http://www.hcfa.gov/stats/nhe-oact/stateestimates/)
*By state of provider.

Percent Change in Expenditures for Hospital Care: 1990 to 1998

National Percent Change = 49.6% Increase*

ALPHA ORDER

RANK	STATE	PERCENT CHANGE
16	Alabama	64.9
8	Alaska	76.7
33	Arizona	54.7
26	Arkansas	57.7
50	California	25.0
28	Colorado	56.3
49	Connecticut	28.1
18	Delaware	64.7
43	Florida	46.7
30	Georgia	55.6
37	Hawaii	54.1
2	Idaho	86.1
44	Illinois	45.2
20	Indiana	61.2
32	Iowa	55.2
29	Kansas	55.8
13	Kentucky	67.0
35	Louisiana	54.4
15	Maine	65.3
27	Maryland	57.0
47	Massachusetts	38.7
36	Michigan	54.2
22	Minnesota	60.2
9	Mississippi	75.9
40	Missouri	47.8
4	Montana	80.5
19	Nebraska	63.7
6	Nevada	78.8
40	New Hampshire	47.8
46	New Jersey	42.5
11	New Mexico	69.9
45	New York	43.7
1	North Carolina	86.3
6	North Dakota	78.8
42	Ohio	46.9
25	Oklahoma	57.8
34	Oregon	54.5
48	Pennsylvania	36.0
31	Rhode Island	55.4
5	South Carolina	80.0
3	South Dakota	81.1
39	Tennessee	50.3
24	Texas	58.9
10	Utah	72.8
23	Vermont	59.3
38	Virginia	53.4
21	Washington	60.5
12	West Virginia	67.8
14	Wisconsin	65.7
16	Wyoming	64.9

RANK ORDER

RANK	STATE	PERCENT CHANGE
1	North Carolina	86.3
2	Idaho	86.1
3	South Dakota	81.1
4	Montana	80.5
5	South Carolina	80.0
6	Nevada	78.8
6	North Dakota	78.8
8	Alaska	76.7
9	Mississippi	75.9
10	Utah	72.8
11	New Mexico	69.9
12	West Virginia	67.8
13	Kentucky	67.0
14	Wisconsin	65.7
15	Maine	65.3
16	Alabama	64.9
16	Wyoming	64.9
18	Delaware	64.7
19	Nebraska	63.7
20	Indiana	61.2
21	Washington	60.5
22	Minnesota	60.2
23	Vermont	59.3
24	Texas	58.9
25	Oklahoma	57.8
26	Arkansas	57.7
27	Maryland	57.0
28	Colorado	56.3
29	Kansas	55.8
30	Georgia	55.6
31	Rhode Island	55.4
32	Iowa	55.2
33	Arizona	54.7
34	Oregon	54.5
35	Louisiana	54.4
36	Michigan	54.2
37	Hawaii	54.1
38	Virginia	53.4
39	Tennessee	50.3
40	Missouri	47.8
40	New Hampshire	47.8
42	Ohio	46.9
43	Florida	46.7
44	Illinois	45.2
45	New York	43.7
46	New Jersey	42.5
47	Massachusetts	38.7
48	Pennsylvania	36.0
49	Connecticut	28.1
50	California	25.0
	District of Columbia	21.0

Source: MQ Press using data from U.S. Dept of Health & Human Services, Centers for Medicare and Medicaid Services "State Health Care Expenditures" (http://www.hcfa.gov/stats/nhe-oact/stateestimates/)
*By state of provider.

Average Annual Change in Expenditures for Hospital Care: 1990 to 1998

National Percent Change = 5.2% Average Annual Increase*

<table>
<tr><td colspan="3">ALPHA ORDER</td><td colspan="3">RANK ORDER</td></tr>
<tr><td>RANK</td><td>STATE</td><td>PERCENT CHANGE</td><td>RANK</td><td>STATE</td><td>PERCENT CHANGE</td></tr>
<tr><td>16</td><td>Alabama</td><td>6.4</td><td>1</td><td>Idaho</td><td>8.1</td></tr>
<tr><td>8</td><td>Alaska</td><td>7.4</td><td>1</td><td>North Carolina</td><td>8.1</td></tr>
<tr><td>32</td><td>Arizona</td><td>5.6</td><td>3</td><td>Montana</td><td>7.7</td></tr>
<tr><td>25</td><td>Arkansas</td><td>5.9</td><td>3</td><td>South Dakota</td><td>7.7</td></tr>
<tr><td>50</td><td>California</td><td>2.8</td><td>5</td><td>South Carolina</td><td>7.6</td></tr>
<tr><td>28</td><td>Colorado</td><td>5.7</td><td>6</td><td>Nevada</td><td>7.5</td></tr>
<tr><td>49</td><td>Connecticut</td><td>3.1</td><td>6</td><td>North Dakota</td><td>7.5</td></tr>
<tr><td>16</td><td>Delaware</td><td>6.4</td><td>8</td><td>Alaska</td><td>7.4</td></tr>
<tr><td>42</td><td>Florida</td><td>4.9</td><td>9</td><td>Mississippi</td><td>7.3</td></tr>
<tr><td>28</td><td>Georgia</td><td>5.7</td><td>10</td><td>Utah</td><td>7.1</td></tr>
<tr><td>32</td><td>Hawaii</td><td>5.6</td><td>11</td><td>New Mexico</td><td>6.8</td></tr>
<tr><td>1</td><td>Idaho</td><td>8.1</td><td>12</td><td>West Virginia</td><td>6.7</td></tr>
<tr><td>44</td><td>Illinois</td><td>4.8</td><td>13</td><td>Kentucky</td><td>6.6</td></tr>
<tr><td>20</td><td>Indiana</td><td>6.1</td><td>14</td><td>Maine</td><td>6.5</td></tr>
<tr><td>32</td><td>Iowa</td><td>5.6</td><td>14</td><td>Wisconsin</td><td>6.5</td></tr>
<tr><td>28</td><td>Kansas</td><td>5.7</td><td>16</td><td>Alabama</td><td>6.4</td></tr>
<tr><td>13</td><td>Kentucky</td><td>6.6</td><td>16</td><td>Delaware</td><td>6.4</td></tr>
<tr><td>32</td><td>Louisiana</td><td>5.6</td><td>16</td><td>Nebraska</td><td>6.4</td></tr>
<tr><td>14</td><td>Maine</td><td>6.5</td><td>16</td><td>Wyoming</td><td>6.4</td></tr>
<tr><td>27</td><td>Maryland</td><td>5.8</td><td>20</td><td>Indiana</td><td>6.1</td></tr>
<tr><td>47</td><td>Massachusetts</td><td>4.2</td><td>20</td><td>Minnesota</td><td>6.1</td></tr>
<tr><td>32</td><td>Michigan</td><td>5.6</td><td>20</td><td>Washington</td><td>6.1</td></tr>
<tr><td>20</td><td>Minnesota</td><td>6.1</td><td>23</td><td>Texas</td><td>6.0</td></tr>
<tr><td>9</td><td>Mississippi</td><td>7.3</td><td>23</td><td>Vermont</td><td>6.0</td></tr>
<tr><td>40</td><td>Missouri</td><td>5.0</td><td>25</td><td>Arkansas</td><td>5.9</td></tr>
<tr><td>3</td><td>Montana</td><td>7.7</td><td>25</td><td>Oklahoma</td><td>5.9</td></tr>
<tr><td>16</td><td>Nebraska</td><td>6.4</td><td>27</td><td>Maryland</td><td>5.8</td></tr>
<tr><td>6</td><td>Nevada</td><td>7.5</td><td>28</td><td>Colorado</td><td>5.7</td></tr>
<tr><td>40</td><td>New Hampshire</td><td>5.0</td><td>28</td><td>Georgia</td><td>5.7</td></tr>
<tr><td>46</td><td>New Jersey</td><td>4.5</td><td>28</td><td>Kansas</td><td>5.7</td></tr>
<tr><td>11</td><td>New Mexico</td><td>6.8</td><td>28</td><td>Rhode Island</td><td>5.7</td></tr>
<tr><td>45</td><td>New York</td><td>4.6</td><td>32</td><td>Arizona</td><td>5.6</td></tr>
<tr><td>1</td><td>North Carolina</td><td>8.1</td><td>32</td><td>Hawaii</td><td>5.6</td></tr>
<tr><td>6</td><td>North Dakota</td><td>7.5</td><td>32</td><td>Iowa</td><td>5.6</td></tr>
<tr><td>42</td><td>Ohio</td><td>4.9</td><td>32</td><td>Louisiana</td><td>5.6</td></tr>
<tr><td>25</td><td>Oklahoma</td><td>5.9</td><td>32</td><td>Michigan</td><td>5.6</td></tr>
<tr><td>32</td><td>Oregon</td><td>5.6</td><td>32</td><td>Oregon</td><td>5.6</td></tr>
<tr><td>48</td><td>Pennsylvania</td><td>3.9</td><td>38</td><td>Virginia</td><td>5.5</td></tr>
<tr><td>28</td><td>Rhode Island</td><td>5.7</td><td>39</td><td>Tennessee</td><td>5.2</td></tr>
<tr><td>5</td><td>South Carolina</td><td>7.6</td><td>40</td><td>Missouri</td><td>5.0</td></tr>
<tr><td>3</td><td>South Dakota</td><td>7.7</td><td>40</td><td>New Hampshire</td><td>5.0</td></tr>
<tr><td>39</td><td>Tennessee</td><td>5.2</td><td>42</td><td>Florida</td><td>4.9</td></tr>
<tr><td>23</td><td>Texas</td><td>6.0</td><td>42</td><td>Ohio</td><td>4.9</td></tr>
<tr><td>10</td><td>Utah</td><td>7.1</td><td>44</td><td>Illinois</td><td>4.8</td></tr>
<tr><td>23</td><td>Vermont</td><td>6.0</td><td>45</td><td>New York</td><td>4.6</td></tr>
<tr><td>38</td><td>Virginia</td><td>5.5</td><td>46</td><td>New Jersey</td><td>4.5</td></tr>
<tr><td>20</td><td>Washington</td><td>6.1</td><td>47</td><td>Massachusetts</td><td>4.2</td></tr>
<tr><td>12</td><td>West Virginia</td><td>6.7</td><td>48</td><td>Pennsylvania</td><td>3.9</td></tr>
<tr><td>14</td><td>Wisconsin</td><td>6.5</td><td>49</td><td>Connecticut</td><td>3.1</td></tr>
<tr><td>16</td><td>Wyoming</td><td>6.4</td><td>50</td><td>California</td><td>2.8</td></tr>
<tr><td></td><td></td><td></td><td></td><td>District of Columbia</td><td>2.4</td></tr>
</table>

Source: U.S. Department of Health and Human Services, Centers for Medicare and Medicaid Services
   "State Health Care Expenditures" (http://www.hcfa.gov/stats/nhe-oact/stateestimates/)
*By state of provider.

Per Capita Expenditures for Hospital Care in 1998

National Per Capita = $1,406*

<table>
<tr><td colspan="3">ALPHA ORDER</td><td colspan="3">RANK ORDER</td></tr>
<tr><td>RANK</td><td>STATE</td><td>PER CAPITA</td><td>RANK</td><td>STATE</td><td>PER CAPITA</td></tr>
<tr><td>14</td><td>Alabama</td><td>$1,521</td><td>1</td><td>North Dakota</td><td>$2,010</td></tr>
<tr><td>10</td><td>Alaska</td><td>1,603</td><td>2</td><td>Massachusetts</td><td>1,840</td></tr>
<tr><td>49</td><td>Arizona</td><td>1,066</td><td>3</td><td>New York</td><td>1,797</td></tr>
<tr><td>37</td><td>Arkansas</td><td>1,310</td><td>4</td><td>Rhode Island</td><td>1,723</td></tr>
<tr><td>48</td><td>California</td><td>1,069</td><td>5</td><td>South Dakota</td><td>1,720</td></tr>
<tr><td>41</td><td>Colorado</td><td>1,222</td><td>6</td><td>Pennsylvania</td><td>1,684</td></tr>
<tr><td>24</td><td>Connecticut</td><td>1,432</td><td>7</td><td>Louisiana</td><td>1,636</td></tr>
<tr><td>11</td><td>Delaware</td><td>1,567</td><td>8</td><td>West Virginia</td><td>1,631</td></tr>
<tr><td>35</td><td>Florida</td><td>1,324</td><td>9</td><td>Missouri</td><td>1,624</td></tr>
<tr><td>32</td><td>Georgia</td><td>1,361</td><td>10</td><td>Alaska</td><td>1,603</td></tr>
<tr><td>16</td><td>Hawaii</td><td>1,491</td><td>11</td><td>Delaware</td><td>1,567</td></tr>
<tr><td>50</td><td>Idaho</td><td>1,004</td><td>12</td><td>Nebraska</td><td>1,564</td></tr>
<tr><td>16</td><td>Illinois</td><td>1,491</td><td>13</td><td>Tennessee</td><td>1,523</td></tr>
<tr><td>23</td><td>Indiana</td><td>1,441</td><td>14</td><td>Alabama</td><td>1,521</td></tr>
<tr><td>25</td><td>Iowa</td><td>1,427</td><td>15</td><td>Ohio</td><td>1,492</td></tr>
<tr><td>33</td><td>Kansas</td><td>1,357</td><td>16</td><td>Hawaii</td><td>1,491</td></tr>
<tr><td>21</td><td>Kentucky</td><td>1,457</td><td>16</td><td>Illinois</td><td>1,491</td></tr>
<tr><td>7</td><td>Louisiana</td><td>1,636</td><td>16</td><td>Michigan</td><td>1,491</td></tr>
<tr><td>19</td><td>Maine</td><td>1,480</td><td>19</td><td>Maine</td><td>1,480</td></tr>
<tr><td>26</td><td>Maryland</td><td>1,426</td><td>20</td><td>South Carolina</td><td>1,458</td></tr>
<tr><td>2</td><td>Massachusetts</td><td>1,840</td><td>21</td><td>Kentucky</td><td>1,457</td></tr>
<tr><td>16</td><td>Michigan</td><td>1,491</td><td>22</td><td>North Carolina</td><td>1,456</td></tr>
<tr><td>30</td><td>Minnesota</td><td>1,384</td><td>23</td><td>Indiana</td><td>1,441</td></tr>
<tr><td>27</td><td>Mississippi</td><td>1,399</td><td>24</td><td>Connecticut</td><td>1,432</td></tr>
<tr><td>9</td><td>Missouri</td><td>1,624</td><td>25</td><td>Iowa</td><td>1,427</td></tr>
<tr><td>28</td><td>Montana</td><td>1,392</td><td>26</td><td>Maryland</td><td>1,426</td></tr>
<tr><td>12</td><td>Nebraska</td><td>1,564</td><td>27</td><td>Mississippi</td><td>1,399</td></tr>
<tr><td>47</td><td>Nevada</td><td>1,070</td><td>28</td><td>Montana</td><td>1,392</td></tr>
<tr><td>36</td><td>New Hampshire</td><td>1,315</td><td>29</td><td>Wisconsin</td><td>1,389</td></tr>
<tr><td>31</td><td>New Jersey</td><td>1,382</td><td>30</td><td>Minnesota</td><td>1,384</td></tr>
<tr><td>34</td><td>New Mexico</td><td>1,337</td><td>31</td><td>New Jersey</td><td>1,382</td></tr>
<tr><td>3</td><td>New York</td><td>1,797</td><td>32</td><td>Georgia</td><td>1,361</td></tr>
<tr><td>22</td><td>North Carolina</td><td>1,456</td><td>33</td><td>Kansas</td><td>1,357</td></tr>
<tr><td>1</td><td>North Dakota</td><td>2,010</td><td>34</td><td>New Mexico</td><td>1,337</td></tr>
<tr><td>15</td><td>Ohio</td><td>1,492</td><td>35</td><td>Florida</td><td>1,324</td></tr>
<tr><td>40</td><td>Oklahoma</td><td>1,263</td><td>36</td><td>New Hampshire</td><td>1,315</td></tr>
<tr><td>46</td><td>Oregon</td><td>1,080</td><td>37</td><td>Arkansas</td><td>1,310</td></tr>
<tr><td>6</td><td>Pennsylvania</td><td>1,684</td><td>38</td><td>Texas</td><td>1,285</td></tr>
<tr><td>4</td><td>Rhode Island</td><td>1,723</td><td>39</td><td>Virginia</td><td>1,280</td></tr>
<tr><td>20</td><td>South Carolina</td><td>1,458</td><td>40</td><td>Oklahoma</td><td>1,263</td></tr>
<tr><td>5</td><td>South Dakota</td><td>1,720</td><td>41</td><td>Colorado</td><td>1,222</td></tr>
<tr><td>13</td><td>Tennessee</td><td>1,523</td><td>42</td><td>Wyoming</td><td>1,212</td></tr>
<tr><td>38</td><td>Texas</td><td>1,285</td><td>43</td><td>Vermont</td><td>1,206</td></tr>
<tr><td>45</td><td>Utah</td><td>1,090</td><td>44</td><td>Washington</td><td>1,119</td></tr>
<tr><td>43</td><td>Vermont</td><td>1,206</td><td>45</td><td>Utah</td><td>1,090</td></tr>
<tr><td>39</td><td>Virginia</td><td>1,280</td><td>46</td><td>Oregon</td><td>1,080</td></tr>
<tr><td>44</td><td>Washington</td><td>1,119</td><td>47</td><td>Nevada</td><td>1,070</td></tr>
<tr><td>8</td><td>West Virginia</td><td>1,631</td><td>48</td><td>California</td><td>1,069</td></tr>
<tr><td>29</td><td>Wisconsin</td><td>1,389</td><td>49</td><td>Arizona</td><td>1,066</td></tr>
<tr><td>42</td><td>Wyoming</td><td>1,212</td><td>50</td><td>Idaho</td><td>1,004</td></tr>
<tr><td></td><td></td><td></td><td></td><td>District of Columbia</td><td>4,958</td></tr>
</table>

Source: MQ Press using data from U.S. Dept of Health & Human Services, Centers for Medicare and Medicaid Services "State Health Care Expenditures" (http://www.hcfa.gov/stats/nhe-oact/stateestimates/)
*By state of provider. Per capita calculated using resident population. These figures may be skewed due to residents crossing state borders for care.

Percent Change in Per Capita Expenditures for Hospital Care: 1990 to 1998

National Percent Change = 38.0% Increase*

ALPHA ORDER			RANK ORDER		
RANK	STATE	PERCENT CHANGE	RANK	STATE	PERCENT CHANGE
15	Alabama	53.5	1	North Dakota	78.7
9	Alaska	58.9	2	South Dakota	72.7
49	Arizona	22.0	3	West Virginia	66.1
27	Arkansas	46.4	4	Mississippi	64.8
50	California	14.6	5	North Carolina	64.3
45	Colorado	30.1	6	Montana	64.2
46	Connecticut	28.8	7	South Carolina	64.0
24	Delaware	48.1	8	Maine	63.2
47	Florida	28.0	9	Alaska	58.9
44	Georgia	32.5	10	Rhode Island	58.1
29	Hawaii	44.1	11	Kentucky	56.8
16	Idaho	53.0	12	Nebraska	55.9
37	Illinois	37.8	13	Wyoming	55.6
18	Indiana	51.5	14	Wisconsin	55.5
19	Iowa	50.7	15	Alabama	53.5
26	Kansas	46.5	16	Idaho	53.0
11	Kentucky	56.8	17	Vermont	52.3
20	Louisiana	49.3	18	Indiana	51.5
8	Maine	63.2	19	Iowa	50.7
25	Maryland	46.9	20	Louisiana	49.3
40	Massachusetts	35.8	21	New Mexico	49.1
28	Michigan	46.2	22	Oklahoma	48.8
23	Minnesota	48.7	23	Minnesota	48.7
4	Mississippi	64.8	24	Delaware	48.1
34	Missouri	39.4	25	Maryland	46.9
6	Montana	64.2	26	Kansas	46.5
12	Nebraska	55.9	27	Arkansas	46.4
48	Nevada	25.0	28	Michigan	46.2
35	New Hampshire	38.6	29	Hawaii	44.1
39	New Jersey	36.6	30	New York	42.4
21	New Mexico	49.1	31	Utah	42.3
30	New York	42.4	32	Ohio	42.0
5	North Carolina	64.3	33	Virginia	40.5
1	North Dakota	78.7	34	Missouri	39.4
32	Ohio	42.0	35	New Hampshire	38.6
22	Oklahoma	48.8	36	Washington	38.3
43	Oregon	34.5	37	Illinois	37.8
42	Pennsylvania	34.8	38	Texas	37.4
10	Rhode Island	58.1	39	New Jersey	36.6
7	South Carolina	64.0	40	Massachusetts	35.8
2	South Dakota	72.7	41	Tennessee	35.3
41	Tennessee	35.3	42	Pennsylvania	34.8
38	Texas	37.4	43	Oregon	34.5
31	Utah	42.3	44	Georgia	32.5
17	Vermont	52.3	45	Colorado	30.1
33	Virginia	40.5	46	Connecticut	28.8
36	Washington	38.3	47	Florida	28.0
3	West Virginia	66.1	48	Nevada	25.0
14	Wisconsin	55.5	49	Arizona	22.0
13	Wyoming	55.6	50	California	14.6
				District of Columbia	40.1

Source: MQ Press using data from U.S. Dept of Health & Human Services, Centers for Medicare and Medicaid Services "State Health Care Expenditures" (http://www.hcfa.gov/stats/nhe-oact/stateestimates/)
*By state of provider. Per capita calculated using resident population. These figures may be skewed due to residents crossing state borders for care.

Average Annual Change in Per Capita Expenditures
For Hospital Care: 1990 to 1998
National Percent Change = 4.1% Average Annual Increase*

ALPHA ORDER

RANK	STATE	PERCENT CHANGE
15	Alabama	5.5
9	Alaska	6.0
49	Arizona	2.5
25	Arkansas	4.9
50	California	1.7
45	Colorado	3.3
46	Connecticut	3.2
24	Delaware	5.0
47	Florida	3.1
44	Georgia	3.6
29	Hawaii	4.7
15	Idaho	5.5
36	Illinois	4.1
18	Indiana	5.3
18	Iowa	5.3
25	Kansas	4.9
11	Kentucky	5.8
20	Louisiana	5.1
8	Maine	6.3
25	Maryland	4.9
40	Massachusetts	3.9
25	Michigan	4.9
20	Minnesota	5.1
4	Mississippi	6.4
34	Missouri	4.2
4	Montana	6.4
12	Nebraska	5.7
48	Nevada	2.8
34	New Hampshire	4.2
39	New Jersey	4.0
20	New Mexico	5.1
30	New York	4.5
4	North Carolina	6.4
1	North Dakota	7.5
30	Ohio	4.5
20	Oklahoma	5.1
41	Oregon	3.8
41	Pennsylvania	3.8
10	Rhode Island	5.9
4	South Carolina	6.4
2	South Dakota	7.1
41	Tennessee	3.8
36	Texas	4.1
30	Utah	4.5
17	Vermont	5.4
33	Virginia	4.3
36	Washington	4.1
3	West Virginia	6.5
12	Wisconsin	5.7
12	Wyoming	5.7

RANK ORDER

RANK	STATE	PERCENT CHANGE
1	North Dakota	7.5
2	South Dakota	7.1
3	West Virginia	6.5
4	Mississippi	6.4
4	Montana	6.4
4	North Carolina	6.4
4	South Carolina	6.4
8	Maine	6.3
9	Alaska	6.0
10	Rhode Island	5.9
11	Kentucky	5.8
12	Nebraska	5.7
12	Wisconsin	5.7
12	Wyoming	5.7
15	Alabama	5.5
15	Idaho	5.5
17	Vermont	5.4
18	Indiana	5.3
18	Iowa	5.3
20	Louisiana	5.1
20	Minnesota	5.1
20	New Mexico	5.1
20	Oklahoma	5.1
24	Delaware	5.0
25	Arkansas	4.9
25	Kansas	4.9
25	Maryland	4.9
25	Michigan	4.9
29	Hawaii	4.7
30	New York	4.5
30	Ohio	4.5
30	Utah	4.5
33	Virginia	4.3
34	Missouri	4.2
34	New Hampshire	4.2
36	Illinois	4.1
36	Texas	4.1
36	Washington	4.1
39	New Jersey	4.0
40	Massachusetts	3.9
41	Oregon	3.8
41	Pennsylvania	3.8
41	Tennessee	3.8
44	Georgia	3.6
45	Colorado	3.3
46	Connecticut	3.2
47	Florida	3.1
48	Nevada	2.8
49	Arizona	2.5
50	California	1.7
	District of Columbia	4.3

Source: MQ Press using data from U.S. Dept of Health & Human Services, Centers for Medicare and Medicaid Services "State Health Care Expenditures" (http://www.hcfa.gov/stats/nhe-oact/stateestimates/)
*By state of provider. Per capita calculated using resident population. These figures may be skewed due to residents crossing state borders for care.

Per Capita Medicare Expenditures for Hospital Care in 1998

National Per Capita = $457*

ALPHA ORDER			RANK ORDER		
RANK	STATE	PER CAPITA	RANK	STATE	PER CAPITA
15	Alabama	$483	1	Pennsylvania	$648
50	Alaska	218	2	Massachusetts	626
41	Arizona	347	3	Louisiana	612
14	Arkansas	494	4	Rhode Island	586
33	California	385	5	West Virginia	579
44	Colorado	317	6	Florida	578
12	Connecticut	496	7	Missouri	564
35	Delaware	371	8	New York	559
6	Florida	578	9	North Dakota	530
38	Georgia	360	10	Mississippi	517
47	Hawaii	272	11	Tennessee	508
46	Idaho	285	12	Connecticut	496
24	Illinois	438	13	New Jersey	495
19	Indiana	460	14	Arkansas	494
27	Iowa	418	15	Alabama	483
30	Kansas	407	16	Michigan	479
17	Kentucky	474	17	Kentucky	474
3	Louisiana	612	18	Oklahoma	468
24	Maine	438	19	Indiana	460
22	Maryland	444	19	Ohio	460
2	Massachusetts	626	21	South Dakota	457
16	Michigan	479	22	Maryland	444
34	Minnesota	382	23	Nebraska	440
10	Mississippi	517	24	Illinois	438
7	Missouri	564	24	Maine	438
32	Montana	391	26	North Carolina	428
23	Nebraska	440	27	Iowa	418
31	Nevada	395	28	South Carolina	414
37	New Hampshire	362	29	Texas	408
13	New Jersey	495	30	Kansas	407
45	New Mexico	299	31	Nevada	395
8	New York	559	32	Montana	391
26	North Carolina	428	33	California	385
9	North Dakota	530	34	Minnesota	382
19	Ohio	460	35	Delaware	371
18	Oklahoma	468	36	Wisconsin	367
39	Oregon	353	37	New Hampshire	362
1	Pennsylvania	648	38	Georgia	360
4	Rhode Island	586	39	Oregon	353
28	South Carolina	414	40	Virginia	352
21	South Dakota	457	41	Arizona	347
11	Tennessee	508	42	Vermont	337
29	Texas	408	43	Washington	327
49	Utah	252	44	Colorado	317
42	Vermont	337	45	New Mexico	299
40	Virginia	352	46	Idaho	285
43	Washington	327	47	Hawaii	272
5	West Virginia	579	48	Wyoming	267
36	Wisconsin	367	49	Utah	252
48	Wyoming	267	50	Alaska	218

District of Columbia   1,105

Source: MQ Press using data from U.S. Dept of Health & Human Services, Centers for Medicare and Medicaid Services "State Health Care Expenditures" (http://www.hcfa.gov/stats/nhe-oact/stateestimates/)

*By state of provider. Per capita calculated using resident population. These figures may be skewed due to residents crossing state borders for care.

Per Capita Medicaid Expenditures for Hospital Care in 1998

National Per Capita = $224*

ALPHA ORDER

ALPHA ORDER

RANK	STATE	PER CAPITA
32	Alabama	$158
16	Alaska	218
8	Arizona	242
27	Arkansas	177
15	California	225
39	Colorado	141
24	Connecticut	195
43	Delaware	125
35	Florida	151
28	Georgia	176
20	Hawaii	205
47	Idaho	106
7	Illinois	266
36	Indiana	146
22	Iowa	199
49	Kansas	100
10	Kentucky	234
2	Louisiana	340
6	Maine	273
17	Maryland	213
4	Massachusetts	302
17	Michigan	213
30	Minnesota	162
13	Mississippi	226
26	Missouri	189
25	Montana	193
37	Nebraska	142
42	Nevada	129
44	New Hampshire	121
13	New Jersey	226
19	New Mexico	209
1	New York	565
12	North Carolina	227
32	North Dakota	158
11	Ohio	229
45	Oklahoma	117
34	Oregon	157
21	Pennsylvania	200
3	Rhode Island	325
9	South Carolina	238
37	South Dakota	142
5	Tennessee	277
31	Texas	161
48	Utah	102
41	Vermont	130
40	Virginia	132
29	Washington	163
23	West Virginia	197
46	Wisconsin	110
50	Wyoming	90

RANK ORDER

RANK	STATE	PER CAPITA
1	New York	$565
2	Louisiana	340
3	Rhode Island	325
4	Massachusetts	302
5	Tennessee	277
6	Maine	273
7	Illinois	266
8	Arizona	242
9	South Carolina	238
10	Kentucky	234
11	Ohio	229
12	North Carolina	227
13	Mississippi	226
13	New Jersey	226
15	California	225
16	Alaska	218
17	Maryland	213
17	Michigan	213
19	New Mexico	209
20	Hawaii	205
21	Pennsylvania	200
22	Iowa	199
23	West Virginia	197
24	Connecticut	195
25	Montana	193
26	Missouri	189
27	Arkansas	177
28	Georgia	176
29	Washington	163
30	Minnesota	162
31	Texas	161
32	Alabama	158
32	North Dakota	158
34	Oregon	157
35	Florida	151
36	Indiana	146
37	Nebraska	142
37	South Dakota	142
39	Colorado	141
40	Virginia	132
41	Vermont	130
42	Nevada	129
43	Delaware	125
44	New Hampshire	121
45	Oklahoma	117
46	Wisconsin	110
47	Idaho	106
48	Utah	102
49	Kansas	100
50	Wyoming	90
	District of Columbia	669

Source: MQ Press using data from U.S. Dept of Health & Human Services, Centers for Medicare and Medicaid Services
"State Health Care Expenditures" (http://www.hcfa.gov/stats/nhe-oact/stateestimates/)
*By state of provider. Per capita calculated using resident population. These figures may be skewed due to
residents crossing state borders for care.

Expenditures for Physician and Other Professional Services in 1998

National Total = $296,102,000,000*

ALPHA ORDER

ALPHA ORDER

RANK	STATE	EXPENDITURES	% of USA
22	Alabama	$4,609,000,000	1.6%
48	Alaska	568,000,000	0.2%
21	Arizona	5,135,000,000	1.7%
32	Arkansas	2,225,000,000	0.8%
1	California	44,239,000,000	14.9%
23	Colorado	4,314,000,000	1.5%
24	Connecticut	4,292,000,000	1.4%
44	Delaware	792,000,000	0.3%
4	Florida	18,985,000,000	6.4%
10	Georgia	8,510,000,000	2.9%
37	Hawaii	1,594,000,000	0.5%
43	Idaho	935,000,000	0.3%
6	Illinois	11,975,000,000	4.0%
19	Indiana	5,613,000,000	1.9%
31	Iowa	2,457,000,000	0.8%
30	Kansas	2,538,000,000	0.9%
26	Kentucky	3,785,000,000	1.3%
25	Louisiana	4,249,000,000	1.4%
41	Maine	1,219,000,000	0.4%
16	Maryland	5,978,000,000	2.0%
11	Massachusetts	8,322,000,000	2.8%
9	Michigan	9,186,000,000	3.1%
12	Minnesota	7,183,000,000	2.4%
33	Mississippi	2,212,000,000	0.7%
20	Missouri	5,310,000,000	1.8%
46	Montana	695,000,000	0.2%
40	Nebraska	1,367,000,000	0.5%
34	Nevada	1,918,000,000	0.6%
39	New Hampshire	1,405,000,000	0.5%
8	New Jersey	9,506,000,000	3.2%
38	New Mexico	1,415,000,000	0.5%
2	New York	20,103,000,000	6.8%
13	North Carolina	7,106,000,000	2.4%
47	North Dakota	612,000,000	0.2%
7	Ohio	11,024,000,000	3.7%
29	Oklahoma	2,978,000,000	1.0%
27	Oregon	3,285,000,000	1.1%
5	Pennsylvania	13,434,000,000	4.5%
42	Rhode Island	1,095,000,000	0.4%
28	South Carolina	3,254,000,000	1.1%
45	South Dakota	747,000,000	0.3%
14	Tennessee	6,719,000,000	2.3%
3	Texas	20,071,000,000	6.8%
36	Utah	1,648,000,000	0.6%
49	Vermont	563,000,000	0.2%
15	Virginia	6,265,000,000	2.1%
17	Washington	5,908,000,000	2.0%
35	West Virginia	1,793,000,000	0.6%
18	Wisconsin	5,844,000,000	2.0%
50	Wyoming	343,000,000	0.1%

RANK ORDER

RANK	STATE	EXPENDITURES	% of USA
1	California	$44,239,000,000	14.9%
2	New York	20,103,000,000	6.8%
3	Texas	20,071,000,000	6.8%
4	Florida	18,985,000,000	6.4%
5	Pennsylvania	13,434,000,000	4.5%
6	Illinois	11,975,000,000	4.0%
7	Ohio	11,024,000,000	3.7%
8	New Jersey	9,506,000,000	3.2%
9	Michigan	9,186,000,000	3.1%
10	Georgia	8,510,000,000	2.9%
11	Massachusetts	8,322,000,000	2.8%
12	Minnesota	7,183,000,000	2.4%
13	North Carolina	7,106,000,000	2.4%
14	Tennessee	6,719,000,000	2.3%
15	Virginia	6,265,000,000	2.1%
16	Maryland	5,978,000,000	2.0%
17	Washington	5,908,000,000	2.0%
18	Wisconsin	5,844,000,000	2.0%
19	Indiana	5,613,000,000	1.9%
20	Missouri	5,310,000,000	1.8%
21	Arizona	5,135,000,000	1.7%
22	Alabama	4,609,000,000	1.6%
23	Colorado	4,314,000,000	1.5%
24	Connecticut	4,292,000,000	1.4%
25	Louisiana	4,249,000,000	1.4%
26	Kentucky	3,785,000,000	1.3%
27	Oregon	3,285,000,000	1.1%
28	South Carolina	3,254,000,000	1.1%
29	Oklahoma	2,978,000,000	1.0%
30	Kansas	2,538,000,000	0.9%
31	Iowa	2,457,000,000	0.8%
32	Arkansas	2,225,000,000	0.8%
33	Mississippi	2,212,000,000	0.7%
34	Nevada	1,918,000,000	0.6%
35	West Virginia	1,793,000,000	0.6%
36	Utah	1,648,000,000	0.6%
37	Hawaii	1,594,000,000	0.5%
38	New Mexico	1,415,000,000	0.5%
39	New Hampshire	1,405,000,000	0.5%
40	Nebraska	1,367,000,000	0.5%
41	Maine	1,219,000,000	0.4%
42	Rhode Island	1,095,000,000	0.4%
43	Idaho	935,000,000	0.3%
44	Delaware	792,000,000	0.3%
45	South Dakota	747,000,000	0.3%
46	Montana	695,000,000	0.2%
47	North Dakota	612,000,000	0.2%
48	Alaska	568,000,000	0.2%
49	Vermont	563,000,000	0.2%
50	Wyoming	343,000,000	0.1%
	District of Columbia	781,000,000	0.3%

Source: U.S. Department of Health and Human Services, Centers for Medicare and Medicaid Services
"State Health Care Expenditures" (http://www.hcfa.gov/stats/nhe-oact/stateestimates/)
By state of provider. Includes "other professional services" previously listed as a separate category. These include services of licensed professionals such as chiropractors, optometrists, podiatrists and independently practicing nurses. Also includes specialty clinics, independently billing laboratories and Medicare ambulance services.

Percent of Total Personal Health Care Expenditures
Spent on Physician and Other Professional Services in 1998
National Percent = 29.1%*

ALPHA ORDER

RANK	STATE	PERCENT
17	Alabama	28.7
42	Alaska	24.7
3	Arizona	34.7
29	Arkansas	26.3
1	California	40.2
7	Colorado	31.6
18	Connecticut	28.2
37	Delaware	25.5
6	Florida	31.8
8	Georgia	31.3
4	Hawaii	34.2
22	Idaho	27.5
25	Illinois	27.0
28	Indiana	26.4
47	Iowa	24.1
25	Kansas	27.0
29	Kentucky	26.3
35	Louisiana	25.8
41	Maine	24.8
11	Maryland	30.4
20	Massachusetts	27.7
35	Michigan	25.8
2	Minnesota	35.4
40	Mississippi	24.9
39	Missouri	25.4
44	Montana	24.5
50	Nebraska	22.4
4	Nevada	34.2
13	New Hampshire	30.2
16	New Jersey	29.1
27	New Mexico	26.5
48	New York	23.4
33	North Carolina	26.0
49	North Dakota	22.8
34	Ohio	25.9
24	Oklahoma	27.1
12	Oregon	30.3
32	Pennsylvania	26.2
46	Rhode Island	24.3
43	South Carolina	24.6
29	South Dakota	26.3
10	Tennessee	30.5
14	Texas	29.6
20	Utah	27.7
23	Vermont	27.3
19	Virginia	28.1
9	Washington	30.6
37	West Virginia	25.5
15	Wisconsin	29.3
45	Wyoming	24.4

RANK ORDER

RANK	STATE	PERCENT
1	California	40.2
2	Minnesota	35.4
3	Arizona	34.7
4	Hawaii	34.2
4	Nevada	34.2
6	Florida	31.8
7	Colorado	31.6
8	Georgia	31.3
9	Washington	30.6
10	Tennessee	30.5
11	Maryland	30.4
12	Oregon	30.3
13	New Hampshire	30.2
14	Texas	29.6
15	Wisconsin	29.3
16	New Jersey	29.1
17	Alabama	28.7
18	Connecticut	28.2
19	Virginia	28.1
20	Massachusetts	27.7
20	Utah	27.7
22	Idaho	27.5
23	Vermont	27.3
24	Oklahoma	27.1
25	Illinois	27.0
25	Kansas	27.0
27	New Mexico	26.5
28	Indiana	26.4
29	Arkansas	26.3
29	Kentucky	26.3
29	South Dakota	26.3
32	Pennsylvania	26.2
33	North Carolina	26.0
34	Ohio	25.9
35	Louisiana	25.8
35	Michigan	25.8
37	Delaware	25.5
37	West Virginia	25.5
39	Missouri	25.4
40	Mississippi	24.9
41	Maine	24.8
42	Alaska	24.7
43	South Carolina	24.6
44	Montana	24.5
45	Wyoming	24.4
46	Rhode Island	24.3
47	Iowa	24.1
48	New York	23.4
49	North Dakota	22.8
50	Nebraska	22.4

| | District of Columbia | 18.3 |

Source: MQ Press using data from U.S. Dept of Health & Human Services, Centers for Medicare and Medicaid Services "State Health Care Expenditures" (http://www.hcfa.gov/stats/nhe-oact/stateestimates/)
By state of provider. Includes "other professional services" previously listed as a separate category. These include services of licensed professionals such as chiropractors, optometrists, podiatrists and independently practicing nurses. Also includes specialty clinics, independently billing laboratories and Medicare ambulance services.

Percent Change in Expenditures for Physician and Other Professional Services: 1990 to 1998
National Percent Change = 63.6% Increase*

ALPHA ORDER				RANK ORDER		
RANK	STATE	PERCENT CHANGE		RANK	STATE	PERCENT CHANGE
22	Alabama	67.1		1	South Dakota	102.4
42	Alaska	57.8		2	Hawaii	102.0
26	Arizona	62.6		3	New Hampshire	100.1
42	Arkansas	57.8		4	Tennessee	96.8
44	California	56.6		5	Minnesota	95.9
18	Colorado	75.1		6	Idaho	95.6
46	Connecticut	52.3		7	South Carolina	92.9
31	Delaware	61.0		8	Mississippi	88.7
48	Florida	48.9		9	Maine	86.1
11	Georgia	84.2		9	North Carolina	86.1
2	Hawaii	102.0		11	Georgia	84.2
6	Idaho	95.6		12	New Mexico	83.1
37	Illinois	59.9		13	Nevada	82.7
33	Indiana	60.7		14	Vermont	81.0
28	Iowa	62.3		15	Wisconsin	79.4
35	Kansas	60.6		16	Kentucky	79.1
16	Kentucky	79.1		17	Utah	77.8
45	Louisiana	55.9		18	Colorado	75.1
9	Maine	86.1		19	Texas	74.2
27	Maryland	62.4		20	Wyoming	71.5
21	Massachusetts	69.6		21	Massachusetts	69.6
47	Michigan	51.8		22	Alabama	67.1
5	Minnesota	95.9		23	Oklahoma	67.0
8	Mississippi	88.7		24	West Virginia	63.7
30	Missouri	61.1		25	Montana	62.8
25	Montana	62.8		26	Arizona	62.6
39	Nebraska	59.0		27	Maryland	62.4
13	Nevada	82.7		28	Iowa	62.3
3	New Hampshire	100.1		29	Oregon	61.9
33	New Jersey	60.7		30	Missouri	61.1
12	New Mexico	83.1		31	Delaware	61.0
35	New York	60.6		32	Washington	60.8
9	North Carolina	86.1		33	Indiana	60.7
50	North Dakota	36.9		33	New Jersey	60.7
49	Ohio	44.6		35	Kansas	60.6
23	Oklahoma	67.0		35	New York	60.6
29	Oregon	61.9		37	Illinois	59.9
38	Pennsylvania	59.4		38	Pennsylvania	59.4
41	Rhode Island	58.0		39	Nebraska	59.0
7	South Carolina	92.9		40	Virginia	58.8
1	South Dakota	102.4		41	Rhode Island	58.0
4	Tennessee	96.8		42	Alaska	57.8
19	Texas	74.2		42	Arkansas	57.8
17	Utah	77.8		44	California	56.6
14	Vermont	81.0		45	Louisiana	55.9
40	Virginia	58.8		46	Connecticut	52.3
32	Washington	60.8		47	Michigan	51.8
24	West Virginia	63.7		48	Florida	48.9
15	Wisconsin	79.4		49	Ohio	44.6
20	Wyoming	71.5		50	North Dakota	36.9

District of Columbia   (11.5)

Source: MQ Press using data from U.S. Dept of Health & Human Services, Centers for Medicare and Medicaid Services "State Health Care Expenditures" (http://www.hcfa.gov/stats/nhe-oact/stateestimates/)

*By state of provider. Includes "other professional services" previously listed as a separate category. These include services of licensed professionals such as chiropractors, optometrists, podiatrists and independently practicing nurses. Also includes specialty clinics, independently billing laboratories and Medicare ambulance services.

Average Annual Change in Expenditures for Physician and Other Professional Services: 1990 to 1998
National Percent Change = 6.3% Average Annual Increase*

ALPHA ORDER

RANK	STATE	PERCENT CHANGE
22	Alabama	6.6
41	Alaska	5.9
25	Arizona	6.3
41	Arkansas	5.9
44	California	5.8
18	Colorado	7.3
46	Connecticut	5.4
30	Delaware	6.1
48	Florida	5.1
11	Georgia	7.9
1	Hawaii	9.2
6	Idaho	8.7
37	Illinois	6.0
30	Indiana	6.1
27	Iowa	6.2
30	Kansas	6.1
15	Kentucky	7.6
45	Louisiana	5.7
9	Maine	8.1
27	Maryland	6.2
21	Massachusetts	6.8
46	Michigan	5.4
4	Minnesota	8.8
8	Mississippi	8.3
30	Missouri	6.1
25	Montana	6.3
37	Nebraska	6.0
13	Nevada	7.8
3	New Hampshire	9.1
30	New Jersey	6.1
11	New Mexico	7.9
30	New York	6.1
9	North Carolina	8.1
50	North Dakota	4.0
49	Ohio	4.7
22	Oklahoma	6.6
27	Oregon	6.2
37	Pennsylvania	6.0
41	Rhode Island	5.9
7	South Carolina	8.6
1	South Dakota	9.2
4	Tennessee	8.8
19	Texas	7.2
17	Utah	7.5
14	Vermont	7.7
37	Virginia	6.0
30	Washington	6.1
24	West Virginia	6.4
15	Wisconsin	7.6
20	Wyoming	7.0

RANK ORDER

RANK	STATE	PERCENT CHANGE
1	Hawaii	9.2
1	South Dakota	9.2
3	New Hampshire	9.1
4	Minnesota	8.8
4	Tennessee	8.8
6	Idaho	8.7
7	South Carolina	8.6
8	Mississippi	8.3
9	Maine	8.1
9	North Carolina	8.1
11	Georgia	7.9
11	New Mexico	7.9
13	Nevada	7.8
14	Vermont	7.7
15	Kentucky	7.6
15	Wisconsin	7.6
17	Utah	7.5
18	Colorado	7.3
19	Texas	7.2
20	Wyoming	7.0
21	Massachusetts	6.8
22	Alabama	6.6
22	Oklahoma	6.6
24	West Virginia	6.4
25	Arizona	6.3
25	Montana	6.3
27	Iowa	6.2
27	Maryland	6.2
27	Oregon	6.2
30	Delaware	6.1
30	Indiana	6.1
30	Kansas	6.1
30	Missouri	6.1
30	New Jersey	6.1
30	New York	6.1
30	Washington	6.1
37	Illinois	6.0
37	Nebraska	6.0
37	Pennsylvania	6.0
37	Virginia	6.0
41	Alaska	5.9
41	Arkansas	5.9
41	Rhode Island	5.9
44	California	5.8
45	Louisiana	5.7
46	Connecticut	5.4
46	Michigan	5.4
48	Florida	5.1
49	Ohio	4.7
50	North Dakota	4.0

District of Columbia (1.5)

Source: U.S. Department of Health and Human Services, Centers for Medicare and Medicaid Services "State Health Care Expenditures" (http://www.hcfa.gov/stats/nhe-oact/stateestimates/)
By state of provider. Includes "other professional services" previously listed as a separate category. These include services of licensed professionals such as chiropractors, optometrists, podiatrists and independently practicing nurses. Also includes specialty clinics, independently billing laboratories and Medicare ambulance services.

Per Capita Expenditures for Physician and Other Professional Services in 1998

National Per Capita = $1,096*

ALPHA ORDER

RANK	STATE	PER CAPITA
20	Alabama	$1,059
38	Alaska	923
16	Arizona	1,100
41	Arkansas	877
2	California	1,354
18	Colorado	1,087
5	Connecticut	1,312
19	Delaware	1,064
6	Florida	1,273
13	Georgia	1,114
4	Hawaii	1,339
49	Idaho	760
25	Illinois	992
35	Indiana	950
42	Iowa	859
31	Kansas	962
31	Kentucky	962
30	Louisiana	974
28	Maine	977
10	Maryland	1,165
2	Massachusetts	1,354
37	Michigan	935
1	Minnesota	1,520
46	Mississippi	804
28	Missouri	977
47	Montana	790
44	Nebraska	823
16	Nevada	1,100
8	New Hampshire	1,185
9	New Jersey	1,174
45	New Mexico	816
15	New York	1,107
36	North Carolina	942
33	North Dakota	960
27	Ohio	981
40	Oklahoma	892
24	Oregon	1,001
11	Pennsylvania	1,119
14	Rhode Island	1,109
43	South Carolina	847
22	South Dakota	1,022
7	Tennessee	1,237
23	Texas	1,018
48	Utah	785
34	Vermont	953
38	Virginia	923
21	Washington	1,039
26	West Virginia	990
11	Wisconsin	1,119
50	Wyoming	715

RANK ORDER

RANK	STATE	PER CAPITA
1	Minnesota	$1,520
2	California	1,354
2	Massachusetts	1,354
4	Hawaii	1,339
5	Connecticut	1,312
6	Florida	1,273
7	Tennessee	1,237
8	New Hampshire	1,185
9	New Jersey	1,174
10	Maryland	1,165
11	Pennsylvania	1,119
11	Wisconsin	1,119
13	Georgia	1,114
14	Rhode Island	1,109
15	New York	1,107
16	Arizona	1,100
16	Nevada	1,100
18	Colorado	1,087
19	Delaware	1,064
20	Alabama	1,059
21	Washington	1,039
22	South Dakota	1,022
23	Texas	1,018
24	Oregon	1,001
25	Illinois	992
26	West Virginia	990
27	Ohio	981
28	Maine	977
28	Missouri	977
30	Louisiana	974
31	Kansas	962
31	Kentucky	962
33	North Dakota	960
34	Vermont	953
35	Indiana	950
36	North Carolina	942
37	Michigan	935
38	Alaska	923
38	Virginia	923
40	Oklahoma	892
41	Arkansas	877
42	Iowa	859
43	South Carolina	847
44	Nebraska	823
45	New Mexico	816
46	Mississippi	804
47	Montana	790
48	Utah	785
49	Idaho	760
50	Wyoming	715

District of Columbia 1,498

Source: MQ Press using data from U.S. Dept of Health & Human Services, Centers for Medicare and Medicaid Services
"State Health Care Expenditures" (http://www.hcfa.gov/stats/nhe-oact/stateestimates/)
*By state of provider. Per capita calculated using resident population. These figures may be skewed due to residents
crossing state borders for care. Includes "other professional services" previously listed as a separate category.
Services include licensed professionals such as chiropractors, optometrists, podiatrists and independently
practicing nurses. Includes specialty clinics, independently billing laboratories and Medicare ambulance services.

Percent Change in Per Capita Expenditures for Physician and Other Professional Services: 1990 to 1998
National Percent Change = 51.0% Increase*

<table>
<tr><td colspan="3">ALPHA ORDER</td><td colspan="3">RANK ORDER</td></tr>
<tr><th>RANK</th><th>STATE</th><th>PERCENT CHANGE</th><th>RANK</th><th>STATE</th><th>PERCENT CHANGE</th></tr>
<tr><td>24</td><td>Alabama</td><td>55.5</td><td>1</td><td>South Dakota</td><td>92.8</td></tr>
<tr><td>43</td><td>Alaska</td><td>41.8</td><td>2</td><td>Hawaii</td><td>88.9</td></tr>
<tr><td>49</td><td>Arizona</td><td>28.2</td><td>3</td><td>New Hampshire</td><td>87.8</td></tr>
<tr><td>37</td><td>Arkansas</td><td>46.4</td><td>4</td><td>Maine</td><td>83.6</td></tr>
<tr><td>42</td><td>California</td><td>43.6</td><td>5</td><td>Minnesota</td><td>81.8</td></tr>
<tr><td>38</td><td>Colorado</td><td>45.7</td><td>6</td><td>Tennessee</td><td>77.2</td></tr>
<tr><td>26</td><td>Connecticut</td><td>53.1</td><td>7</td><td>Mississippi</td><td>76.7</td></tr>
<tr><td>40</td><td>Delaware</td><td>44.8</td><td>8</td><td>South Carolina</td><td>75.7</td></tr>
<tr><td>48</td><td>Florida</td><td>30.0</td><td>9</td><td>Vermont</td><td>73.0</td></tr>
<tr><td>23</td><td>Georgia</td><td>56.9</td><td>10</td><td>Wisconsin</td><td>68.3</td></tr>
<tr><td>2</td><td>Hawaii</td><td>88.9</td><td>11</td><td>Kentucky</td><td>68.2</td></tr>
<tr><td>16</td><td>Idaho</td><td>61.0</td><td>12</td><td>Massachusetts</td><td>66.1</td></tr>
<tr><td>29</td><td>Illinois</td><td>51.7</td><td>13</td><td>North Carolina</td><td>64.1</td></tr>
<tr><td>31</td><td>Indiana</td><td>51.0</td><td>14</td><td>Wyoming</td><td>62.1</td></tr>
<tr><td>21</td><td>Iowa</td><td>57.6</td><td>15</td><td>West Virginia</td><td>62.0</td></tr>
<tr><td>31</td><td>Kansas</td><td>51.0</td><td>16</td><td>Idaho</td><td>61.0</td></tr>
<tr><td>11</td><td>Kentucky</td><td>68.2</td><td>17</td><td>Rhode Island</td><td>60.7</td></tr>
<tr><td>33</td><td>Louisiana</td><td>50.8</td><td>18</td><td>New Mexico</td><td>60.3</td></tr>
<tr><td>4</td><td>Maine</td><td>83.6</td><td>19</td><td>New York</td><td>59.3</td></tr>
<tr><td>27</td><td>Maryland</td><td>51.9</td><td>20</td><td>Pennsylvania</td><td>57.8</td></tr>
<tr><td>12</td><td>Massachusetts</td><td>66.1</td><td>21</td><td>Iowa</td><td>57.6</td></tr>
<tr><td>41</td><td>Michigan</td><td>43.8</td><td>22</td><td>Oklahoma</td><td>57.3</td></tr>
<tr><td>5</td><td>Minnesota</td><td>81.8</td><td>23</td><td>Georgia</td><td>56.9</td></tr>
<tr><td>7</td><td>Mississippi</td><td>76.7</td><td>24</td><td>Alabama</td><td>55.5</td></tr>
<tr><td>27</td><td>Missouri</td><td>51.9</td><td>25</td><td>New Jersey</td><td>53.9</td></tr>
<tr><td>35</td><td>Montana</td><td>47.9</td><td>26</td><td>Connecticut</td><td>53.1</td></tr>
<tr><td>30</td><td>Nebraska</td><td>51.3</td><td>27</td><td>Maryland</td><td>51.9</td></tr>
<tr><td>50</td><td>Nevada</td><td>27.6</td><td>27</td><td>Missouri</td><td>51.9</td></tr>
<tr><td>3</td><td>New Hampshire</td><td>87.8</td><td>29</td><td>Illinois</td><td>51.7</td></tr>
<tr><td>25</td><td>New Jersey</td><td>53.9</td><td>30</td><td>Nebraska</td><td>51.3</td></tr>
<tr><td>18</td><td>New Mexico</td><td>60.3</td><td>31</td><td>Indiana</td><td>51.0</td></tr>
<tr><td>19</td><td>New York</td><td>59.3</td><td>31</td><td>Kansas</td><td>51.0</td></tr>
<tr><td>13</td><td>North Carolina</td><td>64.1</td><td>33</td><td>Louisiana</td><td>50.8</td></tr>
<tr><td>47</td><td>North Dakota</td><td>36.9</td><td>34</td><td>Texas</td><td>50.6</td></tr>
<tr><td>45</td><td>Ohio</td><td>39.7</td><td>35</td><td>Montana</td><td>47.9</td></tr>
<tr><td>22</td><td>Oklahoma</td><td>57.3</td><td>36</td><td>Utah</td><td>46.5</td></tr>
<tr><td>44</td><td>Oregon</td><td>41.0</td><td>37</td><td>Arkansas</td><td>46.4</td></tr>
<tr><td>20</td><td>Pennsylvania</td><td>57.8</td><td>38</td><td>Colorado</td><td>45.7</td></tr>
<tr><td>17</td><td>Rhode Island</td><td>60.7</td><td>39</td><td>Virginia</td><td>45.4</td></tr>
<tr><td>8</td><td>South Carolina</td><td>75.7</td><td>40</td><td>Delaware</td><td>44.8</td></tr>
<tr><td>1</td><td>South Dakota</td><td>92.8</td><td>41</td><td>Michigan</td><td>43.8</td></tr>
<tr><td>6</td><td>Tennessee</td><td>77.2</td><td>42</td><td>California</td><td>43.6</td></tr>
<tr><td>34</td><td>Texas</td><td>50.6</td><td>43</td><td>Alaska</td><td>41.8</td></tr>
<tr><td>36</td><td>Utah</td><td>46.5</td><td>44</td><td>Oregon</td><td>41.0</td></tr>
<tr><td>9</td><td>Vermont</td><td>73.0</td><td>45</td><td>Ohio</td><td>39.7</td></tr>
<tr><td>39</td><td>Virginia</td><td>45.4</td><td>46</td><td>Washington</td><td>38.5</td></tr>
<tr><td>46</td><td>Washington</td><td>38.5</td><td>47</td><td>North Dakota</td><td>36.9</td></tr>
<tr><td>15</td><td>West Virginia</td><td>62.0</td><td>48</td><td>Florida</td><td>30.0</td></tr>
<tr><td>10</td><td>Wisconsin</td><td>68.3</td><td>49</td><td>Arizona</td><td>28.2</td></tr>
<tr><td>14</td><td>Wyoming</td><td>62.1</td><td>50</td><td>Nevada</td><td>27.6</td></tr>
<tr><td></td><td></td><td></td><td></td><td>District of Columbia</td><td>2.5</td></tr>
</table>

Source: MQ Press using data from U.S. Dept of Health & Human Services, Centers for Medicare and Medicaid Services "State Health Care Expenditures" (http://www.hcfa.gov/stats/nhe-oact/stateestimates/)
By state of provider. Per capita calculated using resident population. These figures may be skewed due to residents crossing state borders for care. Includes "other professional services" previously listed as a separate category. Services include licensed professionals such as chiropractors, optometrists, podiatrists and independently practicing nurses. Includes specialty clinics, independently billing laboratories and Medicare ambulance services.

Average Annual Change in Per Capita Expenditures
For Physician Services: 1990 to 1998
National Percent Change = 5.3% Average Annual Increase*

ALPHA ORDER

RANK	STATE	PERCENT CHANGE
24	Alabama	5.7
43	Alaska	4.5
49	Arizona	3.2
36	Arkansas	4.9
41	California	4.6
38	Colorado	4.8
25	Connecticut	5.5
40	Delaware	4.7
48	Florida	3.3
22	Georgia	5.8
2	Hawaii	8.3
16	Idaho	6.1
29	Illinois	5.3
29	Indiana	5.3
20	Iowa	5.9
29	Kansas	5.3
10	Kentucky	6.7
29	Louisiana	5.3
4	Maine	7.9
27	Maryland	5.4
12	Massachusetts	6.6
41	Michigan	4.6
5	Minnesota	7.8
6	Mississippi	7.4
27	Missouri	5.4
35	Montana	5.0
29	Nebraska	5.3
50	Nevada	3.1
3	New Hampshire	8.2
25	New Jersey	5.5
16	New Mexico	6.1
19	New York	6.0
13	North Carolina	6.4
47	North Dakota	4.0
45	Ohio	4.3
22	Oklahoma	5.8
44	Oregon	4.4
20	Pennsylvania	5.9
16	Rhode Island	6.1
8	South Carolina	7.3
1	South Dakota	8.6
6	Tennessee	7.4
29	Texas	5.3
36	Utah	4.9
9	Vermont	7.1
38	Virginia	4.8
46	Washington	4.2
14	West Virginia	6.2
10	Wisconsin	6.7
14	Wyoming	6.2

RANK ORDER

RANK	STATE	PERCENT CHANGE
1	South Dakota	8.6
2	Hawaii	8.3
3	New Hampshire	8.2
4	Maine	7.9
5	Minnesota	7.8
6	Mississippi	7.4
6	Tennessee	7.4
8	South Carolina	7.3
9	Vermont	7.1
10	Kentucky	6.7
10	Wisconsin	6.7
12	Massachusetts	6.6
13	North Carolina	6.4
14	West Virginia	6.2
14	Wyoming	6.2
16	Idaho	6.1
16	New Mexico	6.1
16	Rhode Island	6.1
19	New York	6.0
20	Iowa	5.9
20	Pennsylvania	5.9
22	Georgia	5.8
22	Oklahoma	5.8
24	Alabama	5.7
25	Connecticut	5.5
25	New Jersey	5.5
27	Maryland	5.4
27	Missouri	5.4
29	Illinois	5.3
29	Indiana	5.3
29	Kansas	5.3
29	Louisiana	5.3
29	Nebraska	5.3
29	Texas	5.3
35	Montana	5.0
36	Arkansas	4.9
36	Utah	4.9
38	Colorado	4.8
38	Virginia	4.8
40	Delaware	4.7
41	California	4.6
41	Michigan	4.6
43	Alaska	4.5
44	Oregon	4.4
45	Ohio	4.3
46	Washington	4.2
47	North Dakota	4.0
48	Florida	3.3
49	Arizona	3.2
50	Nevada	3.1
	District of Columbia	0.3

Source: MQ Press using data from U.S. Dept of Health & Human Services, Centers for Medicare and Medicaid Services
"State Health Care Expenditures" (http://www.hcfa.gov/stats/nhe-oact/stateestimates/)
*By state of provider. Per capita calculated using resident population. These figures may be skewed due to residents crossing state borders for care. Includes "other professional services" previously listed as a separate category. Services include licensed professionals such as chiropractors, optometrists, podiatrists and independently practicing nurses. Includes specialty clinics, independently billing laboratories and Medicare ambulance services.

Per Capita Medicare Expenditures for Physician Services in 1998

National Per Capita = $181*

ALPHA ORDER

RANK ORDER

RANK	STATE	PER CAPITA		RANK	STATE	PER CAPITA
14	Alabama	$179		1	Florida	$339
50	Alaska	42		2	Pennsylvania	255
9	Arizona	199		3	Rhode Island	233
18	Arkansas	160		4	New York	227
8	California	204		5	Massachusetts	214
30	Colorado	137		6	New Jersey	210
7	Connecticut	206		7	Connecticut	206
23	Delaware	146		8	California	204
1	Florida	339		9	Arizona	199
37	Georgia	128		10	Nevada	197
44	Hawaii	111		11	Ohio	192
47	Idaho	89		12	Maryland	187
20	Illinois	152		13	Missouri	182
29	Indiana	138		14	Alabama	179
39	Iowa	126		14	Louisiana	179
22	Kansas	150		16	Michigan	174
25	Kentucky	145		17	Tennessee	166
14	Louisiana	179		18	Arkansas	160
32	Maine	135		18	Oregon	160
12	Maryland	187		20	Illinois	152
5	Massachusetts	214		21	North Dakota	151
16	Michigan	174		22	Kansas	150
39	Minnesota	126		23	Delaware	146
35	Mississippi	130		23	West Virginia	146
13	Missouri	182		25	Kentucky	145
41	Montana	118		25	Texas	145
32	Nebraska	135		25	Washington	145
10	Nevada	197		28	Oklahoma	144
45	New Hampshire	108		29	Indiana	138
6	New Jersey	210		30	Colorado	137
41	New Mexico	118		30	North Carolina	137
4	New York	227		32	Maine	135
30	North Carolina	137		32	Nebraska	135
21	North Dakota	151		34	South Dakota	131
11	Ohio	192		35	Mississippi	130
28	Oklahoma	144		36	Wisconsin	129
18	Oregon	160		37	Georgia	128
2	Pennsylvania	255		37	South Carolina	128
3	Rhode Island	233		39	Iowa	126
37	South Carolina	128		39	Minnesota	126
34	South Dakota	131		41	Montana	118
17	Tennessee	166		41	New Mexico	118
25	Texas	145		41	Virginia	118
48	Utah	81		44	Hawaii	111
46	Vermont	97		45	New Hampshire	108
41	Virginia	118		46	Vermont	97
25	Washington	145		47	Idaho	89
23	West Virginia	146		48	Utah	81
36	Wisconsin	129		49	Wyoming	77
49	Wyoming	77		50	Alaska	42

District of Columbia	293

Source: MQ Press using data from U.S. Dept of Health & Human Services, Centers for Medicare and Medicaid Services "State Health Care Expenditures" (http://www.hcfa.gov/stats/nhe-oact/stateestimates/)
*By state of provider. Per capita calculated using resident population. These figures may be skewed due to residents crossing state borders for care.

Per Capita Medicaid Expenditures for Physician Services in 1998

National Per Capita = $55.39*

<table>
<tr><td colspan="3">ALPHA ORDER</td><td colspan="3">RANK ORDER</td></tr>
<tr><th>RANK</th><th>STATE</th><th>PER CAPITA</th><th>RANK</th><th>STATE</th><th>PER CAPITA</th></tr>
<tr><td>16</td><td>Alabama</td><td>$72.86</td><td>1</td><td>Alaska</td><td>$144.67</td></tr>
<tr><td>1</td><td>Alaska</td><td>144.67</td><td>2</td><td>Tennessee</td><td>102.16</td></tr>
<tr><td>6</td><td>Arizona</td><td>88.27</td><td>3</td><td>New York</td><td>101.27</td></tr>
<tr><td>4</td><td>Arkansas</td><td>98.10</td><td>4</td><td>Arkansas</td><td>98.10</td></tr>
<tr><td>23</td><td>California</td><td>56.21</td><td>5</td><td>West Virginia</td><td>91.63</td></tr>
<tr><td>28</td><td>Colorado</td><td>48.12</td><td>6</td><td>Arizona</td><td>88.27</td></tr>
<tr><td>48</td><td>Connecticut</td><td>24.45</td><td>7</td><td>New Hampshire</td><td>86.02</td></tr>
<tr><td>22</td><td>Delaware</td><td>60.48</td><td>8</td><td>North Carolina</td><td>85.88</td></tr>
<tr><td>33</td><td>Florida</td><td>38.37</td><td>9</td><td>Washington</td><td>84.92</td></tr>
<tr><td>19</td><td>Georgia</td><td>66.52</td><td>10</td><td>South Carolina</td><td>84.64</td></tr>
<tr><td>13</td><td>Hawaii</td><td>74.76</td><td>11</td><td>Kentucky</td><td>82.61</td></tr>
<tr><td>32</td><td>Idaho</td><td>39.00</td><td>12</td><td>Massachusetts</td><td>78.77</td></tr>
<tr><td>43</td><td>Illinois</td><td>29.25</td><td>13</td><td>Hawaii</td><td>74.76</td></tr>
<tr><td>45</td><td>Indiana</td><td>27.76</td><td>14</td><td>Utah</td><td>74.27</td></tr>
<tr><td>39</td><td>Iowa</td><td>34.25</td><td>15</td><td>Michigan</td><td>73.32</td></tr>
<tr><td>49</td><td>Kansas</td><td>17.05</td><td>16</td><td>Alabama</td><td>72.86</td></tr>
<tr><td>11</td><td>Kentucky</td><td>82.61</td><td>17</td><td>New Mexico</td><td>68.65</td></tr>
<tr><td>21</td><td>Louisiana</td><td>64.64</td><td>18</td><td>Vermont</td><td>67.73</td></tr>
<tr><td>25</td><td>Maine</td><td>53.71</td><td>19</td><td>Georgia</td><td>66.52</td></tr>
<tr><td>36</td><td>Maryland</td><td>35.48</td><td>20</td><td>Mississippi</td><td>66.15</td></tr>
<tr><td>12</td><td>Massachusetts</td><td>78.77</td><td>21</td><td>Louisiana</td><td>64.64</td></tr>
<tr><td>15</td><td>Michigan</td><td>73.32</td><td>22</td><td>Delaware</td><td>60.48</td></tr>
<tr><td>41</td><td>Minnesota</td><td>33.64</td><td>23</td><td>California</td><td>56.21</td></tr>
<tr><td>20</td><td>Mississippi</td><td>66.15</td><td>24</td><td>Wyoming</td><td>54.16</td></tr>
<tr><td>46</td><td>Missouri</td><td>27.40</td><td>25</td><td>Maine</td><td>53.71</td></tr>
<tr><td>34</td><td>Montana</td><td>37.52</td><td>26</td><td>South Dakota</td><td>50.63</td></tr>
<tr><td>29</td><td>Nebraska</td><td>43.96</td><td>27</td><td>Ohio</td><td>49.39</td></tr>
<tr><td>38</td><td>Nevada</td><td>34.41</td><td>28</td><td>Colorado</td><td>48.12</td></tr>
<tr><td>7</td><td>New Hampshire</td><td>86.02</td><td>29</td><td>Nebraska</td><td>43.96</td></tr>
<tr><td>42</td><td>New Jersey</td><td>32.12</td><td>30</td><td>North Dakota</td><td>43.90</td></tr>
<tr><td>17</td><td>New Mexico</td><td>68.65</td><td>31</td><td>Oregon</td><td>39.91</td></tr>
<tr><td>3</td><td>New York</td><td>101.27</td><td>32</td><td>Idaho</td><td>39.00</td></tr>
<tr><td>8</td><td>North Carolina</td><td>85.88</td><td>33</td><td>Florida</td><td>38.37</td></tr>
<tr><td>30</td><td>North Dakota</td><td>43.90</td><td>34</td><td>Montana</td><td>37.52</td></tr>
<tr><td>27</td><td>Ohio</td><td>49.39</td><td>35</td><td>Texas</td><td>36.58</td></tr>
<tr><td>44</td><td>Oklahoma</td><td>27.85</td><td>36</td><td>Maryland</td><td>35.48</td></tr>
<tr><td>31</td><td>Oregon</td><td>39.91</td><td>37</td><td>Pennsylvania</td><td>34.49</td></tr>
<tr><td>37</td><td>Pennsylvania</td><td>34.49</td><td>38</td><td>Nevada</td><td>34.41</td></tr>
<tr><td>50</td><td>Rhode Island</td><td>15.19</td><td>39</td><td>Iowa</td><td>34.25</td></tr>
<tr><td>10</td><td>South Carolina</td><td>84.64</td><td>40</td><td>Virginia</td><td>33.73</td></tr>
<tr><td>26</td><td>South Dakota</td><td>50.63</td><td>41</td><td>Minnesota</td><td>33.64</td></tr>
<tr><td>2</td><td>Tennessee</td><td>102.16</td><td>42</td><td>New Jersey</td><td>32.12</td></tr>
<tr><td>35</td><td>Texas</td><td>36.58</td><td>43</td><td>Illinois</td><td>29.25</td></tr>
<tr><td>14</td><td>Utah</td><td>74.27</td><td>44</td><td>Oklahoma</td><td>27.85</td></tr>
<tr><td>18</td><td>Vermont</td><td>67.73</td><td>45</td><td>Indiana</td><td>27.76</td></tr>
<tr><td>40</td><td>Virginia</td><td>33.73</td><td>46</td><td>Missouri</td><td>27.40</td></tr>
<tr><td>9</td><td>Washington</td><td>84.92</td><td>47</td><td>Wisconsin</td><td>26.43</td></tr>
<tr><td>5</td><td>West Virginia</td><td>91.63</td><td>48</td><td>Connecticut</td><td>24.45</td></tr>
<tr><td>47</td><td>Wisconsin</td><td>26.43</td><td>49</td><td>Kansas</td><td>17.05</td></tr>
<tr><td>24</td><td>Wyoming</td><td>54.16</td><td>50</td><td>Rhode Island</td><td>15.19</td></tr>
<tr><td></td><td></td><td></td><td></td><td>District of Columbia</td><td>140.00</td></tr>
</table>

Source: MQ Press using data from U.S. Dept of Health & Human Services, Centers for Medicare and Medicaid Services
"State Health Care Expenditures" (http://www.hcfa.gov/stats/nhe-oact/stateestimates/)
*By state of provider. Per capita calculated using resident population. These figures may be skewed due to residents crossing state borders for care.

Expenditures for Prescription Drugs in 1998

National Total = $90,648,000,000*

ALPHA ORDER

RANK ORDER

RANK	STATE	EXPENDITURES	% of USA	RANK	STATE	EXPENDITURES	% of USA
21	Alabama	$1,552,000,000	1.7%	1	California	$7,537,000,000	8.3%
49	Alaska	133,000,000	0.1%	2	New York	7,122,000,000	7.9%
24	Arizona	1,397,000,000	1.5%	3	Florida	6,204,000,000	6.8%
32	Arkansas	903,000,000	1.0%	4	Texas	6,023,000,000	6.6%
1	California	7,537,000,000	8.3%	5	Pennsylvania	5,035,000,000	5.6%
28	Colorado	970,000,000	1.1%	6	Illinois	3,964,000,000	4.4%
25	Connecticut	1,354,000,000	1.5%	7	Ohio	3,898,000,000	4.3%
44	Delaware	300,000,000	0.3%	8	Michigan	3,885,000,000	4.3%
3	Florida	6,204,000,000	6.8%	9	New Jersey	3,545,000,000	3.9%
11	Georgia	2,460,000,000	2.7%	10	North Carolina	2,566,000,000	2.8%
43	Hawaii	311,000,000	0.3%	11	Georgia	2,460,000,000	2.7%
42	Idaho	334,000,000	0.4%	12	Massachusetts	2,172,000,000	2.4%
6	Illinois	3,964,000,000	4.4%	13	Virginia	2,130,000,000	2.3%
15	Indiana	2,058,000,000	2.3%	14	Tennessee	2,129,000,000	2.3%
30	Iowa	945,000,000	1.0%	15	Indiana	2,058,000,000	2.3%
33	Kansas	854,000,000	0.9%	16	Missouri	1,814,000,000	2.0%
20	Kentucky	1,564,000,000	1.7%	17	Wisconsin	1,745,000,000	1.9%
22	Louisiana	1,507,000,000	1.7%	18	Maryland	1,678,000,000	1.9%
38	Maine	456,000,000	0.5%	19	Washington	1,603,000,000	1.8%
18	Maryland	1,678,000,000	1.9%	20	Kentucky	1,564,000,000	1.7%
12	Massachusetts	2,172,000,000	2.4%	21	Alabama	1,552,000,000	1.7%
8	Michigan	3,885,000,000	4.3%	22	Louisiana	1,507,000,000	1.7%
23	Minnesota	1,491,000,000	1.6%	23	Minnesota	1,491,000,000	1.6%
29	Mississippi	962,000,000	1.1%	24	Arizona	1,397,000,000	1.5%
16	Missouri	1,814,000,000	2.0%	25	Connecticut	1,354,000,000	1.5%
45	Montana	234,000,000	0.3%	26	South Carolina	1,315,000,000	1.5%
35	Nebraska	626,000,000	0.7%	27	Oklahoma	1,056,000,000	1.2%
37	Nevada	478,000,000	0.5%	28	Colorado	970,000,000	1.1%
41	New Hampshire	391,000,000	0.4%	29	Mississippi	962,000,000	1.1%
9	New Jersey	3,545,000,000	3.9%	30	Iowa	945,000,000	1.0%
39	New Mexico	402,000,000	0.4%	31	Oregon	918,000,000	1.0%
2	New York	7,122,000,000	7.9%	32	Arkansas	903,000,000	1.0%
10	North Carolina	2,566,000,000	2.8%	33	Kansas	854,000,000	0.9%
47	North Dakota	192,000,000	0.2%	34	West Virginia	776,000,000	0.9%
7	Ohio	3,898,000,000	4.3%	35	Nebraska	626,000,000	0.7%
27	Oklahoma	1,056,000,000	1.2%	36	Utah	564,000,000	0.6%
31	Oregon	918,000,000	1.0%	37	Nevada	478,000,000	0.5%
5	Pennsylvania	5,035,000,000	5.6%	38	Maine	456,000,000	0.5%
40	Rhode Island	400,000,000	0.4%	39	New Mexico	402,000,000	0.4%
26	South Carolina	1,315,000,000	1.5%	40	Rhode Island	400,000,000	0.4%
46	South Dakota	201,000,000	0.2%	41	New Hampshire	391,000,000	0.4%
14	Tennessee	2,129,000,000	2.3%	42	Idaho	334,000,000	0.4%
4	Texas	6,023,000,000	6.6%	43	Hawaii	311,000,000	0.3%
36	Utah	564,000,000	0.6%	44	Delaware	300,000,000	0.3%
48	Vermont	183,000,000	0.2%	45	Montana	234,000,000	0.3%
13	Virginia	2,130,000,000	2.3%	46	South Dakota	201,000,000	0.2%
19	Washington	1,603,000,000	1.8%	47	North Dakota	192,000,000	0.2%
34	West Virginia	776,000,000	0.9%	48	Vermont	183,000,000	0.2%
17	Wisconsin	1,745,000,000	1.9%	49	Alaska	133,000,000	0.1%
49	Wyoming	133,000,000	0.1%	49	Wyoming	133,000,000	0.1%
					District of Columbia	180,000,000	0.2%

Source: U.S. Department of Health and Human Services, Centers for Medicare and Medicaid Services
"State Health Care Expenditures" (http://www.hcfa.gov/stats/nhe-oact/stateestimates/)
*Purchases in retail outlets. By state of outlet.

Percent of Total Personal Health Care Expenditures
Spent on Prescription Drugs in 1998
National Percent = 8.9%*

ALPHA ORDER				RANK ORDER		
RANK	STATE	PERCENT		RANK	STATE	PERCENT
12	Alabama	9.7		1	West Virginia	11.0
50	Alaska	5.8		2	Kentucky	10.9
18	Arizona	9.5		2	Michigan	10.9
6	Arkansas	10.7		4	Mississippi	10.8
48	California	6.8		4	New Jersey	10.8
46	Colorado	7.1		6	Arkansas	10.7
28	Connecticut	8.9		7	Florida	10.4
12	Delaware	9.7		8	Nebraska	10.3
7	Florida	10.4		9	South Carolina	10.0
27	Georgia	9.0		10	Idaho	9.8
49	Hawaii	6.7		10	Pennsylvania	9.8
10	Idaho	9.8		12	Alabama	9.7
28	Illinois	8.9		12	Delaware	9.7
12	Indiana	9.7		12	Indiana	9.7
22	Iowa	9.3		12	Tennessee	9.7
25	Kansas	9.1		16	Oklahoma	9.6
2	Kentucky	10.9		16	Virginia	9.6
25	Louisiana	9.1		18	Arizona	9.5
22	Maine	9.3		18	Utah	9.5
35	Maryland	8.5		18	Wyoming	9.5
44	Massachusetts	7.2		21	North Carolina	9.4
2	Michigan	10.9		22	Iowa	9.3
43	Minnesota	7.3		22	Maine	9.3
4	Mississippi	10.8		24	Ohio	9.2
33	Missouri	8.7		25	Kansas	9.1
41	Montana	8.2		25	Louisiana	9.1
8	Nebraska	10.3		27	Georgia	9.0
35	Nevada	8.5		28	Connecticut	8.9
38	New Hampshire	8.4		28	Illinois	8.9
4	New Jersey	10.8		28	Rhode Island	8.9
42	New Mexico	7.5		28	Texas	8.9
39	New York	8.3		28	Vermont	8.9
21	North Carolina	9.4		33	Missouri	8.7
44	North Dakota	7.2		33	Wisconsin	8.7
24	Ohio	9.2		35	Maryland	8.5
16	Oklahoma	9.6		35	Nevada	8.5
35	Oregon	8.5		35	Oregon	8.5
10	Pennsylvania	9.8		38	New Hampshire	8.4
28	Rhode Island	8.9		39	New York	8.3
9	South Carolina	10.0		39	Washington	8.3
46	South Dakota	7.1		41	Montana	8.2
12	Tennessee	9.7		42	New Mexico	7.5
28	Texas	8.9		43	Minnesota	7.3
18	Utah	9.5		44	Massachusetts	7.2
28	Vermont	8.9		44	North Dakota	7.2
16	Virginia	9.6		46	Colorado	7.1
39	Washington	8.3		46	South Dakota	7.1
1	West Virginia	11.0		48	California	6.8
33	Wisconsin	8.7		49	Hawaii	6.7
18	Wyoming	9.5		50	Alaska	5.8
					District of Columbia	4.2

Source: MQ Press using data from U.S. Dept of Health & Human Services, Centers for Medicare and Medicaid Services
"State Health Care Expenditures" (http://www.hcfa.gov/stats/nhe-oact/stateestimates/)
*Purchases in retail outlets. By state of outlet.

Percent Change in Expenditures for Prescription Drugs: 1990 to 1998

National Percent Change = 140.6% Increase*

ALPHA ORDER				RANK ORDER		
RANK	**STATE**	**PERCENT CHANGE**		**RANK**	**STATE**	**PERCENT CHANGE**
37	Alabama	129.6		1	Nevada	236.6
25	Alaska	141.8		2	Delaware	200.0
4	Arizona	180.0		3	Florida	198.1
30	Arkansas	134.5		4	Arizona	180.0
49	California	98.2		5	Oregon	179.9
8	Colorado	161.5		6	South Carolina	166.7
19	Connecticut	144.8		7	Maine	165.1
2	Delaware	200.0		8	Colorado	161.5
3	Florida	198.1		9	Idaho	160.9
15	Georgia	152.6		10	Minnesota	158.9
50	Hawaii	84.0		11	Utah	157.5
9	Idaho	160.9		12	North Carolina	156.9
46	Illinois	122.9		13	New Jersey	155.6
40	Indiana	127.7		14	New York	152.8
34	Iowa	131.6		15	Georgia	152.6
43	Kansas	124.7		16	Nebraska	152.4
23	Kentucky	142.1		17	Montana	148.9
47	Louisiana	120.3		18	Pennsylvania	146.6
7	Maine	165.1		19	Connecticut	144.8
42	Maryland	125.5		20	Tennessee	144.7
28	Massachusetts	136.6		21	New Hampshire	144.4
27	Michigan	137.0		22	Texas	142.5
10	Minnesota	158.9		23	Kentucky	142.1
29	Mississippi	135.2		23	Washington	142.1
45	Missouri	124.0		25	Alaska	141.8
17	Montana	148.9		26	Wisconsin	141.0
16	Nebraska	152.4		27	Michigan	137.0
1	Nevada	236.6		28	Massachusetts	136.6
21	New Hampshire	144.4		29	Mississippi	135.2
13	New Jersey	155.6		30	Arkansas	134.5
44	New Mexico	124.6		31	Oklahoma	134.1
14	New York	152.8		32	Virginia	133.6
12	North Carolina	156.9		33	Rhode Island	132.6
48	North Dakota	111.0		34	Iowa	131.6
36	Ohio	129.8		35	West Virginia	131.0
31	Oklahoma	134.1		36	Ohio	129.8
5	Oregon	179.9		37	Alabama	129.6
18	Pennsylvania	146.6		38	Wyoming	129.3
33	Rhode Island	132.6		39	Vermont	128.8
6	South Carolina	166.7		40	Indiana	127.7
41	South Dakota	125.8		41	South Dakota	125.8
20	Tennessee	144.7		42	Maryland	125.5
22	Texas	142.5		43	Kansas	124.7
11	Utah	157.5		44	New Mexico	124.6
39	Vermont	128.8		45	Missouri	124.0
32	Virginia	133.6		46	Illinois	122.9
23	Washington	142.1		47	Louisiana	120.3
35	West Virginia	131.0		48	North Dakota	111.0
26	Wisconsin	141.0		49	California	98.2
38	Wyoming	129.3		50	Hawaii	84.0
					District of Columbia	125.0

Source: MQ Press using data from U.S. Dept of Health & Human Services, Centers for Medicare and Medicaid Services "State Health Care Expenditures" (http://www.hcfa.gov/stats/nhe-oact/stateestimates/)
*Purchases in retail outlets. By state of outlet.

Average Annual Change in Expenditures for Prescription Drugs: 1990 to 1998

National Percent Change = 11.6% Average Annual Increase*

ALPHA ORDER			RANK ORDER		
RANK	**STATE**	**PERCENT CHANGE**	**RANK**	**STATE**	**PERCENT CHANGE**
37	Alabama	10.9	1	Nevada	16.4
22	Alaska	11.7	2	Delaware	14.7
4	Arizona	13.7	3	Florida	14.6
30	Arkansas	11.2	4	Arizona	13.7
49	California	8.9	4	Oregon	13.7
8	Colorado	12.8	6	Maine	13.0
19	Connecticut	11.8	6	South Carolina	13.0
2	Delaware	14.7	8	Colorado	12.8
3	Florida	14.6	9	Idaho	12.7
14	Georgia	12.3	10	Minnesota	12.6
50	Hawaii	7.9	10	Utah	12.6
9	Idaho	12.7	12	North Carolina	12.5
46	Illinois	10.5	13	New Jersey	12.4
40	Indiana	10.8	14	Georgia	12.3
33	Iowa	11.1	14	Nebraska	12.3
41	Kansas	10.7	14	New York	12.3
22	Kentucky	11.7	17	Montana	12.1
47	Louisiana	10.4	18	Pennsylvania	11.9
6	Maine	13.0	19	Connecticut	11.8
41	Maryland	10.7	19	New Hampshire	11.8
27	Massachusetts	11.4	19	Tennessee	11.8
27	Michigan	11.4	22	Alaska	11.7
10	Minnesota	12.6	22	Kentucky	11.7
29	Mississippi	11.3	22	Texas	11.7
44	Missouri	10.6	22	Washington	11.7
17	Montana	12.1	26	Wisconsin	11.6
14	Nebraska	12.3	27	Massachusetts	11.4
1	Nevada	16.4	27	Michigan	11.4
19	New Hampshire	11.8	29	Mississippi	11.3
13	New Jersey	12.4	30	Arkansas	11.2
44	New Mexico	10.6	30	Oklahoma	11.2
14	New York	12.3	30	Virginia	11.2
12	North Carolina	12.5	33	Iowa	11.1
48	North Dakota	9.8	33	Rhode Island	11.1
35	Ohio	11.0	35	Ohio	11.0
30	Oklahoma	11.2	35	West Virginia	11.0
4	Oregon	13.7	37	Alabama	10.9
18	Pennsylvania	11.9	37	Vermont	10.9
33	Rhode Island	11.1	37	Wyoming	10.9
6	South Carolina	13.0	40	Indiana	10.8
41	South Dakota	10.7	41	Kansas	10.7
19	Tennessee	11.8	41	Maryland	10.7
22	Texas	11.7	41	South Dakota	10.7
10	Utah	12.6	44	Missouri	10.6
37	Vermont	10.9	44	New Mexico	10.6
30	Virginia	11.2	46	Illinois	10.5
22	Washington	11.7	47	Louisiana	10.4
35	West Virginia	11.0	48	North Dakota	9.8
26	Wisconsin	11.6	49	California	8.9
37	Wyoming	10.9	50	Hawaii	7.9
				District of Columbia	10.7

Source: U.S. Department of Health and Human Services, Centers for Medicare and Medicaid Services
   "State Health Care Expenditures" (http://www.hcfa.gov/stats/nhe-oact/stateestimates/)
*Purchases in retail outlets. By state of outlet.

Per Capita Expenditures for Prescription Drugs in 1998

National Per Capita = $335*

<u>ALPHA ORDER</u>

RANK	STATE	PER CAPITA
14	Alabama	$357
50	Alaska	216
37	Arizona	299
15	Arkansas	356
49	California	231
47	Colorado	244
5	Connecticut	414
7	Delaware	403
4	Florida	416
30	Georgia	322
46	Hawaii	261
43	Idaho	271
27	Illinois	328
18	Indiana	348
25	Iowa	330
29	Kansas	324
8	Kentucky	398
20	Louisiana	345
13	Maine	366
28	Maryland	327
16	Massachusetts	353
9	Michigan	396
32	Minnesota	315
17	Mississippi	350
23	Missouri	334
45	Montana	266
12	Nebraska	377
42	Nevada	274
25	New Hampshire	330
1	New Jersey	438
48	New Mexico	232
10	New York	392
22	North Carolina	340
36	North Dakota	301
19	Ohio	347
31	Oklahoma	316
39	Oregon	280
3	Pennsylvania	420
6	Rhode Island	405
21	South Carolina	342
41	South Dakota	275
10	Tennessee	392
35	Texas	306
44	Utah	268
34	Vermont	310
33	Virginia	314
38	Washington	282
2	West Virginia	428
23	Wisconsin	334
40	Wyoming	277

<u>RANK ORDER</u>

RANK	STATE	PER CAPITA
1	New Jersey	$438
2	West Virginia	428
3	Pennsylvania	420
4	Florida	416
5	Connecticut	414
6	Rhode Island	405
7	Delaware	403
8	Kentucky	398
9	Michigan	396
10	New York	392
10	Tennessee	392
12	Nebraska	377
13	Maine	366
14	Alabama	357
15	Arkansas	356
16	Massachusetts	353
17	Mississippi	350
18	Indiana	348
19	Ohio	347
20	Louisiana	345
21	South Carolina	342
22	North Carolina	340
23	Missouri	334
23	Wisconsin	334
25	Iowa	330
25	New Hampshire	330
27	Illinois	328
28	Maryland	327
29	Kansas	324
30	Georgia	322
31	Oklahoma	316
32	Minnesota	315
33	Virginia	314
34	Vermont	310
35	Texas	306
36	North Dakota	301
37	Arizona	299
38	Washington	282
39	Oregon	280
40	Wyoming	277
41	South Dakota	275
42	Nevada	274
43	Idaho	271
44	Utah	268
45	Montana	266
46	Hawaii	261
47	Colorado	244
48	New Mexico	232
49	California	231
50	Alaska	216

| | District of Columbia | 345 |

Source: MQ Press using data from U.S. Dept of Health & Human Services, Centers for Medicare and Medicaid Services "State Health Care Expenditures" (http://www.hcfa.gov/stats/nhe-oact/stateestimates/)
Purchases in retail outlets. By state of outlet.

Percent Change in Per Capita Expenditures for Prescription Drugs: 1990 to 1998

National Percent Change = 121.9% Increase*

ALPHA ORDER			RANK ORDER		
RANK	STATE	PERCENT CHANGE	RANK	STATE	PERCENT CHANGE
36	Alabama	113.8	1	Delaware	170.5
29	Alaska	118.2	2	Maine	161.4
27	Arizona	119.9	3	Florida	160.0
31	Arkansas	117.1	4	New York	151.3
49	California	81.9	5	Connecticut	146.4
30	Colorado	117.9	6	New Jersey	144.7
5	Connecticut	146.4	7	Pennsylvania	144.2
1	Delaware	170.5	8	Oregon	143.5
3	Florida	160.0	9	South Carolina	142.6
35	Georgia	114.7	10	Minnesota	140.5
50	Hawaii	71.7	11	Nebraska	140.1
33	Idaho	115.1	12	Rhode Island	136.8
41	Illinois	111.6	13	Nevada	134.2
38	Indiana	113.5	14	Massachusetts	130.7
22	Iowa	124.5	15	New Hampshire	129.2
40	Kansas	111.8	16	West Virginia	128.9
17	Kentucky	127.4	17	Kentucky	127.4
39	Louisiana	113.0	18	North Carolina	126.7
2	Maine	161.4	19	Wisconsin	125.7
43	Maryland	111.0	20	Montana	125.4
14	Massachusetts	130.7	21	Michigan	125.0
21	Michigan	125.0	22	Iowa	124.5
10	Minnesota	140.5	23	Ohio	122.4
26	Mississippi	120.1	24	Oklahoma	121.0
42	Missouri	111.4	25	Tennessee	120.2
20	Montana	125.4	26	Mississippi	120.1
11	Nebraska	140.1	27	Arizona	119.9
13	Nevada	134.2	28	Vermont	118.3
15	New Hampshire	129.2	29	Alaska	118.2
6	New Jersey	144.7	30	Colorado	117.9
48	New Mexico	96.6	31	Arkansas	117.1
4	New York	151.3	32	Wyoming	116.4
18	North Carolina	126.7	33	Idaho	115.1
45	North Dakota	110.5	34	South Dakota	114.8
23	Ohio	122.4	35	Georgia	114.7
24	Oklahoma	121.0	36	Alabama	113.8
8	Oregon	143.5	37	Virginia	113.6
7	Pennsylvania	144.2	38	Indiana	113.5
12	Rhode Island	136.8	39	Louisiana	113.0
9	South Carolina	142.6	40	Kansas	111.8
34	South Dakota	114.8	41	Illinois	111.6
25	Tennessee	120.2	42	Missouri	111.4
46	Texas	109.6	43	Maryland	111.0
43	Utah	111.0	43	Utah	111.0
28	Vermont	118.3	45	North Dakota	110.5
37	Virginia	113.6	46	Texas	109.6
47	Washington	108.9	47	Washington	108.9
16	West Virginia	128.9	48	New Mexico	96.6
19	Wisconsin	125.7	49	California	81.9
32	Wyoming	116.4	50	Hawaii	71.7

			District of Columbia	161.4

Source: MQ Press using data from U.S. Dept of Health & Human Services, Centers for Medicare and Medicaid Services
"State Health Care Expenditures" (http://www.hcfa.gov/stats/nhe-oact/stateestimates/)
*Purchases in retail outlets. By state of outlet.

Average Annual Change in Per Capita Expenditures
For Prescription Drugs: 1990 to 1998
National Percent Change = 10.5% Average Annual Increase*

ALPHA ORDER

RANK	STATE	PERCENT CHANGE
33	Alabama	10.0
29	Alaska	10.2
27	Arizona	10.3
29	Arkansas	10.2
49	California	7.8
29	Colorado	10.2
5	Connecticut	11.9
1	Delaware	13.2
3	Florida	12.7
33	Georgia	10.0
50	Hawaii	7.0
33	Idaho	10.0
40	Illinois	9.8
38	Indiana	9.9
22	Iowa	10.6
40	Kansas	9.8
17	Kentucky	10.8
38	Louisiana	9.9
2	Maine	12.8
40	Maryland	9.8
14	Massachusetts	11.0
19	Michigan	10.7
10	Minnesota	11.6
24	Mississippi	10.4
40	Missouri	9.8
19	Montana	10.7
10	Nebraska	11.6
13	Nevada	11.2
15	New Hampshire	10.9
6	New Jersey	11.8
48	New Mexico	8.8
4	New York	12.2
17	North Carolina	10.8
45	North Dakota	9.7
23	Ohio	10.5
24	Oklahoma	10.4
6	Oregon	11.8
6	Pennsylvania	11.8
12	Rhode Island	11.4
9	South Carolina	11.7
33	South Dakota	10.0
24	Tennessee	10.4
45	Texas	9.7
40	Utah	9.8
27	Vermont	10.3
33	Virginia	10.0
47	Washington	9.6
15	West Virginia	10.9
19	Wisconsin	10.7
32	Wyoming	10.1

RANK ORDER

RANK	STATE	PERCENT CHANGE
1	Delaware	13.2
2	Maine	12.8
3	Florida	12.7
4	New York	12.2
5	Connecticut	11.9
6	New Jersey	11.8
6	Oregon	11.8
6	Pennsylvania	11.8
9	South Carolina	11.7
10	Minnesota	11.6
10	Nebraska	11.6
12	Rhode Island	11.4
13	Nevada	11.2
14	Massachusetts	11.0
15	New Hampshire	10.9
15	West Virginia	10.9
17	Kentucky	10.8
17	North Carolina	10.8
19	Michigan	10.7
19	Montana	10.7
19	Wisconsin	10.7
22	Iowa	10.6
23	Ohio	10.5
24	Mississippi	10.4
24	Oklahoma	10.4
24	Tennessee	10.4
27	Arizona	10.3
27	Vermont	10.3
29	Alaska	10.2
29	Arkansas	10.2
29	Colorado	10.2
32	Wyoming	10.1
33	Alabama	10.0
33	Georgia	10.0
33	Idaho	10.0
33	South Dakota	10.0
33	Virginia	10.0
38	Indiana	9.9
38	Louisiana	9.9
40	Illinois	9.8
40	Kansas	9.8
40	Maryland	9.8
40	Missouri	9.8
40	Utah	9.8
45	North Dakota	9.7
45	Texas	9.7
47	Washington	9.6
48	New Mexico	8.8
49	California	7.8
50	Hawaii	7.0

| District of Columbia | 12.8 |

Source: MQ Press using data from U.S. Dept of Health & Human Services, Centers for Medicare and Medicaid Services "State Health Care Expenditures" (http://www.hcfa.gov/stats/nhe-oact/stateestimates/)
*Purchases in retail outlets. By state of outlet.

Expenditures for Dental Services in 1998

National Total = $53,829,000,000*

ALPHA ORDER

RANK	STATE	EXPENDITURES	% of USA
26	Alabama	$652,000,000	1.2%
44	Alaska	173,000,000	0.3%
24	Arizona	867,000,000	1.6%
33	Arkansas	392,000,000	0.7%
1	California	7,999,000,000	14.9%
19	Colorado	944,000,000	1.8%
22	Connecticut	896,000,000	1.7%
45	Delaware	155,000,000	0.3%
4	Florida	2,957,000,000	5.5%
12	Georgia	1,381,000,000	2.6%
36	Hawaii	284,000,000	0.5%
40	Idaho	253,000,000	0.5%
5	Illinois	2,283,000,000	4.2%
18	Indiana	1,021,000,000	1.9%
31	Iowa	482,000,000	0.9%
30	Kansas	484,000,000	0.9%
28	Kentucky	533,000,000	1.0%
25	Louisiana	703,000,000	1.3%
41	Maine	233,000,000	0.4%
17	Maryland	1,047,000,000	1.9%
11	Massachusetts	1,472,000,000	2.7%
7	Michigan	2,141,000,000	4.0%
16	Minnesota	1,052,000,000	2.0%
35	Mississippi	317,000,000	0.6%
23	Missouri	877,000,000	1.6%
46	Montana	151,000,000	0.3%
38	Nebraska	274,000,000	0.5%
34	Nevada	391,000,000	0.7%
37	New Hampshire	283,000,000	0.5%
9	New Jersey	1,917,000,000	3.6%
39	New Mexico	268,000,000	0.5%
2	New York	3,698,000,000	6.9%
13	North Carolina	1,323,000,000	2.5%
49	North Dakota	110,000,000	0.2%
8	Ohio	1,978,000,000	3.7%
29	Oklahoma	505,000,000	0.9%
21	Oregon	902,000,000	1.7%
6	Pennsylvania	2,237,000,000	4.2%
43	Rhode Island	217,000,000	0.4%
27	South Carolina	591,000,000	1.1%
48	South Dakota	121,000,000	0.2%
20	Tennessee	927,000,000	1.7%
3	Texas	3,218,000,000	6.0%
32	Utah	461,000,000	0.9%
47	Vermont	127,000,000	0.2%
14	Virginia	1,272,000,000	2.4%
10	Washington	1,722,000,000	3.2%
42	West Virginia	221,000,000	0.4%
15	Wisconsin	1,089,000,000	2.0%
50	Wyoming	76,000,000	0.1%

RANK ORDER

RANK	STATE	EXPENDITURES	% of USA
1	California	$7,999,000,000	14.9%
2	New York	3,698,000,000	6.9%
3	Texas	3,218,000,000	6.0%
4	Florida	2,957,000,000	5.5%
5	Illinois	2,283,000,000	4.2%
6	Pennsylvania	2,237,000,000	4.2%
7	Michigan	2,141,000,000	4.0%
8	Ohio	1,978,000,000	3.7%
9	New Jersey	1,917,000,000	3.6%
10	Washington	1,722,000,000	3.2%
11	Massachusetts	1,472,000,000	2.7%
12	Georgia	1,381,000,000	2.6%
13	North Carolina	1,323,000,000	2.5%
14	Virginia	1,272,000,000	2.4%
15	Wisconsin	1,089,000,000	2.0%
16	Minnesota	1,052,000,000	2.0%
17	Maryland	1,047,000,000	1.9%
18	Indiana	1,021,000,000	1.9%
19	Colorado	944,000,000	1.8%
20	Tennessee	927,000,000	1.7%
21	Oregon	902,000,000	1.7%
22	Connecticut	896,000,000	1.7%
23	Missouri	877,000,000	1.6%
24	Arizona	867,000,000	1.6%
25	Louisiana	703,000,000	1.3%
26	Alabama	652,000,000	1.2%
27	South Carolina	591,000,000	1.1%
28	Kentucky	533,000,000	1.0%
29	Oklahoma	505,000,000	0.9%
30	Kansas	484,000,000	0.9%
31	Iowa	482,000,000	0.9%
32	Utah	461,000,000	0.9%
33	Arkansas	392,000,000	0.7%
34	Nevada	391,000,000	0.7%
35	Mississippi	317,000,000	0.6%
36	Hawaii	284,000,000	0.5%
37	New Hampshire	283,000,000	0.5%
38	Nebraska	274,000,000	0.5%
39	New Mexico	268,000,000	0.5%
40	Idaho	253,000,000	0.5%
41	Maine	233,000,000	0.4%
42	West Virginia	221,000,000	0.4%
43	Rhode Island	217,000,000	0.4%
44	Alaska	173,000,000	0.3%
45	Delaware	155,000,000	0.3%
46	Montana	151,000,000	0.3%
47	Vermont	127,000,000	0.2%
48	South Dakota	121,000,000	0.2%
49	North Dakota	110,000,000	0.2%
50	Wyoming	76,000,000	0.1%
	District of Columbia	151,000,000	0.3%

Source: U.S. Department of Health and Human Services, Centers for Medicare and Medicaid Services
"State Health Care Expenditures" (http://www.hcfa.gov/stats/nhe-oact/stateestimates/)
*By state of provider.

Percent of Total Personal Health Care Expenditures
Spent on Dental Services in 1998
National Percent = 5.3%*

ALPHA ORDER

RANK	STATE	PERCENT
46	Alabama	4.1
4	Alaska	7.5
13	Arizona	5.9
35	Arkansas	4.6
6	California	7.3
8	Colorado	6.9
13	Connecticut	5.9
25	Delaware	5.0
25	Florida	5.0
24	Georgia	5.1
9	Hawaii	6.1
5	Idaho	7.4
21	Illinois	5.2
29	Indiana	4.8
32	Iowa	4.7
21	Kansas	5.2
48	Kentucky	3.7
41	Louisiana	4.3
32	Maine	4.7
19	Maryland	5.3
28	Massachusetts	4.9
12	Michigan	6.0
21	Minnesota	5.2
49	Mississippi	3.6
44	Missouri	4.2
19	Montana	5.3
38	Nebraska	4.5
7	Nevada	7.0
9	New Hampshire	6.1
13	New Jersey	5.9
25	New Mexico	5.0
41	New York	4.3
29	North Carolina	4.8
46	North Dakota	4.1
35	Ohio	4.6
35	Oklahoma	4.6
2	Oregon	8.3
40	Pennsylvania	4.4
29	Rhode Island	4.8
38	South Carolina	4.5
41	South Dakota	4.3
44	Tennessee	4.2
32	Texas	4.7
3	Utah	7.8
9	Vermont	6.1
16	Virginia	5.7
1	Washington	8.9
50	West Virginia	3.1
17	Wisconsin	5.5
18	Wyoming	5.4

RANK ORDER

RANK	STATE	PERCENT
1	Washington	8.9
2	Oregon	8.3
3	Utah	7.8
4	Alaska	7.5
5	Idaho	7.4
6	California	7.3
7	Nevada	7.0
8	Colorado	6.9
9	Hawaii	6.1
9	New Hampshire	6.1
9	Vermont	6.1
12	Michigan	6.0
13	Arizona	5.9
13	Connecticut	5.9
13	New Jersey	5.9
16	Virginia	5.7
17	Wisconsin	5.5
18	Wyoming	5.4
19	Maryland	5.3
19	Montana	5.3
21	Illinois	5.2
21	Kansas	5.2
21	Minnesota	5.2
24	Georgia	5.1
25	Delaware	5.0
25	Florida	5.0
25	New Mexico	5.0
28	Massachusetts	4.9
29	Indiana	4.8
29	North Carolina	4.8
29	Rhode Island	4.8
32	Iowa	4.7
32	Maine	4.7
32	Texas	4.7
35	Arkansas	4.6
35	Ohio	4.6
35	Oklahoma	4.6
38	Nebraska	4.5
38	South Carolina	4.5
40	Pennsylvania	4.4
41	Louisiana	4.3
41	New York	4.3
41	South Dakota	4.3
44	Missouri	4.2
44	Tennessee	4.2
46	Alabama	4.1
46	North Dakota	4.1
48	Kentucky	3.7
49	Mississippi	3.6
50	West Virginia	3.1
	District of Columbia	3.5

Source: MQ Press using data from U.S. Dept of Health & Human Services, Centers for Medicare and Medicaid Services "State Health Care Expenditures" (http://www.hcfa.gov/stats/nhe-oact/stateestimates/)
*By state of provider.

Average Annual Change in Expenditures for Dental Services: 1990 to 1998

National Percent Change = 6.9% Average Annual Increase*

<table>
<tr><td colspan="3">ALPHA ORDER</td><td colspan="3">RANK ORDER</td></tr>
<tr><td>RANK</td><td>STATE</td><td>PERCENT CHANGE</td><td>RANK</td><td>STATE</td><td>PERCENT CHANGE</td></tr>
<tr><td>26</td><td>Alabama</td><td>7.4</td><td>1</td><td>Nevada</td><td>11.1</td></tr>
<tr><td>20</td><td>Alaska</td><td>7.8</td><td>2</td><td>Idaho</td><td>9.3</td></tr>
<tr><td>6</td><td>Arizona</td><td>8.6</td><td>3</td><td>North Carolina</td><td>9.0</td></tr>
<tr><td>11</td><td>Arkansas</td><td>8.4</td><td>3</td><td>Utah</td><td>9.0</td></tr>
<tr><td>39</td><td>California</td><td>6.5</td><td>5</td><td>Louisiana</td><td>8.8</td></tr>
<tr><td>6</td><td>Colorado</td><td>8.6</td><td>6</td><td>Arizona</td><td>8.6</td></tr>
<tr><td>50</td><td>Connecticut</td><td>4.3</td><td>6</td><td>Colorado</td><td>8.6</td></tr>
<tr><td>12</td><td>Delaware</td><td>8.3</td><td>6</td><td>Oregon</td><td>8.6</td></tr>
<tr><td>28</td><td>Florida</td><td>7.3</td><td>6</td><td>Texas</td><td>8.6</td></tr>
<tr><td>17</td><td>Georgia</td><td>7.9</td><td>10</td><td>New Mexico</td><td>8.5</td></tr>
<tr><td>49</td><td>Hawaii</td><td>4.8</td><td>11</td><td>Arkansas</td><td>8.4</td></tr>
<tr><td>2</td><td>Idaho</td><td>9.3</td><td>12</td><td>Delaware</td><td>8.3</td></tr>
<tr><td>39</td><td>Illinois</td><td>6.5</td><td>12</td><td>Kentucky</td><td>8.3</td></tr>
<tr><td>14</td><td>Indiana</td><td>8.2</td><td>14</td><td>Indiana</td><td>8.2</td></tr>
<tr><td>28</td><td>Iowa</td><td>7.3</td><td>15</td><td>Washington</td><td>8.1</td></tr>
<tr><td>24</td><td>Kansas</td><td>7.5</td><td>16</td><td>South Carolina</td><td>8.0</td></tr>
<tr><td>12</td><td>Kentucky</td><td>8.3</td><td>17</td><td>Georgia</td><td>7.9</td></tr>
<tr><td>5</td><td>Louisiana</td><td>8.8</td><td>17</td><td>Mississippi</td><td>7.9</td></tr>
<tr><td>31</td><td>Maine</td><td>7.2</td><td>17</td><td>Tennessee</td><td>7.9</td></tr>
<tr><td>37</td><td>Maryland</td><td>6.6</td><td>20</td><td>Alaska</td><td>7.8</td></tr>
<tr><td>42</td><td>Massachusetts</td><td>6.3</td><td>20</td><td>Montana</td><td>7.8</td></tr>
<tr><td>43</td><td>Michigan</td><td>6.1</td><td>20</td><td>New Hampshire</td><td>7.8</td></tr>
<tr><td>37</td><td>Minnesota</td><td>6.6</td><td>23</td><td>South Dakota</td><td>7.7</td></tr>
<tr><td>17</td><td>Mississippi</td><td>7.9</td><td>24</td><td>Kansas</td><td>7.5</td></tr>
<tr><td>35</td><td>Missouri</td><td>6.9</td><td>24</td><td>Vermont</td><td>7.5</td></tr>
<tr><td>20</td><td>Montana</td><td>7.8</td><td>26</td><td>Alabama</td><td>7.4</td></tr>
<tr><td>33</td><td>Nebraska</td><td>7.0</td><td>26</td><td>Virginia</td><td>7.4</td></tr>
<tr><td>1</td><td>Nevada</td><td>11.1</td><td>28</td><td>Florida</td><td>7.3</td></tr>
<tr><td>20</td><td>New Hampshire</td><td>7.8</td><td>28</td><td>Iowa</td><td>7.3</td></tr>
<tr><td>45</td><td>New Jersey</td><td>5.4</td><td>28</td><td>Wisconsin</td><td>7.3</td></tr>
<tr><td>10</td><td>New Mexico</td><td>8.5</td><td>31</td><td>Maine</td><td>7.2</td></tr>
<tr><td>47</td><td>New York</td><td>5.0</td><td>31</td><td>North Dakota</td><td>7.2</td></tr>
<tr><td>3</td><td>North Carolina</td><td>9.0</td><td>33</td><td>Nebraska</td><td>7.0</td></tr>
<tr><td>31</td><td>North Dakota</td><td>7.2</td><td>33</td><td>West Virginia</td><td>7.0</td></tr>
<tr><td>39</td><td>Ohio</td><td>6.5</td><td>35</td><td>Missouri</td><td>6.9</td></tr>
<tr><td>36</td><td>Oklahoma</td><td>6.8</td><td>36</td><td>Oklahoma</td><td>6.8</td></tr>
<tr><td>6</td><td>Oregon</td><td>8.6</td><td>37</td><td>Maryland</td><td>6.6</td></tr>
<tr><td>48</td><td>Pennsylvania</td><td>4.9</td><td>37</td><td>Minnesota</td><td>6.6</td></tr>
<tr><td>46</td><td>Rhode Island</td><td>5.1</td><td>39</td><td>California</td><td>6.5</td></tr>
<tr><td>16</td><td>South Carolina</td><td>8.0</td><td>39</td><td>Illinois</td><td>6.5</td></tr>
<tr><td>23</td><td>South Dakota</td><td>7.7</td><td>39</td><td>Ohio</td><td>6.5</td></tr>
<tr><td>17</td><td>Tennessee</td><td>7.9</td><td>42</td><td>Massachusetts</td><td>6.3</td></tr>
<tr><td>6</td><td>Texas</td><td>8.6</td><td>43</td><td>Michigan</td><td>6.1</td></tr>
<tr><td>3</td><td>Utah</td><td>9.0</td><td>44</td><td>Wyoming</td><td>5.6</td></tr>
<tr><td>24</td><td>Vermont</td><td>7.5</td><td>45</td><td>New Jersey</td><td>5.4</td></tr>
<tr><td>26</td><td>Virginia</td><td>7.4</td><td>46</td><td>Rhode Island</td><td>5.1</td></tr>
<tr><td>15</td><td>Washington</td><td>8.1</td><td>47</td><td>New York</td><td>5.0</td></tr>
<tr><td>33</td><td>West Virginia</td><td>7.0</td><td>48</td><td>Pennsylvania</td><td>4.9</td></tr>
<tr><td>28</td><td>Wisconsin</td><td>7.3</td><td>49</td><td>Hawaii</td><td>4.8</td></tr>
<tr><td>44</td><td>Wyoming</td><td>5.6</td><td>50</td><td>Connecticut</td><td>4.3</td></tr>
<tr><td></td><td></td><td></td><td></td><td>District of Columbia</td><td>5.3</td></tr>
</table>

Source: U.S. Department of Health and Human Services, Centers for Medicare and Medicaid Services
"State Health Care Expenditures" (http://www.hcfa.gov/stats/nhe-oact/stateestimates/)
*Purchases in retail outlets. By state of outlet. Includes over-the-counter drugs and sundries.

Per Capita Expenditures for Dental Services in 1998

National Per Capita = $199*

ALPHA ORDER				RANK ORDER		
RANK	STATE	PER CAPITA		RANK	STATE	PER CAPITA
47	Alabama	$150		1	Washington	$303
2	Alaska	281		2	Alaska	281
26	Arizona	186		3	Oregon	275
44	Arkansas	154		4	Connecticut	274
5	California	245		5	California	245
9	Colorado	238		6	Massachusetts	240
4	Connecticut	274		7	Hawaii	239
18	Delaware	208		7	New Hampshire	239
22	Florida	198		9	Colorado	238
29	Georgia	181		10	New Jersey	237
7	Hawaii	239		11	Nevada	224
19	Idaho	206		12	Minnesota	223
23	Illinois	189		13	Rhode Island	220
32	Indiana	173		14	Utah	219
36	Iowa	168		15	Michigan	218
28	Kansas	183		16	Vermont	215
48	Kentucky	135		17	Wisconsin	209
40	Louisiana	161		18	Delaware	208
24	Maine	187		19	Idaho	206
20	Maryland	204		20	Maryland	204
6	Massachusetts	240		20	New York	204
15	Michigan	218		22	Florida	198
12	Minnesota	223		23	Illinois	189
50	Mississippi	115		24	Maine	187
40	Missouri	161		24	Virginia	187
33	Montana	172		26	Arizona	186
38	Nebraska	165		26	Pennsylvania	186
11	Nevada	224		28	Kansas	183
7	New Hampshire	239		29	Georgia	181
10	New Jersey	237		30	Ohio	176
43	New Mexico	155		31	North Carolina	175
20	New York	204		32	Indiana	173
31	North Carolina	175		33	Montana	172
33	North Dakota	172		33	North Dakota	172
30	Ohio	176		35	Tennessee	171
46	Oklahoma	151		36	Iowa	168
3	Oregon	275		37	South Dakota	166
26	Pennsylvania	186		38	Nebraska	165
13	Rhode Island	220		39	Texas	163
44	South Carolina	154		40	Louisiana	161
37	South Dakota	166		40	Missouri	161
35	Tennessee	171		42	Wyoming	158
39	Texas	163		43	New Mexico	155
14	Utah	219		44	Arkansas	154
16	Vermont	215		44	South Carolina	154
24	Virginia	187		46	Oklahoma	151
1	Washington	303		47	Alabama	150
49	West Virginia	122		48	Kentucky	135
17	Wisconsin	209		49	West Virginia	122
42	Wyoming	158		50	Mississippi	115
					District of Columbia	290

Source: MQ Press using data from U.S. Dept of Health & Human Services, Centers for Medicare and Medicaid Services
"State Health Care Expenditures" (http://www.hcfa.gov/stats/nhe-oact/stateestimates/)
*By state of provider. Per capita calculated using resident population. These figures may be skewed due to
residents crossing state borders for care.

Per Capita Medicaid Expenditures for Dental Services in 1998

National Per Capita = $7.37*

ALPHA ORDER

RANK	STATE	PER CAPITA
40	Alabama	$2.99
5	Alaska	13.00
6	Arizona	12.43
31	Arkansas	4.33
1	California	20.47
39	Colorado	3.02
42	Connecticut	2.75
35	Delaware	4.03
25	Florida	4.96
29	Georgia	4.58
49	Hawaii	0.84
12	Idaho	8.12
41	Illinois	2.90
30	Indiana	4.57
9	Iowa	9.44
37	Kansas	3.79
10	Kentucky	8.64
34	Louisiana	4.13
18	Maine	6.41
50	Maryland	0.39
3	Massachusetts	14.00
22	Michigan	5.50
27	Minnesota	4.65
48	Mississippi	1.09
43	Missouri	2.39
14	Montana	7.96
15	Nebraska	7.83
13	Nevada	8.03
32	New Hampshire	4.22
44	New Jersey	2.22
28	New Mexico	4.61
17	New York	6.61
20	North Carolina	5.96
19	North Dakota	6.27
36	Ohio	3.83
45	Oklahoma	2.10
47	Oregon	1.52
24	Pennsylvania	5.17
7	Rhode Island	12.15
26	South Carolina	4.69
23	South Dakota	5.47
21	Tennessee	5.89
16	Texas	6.90
11	Utah	8.57
4	Vermont	13.55
46	Virginia	1.91
2	Washington	20.22
8	West Virginia	11.59
38	Wisconsin	3.64
33	Wyoming	4.17

RANK ORDER

RANK	STATE	PER CAPITA
1	California	$20.47
2	Washington	20.22
3	Massachusetts	14.00
4	Vermont	13.55
5	Alaska	13.00
6	Arizona	12.43
7	Rhode Island	12.15
8	West Virginia	11.59
9	Iowa	9.44
10	Kentucky	8.64
11	Utah	8.57
12	Idaho	8.12
13	Nevada	8.03
14	Montana	7.96
15	Nebraska	7.83
16	Texas	6.90
17	New York	6.61
18	Maine	6.41
19	North Dakota	6.27
20	North Carolina	5.96
21	Tennessee	5.89
22	Michigan	5.50
23	South Dakota	5.47
24	Pennsylvania	5.17
25	Florida	4.96
26	South Carolina	4.69
27	Minnesota	4.65
28	New Mexico	4.61
29	Georgia	4.58
30	Indiana	4.57
31	Arkansas	4.33
32	New Hampshire	4.22
33	Wyoming	4.17
34	Louisiana	4.13
35	Delaware	4.03
36	Ohio	3.83
37	Kansas	3.79
38	Wisconsin	3.64
39	Colorado	3.02
40	Alabama	2.99
41	Illinois	2.90
42	Connecticut	2.75
43	Missouri	2.39
44	New Jersey	2.22
45	Oklahoma	2.10
46	Virginia	1.91
47	Oregon	1.52
48	Mississippi	1.09
49	Hawaii	0.84
50	Maryland	0.39
	District of Columbia	3.84

Source: MQ Press using data from U.S. Dept of Health & Human Services, Centers for Medicare and Medicaid Services
"State Health Care Expenditures" (http://www.hcfa.gov/stats/nhe-oact/stateestimates/)
*By state of provider. Per capita calculated using resident population. These figures may be skewed due to residents crossing state borders for care.

Expenditures for Other Personal Health Care Services in 1998

National Total = $31,917,000,000*

ALPHA ORDER

RANK	STATE	EXPENDITURES	% of USA
26	Alabama	$407,000,000	1.3%
35	Alaska	262,000,000	0.8%
34	Arizona	300,000,000	0.9%
36	Arkansas	240,000,000	0.8%
3	California	2,033,000,000	6.4%
22	Colorado	464,000,000	1.5%
21	Connecticut	548,000,000	1.7%
43	Delaware	153,000,000	0.5%
5	Florida	1,525,000,000	4.8%
13	Georgia	778,000,000	2.4%
44	Hawaii	149,000,000	0.5%
46	Idaho	116,000,000	0.4%
6	Illinois	1,320,000,000	4.1%
28	Indiana	381,000,000	1.2%
31	Iowa	344,000,000	1.1%
24	Kansas	437,000,000	1.4%
25	Kentucky	425,000,000	1.3%
32	Louisiana	342,000,000	1.1%
30	Maine	345,000,000	1.1%
18	Maryland	598,000,000	1.9%
7	Massachusetts	1,144,000,000	3.6%
10	Michigan	868,000,000	2.7%
11	Minnesota	808,000,000	2.5%
39	Mississippi	211,000,000	0.7%
17	Missouri	644,000,000	2.0%
48	Montana	99,000,000	0.3%
40	Nebraska	179,000,000	0.6%
45	Nevada	140,000,000	0.4%
38	New Hampshire	234,000,000	0.7%
12	New Jersey	793,000,000	2.5%
37	New Mexico	238,000,000	0.7%
1	New York	4,431,000,000	13.9%
9	North Carolina	880,000,000	2.8%
49	North Dakota	83,000,000	0.3%
8	Ohio	940,000,000	2.9%
27	Oklahoma	383,000,000	1.2%
20	Oregon	563,000,000	1.8%
4	Pennsylvania	1,596,000,000	5.0%
29	Rhode Island	358,000,000	1.1%
19	South Carolina	576,000,000	1.8%
47	South Dakota	113,000,000	0.4%
23	Tennessee	459,000,000	1.4%
2	Texas	2,083,000,000	6.5%
41	Utah	160,000,000	0.5%
42	Vermont	155,000,000	0.5%
15	Virginia	666,000,000	2.1%
14	Washington	732,000,000	2.3%
33	West Virginia	331,000,000	1.0%
16	Wisconsin	656,000,000	2.1%
50	Wyoming	69,000,000	0.2%

RANK ORDER

RANK	STATE	EXPENDITURES	% of USA
1	New York	$4,431,000,000	13.9%
2	Texas	2,083,000,000	6.5%
3	California	2,033,000,000	6.4%
4	Pennsylvania	1,596,000,000	5.0%
5	Florida	1,525,000,000	4.8%
6	Illinois	1,320,000,000	4.1%
7	Massachusetts	1,144,000,000	3.6%
8	Ohio	940,000,000	2.9%
9	North Carolina	880,000,000	2.8%
10	Michigan	868,000,000	2.7%
11	Minnesota	808,000,000	2.5%
12	New Jersey	793,000,000	2.5%
13	Georgia	778,000,000	2.4%
14	Washington	732,000,000	2.3%
15	Virginia	666,000,000	2.1%
16	Wisconsin	656,000,000	2.1%
17	Missouri	644,000,000	2.0%
18	Maryland	598,000,000	1.9%
19	South Carolina	576,000,000	1.8%
20	Oregon	563,000,000	1.8%
21	Connecticut	548,000,000	1.7%
22	Colorado	464,000,000	1.5%
23	Tennessee	459,000,000	1.4%
24	Kansas	437,000,000	1.4%
25	Kentucky	425,000,000	1.3%
26	Alabama	407,000,000	1.3%
27	Oklahoma	383,000,000	1.2%
28	Indiana	381,000,000	1.2%
29	Rhode Island	358,000,000	1.1%
30	Maine	345,000,000	1.1%
31	Iowa	344,000,000	1.1%
32	Louisiana	342,000,000	1.1%
33	West Virginia	331,000,000	1.0%
34	Arizona	300,000,000	0.9%
35	Alaska	262,000,000	0.8%
36	Arkansas	240,000,000	0.8%
37	New Mexico	238,000,000	0.7%
38	New Hampshire	234,000,000	0.7%
39	Mississippi	211,000,000	0.7%
40	Nebraska	179,000,000	0.6%
41	Utah	160,000,000	0.5%
42	Vermont	155,000,000	0.5%
43	Delaware	153,000,000	0.5%
44	Hawaii	149,000,000	0.5%
45	Nevada	140,000,000	0.4%
46	Idaho	116,000,000	0.4%
47	South Dakota	113,000,000	0.4%
48	Montana	99,000,000	0.3%
49	North Dakota	83,000,000	0.3%
50	Wyoming	69,000,000	0.2%
	District of Columbia	161,000,000	0.5%

Source: U.S. Department of Health and Human Services, Centers for Medicare and Medicaid Services
"State Health Care Expenditures" (http://www.hcfa.gov/stats/nhe-oact/stateestimates/)
*By state of provider. Includes on-site services provided by employers for the health care needs of their employees.
Also includes shipboard facilities and field stations operated by the U.S. Department of Defense; certain state and
local maternal and child health programs; school health programs and federal agency programs targeting veterans,
military personnel, Native Americans and persons with dependency and mental-health-related problems.

Percent of Total Personal Health Care Expenditures
Spent on Other Personal Health Care Services in 1998
National Percent = 3.1%*

ALPHA ORDER

RANK	STATE	PERCENT
40	Alabama	2.5
1	Alaska	11.4
48	Arizona	2.0
37	Arkansas	2.8
49	California	1.8
21	Colorado	3.4
18	Connecticut	3.6
8	Delaware	4.9
39	Florida	2.6
34	Georgia	2.9
25	Hawaii	3.2
21	Idaho	3.4
31	Illinois	3.0
49	Indiana	1.8
21	Iowa	3.4
10	Kansas	4.7
34	Kentucky	2.9
46	Louisiana	2.1
4	Maine	7.0
31	Maryland	3.0
16	Massachusetts	3.8
42	Michigan	2.4
14	Minnesota	4.0
42	Mississippi	2.4
27	Missouri	3.1
19	Montana	3.5
34	Nebraska	2.9
40	Nevada	2.5
7	New Hampshire	5.0
42	New Jersey	2.4
12	New Mexico	4.5
5	New York	5.2
25	North Carolina	3.2
27	North Dakota	3.1
45	Ohio	2.2
19	Oklahoma	3.5
5	Oregon	5.2
27	Pennsylvania	3.1
2	Rhode Island	7.9
13	South Carolina	4.4
14	South Dakota	4.0
46	Tennessee	2.1
27	Texas	3.1
38	Utah	2.7
3	Vermont	7.5
31	Virginia	3.0
16	Washington	3.8
10	West Virginia	4.7
24	Wisconsin	3.3
8	Wyoming	4.9

RANK ORDER

RANK	STATE	PERCENT
1	Alaska	11.4
2	Rhode Island	7.9
3	Vermont	7.5
4	Maine	7.0
5	New York	5.2
5	Oregon	5.2
7	New Hampshire	5.0
8	Delaware	4.9
8	Wyoming	4.9
10	Kansas	4.7
10	West Virginia	4.7
12	New Mexico	4.5
13	South Carolina	4.4
14	Minnesota	4.0
14	South Dakota	4.0
16	Massachusetts	3.8
16	Washington	3.8
18	Connecticut	3.6
19	Montana	3.5
19	Oklahoma	3.5
21	Colorado	3.4
21	Idaho	3.4
21	Iowa	3.4
24	Wisconsin	3.3
25	Hawaii	3.2
25	North Carolina	3.2
27	Missouri	3.1
27	North Dakota	3.1
27	Pennsylvania	3.1
27	Texas	3.1
31	Illinois	3.0
31	Maryland	3.0
31	Virginia	3.0
34	Georgia	2.9
34	Kentucky	2.9
34	Nebraska	2.9
37	Arkansas	2.8
38	Utah	2.7
39	Florida	2.6
40	Alabama	2.5
40	Nevada	2.5
42	Michigan	2.4
42	Mississippi	2.4
42	New Jersey	2.4
45	Ohio	2.2
46	Louisiana	2.1
46	Tennessee	2.1
48	Arizona	2.0
49	California	1.8
49	Indiana	1.8
	District of Columbia	3.8

Source: MQ Press using data from U.S. Dept of Health & Human Services, Centers for Medicare and Medicaid Services
"State Health Care Expenditures" (http://www.hcfa.gov/stats/nhe-oact/stateestimates/)
*By state of provider. Includes on-site services provided by employers for the health care needs of their employees.
Also includes shipboard facilities and field stations operated by the U.S. Department of Defense; certain state and
local maternal and child health programs; school health programs and federal agency programs targeting veterans,
military personnel, Native Americans and persons with dependency and mental-health-related problems.

Average Annual Change in Expenditures for
Other Personal Health Care Services: 1990 to 1998
National Percent Change = 14.1% Average Annual Increase*

ALPHA ORDER				RANK ORDER		
RANK	STATE	PERCENT CHANGE		RANK	STATE	PERCENT CHANGE
44	Alabama	10.1		1	Kansas	22.7
48	Alaska	7.9		2	Maine	22.3
42	Arizona	11.1		3	Rhode Island	21.8
11	Arkansas	17.5		4	West Virginia	20.4
50	California	6.9		5	New York	20.2
34	Colorado	12.7		6	Wyoming	20.0
31	Connecticut	12.9		7	Iowa	19.4
15	Delaware	16.5		8	Oklahoma	19.2
29	Florida	13.1		9	North Carolina	18.1
40	Georgia	11.6		9	Vermont	18.1
45	Hawaii	9.3		11	Arkansas	17.5
26	Idaho	14.2		11	Oregon	17.5
20	Illinois	15.0		13	Missouri	17.0
46	Indiana	9.1		14	Minnesota	16.9
7	Iowa	19.4		15	Delaware	16.5
1	Kansas	22.7		16	Nevada	15.9
25	Kentucky	14.4		16	New Hampshire	15.9
43	Louisiana	10.8		18	Texas	15.7
2	Maine	22.3		19	New Mexico	15.3
34	Maryland	12.7		20	Illinois	15.0
24	Massachusetts	14.8		20	Pennsylvania	15.0
37	Michigan	12.1		20	Washington	15.0
14	Minnesota	16.9		23	South Carolina	14.9
41	Mississippi	11.2		24	Massachusetts	14.8
13	Missouri	17.0		25	Kentucky	14.4
48	Montana	7.9		26	Idaho	14.2
28	Nebraska	13.3		27	Tennessee	13.6
16	Nevada	15.9		28	Nebraska	13.3
16	New Hampshire	15.9		29	Florida	13.1
47	New Jersey	8.2		30	Virginia	13.0
19	New Mexico	15.3		31	Connecticut	12.9
5	New York	20.2		32	South Dakota	12.8
9	North Carolina	18.1		32	Utah	12.8
38	North Dakota	11.8		34	Colorado	12.7
39	Ohio	11.7		34	Maryland	12.7
8	Oklahoma	19.2		36	Wisconsin	12.2
11	Oregon	17.5		37	Michigan	12.1
20	Pennsylvania	15.0		38	North Dakota	11.8
3	Rhode Island	21.8		39	Ohio	11.7
23	South Carolina	14.9		40	Georgia	11.6
32	South Dakota	12.8		41	Mississippi	11.2
27	Tennessee	13.6		42	Arizona	11.1
18	Texas	15.7		43	Louisiana	10.8
32	Utah	12.8		44	Alabama	10.1
9	Vermont	18.1		45	Hawaii	9.3
30	Virginia	13.0		46	Indiana	9.1
20	Washington	15.0		47	New Jersey	8.2
4	West Virginia	20.4		48	Alaska	7.9
36	Wisconsin	12.2		48	Montana	7.9
6	Wyoming	20.0		50	California	6.9
					District of Columbia	7.1

Source: U.S. Department of Health and Human Services, Centers for Medicare and Medicaid Services
"State Health Care Expenditures" (http://www.hcfa.gov/stats/nhe-oact/stateestimates/)
*By state of provider. Includes on-site services provided by employers for the health care needs of their employees.
Also includes shipboard facilities and field stations operated by the U.S. Department of Defense; certain state and
local maternal and child health programs; school health programs and federal agency programs targeting veterans,
military personnel, Native Americans and persons with dependency and mental-health-related problems.

Per Capita Expenditures for Other Personal Health Care Services in 1998

National Per Capita = $118*

ALPHA ORDER

RANK	STATE	PER CAPITA
39	Alabama	$94
1	Alaska	426
48	Arizona	64
38	Arkansas	95
50	California	62
25	Colorado	117
12	Connecticut	167
6	Delaware	206
34	Florida	102
34	Georgia	102
22	Hawaii	125
39	Idaho	94
30	Illinois	109
48	Indiana	64
23	Iowa	120
13	Kansas	166
31	Kentucky	108
45	Louisiana	78
3	Maine	277
25	Maryland	117
8	Massachusetts	186
41	Michigan	88
11	Minnesota	171
46	Mississippi	77
24	Missouri	118
29	Montana	113
31	Nebraska	108
44	Nevada	80
7	New Hampshire	197
36	New Jersey	98
17	New Mexico	137
5	New York	244
25	North Carolina	117
19	North Dakota	130
42	Ohio	84
28	Oklahoma	115
10	Oregon	172
18	Pennsylvania	133
2	Rhode Island	362
15	South Carolina	150
14	South Dakota	155
42	Tennessee	84
33	Texas	106
47	Utah	76
4	Vermont	262
36	Virginia	98
20	Washington	129
9	West Virginia	183
21	Wisconsin	126
16	Wyoming	144

RANK ORDER

RANK	STATE	PER CAPITA
1	Alaska	$426
2	Rhode Island	362
3	Maine	277
4	Vermont	262
5	New York	244
6	Delaware	206
7	New Hampshire	197
8	Massachusetts	186
9	West Virginia	183
10	Oregon	172
11	Minnesota	171
12	Connecticut	167
13	Kansas	166
14	South Dakota	155
15	South Carolina	150
16	Wyoming	144
17	New Mexico	137
18	Pennsylvania	133
19	North Dakota	130
20	Washington	129
21	Wisconsin	126
22	Hawaii	125
23	Iowa	120
24	Missouri	118
25	Colorado	117
25	Maryland	117
25	North Carolina	117
28	Oklahoma	115
29	Montana	113
30	Illinois	109
31	Kentucky	108
31	Nebraska	108
33	Texas	106
34	Florida	102
34	Georgia	102
36	New Jersey	98
36	Virginia	98
38	Arkansas	95
39	Alabama	94
39	Idaho	94
41	Michigan	88
42	Ohio	84
42	Tennessee	84
44	Nevada	80
45	Louisiana	78
46	Mississippi	77
47	Utah	76
48	Arizona	64
48	Indiana	64
50	California	62

District of Columbia 309

Source: MQ Press using data from U.S. Dept of Health & Human Services, Centers for Medicare and Medicaid Services
"State Health Care Expenditures" (http://www.hcfa.gov/stats/nhe-oact/stateestimates/)
*By state of provider. Includes on-site services provided by employers for the health care needs of their employees.
Also includes shipboard facilities and field stations operated by the U.S. Department of Defense; certain state and
local maternal and child health programs; school health programs and federal agency programs targeting veterans,
military personnel, Native Americans and persons with dependency and mental-health-related problems.

Expenditures for Home Health Care in 1998

National Total = $29,255,000,000*

ALPHA ORDER					RANK ORDER			

RANK	STATE	EXPENDITURES	% of USA	RANK	STATE	EXPENDITURES	% of USA
19	Alabama	$470,000,000	1.6%	1	New York	$4,292,000,000	14.7%
50	Alaska	9,000,000	0.0%	2	Texas	2,862,000,000	9.8%
27	Arizona	331,000,000	1.1%	3	Florida	2,225,000,000	7.6%
31	Arkansas	242,000,000	0.8%	4	California	1,951,000,000	6.7%
4	California	1,951,000,000	6.7%	5	Ohio	1,224,000,000	4.2%
28	Colorado	324,000,000	1.1%	6	Pennsylvania	1,109,000,000	3.8%
15	Connecticut	599,000,000	2.0%	7	Massachusetts	999,000,000	3.4%
41	Delaware	110,000,000	0.4%	8	Illinois	972,000,000	3.3%
3	Florida	2,225,000,000	7.6%	9	New Jersey	938,000,000	3.2%
12	Georgia	810,000,000	2.8%	10	North Carolina	934,000,000	3.2%
44	Hawaii	60,000,000	0.2%	11	Michigan	841,000,000	2.9%
44	Idaho	60,000,000	0.2%	12	Georgia	810,000,000	2.8%
8	Illinois	972,000,000	3.3%	13	Louisiana	629,000,000	2.2%
21	Indiana	415,000,000	1.4%	14	Tennessee	617,000,000	2.1%
30	Iowa	248,000,000	0.8%	15	Connecticut	599,000,000	2.0%
32	Kansas	220,000,000	0.8%	16	Missouri	567,000,000	1.9%
17	Kentucky	506,000,000	1.7%	17	Kentucky	506,000,000	1.7%
13	Louisiana	629,000,000	2.2%	18	Virginia	484,000,000	1.7%
33	Maine	188,000,000	0.6%	19	Alabama	470,000,000	1.6%
25	Maryland	390,000,000	1.3%	20	Minnesota	419,000,000	1.4%
7	Massachusetts	999,000,000	3.4%	21	Indiana	415,000,000	1.4%
11	Michigan	841,000,000	2.9%	22	Wisconsin	393,000,000	1.3%
20	Minnesota	419,000,000	1.4%	23	Oklahoma	391,000,000	1.3%
29	Mississippi	293,000,000	1.0%	23	South Carolina	391,000,000	1.3%
16	Missouri	567,000,000	1.9%	25	Maryland	390,000,000	1.3%
46	Montana	56,000,000	0.2%	26	Washington	365,000,000	1.2%
42	Nebraska	71,000,000	0.2%	27	Arizona	331,000,000	1.1%
35	Nevada	180,000,000	0.6%	28	Colorado	324,000,000	1.1%
37	New Hampshire	145,000,000	0.5%	29	Mississippi	293,000,000	1.0%
9	New Jersey	938,000,000	3.2%	30	Iowa	248,000,000	0.8%
38	New Mexico	143,000,000	0.5%	31	Arkansas	242,000,000	0.8%
1	New York	4,292,000,000	14.7%	32	Kansas	220,000,000	0.8%
10	North Carolina	934,000,000	3.2%	33	Maine	188,000,000	0.6%
48	North Dakota	20,000,000	0.1%	34	West Virginia	187,000,000	0.6%
5	Ohio	1,224,000,000	4.2%	35	Nevada	180,000,000	0.6%
23	Oklahoma	391,000,000	1.3%	36	Oregon	151,000,000	0.5%
36	Oregon	151,000,000	0.5%	37	New Hampshire	145,000,000	0.5%
6	Pennsylvania	1,109,000,000	3.8%	38	New Mexico	143,000,000	0.5%
40	Rhode Island	134,000,000	0.5%	39	Utah	136,000,000	0.5%
23	South Carolina	391,000,000	1.3%	40	Rhode Island	134,000,000	0.5%
49	South Dakota	11,000,000	0.0%	41	Delaware	110,000,000	0.4%
14	Tennessee	617,000,000	2.1%	42	Nebraska	71,000,000	0.2%
2	Texas	2,862,000,000	9.8%	43	Vermont	68,000,000	0.2%
39	Utah	136,000,000	0.5%	44	Hawaii	60,000,000	0.2%
43	Vermont	68,000,000	0.2%	44	Idaho	60,000,000	0.2%
18	Virginia	484,000,000	1.7%	46	Montana	56,000,000	0.2%
26	Washington	365,000,000	1.2%	47	Wyoming	24,000,000	0.1%
34	West Virginia	187,000,000	0.6%	48	North Dakota	20,000,000	0.1%
22	Wisconsin	393,000,000	1.3%	49	South Dakota	11,000,000	0.0%
47	Wyoming	24,000,000	0.1%	50	Alaska	9,000,000	0.0%
					District of Columbia	54,000,000	0.2%

Source: U.S. Department of Health and Human Services, Centers for Medicare and Medicaid Services "State Health Care Expenditures" (http://www.hcfa.gov/stats/nhe-oact/stateestimates/)
By state of provider. Includes spending for services and products by public and private freestanding home health agencies. Excludes home health care services provided by hospital-based agencies which are included in hospital expenditures.

Percent of Total Personal Health Care Expenditures
Spent on Home Health Care in 1998
National Percent = 2.9%*

ALPHA ORDER

RANK	STATE	PERCENT
19	Alabama	2.9
49	Alaska	0.4
32	Arizona	2.2
19	Arkansas	2.9
42	California	1.8
27	Colorado	2.4
3	Connecticut	3.9
8	Delaware	3.5
6	Florida	3.7
16	Georgia	3.0
46	Hawaii	1.3
42	Idaho	1.8
32	Illinois	2.2
37	Indiana	2.0
27	Iowa	2.4
30	Kansas	2.3
8	Kentucky	3.5
4	Louisiana	3.8
4	Maine	3.8
37	Maryland	2.0
11	Massachusetts	3.3
27	Michigan	2.4
36	Minnesota	2.1
11	Mississippi	3.3
24	Missouri	2.7
37	Montana	2.0
47	Nebraska	1.2
14	Nevada	3.2
15	New Hampshire	3.1
19	New Jersey	2.9
24	New Mexico	2.7
1	New York	5.0
10	North Carolina	3.4
48	North Dakota	0.7
19	Ohio	2.9
7	Oklahoma	3.6
45	Oregon	1.4
32	Pennsylvania	2.2
16	Rhode Island	3.0
16	South Carolina	3.0
49	South Dakota	0.4
23	Tennessee	2.8
2	Texas	4.2
30	Utah	2.3
11	Vermont	3.3
32	Virginia	2.2
41	Washington	1.9
24	West Virginia	2.7
37	Wisconsin	2.0
44	Wyoming	1.7

RANK ORDER

RANK	STATE	PERCENT
1	New York	5.0
2	Texas	4.2
3	Connecticut	3.9
4	Louisiana	3.8
4	Maine	3.8
6	Florida	3.7
7	Oklahoma	3.6
8	Delaware	3.5
8	Kentucky	3.5
10	North Carolina	3.4
11	Massachusetts	3.3
11	Mississippi	3.3
11	Vermont	3.3
14	Nevada	3.2
15	New Hampshire	3.1
16	Georgia	3.0
16	Rhode Island	3.0
16	South Carolina	3.0
19	Alabama	2.9
19	Arkansas	2.9
19	New Jersey	2.9
19	Ohio	2.9
23	Tennessee	2.8
24	Missouri	2.7
24	New Mexico	2.7
24	West Virginia	2.7
27	Colorado	2.4
27	Iowa	2.4
27	Michigan	2.4
30	Kansas	2.3
30	Utah	2.3
32	Arizona	2.2
32	Illinois	2.2
32	Pennsylvania	2.2
32	Virginia	2.2
36	Minnesota	2.1
37	Indiana	2.0
37	Maryland	2.0
37	Montana	2.0
37	Wisconsin	2.0
41	Washington	1.9
42	California	1.8
42	Idaho	1.8
44	Wyoming	1.7
45	Oregon	1.4
46	Hawaii	1.3
47	Nebraska	1.2
48	North Dakota	0.7
49	Alaska	0.4
49	South Dakota	0.4

District of Columbia 1.3

Source: MQ Press using data from U.S. Dept of Health & Human Services, Centers for Medicare and Medicaid Services "State Health Care Expenditures" (http://www.hcfa.gov/stats/nhe-oact/stateestimates/)
*By state of provider. Includes spending for services and products by public and private freestanding home health agencies. Excludes home health care services provided by hospital-based agencies which are included in hospital expenditures.

Average Annual Change in Expenditures for Home Health Care: 1990 to 1998

National Percent Change = 10.5% Average Annual Increase*

ALPHA ORDER			RANK ORDER		
RANK	STATE	PERCENT CHANGE	RANK	STATE	PERCENT CHANGE
31	Alabama	10.8	1	Hawaii	25.1
4	Alaska	20.7	2	Louisiana	21.3
25	Arizona	12.3	3	Utah	20.8
14	Arkansas	15.0	4	Alaska	20.7
33	California	10.5	5	New Mexico	20.1
17	Colorado	14.3	6	Idaho	18.9
32	Connecticut	10.7	7	Nevada	18.6
10	Delaware	17.2	8	Oklahoma	18.1
30	Florida	11.3	9	Texas	17.6
28	Georgia	11.5	10	Delaware	17.2
1	Hawaii	25.1	11	Ohio	15.7
6	Idaho	18.9	12	North Carolina	15.3
34	Illinois	10.4	13	Kentucky	15.2
21	Indiana	13.8	14	Arkansas	15.0
20	Iowa	14.0	15	New Hampshire	14.5
21	Kansas	13.8	16	Maine	14.4
13	Kentucky	15.2	17	Colorado	14.3
2	Louisiana	21.3	17	South Carolina	14.3
16	Maine	14.4	17	West Virginia	14.3
39	Maryland	9.5	20	Iowa	14.0
43	Massachusetts	8.5	21	Indiana	13.8
50	Michigan	4.6	21	Kansas	13.8
42	Minnesota	9.2	23	Missouri	13.6
41	Mississippi	9.4	24	Oregon	13.2
23	Missouri	13.6	25	Arizona	12.3
46	Montana	7.7	26	Virginia	11.8
36	Nebraska	10.1	27	Wyoming	11.6
7	Nevada	18.6	28	Georgia	11.5
15	New Hampshire	14.5	28	Rhode Island	11.5
38	New Jersey	9.6	30	Florida	11.3
5	New Mexico	20.1	31	Alabama	10.8
49	New York	4.7	32	Connecticut	10.7
12	North Carolina	15.3	33	California	10.5
45	North Dakota	7.8	34	Illinois	10.4
11	Ohio	15.7	34	South Dakota	10.4
8	Oklahoma	18.1	36	Nebraska	10.1
24	Oregon	13.2	37	Pennsylvania	9.9
37	Pennsylvania	9.9	38	New Jersey	9.6
28	Rhode Island	11.5	39	Maryland	9.5
17	South Carolina	14.3	39	Vermont	9.5
34	South Dakota	10.4	41	Mississippi	9.4
48	Tennessee	6.0	42	Minnesota	9.2
9	Texas	17.6	43	Massachusetts	8.5
3	Utah	20.8	43	Washington	8.5
39	Vermont	9.5	45	North Dakota	7.8
26	Virginia	11.8	46	Montana	7.7
43	Washington	8.5	47	Wisconsin	6.8
17	West Virginia	14.3	48	Tennessee	6.0
47	Wisconsin	6.8	49	New York	4.7
27	Wyoming	11.6	50	Michigan	4.6
				District of Columbia	6.0

Source: U.S. Department of Health and Human Services, Centers for Medicare and Medicaid Services "State Health Care Expenditures" (http://www.hcfa.gov/stats/nhe-oact/stateestimates/)

By state of provider. Includes spending for services and products by public and private freestanding home health agencies. Excludes home health care services provided by hospital-based agencies which are included in hospital expenditures.

Per Capita Expenditures for Home Health Care in 1998

National Per Capita = $108*

ALPHA ORDER

RANK	STATE	PER CAPITA
18	Alabama	$108
49	Alaska	15
36	Arizona	71
25	Arkansas	95
42	California	60
31	Colorado	82
2	Connecticut	183
6	Delaware	148
5	Florida	149
19	Georgia	106
43	Hawaii	50
45	Idaho	49
33	Illinois	81
38	Indiana	70
28	Iowa	87
30	Kansas	83
10	Kentucky	129
8	Louisiana	144
4	Maine	151
34	Maryland	76
3	Massachusetts	163
29	Michigan	86
27	Minnesota	89
19	Mississippi	106
21	Missouri	104
40	Montana	64
47	Nebraska	43
22	Nevada	103
12	New Hampshire	122
14	New Jersey	116
31	New Mexico	82
1	New York	236
11	North Carolina	124
48	North Dakota	31
17	Ohio	109
13	Oklahoma	117
46	Oregon	46
26	Pennsylvania	92
9	Rhode Island	136
24	South Carolina	102
49	South Dakota	15
16	Tennessee	114
7	Texas	145
39	Utah	65
15	Vermont	115
36	Virginia	71
40	Washington	64
22	West Virginia	103
35	Wisconsin	75
43	Wyoming	50

RANK ORDER

RANK	STATE	PER CAPITA
1	New York	$236
2	Connecticut	183
3	Massachusetts	163
4	Maine	151
5	Florida	149
6	Delaware	148
7	Texas	145
8	Louisiana	144
9	Rhode Island	136
10	Kentucky	129
11	North Carolina	124
12	New Hampshire	122
13	Oklahoma	117
14	New Jersey	116
15	Vermont	115
16	Tennessee	114
17	Ohio	109
18	Alabama	108
19	Georgia	106
19	Mississippi	106
21	Missouri	104
22	Nevada	103
22	West Virginia	103
24	South Carolina	102
25	Arkansas	95
26	Pennsylvania	92
27	Minnesota	89
28	Iowa	87
29	Michigan	86
30	Kansas	83
31	Colorado	82
31	New Mexico	82
33	Illinois	81
34	Maryland	76
35	Wisconsin	75
36	Arizona	71
36	Virginia	71
38	Indiana	70
39	Utah	65
40	Montana	64
40	Washington	64
42	California	60
43	Hawaii	50
43	Wyoming	50
45	Idaho	49
46	Oregon	46
47	Nebraska	43
48	North Dakota	31
49	Alaska	15
49	South Dakota	15
	District of Columbia	104

Source: MQ Press using data from U.S. Dept of Health & Human Services, Centers for Medicare and Medicaid Services
"State Health Care Expenditures" (http://www.hcfa.gov/stats/nhe-oact/stateestimates/)
*By state of provider. Includes spending for services and products by public and private freestanding home health agencies. Excludes home health care services provided by hospital-based agencies which are included in hospital expenditures.

Per Capita Medicare Expenditures for Home Health Care in 1998

National Per Capita = $38.27*

ALPHA ORDER

RANK	STATE	PER CAPITA
12	Alabama	$44.82
49	Alaska	6.50
38	Arizona	19.07
32	Arkansas	23.24
29	California	26.37
39	Colorado	18.90
4	Connecticut	75.78
20	Delaware	32.26
11	Florida	46.15
21	Georgia	31.82
45	Hawaii	8.40
37	Idaho	20.31
31	Illinois	25.02
27	Indiana	26.91
43	Iowa	13.28
35	Kansas	22.74
18	Kentucky	32.53
1	Louisiana	129.05
7	Maine	72.14
24	Maryland	30.60
10	Massachusetts	66.73
13	Michigan	39.00
42	Minnesota	13.96
8	Mississippi	71.24
33	Missouri	23.17
41	Montana	18.19
48	Nebraska	6.62
28	Nevada	26.38
14	New Hampshire	38.79
23	New Jersey	31.38
25	New Mexico	29.42
22	New York	31.44
17	North Carolina	33.26
50	North Dakota	6.27
26	Ohio	27.50
2	Oklahoma	89.83
46	Oregon	8.23
15	Pennsylvania	38.49
6	Rhode Island	72.90
19	South Carolina	32.30
47	South Dakota	8.21
5	Tennessee	73.63
3	Texas	85.02
30	Utah	26.18
9	Vermont	71.12
34	Virginia	23.12
44	Washington	9.85
16	West Virginia	34.77
36	Wisconsin	20.68
40	Wyoming	18.75

RANK ORDER

RANK	STATE	PER CAPITA
1	Louisiana	$129.05
2	Oklahoma	89.83
3	Texas	85.02
4	Connecticut	75.78
5	Tennessee	73.63
6	Rhode Island	72.90
7	Maine	72.14
8	Mississippi	71.24
9	Vermont	71.12
10	Massachusetts	66.73
11	Florida	46.15
12	Alabama	44.82
13	Michigan	39.00
14	New Hampshire	38.79
15	Pennsylvania	38.49
16	West Virginia	34.77
17	North Carolina	33.26
18	Kentucky	32.53
19	South Carolina	32.30
20	Delaware	32.26
21	Georgia	31.82
22	New York	31.44
23	New Jersey	31.38
24	Maryland	30.60
25	New Mexico	29.42
26	Ohio	27.50
27	Indiana	26.91
28	Nevada	26.38
29	California	26.37
30	Utah	26.18
31	Illinois	25.02
32	Arkansas	23.24
33	Missouri	23.17
34	Virginia	23.12
35	Kansas	22.74
36	Wisconsin	20.68
37	Idaho	20.31
38	Arizona	19.07
39	Colorado	18.90
40	Wyoming	18.75
41	Montana	18.19
42	Minnesota	13.96
43	Iowa	13.28
44	Washington	9.85
45	Hawaii	8.40
46	Oregon	8.23
47	South Dakota	8.21
48	Nebraska	6.62
49	Alaska	6.50
50	North Dakota	6.27

District of Columbia 51.78

Source: MQ Press using data from U.S. Dept of Health & Human Services, Centers for Medicare and Medicaid Services
"State Health Care Expenditures" (http://www.hcfa.gov/stats/nhe-oact/stateestimates/)
*By state of provider. Includes spending for services and products by public and private freestanding home health agencies. Excludes home health care services provided by hospital-based agencies which are included in hospital expenditures.

Per Capita Medicaid Expenditures for Home Health Care in 1998

National Per Capita = $18.48*

ALPHA ORDER				RANK ORDER		
RANK	STATE	PER CAPITA		RANK	STATE	PER CAPITA
34	Alabama	$4.37		1	New York	$102.10
40	Alaska	3.25		2	Connecticut	58.98
44	Arizona	1.93		3	Massachusetts	45.08
17	Arkansas	12.61		4	Minnesota	30.68
18	California	11.60		5	New Jersey	27.55
19	Colorado	11.59		6	Wisconsin	25.47
2	Connecticut	58.98		7	Michigan	24.03
9	Delaware	21.50		8	Maryland	23.78
26	Florida	5.77		9	Delaware	21.50
37	Georgia	3.54		10	Texas	21.36
45	Hawaii	1.68		11	West Virginia	20.42
23	Idaho	8.94		12	North Carolina	18.02
49	Illinois	0.66		13	Vermont	16.93
29	Indiana	5.08		14	Kentucky	15.25
21	Iowa	10.14		15	Maine	15.23
27	Kansas	5.31		16	Washington	13.89
14	Kentucky	15.25		17	Arkansas	12.61
32	Louisiana	4.81		18	California	11.60
15	Maine	15.23		19	Colorado	11.59
8	Maryland	23.78		20	Missouri	10.30
3	Massachusetts	45.08		21	Iowa	10.14
7	Michigan	24.03		22	Montana	9.10
4	Minnesota	30.68		23	Idaho	8.94
39	Mississippi	3.27		24	Oklahoma	7.49
20	Missouri	10.30		25	Pennsylvania	6.42
22	Montana	9.10		26	Florida	5.77
42	Nebraska	3.01		27	Kansas	5.31
33	Nevada	4.59		28	Oregon	5.18
30	New Hampshire	5.06		29	Indiana	5.08
5	New Jersey	27.55		30	New Hampshire	5.06
38	New Mexico	3.46		30	Rhode Island	5.06
1	New York	102.10		32	Louisiana	4.81
12	North Carolina	18.02		33	Nevada	4.59
50	North Dakota	0.00		34	Alabama	4.37
41	Ohio	3.03		35	Wyoming	4.17
24	Oklahoma	7.49		36	Tennessee	3.87
28	Oregon	5.18		37	Georgia	3.54
25	Pennsylvania	6.42		38	New Mexico	3.46
30	Rhode Island	5.06		39	Mississippi	3.27
43	South Carolina	2.86		40	Alaska	3.25
47	South Dakota	1.37		41	Ohio	3.03
36	Tennessee	3.87		42	Nebraska	3.01
10	Texas	21.36		43	South Carolina	2.86
46	Utah	1.43		44	Arizona	1.93
13	Vermont	16.93		45	Hawaii	1.68
48	Virginia	0.74		46	Utah	1.43
16	Washington	13.89		47	South Dakota	1.37
11	West Virginia	20.42		48	Virginia	0.74
6	Wisconsin	25.47		49	Illinois	0.66
35	Wyoming	4.17		50	North Dakota	0.00
					District of Columbia	30.69

Source: MQ Press using data from U.S. Dept of Health & Human Services, Centers for Medicare and Medicaid Services
  "State Health Care Expenditures" (http://www.hcfa.gov/stats/nhe-oact/stateestimates/)
*By state of provider. Includes spending for services and products by public and private freestanding home health
agencies. Excludes home health care services provided by hospital-based agencies which are included in hospital
expenditures.

Expenditures for Over-the-Counter Drugs and Other Medical Non-Durables in 1998
National Total = $121,906,000,000*

ALPHA ORDER

RANK ORDER

RANK	STATE	EXPENDITURES	% of USA	RANK	STATE	EXPENDITURES	% of USA
21	Alabama	$2,049,000,000	1.7%	1	California	$11,604,000,000	9.5%
49	Alaska	221,000,000	0.2%	2	New York	8,940,000,000	7.3%
20	Arizona	2,066,000,000	1.7%	3	Texas	8,672,000,000	7.1%
32	Arkansas	1,177,000,000	1.0%	4	Florida	8,226,000,000	6.7%
1	California	11,604,000,000	9.5%	5	Pennsylvania	6,162,000,000	5.1%
27	Colorado	1,546,000,000	1.3%	6	Illinois	5,174,000,000	4.2%
26	Connecticut	1,705,000,000	1.4%	7	Ohio	5,027,000,000	4.1%
44	Delaware	390,000,000	0.3%	8	Michigan	4,884,000,000	4.0%
4	Florida	8,226,000,000	6.7%	9	New Jersey	4,564,000,000	3.7%
11	Georgia	3,367,000,000	2.8%	10	North Carolina	3,411,000,000	2.8%
41	Hawaii	514,000,000	0.4%	11	Georgia	3,367,000,000	2.8%
43	Idaho	474,000,000	0.4%	12	Virginia	2,947,000,000	2.4%
6	Illinois	5,174,000,000	4.2%	13	Massachusetts	2,882,000,000	2.4%
15	Indiana	2,649,000,000	2.2%	14	Tennessee	2,751,000,000	2.3%
31	Iowa	1,219,000,000	1.0%	15	Indiana	2,649,000,000	2.2%
33	Kansas	1,087,000,000	0.9%	16	Missouri	2,403,000,000	2.0%
24	Kentucky	1,966,000,000	1.6%	17	Washington	2,365,000,000	1.9%
23	Louisiana	1,992,000,000	1.6%	18	Maryland	2,304,000,000	1.9%
39	Maine	559,000,000	0.5%	19	Wisconsin	2,269,000,000	1.9%
18	Maryland	2,304,000,000	1.9%	20	Arizona	2,066,000,000	1.7%
13	Massachusetts	2,882,000,000	2.4%	21	Alabama	2,049,000,000	1.7%
8	Michigan	4,884,000,000	4.0%	22	Minnesota	2,004,000,000	1.6%
22	Minnesota	2,004,000,000	1.6%	23	Louisiana	1,992,000,000	1.6%
30	Mississippi	1,222,000,000	1.0%	24	Kentucky	1,966,000,000	1.6%
16	Missouri	2,403,000,000	2.0%	25	South Carolina	1,721,000,000	1.4%
45	Montana	349,000,000	0.3%	26	Connecticut	1,705,000,000	1.4%
37	Nebraska	791,000,000	0.6%	27	Colorado	1,546,000,000	1.3%
36	Nevada	825,000,000	0.7%	28	Oklahoma	1,418,000,000	1.2%
40	New Hampshire	539,000,000	0.4%	29	Oregon	1,386,000,000	1.1%
9	New Jersey	4,564,000,000	3.7%	30	Mississippi	1,222,000,000	1.0%
38	New Mexico	630,000,000	0.5%	31	Iowa	1,219,000,000	1.0%
2	New York	8,940,000,000	7.3%	32	Arkansas	1,177,000,000	1.0%
10	North Carolina	3,411,000,000	2.8%	33	Kansas	1,087,000,000	0.9%
47	North Dakota	250,000,000	0.2%	34	West Virginia	949,000,000	0.8%
7	Ohio	5,027,000,000	4.1%	35	Utah	828,000,000	0.7%
28	Oklahoma	1,418,000,000	1.2%	36	Nevada	825,000,000	0.7%
29	Oregon	1,386,000,000	1.1%	37	Nebraska	791,000,000	0.6%
5	Pennsylvania	6,162,000,000	5.1%	38	New Mexico	630,000,000	0.5%
42	Rhode Island	505,000,000	0.4%	39	Maine	559,000,000	0.5%
25	South Carolina	1,721,000,000	1.4%	40	New Hampshire	539,000,000	0.4%
46	South Dakota	268,000,000	0.2%	41	Hawaii	514,000,000	0.4%
14	Tennessee	2,751,000,000	2.3%	42	Rhode Island	505,000,000	0.4%
3	Texas	8,672,000,000	7.1%	43	Idaho	474,000,000	0.4%
35	Utah	828,000,000	0.7%	44	Delaware	390,000,000	0.3%
48	Vermont	237,000,000	0.2%	45	Montana	349,000,000	0.3%
12	Virginia	2,947,000,000	2.4%	46	South Dakota	268,000,000	0.2%
17	Washington	2,365,000,000	1.9%	47	North Dakota	250,000,000	0.2%
34	West Virginia	949,000,000	0.8%	48	Vermont	237,000,000	0.2%
19	Wisconsin	2,269,000,000	1.9%	49	Alaska	221,000,000	0.2%
50	Wyoming	178,000,000	0.1%	50	Wyoming	178,000,000	0.1%
					District of Columbia	239,000,000	0.2%

Source: U.S. Department of Health and Human Services, Centers for Medicare and Medicaid Services
"State Health Care Expenditures" (http://www.hcfa.gov/stats/nhe-oact/stateestimates/)
*Purchases in retail outlets. By state of outlet. Includes over-the-counter drugs and sundries.

Percent of Total Personal Health Care Expenditures
Spent on Over-the-Counter Drugs and Other Medical Non-Durables in 1998
National Percent = 12.0%*

ALPHA ORDER

RANK	STATE	PERCENT
16	Alabama	12.8
47	Alaska	9.6
2	Arizona	14.0
5	Arkansas	13.9
44	California	10.5
40	Colorado	11.3
41	Connecticut	11.2
20	Delaware	12.6
7	Florida	13.8
24	Georgia	12.4
43	Hawaii	11.0
2	Idaho	14.0
32	Illinois	11.7
21	Indiana	12.5
28	Iowa	12.0
34	Kansas	11.6
10	Kentucky	13.6
27	Louisiana	12.1
38	Maine	11.4
32	Maryland	11.7
47	Massachusetts	9.6
9	Michigan	13.7
46	Minnesota	9.9
7	Mississippi	13.8
36	Missouri	11.5
25	Montana	12.3
13	Nebraska	13.0
1	Nevada	14.7
34	New Hampshire	11.6
2	New Jersey	14.0
30	New Mexico	11.8
45	New York	10.4
21	North Carolina	12.5
50	North Dakota	9.3
30	Ohio	11.8
15	Oklahoma	12.9
16	Oregon	12.8
28	Pennsylvania	12.0
41	Rhode Island	11.2
13	South Carolina	13.0
49	South Dakota	9.4
21	Tennessee	12.5
16	Texas	12.8
5	Utah	13.9
36	Vermont	11.5
12	Virginia	13.2
25	Washington	12.3
11	West Virginia	13.5
38	Wisconsin	11.4
19	Wyoming	12.7

RANK ORDER

RANK	STATE	PERCENT
1	Nevada	14.7
2	Arizona	14.0
2	Idaho	14.0
2	New Jersey	14.0
5	Arkansas	13.9
5	Utah	13.9
7	Florida	13.8
7	Mississippi	13.8
9	Michigan	13.7
10	Kentucky	13.6
11	West Virginia	13.5
12	Virginia	13.2
13	Nebraska	13.0
13	South Carolina	13.0
15	Oklahoma	12.9
16	Alabama	12.8
16	Oregon	12.8
16	Texas	12.8
19	Wyoming	12.7
20	Delaware	12.6
21	Indiana	12.5
21	North Carolina	12.5
21	Tennessee	12.5
24	Georgia	12.4
25	Montana	12.3
25	Washington	12.3
27	Louisiana	12.1
28	Iowa	12.0
28	Pennsylvania	12.0
30	New Mexico	11.8
30	Ohio	11.8
32	Illinois	11.7
32	Maryland	11.7
34	Kansas	11.6
34	New Hampshire	11.6
36	Missouri	11.5
36	Vermont	11.5
38	Maine	11.4
38	Wisconsin	11.4
40	Colorado	11.3
41	Connecticut	11.2
41	Rhode Island	11.2
43	Hawaii	11.0
44	California	10.5
45	New York	10.4
46	Minnesota	9.9
47	Alaska	9.6
47	Massachusetts	9.6
49	South Dakota	9.4
50	North Dakota	9.3

District of Columbia 5.6

Source: MQ Press using data from U.S. Dept of Health & Human Services, Centers for Medicare and Medicaid Services
"State Health Care Expenditures" (http://www.hcfa.gov/stats/nhe-oact/stateestimates/)
*Purchases in retail outlets. By state of outlet. Includes over-the-counter drugs and sundries.

Average Annual Change in Expenditures for Over-the-Counter Drugs and Other Medical Non-Durables: 1990 to 1998
National Percent Change = 9.3% Average Annual Increase*

<table>
<tr><td colspan="3">ALPHA ORDER</td><td colspan="3">RANK ORDER</td></tr>
<tr><td>RANK</td><td>STATE</td><td>PERCENT CHANGE</td><td>RANK</td><td>STATE</td><td>PERCENT CHANGE</td></tr>
<tr><td>23</td><td>Alabama</td><td>9.3</td><td>1</td><td>Nevada</td><td>14.3</td></tr>
<tr><td>47</td><td>Alaska</td><td>8.0</td><td>2</td><td>Florida</td><td>11.6</td></tr>
<tr><td>3</td><td>Arizona</td><td>11.4</td><td>3</td><td>Arizona</td><td>11.4</td></tr>
<tr><td>20</td><td>Arkansas</td><td>9.5</td><td>3</td><td>Delaware</td><td>11.4</td></tr>
<tr><td>49</td><td>California</td><td>7.1</td><td>5</td><td>Idaho</td><td>10.6</td></tr>
<tr><td>8</td><td>Colorado</td><td>10.4</td><td>5</td><td>Oregon</td><td>10.6</td></tr>
<tr><td>29</td><td>Connecticut</td><td>9.1</td><td>5</td><td>South Carolina</td><td>10.6</td></tr>
<tr><td>3</td><td>Delaware</td><td>11.4</td><td>8</td><td>Colorado</td><td>10.4</td></tr>
<tr><td>2</td><td>Florida</td><td>11.6</td><td>8</td><td>Maine</td><td>10.4</td></tr>
<tr><td>12</td><td>Georgia</td><td>10.2</td><td>8</td><td>North Carolina</td><td>10.4</td></tr>
<tr><td>50</td><td>Hawaii</td><td>5.6</td><td>11</td><td>Utah</td><td>10.3</td></tr>
<tr><td>5</td><td>Idaho</td><td>10.6</td><td>12</td><td>Georgia</td><td>10.2</td></tr>
<tr><td>40</td><td>Illinois</td><td>8.5</td><td>13</td><td>Nebraska</td><td>10.1</td></tr>
<tr><td>31</td><td>Indiana</td><td>8.9</td><td>14</td><td>Minnesota</td><td>10.0</td></tr>
<tr><td>31</td><td>Iowa</td><td>8.9</td><td>14</td><td>Tennessee</td><td>10.0</td></tr>
<tr><td>39</td><td>Kansas</td><td>8.6</td><td>16</td><td>New Jersey</td><td>9.9</td></tr>
<tr><td>17</td><td>Kentucky</td><td>9.6</td><td>17</td><td>Kentucky</td><td>9.6</td></tr>
<tr><td>44</td><td>Louisiana</td><td>8.2</td><td>17</td><td>Texas</td><td>9.6</td></tr>
<tr><td>8</td><td>Maine</td><td>10.4</td><td>17</td><td>Wisconsin</td><td>9.6</td></tr>
<tr><td>44</td><td>Maryland</td><td>8.2</td><td>20</td><td>Arkansas</td><td>9.5</td></tr>
<tr><td>37</td><td>Massachusetts</td><td>8.8</td><td>20</td><td>Pennsylvania</td><td>9.5</td></tr>
<tr><td>23</td><td>Michigan</td><td>9.3</td><td>22</td><td>New York</td><td>9.4</td></tr>
<tr><td>14</td><td>Minnesota</td><td>10.0</td><td>23</td><td>Alabama</td><td>9.3</td></tr>
<tr><td>23</td><td>Mississippi</td><td>9.3</td><td>23</td><td>Michigan</td><td>9.3</td></tr>
<tr><td>37</td><td>Missouri</td><td>8.8</td><td>23</td><td>Mississippi</td><td>9.3</td></tr>
<tr><td>27</td><td>Montana</td><td>9.2</td><td>23</td><td>Washington</td><td>9.3</td></tr>
<tr><td>13</td><td>Nebraska</td><td>10.1</td><td>27</td><td>Montana</td><td>9.2</td></tr>
<tr><td>1</td><td>Nevada</td><td>14.3</td><td>27</td><td>New Hampshire</td><td>9.2</td></tr>
<tr><td>27</td><td>New Hampshire</td><td>9.2</td><td>29</td><td>Connecticut</td><td>9.1</td></tr>
<tr><td>16</td><td>New Jersey</td><td>9.9</td><td>30</td><td>West Virginia</td><td>9.0</td></tr>
<tr><td>31</td><td>New Mexico</td><td>8.9</td><td>31</td><td>Indiana</td><td>8.9</td></tr>
<tr><td>22</td><td>New York</td><td>9.4</td><td>31</td><td>Iowa</td><td>8.9</td></tr>
<tr><td>8</td><td>North Carolina</td><td>10.4</td><td>31</td><td>New Mexico</td><td>8.9</td></tr>
<tr><td>48</td><td>North Dakota</td><td>7.6</td><td>31</td><td>Oklahoma</td><td>8.9</td></tr>
<tr><td>40</td><td>Ohio</td><td>8.5</td><td>31</td><td>Vermont</td><td>8.9</td></tr>
<tr><td>31</td><td>Oklahoma</td><td>8.9</td><td>31</td><td>Virginia</td><td>8.9</td></tr>
<tr><td>5</td><td>Oregon</td><td>10.6</td><td>37</td><td>Massachusetts</td><td>8.8</td></tr>
<tr><td>20</td><td>Pennsylvania</td><td>9.5</td><td>37</td><td>Missouri</td><td>8.8</td></tr>
<tr><td>40</td><td>Rhode Island</td><td>8.5</td><td>39</td><td>Kansas</td><td>8.6</td></tr>
<tr><td>5</td><td>South Carolina</td><td>10.6</td><td>40</td><td>Illinois</td><td>8.5</td></tr>
<tr><td>40</td><td>South Dakota</td><td>8.5</td><td>40</td><td>Ohio</td><td>8.5</td></tr>
<tr><td>14</td><td>Tennessee</td><td>10.0</td><td>40</td><td>Rhode Island</td><td>8.5</td></tr>
<tr><td>17</td><td>Texas</td><td>9.6</td><td>40</td><td>South Dakota</td><td>8.5</td></tr>
<tr><td>11</td><td>Utah</td><td>10.3</td><td>44</td><td>Louisiana</td><td>8.2</td></tr>
<tr><td>31</td><td>Vermont</td><td>8.9</td><td>44</td><td>Maryland</td><td>8.2</td></tr>
<tr><td>31</td><td>Virginia</td><td>8.9</td><td>44</td><td>Wyoming</td><td>8.2</td></tr>
<tr><td>23</td><td>Washington</td><td>9.3</td><td>47</td><td>Alaska</td><td>8.0</td></tr>
<tr><td>30</td><td>West Virginia</td><td>9.0</td><td>48</td><td>North Dakota</td><td>7.6</td></tr>
<tr><td>17</td><td>Wisconsin</td><td>9.6</td><td>49</td><td>California</td><td>7.1</td></tr>
<tr><td>44</td><td>Wyoming</td><td>8.2</td><td>50</td><td>Hawaii</td><td>5.6</td></tr>
<tr><td></td><td></td><td></td><td></td><td>District of Columbia</td><td>6.5</td></tr>
</table>

Source: U.S. Department of Health and Human Services, Centers for Medicare and Medicaid Services
"State Health Care Expenditures" (http://www.hcfa.gov/stats/nhe-oact/stateestimates/)
*Purchases in retail outlets. By state of outlet. Includes over-the-counter drugs and sundries.

Per Capita Expenditures for Over-the-Counter Drugs and Other Medical Non-Durables in 1998
National Per Capita = $451*

ALPHA ORDER

RANK	STATE	PER CAPITA
14	Alabama	$471
49	Alaska	359
26	Arizona	443
16	Arkansas	464
50	California	355
44	Colorado	390
5	Connecticut	521
3	Delaware	524
2	Florida	552
28	Georgia	441
32	Hawaii	432
45	Idaho	385
33	Illinois	429
21	Indiana	448
34	Iowa	426
39	Kansas	412
9	Kentucky	500
17	Louisiana	457
21	Maine	448
20	Maryland	449
15	Massachusetts	469
10	Michigan	497
36	Minnesota	424
25	Mississippi	444
27	Missouri	442
41	Montana	397
12	Nebraska	476
13	Nevada	473
18	New Hampshire	455
1	New Jersey	564
48	New Mexico	363
11	New York	492
19	North Carolina	452
43	North Dakota	392
24	Ohio	447
35	Oklahoma	425
37	Oregon	422
6	Pennsylvania	513
7	Rhode Island	511
21	South Carolina	448
47	South Dakota	367
8	Tennessee	506
29	Texas	440
42	Utah	394
40	Vermont	401
30	Virginia	434
38	Washington	416
3	West Virginia	524
30	Wisconsin	434
46	Wyoming	371

RANK ORDER

RANK	STATE	PER CAPITA
1	New Jersey	$564
2	Florida	552
3	Delaware	524
3	West Virginia	524
5	Connecticut	521
6	Pennsylvania	513
7	Rhode Island	511
8	Tennessee	506
9	Kentucky	500
10	Michigan	497
11	New York	492
12	Nebraska	476
13	Nevada	473
14	Alabama	471
15	Massachusetts	469
16	Arkansas	464
17	Louisiana	457
18	New Hampshire	455
19	North Carolina	452
20	Maryland	449
21	Indiana	448
21	Maine	448
21	South Carolina	448
24	Ohio	447
25	Mississippi	444
26	Arizona	443
27	Missouri	442
28	Georgia	441
29	Texas	440
30	Virginia	434
30	Wisconsin	434
32	Hawaii	432
33	Illinois	429
34	Iowa	426
35	Oklahoma	425
36	Minnesota	424
37	Oregon	422
38	Washington	416
39	Kansas	412
40	Vermont	401
41	Montana	397
42	Utah	394
43	North Dakota	392
44	Colorado	390
45	Idaho	385
46	Wyoming	371
47	South Dakota	367
48	New Mexico	363
49	Alaska	359
50	California	355
	District of Columbia	458

Source: MQ Press using data from U.S. Dept of Health & Human Services, Centers for Medicare and Medicaid Services "State Health Care Expenditures" (http://www.hcfa.gov/stats/nhe-oact/stateestimates/)
*Purchases in retail outlets. By state of outlet. Includes over-the-counter drugs and sundries. Per capita calculated using resident population. These figures may be skewed due to residents crossing state borders to make purchases.

Expenditures for Vision Products and Other Medical Durables in 1998

National Total = $15,499,000,000*

ALPHA ORDER

RANK	STATE	EXPENDITURES	% of USA
25	Alabama	$186,000,000	1.2%
46	Alaska	38,000,000	0.2%
22	Arizona	267,000,000	1.7%
36	Arkansas	87,000,000	0.6%
1	California	1,656,000,000	10.7%
18	Colorado	323,000,000	2.1%
23	Connecticut	231,000,000	1.5%
43	Delaware	49,000,000	0.3%
2	Florida	1,184,000,000	7.6%
10	Georgia	432,000,000	2.8%
38	Hawaii	78,000,000	0.5%
41	Idaho	59,000,000	0.4%
6	Illinois	662,000,000	4.3%
17	Indiana	328,000,000	2.1%
27	Iowa	177,000,000	1.1%
31	Kansas	128,000,000	0.8%
26	Kentucky	185,000,000	1.2%
24	Louisiana	198,000,000	1.3%
42	Maine	58,000,000	0.4%
19	Maryland	322,000,000	2.1%
12	Massachusetts	347,000,000	2.2%
8	Michigan	626,000,000	4.0%
14	Minnesota	343,000,000	2.2%
35	Mississippi	93,000,000	0.6%
20	Missouri	280,000,000	1.8%
44	Montana	41,000,000	0.3%
34	Nebraska	119,000,000	0.8%
32	Nevada	123,000,000	0.8%
40	New Hampshire	68,000,000	0.4%
9	New Jersey	552,000,000	3.6%
39	New Mexico	77,000,000	0.5%
4	New York	1,099,000,000	7.1%
15	North Carolina	338,000,000	2.2%
47	North Dakota	35,000,000	0.2%
7	Ohio	647,000,000	4.2%
30	Oklahoma	142,000,000	0.9%
28	Oregon	169,000,000	1.1%
5	Pennsylvania	688,000,000	4.4%
47	Rhode Island	35,000,000	0.2%
29	South Carolina	168,000,000	1.1%
45	South Dakota	40,000,000	0.3%
21	Tennessee	271,000,000	1.7%
3	Texas	1,176,000,000	7.6%
33	Utah	121,000,000	0.8%
49	Vermont	29,000,000	0.2%
11	Virginia	392,000,000	2.5%
13	Washington	346,000,000	2.2%
36	West Virginia	87,000,000	0.6%
16	Wisconsin	333,000,000	2.1%
50	Wyoming	22,000,000	0.1%

RANK ORDER

RANK	STATE	EXPENDITURES	% of USA
1	California	$1,656,000,000	10.7%
2	Florida	1,184,000,000	7.6%
3	Texas	1,176,000,000	7.6%
4	New York	1,099,000,000	7.1%
5	Pennsylvania	688,000,000	4.4%
6	Illinois	662,000,000	4.3%
7	Ohio	647,000,000	4.2%
8	Michigan	626,000,000	4.0%
9	New Jersey	552,000,000	3.6%
10	Georgia	432,000,000	2.8%
11	Virginia	392,000,000	2.5%
12	Massachusetts	347,000,000	2.2%
13	Washington	346,000,000	2.2%
14	Minnesota	343,000,000	2.2%
15	North Carolina	338,000,000	2.2%
16	Wisconsin	333,000,000	2.1%
17	Indiana	328,000,000	2.1%
18	Colorado	323,000,000	2.1%
19	Maryland	322,000,000	2.1%
20	Missouri	280,000,000	1.8%
21	Tennessee	271,000,000	1.7%
22	Arizona	267,000,000	1.7%
23	Connecticut	231,000,000	1.5%
24	Louisiana	198,000,000	1.3%
25	Alabama	186,000,000	1.2%
26	Kentucky	185,000,000	1.2%
27	Iowa	177,000,000	1.1%
28	Oregon	169,000,000	1.1%
29	South Carolina	168,000,000	1.1%
30	Oklahoma	142,000,000	0.9%
31	Kansas	128,000,000	0.8%
32	Nevada	123,000,000	0.8%
33	Utah	121,000,000	0.8%
34	Nebraska	119,000,000	0.8%
35	Mississippi	93,000,000	0.6%
36	Arkansas	87,000,000	0.6%
36	West Virginia	87,000,000	0.6%
38	Hawaii	78,000,000	0.5%
39	New Mexico	77,000,000	0.5%
40	New Hampshire	68,000,000	0.4%
41	Idaho	59,000,000	0.4%
42	Maine	58,000,000	0.4%
43	Delaware	49,000,000	0.3%
44	Montana	41,000,000	0.3%
45	South Dakota	40,000,000	0.3%
46	Alaska	38,000,000	0.2%
47	North Dakota	35,000,000	0.2%
47	Rhode Island	35,000,000	0.2%
49	Vermont	29,000,000	0.2%
50	Wyoming	22,000,000	0.1%
	District of Columbia	42,000,000	0.3%

Source: U.S. Department of Health and Human Services, Centers for Medicare and Medicaid Services
"State Health Care Expenditures" (http://www.hcfa.gov/stats/nhe-oact/stateestimates/)
*By state of provider. Includes eyeglasses, hearing aids, surgical appliances and supplies, bulk and cylinder oxygen and medical equipment rentals.

Percent of Total Personal Health Care Expenditures Spent on Vision Products and Other Medical Durables in 1998
National Percent = 1.5%*

ALPHA ORDER

RANK	STATE	PERCENT
41	Alabama	1.2
10	Alaska	1.7
6	Arizona	1.8
48	Arkansas	1.0
23	California	1.5
1	Colorado	2.4
23	Connecticut	1.5
18	Delaware	1.6
3	Florida	2.0
18	Georgia	1.6
10	Hawaii	1.7
10	Idaho	1.7
23	Illinois	1.5
23	Indiana	1.5
10	Iowa	1.7
29	Kansas	1.4
34	Kentucky	1.3
41	Louisiana	1.2
41	Maine	1.2
18	Maryland	1.6
41	Massachusetts	1.2
6	Michigan	1.8
10	Minnesota	1.7
48	Mississippi	1.0
34	Missouri	1.3
29	Montana	1.4
3	Nebraska	2.0
2	Nevada	2.2
23	New Hampshire	1.5
10	New Jersey	1.7
29	New Mexico	1.4
34	New York	1.3
41	North Carolina	1.2
34	North Dakota	1.3
23	Ohio	1.5
34	Oklahoma	1.3
18	Oregon	1.6
34	Pennsylvania	1.3
50	Rhode Island	0.8
34	South Carolina	1.3
29	South Dakota	1.4
41	Tennessee	1.2
10	Texas	1.7
3	Utah	2.0
29	Vermont	1.4
6	Virginia	1.8
6	Washington	1.8
41	West Virginia	1.2
10	Wisconsin	1.7
18	Wyoming	1.6

RANK ORDER

RANK	STATE	PERCENT
1	Colorado	2.4
2	Nevada	2.2
3	Florida	2.0
3	Nebraska	2.0
3	Utah	2.0
6	Arizona	1.8
6	Michigan	1.8
6	Virginia	1.8
6	Washington	1.8
10	Alaska	1.7
10	Hawaii	1.7
10	Idaho	1.7
10	Iowa	1.7
10	Minnesota	1.7
10	New Jersey	1.7
10	Texas	1.7
10	Wisconsin	1.7
18	Delaware	1.6
18	Georgia	1.6
18	Maryland	1.6
18	Oregon	1.6
18	Wyoming	1.6
23	California	1.5
23	Connecticut	1.5
23	Illinois	1.5
23	Indiana	1.5
23	New Hampshire	1.5
23	Ohio	1.5
29	Kansas	1.4
29	Montana	1.4
29	New Mexico	1.4
29	South Dakota	1.4
29	Vermont	1.4
34	Kentucky	1.3
34	Missouri	1.3
34	New York	1.3
34	North Dakota	1.3
34	Oklahoma	1.3
34	Pennsylvania	1.3
34	South Carolina	1.3
41	Alabama	1.2
41	Louisiana	1.2
41	Maine	1.2
41	Massachusetts	1.2
41	North Carolina	1.2
41	Tennessee	1.2
41	West Virginia	1.2
48	Arkansas	1.0
48	Mississippi	1.0
50	Rhode Island	0.8

| | District of Columbia | 1.0 |

Source: MQ Press using data from U.S. Dept of Health & Human Services, Centers for Medicare and Medicaid Services "State Health Care Expenditures" (http://www.hcfa.gov/stats/nhe-oact/stateestimates/)
*By state of provider. Includes eyeglasses, hearing aids, surgical appliances and supplies, bulk and cylinder oxygen and medical equipment rentals.

Average Annual Change in Expenditures for Vision Products and Other Medical Durables: 1990 to 1998
National Percent Change = 5.0% Average Annual Increase*

ALPHA ORDER

RANK	STATE	PERCENT CHANGE	RANK	STATE	PERCENT CHANGE
22	Alabama	5.2	1	Nevada	8.9
19	Alaska	5.4	2	Colorado	7.5
8	Arizona	6.4	2	Idaho	7.5
16	Arkansas	5.9	4	Oregon	7.0
45	California	4.0	5	Washington	6.6
2	Colorado	7.5	6	Mississippi	6.5
38	Connecticut	4.3	6	Utah	6.5
10	Delaware	6.3	8	Arizona	6.4
10	Florida	6.3	8	Georgia	6.4
8	Georgia	6.4	10	Delaware	6.3
41	Hawaii	4.2	10	Florida	6.3
2	Idaho	7.5	10	Texas	6.3
41	Illinois	4.2	13	New Hampshire	6.2
31	Indiana	4.7	13	South Carolina	6.2
38	Iowa	4.3	15	North Carolina	6.0
33	Kansas	4.5	16	Arkansas	5.9
17	Kentucky	5.6	17	Kentucky	5.6
27	Louisiana	4.9	17	Virginia	5.6
43	Maine	4.1	19	Alaska	5.4
32	Maryland	4.6	19	Wisconsin	5.4
29	Massachusetts	4.8	21	Tennessee	5.3
22	Michigan	5.2	22	Alabama	5.2
22	Minnesota	5.2	22	Michigan	5.2
6	Mississippi	6.5	22	Minnesota	5.2
35	Missouri	4.4	25	New Mexico	5.0
45	Montana	4.0	25	South Dakota	5.0
27	Nebraska	4.9	27	Louisiana	4.9
1	Nevada	8.9	27	Nebraska	4.9
13	New Hampshire	6.2	29	Massachusetts	4.8
33	New Jersey	4.5	29	Vermont	4.8
25	New Mexico	5.0	31	Indiana	4.7
49	New York	3.4	32	Maryland	4.6
15	North Carolina	6.0	33	Kansas	4.5
38	North Dakota	4.3	33	New Jersey	4.5
35	Ohio	4.4	35	Missouri	4.4
35	Oklahoma	4.4	35	Ohio	4.4
4	Oregon	7.0	35	Oklahoma	4.4
47	Pennsylvania	3.9	38	Connecticut	4.3
50	Rhode Island	3.3	38	Iowa	4.3
13	South Carolina	6.2	38	North Dakota	4.3
25	South Dakota	5.0	41	Hawaii	4.2
21	Tennessee	5.3	41	Illinois	4.2
10	Texas	6.3	43	Maine	4.1
6	Utah	6.5	43	Wyoming	4.1
29	Vermont	4.8	45	California	4.0
17	Virginia	5.6	45	Montana	4.0
5	Washington	6.6	47	Pennsylvania	3.9
48	West Virginia	3.7	48	West Virginia	3.7
19	Wisconsin	5.4	49	New York	3.4
43	Wyoming	4.1	50	Rhode Island	3.3
				District of Columbia	3.5

Source: U.S. Department of Health and Human Services, Centers for Medicare and Medicaid Services
    "State Health Care Expenditures" (http://www.hcfa.gov/stats/nhe-oact/stateestimates/)
*By state of provider. Includes eyeglasses, hearing aids, surgical appliances and supplies, bulk and cylinder oxygen and medical equipment rentals.

Per Capita Expenditures for Vision Products and Other Medical Durables in 1998

National Per Capita = $57*

<table>
<tr><th colspan="3">ALPHA ORDER</th><th colspan="3">RANK ORDER</th></tr>
<tr><th>RANK</th><th>STATE</th><th>PER CAPITA</th><th>RANK</th><th>STATE</th><th>PER CAPITA</th></tr>
<tr><td>46</td><td>Alabama</td><td>$43</td><td>1</td><td>Colorado</td><td>$81</td></tr>
<tr><td>13</td><td>Alaska</td><td>62</td><td>2</td><td>Florida</td><td>79</td></tr>
<tr><td>21</td><td>Arizona</td><td>57</td><td>3</td><td>Minnesota</td><td>73</td></tr>
<tr><td>49</td><td>Arkansas</td><td>34</td><td>4</td><td>Nebraska</td><td>72</td></tr>
<tr><td>30</td><td>California</td><td>51</td><td>5</td><td>Connecticut</td><td>71</td></tr>
<tr><td>1</td><td>Colorado</td><td>81</td><td>5</td><td>Nevada</td><td>71</td></tr>
<tr><td>5</td><td>Connecticut</td><td>71</td><td>7</td><td>New Jersey</td><td>68</td></tr>
<tr><td>8</td><td>Delaware</td><td>66</td><td>8</td><td>Delaware</td><td>66</td></tr>
<tr><td>2</td><td>Florida</td><td>79</td><td>8</td><td>Hawaii</td><td>66</td></tr>
<tr><td>21</td><td>Georgia</td><td>57</td><td>10</td><td>Michigan</td><td>64</td></tr>
<tr><td>8</td><td>Hawaii</td><td>66</td><td>10</td><td>Wisconsin</td><td>64</td></tr>
<tr><td>36</td><td>Idaho</td><td>48</td><td>12</td><td>Maryland</td><td>63</td></tr>
<tr><td>27</td><td>Illinois</td><td>55</td><td>13</td><td>Alaska</td><td>62</td></tr>
<tr><td>25</td><td>Indiana</td><td>56</td><td>13</td><td>Iowa</td><td>62</td></tr>
<tr><td>13</td><td>Iowa</td><td>62</td><td>15</td><td>New York</td><td>61</td></tr>
<tr><td>34</td><td>Kansas</td><td>49</td><td>15</td><td>Washington</td><td>61</td></tr>
<tr><td>38</td><td>Kentucky</td><td>47</td><td>17</td><td>Texas</td><td>60</td></tr>
<tr><td>42</td><td>Louisiana</td><td>45</td><td>18</td><td>Ohio</td><td>58</td></tr>
<tr><td>40</td><td>Maine</td><td>46</td><td>18</td><td>Utah</td><td>58</td></tr>
<tr><td>12</td><td>Maryland</td><td>63</td><td>18</td><td>Virginia</td><td>58</td></tr>
<tr><td>25</td><td>Massachusetts</td><td>56</td><td>21</td><td>Arizona</td><td>57</td></tr>
<tr><td>10</td><td>Michigan</td><td>64</td><td>21</td><td>Georgia</td><td>57</td></tr>
<tr><td>3</td><td>Minnesota</td><td>73</td><td>21</td><td>New Hampshire</td><td>57</td></tr>
<tr><td>49</td><td>Mississippi</td><td>34</td><td>21</td><td>Pennsylvania</td><td>57</td></tr>
<tr><td>30</td><td>Missouri</td><td>51</td><td>25</td><td>Indiana</td><td>56</td></tr>
<tr><td>38</td><td>Montana</td><td>47</td><td>25</td><td>Massachusetts</td><td>56</td></tr>
<tr><td>4</td><td>Nebraska</td><td>72</td><td>27</td><td>Illinois</td><td>55</td></tr>
<tr><td>5</td><td>Nevada</td><td>71</td><td>27</td><td>North Dakota</td><td>55</td></tr>
<tr><td>21</td><td>New Hampshire</td><td>57</td><td>27</td><td>South Dakota</td><td>55</td></tr>
<tr><td>7</td><td>New Jersey</td><td>68</td><td>30</td><td>California</td><td>51</td></tr>
<tr><td>44</td><td>New Mexico</td><td>44</td><td>30</td><td>Missouri</td><td>51</td></tr>
<tr><td>15</td><td>New York</td><td>61</td><td>30</td><td>Oregon</td><td>51</td></tr>
<tr><td>42</td><td>North Carolina</td><td>45</td><td>33</td><td>Tennessee</td><td>50</td></tr>
<tr><td>27</td><td>North Dakota</td><td>55</td><td>34</td><td>Kansas</td><td>49</td></tr>
<tr><td>18</td><td>Ohio</td><td>58</td><td>34</td><td>Vermont</td><td>49</td></tr>
<tr><td>46</td><td>Oklahoma</td><td>43</td><td>36</td><td>Idaho</td><td>48</td></tr>
<tr><td>30</td><td>Oregon</td><td>51</td><td>36</td><td>West Virginia</td><td>48</td></tr>
<tr><td>21</td><td>Pennsylvania</td><td>57</td><td>38</td><td>Kentucky</td><td>47</td></tr>
<tr><td>48</td><td>Rhode Island</td><td>35</td><td>38</td><td>Montana</td><td>47</td></tr>
<tr><td>44</td><td>South Carolina</td><td>44</td><td>40</td><td>Maine</td><td>46</td></tr>
<tr><td>27</td><td>South Dakota</td><td>55</td><td>40</td><td>Wyoming</td><td>46</td></tr>
<tr><td>33</td><td>Tennessee</td><td>50</td><td>42</td><td>Louisiana</td><td>45</td></tr>
<tr><td>17</td><td>Texas</td><td>60</td><td>42</td><td>North Carolina</td><td>45</td></tr>
<tr><td>18</td><td>Utah</td><td>58</td><td>44</td><td>New Mexico</td><td>44</td></tr>
<tr><td>34</td><td>Vermont</td><td>49</td><td>44</td><td>South Carolina</td><td>44</td></tr>
<tr><td>18</td><td>Virginia</td><td>58</td><td>46</td><td>Alabama</td><td>43</td></tr>
<tr><td>15</td><td>Washington</td><td>61</td><td>46</td><td>Oklahoma</td><td>43</td></tr>
<tr><td>36</td><td>West Virginia</td><td>48</td><td>48</td><td>Rhode Island</td><td>35</td></tr>
<tr><td>10</td><td>Wisconsin</td><td>64</td><td>49</td><td>Arkansas</td><td>34</td></tr>
<tr><td>40</td><td>Wyoming</td><td>46</td><td>49</td><td>Mississippi</td><td>34</td></tr>
<tr><td></td><td></td><td></td><td></td><td>District of Columbia</td><td>81</td></tr>
</table>

Source: MQ Press using data from U.S. Dept of Health & Human Services, Centers for Medicare and Medicaid Services
"State Health Care Expenditures" (http://www.hcfa.gov/stats/nhe-oact/stateestimates/)
*By state of provider. Includes eyeglasses, hearing aids, surgical appliances and supplies, bulk and cylinder
oxygen and medical equipment rentals.

Expenditures for Nursing Home Care in 1998

National Total = $87,826,000,000*

<table>
<tr><td colspan="4">ALPHA ORDER</td><td colspan="4">RANK ORDER</td></tr>
<tr><td>RANK</td><td>STATE</td><td>EXPENDITURES</td><td>% of USA</td><td>RANK</td><td>STATE</td><td>EXPENDITURES</td><td>% of USA</td></tr>
<tr><td>25</td><td>Alabama</td><td>$1,064,000,000</td><td>1.2%</td><td>1</td><td>New York</td><td>$10,586,000,000</td><td>12.1%</td></tr>
<tr><td>50</td><td>Alaska</td><td>42,000,000</td><td>0.0%</td><td>2</td><td>Pennsylvania</td><td>5,883,000,000</td><td>6.7%</td></tr>
<tr><td>30</td><td>Arizona</td><td>839,000,000</td><td>1.0%</td><td>3</td><td>California</td><td>5,626,000,000</td><td>6.4%</td></tr>
<tr><td>32</td><td>Arkansas</td><td>776,000,000</td><td>0.9%</td><td>4</td><td>Ohio</td><td>4,978,000,000</td><td>5.7%</td></tr>
<tr><td>3</td><td>California</td><td>5,626,000,000</td><td>6.4%</td><td>5</td><td>Florida</td><td>4,880,000,000</td><td>5.6%</td></tr>
<tr><td>29</td><td>Colorado</td><td>904,000,000</td><td>1.0%</td><td>6</td><td>Texas</td><td>4,346,000,000</td><td>4.9%</td></tr>
<tr><td>13</td><td>Connecticut</td><td>2,264,000,000</td><td>2.6%</td><td>7</td><td>Illinois</td><td>3,924,000,000</td><td>4.5%</td></tr>
<tr><td>40</td><td>Delaware</td><td>290,000,000</td><td>0.3%</td><td>8</td><td>Massachusetts</td><td>3,568,000,000</td><td>4.1%</td></tr>
<tr><td>5</td><td>Florida</td><td>4,880,000,000</td><td>5.6%</td><td>9</td><td>New Jersey</td><td>3,233,000,000</td><td>3.7%</td></tr>
<tr><td>20</td><td>Georgia</td><td>1,545,000,000</td><td>1.8%</td><td>10</td><td>Michigan</td><td>2,459,000,000</td><td>2.8%</td></tr>
<tr><td>46</td><td>Hawaii</td><td>204,000,000</td><td>0.2%</td><td>11</td><td>North Carolina</td><td>2,347,000,000</td><td>2.7%</td></tr>
<tr><td>43</td><td>Idaho</td><td>264,000,000</td><td>0.3%</td><td>12</td><td>Indiana</td><td>2,337,000,000</td><td>2.7%</td></tr>
<tr><td>7</td><td>Illinois</td><td>3,924,000,000</td><td>4.5%</td><td>13</td><td>Connecticut</td><td>2,264,000,000</td><td>2.6%</td></tr>
<tr><td>12</td><td>Indiana</td><td>2,337,000,000</td><td>2.7%</td><td>14</td><td>Wisconsin</td><td>2,110,000,000</td><td>2.4%</td></tr>
<tr><td>24</td><td>Iowa</td><td>1,186,000,000</td><td>1.4%</td><td>15</td><td>Missouri</td><td>2,002,000,000</td><td>2.3%</td></tr>
<tr><td>27</td><td>Kansas</td><td>920,000,000</td><td>1.0%</td><td>16</td><td>Tennessee</td><td>2,001,000,000</td><td>2.3%</td></tr>
<tr><td>22</td><td>Kentucky</td><td>1,283,000,000</td><td>1.5%</td><td>17</td><td>Minnesota</td><td>1,964,000,000</td><td>2.2%</td></tr>
<tr><td>23</td><td>Louisiana</td><td>1,248,000,000</td><td>1.4%</td><td>18</td><td>Maryland</td><td>1,695,000,000</td><td>1.9%</td></tr>
<tr><td>36</td><td>Maine</td><td>476,000,000</td><td>0.5%</td><td>19</td><td>Virginia</td><td>1,546,000,000</td><td>1.8%</td></tr>
<tr><td>18</td><td>Maryland</td><td>1,695,000,000</td><td>1.9%</td><td>20</td><td>Georgia</td><td>1,545,000,000</td><td>1.8%</td></tr>
<tr><td>8</td><td>Massachusetts</td><td>3,568,000,000</td><td>4.1%</td><td>21</td><td>Washington</td><td>1,492,000,000</td><td>1.7%</td></tr>
<tr><td>10</td><td>Michigan</td><td>2,459,000,000</td><td>2.8%</td><td>22</td><td>Kentucky</td><td>1,283,000,000</td><td>1.5%</td></tr>
<tr><td>17</td><td>Minnesota</td><td>1,964,000,000</td><td>2.2%</td><td>23</td><td>Louisiana</td><td>1,248,000,000</td><td>1.4%</td></tr>
<tr><td>34</td><td>Mississippi</td><td>687,000,000</td><td>0.8%</td><td>24</td><td>Iowa</td><td>1,186,000,000</td><td>1.4%</td></tr>
<tr><td>15</td><td>Missouri</td><td>2,002,000,000</td><td>2.3%</td><td>25</td><td>Alabama</td><td>1,064,000,000</td><td>1.2%</td></tr>
<tr><td>45</td><td>Montana</td><td>222,000,000</td><td>0.3%</td><td>26</td><td>Oklahoma</td><td>954,000,000</td><td>1.1%</td></tr>
<tr><td>33</td><td>Nebraska</td><td>697,000,000</td><td>0.8%</td><td>27</td><td>Kansas</td><td>920,000,000</td><td>1.0%</td></tr>
<tr><td>48</td><td>Nevada</td><td>164,000,000</td><td>0.2%</td><td>28</td><td>South Carolina</td><td>907,000,000</td><td>1.0%</td></tr>
<tr><td>38</td><td>New Hampshire</td><td>425,000,000</td><td>0.5%</td><td>29</td><td>Colorado</td><td>904,000,000</td><td>1.0%</td></tr>
<tr><td>9</td><td>New Jersey</td><td>3,233,000,000</td><td>3.7%</td><td>30</td><td>Arizona</td><td>839,000,000</td><td>1.0%</td></tr>
<tr><td>44</td><td>New Mexico</td><td>257,000,000</td><td>0.3%</td><td>31</td><td>Oregon</td><td>838,000,000</td><td>1.0%</td></tr>
<tr><td>1</td><td>New York</td><td>10,586,000,000</td><td>12.1%</td><td>32</td><td>Arkansas</td><td>776,000,000</td><td>0.9%</td></tr>
<tr><td>11</td><td>North Carolina</td><td>2,347,000,000</td><td>2.7%</td><td>33</td><td>Nebraska</td><td>697,000,000</td><td>0.8%</td></tr>
<tr><td>41</td><td>North Dakota</td><td>287,000,000</td><td>0.3%</td><td>34</td><td>Mississippi</td><td>687,000,000</td><td>0.8%</td></tr>
<tr><td>4</td><td>Ohio</td><td>4,978,000,000</td><td>5.7%</td><td>35</td><td>West Virginia</td><td>515,000,000</td><td>0.6%</td></tr>
<tr><td>26</td><td>Oklahoma</td><td>954,000,000</td><td>1.1%</td><td>36</td><td>Maine</td><td>476,000,000</td><td>0.5%</td></tr>
<tr><td>31</td><td>Oregon</td><td>838,000,000</td><td>1.0%</td><td>37</td><td>Rhode Island</td><td>468,000,000</td><td>0.5%</td></tr>
<tr><td>2</td><td>Pennsylvania</td><td>5,883,000,000</td><td>6.7%</td><td>38</td><td>New Hampshire</td><td>425,000,000</td><td>0.5%</td></tr>
<tr><td>37</td><td>Rhode Island</td><td>468,000,000</td><td>0.5%</td><td>39</td><td>Utah</td><td>300,000,000</td><td>0.3%</td></tr>
<tr><td>28</td><td>South Carolina</td><td>907,000,000</td><td>1.0%</td><td>40</td><td>Delaware</td><td>290,000,000</td><td>0.3%</td></tr>
<tr><td>42</td><td>South Dakota</td><td>286,000,000</td><td>0.3%</td><td>41</td><td>North Dakota</td><td>287,000,000</td><td>0.3%</td></tr>
<tr><td>16</td><td>Tennessee</td><td>2,001,000,000</td><td>2.3%</td><td>42</td><td>South Dakota</td><td>286,000,000</td><td>0.3%</td></tr>
<tr><td>6</td><td>Texas</td><td>4,346,000,000</td><td>4.9%</td><td>43</td><td>Idaho</td><td>264,000,000</td><td>0.3%</td></tr>
<tr><td>39</td><td>Utah</td><td>300,000,000</td><td>0.3%</td><td>44</td><td>New Mexico</td><td>257,000,000</td><td>0.3%</td></tr>
<tr><td>47</td><td>Vermont</td><td>177,000,000</td><td>0.2%</td><td>45</td><td>Montana</td><td>222,000,000</td><td>0.3%</td></tr>
<tr><td>19</td><td>Virginia</td><td>1,546,000,000</td><td>1.8%</td><td>46</td><td>Hawaii</td><td>204,000,000</td><td>0.2%</td></tr>
<tr><td>21</td><td>Washington</td><td>1,492,000,000</td><td>1.7%</td><td>47</td><td>Vermont</td><td>177,000,000</td><td>0.2%</td></tr>
<tr><td>35</td><td>West Virginia</td><td>515,000,000</td><td>0.6%</td><td>48</td><td>Nevada</td><td>164,000,000</td><td>0.2%</td></tr>
<tr><td>14</td><td>Wisconsin</td><td>2,110,000,000</td><td>2.4%</td><td>49</td><td>Wyoming</td><td>113,000,000</td><td>0.1%</td></tr>
<tr><td>49</td><td>Wyoming</td><td>113,000,000</td><td>0.1%</td><td>50</td><td>Alaska</td><td>42,000,000</td><td>0.0%</td></tr>
<tr><td></td><td></td><td></td><td></td><td></td><td>District of Columbia</td><td>245,000,000</td><td>0.3%</td></tr>
</table>

Source: U.S. Department of Health and Human Services, Centers for Medicare and Medicaid Services
"State Health Care Expenditures" (http://www.hcfa.gov/stats/nhe-oact/stateestimates/)
*By state of provider. Includes freestanding nursing and personal-care facilities. Includes Medicare- and Medicaid-certified skilled nursing and intermediate care facilities as well as facilities that are not certified. Excludes hospital-based facilities as they are counted in hospital care expenditures.

Percent of Total Personal Health Care Expenditures
Spent on Nursing Home Care in 1998
National Percent = 8.6%*

RANK	STATE	PERCENT
40	Alabama	6.6
50	Alaska	1.8
43	Arizona	5.7
19	Arkansas	9.2
45	California	5.1
40	Colorado	6.6
1	Connecticut	14.9
18	Delaware	9.3
28	Florida	8.2
43	Georgia	5.7
48	Hawaii	4.4
30	Idaho	7.8
22	Illinois	8.9
8	Indiana	11.0
5	Iowa	11.6
14	Kansas	9.8
22	Kentucky	8.9
35	Louisiana	7.6
15	Maine	9.7
25	Maryland	8.6
3	Massachusetts	11.9
37	Michigan	6.9
15	Minnesota	9.7
32	Mississippi	7.7
17	Missouri	9.6
30	Montana	7.8
7	Nebraska	11.4
49	Nevada	2.9
20	New Hampshire	9.1
13	New Jersey	9.9
47	New Mexico	4.8
2	New York	12.3
25	North Carolina	8.6
9	North Dakota	10.7
4	Ohio	11.7
24	Oklahoma	8.7
32	Oregon	7.7
6	Pennsylvania	11.5
11	Rhode Island	10.4
37	South Carolina	6.9
12	South Dakota	10.1
20	Tennessee	9.1
42	Texas	6.4
46	Utah	5.0
25	Vermont	8.6
37	Virginia	6.9
32	Washington	7.7
36	West Virginia	7.3
10	Wisconsin	10.6
29	Wyoming	8.0

RANK	STATE	PERCENT
1	Connecticut	14.9
2	New York	12.3
3	Massachusetts	11.9
4	Ohio	11.7
5	Iowa	11.6
6	Pennsylvania	11.5
7	Nebraska	11.4
8	Indiana	11.0
9	North Dakota	10.7
10	Wisconsin	10.6
11	Rhode Island	10.4
12	South Dakota	10.1
13	New Jersey	9.9
14	Kansas	9.8
15	Maine	9.7
15	Minnesota	9.7
17	Missouri	9.6
18	Delaware	9.3
19	Arkansas	9.2
20	New Hampshire	9.1
20	Tennessee	9.1
22	Illinois	8.9
22	Kentucky	8.9
24	Oklahoma	8.7
25	Maryland	8.6
25	North Carolina	8.6
25	Vermont	8.6
28	Florida	8.2
29	Wyoming	8.0
30	Idaho	7.8
30	Montana	7.8
32	Mississippi	7.7
32	Oregon	7.7
32	Washington	7.7
35	Louisiana	7.6
36	West Virginia	7.3
37	Michigan	6.9
37	South Carolina	6.9
37	Virginia	6.9
40	Alabama	6.6
40	Colorado	6.6
42	Texas	6.4
43	Arizona	5.7
43	Georgia	5.7
45	California	5.1
46	Utah	5.0
47	New Mexico	4.8
48	Hawaii	4.4
49	Nevada	2.9
50	Alaska	1.8

District of Columbia 5.8

Source: MQ Press using data from U.S. Dept of Health & Human Services, Centers for Medicare and Medicaid Services "State Health Care Expenditures" (http://www.hcfa.gov/stats/nhe-oact/stateestimates/)
By state of provider. Includes freestanding nursing and personal-care facilities. Includes Medicare- and Medicaid-certified skilled nursing and intermediate care facilities as well as facilities that are not certified. Excludes hospital-based facilities as they are counted in hospital care expenditures.

Average Annual Change in Expenditures for Nursing Home Care: 1990 to 1998

National Percent Change = 7.1% Average Annual Increase*

ALPHA ORDER

RANK	STATE	PERCENT CHANGE
5	Alabama	10.1
50	Alaska	(0.9)
14	Arizona	8.2
20	Arkansas	7.7
24	California	6.8
22	Colorado	7.3
32	Connecticut	6.1
27	Delaware	6.7
3	Florida	10.2
10	Georgia	9.0
41	Hawaii	4.9
9	Idaho	9.2
24	Illinois	6.8
36	Indiana	5.9
29	Iowa	6.2
32	Kansas	6.1
8	Kentucky	9.5
36	Louisiana	5.9
47	Maine	3.6
16	Maryland	7.9
42	Massachusetts	4.8
28	Michigan	6.4
47	Minnesota	3.6
2	Mississippi	10.5
19	Missouri	7.8
42	Montana	4.8
16	Nebraska	7.9
40	Nevada	5.0
11	New Hampshire	8.8
15	New Jersey	8.1
34	New Mexico	6.0
39	New York	5.3
3	North Carolina	10.2
45	North Dakota	4.6
22	Ohio	7.3
29	Oklahoma	6.2
34	Oregon	6.0
21	Pennsylvania	7.6
49	Rhode Island	2.8
16	South Carolina	7.9
24	South Dakota	6.8
1	Tennessee	12.7
13	Texas	8.4
44	Utah	4.7
46	Vermont	3.9
6	Virginia	9.7
29	Washington	6.2
12	West Virginia	8.7
38	Wisconsin	5.4
6	Wyoming	9.7

RANK ORDER

RANK	STATE	PERCENT CHANGE
1	Tennessee	12.7
2	Mississippi	10.5
3	Florida	10.2
3	North Carolina	10.2
5	Alabama	10.1
6	Virginia	9.7
6	Wyoming	9.7
8	Kentucky	9.5
9	Idaho	9.2
10	Georgia	9.0
11	New Hampshire	8.8
12	West Virginia	8.7
13	Texas	8.4
14	Arizona	8.2
15	New Jersey	8.1
16	Maryland	7.9
16	Nebraska	7.9
16	South Carolina	7.9
19	Missouri	7.8
20	Arkansas	7.7
21	Pennsylvania	7.6
22	Colorado	7.3
22	Ohio	7.3
24	California	6.8
24	Illinois	6.8
24	South Dakota	6.8
27	Delaware	6.7
28	Michigan	6.4
29	Iowa	6.2
29	Oklahoma	6.2
29	Washington	6.2
32	Connecticut	6.1
32	Kansas	6.1
34	New Mexico	6.0
34	Oregon	6.0
36	Indiana	5.9
36	Louisiana	5.9
38	Wisconsin	5.4
39	New York	5.3
40	Nevada	5.0
41	Hawaii	4.9
42	Massachusetts	4.8
42	Montana	4.8
44	Utah	4.7
45	North Dakota	4.6
46	Vermont	3.9
47	Maine	3.6
47	Minnesota	3.6
49	Rhode Island	2.8
50	Alaska	(0.9)
	District of Columbia	7.2

Source: U.S. Department of Health and Human Services, Centers for Medicare and Medicaid Services "State Health Care Expenditures" (http://www.hcfa.gov/stats/nhe-oact/stateestimates/)
By state of provider. Includes freestanding nursing and personal-care facilities. Includes Medicare- and Medicaid-certified skilled nursing and intermediate care facilities as well as facilities that are not certified. Excludes hospital-based facilities as they are counted in hospital care expenditures.

Per Capita Expenditures for Nursing Home Care in 1998

National Per Capita = $325*

ALPHA ORDER

RANK	STATE	PER CAPITA
36	Alabama	$245
50	Alaska	68
44	Arizona	180
26	Arkansas	306
45	California	172
39	Colorado	228
1	Connecticut	692
15	Delaware	390
22	Florida	327
43	Georgia	202
46	Hawaii	171
42	Idaho	214
24	Illinois	325
13	Indiana	396
10	Iowa	415
20	Kansas	349
23	Kentucky	326
28	Louisiana	286
16	Maine	382
21	Maryland	330
3	Massachusetts	581
34	Michigan	250
9	Minnesota	416
34	Mississippi	250
17	Missouri	368
33	Montana	252
8	Nebraska	420
49	Nevada	94
19	New Hampshire	358
12	New Jersey	399
47	New Mexico	148
2	New York	583
25	North Carolina	311
6	North Dakota	450
7	Ohio	443
28	Oklahoma	286
32	Oregon	255
4	Pennsylvania	490
5	Rhode Island	474
37	South Carolina	236
14	South Dakota	391
17	Tennessee	368
41	Texas	220
48	Utah	143
27	Vermont	300
39	Virginia	228
31	Washington	262
30	West Virginia	284
11	Wisconsin	404
38	Wyoming	235

RANK ORDER

RANK	STATE	PER CAPITA
1	Connecticut	$692
2	New York	583
3	Massachusetts	581
4	Pennsylvania	490
5	Rhode Island	474
6	North Dakota	450
7	Ohio	443
8	Nebraska	420
9	Minnesota	416
10	Iowa	415
11	Wisconsin	404
12	New Jersey	399
13	Indiana	396
14	South Dakota	391
15	Delaware	390
16	Maine	382
17	Missouri	368
17	Tennessee	368
19	New Hampshire	358
20	Kansas	349
21	Maryland	330
22	Florida	327
23	Kentucky	326
24	Illinois	325
25	North Carolina	311
26	Arkansas	306
27	Vermont	300
28	Louisiana	286
28	Oklahoma	286
30	West Virginia	284
31	Washington	262
32	Oregon	255
33	Montana	252
34	Michigan	250
34	Mississippi	250
36	Alabama	245
37	South Carolina	236
38	Wyoming	235
39	Colorado	228
39	Virginia	228
41	Texas	220
42	Idaho	214
43	Georgia	202
44	Arizona	180
45	California	172
46	Hawaii	171
47	New Mexico	148
48	Utah	143
49	Nevada	94
50	Alaska	68
	District of Columbia	470

Source: MQ Press using data from U.S. Dept of Health & Human Services, Centers for Medicare and Medicaid Services "State Health Care Expenditures" (http://www.hcfa.gov/stats/nhe-oact/stateestimates/)
*By state of provider. Includes freestanding nursing and personal-care facilities. Includes Medicare- and Medicaid-certified skilled nursing and intermediate care facilities as well as facilities that are not certified. Excludes hospital-based facilities as they are counted in hospital care expenditures.

Per Capita Medicare Expenditures for Nursing Home Care in 1998

National Per Capita = $38.62*

ALPHA ORDER

RANK	STATE	PER CAPITA
14	Alabama	$39.07
50	Alaska	3.25
26	Arizona	31.71
30	Arkansas	29.15
27	California	30.66
17	Colorado	37.04
1	Connecticut	89.84
23	Delaware	33.60
4	Florida	67.81
35	Georgia	27.63
49	Hawaii	10.92
21	Idaho	34.12
33	Illinois	28.50
6	Indiana	49.43
44	Iowa	22.02
37	Kansas	26.91
34	Kentucky	28.47
46	Louisiana	20.86
11	Maine	44.89
20	Maryland	34.50
2	Massachusetts	71.12
16	Michigan	37.37
24	Minnesota	33.01
40	Mississippi	25.08
19	Missouri	35.13
42	Montana	22.74
39	Nebraska	25.89
47	Nevada	20.64
12	New Hampshire	43.01
9	New Jersey	47.43
45	New Mexico	21.92
10	New York	47.41
22	North Carolina	33.66
48	North Dakota	15.68
8	Ohio	47.70
43	Oklahoma	22.46
36	Oregon	27.42
7	Pennsylvania	48.16
3	Rhode Island	70.87
28	South Carolina	29.69
18	South Dakota	35.58
15	Tennessee	38.84
25	Texas	32.01
41	Utah	23.33
31	Vermont	28.79
38	Virginia	26.81
13	Washington	41.84
32	West Virginia	28.70
5	Wisconsin	54.00
29	Wyoming	29.16

RANK ORDER

RANK	STATE	PER CAPITA
1	Connecticut	$89.84
2	Massachusetts	71.12
3	Rhode Island	70.87
4	Florida	67.81
5	Wisconsin	54.00
6	Indiana	49.43
7	Pennsylvania	48.16
8	Ohio	47.70
9	New Jersey	47.43
10	New York	47.41
11	Maine	44.89
12	New Hampshire	43.01
13	Washington	41.84
14	Alabama	39.07
15	Tennessee	38.84
16	Michigan	37.37
17	Colorado	37.04
18	South Dakota	35.58
19	Missouri	35.13
20	Maryland	34.50
21	Idaho	34.12
22	North Carolina	33.66
23	Delaware	33.60
24	Minnesota	33.01
25	Texas	32.01
26	Arizona	31.71
27	California	30.66
28	South Carolina	29.69
29	Wyoming	29.16
30	Arkansas	29.15
31	Vermont	28.79
32	West Virginia	28.70
33	Illinois	28.50
34	Kentucky	28.47
35	Georgia	27.63
36	Oregon	27.42
37	Kansas	26.91
38	Virginia	26.81
39	Nebraska	25.89
40	Mississippi	25.08
41	Utah	23.33
42	Montana	22.74
43	Oklahoma	22.46
44	Iowa	22.02
45	New Mexico	21.92
46	Louisiana	20.86
47	Nevada	20.64
48	North Dakota	15.68
49	Hawaii	10.92
50	Alaska	3.25

District of Columbia   23.01

Source: MQ Press using data from U.S. Dept of Health & Human Services, Centers for Medicare and Medicaid Services "State Health Care Expenditures" (http://www.hcfa.gov/stats/nhe-oact/stateestimates/)
*By state of provider. Includes freestanding nursing and personal-care facilities. Includes Medicare-certified skilled nursing and intermediate care facilities as well as facilities that are not certified. Excludes hospital-based facilities as they are counted in hospital care expenditures.

Per Capita Medicaid Expenditures for Nursing Home Care in 1998

National Per Capita = $150*

<table>
<tr><td colspan="3"><u>ALPHA ORDER</u></td><td colspan="3"><u>RANK ORDER</u></td></tr>
<tr><th>RANK</th><th>STATE</th><th>PER CAPITA</th><th>RANK</th><th>STATE</th><th>PER CAPITA</th></tr>
<tr><td>31</td><td>Alabama</td><td>$128</td><td>1</td><td>New York</td><td>$417</td></tr>
<tr><td>47</td><td>Alaska</td><td>60</td><td>2</td><td>Connecticut</td><td>317</td></tr>
<tr><td>50</td><td>Arizona</td><td>3</td><td>3</td><td>Pennsylvania</td><td>275</td></tr>
<tr><td>24</td><td>Arkansas</td><td>136</td><td>4</td><td>Massachusetts</td><td>239</td></tr>
<tr><td>49</td><td>California</td><td>46</td><td>5</td><td>Rhode Island</td><td>227</td></tr>
<tr><td>44</td><td>Colorado</td><td>73</td><td>6</td><td>North Dakota</td><td>198</td></tr>
<tr><td>2</td><td>Connecticut</td><td>317</td><td>7</td><td>Ohio</td><td>194</td></tr>
<tr><td>20</td><td>Delaware</td><td>155</td><td>8</td><td>Minnesota</td><td>189</td></tr>
<tr><td>38</td><td>Florida</td><td>104</td><td>8</td><td>Wisconsin</td><td>189</td></tr>
<tr><td>41</td><td>Georgia</td><td>86</td><td>10</td><td>Louisiana</td><td>188</td></tr>
<tr><td>28</td><td>Hawaii</td><td>131</td><td>10</td><td>Nebraska</td><td>188</td></tr>
<tr><td>36</td><td>Idaho</td><td>107</td><td>12</td><td>New Jersey</td><td>185</td></tr>
<tr><td>22</td><td>Illinois</td><td>146</td><td>13</td><td>Maine</td><td>180</td></tr>
<tr><td>19</td><td>Indiana</td><td>159</td><td>14</td><td>New Hampshire</td><td>175</td></tr>
<tr><td>15</td><td>Iowa</td><td>174</td><td>15</td><td>Iowa</td><td>174</td></tr>
<tr><td>36</td><td>Kansas</td><td>107</td><td>16</td><td>Tennessee</td><td>172</td></tr>
<tr><td>27</td><td>Kentucky</td><td>133</td><td>17</td><td>South Dakota</td><td>170</td></tr>
<tr><td>10</td><td>Louisiana</td><td>188</td><td>18</td><td>West Virginia</td><td>166</td></tr>
<tr><td>13</td><td>Maine</td><td>180</td><td>19</td><td>Indiana</td><td>159</td></tr>
<tr><td>33</td><td>Maryland</td><td>116</td><td>20</td><td>Delaware</td><td>155</td></tr>
<tr><td>4</td><td>Massachusetts</td><td>239</td><td>21</td><td>Missouri</td><td>153</td></tr>
<tr><td>25</td><td>Michigan</td><td>135</td><td>22</td><td>Illinois</td><td>146</td></tr>
<tr><td>8</td><td>Minnesota</td><td>189</td><td>23</td><td>North Carolina</td><td>137</td></tr>
<tr><td>25</td><td>Mississippi</td><td>135</td><td>24</td><td>Arkansas</td><td>136</td></tr>
<tr><td>21</td><td>Missouri</td><td>153</td><td>25</td><td>Michigan</td><td>135</td></tr>
<tr><td>42</td><td>Montana</td><td>80</td><td>25</td><td>Mississippi</td><td>135</td></tr>
<tr><td>10</td><td>Nebraska</td><td>188</td><td>27</td><td>Kentucky</td><td>133</td></tr>
<tr><td>48</td><td>Nevada</td><td>53</td><td>28</td><td>Hawaii</td><td>131</td></tr>
<tr><td>14</td><td>New Hampshire</td><td>175</td><td>28</td><td>Wyoming</td><td>131</td></tr>
<tr><td>12</td><td>New Jersey</td><td>185</td><td>30</td><td>Vermont</td><td>129</td></tr>
<tr><td>40</td><td>New Mexico</td><td>88</td><td>31</td><td>Alabama</td><td>128</td></tr>
<tr><td>1</td><td>New York</td><td>417</td><td>31</td><td>Oklahoma</td><td>128</td></tr>
<tr><td>23</td><td>North Carolina</td><td>137</td><td>33</td><td>Maryland</td><td>116</td></tr>
<tr><td>6</td><td>North Dakota</td><td>198</td><td>34</td><td>South Carolina</td><td>115</td></tr>
<tr><td>7</td><td>Ohio</td><td>194</td><td>35</td><td>Washington</td><td>111</td></tr>
<tr><td>31</td><td>Oklahoma</td><td>128</td><td>36</td><td>Idaho</td><td>107</td></tr>
<tr><td>43</td><td>Oregon</td><td>79</td><td>36</td><td>Kansas</td><td>107</td></tr>
<tr><td>3</td><td>Pennsylvania</td><td>275</td><td>38</td><td>Florida</td><td>104</td></tr>
<tr><td>5</td><td>Rhode Island</td><td>227</td><td>39</td><td>Texas</td><td>97</td></tr>
<tr><td>34</td><td>South Carolina</td><td>115</td><td>40</td><td>New Mexico</td><td>88</td></tr>
<tr><td>17</td><td>South Dakota</td><td>170</td><td>41</td><td>Georgia</td><td>86</td></tr>
<tr><td>16</td><td>Tennessee</td><td>172</td><td>42</td><td>Montana</td><td>80</td></tr>
<tr><td>39</td><td>Texas</td><td>97</td><td>43</td><td>Oregon</td><td>79</td></tr>
<tr><td>46</td><td>Utah</td><td>62</td><td>44</td><td>Colorado</td><td>73</td></tr>
<tr><td>30</td><td>Vermont</td><td>129</td><td>45</td><td>Virginia</td><td>68</td></tr>
<tr><td>45</td><td>Virginia</td><td>68</td><td>46</td><td>Utah</td><td>62</td></tr>
<tr><td>35</td><td>Washington</td><td>111</td><td>47</td><td>Alaska</td><td>60</td></tr>
<tr><td>18</td><td>West Virginia</td><td>166</td><td>48</td><td>Nevada</td><td>53</td></tr>
<tr><td>8</td><td>Wisconsin</td><td>189</td><td>49</td><td>California</td><td>46</td></tr>
<tr><td>28</td><td>Wyoming</td><td>131</td><td>50</td><td>Arizona</td><td>3</td></tr>
<tr><td></td><td></td><td></td><td></td><td>District of Columbia</td><td>407</td></tr>
</table>

Source: MQ Press using data from U.S. Dept of Health & Human Services, Centers for Medicare and Medicaid Services "State Health Care Expenditures" (http://www.hcfa.gov/stats/nhe-oact/stateestimates/)

*By state of provider. Includes freestanding nursing and personal-care facilities. Includes Medicaid-certified skilled nursing and intermediate care facilities as well as facilities that are not certified. Excludes hospital-based facilities as they are counted in hospital care expenditures.

Estimated State Funds from the Tobacco Settlement Through 2025

National Total = $195,918,675,920*

ALPHA ORDER

RANK	STATE	FUNDS	% of USA
21	Alabama	$3,166,302,119	1.6%
45	Alaska	668,903,057	0.3%
22	Arizona	2,887,614,909	1.5%
30	Arkansas	1,622,336,126	0.8%
1	California	25,006,972,511	12.8%
23	Colorado	2,685,773,549	1.4%
19	Connecticut	3,637,303,382	1.9%
41	Delaware	774,798,677	0.4%
NA	Florida**	NA	NA
9	Georgia	4,808,740,669	2.5%
35	Hawaii	1,179,165,923	0.6%
43	Idaho	711,700,479	0.4%
5	Illinois	9,118,539,559	4.7%
18	Indiana	3,996,355,551	2.0%
28	Iowa	1,703,839,986	0.9%
29	Kansas	1,633,317,646	0.8%
20	Kentucky	3,450,438,586	1.8%
14	Louisiana	4,418,657,915	2.3%
31	Maine	1,507,301,276	0.8%
13	Maryland	4,428,657,384	2.3%
7	Massachusetts	7,913,114,213	4.0%
6	Michigan	8,526,278,034	4.4%
NA	Minnesota**	NA	NA
NA	Mississippi**	NA	NA
12	Missouri	4,456,368,286	2.3%
39	Montana	832,182,431	0.4%
37	Nebraska	1,165,683,457	0.6%
34	Nevada	1,194,976,855	0.6%
33	New Hampshire	1,304,689,150	0.7%
8	New Jersey	7,576,167,918	3.9%
36	New Mexico	1,168,438,809	0.6%
2	New York	25,003,202,243	12.8%
11	North Carolina	4,569,381,898	2.3%
42	North Dakota	717,089,369	0.4%
4	Ohio	9,869,422,449	5.0%
26	Oklahoma	2,029,985,862	1.0%
25	Oregon	2,248,476,833	1.1%
3	Pennsylvania	11,259,169,603	5.7%
32	Rhode Island	1,408,469,747	0.7%
24	South Carolina	2,304,693,120	1.2%
44	South Dakota	683,650,009	0.3%
10	Tennessee	4,782,168,127	2.4%
NA	Texas**	NA	NA
38	Utah	871,616,513	0.4%
40	Vermont	805,588,329	0.4%
17	Virginia	4,006,037,550	2.0%
16	Washington	4,022,716,267	2.1%
27	West Virginia	1,736,741,427	0.9%
15	Wisconsin	4,059,511,421	2.1%
46	Wyoming	486,553,976	0.2%

RANK ORDER

RANK	STATE	FUNDS	% of USA
1	California	$25,006,972,511	12.8%
2	New York	25,003,202,243	12.8%
3	Pennsylvania	11,259,169,603	5.7%
4	Ohio	9,869,422,449	5.0%
5	Illinois	9,118,539,559	4.7%
6	Michigan	8,526,278,034	4.4%
7	Massachusetts	7,913,114,213	4.0%
8	New Jersey	7,576,167,918	3.9%
9	Georgia	4,808,740,669	2.5%
10	Tennessee	4,782,168,127	2.4%
11	North Carolina	4,569,381,898	2.3%
12	Missouri	4,456,368,286	2.3%
13	Maryland	4,428,657,384	2.3%
14	Louisiana	4,418,657,915	2.3%
15	Wisconsin	4,059,511,421	2.1%
16	Washington	4,022,716,267	2.1%
17	Virginia	4,006,037,550	2.0%
18	Indiana	3,996,355,551	2.0%
19	Connecticut	3,637,303,382	1.9%
20	Kentucky	3,450,438,586	1.8%
21	Alabama	3,166,302,119	1.6%
22	Arizona	2,887,614,909	1.5%
23	Colorado	2,685,773,549	1.4%
24	South Carolina	2,304,693,120	1.2%
25	Oregon	2,248,476,833	1.1%
26	Oklahoma	2,029,985,862	1.0%
27	West Virginia	1,736,741,427	0.9%
28	Iowa	1,703,839,986	0.9%
29	Kansas	1,633,317,646	0.8%
30	Arkansas	1,622,336,126	0.8%
31	Maine	1,507,301,276	0.8%
32	Rhode Island	1,408,469,747	0.7%
33	New Hampshire	1,304,689,150	0.7%
34	Nevada	1,194,976,855	0.6%
35	Hawaii	1,179,165,923	0.6%
36	New Mexico	1,168,438,809	0.6%
37	Nebraska	1,165,683,457	0.6%
38	Utah	871,616,513	0.4%
39	Montana	832,182,431	0.4%
40	Vermont	805,588,329	0.4%
41	Delaware	774,798,677	0.4%
42	North Dakota	717,089,369	0.4%
43	Idaho	711,700,479	0.4%
44	South Dakota	683,650,009	0.3%
45	Alaska	668,903,057	0.3%
46	Wyoming	486,553,976	0.2%
NA	Florida**	NA	NA
NA	Minnesota**	NA	NA
NA	Mississippi**	NA	NA
NA	Texas**	NA	NA
	District of Columbia	1,189,458,106	0.6%

Source: National Association of Attorneys General
"Attorneys General Announce Tobacco Settlement Proposal" (News release, http://www.naag.org/tob2.htm)
*This settlement was reached in November 1998. National total includes $4,640,249,229 for U.S. territories.
**Total does not include $40 billion in previous settlements with Florida, Minnesota, Mississippi and Texas.

State Government Expenditures for Health Programs in 1999

National Total = $38,008,201,000*

ALPHA ORDER

RANK	STATE	EXPENDITURES	% of USA
18	Alabama	$588,248,000	1.5%
41	Alaska	159,419,000	0.4%
14	Arizona	737,725,000	1.9%
32	Arkansas	289,496,000	0.8%
1	California	6,960,201,000	18.3%
31	Colorado	292,724,000	0.8%
22	Connecticut	446,067,000	1.2%
38	Delaware	199,834,000	0.5%
4	Florida	2,328,849,000	6.1%
13	Georgia	750,905,000	2.0%
29	Hawaii	354,006,000	0.9%
45	Idaho	98,227,000	0.3%
5	Illinois	1,947,604,000	5.1%
23	Indiana	445,593,000	1.2%
37	Iowa	208,163,000	0.5%
30	Kansas	342,450,000	0.9%
27	Kentucky	374,092,000	1.0%
26	Louisiana	385,848,000	1.0%
33	Maine	278,012,000	0.7%
12	Maryland	927,747,000	2.4%
9	Massachusetts	1,374,227,000	3.6%
3	Michigan	2,408,275,000	6.3%
25	Minnesota	425,013,000	1.1%
35	Mississippi	269,645,000	0.7%
17	Missouri	619,811,000	1.6%
39	Montana	198,222,000	0.5%
36	Nebraska	229,902,000	0.6%
46	Nevada	93,834,000	0.2%
44	New Hampshire	122,937,000	0.3%
15	New Jersey	698,841,000	1.8%
34	New Mexico	274,677,000	0.7%
2	New York	2,794,231,000	7.4%
11	North Carolina	940,239,000	2.5%
50	North Dakota	46,325,000	0.1%
6	Ohio	1,530,380,000	4.0%
28	Oklahoma	362,693,000	1.0%
24	Oregon	436,449,000	1.1%
8	Pennsylvania	1,423,139,000	3.7%
43	Rhode Island	128,116,000	0.3%
16	South Carolina	647,803,000	1.7%
48	South Dakota	61,721,000	0.2%
20	Tennessee	581,469,000	1.5%
7	Texas	1,473,317,000	3.9%
40	Utah	191,247,000	0.5%
49	Vermont	50,557,000	0.1%
19	Virginia	581,676,000	1.5%
10	Washington	1,152,418,000	3.0%
42	West Virginia	139,895,000	0.4%
21	Wisconsin	546,479,000	1.4%
47	Wyoming	89,453,000	0.2%

RANK ORDER

RANK	STATE	EXPENDITURES	% of USA
1	California	$6,960,201,000	18.3%
2	New York	2,794,231,000	7.4%
3	Michigan	2,408,275,000	6.3%
4	Florida	2,328,849,000	6.1%
5	Illinois	1,947,604,000	5.1%
6	Ohio	1,530,380,000	4.0%
7	Texas	1,473,317,000	3.9%
8	Pennsylvania	1,423,139,000	3.7%
9	Massachusetts	1,374,227,000	3.6%
10	Washington	1,152,418,000	3.0%
11	North Carolina	940,239,000	2.5%
12	Maryland	927,747,000	2.4%
13	Georgia	750,905,000	2.0%
14	Arizona	737,725,000	1.9%
15	New Jersey	698,841,000	1.8%
16	South Carolina	647,803,000	1.7%
17	Missouri	619,811,000	1.6%
18	Alabama	588,248,000	1.5%
19	Virginia	581,676,000	1.5%
20	Tennessee	581,469,000	1.5%
21	Wisconsin	546,479,000	1.4%
22	Connecticut	446,067,000	1.2%
23	Indiana	445,593,000	1.2%
24	Oregon	436,449,000	1.1%
25	Minnesota	425,013,000	1.1%
26	Louisiana	385,848,000	1.0%
27	Kentucky	374,092,000	1.0%
28	Oklahoma	362,693,000	1.0%
29	Hawaii	354,006,000	0.9%
30	Kansas	342,450,000	0.9%
31	Colorado	292,724,000	0.8%
32	Arkansas	289,496,000	0.8%
33	Maine	278,012,000	0.7%
34	New Mexico	274,677,000	0.7%
35	Mississippi	269,645,000	0.7%
36	Nebraska	229,902,000	0.6%
37	Iowa	208,163,000	0.5%
38	Delaware	199,834,000	0.5%
39	Montana	198,222,000	0.5%
40	Utah	191,247,000	0.5%
41	Alaska	159,419,000	0.4%
42	West Virginia	139,895,000	0.4%
43	Rhode Island	128,116,000	0.3%
44	New Hampshire	122,937,000	0.3%
45	Idaho	98,227,000	0.3%
46	Nevada	93,834,000	0.2%
47	Wyoming	89,453,000	0.2%
48	South Dakota	61,721,000	0.2%
49	Vermont	50,557,000	0.1%
50	North Dakota	46,325,000	0.1%
	District of Columbia**	NA	NA

Source: U.S. Bureau of the Census, Governments Division
"1999 State Government Finance Data" (http://www.census.gov/govs/www/state99.html)
*Includes outpatient health services other than hospital care, research and education, categorical health programs, treatment and immunization clinics, nursing and environmental health activities. Includes capital expenditures.
**Not applicable.

Per Capita State Government Expenditures for Health Programs in 1999

National Per Capita = $140*

ALPHA ORDER

RANK ORDER

RANK	STATE	PER CAPITA		RANK	STATE	PER CAPITA
21	Alabama	$135		1	Hawaii	$299
3	Alaska	257		2	Delaware	265
15	Arizona	154		3	Alaska	257
27	Arkansas	113		4	Michigan	244
8	California	210		5	Montana	225
49	Colorado	72		6	Massachusetts	223
19	Connecticut	136		7	Maine	222
2	Delaware	265		8	California	210
15	Florida	154		9	Washington	200
34	Georgia	96		10	Wyoming	187
1	Hawaii	299		11	Maryland	179
43	Idaho	78		12	South Carolina	167
13	Illinois	161		13	Illinois	161
45	Indiana	75		14	New Mexico	158
47	Iowa	73		15	Arizona	154
23	Kansas	129		15	Florida	154
35	Kentucky	94		15	New York	154
38	Louisiana	88		18	Nebraska	138
7	Maine	222		19	Connecticut	136
11	Maryland	179		19	Ohio	136
6	Massachusetts	223		21	Alabama	135
4	Michigan	244		22	Oregon	132
37	Minnesota	89		23	Kansas	129
33	Mississippi	97		23	Rhode Island	129
27	Missouri	113		25	North Carolina	123
5	Montana	225		26	Pennsylvania	119
18	Nebraska	138		27	Arkansas	113
50	Nevada	52		27	Missouri	113
32	New Hampshire	102		29	Oklahoma	108
39	New Jersey	86		30	Tennessee	106
14	New Mexico	158		31	Wisconsin	104
15	New York	154		32	New Hampshire	102
25	North Carolina	123		33	Mississippi	97
47	North Dakota	73		34	Georgia	96
19	Ohio	136		35	Kentucky	94
29	Oklahoma	108		36	Utah	90
22	Oregon	132		37	Minnesota	89
26	Pennsylvania	119		38	Louisiana	88
23	Rhode Island	129		39	New Jersey	86
12	South Carolina	167		40	Vermont	85
42	South Dakota	84		40	Virginia	85
30	Tennessee	106		42	South Dakota	84
46	Texas	74		43	Idaho	78
36	Utah	90		44	West Virginia	77
40	Vermont	85		45	Indiana	75
40	Virginia	85		46	Texas	74
9	Washington	200		47	Iowa	73
44	West Virginia	77		47	North Dakota	73
31	Wisconsin	104		49	Colorado	72
10	Wyoming	187		50	Nevada	52
					District of Columbia**	NA

Source: Morgan Quitno Press using data from U.S. Bureau of the Census, Governments Division
    "1999 State Government Finance Data" (http://www.census.gov/govs/www/state99.html)
*Includes outpatient health services other than hospital care, research and education, categorical health programs,
treatment and immunization clinics, nursing and environmental health activities. Includes capital expenditures.
**Not applicable.

State Government Expenditures for Hospitals in 1999

National Total = $29,994,422,000*

ALPHA ORDER

RANK	STATE	EXPENDITURES	% of USA
10	Alabama	$1,027,751,000	3.4%
48	Alaska	22,105,000	0.1%
40	Arizona	66,505,000	0.2%
26	Arkansas	401,888,000	1.3%
2	California	2,918,092,000	9.7%
35	Colorado	155,212,000	0.5%
7	Connecticut	1,134,791,000	3.8%
41	Delaware	58,678,000	0.2%
19	Florida	552,054,000	1.8%
15	Georgia	664,650,000	2.2%
32	Hawaii	184,901,000	0.6%
45	Idaho	40,810,000	0.1%
13	Illinois	854,257,000	2.8%
30	Indiana	217,824,000	0.7%
17	Iowa	576,783,000	1.9%
34	Kansas	163,038,000	0.5%
24	Kentucky	454,184,000	1.5%
6	Louisiana	1,282,421,000	4.3%
43	Maine	44,171,000	0.1%
28	Maryland	339,426,000	1.1%
22	Massachusetts	518,146,000	1.7%
8	Michigan	1,053,030,000	3.5%
31	Minnesota	213,596,000	0.7%
25	Mississippi	433,410,000	1.4%
21	Missouri	526,665,000	1.8%
46	Montana	38,939,000	0.1%
36	Nebraska	154,532,000	0.5%
38	Nevada	91,600,000	0.3%
44	New Hampshire	41,047,000	0.1%
11	New Jersey	964,339,000	3.2%
29	New Mexico	332,311,000	1.1%
1	New York	3,143,808,000	10.5%
12	North Carolina	895,878,000	3.0%
NA	North Dakota**	NA	NA
9	Ohio	1,043,969,000	3.5%
33	Oklahoma	170,103,000	0.6%
23	Oregon	513,180,000	1.7%
4	Pennsylvania	1,616,407,000	5.4%
37	Rhode Island	109,926,000	0.4%
14	South Carolina	731,431,000	2.4%
42	South Dakota	44,671,000	0.1%
18	Tennessee	564,071,000	1.9%
3	Texas	2,614,904,000	8.7%
27	Utah	397,158,000	1.3%
49	Vermont	5,370,000	0.0%
5	Virginia	1,358,220,000	4.5%
16	Washington	600,142,000	2.0%
39	West Virginia	83,012,000	0.3%
20	Wisconsin	536,748,000	1.8%
47	Wyoming	38,268,000	0.1%

RANK ORDER

RANK	STATE	EXPENDITURES	% of USA
1	New York	$3,143,808,000	10.5%
2	California	2,918,092,000	9.7%
3	Texas	2,614,904,000	8.7%
4	Pennsylvania	1,616,407,000	5.4%
5	Virginia	1,358,220,000	4.5%
6	Louisiana	1,282,421,000	4.3%
7	Connecticut	1,134,791,000	3.8%
8	Michigan	1,053,030,000	3.5%
9	Ohio	1,043,969,000	3.5%
10	Alabama	1,027,751,000	3.4%
11	New Jersey	964,339,000	3.2%
12	North Carolina	895,878,000	3.0%
13	Illinois	854,257,000	2.8%
14	South Carolina	731,431,000	2.4%
15	Georgia	664,650,000	2.2%
16	Washington	600,142,000	2.0%
17	Iowa	576,783,000	1.9%
18	Tennessee	564,071,000	1.9%
19	Florida	552,054,000	1.8%
20	Wisconsin	536,748,000	1.8%
21	Missouri	526,665,000	1.8%
22	Massachusetts	518,146,000	1.7%
23	Oregon	513,180,000	1.7%
24	Kentucky	454,184,000	1.5%
25	Mississippi	433,410,000	1.4%
26	Arkansas	401,888,000	1.3%
27	Utah	397,158,000	1.3%
28	Maryland	339,426,000	1.1%
29	New Mexico	332,311,000	1.1%
30	Indiana	217,824,000	0.7%
31	Minnesota	213,596,000	0.7%
32	Hawaii	184,901,000	0.6%
33	Oklahoma	170,103,000	0.6%
34	Kansas	163,038,000	0.5%
35	Colorado	155,212,000	0.5%
36	Nebraska	154,532,000	0.5%
37	Rhode Island	109,926,000	0.4%
38	Nevada	91,600,000	0.3%
39	West Virginia	83,012,000	0.3%
40	Arizona	66,505,000	0.2%
41	Delaware	58,678,000	0.2%
42	South Dakota	44,671,000	0.1%
43	Maine	44,171,000	0.1%
44	New Hampshire	41,047,000	0.1%
45	Idaho	40,810,000	0.1%
46	Montana	38,939,000	0.1%
47	Wyoming	38,268,000	0.1%
48	Alaska	22,105,000	0.1%
49	Vermont	5,370,000	0.0%
NA	North Dakota**	NA	NA
	District of Columbia**	NA	NA

Source: U.S. Bureau of the Census, Governments Division
   "1999 State Government Finance Data" (http://www.census.gov/govs/www/state99.html)
*Financing, construction, acquisition, maintenance or operation of hospital facilities, provision of hospital care and support of public or private hospitals.
**Not available or not applicable.

Per Capita State Government Expenditures for Hospitals in 1999

National Per Capita = $110*

<u>ALPHA ORDER</u>

RANK	STATE	PER CAPITA
3	Alabama	$235
44	Alaska	36
48	Arizona	14
10	Arkansas	158
27	California	88
41	Colorado	38
1	Connecticut	346
31	Delaware	78
42	Florida	37
28	Georgia	85
12	Hawaii	156
47	Idaho	33
32	Illinois	70
42	Indiana	37
4	Iowa	201
34	Kansas	61
18	Kentucky	115
2	Louisiana	293
45	Maine	35
33	Maryland	66
29	Massachusetts	84
20	Michigan	107
39	Minnesota	45
11	Mississippi	157
24	Missouri	96
40	Montana	44
25	Nebraska	93
36	Nevada	51
46	New Hampshire	34
16	New Jersey	118
6	New Mexico	191
9	New York	173
17	North Carolina	117
NA	North Dakota**	NA
25	Ohio	93
36	Oklahoma	51
13	Oregon	155
14	Pennsylvania	135
19	Rhode Island	111
7	South Carolina	188
34	South Dakota	61
22	Tennessee	103
15	Texas	130
8	Utah	186
49	Vermont	9
5	Virginia	198
21	Washington	104
38	West Virginia	46
23	Wisconsin	102
30	Wyoming	80

<u>RANK ORDER</u>

RANK	STATE	PER CAPITA
1	Connecticut	$346
2	Louisiana	293
3	Alabama	235
4	Iowa	201
5	Virginia	198
6	New Mexico	191
7	South Carolina	188
8	Utah	186
9	New York	173
10	Arkansas	158
11	Mississippi	157
12	Hawaii	156
13	Oregon	155
14	Pennsylvania	135
15	Texas	130
16	New Jersey	118
17	North Carolina	117
18	Kentucky	115
19	Rhode Island	111
20	Michigan	107
21	Washington	104
22	Tennessee	103
23	Wisconsin	102
24	Missouri	96
25	Nebraska	93
25	Ohio	93
27	California	88
28	Georgia	85
29	Massachusetts	84
30	Wyoming	80
31	Delaware	78
32	Illinois	70
33	Maryland	66
34	Kansas	61
34	South Dakota	61
36	Nevada	51
36	Oklahoma	51
38	West Virginia	46
39	Minnesota	45
40	Montana	44
41	Colorado	38
42	Florida	37
42	Indiana	37
44	Alaska	36
45	Maine	35
46	New Hampshire	34
47	Idaho	33
48	Arizona	14
49	Vermont	9
NA	North Dakota**	NA
	District of Columbia**	NA

Source: Morgan Quitno Press using data from U.S. Bureau of the Census, Governments Division
   "1999 State Government Finance Data" (http://www.census.gov/govs/www/state99.html)
*Financing, construction, acquisition, maintenance or operation of hospital facilities, provision of hospital care and support of public or private hospitals.
**Not available or not applicable.

Payroll of Health Care Establishments in 1999

National Total = $380,895,210,000*

ALPHA ORDER

RANK	STATE	PAYROLL	% of USA
23	Alabama	$5,576,695,000	1.5%
46	Alaska	987,326,000	0.3%
24	Arizona	5,481,570,000	1.4%
33	Arkansas	3,075,156,000	0.8%
1	California	37,672,551,000	9.9%
25	Colorado	5,136,413,000	1.3%
21	Connecticut	6,359,842,000	1.7%
44	Delaware	1,219,864,000	0.3%
4	Florida	20,877,067,000	5.5%
12	Georgia	9,529,843,000	2.5%
42	Hawaii	1,563,851,000	0.4%
43	Idaho	1,273,268,000	0.3%
6	Illinois	17,219,507,000	4.5%
15	Indiana	8,196,356,000	2.2%
28	Iowa	4,081,042,000	1.1%
31	Kansas	3,608,586,000	0.9%
26	Kentucky	5,056,678,000	1.3%
22	Louisiana	5,684,285,000	1.5%
38	Maine	1,959,853,000	0.5%
20	Maryland	7,178,774,000	1.9%
10	Massachusetts	12,492,100,000	3.3%
8	Michigan	13,942,598,000	3.7%
14	Minnesota	8,217,295,000	2.2%
32	Mississippi	3,194,215,000	0.8%
13	Missouri	8,224,466,000	2.2%
45	Montana	1,050,909,000	0.3%
34	Nebraska	2,497,345,000	0.7%
37	Nevada	2,011,083,000	0.5%
40	New Hampshire	1,756,912,000	0.5%
9	New Jersey	12,730,663,000	3.3%
39	New Mexico	1,883,380,000	0.5%
2	New York	33,776,122,000	8.9%
11	North Carolina	10,463,525,000	2.7%
NA	North Dakota**	NA	NA
7	Ohio	16,971,441,000	4.5%
30	Oklahoma	3,919,968,000	1.0%
29	Oregon	4,057,552,000	1.1%
5	Pennsylvania	19,711,669,000	5.2%
41	Rhode Island	1,733,512,000	0.5%
27	South Carolina	4,700,856,000	1.2%
NA	South Dakota**	NA	NA
17	Tennessee	8,102,722,000	2.1%
3	Texas	24,344,731,000	6.4%
36	Utah	2,176,282,000	0.6%
NA	Vermont**	NA	NA
16	Virginia	8,110,145,000	2.1%
19	Washington	7,555,013,000	2.0%
35	West Virginia	2,409,131,000	0.6%
18	Wisconsin	7,682,553,000	2.0%
NA	Wyoming**	NA	NA

RANK ORDER

RANK	STATE	PAYROLL	% of USA
1	California	$37,672,551,000	9.9%
2	New York	33,776,122,000	8.9%
3	Texas	24,344,731,000	6.4%
4	Florida	20,877,067,000	5.5%
5	Pennsylvania	19,711,669,000	5.2%
6	Illinois	17,219,507,000	4.5%
7	Ohio	16,971,441,000	4.5%
8	Michigan	13,942,598,000	3.7%
9	New Jersey	12,730,663,000	3.3%
10	Massachusetts	12,492,100,000	3.3%
11	North Carolina	10,463,525,000	2.7%
12	Georgia	9,529,843,000	2.5%
13	Missouri	8,224,466,000	2.2%
14	Minnesota	8,217,295,000	2.2%
15	Indiana	8,196,356,000	2.2%
16	Virginia	8,110,145,000	2.1%
17	Tennessee	8,102,722,000	2.1%
18	Wisconsin	7,682,553,000	2.0%
19	Washington	7,555,013,000	2.0%
20	Maryland	7,178,774,000	1.9%
21	Connecticut	6,359,842,000	1.7%
22	Louisiana	5,684,285,000	1.5%
23	Alabama	5,576,695,000	1.5%
24	Arizona	5,481,570,000	1.4%
25	Colorado	5,136,413,000	1.3%
26	Kentucky	5,056,678,000	1.3%
27	South Carolina	4,700,856,000	1.2%
28	Iowa	4,081,042,000	1.1%
29	Oregon	4,057,552,000	1.1%
30	Oklahoma	3,919,968,000	1.0%
31	Kansas	3,608,586,000	0.9%
32	Mississippi	3,194,215,000	0.8%
33	Arkansas	3,075,156,000	0.8%
34	Nebraska	2,497,345,000	0.7%
35	West Virginia	2,409,131,000	0.6%
36	Utah	2,176,282,000	0.6%
37	Nevada	2,011,083,000	0.5%
38	Maine	1,959,853,000	0.5%
39	New Mexico	1,883,380,000	0.5%
40	New Hampshire	1,756,912,000	0.5%
41	Rhode Island	1,733,512,000	0.5%
42	Hawaii	1,563,851,000	0.4%
43	Idaho	1,273,268,000	0.3%
44	Delaware	1,219,864,000	0.3%
45	Montana	1,050,909,000	0.3%
46	Alaska	987,326,000	0.3%
NA	North Dakota**	NA	NA
NA	South Dakota**	NA	NA
NA	Vermont**	NA	NA
NA	Wyoming**	NA	NA
	District of Columbia	1,853,007,000	0.5%

Source: U.S. Bureau of the Census
   "County Business Patterns 1999 (NAICS)" (http://tier2.census.gov/cbp_naics/index.html)
*Includes establishments exempt from as well as subject to the federal income tax. Includes those establishments within the North American Industry Classification System (NAICS) classifications 621 (ambulatory health care services), 622 (hospitals) and 623 (nursing and residential care facilities). See Facilities Chapter for establishments.
**Not available.

Average Pay per Health Care Establishment Employee in 1999

National Average = $31,650 per Employee*

RANK	STATE	AVERAGE PAY		RANK	STATE	AVERAGE PAY
30	Alabama	$30,282		1	Alaska	$42,610
1	Alaska	42,610		2	Hawaii	37,663
10	Arizona	32,766		3	Nevada	37,352
42	Arkansas	27,680		4	Delaware	35,377
8	California	33,885		5	New Jersey	35,236
17	Colorado	32,023		6	Connecticut	34,710
6	Connecticut	34,710		7	New York	34,463
4	Delaware	35,377		8	California	33,885
18	Florida	31,955		9	Massachusetts	33,034
12	Georgia	32,522		10	Arizona	32,766
2	Hawaii	37,663		11	Washington	32,755
38	Idaho	28,396		12	Georgia	32,522
15	Illinois	32,145		13	Tennessee	32,483
33	Indiana	29,622		14	Maryland	32,177
46	Iowa	26,713		15	Illinois	32,145
43	Kansas	27,559		16	Michigan	32,091
34	Kentucky	29,023		17	Colorado	32,023
41	Louisiana	27,913		18	Florida	31,955
39	Maine	28,319		19	Virginia	31,908
14	Maryland	32,177		20	South Carolina	31,622
9	Massachusetts	33,034		21	Rhode Island	31,524
16	Michigan	32,091		22	Oregon	31,428
24	Minnesota	30,953		23	New Hampshire	31,210
37	Mississippi	28,618		24	Minnesota	30,953
32	Missouri	29,633		25	North Carolina	30,947
45	Montana	26,800		26	Pennsylvania	30,796
36	Nebraska	28,638		27	Wisconsin	30,594
3	Nevada	37,352		28	Ohio	30,383
23	New Hampshire	31,210		29	New Mexico	30,348
5	New Jersey	35,236		30	Alabama	30,282
29	New Mexico	30,348		31	Texas	29,848
7	New York	34,463		32	Missouri	29,633
25	North Carolina	30,947		33	Indiana	29,622
NA	North Dakota**	NA		34	Kentucky	29,023
28	Ohio	30,383		35	Utah	28,922
44	Oklahoma	27,436		36	Nebraska	28,638
22	Oregon	31,428		37	Mississippi	28,618
26	Pennsylvania	30,796		38	Idaho	28,396
21	Rhode Island	31,524		39	Maine	28,319
20	South Carolina	31,622		40	West Virginia	28,036
NA	South Dakota**	NA		41	Louisiana	27,913
13	Tennessee	32,483		42	Arkansas	27,680
31	Texas	29,848		43	Kansas	27,559
35	Utah	28,922		44	Oklahoma	27,436
NA	Vermont**	NA		45	Montana	26,800
19	Virginia	31,908		46	Iowa	26,713
11	Washington	32,755		NA	North Dakota**	NA
40	West Virginia	28,036		NA	South Dakota**	NA
27	Wisconsin	30,594		NA	Vermont**	NA
NA	Wyoming**	NA		NA	Wyoming**	NA
					District of Columbia	39,036

Source: Morgan Quitno Press using data from U.S. Bureau of the Census
"County Business Patterns 1999 (NAICS)" (http://tier2.census.gov/cbp_naics/index.html)
*Includes establishments exempt from as well as subject to the federal income tax. Includes those establishments within the North American Industry Classification System (NAICS) classifications 621 (ambulatory health care services), 622 (hospitals) and 623 (nursing and residential care facilities). See Facilities Chapter for establishments.
**Not available.

Receipts per Health Service Establishment in 1997

National Rate = $1,370,364 per Establishment*

ALPHA ORDER

RANK	STATE	PER ESTABLISHMENT
5	Alabama	$1,552,760
32	Alaska	1,300,158
38	Arizona	1,220,528
35	Arkansas	1,263,342
36	California	1,250,395
42	Colorado	1,129,615
10	Connecticut	1,488,600
15	Delaware	1,438,157
28	Florida	1,307,922
11	Georgia	1,483,086
22	Hawaii	1,351,688
48	Idaho	923,630
7	Illinois	1,527,359
19	Indiana	1,409,495
39	Iowa	1,218,292
34	Kansas	1,278,185
18	Kentucky	1,426,882
17	Louisiana	1,432,178
44	Maine	1,117,962
23	Maryland	1,341,244
1	Massachusetts	1,671,512
26	Michigan	1,323,486
6	Minnesota	1,535,255
3	Mississippi	1,580,683
14	Missouri	1,439,935
50	Montana	869,357
33	Nebraska	1,284,942
31	Nevada	1,301,387
37	New Hampshire	1,241,136
27	New Jersey	1,318,017
40	New Mexico	1,207,674
2	New York	1,627,723
9	North Carolina	1,502,931
8	North Dakota	1,525,628
12	Ohio	1,464,119
45	Oklahoma	1,105,388
46	Oregon	1,020,240
16	Pennsylvania	1,436,074
13	Rhode Island	1,456,061
24	South Carolina	1,334,095
29	South Dakota	1,305,312
4	Tennessee	1,562,915
30	Texas	1,304,200
41	Utah	1,157,153
47	Vermont	949,657
25	Virginia	1,330,452
43	Washington	1,127,303
20	West Virginia	1,374,164
21	Wisconsin	1,353,159
49	Wyoming	877,211

RANK ORDER

RANK	STATE	PER ESTABLISHMENT
1	Massachusetts	$1,671,512
2	New York	1,627,723
3	Mississippi	1,580,683
4	Tennessee	1,562,915
5	Alabama	1,552,760
6	Minnesota	1,535,255
7	Illinois	1,527,359
8	North Dakota	1,525,628
9	North Carolina	1,502,931
10	Connecticut	1,488,600
11	Georgia	1,483,086
12	Ohio	1,464,119
13	Rhode Island	1,456,061
14	Missouri	1,439,935
15	Delaware	1,438,157
16	Pennsylvania	1,436,074
17	Louisiana	1,432,178
18	Kentucky	1,426,882
19	Indiana	1,409,495
20	West Virginia	1,374,164
21	Wisconsin	1,353,159
22	Hawaii	1,351,688
23	Maryland	1,341,244
24	South Carolina	1,334,095
25	Virginia	1,330,452
26	Michigan	1,323,486
27	New Jersey	1,318,017
28	Florida	1,307,922
29	South Dakota	1,305,312
30	Texas	1,304,200
31	Nevada	1,301,387
32	Alaska	1,300,158
33	Nebraska	1,284,942
34	Kansas	1,278,185
35	Arkansas	1,263,342
36	California	1,250,395
37	New Hampshire	1,241,136
38	Arizona	1,220,528
39	Iowa	1,218,292
40	New Mexico	1,207,674
41	Utah	1,157,153
42	Colorado	1,129,615
43	Washington	1,127,303
44	Maine	1,117,962
45	Oklahoma	1,105,388
46	Oregon	1,020,240
47	Vermont	949,657
48	Idaho	923,630
49	Wyoming	877,211
50	Montana	869,357
	District of Columbia	2,303,504

Source: Morgan Quitno Press using data from U.S. Bureau of the Census
  "1997 Economic Census, Health Care and Social Assistance" (EC97562A, October 1999)
*Includes establishments exempt from as well as subject to the federal income tax. These include those primarily engaged in furnishing medical, surgical and other health services to persons. See Facilities Chapter for establishments.

Receipts per Hospital in 1997

National Rate = $56,720,765 per Hospital*

ALPHA ORDER

RANK ORDER

RANK	STATE	PER HOSPITAL		RANK	STATE	PER HOSPITAL
27	Alabama	$46,379,759		1	New York	$108,392,790
39	Alaska	37,239,815		2	Delaware**	96,436,417
22	Arizona	52,040,783		3	Connecticut**	95,949,720
40	Arkansas	36,040,724		4	New Jersey	91,948,488
13	California	66,287,980		5	Rhode Island**	90,917,684
23	Colorado	51,659,640		6	Maryland	79,089,326
3	Connecticut**	95,949,720		7	Massachusetts	76,688,105
2	Delaware**	96,436,417		8	Illinois	75,884,574
11	Florida	69,236,515		9	Ohio	73,910,477
24	Georgia	51,572,257		10	Michigan	71,471,490
20	Hawaii**	54,566,500		11	Florida	69,236,515
44	Idaho	23,503,453		12	Pennsylvania	68,141,057
8	Illinois	75,884,574		13	California	66,287,980
26	Indiana	49,140,018		14	North Carolina	65,828,184
42	Iowa**	31,905,866		15	Virginia	61,573,103
46	Kansas**	21,895,715		16	South Carolina	58,809,779
30	Kentucky	43,779,008		17	Missouri	56,331,463
36	Louisiana	38,533,383		18	Nevada	55,369,912
35	Maine**	40,535,310		19	Washington	54,844,681
6	Maryland	79,089,326		20	Hawaii**	54,566,500
7	Massachusetts	76,688,105		21	Tennessee	52,581,945
10	Michigan	71,471,490		22	Arizona	52,040,783
37	Minnesota**	37,758,312		23	Colorado	51,659,640
38	Mississippi	37,329,017		24	Georgia	51,572,257
17	Missouri	56,331,463		25	Oregon	50,952,235
49	Montana**	19,658,964		26	Indiana	49,140,018
45	Nebraska**	23,468,970		27	Alabama	46,379,759
18	Nevada	55,369,912		28	Wisconsin	46,319,112
31	New Hampshire	42,421,139		29	Texas	45,460,076
4	New Jersey	91,948,488		30	Kentucky	43,779,008
41	New Mexico	32,234,111		31	New Hampshire	42,421,139
1	New York	108,392,790		32	Utah	41,733,547
14	North Carolina	65,828,184		33	West Virginia	41,705,324
47	North Dakota**	21,463,041		34	Vermont	40,584,059
9	Ohio	73,910,477		35	Maine**	40,535,310
43	Oklahoma	28,186,912		36	Louisiana	38,533,383
25	Oregon	50,952,235		37	Minnesota**	37,758,312
12	Pennsylvania	68,141,057		38	Mississippi	37,329,017
5	Rhode Island**	90,917,684		39	Alaska	37,239,815
16	South Carolina	58,809,779		40	Arkansas	36,040,724
48	South Dakota	20,518,032		41	New Mexico	32,234,111
21	Tennessee	52,581,945		42	Iowa**	31,905,866
29	Texas	45,460,076		43	Oklahoma	28,186,912
32	Utah	41,733,547		44	Idaho	23,503,453
34	Vermont	40,584,059		45	Nebraska**	23,468,970
15	Virginia	61,573,103		46	Kansas**	21,895,715
19	Washington	54,844,681		47	North Dakota**	21,463,041
33	West Virginia	41,705,324		48	South Dakota	20,518,032
28	Wisconsin	46,319,112		49	Montana**	19,658,964
50	Wyoming	18,252,742		50	Wyoming	18,252,742
					District of Columbia	165,478,889

Source: Morgan Quitno Press using data from U.S. Bureau of the Census
   "1997 Economic Census, Health Care and Social Assistance" (EC97562A, October 1999)
*Includes establishments exempt from as well as subject to the federal income tax. Includes general medical and surgical hospitals, psychiatric hospitals and other specialty hospitals. Includes government owned hospitals.
**Amounts shown for these states are only for establishments exempt from federal income tax.

Receipts per Office or Clinic of Doctors of Medicine in 1997

National Rate = $909,008 per Establishment*

<table>
<tr><td colspan="3">ALPHA ORDER</td><td colspan="3">RANK ORDER</td></tr>
<tr><td>RANK</td><td>STATE</td><td>PER ESTABLISHMENT</td><td>RANK</td><td>STATE</td><td>PER ESTABLISHMENT</td></tr>
<tr><td>10</td><td>Alabama</td><td>$1,032,237</td><td>1</td><td>North Dakota</td><td>$2,239,607</td></tr>
<tr><td>28</td><td>Alaska</td><td>889,371</td><td>2</td><td>Minnesota</td><td>1,945,223</td></tr>
<tr><td>38</td><td>Arizona</td><td>821,155</td><td>3</td><td>Wisconsin</td><td>1,387,465</td></tr>
<tr><td>33</td><td>Arkansas</td><td>852,739</td><td>4</td><td>South Dakota</td><td>1,277,780</td></tr>
<tr><td>21</td><td>California</td><td>926,843</td><td>5</td><td>Kansas</td><td>1,145,207</td></tr>
<tr><td>30</td><td>Colorado</td><td>884,159</td><td>6</td><td>Tennessee</td><td>1,142,983</td></tr>
<tr><td>13</td><td>Connecticut</td><td>983,190</td><td>7</td><td>Iowa</td><td>1,141,907</td></tr>
<tr><td>31</td><td>Delaware</td><td>875,135</td><td>8</td><td>Nebraska</td><td>1,139,752</td></tr>
<tr><td>34</td><td>Florida</td><td>847,079</td><td>9</td><td>North Carolina</td><td>1,107,277</td></tr>
<tr><td>16</td><td>Georgia</td><td>941,810</td><td>10</td><td>Alabama</td><td>1,032,237</td></tr>
<tr><td>47</td><td>Hawaii</td><td>705,161</td><td>11</td><td>Indiana</td><td>1,026,262</td></tr>
<tr><td>39</td><td>Idaho</td><td>798,831</td><td>12</td><td>Missouri</td><td>991,859</td></tr>
<tr><td>14</td><td>Illinois</td><td>972,190</td><td>13</td><td>Connecticut</td><td>983,190</td></tr>
<tr><td>11</td><td>Indiana</td><td>1,026,262</td><td>14</td><td>Illinois</td><td>972,190</td></tr>
<tr><td>7</td><td>Iowa</td><td>1,141,907</td><td>15</td><td>Kentucky</td><td>946,675</td></tr>
<tr><td>5</td><td>Kansas</td><td>1,145,207</td><td>16</td><td>Georgia</td><td>941,810</td></tr>
<tr><td>15</td><td>Kentucky</td><td>946,675</td><td>17</td><td>New Hampshire</td><td>935,678</td></tr>
<tr><td>26</td><td>Louisiana</td><td>898,652</td><td>18</td><td>Virginia</td><td>931,328</td></tr>
<tr><td>45</td><td>Maine</td><td>757,973</td><td>19</td><td>Massachusetts</td><td>929,882</td></tr>
<tr><td>44</td><td>Maryland</td><td>772,308</td><td>20</td><td>South Carolina</td><td>927,371</td></tr>
<tr><td>19</td><td>Massachusetts</td><td>929,882</td><td>21</td><td>California</td><td>926,843</td></tr>
<tr><td>37</td><td>Michigan</td><td>824,127</td><td>22</td><td>Washington</td><td>921,563</td></tr>
<tr><td>2</td><td>Minnesota</td><td>1,945,223</td><td>23</td><td>Mississippi</td><td>916,212</td></tr>
<tr><td>23</td><td>Mississippi</td><td>916,212</td><td>24</td><td>Nevada</td><td>914,356</td></tr>
<tr><td>12</td><td>Missouri</td><td>991,859</td><td>25</td><td>Oregon</td><td>912,940</td></tr>
<tr><td>46</td><td>Montana</td><td>748,833</td><td>26</td><td>Louisiana</td><td>898,652</td></tr>
<tr><td>8</td><td>Nebraska</td><td>1,139,752</td><td>27</td><td>Ohio</td><td>896,004</td></tr>
<tr><td>24</td><td>Nevada</td><td>914,356</td><td>28</td><td>Alaska</td><td>889,371</td></tr>
<tr><td>17</td><td>New Hampshire</td><td>935,678</td><td>29</td><td>Texas</td><td>885,931</td></tr>
<tr><td>40</td><td>New Jersey</td><td>796,404</td><td>30</td><td>Colorado</td><td>884,159</td></tr>
<tr><td>49</td><td>New Mexico</td><td>665,430</td><td>31</td><td>Delaware</td><td>875,135</td></tr>
<tr><td>42</td><td>New York</td><td>790,511</td><td>32</td><td>Utah</td><td>853,007</td></tr>
<tr><td>9</td><td>North Carolina</td><td>1,107,277</td><td>33</td><td>Arkansas</td><td>852,739</td></tr>
<tr><td>1</td><td>North Dakota</td><td>2,239,607</td><td>34</td><td>Florida</td><td>847,079</td></tr>
<tr><td>27</td><td>Ohio</td><td>896,004</td><td>35</td><td>Pennsylvania</td><td>836,601</td></tr>
<tr><td>36</td><td>Oklahoma</td><td>828,010</td><td>36</td><td>Oklahoma</td><td>828,010</td></tr>
<tr><td>25</td><td>Oregon</td><td>912,940</td><td>37</td><td>Michigan</td><td>824,127</td></tr>
<tr><td>35</td><td>Pennsylvania</td><td>836,601</td><td>38</td><td>Arizona</td><td>821,155</td></tr>
<tr><td>48</td><td>Rhode Island</td><td>687,948</td><td>39</td><td>Idaho</td><td>798,831</td></tr>
<tr><td>20</td><td>South Carolina</td><td>927,371</td><td>40</td><td>New Jersey</td><td>796,404</td></tr>
<tr><td>4</td><td>South Dakota</td><td>1,277,780</td><td>41</td><td>West Virginia</td><td>794,372</td></tr>
<tr><td>6</td><td>Tennessee</td><td>1,142,983</td><td>42</td><td>New York</td><td>790,511</td></tr>
<tr><td>29</td><td>Texas</td><td>885,931</td><td>43</td><td>Vermont</td><td>774,319</td></tr>
<tr><td>32</td><td>Utah</td><td>853,007</td><td>44</td><td>Maryland</td><td>772,308</td></tr>
<tr><td>43</td><td>Vermont</td><td>774,319</td><td>45</td><td>Maine</td><td>757,973</td></tr>
<tr><td>18</td><td>Virginia</td><td>931,328</td><td>46</td><td>Montana</td><td>748,833</td></tr>
<tr><td>22</td><td>Washington</td><td>921,563</td><td>47</td><td>Hawaii</td><td>705,161</td></tr>
<tr><td>41</td><td>West Virginia</td><td>794,372</td><td>48</td><td>Rhode Island</td><td>687,948</td></tr>
<tr><td>3</td><td>Wisconsin</td><td>1,387,465</td><td>49</td><td>New Mexico</td><td>665,430</td></tr>
<tr><td>50</td><td>Wyoming</td><td>624,939</td><td>50</td><td>Wyoming</td><td>624,939</td></tr>
<tr><td></td><td></td><td></td><td></td><td>District of Columbia</td><td>787,712</td></tr>
</table>

Source: Morgan Quitno Press using data from U.S. Bureau of the Census
   "1997 Economic Census, Health Care and Social Assistance" (EC97562A, October 1999)
*Includes only establishments subject to the federal income tax. See Facilities Chapter for establishments.

Receipts per Office or Clinic of Dentists in 1997

National Rate = $424,618 per Establishment*

<table>
<tr><td colspan="3">ALPHA ORDER</td><td colspan="3">RANK ORDER</td></tr>
<tr><th>RANK</th><th>STATE</th><th>PER ESTABLISHMENT</th><th>RANK</th><th>STATE</th><th>PER ESTABLISHMENT</th></tr>
<tr><td>22</td><td>Alabama</td><td>$431,956</td><td>1</td><td>Delaware</td><td>$652,550</td></tr>
<tr><td>4</td><td>Alaska</td><td>542,873</td><td>2</td><td>Nevada</td><td>571,610</td></tr>
<tr><td>12</td><td>Arizona</td><td>462,255</td><td>3</td><td>Washington</td><td>549,787</td></tr>
<tr><td>37</td><td>Arkansas</td><td>387,532</td><td>4</td><td>Alaska</td><td>542,873</td></tr>
<tr><td>16</td><td>California</td><td>446,376</td><td>5</td><td>North Carolina</td><td>504,422</td></tr>
<tr><td>31</td><td>Colorado</td><td>408,087</td><td>6</td><td>Oregon</td><td>482,404</td></tr>
<tr><td>10</td><td>Connecticut</td><td>465,831</td><td>7</td><td>Georgia</td><td>477,108</td></tr>
<tr><td>1</td><td>Delaware</td><td>652,550</td><td>8</td><td>Rhode Island</td><td>471,659</td></tr>
<tr><td>21</td><td>Florida</td><td>433,095</td><td>9</td><td>Minnesota</td><td>470,948</td></tr>
<tr><td>7</td><td>Georgia</td><td>477,108</td><td>10</td><td>Connecticut</td><td>465,831</td></tr>
<tr><td>32</td><td>Hawaii</td><td>407,301</td><td>11</td><td>New Hampshire</td><td>465,538</td></tr>
<tr><td>14</td><td>Idaho</td><td>451,837</td><td>12</td><td>Arizona</td><td>462,255</td></tr>
<tr><td>41</td><td>Illinois</td><td>377,649</td><td>13</td><td>Massachusetts</td><td>458,523</td></tr>
<tr><td>30</td><td>Indiana</td><td>408,918</td><td>14</td><td>Idaho</td><td>451,837</td></tr>
<tr><td>39</td><td>Iowa</td><td>387,052</td><td>15</td><td>Michigan</td><td>450,436</td></tr>
<tr><td>24</td><td>Kansas</td><td>423,526</td><td>16</td><td>California</td><td>446,376</td></tr>
<tr><td>50</td><td>Kentucky</td><td>316,495</td><td>17</td><td>Wisconsin</td><td>444,465</td></tr>
<tr><td>28</td><td>Louisiana</td><td>417,048</td><td>18</td><td>Maine</td><td>444,325</td></tr>
<tr><td>18</td><td>Maine</td><td>444,325</td><td>19</td><td>South Carolina</td><td>437,257</td></tr>
<tr><td>33</td><td>Maryland</td><td>401,741</td><td>20</td><td>Vermont</td><td>433,270</td></tr>
<tr><td>13</td><td>Massachusetts</td><td>458,523</td><td>21</td><td>Florida</td><td>433,095</td></tr>
<tr><td>15</td><td>Michigan</td><td>450,436</td><td>22</td><td>Alabama</td><td>431,956</td></tr>
<tr><td>9</td><td>Minnesota</td><td>470,948</td><td>23</td><td>Virginia</td><td>429,474</td></tr>
<tr><td>43</td><td>Mississippi</td><td>371,849</td><td>24</td><td>Kansas</td><td>423,526</td></tr>
<tr><td>40</td><td>Missouri</td><td>381,919</td><td>25</td><td>New Jersey</td><td>422,076</td></tr>
<tr><td>49</td><td>Montana</td><td>331,012</td><td>26</td><td>Texas</td><td>420,133</td></tr>
<tr><td>47</td><td>Nebraska</td><td>334,887</td><td>27</td><td>New Mexico</td><td>418,052</td></tr>
<tr><td>2</td><td>Nevada</td><td>571,610</td><td>28</td><td>Louisiana</td><td>417,048</td></tr>
<tr><td>11</td><td>New Hampshire</td><td>465,538</td><td>29</td><td>South Dakota</td><td>410,041</td></tr>
<tr><td>25</td><td>New Jersey</td><td>422,076</td><td>30</td><td>Indiana</td><td>408,918</td></tr>
<tr><td>27</td><td>New Mexico</td><td>418,052</td><td>31</td><td>Colorado</td><td>408,087</td></tr>
<tr><td>38</td><td>New York</td><td>387,060</td><td>32</td><td>Hawaii</td><td>407,301</td></tr>
<tr><td>5</td><td>North Carolina</td><td>504,422</td><td>33</td><td>Maryland</td><td>401,741</td></tr>
<tr><td>34</td><td>North Dakota</td><td>401,634</td><td>34</td><td>North Dakota</td><td>401,634</td></tr>
<tr><td>36</td><td>Ohio</td><td>393,602</td><td>35</td><td>Tennessee</td><td>397,068</td></tr>
<tr><td>45</td><td>Oklahoma</td><td>359,185</td><td>36</td><td>Ohio</td><td>393,602</td></tr>
<tr><td>6</td><td>Oregon</td><td>482,404</td><td>37</td><td>Arkansas</td><td>387,532</td></tr>
<tr><td>42</td><td>Pennsylvania</td><td>375,515</td><td>38</td><td>New York</td><td>387,060</td></tr>
<tr><td>8</td><td>Rhode Island</td><td>471,659</td><td>39</td><td>Iowa</td><td>387,052</td></tr>
<tr><td>19</td><td>South Carolina</td><td>437,257</td><td>40</td><td>Missouri</td><td>381,919</td></tr>
<tr><td>29</td><td>South Dakota</td><td>410,041</td><td>41</td><td>Illinois</td><td>377,649</td></tr>
<tr><td>35</td><td>Tennessee</td><td>397,068</td><td>42</td><td>Pennsylvania</td><td>375,515</td></tr>
<tr><td>26</td><td>Texas</td><td>420,133</td><td>43</td><td>Mississippi</td><td>371,849</td></tr>
<tr><td>44</td><td>Utah</td><td>369,642</td><td>44</td><td>Utah</td><td>369,642</td></tr>
<tr><td>20</td><td>Vermont</td><td>433,270</td><td>45</td><td>Oklahoma</td><td>359,185</td></tr>
<tr><td>23</td><td>Virginia</td><td>429,474</td><td>46</td><td>West Virginia</td><td>340,733</td></tr>
<tr><td>3</td><td>Washington</td><td>549,787</td><td>47</td><td>Nebraska</td><td>334,887</td></tr>
<tr><td>46</td><td>West Virginia</td><td>340,733</td><td>48</td><td>Wyoming</td><td>331,732</td></tr>
<tr><td>17</td><td>Wisconsin</td><td>444,465</td><td>49</td><td>Montana</td><td>331,012</td></tr>
<tr><td>48</td><td>Wyoming</td><td>331,732</td><td>50</td><td>Kentucky</td><td>316,495</td></tr>
<tr><td></td><td></td><td></td><td></td><td>District of Columbia</td><td>412,602</td></tr>
</table>

Source: Morgan Quitno Press using data from U.S. Bureau of the Census
"1997 Economic Census, Health Care and Social Assistance" (EC97562A, October 1999)
*Includes only establishments subject to the federal income tax. See Facilities Chapter for establishments.

V. INCIDENCE OF DISEASE

353   Estimated New Cancer Cases in 2002
354   Estimated Rate of New Cancer Cases in 2002
355   Age-Adjusted Rate of New Cancer Cases for Males in 1998
356   Age-Adjusted Rate of New Cancer Cases for Females in 1998
357   Estimated New Cases of Bladder Cancer in 2002
358   Estimated Rate of New Bladder Cancer Cases in 2002
359   Estimated New Female Breast Cancer Cases in 2002
360   Estimated Rate of New Female Breast Cancer Cases in 2002
361   Percent of Women 40 and Older Who Have Ever Had a Mammogram: 2000
362   Estimated New Colon and Rectum Cancer Cases in 2002
363   Estimated Rate of New Colon and Rectum Cancer Cases in 2002
364   Estimated New Leukemia Cases in 2002
365   Estimated Rate of New Leukemia Cases in 2002
366   Estimated New Lung Cancer Cases in 2002
367   Estimated Rate of New Lung Cancer Cases in 2002
368   Estimated New Non-Hodgkin's Lymphoma Cases in 2002
369   Estimated Rate of New Non-Hodgkin's Lymphoma Cases in 2002
370   Estimated New Prostate Cancer Cases in 2002
371   Estimated Rate of New Prostate Cancer Cases in 2002
372   Estimated New Skin Melanoma Cases in 2002
373   Estimated Rate of New Skin Melanoma Cases in 2002
374   Estimated New Cervical Cancer Cases in 2002
375   Estimated Rate of New Cervical Cancer Cases in 2002
376   Percent of Women 18 Years Old and Older Who Had a Pap Smear Within the Past Three Years: 2000
377   AIDS Cases Reported in 2001
378   AIDS Rate in 2001
379   AIDS Cases Reported Through June 2001
380   AIDS Cases in Children 12 Years and Younger Through June 2001
381   E-Coli Cases Reported in 2001
382   E-Coli Rate in 2001
383   German Measles (Rubella) Cases Reported in 2001
384   German Measles (Rubella) Rate in 2001
385   Hepatitis A and B Cases Reported in 2001
386   Hepatitis A and B Rate in 2001
387   Hepatitis C Cases Reported in 2001
388   Hepatitis C Rate in 2001
389   Legionellosis Cases Reported in 2001
390   Legionellosis Rate in 2001
391   Lyme Disease Cases in 2001
392   Lyme Disease Rate in 2001
393   Malaria Cases Reported in 2001
394   Malaria Rate in 2001
395   Measles (Rubeola) Cases Reported in 2001
396   Measles (Rubeola) Rate in 2001
397   Meningococcal Infections Reported in 2001
398   Meningococcal Infection Rate in 2001
399   Mumps Cases Reported in 2001
400   Mumps Rate in 2001
401   Rabies (Animal) Cases Reported in 2001
402   Rabies (Animal) Rate in 2001
403   Salmonellosis Cases Reported in 2001
404   Salmonellosis Rate in 2001
405   Shigellosis Cases Reported in 2001
406   Shigellosis Rate in 2001
407   Tuberculosis Cases Reported in 2001
408   Tuberculosis Rate in 2001
409   Whooping Cough (Pertussis) Cases Reported in 2001
410   Whooping Cough (Pertussis) Rate in 2001
411   Percent of Children Aged 19 to 35 Months Fully Immunized in 2000
412   Sexually Transmitted Diseases in 2000
413   Sexually Transmitted Disease Rate in 2000

V. INCIDENCE OF DISEASE (Continued)

414   Chancroid Cases in 2000
415   Chancroid Rate in 2000
416   Chlamydia Cases Reported in 2000
417   Chlamydia Rate in 2000
418   Gonorrhea Cases Reported in 2000
419   Gonorrhea Rate in 2000
420   Syphilis Cases Reported in 2000
421   Syphilis Rate in 2000

Estimated New Cancer Cases in 2002

National Estimated Total = 1,284,900 New Cases*

ALPHA ORDER

RANK	STATE	CASES	% of USA
20	Alabama	22,600	1.8%
50	Alaska	1,600	0.1%
21	Arizona	22,100	1.7%
32	Arkansas	14,200	1.1%
1	California	119,900	9.3%
30	Colorado	14,500	1.1%
28	Connecticut	16,100	1.3%
45	Delaware	4,100	0.3%
2	Florida	92,200	7.2%
12	Georgia	31,600	2.5%
43	Hawaii	4,700	0.4%
42	Idaho	5,200	0.4%
7	Illinois	57,400	4.5%
14	Indiana	30,000	2.3%
29	Iowa	14,800	1.2%
33	Kansas	12,300	1.0%
23	Kentucky	21,100	1.6%
22	Louisiana	21,900	1.7%
38	Maine	7,000	0.5%
19	Maryland	23,500	1.8%
11	Massachusetts	31,700	2.5%
8	Michigan	45,800	3.6%
24	Minnesota	20,800	1.6%
31	Mississippi	14,400	1.1%
16	Missouri	28,600	2.2%
44	Montana	4,400	0.3%
36	Nebraska	7,700	0.6%
35	Nevada	9,500	0.7%
40	New Hampshire	5,800	0.5%
9	New Jersey	41,100	3.2%
37	New Mexico	7,100	0.6%
3	New York	83,700	6.5%
10	North Carolina	38,200	3.0%
47	North Dakota	3,100	0.2%
6	Ohio	58,700	4.6%
26	Oklahoma	16,900	1.3%
27	Oregon	16,800	1.3%
5	Pennsylvania	68,900	5.4%
41	Rhode Island	5,600	0.4%
25	South Carolina	19,500	1.5%
46	South Dakota	3,700	0.3%
15	Tennessee	29,100	2.3%
4	Texas	79,700	6.2%
39	Utah	5,900	0.5%
48	Vermont	2,900	0.2%
13	Virginia	31,300	2.4%
17	Washington	25,600	2.0%
34	West Virginia	11,000	0.9%
18	Wisconsin	25,300	2.0%
49	Wyoming	2,300	0.2%

RANK ORDER

RANK	STATE	CASES	% of USA
1	California	119,900	9.3%
2	Florida	92,200	7.2%
3	New York	83,700	6.5%
4	Texas	79,700	6.2%
5	Pennsylvania	68,900	5.4%
6	Ohio	58,700	4.6%
7	Illinois	57,400	4.5%
8	Michigan	45,800	3.6%
9	New Jersey	41,100	3.2%
10	North Carolina	38,200	3.0%
11	Massachusetts	31,700	2.5%
12	Georgia	31,600	2.5%
13	Virginia	31,300	2.4%
14	Indiana	30,000	2.3%
15	Tennessee	29,100	2.3%
16	Missouri	28,600	2.2%
17	Washington	25,600	2.0%
18	Wisconsin	25,300	2.0%
19	Maryland	23,500	1.8%
20	Alabama	22,600	1.8%
21	Arizona	22,100	1.7%
22	Louisiana	21,900	1.7%
23	Kentucky	21,100	1.6%
24	Minnesota	20,800	1.6%
25	South Carolina	19,500	1.5%
26	Oklahoma	16,900	1.3%
27	Oregon	16,800	1.3%
28	Connecticut	16,100	1.3%
29	Iowa	14,800	1.2%
30	Colorado	14,500	1.1%
31	Mississippi	14,400	1.1%
32	Arkansas	14,200	1.1%
33	Kansas	12,300	1.0%
34	West Virginia	11,000	0.9%
35	Nevada	9,500	0.7%
36	Nebraska	7,700	0.6%
37	New Mexico	7,100	0.6%
38	Maine	7,000	0.5%
39	Utah	5,900	0.5%
40	New Hampshire	5,800	0.5%
41	Rhode Island	5,600	0.4%
42	Idaho	5,200	0.4%
43	Hawaii	4,700	0.4%
44	Montana	4,400	0.3%
45	Delaware	4,100	0.3%
46	South Dakota	3,700	0.3%
47	North Dakota	3,100	0.2%
48	Vermont	2,900	0.2%
49	Wyoming	2,300	0.2%
50	Alaska	1,600	0.1%
	District of Columbia	2,700	0.2%

Source: American Cancer Society

"Cancer Facts & Figures 2002" (Copyright 2002, Reprinted with permission from the American Cancer Society)
These estimates are offered as a rough guide and should not be regarded as definitive. They are calculated according to the distribution of estimated 2002 cancer deaths by state. Totals do not include basal and squamous cell skin cancers or in situ carcinomas except urinary bladder.

Estimated Rate of New Cancer Cases in 2002

National Estimated Rate = 451.2 New Cases per 100,000 Population*

ALPHA ORDER

RANK	STATE	RATE
13	Alabama	506.2
50	Alaska	252.0
41	Arizona	416.4
6	Arkansas	527.5
47	California	347.5
48	Colorado	328.2
26	Connecticut	470.1
9	Delaware	515.0
2	Florida	562.3
45	Georgia	376.9
44	Hawaii	383.9
42	Idaho	393.6
31	Illinois	459.9
16	Indiana	490.6
12	Iowa	506.3
33	Kansas	456.5
7	Kentucky	519.0
17	Louisiana	490.4
4	Maine	544.0
37	Maryland	437.2
15	Massachusetts	496.9
32	Michigan	458.4
40	Minnesota	418.3
14	Mississippi	503.8
10	Missouri	508.0
21	Montana	486.5
35	Nebraska	449.4
34	Nevada	451.1
30	New Hampshire	460.6
22	New Jersey	484.4
43	New Mexico	388.2
36	New York	440.3
28	North Carolina	466.6
19	North Dakota	488.6
8	Ohio	516.1
20	Oklahoma	488.4
23	Oregon	483.8
3	Pennsylvania	560.7
5	Rhode Island	528.8
24	South Carolina	479.9
18	South Dakota	489.0
11	Tennessee	507.0
46	Texas	373.7
49	Utah	259.9
25	Vermont	473.0
38	Virginia	435.5
39	Washington	427.5
1	West Virginia	610.5
27	Wisconsin	468.4
29	Wyoming	465.2

RANK ORDER

RANK	STATE	RATE
1	West Virginia	610.5
2	Florida	562.3
3	Pennsylvania	560.7
4	Maine	544.0
5	Rhode Island	528.8
6	Arkansas	527.5
7	Kentucky	519.0
8	Ohio	516.1
9	Delaware	515.0
10	Missouri	508.0
11	Tennessee	507.0
12	Iowa	506.3
13	Alabama	506.2
14	Mississippi	503.8
15	Massachusetts	496.9
16	Indiana	490.6
17	Louisiana	490.4
18	South Dakota	489.0
19	North Dakota	488.6
20	Oklahoma	488.4
21	Montana	486.5
22	New Jersey	484.4
23	Oregon	483.8
24	South Carolina	479.9
25	Vermont	473.0
26	Connecticut	470.1
27	Wisconsin	468.4
28	North Carolina	466.6
29	Wyoming	465.2
30	New Hampshire	460.6
31	Illinois	459.9
32	Michigan	458.4
33	Kansas	456.5
34	Nevada	451.1
35	Nebraska	449.4
36	New York	440.3
37	Maryland	437.2
38	Virginia	435.5
39	Washington	427.5
40	Minnesota	418.3
41	Arizona	416.4
42	Idaho	393.6
43	New Mexico	388.2
44	Hawaii	383.9
45	Georgia	376.9
46	Texas	373.7
47	California	347.5
48	Colorado	328.2
49	Utah	259.9
50	Alaska	252.0

District of Columbia 472.2

Source: Morgan Quitno Press using data from American Cancer Society
"Cancer Facts & Figures 2002" (Copyright 2002, Reprinted with permission from the American Cancer Society)
*These estimates are offered as a rough guide and should not be regarded as definitive. They are calculated according to the distribution of estimated 2002 cancer deaths by state. Totals do not include basal and squamous cell skin cancers or in situ carcinomas except urinary bladder. Rates calculated using 2001 Census resident population estimates.

Age-Adjusted Rate of New Cancer Cases for Males in 1998

National Rate = 468.5 New Cases per 100,000 Male Population*

ALPHA ORDER				RANK ORDER		
RANK	STATE	RATE		RANK	STATE	RATE
43	Alabama	334.7		1	Rhode Island	526.3
32	Alaska	419.2		2	Maryland	519.2
35	Arizona	406.5		3	New Jersey	513.4
NA	Arkansas**	NA		4	Delaware	500.4
25	California	441.9		5	Michigan	499.4
30	Colorado	423.6		6	Louisiana	495.2
8	Connecticut	492.9		7	Florida	494.6
4	Delaware	500.4		8	Connecticut	492.9
7	Florida	494.6		9	Massachusetts	488.5
41	Georgia	365.1		10	Kentucky	487.1
38	Hawaii	391.4		11	Pennsylvania	485.4
33	Idaho	418.0		12	South Carolina	469.7
13	Illinois	469.1		13	Illinois	469.1
34	Indiana	410.3		14	Wisconsin	468.4
19	Iowa	459.0		15	New Hampshire	467.5
NA	Kansas**	NA		16	Missouri	464.3
10	Kentucky	487.1		17	Washington	463.7
6	Louisiana	495.2		18	New York	461.7
NA	Maine**	NA		19	Iowa	459.0
2	Maryland	519.2		20	West Virginia	458.3
9	Massachusetts	488.5		21	Minnesota	453.5
5	Michigan	499.4		22	North Dakota	447.8
21	Minnesota	453.5		23	Nebraska	446.0
40	Mississippi	383.2		24	Texas	445.2
16	Missouri	464.3		25	California	441.9
31	Montana	419.6		26	North Carolina	441.8
23	Nebraska	446.0		27	Oregon	436.3
42	Nevada	360.3		28	Ohio	431.2
15	New Hampshire	467.5		29	Wyoming	423.8
3	New Jersey	513.4		30	Colorado	423.6
37	New Mexico	392.7		31	Montana	419.6
18	New York	461.7		32	Alaska	419.2
26	North Carolina	441.8		33	Idaho	418.0
22	North Dakota	447.8		34	Indiana	410.3
28	Ohio	431.2		35	Arizona	406.5
NA	Oklahoma**	NA		36	Virginia	404.8
27	Oregon	436.3		37	New Mexico	392.7
11	Pennsylvania	485.4		38	Hawaii	391.4
1	Rhode Island	526.3		39	Utah	385.8
12	South Carolina	469.7		40	Mississippi	383.2
NA	South Dakota**	NA		41	Georgia	365.1
NA	Tennessee**	NA		42	Nevada	360.3
24	Texas	445.2		43	Alabama	334.7
39	Utah	385.8		NA	Arkansas**	NA
NA	Vermont**	NA		NA	Kansas**	NA
36	Virginia	404.8		NA	Maine**	NA
17	Washington	463.7		NA	Oklahoma**	NA
20	West Virginia	458.3		NA	South Dakota**	NA
14	Wisconsin	468.4		NA	Tennessee**	NA
29	Wyoming	423.8		NA	Vermont**	NA
					District of Columbia	606.9

Source: American Cancer Society

"Cancer Facts & Figures 2002" (Copyright 2002, Reprinted with permission from the American Cancer Society)
*For 1994 to 1998. Age-adjusted to the 1970 U.S. standard population.
**Not available.

Age-Adjusted Rate of New Cancer Cases for Females in 1998

National Rate = 352.8 New Cases per 100,000 Female Population*

ALPHA ORDER

RANK	STATE	RATE
43	Alabama	246.8
9	Alaska	362.8
34	Arizona	313.9
NA	Arkansas**	NA
21	California	343.2
25	Colorado	324.8
2	Connecticut	379.9
4	Delaware	375.6
7	Florida	366.1
41	Georgia	261.2
33	Hawaii	315.8
27	Idaho	323.4
15	Illinois	353.2
28	Indiana	323.0
19	Iowa	349.0
NA	Kansas**	NA
13	Kentucky	354.8
30	Louisiana	319.9
NA	Maine**	NA
5	Maryland	374.2
8	Massachusetts	365.7
12	Michigan	358.7
23	Minnesota	336.5
42	Mississippi	253.7
16	Missouri	352.7
26	Montana	323.9
24	Nebraska	334.5
37	Nevada	307.2
11	New Hampshire	359.3
3	New Jersey	377.3
38	New Mexico	301.4
10	New York	360.4
36	North Carolina	308.8
35	North Dakota	311.4
22	Ohio	341.0
NA	Oklahoma**	NA
14	Oregon	354.2
17	Pennsylvania	352.6
1	Rhode Island	388.3
29	South Carolina	321.0
NA	South Dakota**	NA
NA	Tennessee**	NA
31	Texas	316.6
40	Utah	286.1
NA	Vermont**	NA
39	Virginia	297.9
6	Washington	371.7
20	West Virginia	346.1
18	Wisconsin	351.5
32	Wyoming	316.5

RANK ORDER

RANK	STATE	RATE
1	Rhode Island	388.3
2	Connecticut	379.9
3	New Jersey	377.3
4	Delaware	375.6
5	Maryland	374.2
6	Washington	371.7
7	Florida	366.1
8	Massachusetts	365.7
9	Alaska	362.8
10	New York	360.4
11	New Hampshire	359.3
12	Michigan	358.7
13	Kentucky	354.8
14	Oregon	354.2
15	Illinois	353.2
16	Missouri	352.7
17	Pennsylvania	352.6
18	Wisconsin	351.5
19	Iowa	349.0
20	West Virginia	346.1
21	California	343.2
22	Ohio	341.0
23	Minnesota	336.5
24	Nebraska	334.5
25	Colorado	324.8
26	Montana	323.9
27	Idaho	323.4
28	Indiana	323.0
29	South Carolina	321.0
30	Louisiana	319.9
31	Texas	316.6
32	Wyoming	316.5
33	Hawaii	315.8
34	Arizona	313.9
35	North Dakota	311.4
36	North Carolina	308.8
37	Nevada	307.2
38	New Mexico	301.4
39	Virginia	297.9
40	Utah	286.1
41	Georgia	261.2
42	Mississippi	253.7
43	Alabama	246.8
NA	Arkansas**	NA
NA	Kansas**	NA
NA	Maine**	NA
NA	Oklahoma**	NA
NA	South Dakota**	NA
NA	Tennessee**	NA
NA	Vermont**	NA
	District of Columbia	374.1

Source: American Cancer Society
    "Cancer Facts & Figures 2002" (Copyright 2002, Reprinted with permission from the American Cancer Society)
*For 1994 to 1998. Age-adjusted to the 1970 U.S. standard population.
**Not available.

Estimated New Cases of Bladder Cancer in 2002

National Estimated Total = 56,500 New Cases*

ALPHA ORDER

RANK	STATE	CASES	% of USA
22	Alabama	800	1.4%
46	Alaska	100	0.2%
19	Arizona	1,000	1.8%
31	Arkansas	500	0.9%
1	California	5,600	9.9%
29	Colorado	600	1.1%
22	Connecticut	800	1.4%
37	Delaware	300	0.5%
2	Florida	4,300	7.6%
15	Georgia	1,100	1.9%
46	Hawaii	100	0.2%
37	Idaho	300	0.5%
7	Illinois	2,500	4.4%
12	Indiana	1,300	2.3%
29	Iowa	600	1.1%
31	Kansas	500	0.9%
22	Kentucky	800	1.4%
27	Louisiana	700	1.2%
35	Maine	400	0.7%
15	Maryland	1,100	1.9%
10	Massachusetts	1,700	3.0%
8	Michigan	2,100	3.7%
19	Minnesota	1,000	1.8%
31	Mississippi	500	0.9%
15	Missouri	1,100	1.9%
44	Montana	200	0.4%
37	Nebraska	300	0.5%
35	Nevada	400	0.7%
37	New Hampshire	300	0.5%
8	New Jersey	2,100	3.7%
37	New Mexico	300	0.5%
2	New York	4,300	7.6%
11	North Carolina	1,500	2.7%
44	North Dakota	200	0.4%
6	Ohio	2,700	4.8%
27	Oklahoma	700	1.2%
22	Oregon	800	1.4%
4	Pennsylvania	3,300	5.8%
37	Rhode Island	300	0.5%
22	South Carolina	800	1.4%
46	South Dakota	100	0.2%
19	Tennessee	1,000	1.8%
5	Texas	3,000	5.3%
37	Utah	300	0.5%
46	Vermont	100	0.2%
13	Virginia	1,200	2.1%
15	Washington	1,100	1.9%
31	West Virginia	500	0.9%
13	Wisconsin	1,200	2.1%
46	Wyoming	100	0.2%

RANK ORDER

RANK	STATE	CASES	% of USA
1	California	5,600	9.9%
2	Florida	4,300	7.6%
2	New York	4,300	7.6%
4	Pennsylvania	3,300	5.8%
5	Texas	3,000	5.3%
6	Ohio	2,700	4.8%
7	Illinois	2,500	4.4%
8	Michigan	2,100	3.7%
8	New Jersey	2,100	3.7%
10	Massachusetts	1,700	3.0%
11	North Carolina	1,500	2.7%
12	Indiana	1,300	2.3%
13	Virginia	1,200	2.1%
13	Wisconsin	1,200	2.1%
15	Georgia	1,100	1.9%
15	Maryland	1,100	1.9%
15	Missouri	1,100	1.9%
15	Washington	1,100	1.9%
19	Arizona	1,000	1.8%
19	Minnesota	1,000	1.8%
19	Tennessee	1,000	1.8%
22	Alabama	800	1.4%
22	Connecticut	800	1.4%
22	Kentucky	800	1.4%
22	Oregon	800	1.4%
22	South Carolina	800	1.4%
27	Louisiana	700	1.2%
27	Oklahoma	700	1.2%
29	Colorado	600	1.1%
29	Iowa	600	1.1%
31	Arkansas	500	0.9%
31	Kansas	500	0.9%
31	Mississippi	500	0.9%
31	West Virginia	500	0.9%
35	Maine	400	0.7%
35	Nevada	400	0.7%
37	Delaware	300	0.5%
37	Idaho	300	0.5%
37	Nebraska	300	0.5%
37	New Hampshire	300	0.5%
37	New Mexico	300	0.5%
37	Rhode Island	300	0.5%
37	Utah	300	0.5%
44	Montana	200	0.4%
44	North Dakota	200	0.4%
46	Alaska	100	0.2%
46	Hawaii	100	0.2%
46	South Dakota	100	0.2%
46	Vermont	100	0.2%
46	Wyoming	100	0.2%
	District of Columbia	100	0.2%

Source: American Cancer Society
    "Cancer Facts & Figures 2002" (Copyright 2002, Reprinted with permission from the American Cancer Society)
*These estimates are offered as a rough guide and should be interpreted with caution. They are calculated
according to the distribution of estimated 2002 cancer deaths by state.

Estimated Rate of New Bladder Cancer Cases in 2002

National Estimated Rate = 19.8 New Cases per 100,000 Population*

ALPHA ORDER

RANK	STATE	RATE
35	Alabama	17.9
43	Alaska	15.8
30	Arizona	18.8
31	Arkansas	18.6
42	California	16.2
46	Colorado	13.6
12	Connecticut	23.4
1	Delaware	37.7
8	Florida	26.2
49	Georgia	13.1
50	Hawaii	8.2
14	Idaho	22.7
25	Illinois	20.0
18	Indiana	21.3
20	Iowa	20.5
31	Kansas	18.6
26	Kentucky	19.7
44	Louisiana	15.7
3	Maine	31.1
20	Maryland	20.5
7	Massachusetts	26.6
19	Michigan	21.0
24	Minnesota	20.1
36	Mississippi	17.5
28	Missouri	19.5
17	Montana	22.1
36	Nebraska	17.5
29	Nevada	19.0
10	New Hampshire	23.8
9	New Jersey	24.8
40	New Mexico	16.4
15	New York	22.6
34	North Carolina	18.3
2	North Dakota	31.5
11	Ohio	23.7
22	Oklahoma	20.2
13	Oregon	23.0
6	Pennsylvania	26.9
4	Rhode Island	28.3
26	South Carolina	19.7
47	South Dakota	13.2
38	Tennessee	17.4
45	Texas	14.1
47	Utah	13.2
41	Vermont	16.3
39	Virginia	16.7
33	Washington	18.4
5	West Virginia	27.7
16	Wisconsin	22.2
22	Wyoming	20.2

RANK ORDER

RANK	STATE	RATE
1	Delaware	37.7
2	North Dakota	31.5
3	Maine	31.1
4	Rhode Island	28.3
5	West Virginia	27.7
6	Pennsylvania	26.9
7	Massachusetts	26.6
8	Florida	26.2
9	New Jersey	24.8
10	New Hampshire	23.8
11	Ohio	23.7
12	Connecticut	23.4
13	Oregon	23.0
14	Idaho	22.7
15	New York	22.6
16	Wisconsin	22.2
17	Montana	22.1
18	Indiana	21.3
19	Michigan	21.0
20	Iowa	20.5
20	Maryland	20.5
22	Oklahoma	20.2
22	Wyoming	20.2
24	Minnesota	20.1
25	Illinois	20.0
26	Kentucky	19.7
26	South Carolina	19.7
28	Missouri	19.5
29	Nevada	19.0
30	Arizona	18.8
31	Arkansas	18.6
31	Kansas	18.6
33	Washington	18.4
34	North Carolina	18.3
35	Alabama	17.9
36	Mississippi	17.5
36	Nebraska	17.5
38	Tennessee	17.4
39	Virginia	16.7
40	New Mexico	16.4
41	Vermont	16.3
42	California	16.2
43	Alaska	15.8
44	Louisiana	15.7
45	Texas	14.1
46	Colorado	13.6
47	South Dakota	13.2
47	Utah	13.2
49	Georgia	13.1
50	Hawaii	8.2
	District of Columbia	17.5

Source: Morgan Quitno Press using data from American Cancer Society
    "Cancer Facts & Figures 2002" (Copyright 2002, Reprinted with permission from the American Cancer Society)
*These estimates are offered as a rough guide and should be interpreted with caution. They are calculated according to the distribution of estimated 2002 cancer deaths by state. Rates calculated using 2001 Census resident population estimates.

Estimated New Female Breast Cancer Cases in 2002

National Estimated Total = 203,500 New Cases*

ALPHA ORDER					RANK ORDER				
RANK	STATE		CASES	% of USA	RANK	STATE		CASES	% of USA
23	Alabama		3,100	1.5%	1	California		19,900	9.8%
49	Alaska		300	0.1%	2	New York		14,700	7.2%
20	Arizona		3,500	1.7%	3	Florida		13,100	6.4%
32	Arkansas		2,000	1.0%	3	Texas		13,100	6.4%
1	California		19,900	9.8%	5	Pennsylvania		11,000	5.4%
29	Colorado		2,400	1.2%	6	Illinois		9,700	4.8%
27	Connecticut		2,600	1.3%	7	Ohio		9,500	4.7%
44	Delaware		600	0.3%	8	Michigan		7,300	3.6%
3	Florida		13,100	6.4%	9	New Jersey		6,900	3.4%
11	Georgia		5,200	2.6%	10	North Carolina		5,900	2.9%
43	Hawaii		700	0.3%	11	Georgia		5,200	2.6%
40	Idaho		900	0.4%	12	Virginia		5,000	2.5%
6	Illinois		9,700	4.8%	13	Massachusetts		4,700	2.3%
14	Indiana		4,600	2.3%	14	Indiana		4,600	2.3%
29	Iowa		2,400	1.2%	15	Tennessee		4,400	2.2%
33	Kansas		1,800	0.9%	16	Maryland		4,100	2.0%
23	Kentucky		3,100	1.5%	17	Missouri		4,000	2.0%
20	Louisiana		3,500	1.7%	18	Wisconsin		3,900	1.9%
39	Maine		1,000	0.5%	19	Washington		3,700	1.8%
16	Maryland		4,100	2.0%	20	Arizona		3,500	1.7%
13	Massachusetts		4,700	2.3%	20	Louisiana		3,500	1.7%
8	Michigan		7,300	3.6%	22	Minnesota		3,200	1.6%
22	Minnesota		3,200	1.6%	23	Alabama		3,100	1.5%
31	Mississippi		2,200	1.1%	23	Kentucky		3,100	1.5%
17	Missouri		4,000	2.0%	23	South Carolina		3,100	1.5%
44	Montana		600	0.3%	26	Oklahoma		2,700	1.3%
36	Nebraska		1,200	0.6%	27	Connecticut		2,600	1.3%
35	Nevada		1,300	0.6%	27	Oregon		2,600	1.3%
41	New Hampshire		800	0.4%	29	Colorado		2,400	1.2%
9	New Jersey		6,900	3.4%	29	Iowa		2,400	1.2%
36	New Mexico		1,200	0.6%	31	Mississippi		2,200	1.1%
2	New York		14,700	7.2%	32	Arkansas		2,000	1.0%
10	North Carolina		5,900	2.9%	33	Kansas		1,800	0.9%
46	North Dakota		500	0.2%	34	West Virginia		1,500	0.7%
7	Ohio		9,500	4.7%	35	Nevada		1,300	0.6%
26	Oklahoma		2,700	1.3%	36	Nebraska		1,200	0.6%
27	Oregon		2,600	1.3%	36	New Mexico		1,200	0.6%
5	Pennsylvania		11,000	5.4%	38	Utah		1,100	0.5%
41	Rhode Island		800	0.4%	39	Maine		1,000	0.5%
23	South Carolina		3,100	1.5%	40	Idaho		900	0.4%
46	South Dakota		500	0.2%	41	New Hampshire		800	0.4%
15	Tennessee		4,400	2.2%	41	Rhode Island		800	0.4%
3	Texas		13,100	6.4%	43	Hawaii		700	0.3%
38	Utah		1,100	0.5%	44	Delaware		600	0.3%
48	Vermont		400	0.2%	44	Montana		600	0.3%
12	Virginia		5,000	2.5%	46	North Dakota		500	0.2%
19	Washington		3,700	1.8%	46	South Dakota		500	0.2%
34	West Virginia		1,500	0.7%	48	Vermont		400	0.2%
18	Wisconsin		3,900	1.9%	49	Alaska		300	0.1%
49	Wyoming		300	0.1%	49	Wyoming		300	0.1%
						District of Columbia		600	0.3%

Source: American Cancer Society

"Cancer Facts & Figures 2002" (Copyright 2002, Reprinted with permission from the American Cancer Society)
*These estimates are offered as a rough guide and should be interpreted with caution. They are calculated according to the distribution of estimated 2002 cancer deaths by state.

Estimated Rate of New Female Breast Cancer Cases in 2002

National Estimated Rate = 141.9 New Cases per 100,000 Female Population*

ALPHA ORDER			RANK ORDER		
RANK	STATE	RATE	RANK	STATE	RATE
33	Alabama	134.7	1	Pennsylvania	173.2
49	Alaska	99.1	2	Ohio	162.6
32	Arizona	136.2	3	West Virginia	161.4
23	Arkansas	146.1	4	Iowa	161.0
46	California	117.1	5	Florida	160.1
48	Colorado	112.4	6	New Jersey	159.3
21	Connecticut	148.0	7	North Dakota	155.4
19	Delaware	148.9	8	Oklahoma	153.9
5	Florida	160.1	9	Illinois	153.0
42	Georgia	125.0	10	Maine	152.8
47	Hawaii	116.1	11	Louisiana	151.8
28	Idaho	139.5	12	Oregon	150.7
9	Illinois	153.0	12	Tennessee	150.7
20	Indiana	148.5	14	South Carolina	150.3
4	Iowa	161.0	15	Kentucky	150.0
36	Kansas	132.4	16	Maryland	149.7
15	Kentucky	150.0	17	Mississippi	149.5
11	Louisiana	151.8	17	New York	149.5
10	Maine	152.8	19	Delaware	148.9
16	Maryland	149.7	20	Indiana	148.5
27	Massachusetts	142.8	21	Connecticut	148.0
24	Michigan	144.1	22	Rhode Island	146.9
39	Minnesota	128.8	23	Arkansas	146.1
17	Mississippi	149.5	24	Michigan	144.1
29	Missouri	139.1	25	North Carolina	143.7
35	Montana	132.5	25	Wisconsin	143.7
31	Nebraska	138.3	27	Massachusetts	142.8
34	Nevada	132.6	28	Idaho	139.5
41	New Hampshire	127.4	29	Missouri	139.1
6	New Jersey	159.3	30	Virginia	138.6
38	New Mexico	129.8	31	Nebraska	138.3
17	New York	149.5	32	Arizona	136.2
25	North Carolina	143.7	33	Alabama	134.7
7	North Dakota	155.4	34	Nevada	132.6
2	Ohio	162.6	35	Montana	132.5
8	Oklahoma	153.9	36	Kansas	132.4
12	Oregon	150.7	37	South Dakota	131.5
1	Pennsylvania	173.2	38	New Mexico	129.8
22	Rhode Island	146.9	39	Minnesota	128.8
14	South Carolina	150.3	39	Vermont	128.8
37	South Dakota	131.5	41	New Hampshire	127.4
12	Tennessee	150.7	42	Georgia	125.0
44	Texas	124.8	42	Washington	125.0
50	Utah	98.7	44	Texas	124.8
39	Vermont	128.8	45	Wyoming	122.2
30	Virginia	138.6	46	California	117.1
42	Washington	125.0	47	Hawaii	116.1
3	West Virginia	161.4	48	Colorado	112.4
25	Wisconsin	143.7	49	Alaska	99.1
45	Wyoming	122.2	50	Utah	98.7
				District of Columbia	198.2

Source: Morgan Quitno Press using data from American Cancer Society
"Cancer Facts & Figures 2002" (Copyright 2002, Reprinted with permission from the American Cancer Society)
*These estimates are offered as a rough guide and should be interpreted with caution. They are calculated according to the distribution of estimated 2002 cancer deaths by state. Rates calculated using 2000 Census female resident population figures.

Percent of Women 40 and Older
Who Have Ever Had a Mammogram: 2000
National Percent = 88.0% of Women 40 and Older

ALPHA ORDER

RANK	STATE	PERCENT
20	Alabama	88.7
41	Alaska	86.2
14	Arizona	89.5
44	Arkansas	85.3
NA	California*	NA
26	Colorado	87.6
2	Connecticut	92.7
1	Delaware	92.9
19	Florida	88.9
27	Georgia	87.4
14	Hawaii	89.5
47	Idaho	84.1
27	Illinois	87.4
36	Indiana	86.5
35	Iowa	86.9
22	Kansas	88.3
33	Kentucky	87.1
43	Louisiana	85.8
8	Maine	90.7
7	Maryland	90.8
3	Massachusetts	92.1
5	Michigan	91.2
31	Minnesota	87.3
48	Mississippi	83.6
44	Missouri	85.3
27	Montana	87.4
37	Nebraska	86.4
17	Nevada	89.1
6	New Hampshire	91.0
42	New Jersey	86.0
31	New Mexico	87.3
10	New York	90.2
17	North Carolina	89.1
25	North Dakota	88.0
13	Ohio	89.6
49	Oklahoma	82.3
9	Oregon	90.6
11	Pennsylvania	90.0
4	Rhode Island	91.9
11	South Carolina	90.0
34	South Dakota	87.0
24	Tennessee	88.1
46	Texas	84.9
37	Utah	86.4
27	Vermont	87.4
21	Virginia	88.6
16	Washington	89.3
37	West Virginia	86.4
23	Wisconsin	88.2
37	Wyoming	86.4

RANK ORDER

RANK	STATE	PERCENT
1	Delaware	92.9
2	Connecticut	92.7
3	Massachusetts	92.1
4	Rhode Island	91.9
5	Michigan	91.2
6	New Hampshire	91.0
7	Maryland	90.8
8	Maine	90.7
9	Oregon	90.6
10	New York	90.2
11	Pennsylvania	90.0
11	South Carolina	90.0
13	Ohio	89.6
14	Arizona	89.5
14	Hawaii	89.5
16	Washington	89.3
17	Nevada	89.1
17	North Carolina	89.1
19	Florida	88.9
20	Alabama	88.7
21	Virginia	88.6
22	Kansas	88.3
23	Wisconsin	88.2
24	Tennessee	88.1
25	North Dakota	88.0
26	Colorado	87.6
27	Georgia	87.4
27	Illinois	87.4
27	Montana	87.4
27	Vermont	87.4
31	Minnesota	87.3
31	New Mexico	87.3
33	Kentucky	87.1
34	South Dakota	87.0
35	Iowa	86.9
36	Indiana	86.5
37	Nebraska	86.4
37	Utah	86.4
37	West Virginia	86.4
37	Wyoming	86.4
41	Alaska	86.2
42	New Jersey	86.0
43	Louisiana	85.8
44	Arkansas	85.3
44	Missouri	85.3
46	Texas	84.9
47	Idaho	84.1
48	Mississippi	83.6
49	Oklahoma	82.3
NA	California*	NA
	District of Columbia	93.0

Source: U.S. Department of Health and Human Services, Centers for Disease Control and Prevention
"2000 Behavioral Risk Factor Surveillance Summary Prevalence Report" (May 3, 2001)
*Not available.

Estimated New Colon and Rectum Cancer Cases in 2002

National Estimated Total = 148,300 New Cases*

ALPHA ORDER

RANK ORDER

RANK	STATE	CASES	% of USA
24	Alabama	2,200	1.5%
50	Alaska	200	0.1%
21	Arizona	2,400	1.6%
31	Arkansas	1,500	1.0%
1	California	12,900	8.7%
30	Colorado	1,600	1.1%
28	Connecticut	1,800	1.2%
46	Delaware	400	0.3%
2	Florida	10,400	7.0%
15	Georgia	3,200	2.2%
43	Hawaii	500	0.3%
42	Idaho	600	0.4%
7	Illinois	6,800	4.6%
12	Indiana	3,600	2.4%
26	Iowa	2,000	1.3%
33	Kansas	1,400	0.9%
22	Kentucky	2,300	1.6%
20	Louisiana	2,600	1.8%
37	Maine	800	0.5%
17	Maryland	2,900	2.0%
11	Massachusetts	3,800	2.6%
8	Michigan	5,300	3.6%
22	Minnesota	2,300	1.6%
31	Mississippi	1,500	1.0%
14	Missouri	3,300	2.2%
43	Montana	500	0.3%
36	Nebraska	1,100	0.7%
35	Nevada	1,200	0.8%
39	New Hampshire	700	0.5%
9	New Jersey	4,900	3.3%
37	New Mexico	800	0.5%
2	New York	10,400	7.0%
10	North Carolina	4,200	2.8%
46	North Dakota	400	0.3%
6	Ohio	7,200	4.9%
26	Oklahoma	2,000	1.3%
28	Oregon	1,800	1.2%
5	Pennsylvania	8,700	5.9%
39	Rhode Island	700	0.5%
24	South Carolina	2,200	1.5%
43	South Dakota	500	0.3%
16	Tennessee	3,100	2.1%
4	Texas	9,500	6.4%
39	Utah	700	0.5%
46	Vermont	400	0.3%
13	Virginia	3,500	2.4%
19	Washington	2,700	1.8%
34	West Virginia	1,300	0.9%
17	Wisconsin	2,900	2.0%
49	Wyoming	300	0.2%

RANK	STATE	CASES	% of USA
1	California	12,900	8.7%
2	Florida	10,400	7.0%
2	New York	10,400	7.0%
4	Texas	9,500	6.4%
5	Pennsylvania	8,700	5.9%
6	Ohio	7,200	4.9%
7	Illinois	6,800	4.6%
8	Michigan	5,300	3.6%
9	New Jersey	4,900	3.3%
10	North Carolina	4,200	2.8%
11	Massachusetts	3,800	2.6%
12	Indiana	3,600	2.4%
13	Virginia	3,500	2.4%
14	Missouri	3,300	2.2%
15	Georgia	3,200	2.2%
16	Tennessee	3,100	2.1%
17	Maryland	2,900	2.0%
17	Wisconsin	2,900	2.0%
19	Washington	2,700	1.8%
20	Louisiana	2,600	1.8%
21	Arizona	2,400	1.6%
22	Kentucky	2,300	1.6%
22	Minnesota	2,300	1.6%
24	Alabama	2,200	1.5%
24	South Carolina	2,200	1.5%
26	Iowa	2,000	1.3%
26	Oklahoma	2,000	1.3%
28	Connecticut	1,800	1.2%
28	Oregon	1,800	1.2%
30	Colorado	1,600	1.1%
31	Arkansas	1,500	1.0%
31	Mississippi	1,500	1.0%
33	Kansas	1,400	0.9%
34	West Virginia	1,300	0.9%
35	Nevada	1,200	0.8%
36	Nebraska	1,100	0.7%
37	Maine	800	0.5%
37	New Mexico	800	0.5%
39	New Hampshire	700	0.5%
39	Rhode Island	700	0.5%
39	Utah	700	0.5%
42	Idaho	600	0.4%
43	Hawaii	500	0.3%
43	Montana	500	0.3%
43	South Dakota	500	0.3%
46	Delaware	400	0.3%
46	North Dakota	400	0.3%
46	Vermont	400	0.3%
49	Wyoming	300	0.2%
50	Alaska	200	0.1%
	District of Columbia	300	0.2%

Source: American Cancer Society
    "Cancer Facts & Figures 2002" (Copyright 2002, Reprinted with permission from the American Cancer Society)
*These estimates are offered as a rough guide and should be interpreted with caution. They are calculated according to the distribution of estimated 2002 cancer deaths by state.

Estimated Rate of New Colon and Rectum Cancer Cases in 2002

National Estimated Rate = 52.1 New Cases per 100,000 Population*

ALPHA ORDER

RANK	STATE	RATE
37	Alabama	49.3
49	Alaska	31.5
41	Arizona	45.2
21	Arkansas	55.7
47	California	37.4
48	Colorado	36.2
31	Connecticut	52.6
36	Delaware	50.2
8	Florida	63.4
46	Georgia	38.2
45	Hawaii	40.8
40	Idaho	45.4
25	Illinois	54.5
14	Indiana	58.9
3	Iowa	68.4
33	Kansas	52.0
20	Kentucky	56.6
16	Louisiana	58.2
11	Maine	62.2
27	Maryland	54.0
13	Massachusetts	59.6
30	Michigan	53.0
39	Minnesota	46.3
32	Mississippi	52.5
15	Missouri	58.6
23	Montana	55.3
7	Nebraska	64.2
19	Nevada	57.0
22	New Hampshire	55.6
17	New Jersey	57.8
44	New Mexico	43.7
24	New York	54.7
35	North Carolina	51.3
10	North Dakota	63.0
9	Ohio	63.3
17	Oklahoma	57.8
34	Oregon	51.8
2	Pennsylvania	70.8
4	Rhode Island	66.1
26	South Carolina	54.1
4	South Dakota	66.1
27	Tennessee	54.0
43	Texas	44.5
50	Utah	30.8
6	Vermont	65.2
38	Virginia	48.7
42	Washington	45.1
1	West Virginia	72.1
29	Wisconsin	53.7
12	Wyoming	60.7

RANK ORDER

RANK	STATE	RATE
1	West Virginia	72.1
2	Pennsylvania	70.8
3	Iowa	68.4
4	Rhode Island	66.1
4	South Dakota	66.1
6	Vermont	65.2
7	Nebraska	64.2
8	Florida	63.4
9	Ohio	63.3
10	North Dakota	63.0
11	Maine	62.2
12	Wyoming	60.7
13	Massachusetts	59.6
14	Indiana	58.9
15	Missouri	58.6
16	Louisiana	58.2
17	New Jersey	57.8
17	Oklahoma	57.8
19	Nevada	57.0
20	Kentucky	56.6
21	Arkansas	55.7
22	New Hampshire	55.6
23	Montana	55.3
24	New York	54.7
25	Illinois	54.5
26	South Carolina	54.1
27	Maryland	54.0
27	Tennessee	54.0
29	Wisconsin	53.7
30	Michigan	53.0
31	Connecticut	52.6
32	Mississippi	52.5
33	Kansas	52.0
34	Oregon	51.8
35	North Carolina	51.3
36	Delaware	50.2
37	Alabama	49.3
38	Virginia	48.7
39	Minnesota	46.3
40	Idaho	45.4
41	Arizona	45.2
42	Washington	45.1
43	Texas	44.5
44	New Mexico	43.7
45	Hawaii	40.8
46	Georgia	38.2
47	California	37.4
48	Colorado	36.2
49	Alaska	31.5
50	Utah	30.8
	District of Columbia	52.5

Source: Morgan Quitno Press using data from American Cancer Society
   "Cancer Facts & Figures 2002" (Copyright 2002, Reprinted with permission from the American Cancer Society)
*These estimates are offered as a rough guide and should be interpreted with caution. They are calculated
according to the distribution of estimated 2002 cancer deaths by state. Rates calculated using 2001 Census
resident population estimates.

Estimated New Leukemia Cases in 2002

National Estimated Total = 30,800 New Cases*

ALPHA ORDER

RANK	STATE	CASES	% of USA
20	Alabama	500	1.6%
NA	Alaska**	NA	NA
20	Arizona	500	1.6%
31	Arkansas	300	1.0%
1	California	3,000	9.7%
24	Colorado	400	1.3%
24	Connecticut	400	1.3%
39	Delaware	100	0.3%
2	Florida	2,200	7.1%
11	Georgia	700	2.3%
39	Hawaii	100	0.3%
39	Idaho	100	0.3%
6	Illinois	1,400	4.5%
11	Indiana	700	2.3%
24	Iowa	400	1.3%
31	Kansas	300	1.0%
24	Kentucky	400	1.3%
20	Louisiana	500	1.6%
39	Maine	100	0.3%
20	Maryland	500	1.6%
11	Massachusetts	700	2.3%
9	Michigan	1,000	3.2%
19	Minnesota	600	1.9%
31	Mississippi	300	1.0%
11	Missouri	700	2.3%
39	Montana	100	0.3%
35	Nebraska	200	0.6%
35	Nevada	200	0.6%
39	New Hampshire	100	0.3%
8	New Jersey	1,100	3.6%
35	New Mexico	200	0.6%
3	New York	2,000	6.5%
10	North Carolina	900	2.9%
39	North Dakota	100	0.3%
6	Ohio	1,400	4.5%
24	Oklahoma	400	1.3%
24	Oregon	400	1.3%
5	Pennsylvania	1,600	5.2%
39	Rhode Island	100	0.3%
24	South Carolina	400	1.3%
39	South Dakota	100	0.3%
11	Tennessee	700	2.3%
4	Texas	1,900	6.2%
35	Utah	200	0.6%
39	Vermont	100	0.3%
11	Virginia	700	2.3%
11	Washington	700	2.3%
31	West Virginia	300	1.0%
11	Wisconsin	700	2.3%
39	Wyoming	100	0.3%

RANK ORDER

RANK	STATE	CASES	% of USA
1	California	3,000	9.7%
2	Florida	2,200	7.1%
3	New York	2,000	6.5%
4	Texas	1,900	6.2%
5	Pennsylvania	1,600	5.2%
6	Illinois	1,400	4.5%
6	Ohio	1,400	4.5%
8	New Jersey	1,100	3.6%
9	Michigan	1,000	3.2%
10	North Carolina	900	2.9%
11	Georgia	700	2.3%
11	Indiana	700	2.3%
11	Massachusetts	700	2.3%
11	Missouri	700	2.3%
11	Tennessee	700	2.3%
11	Virginia	700	2.3%
11	Washington	700	2.3%
11	Wisconsin	700	2.3%
19	Minnesota	600	1.9%
20	Alabama	500	1.6%
20	Arizona	500	1.6%
20	Louisiana	500	1.6%
20	Maryland	500	1.6%
24	Colorado	400	1.3%
24	Connecticut	400	1.3%
24	Iowa	400	1.3%
24	Kentucky	400	1.3%
24	Oklahoma	400	1.3%
24	Oregon	400	1.3%
24	South Carolina	400	1.3%
31	Arkansas	300	1.0%
31	Kansas	300	1.0%
31	Mississippi	300	1.0%
31	West Virginia	300	1.0%
35	Nebraska	200	0.6%
35	Nevada	200	0.6%
35	New Mexico	200	0.6%
35	Utah	200	0.6%
39	Delaware	100	0.3%
39	Hawaii	100	0.3%
39	Idaho	100	0.3%
39	Maine	100	0.3%
39	Montana	100	0.3%
39	New Hampshire	100	0.3%
39	North Dakota	100	0.3%
39	Rhode Island	100	0.3%
39	South Dakota	100	0.3%
39	Vermont	100	0.3%
39	Wyoming	100	0.3%
NA	Alaska**	NA	NA
	District of Columbia**	NA	NA

Source: American Cancer Society
"Cancer Facts & Figures 2002" (Copyright 2002, Reprinted with permission from the American Cancer Society)
*These estimates are offered as a rough guide and should be interpreted with caution. They are calculated according to the distribution of estimated 2002 cancer deaths by state.
**Not available.

Estimated Rate of New Leukemia Cases in 2002

National Estimated Rate = 10.8 New Cases per 100,000 Population*

ALPHA ORDER

RANK	STATE	RATE
22	Alabama	11.2
NA	Alaska**	NA
38	Arizona	9.4
25	Arkansas	11.1
44	California	8.7
41	Colorado	9.1
16	Connecticut	11.7
11	Delaware	12.6
6	Florida	13.4
45	Georgia	8.3
46	Hawaii	8.2
49	Idaho	7.6
22	Illinois	11.2
21	Indiana	11.4
5	Iowa	13.7
25	Kansas	11.1
34	Kentucky	9.8
22	Louisiana	11.2
48	Maine	7.8
40	Maryland	9.3
28	Massachusetts	11.0
33	Michigan	10.0
15	Minnesota	12.1
31	Mississippi	10.5
12	Missouri	12.4
25	Montana	11.1
16	Nebraska	11.7
37	Nevada	9.5
47	New Hampshire	7.9
8	New Jersey	13.0
30	New Mexico	10.9
31	New York	10.5
28	North Carolina	11.0
4	North Dakota	15.8
13	Ohio	12.3
19	Oklahoma	11.6
20	Oregon	11.5
8	Pennsylvania	13.0
38	Rhode Island	9.4
34	South Carolina	9.8
7	South Dakota	13.2
14	Tennessee	12.2
42	Texas	8.9
43	Utah	8.8
3	Vermont	16.3
36	Virginia	9.7
16	Washington	11.7
2	West Virginia	16.6
8	Wisconsin	13.0
1	Wyoming	20.2

RANK ORDER

RANK	STATE	RATE
1	Wyoming	20.2
2	West Virginia	16.6
3	Vermont	16.3
4	North Dakota	15.8
5	Iowa	13.7
6	Florida	13.4
7	South Dakota	13.2
8	New Jersey	13.0
8	Pennsylvania	13.0
8	Wisconsin	13.0
11	Delaware	12.6
12	Missouri	12.4
13	Ohio	12.3
14	Tennessee	12.2
15	Minnesota	12.1
16	Connecticut	11.7
16	Nebraska	11.7
16	Washington	11.7
19	Oklahoma	11.6
20	Oregon	11.5
21	Indiana	11.4
22	Alabama	11.2
22	Illinois	11.2
22	Louisiana	11.2
25	Arkansas	11.1
25	Kansas	11.1
25	Montana	11.1
28	Massachusetts	11.0
28	North Carolina	11.0
30	New Mexico	10.9
31	Mississippi	10.5
31	New York	10.5
33	Michigan	10.0
34	Kentucky	9.8
34	South Carolina	9.8
36	Virginia	9.7
37	Nevada	9.5
38	Arizona	9.4
38	Rhode Island	9.4
40	Maryland	9.3
41	Colorado	9.1
42	Texas	8.9
43	Utah	8.8
44	California	8.7
45	Georgia	8.3
46	Hawaii	8.2
47	New Hampshire	7.9
48	Maine	7.8
49	Idaho	7.6
NA	Alaska**	NA
	District of Columbia**	NA

Source: Morgan Quitno Press using data from American Cancer Society
"Cancer Facts & Figures 2002" (Copyright 2002, Reprinted with permission from the American Cancer Society)
*These estimates are offered as a rough guide and should be interpreted with caution. They are calculated according to the distribution of estimated 2002 cancer deaths by state. Rates calculated using 2001 Census resident population estimates.
**Not available.

Estimated New Lung Cancer Cases in 2002

National Estimated Total = 169,400 New Cases*

ALPHA ORDER

RANK	STATE	CASES	% of USA
19	Alabama	3,200	1.9%
50	Alaska	200	0.1%
22	Arizona	2,900	1.7%
27	Arkansas	2,200	1.3%
1	California	14,300	8.4%
34	Colorado	1,600	0.9%
30	Connecticut	2,000	1.2%
41	Delaware	600	0.4%
2	Florida	13,000	7.7%
11	Georgia	4,400	2.6%
41	Hawaii	600	0.4%
41	Idaho	600	0.4%
7	Illinois	7,400	4.4%
13	Indiana	4,300	2.5%
31	Iowa	1,900	1.1%
32	Kansas	1,700	1.0%
17	Kentucky	3,400	2.0%
22	Louisiana	2,900	1.7%
36	Maine	1,000	0.6%
19	Maryland	3,200	1.9%
16	Massachusetts	4,000	2.4%
8	Michigan	6,100	3.6%
25	Minnesota	2,500	1.5%
29	Mississippi	2,100	1.2%
14	Missouri	4,200	2.5%
41	Montana	600	0.4%
36	Nebraska	1,000	0.6%
35	Nevada	1,400	0.8%
38	New Hampshire	800	0.5%
10	New Jersey	4,900	2.9%
38	New Mexico	800	0.5%
4	New York	10,000	5.9%
9	North Carolina	5,500	3.2%
48	North Dakota	300	0.2%
6	Ohio	7,900	4.7%
25	Oklahoma	2,500	1.5%
27	Oregon	2,200	1.3%
5	Pennsylvania	8,700	5.1%
38	Rhode Island	800	0.5%
24	South Carolina	2,600	1.5%
46	South Dakota	400	0.2%
11	Tennessee	4,400	2.6%
3	Texas	10,800	6.4%
45	Utah	500	0.3%
46	Vermont	400	0.2%
14	Virginia	4,200	2.5%
17	Washington	3,400	2.0%
32	West Virginia	1,700	1.0%
21	Wisconsin	3,000	1.8%
48	Wyoming	300	0.2%

RANK ORDER

RANK	STATE	CASES	% of USA
1	California	14,300	8.4%
2	Florida	13,000	7.7%
3	Texas	10,800	6.4%
4	New York	10,000	5.9%
5	Pennsylvania	8,700	5.1%
6	Ohio	7,900	4.7%
7	Illinois	7,400	4.4%
8	Michigan	6,100	3.6%
9	North Carolina	5,500	3.2%
10	New Jersey	4,900	2.9%
11	Georgia	4,400	2.6%
11	Tennessee	4,400	2.6%
13	Indiana	4,300	2.5%
14	Missouri	4,200	2.5%
14	Virginia	4,200	2.5%
16	Massachusetts	4,000	2.4%
17	Kentucky	3,400	2.0%
17	Washington	3,400	2.0%
19	Alabama	3,200	1.9%
19	Maryland	3,200	1.9%
21	Wisconsin	3,000	1.8%
22	Arizona	2,900	1.7%
22	Louisiana	2,900	1.7%
24	South Carolina	2,600	1.5%
25	Minnesota	2,500	1.5%
25	Oklahoma	2,500	1.5%
27	Arkansas	2,200	1.3%
27	Oregon	2,200	1.3%
29	Mississippi	2,100	1.2%
30	Connecticut	2,000	1.2%
31	Iowa	1,900	1.1%
32	Kansas	1,700	1.0%
32	West Virginia	1,700	1.0%
34	Colorado	1,600	0.9%
35	Nevada	1,400	0.8%
36	Maine	1,000	0.6%
36	Nebraska	1,000	0.6%
38	New Hampshire	800	0.5%
38	New Mexico	800	0.5%
38	Rhode Island	800	0.5%
41	Delaware	600	0.4%
41	Hawaii	600	0.4%
41	Idaho	600	0.4%
41	Montana	600	0.4%
45	Utah	500	0.3%
46	South Dakota	400	0.2%
46	Vermont	400	0.2%
48	North Dakota	300	0.2%
48	Wyoming	300	0.2%
50	Alaska	200	0.1%
	District of Columbia	300	0.2%

Source: American Cancer Society
"Cancer Facts & Figures 2002" (Copyright 2002, Reprinted with permission from the American Cancer Society)
*These estimates are offered as a rough guide and should be interpreted with caution. They are calculated according to the distribution of estimated 2002 cancer deaths by state.

Estimated Rate of New Lung Cancer Cases in 2002

National Estimated Rate = 59.5 New Cases per 100,000 Population*

ALPHA ORDER			RANK ORDER		
RANK	**STATE**	**RATE**	**RANK**	**STATE**	**RATE**
12	Alabama	71.7	1	West Virginia	94.3
49	Alaska	31.5	2	Kentucky	83.6
37	Arizona	54.6	3	Arkansas	81.7
3	Arkansas	81.7	4	Florida	79.3
47	California	41.4	5	Maine	77.7
48	Colorado	36.2	6	Tennessee	76.7
31	Connecticut	58.4	7	Rhode Island	75.5
8	Delaware	75.4	8	Delaware	75.4
4	Florida	79.3	9	Missouri	74.6
40	Georgia	52.5	10	Mississippi	73.5
43	Hawaii	49.0	11	Oklahoma	72.3
45	Idaho	45.4	12	Alabama	71.7
30	Illinois	59.3	13	Pennsylvania	70.8
14	Indiana	70.3	14	Indiana	70.3
20	Iowa	65.0	15	Ohio	69.5
25	Kansas	63.1	16	North Carolina	67.2
2	Kentucky	83.6	17	Nevada	66.5
21	Louisiana	64.9	18	Montana	66.3
5	Maine	77.7	19	Vermont	65.2
29	Maryland	59.5	20	Iowa	65.0
26	Massachusetts	62.7	21	Louisiana	64.9
27	Michigan	61.1	22	South Carolina	64.0
42	Minnesota	50.3	23	New Hampshire	63.5
10	Mississippi	73.5	24	Oregon	63.3
9	Missouri	74.6	25	Kansas	63.1
18	Montana	66.3	26	Massachusetts	62.7
31	Nebraska	58.4	27	Michigan	61.1
17	Nevada	66.5	28	Wyoming	60.7
23	New Hampshire	63.5	29	Maryland	59.5
34	New Jersey	57.8	30	Illinois	59.3
46	New Mexico	43.7	31	Connecticut	58.4
39	New York	52.6	31	Nebraska	58.4
16	North Carolina	67.2	31	Virginia	58.4
44	North Dakota	47.3	34	New Jersey	57.8
15	Ohio	69.5	35	Washington	56.8
11	Oklahoma	72.3	36	Wisconsin	55.5
24	Oregon	63.3	37	Arizona	54.6
13	Pennsylvania	70.8	38	South Dakota	52.9
7	Rhode Island	75.5	39	New York	52.6
22	South Carolina	64.0	40	Georgia	52.5
38	South Dakota	52.9	41	Texas	50.6
6	Tennessee	76.7	42	Minnesota	50.3
41	Texas	50.6	43	Hawaii	49.0
50	Utah	22.0	44	North Dakota	47.3
19	Vermont	65.2	45	Idaho	45.4
31	Virginia	58.4	46	New Mexico	43.7
35	Washington	56.8	47	California	41.4
1	West Virginia	94.3	48	Colorado	36.2
36	Wisconsin	55.5	49	Alaska	31.5
28	Wyoming	60.7	50	Utah	22.0
				District of Columbia	52.5

Source: Morgan Quitno Press using data from American Cancer Society
"Cancer Facts & Figures 2002" (Copyright 2002, Reprinted with permission from the American Cancer Society)
*These estimates are offered as a rough guide and should be interpreted with caution. They are calculated according to the distribution of estimated 2002 cancer deaths by state. Rates calculated using 2001 Census resident population estimates.

Estimated New Non-Hodgkin's Lymphoma Cases in 2002

National Estimated Total = 53,900 New Cases*

ALPHA ORDER

RANK	STATE	CASES	% of USA
22	Alabama	800	1.5%
46	Alaska	100	0.2%
20	Arizona	1,000	1.9%
30	Arkansas	600	1.1%
1	California	5,100	9.5%
25	Colorado	700	1.3%
25	Connecticut	700	1.3%
46	Delaware	100	0.2%
2	Florida	3,900	7.2%
16	Georgia	1,100	2.0%
39	Hawaii	200	0.4%
39	Idaho	200	0.4%
7	Illinois	2,400	4.5%
13	Indiana	1,200	2.2%
30	Iowa	600	1.1%
32	Kansas	500	0.9%
22	Kentucky	800	1.5%
22	Louisiana	800	1.5%
35	Maine	300	0.6%
21	Maryland	900	1.7%
10	Massachusetts	1,400	2.6%
8	Michigan	2,100	3.9%
16	Minnesota	1,100	2.0%
32	Mississippi	500	0.9%
16	Missouri	1,100	2.0%
39	Montana	200	0.4%
35	Nebraska	300	0.6%
35	Nevada	300	0.6%
39	New Hampshire	200	0.4%
9	New Jersey	1,900	3.5%
39	New Mexico	200	0.4%
3	New York	3,400	6.3%
10	North Carolina	1,400	2.6%
46	North Dakota	100	0.2%
6	Ohio	2,600	4.8%
25	Oklahoma	700	1.3%
25	Oregon	700	1.3%
5	Pennsylvania	3,000	5.6%
39	Rhode Island	200	0.4%
25	South Carolina	700	1.3%
39	South Dakota	200	0.4%
13	Tennessee	1,200	2.2%
3	Texas	3,400	6.3%
35	Utah	300	0.6%
46	Vermont	100	0.2%
13	Virginia	1,200	2.2%
16	Washington	1,100	2.0%
34	West Virginia	400	0.7%
12	Wisconsin	1,300	2.4%
46	Wyoming	100	0.2%

RANK ORDER

RANK	STATE	CASES	% of USA
1	California	5,100	9.5%
2	Florida	3,900	7.2%
3	New York	3,400	6.3%
3	Texas	3,400	6.3%
5	Pennsylvania	3,000	5.6%
6	Ohio	2,600	4.8%
7	Illinois	2,400	4.5%
8	Michigan	2,100	3.9%
9	New Jersey	1,900	3.5%
10	Massachusetts	1,400	2.6%
10	North Carolina	1,400	2.6%
12	Wisconsin	1,300	2.4%
13	Indiana	1,200	2.2%
13	Tennessee	1,200	2.2%
13	Virginia	1,200	2.2%
16	Georgia	1,100	2.0%
16	Minnesota	1,100	2.0%
16	Missouri	1,100	2.0%
16	Washington	1,100	2.0%
20	Arizona	1,000	1.9%
21	Maryland	900	1.7%
22	Alabama	800	1.5%
22	Kentucky	800	1.5%
22	Louisiana	800	1.5%
25	Colorado	700	1.3%
25	Connecticut	700	1.3%
25	Oklahoma	700	1.3%
25	Oregon	700	1.3%
25	South Carolina	700	1.3%
30	Arkansas	600	1.1%
30	Iowa	600	1.1%
32	Kansas	500	0.9%
32	Mississippi	500	0.9%
34	West Virginia	400	0.7%
35	Maine	300	0.6%
35	Nebraska	300	0.6%
35	Nevada	300	0.6%
35	Utah	300	0.6%
39	Hawaii	200	0.4%
39	Idaho	200	0.4%
39	Montana	200	0.4%
39	New Hampshire	200	0.4%
39	New Mexico	200	0.4%
39	Rhode Island	200	0.4%
39	South Dakota	200	0.4%
46	Alaska	100	0.2%
46	Delaware	100	0.2%
46	North Dakota	100	0.2%
46	Vermont	100	0.2%
46	Wyoming	100	0.2%
	District of Columbia**	NA	NA

Source: American Cancer Society
"Cancer Facts & Figures 2002" (Copyright 2002, Reprinted with permission from the American Cancer Society)
*These estimates are offered as a rough guide and should be interpreted with caution. They are calculated according to the distribution of estimated 2002 cancer deaths by state.
**Not available.

Estimated Rate of New Non-Hodgkin's Lymphoma Cases in 2002

National Estimated Rate = 18.9 New Cases per 100,000 Population*

ALPHA ORDER

RANK	STATE	RATE
28	Alabama	17.9
41	Alaska	15.8
25	Arizona	18.8
8	Arkansas	22.3
45	California	14.8
41	Colorado	15.8
16	Connecticut	20.4
49	Delaware	12.6
4	Florida	23.8
48	Georgia	13.1
37	Hawaii	16.3
44	Idaho	15.1
23	Illinois	19.2
21	Indiana	19.6
15	Iowa	20.5
26	Kansas	18.6
20	Kentucky	19.7
28	Louisiana	17.9
5	Maine	23.3
35	Maryland	16.7
12	Massachusetts	21.9
13	Michigan	21.0
10	Minnesota	22.1
31	Mississippi	17.5
22	Missouri	19.5
10	Montana	22.1
31	Nebraska	17.5
46	Nevada	14.2
39	New Hampshire	15.9
7	New Jersey	22.4
50	New Mexico	10.9
28	New York	17.9
34	North Carolina	17.1
41	North Dakota	15.8
6	Ohio	22.9
17	Oklahoma	20.2
17	Oregon	20.2
2	Pennsylvania	24.4
24	Rhode Island	18.9
33	South Carolina	17.2
1	South Dakota	26.4
14	Tennessee	20.9
39	Texas	15.9
47	Utah	13.2
37	Vermont	16.3
35	Virginia	16.7
27	Washington	18.4
9	West Virginia	22.2
3	Wisconsin	24.1
17	Wyoming	20.2

RANK ORDER

RANK	STATE	RATE
1	South Dakota	26.4
2	Pennsylvania	24.4
3	Wisconsin	24.1
4	Florida	23.8
5	Maine	23.3
6	Ohio	22.9
7	New Jersey	22.4
8	Arkansas	22.3
9	West Virginia	22.2
10	Minnesota	22.1
10	Montana	22.1
12	Massachusetts	21.9
13	Michigan	21.0
14	Tennessee	20.9
15	Iowa	20.5
16	Connecticut	20.4
17	Oklahoma	20.2
17	Oregon	20.2
17	Wyoming	20.2
20	Kentucky	19.7
21	Indiana	19.6
22	Missouri	19.5
23	Illinois	19.2
24	Rhode Island	18.9
25	Arizona	18.8
26	Kansas	18.6
27	Washington	18.4
28	Alabama	17.9
28	Louisiana	17.9
28	New York	17.9
31	Mississippi	17.5
31	Nebraska	17.5
33	South Carolina	17.2
34	North Carolina	17.1
35	Maryland	16.7
35	Virginia	16.7
37	Hawaii	16.3
37	Vermont	16.3
39	New Hampshire	15.9
39	Texas	15.9
41	Alaska	15.8
41	Colorado	15.8
41	North Dakota	15.8
44	Idaho	15.1
45	California	14.8
46	Nevada	14.2
47	Utah	13.2
48	Georgia	13.1
49	Delaware	12.6
50	New Mexico	10.9

District of Columbia** NA

Source: Morgan Quitno Press using data from American Cancer Society
"Cancer Facts & Figures 2002" (Copyright 2002, Reprinted with permission from the American Cancer Society)
*These estimates are offered as a rough guide and should be interpreted with caution. They are calculated according to the distribution of estimated 2002 cancer deaths by state. Rates calculated using 2001 Census resident population estimates.
**Not available.

Estimated New Prostate Cancer Cases in 2002

National Estimated Total = 189,000 New Cases*

ALPHA ORDER

RANK	STATE	CASES	% of USA
16	Alabama	3,900	2.1%
50	Alaska	100	0.1%
22	Arizona	3,300	1.7%
30	Arkansas	2,300	1.2%
1	California	17,300	9.2%
31	Colorado	2,200	1.2%
28	Connecticut	2,400	1.3%
45	Delaware	600	0.3%
2	Florida	13,600	7.2%
11	Georgia	4,800	2.5%
43	Hawaii	700	0.4%
39	Idaho	900	0.5%
6	Illinois	8,500	4.5%
14	Indiana	4,400	2.3%
28	Iowa	2,400	1.3%
33	Kansas	1,900	1.0%
26	Kentucky	2,700	1.4%
19	Louisiana	3,400	1.8%
40	Maine	800	0.4%
19	Maryland	3,400	1.8%
13	Massachusetts	4,600	2.4%
8	Michigan	6,700	3.5%
19	Minnesota	3,400	1.8%
27	Mississippi	2,500	1.3%
16	Missouri	3,900	2.1%
40	Montana	800	0.4%
38	Nebraska	1,000	0.5%
34	Nevada	1,400	0.7%
43	New Hampshire	700	0.4%
9	New Jersey	5,700	3.0%
37	New Mexico	1,200	0.6%
3	New York	11,800	6.2%
10	North Carolina	5,600	3.0%
47	North Dakota	400	0.2%
7	Ohio	8,100	4.3%
32	Oklahoma	2,100	1.1%
25	Oregon	2,800	1.5%
5	Pennsylvania	10,300	5.4%
40	Rhode Island	800	0.4%
24	South Carolina	3,100	1.6%
45	South Dakota	600	0.3%
16	Tennessee	3,900	2.1%
4	Texas	11,700	6.2%
36	Utah	1,300	0.7%
47	Vermont	400	0.2%
12	Virginia	4,700	2.5%
22	Washington	3,300	1.7%
34	West Virginia	1,400	0.7%
15	Wisconsin	4,000	2.1%
47	Wyoming	400	0.2%

RANK ORDER

RANK	STATE	CASES	% of USA
1	California	17,300	9.2%
2	Florida	13,600	7.2%
3	New York	11,800	6.2%
4	Texas	11,700	6.2%
5	Pennsylvania	10,300	5.4%
6	Illinois	8,500	4.5%
7	Ohio	8,100	4.3%
8	Michigan	6,700	3.5%
9	New Jersey	5,700	3.0%
10	North Carolina	5,600	3.0%
11	Georgia	4,800	2.5%
12	Virginia	4,700	2.5%
13	Massachusetts	4,600	2.4%
14	Indiana	4,400	2.3%
15	Wisconsin	4,000	2.1%
16	Alabama	3,900	2.1%
16	Missouri	3,900	2.1%
16	Tennessee	3,900	2.1%
19	Louisiana	3,400	1.8%
19	Maryland	3,400	1.8%
19	Minnesota	3,400	1.8%
22	Arizona	3,300	1.7%
22	Washington	3,300	1.7%
24	South Carolina	3,100	1.6%
25	Oregon	2,800	1.5%
26	Kentucky	2,700	1.4%
27	Mississippi	2,500	1.3%
28	Connecticut	2,400	1.3%
28	Iowa	2,400	1.3%
30	Arkansas	2,300	1.2%
31	Colorado	2,200	1.2%
32	Oklahoma	2,100	1.1%
33	Kansas	1,900	1.0%
34	Nevada	1,400	0.7%
34	West Virginia	1,400	0.7%
36	Utah	1,300	0.7%
37	New Mexico	1,200	0.6%
38	Nebraska	1,000	0.5%
39	Idaho	900	0.5%
40	Maine	800	0.4%
40	Montana	800	0.4%
40	Rhode Island	800	0.4%
43	Hawaii	700	0.4%
43	New Hampshire	700	0.4%
45	Delaware	600	0.3%
45	South Dakota	600	0.3%
47	North Dakota	400	0.2%
47	Vermont	400	0.2%
47	Wyoming	400	0.2%
50	Alaska	100	0.1%
	District of Columbia	500	0.3%

Source: American Cancer Society
  "Cancer Facts & Figures 2002" (Copyright 2002, Reprinted with permission from the American Cancer Society)
These estimates are offered as a rough guide and should be interpreted with caution. They are calculated according to the distribution of estimated 2002 cancer deaths by state.

Estimated Rate of New Prostate Cancer Cases in 2002

National Estimated Rate = 136.9 New Cases per 100,000 Male Population*

ALPHA ORDER

RANK ORDER

RANK	STATE	RATE		RANK	STATE	RATE
2	Alabama	181.7		1	Mississippi	182.0
50	Alaska	30.9		2	Alabama	181.7
38	Arizona	128.9		3	Montana	178.0
4	Arkansas	176.3		4	Arkansas	176.3
48	California	102.5		5	Florida	174.4
49	Colorado	101.6		6	Pennsylvania	173.7
20	Connecticut	145.5		7	Iowa	167.2
14	Delaware	157.7		8	Oregon	165.0
5	Florida	174.4		9	Wyoming	161.0
41	Georgia	119.2		10	South Dakota	160.2
45	Hawaii	115.0		11	West Virginia	159.2
28	Idaho	138.7		12	South Carolina	159.1
25	Illinois	139.8		13	Rhode Island	158.8
18	Indiana	147.5		14	Delaware	157.7
7	Iowa	167.2		15	Louisiana	157.2
22	Kansas	143.0		16	Wisconsin	151.0
31	Kentucky	136.7		17	Massachusetts	150.4
15	Louisiana	157.2		18	Indiana	147.5
36	Maine	129.0		19	Ohio	146.9
35	Maryland	132.9		20	Connecticut	145.5
17	Massachusetts	150.4		21	Missouri	143.4
29	Michigan	137.5		22	Kansas	143.0
26	Minnesota	139.6		23	North Carolina	142.0
1	Mississippi	182.0		24	Tennessee	140.8
21	Missouri	143.4		25	Illinois	139.8
3	Montana	178.0		26	Minnesota	139.6
42	Nebraska	118.6		26	New Jersey	139.6
29	Nevada	137.5		28	Idaho	138.7
44	New Hampshire	115.2		29	Michigan	137.5
26	New Jersey	139.6		29	Nevada	137.5
33	New Mexico	134.2		31	Kentucky	136.7
36	New York	129.0		32	Virginia	135.4
23	North Carolina	142.0		33	New Mexico	134.2
39	North Dakota	124.8		34	Vermont	134.1
19	Ohio	146.9		35	Maryland	132.9
40	Oklahoma	123.8		36	Maine	129.0
8	Oregon	165.0		36	New York	129.0
6	Pennsylvania	173.7		38	Arizona	128.9
13	Rhode Island	158.8		39	North Dakota	124.8
12	South Carolina	159.1		40	Oklahoma	123.8
10	South Dakota	160.2		41	Georgia	119.2
24	Tennessee	140.8		42	Nebraska	118.6
46	Texas	113.0		43	Utah	116.2
43	Utah	116.2		44	New Hampshire	115.2
34	Vermont	134.1		45	Hawaii	115.0
32	Virginia	135.4		46	Texas	113.0
47	Washington	112.5		47	Washington	112.5
11	West Virginia	159.2		48	California	102.5
16	Wisconsin	151.0		49	Colorado	101.6
9	Wyoming	161.0		50	Alaska	30.9
					District of Columbia	185.6

Source: Morgan Quitno Press using data from American Cancer Society
    "Cancer Facts & Figures 2002" (Copyright 2002, Reprinted with permission from the American Cancer Society)
These estimates are offered as a rough guide and should be interpreted with caution. They are calculated according to the distribution of estimated 2002 cancer deaths by state. Rates calculated using 2000 Census male resident population figures.

Estimated New Skin Melanoma Cases in 2002

National Estimated Total = 53,600 New Cases*

ALPHA ORDER

RANK	STATE	CASES	% of USA
20	Alabama	900	1.7%
47	Alaska	100	0.2%
18	Arizona	1,200	2.2%
32	Arkansas	500	0.9%
1	California	5,300	9.9%
24	Colorado	800	1.5%
29	Connecticut	600	1.1%
42	Delaware	200	0.4%
2	Florida	4,100	7.6%
13	Georgia	1,300	2.4%
47	Hawaii	100	0.2%
38	Idaho	300	0.6%
7	Illinois	2,200	4.1%
13	Indiana	1,300	2.4%
29	Iowa	600	1.1%
29	Kansas	600	1.1%
20	Kentucky	900	1.7%
27	Louisiana	700	1.3%
38	Maine	300	0.6%
24	Maryland	800	1.5%
11	Massachusetts	1,400	2.6%
9	Michigan	1,700	3.2%
20	Minnesota	900	1.7%
32	Mississippi	500	0.9%
13	Missouri	1,300	2.4%
42	Montana	200	0.4%
38	Nebraska	300	0.6%
32	Nevada	500	0.9%
38	New Hampshire	300	0.6%
8	New Jersey	1,800	3.4%
35	New Mexico	400	0.7%
4	New York	2,800	5.2%
10	North Carolina	1,500	2.8%
47	North Dakota	100	0.2%
6	Ohio	2,300	4.3%
20	Oklahoma	900	1.7%
24	Oregon	800	1.5%
5	Pennsylvania	2,700	5.0%
42	Rhode Island	200	0.4%
27	South Carolina	700	1.3%
42	South Dakota	200	0.4%
11	Tennessee	1,400	2.6%
3	Texas	3,600	6.7%
35	Utah	400	0.7%
42	Vermont	200	0.4%
13	Virginia	1,300	2.4%
13	Washington	1,300	2.4%
35	West Virginia	400	0.7%
19	Wisconsin	1,100	2.1%
47	Wyoming	100	0.2%

RANK ORDER

RANK	STATE	CASES	% of USA
1	California	5,300	9.9%
2	Florida	4,100	7.6%
3	Texas	3,600	6.7%
4	New York	2,800	5.2%
5	Pennsylvania	2,700	5.0%
6	Ohio	2,300	4.3%
7	Illinois	2,200	4.1%
8	New Jersey	1,800	3.4%
9	Michigan	1,700	3.2%
10	North Carolina	1,500	2.8%
11	Massachusetts	1,400	2.6%
11	Tennessee	1,400	2.6%
13	Georgia	1,300	2.4%
13	Indiana	1,300	2.4%
13	Missouri	1,300	2.4%
13	Virginia	1,300	2.4%
13	Washington	1,300	2.4%
18	Arizona	1,200	2.2%
19	Wisconsin	1,100	2.1%
20	Alabama	900	1.7%
20	Kentucky	900	1.7%
20	Minnesota	900	1.7%
20	Oklahoma	900	1.7%
24	Colorado	800	1.5%
24	Maryland	800	1.5%
24	Oregon	800	1.5%
27	Louisiana	700	1.3%
27	South Carolina	700	1.3%
29	Connecticut	600	1.1%
29	Iowa	600	1.1%
29	Kansas	600	1.1%
32	Arkansas	500	0.9%
32	Mississippi	500	0.9%
32	Nevada	500	0.9%
35	New Mexico	400	0.7%
35	Utah	400	0.7%
35	West Virginia	400	0.7%
38	Idaho	300	0.6%
38	Maine	300	0.6%
38	Nebraska	300	0.6%
38	New Hampshire	300	0.6%
42	Delaware	200	0.4%
42	Montana	200	0.4%
42	Rhode Island	200	0.4%
42	South Dakota	200	0.4%
42	Vermont	200	0.4%
47	Alaska	100	0.2%
47	Hawaii	100	0.2%
47	North Dakota	100	0.2%
47	Wyoming	100	0.2%
	District of Columbia**	NA	NA

Source: American Cancer Society
"Cancer Facts & Figures 2002" (Copyright 2002, Reprinted with permission from the American Cancer Society)
*These estimates are offered as a rough guide and should be interpreted with caution. They are calculated according to the distribution of estimated 2002 cancer deaths by state.
**Not available.

Estimated Rate of New Skin Melanoma Cases in 2002

National Estimated Rate = 18.8 New Cases per 100,000 Population*

ALPHA ORDER

RANK	STATE	RATE
26	Alabama	20.2
43	Alaska	15.8
13	Arizona	22.6
30	Arkansas	18.6
47	California	15.4
32	Colorado	18.1
37	Connecticut	17.5
4	Delaware	25.1
5	Florida	25.0
46	Georgia	15.5
50	Hawaii	8.2
12	Idaho	22.7
35	Illinois	17.6
22	Indiana	21.3
24	Iowa	20.5
14	Kansas	22.3
16	Kentucky	22.1
45	Louisiana	15.7
9	Maine	23.3
48	Maryland	14.9
19	Massachusetts	21.9
41	Michigan	17.0
32	Minnesota	18.1
37	Mississippi	17.5
10	Missouri	23.1
16	Montana	22.1
37	Nebraska	17.5
8	Nevada	23.7
7	New Hampshire	23.8
23	New Jersey	21.2
19	New Mexico	21.9
49	New York	14.7
31	North Carolina	18.3
43	North Dakota	15.8
26	Ohio	20.2
3	Oklahoma	26.0
11	Oregon	23.0
18	Pennsylvania	22.0
29	Rhode Island	18.9
40	South Carolina	17.2
2	South Dakota	26.4
6	Tennessee	24.4
42	Texas	16.9
35	Utah	17.6
1	Vermont	32.6
32	Virginia	18.1
21	Washington	21.7
15	West Virginia	22.2
25	Wisconsin	20.4
26	Wyoming	20.2

RANK ORDER

RANK	STATE	RATE
1	Vermont	32.6
2	South Dakota	26.4
3	Oklahoma	26.0
4	Delaware	25.1
5	Florida	25.0
6	Tennessee	24.4
7	New Hampshire	23.8
8	Nevada	23.7
9	Maine	23.3
10	Missouri	23.1
11	Oregon	23.0
12	Idaho	22.7
13	Arizona	22.6
14	Kansas	22.3
15	West Virginia	22.2
16	Kentucky	22.1
16	Montana	22.1
18	Pennsylvania	22.0
19	Massachusetts	21.9
19	New Mexico	21.9
21	Washington	21.7
22	Indiana	21.3
23	New Jersey	21.2
24	Iowa	20.5
25	Wisconsin	20.4
26	Alabama	20.2
26	Ohio	20.2
26	Wyoming	20.2
29	Rhode Island	18.9
30	Arkansas	18.6
31	North Carolina	18.3
32	Colorado	18.1
32	Minnesota	18.1
32	Virginia	18.1
35	Illinois	17.6
35	Utah	17.6
37	Connecticut	17.5
37	Mississippi	17.5
37	Nebraska	17.5
40	South Carolina	17.2
41	Michigan	17.0
42	Texas	16.9
43	Alaska	15.8
43	North Dakota	15.8
45	Louisiana	15.7
46	Georgia	15.5
47	California	15.4
48	Maryland	14.9
49	New York	14.7
50	Hawaii	8.2

District of Columbia**   NA

Source: Morgan Quitno Press using data from American Cancer Society
    "Cancer Facts & Figures 2002" (Copyright 2002, Reprinted with permission from the American Cancer Society)
*These estimates are offered as a rough guide and should be interpreted with caution. They are calculated
according to the distribution of estimated 2002 cancer deaths by state. Rates calculated using 2001 Census
resident population estimates.
**Not available.

Estimated New Cervical Cancer Cases in 2002

National Estimated Total = 13,000 New Cases*

ALPHA ORDER

RANK	STATE	CASES	% of USA
18	Alabama	200	1.5%
50	Alaska	10	0.1%
18	Arizona	200	1.5%
18	Arkansas	200	1.5%
1	California	1,400	10.8%
29	Colorado	100	0.8%
29	Connecticut	100	0.8%
29	Delaware	100	0.8%
4	Florida	900	6.9%
8	Georgia	400	3.1%
46	Hawaii	30	0.2%
41	Idaho	40	0.3%
5	Illinois	700	5.4%
13	Indiana	300	2.3%
29	Iowa	100	0.8%
29	Kansas	100	0.8%
13	Kentucky	300	2.3%
18	Louisiana	200	1.5%
29	Maine	100	0.8%
13	Maryland	300	2.3%
18	Massachusetts	200	1.5%
8	Michigan	400	3.1%
18	Minnesota	200	1.5%
18	Mississippi	200	1.5%
13	Missouri	300	2.3%
41	Montana	40	0.3%
29	Nebraska	100	0.8%
29	Nevada	100	0.8%
41	New Hampshire	40	0.3%
8	New Jersey	400	3.1%
29	New Mexico	100	0.8%
2	New York	1,000	7.7%
8	North Carolina	400	3.1%
46	North Dakota	30	0.2%
6	Ohio	600	4.6%
18	Oklahoma	200	1.5%
29	Oregon	100	0.8%
6	Pennsylvania	600	4.6%
29	Rhode Island	100	0.8%
18	South Carolina	200	1.5%
48	South Dakota	20	0.2%
8	Tennessee	400	3.1%
2	Texas	1,000	7.7%
41	Utah	40	0.3%
41	Vermont	40	0.3%
13	Virginia	300	2.3%
18	Washington	200	1.5%
29	West Virginia	100	0.8%
18	Wisconsin	200	1.5%
48	Wyoming	20	0.2%

RANK ORDER

RANK	STATE	CASES	% of USA
1	California	1,400	10.8%
2	New York	1,000	7.7%
2	Texas	1,000	7.7%
4	Florida	900	6.9%
5	Illinois	700	5.4%
6	Ohio	600	4.6%
6	Pennsylvania	600	4.6%
8	Georgia	400	3.1%
8	Michigan	400	3.1%
8	New Jersey	400	3.1%
8	North Carolina	400	3.1%
8	Tennessee	400	3.1%
13	Indiana	300	2.3%
13	Kentucky	300	2.3%
13	Maryland	300	2.3%
13	Missouri	300	2.3%
13	Virginia	300	2.3%
18	Alabama	200	1.5%
18	Arizona	200	1.5%
18	Arkansas	200	1.5%
18	Louisiana	200	1.5%
18	Massachusetts	200	1.5%
18	Minnesota	200	1.5%
18	Mississippi	200	1.5%
18	Oklahoma	200	1.5%
18	South Carolina	200	1.5%
18	Washington	200	1.5%
18	Wisconsin	200	1.5%
29	Colorado	100	0.8%
29	Connecticut	100	0.8%
29	Delaware	100	0.8%
29	Iowa	100	0.8%
29	Kansas	100	0.8%
29	Maine	100	0.8%
29	Nebraska	100	0.8%
29	Nevada	100	0.8%
29	New Mexico	100	0.8%
29	Oregon	100	0.8%
29	Rhode Island	100	0.8%
29	West Virginia	100	0.8%
41	Idaho	40	0.3%
41	Montana	40	0.3%
41	New Hampshire	40	0.3%
41	Utah	40	0.3%
41	Vermont	40	0.3%
46	Hawaii	30	0.2%
46	North Dakota	30	0.2%
48	South Dakota	20	0.2%
48	Wyoming	20	0.2%
50	Alaska	10	0.1%
	District of Columbia	40	0.3%

Source: American Cancer Society
"Cancer Facts & Figures 2002" (Copyright 2002, Reprinted with permission from the American Cancer Society)
*These estimates are offered as a rough guide and should be interpreted with caution. They are calculated
according to the distribution of estimated 2002 cancer deaths by state.

Estimated Rate of New Cervical Cancer Cases in 2002

National Estimated Rate = 9.1 New Cases per 100,000 Population*

ALPHA ORDER

RANK	STATE	RATE
29	Alabama	8.7
50	Alaska	3.3
36	Arizona	7.8
4	Arkansas	14.6
32	California	8.2
48	Colorado	4.7
45	Connecticut	5.7
1	Delaware	24.8
11	Florida	11.0
23	Georgia	9.6
47	Hawaii	5.0
42	Idaho	6.2
11	Illinois	11.0
20	Indiana	9.7
40	Iowa	6.7
37	Kansas	7.4
5	Kentucky	14.5
29	Louisiana	8.7
3	Maine	15.3
11	Maryland	11.0
43	Massachusetts	6.1
35	Michigan	7.9
33	Minnesota	8.1
7	Mississippi	13.6
16	Missouri	10.4
28	Montana	8.8
9	Nebraska	11.5
18	Nevada	10.2
41	New Hampshire	6.4
27	New Jersey	9.2
14	New Mexico	10.8
18	New York	10.2
20	North Carolina	9.7
26	North Dakota	9.3
17	Ohio	10.3
10	Oklahoma	11.4
44	Oregon	5.8
25	Pennsylvania	9.4
2	Rhode Island	18.4
20	South Carolina	9.7
46	South Dakota	5.3
6	Tennessee	13.7
24	Texas	9.5
49	Utah	3.6
8	Vermont	12.9
31	Virginia	8.3
39	Washington	6.8
14	West Virginia	10.8
37	Wisconsin	7.4
33	Wyoming	8.1

RANK ORDER

RANK	STATE	RATE
1	Delaware	24.8
2	Rhode Island	18.4
3	Maine	15.3
4	Arkansas	14.6
5	Kentucky	14.5
6	Tennessee	13.7
7	Mississippi	13.6
8	Vermont	12.9
9	Nebraska	11.5
10	Oklahoma	11.4
11	Florida	11.0
11	Illinois	11.0
11	Maryland	11.0
14	New Mexico	10.8
14	West Virginia	10.8
16	Missouri	10.4
17	Ohio	10.3
18	Nevada	10.2
18	New York	10.2
20	Indiana	9.7
20	North Carolina	9.7
20	South Carolina	9.7
23	Georgia	9.6
24	Texas	9.5
25	Pennsylvania	9.4
26	North Dakota	9.3
27	New Jersey	9.2
28	Montana	8.8
29	Alabama	8.7
29	Louisiana	8.7
31	Virginia	8.3
32	California	8.2
33	Minnesota	8.1
33	Wyoming	8.1
35	Michigan	7.9
36	Arizona	7.8
37	Kansas	7.4
37	Wisconsin	7.4
39	Washington	6.8
40	Iowa	6.7
41	New Hampshire	6.4
42	Idaho	6.2
43	Massachusetts	6.1
44	Oregon	5.8
45	Connecticut	5.7
46	South Dakota	5.3
47	Hawaii	5.0
48	Colorado	4.7
49	Utah	3.6
50	Alaska	3.3

District of Columbia 13.2

Source: Morgan Quitno Press using data from American Cancer Society
    "Cancer Facts & Figures 2002" (Copyright 2002, Reprinted with permission from the American Cancer Society)
*These estimates are offered as a rough guide and should be interpreted with caution. They are calculated
according to the distribution of estimated 2002 cancer deaths by state. Rates calculated using 2000 Census female
resident population figures.

Percent of Women 18 Years Old and Older
Who Had a Pap Smear Within the Past Three Years: 2000
National Median = 86.8% of Women 18 Years and Older*

ALPHA ORDER

RANK	STATE	PERCENT
30	Alabama	86.3
3	Alaska	90.1
19	Arizona	87.9
43	Arkansas	83.6
NA	California**	NA
22	Colorado	87.6
16	Connecticut	88.0
1	Delaware	92.0
39	Florida	84.5
8	Georgia	89.1
20	Hawaii	87.8
45	Idaho	83.1
39	Illinois	84.5
37	Indiana	84.7
24	Iowa	86.8
16	Kansas	88.0
29	Kentucky	86.4
21	Louisiana	87.7
9	Maine	89.0
5	Maryland	89.9
6	Massachusetts	89.6
27	Michigan	86.7
31	Minnesota	86.0
13	Mississippi	88.1
37	Missouri	84.7
10	Montana	88.8
31	Nebraska	86.0
42	Nevada	83.8
3	New Hampshire	90.1
48	New Jersey	81.9
36	New Mexico	85.1
33	New York	85.6
7	North Carolina	89.3
41	North Dakota	84.1
28	Ohio	86.5
33	Oklahoma	85.6
16	Oregon	88.0
35	Pennsylvania	85.5
11	Rhode Island	88.5
2	South Carolina	90.8
11	South Dakota	88.5
13	Tennessee	88.1
46	Texas	82.5
44	Utah	83.4
13	Vermont	88.1
24	Virginia	86.8
23	Washington	87.3
47	West Virginia	82.1
24	Wisconsin	86.8
49	Wyoming	81.3

RANK ORDER

RANK	STATE	PERCENT
1	Delaware	92.0
2	South Carolina	90.8
3	Alaska	90.1
3	New Hampshire	90.1
5	Maryland	89.9
6	Massachusetts	89.6
7	North Carolina	89.3
8	Georgia	89.1
9	Maine	89.0
10	Montana	88.8
11	Rhode Island	88.5
11	South Dakota	88.5
13	Mississippi	88.1
13	Tennessee	88.1
13	Vermont	88.1
16	Connecticut	88.0
16	Kansas	88.0
16	Oregon	88.0
19	Arizona	87.9
20	Hawaii	87.8
21	Louisiana	87.7
22	Colorado	87.6
23	Washington	87.3
24	Iowa	86.8
24	Virginia	86.8
24	Wisconsin	86.8
27	Michigan	86.7
28	Ohio	86.5
29	Kentucky	86.4
30	Alabama	86.3
31	Minnesota	86.0
31	Nebraska	86.0
33	New York	85.6
33	Oklahoma	85.6
35	Pennsylvania	85.5
36	New Mexico	85.1
37	Indiana	84.7
37	Missouri	84.7
39	Florida	84.5
39	Illinois	84.5
41	North Dakota	84.1
42	Nevada	83.8
43	Arkansas	83.6
44	Utah	83.4
45	Idaho	83.1
46	Texas	82.5
47	West Virginia	82.1
48	New Jersey	81.9
49	Wyoming	81.3
NA	California**	NA

District of Columbia	88.7

*Source: U.S. Department of Health and Human Services, Centers for Disease Control and Prevention
"2000 Behavioral Risk Factor Surveillance Summary Prevalence Report" (May 3, 2001)*

*Of women with intact cervix. Pap smear is a test for cancer, especially of the female genital tract. Named after George Papanicolaou (1883-1962), American anatomist.
**Not available.*

AIDS Cases Reported in 2001

National Total = 42,008 New AIDS Cases*

ALPHA ORDER

RANK	STATE	CASES	% of USA
22	Alabama	438	1.0%
47	Alaska	18	0.0%
19	Arizona	541	1.3%
31	Arkansas	200	0.5%
3	California	4,315	10.3%
26	Colorado	288	0.7%
16	Connecticut	584	1.4%
29	Delaware	248	0.6%
2	Florida	5,139	12.2%
8	Georgia	1,750	4.2%
35	Hawaii	124	0.3%
46	Idaho	19	0.0%
9	Illinois	1,327	3.2%
24	Indiana	378	0.9%
40	Iowa	90	0.2%
39	Kansas	98	0.2%
25	Kentucky	333	0.8%
12	Louisiana	861	2.0%
42	Maine	48	0.1%
5	Maryland	1,860	4.4%
13	Massachusetts	765	1.8%
18	Michigan	549	1.3%
33	Minnesota	157	0.4%
23	Mississippi	420	1.0%
21	Missouri	445	1.1%
48	Montana	15	0.0%
41	Nebraska	74	0.2%
28	Nevada	252	0.6%
43	New Hampshire	40	0.1%
7	New Jersey	1,761	4.2%
34	New Mexico	143	0.3%
1	New York	7,699	18.3%
11	North Carolina	947	2.3%
50	North Dakota	3	0.0%
16	Ohio	584	1.4%
30	Oklahoma	243	0.6%
27	Oregon	259	0.6%
6	Pennsylvania	1,841	4.4%
37	Rhode Island	103	0.2%
14	South Carolina	729	1.7%
44	South Dakota	25	0.1%
15	Tennessee	602	1.4%
4	Texas	2,892	6.9%
35	Utah	124	0.3%
44	Vermont	25	0.1%
10	Virginia	951	2.3%
20	Washington	533	1.3%
38	West Virginia	100	0.2%
32	Wisconsin	193	0.5%
49	Wyoming	5	0.0%

RANK ORDER

RANK	STATE	CASES	% of USA
1	New York	7,699	18.3%
2	Florida	5,139	12.2%
3	California	4,315	10.3%
4	Texas	2,892	6.9%
5	Maryland	1,860	4.4%
6	Pennsylvania	1,841	4.4%
7	New Jersey	1,761	4.2%
8	Georgia	1,750	4.2%
9	Illinois	1,327	3.2%
10	Virginia	951	2.3%
11	North Carolina	947	2.3%
12	Louisiana	861	2.0%
13	Massachusetts	765	1.8%
14	South Carolina	729	1.7%
15	Tennessee	602	1.4%
16	Connecticut	584	1.4%
16	Ohio	584	1.4%
18	Michigan	549	1.3%
19	Arizona	541	1.3%
20	Washington	533	1.3%
21	Missouri	445	1.1%
22	Alabama	438	1.0%
23	Mississippi	420	1.0%
24	Indiana	378	0.9%
25	Kentucky	333	0.8%
26	Colorado	288	0.7%
27	Oregon	259	0.6%
28	Nevada	252	0.6%
29	Delaware	248	0.6%
30	Oklahoma	243	0.6%
31	Arkansas	200	0.5%
32	Wisconsin	193	0.5%
33	Minnesota	157	0.4%
34	New Mexico	143	0.3%
35	Hawaii	124	0.3%
35	Utah	124	0.3%
37	Rhode Island	103	0.2%
38	West Virginia	100	0.2%
39	Kansas	98	0.2%
40	Iowa	90	0.2%
41	Nebraska	74	0.2%
42	Maine	48	0.1%
43	New Hampshire	40	0.1%
44	South Dakota	25	0.1%
44	Vermont	25	0.1%
46	Idaho	19	0.0%
47	Alaska	18	0.0%
48	Montana	15	0.0%
49	Wyoming	5	0.0%
50	North Dakota	3	0.0%
	District of Columbia	870	2.1%

Source: U.S. Department of Health and Human Services, National Center for Health Statistics
"Morbidity and Mortality Weekly Report" (January 4, 2002, Vol. 50, No. 51)
*Provisional data. AIDS is Acquired Immunodeficiency Syndrome. It is a specific group of diseases or conditions which are indicative of severe immunosuppression related to infection with the Human Immunodeficiency Virus (HIV). National total does not include 1,242 cases in Puerto Rico.

AIDS Rate in 2001

National Rate = 14.8 New AIDS Cases Reported per 100,000 Population*

ALPHA ORDER

RANK	STATE	RATE
22	Alabama	9.8
46	Alaska	2.8
20	Arizona	10.2
29	Arkansas	7.4
14	California	12.5
31	Colorado	6.5
9	Connecticut	17.1
4	Delaware	31.1
3	Florida	31.3
5	Georgia	20.9
21	Hawaii	10.1
48	Idaho	1.4
18	Illinois	10.6
32	Indiana	6.2
45	Iowa	3.1
40	Kansas	3.6
25	Kentucky	8.2
7	Louisiana	19.3
39	Maine	3.7
2	Maryland	34.6
15	Massachusetts	12.0
33	Michigan	5.5
43	Minnesota	3.2
11	Mississippi	14.7
26	Missouri	7.9
47	Montana	1.7
37	Nebraska	4.3
15	Nevada	12.0
43	New Hampshire	3.2
6	New Jersey	20.8
27	New Mexico	7.8
1	New York	40.5
17	North Carolina	11.6
50	North Dakota	0.5
36	Ohio	5.1
30	Oklahoma	7.0
28	Oregon	7.5
10	Pennsylvania	15.0
23	Rhode Island	9.7
8	South Carolina	17.9
42	South Dakota	3.3
19	Tennessee	10.5
12	Texas	13.6
33	Utah	5.5
38	Vermont	4.1
13	Virginia	13.2
24	Washington	8.9
33	West Virginia	5.5
40	Wisconsin	3.6
49	Wyoming	1.0

RANK ORDER

RANK	STATE	RATE
1	New York	40.5
2	Maryland	34.6
3	Florida	31.3
4	Delaware	31.1
5	Georgia	20.9
6	New Jersey	20.8
7	Louisiana	19.3
8	South Carolina	17.9
9	Connecticut	17.1
10	Pennsylvania	15.0
11	Mississippi	14.7
12	Texas	13.6
13	Virginia	13.2
14	California	12.5
15	Massachusetts	12.0
15	Nevada	12.0
17	North Carolina	11.6
18	Illinois	10.6
19	Tennessee	10.5
20	Arizona	10.2
21	Hawaii	10.1
22	Alabama	9.8
23	Rhode Island	9.7
24	Washington	8.9
25	Kentucky	8.2
26	Missouri	7.9
27	New Mexico	7.8
28	Oregon	7.5
29	Arkansas	7.4
30	Oklahoma	7.0
31	Colorado	6.5
32	Indiana	6.2
33	Michigan	5.5
33	Utah	5.5
33	West Virginia	5.5
36	Ohio	5.1
37	Nebraska	4.3
38	Vermont	4.1
39	Maine	3.7
40	Kansas	3.6
40	Wisconsin	3.6
42	South Dakota	3.3
43	Minnesota	3.2
43	New Hampshire	3.2
45	Iowa	3.1
46	Alaska	2.8
47	Montana	1.7
48	Idaho	1.4
49	Wyoming	1.0
50	North Dakota	0.5

District of Columbia 152.1

Source: Morgan Quitno Press using data from U.S. Dept. of Health & Human Serv's, National Center for Health Statistics
"Morbidity and Mortality Weekly Report" (January 4, 2002, Vol. 50, No. 51)
*Provisional data. AIDS is Acquired Immunodeficiency Syndrome. It is a specific group of diseases or conditions
which are indicative of severe immunosuppression related to infection with the Human Immunodeficiency Virus
(HIV). National rate does not include cases or population in U.S. territories.

AIDS Cases Reported Through June 2001

National Total = 766,289 Reported AIDS Cases*

RANK	STATE	CASES	% of USA
23	Alabama	6,492	0.8%
45	Alaska	490	0.1%
21	Arizona	7,722	1.0%
32	Arkansas	3,081	0.4%
2	California	121,831	15.9%
22	Colorado	7,235	0.9%
13	Connecticut	11,798	1.5%
33	Delaware	2,696	0.4%
3	Florida	83,005	10.8%
8	Georgia	23,575	3.1%
34	Hawaii	2,489	0.3%
44	Idaho	512	0.1%
6	Illinois	25,665	3.3%
24	Indiana	6,303	0.8%
39	Iowa	1,363	0.2%
35	Kansas	2,412	0.3%
31	Kentucky	3,544	0.5%
12	Louisiana	13,090	1.7%
42	Maine	976	0.1%
9	Maryland	22,432	2.9%
10	Massachusetts	16,662	2.2%
15	Michigan	11,573	1.5%
29	Minnesota	3,847	0.5%
26	Mississippi	4,718	0.6%
19	Missouri	9,429	1.2%
47	Montana	338	0.0%
40	Nebraska	1,133	0.1%
27	Nevada	4,545	0.6%
43	New Hampshire	897	0.1%
5	New Jersey	43,017	5.6%
37	New Mexico	2,101	0.3%
1	New York	144,106	18.8%
16	North Carolina	10,809	1.4%
50	North Dakota	108	0.0%
14	Ohio	11,609	1.5%
28	Oklahoma	3,895	0.5%
25	Oregon	4,910	0.6%
7	Pennsylvania	25,264	3.3%
36	Rhode Island	2,105	0.3%
17	South Carolina	9,857	1.3%
49	South Dakota	184	0.0%
20	Tennessee	8,858	1.2%
4	Texas	55,292	7.2%
38	Utah	2,036	0.3%
46	Vermont	413	0.1%
11	Virginia	13,569	1.8%
18	Washington	9,767	1.3%
41	West Virginia	1,126	0.1%
30	Wisconsin	3,656	0.5%
48	Wyoming	188	0.0%

RANK	STATE	CASES	% of USA
1	New York	144,106	18.8%
2	California	121,831	15.9%
3	Florida	83,005	10.8%
4	Texas	55,292	7.2%
5	New Jersey	43,017	5.6%
6	Illinois	25,665	3.3%
7	Pennsylvania	25,264	3.3%
8	Georgia	23,575	3.1%
9	Maryland	22,432	2.9%
10	Massachusetts	16,662	2.2%
11	Virginia	13,569	1.8%
12	Louisiana	13,090	1.7%
13	Connecticut	11,798	1.5%
14	Ohio	11,609	1.5%
15	Michigan	11,573	1.5%
16	North Carolina	10,809	1.4%
17	South Carolina	9,857	1.3%
18	Washington	9,767	1.3%
19	Missouri	9,429	1.2%
20	Tennessee	8,858	1.2%
21	Arizona	7,722	1.0%
22	Colorado	7,235	0.9%
23	Alabama	6,492	0.8%
24	Indiana	6,303	0.8%
25	Oregon	4,910	0.6%
26	Mississippi	4,718	0.6%
27	Nevada	4,545	0.6%
28	Oklahoma	3,895	0.5%
29	Minnesota	3,847	0.5%
30	Wisconsin	3,656	0.5%
31	Kentucky	3,544	0.5%
32	Arkansas	3,081	0.4%
33	Delaware	2,696	0.4%
34	Hawaii	2,489	0.3%
35	Kansas	2,412	0.3%
36	Rhode Island	2,105	0.3%
37	New Mexico	2,101	0.3%
38	Utah	2,036	0.3%
39	Iowa	1,363	0.2%
40	Nebraska	1,133	0.1%
41	West Virginia	1,126	0.1%
42	Maine	976	0.1%
43	New Hampshire	897	0.1%
44	Idaho	512	0.1%
45	Alaska	490	0.1%
46	Vermont	413	0.1%
47	Montana	338	0.0%
48	Wyoming	188	0.0%
49	South Dakota	184	0.0%
50	North Dakota	108	0.0%
	District of Columbia	13,566	1.8%

Source: U.S. Department of Health and Human Services, Centers for Disease Control and Prevention "HIV/AIDS Surveillance Report, 2001" (Mid-year Edition, Vol. 13, No. 1)

*Cumulative through June 2001. AIDS is Acquired Immunodeficiency Syndrome. It is a specific group of diseases or conditions which are indicative of severe immunosuppression related to infection with the Human Immunodeficiency Virus (HIV). National total does not include 25,459 cases in Puerto Rico, 485 cases in the Virgin Islands and 59 cases in other U.S. territories.

AIDS Cases in Children 12 Years and Younger Through June 2001

National Total = 8,582 Juvenile AIDS Cases*

ALPHA ORDER

RANK	STATE	CASES	% of USA
18	Alabama	72	0.8%
45	Alaska	5	0.1%
23	Arizona	40	0.5%
24	Arkansas	38	0.4%
4	California	613	7.1%
26	Colorado	30	0.3%
11	Connecticut	176	2.1%
33	Delaware	22	0.3%
2	Florida	1,414	16.5%
9	Georgia	213	2.5%
36	Hawaii	16	0.2%
49	Idaho	2	0.0%
8	Illinois	272	3.2%
22	Indiana	42	0.5%
38	Iowa	10	0.1%
37	Kansas	12	0.1%
29	Kentucky	26	0.3%
13	Louisiana	125	1.5%
41	Maine	9	0.1%
7	Maryland	304	3.5%
10	Massachusetts	207	2.4%
16	Michigan	107	1.2%
31	Minnesota	23	0.3%
20	Mississippi	56	0.7%
19	Missouri	59	0.7%
47	Montana	3	0.0%
38	Nebraska	10	0.1%
28	Nevada	28	0.3%
41	New Hampshire	9	0.1%
3	New Jersey	754	8.8%
43	New Mexico	8	0.1%
1	New York	2,267	26.4%
15	North Carolina	116	1.4%
50	North Dakota	1	0.0%
14	Ohio	123	1.4%
29	Oklahoma	26	0.3%
35	Oregon	17	0.2%
6	Pennsylvania	333	3.9%
31	Rhode Island	23	0.3%
17	South Carolina	80	0.9%
46	South Dakota	4	0.0%
21	Tennessee	52	0.6%
5	Texas	386	4.5%
34	Utah	21	0.2%
44	Vermont	6	0.1%
12	Virginia	174	2.0%
25	Washington	35	0.4%
38	West Virginia	10	0.1%
27	Wisconsin	29	0.3%
47	Wyoming	3	0.0%

RANK ORDER

RANK	STATE	CASES	% of USA
1	New York	2,267	26.4%
2	Florida	1,414	16.5%
3	New Jersey	754	8.8%
4	California	613	7.1%
5	Texas	386	4.5%
6	Pennsylvania	333	3.9%
7	Maryland	304	3.5%
8	Illinois	272	3.2%
9	Georgia	213	2.5%
10	Massachusetts	207	2.4%
11	Connecticut	176	2.1%
12	Virginia	174	2.0%
13	Louisiana	125	1.5%
14	Ohio	123	1.4%
15	North Carolina	116	1.4%
16	Michigan	107	1.2%
17	South Carolina	80	0.9%
18	Alabama	72	0.8%
19	Missouri	59	0.7%
20	Mississippi	56	0.7%
21	Tennessee	52	0.6%
22	Indiana	42	0.5%
23	Arizona	40	0.5%
24	Arkansas	38	0.4%
25	Washington	35	0.4%
26	Colorado	30	0.3%
27	Wisconsin	29	0.3%
28	Nevada	28	0.3%
29	Kentucky	26	0.3%
29	Oklahoma	26	0.3%
31	Minnesota	23	0.3%
31	Rhode Island	23	0.3%
33	Delaware	22	0.3%
34	Utah	21	0.2%
35	Oregon	17	0.2%
36	Hawaii	16	0.2%
37	Kansas	12	0.1%
38	Iowa	10	0.1%
38	Nebraska	10	0.1%
38	West Virginia	10	0.1%
41	Maine	9	0.1%
41	New Hampshire	9	0.1%
43	New Mexico	8	0.1%
44	Vermont	6	0.1%
45	Alaska	5	0.1%
46	South Dakota	4	0.0%
47	Montana	3	0.0%
47	Wyoming	3	0.0%
49	Idaho	2	0.0%
50	North Dakota	1	0.0%
	District of Columbia	171	2.0%

*Source: U.S. Department of Health and Human Services, Centers for Disease Control and Prevention
"HIV/AIDS Surveillance Report, 2001" (Mid-year Edition, Vol. 13, No. 1)*
Cumulative through June 2001. AIDS is Acquired Immunodeficiency Syndrome. It is a specific group of diseases or conditions which are indicative of severe immunosuppression related to infection with the Human Immunodeficiency Virus (HIV). National total does not include 388 cases in Puerto Rico and 17 cases in the Virgin Islands.

E-Coli Cases Reported in 2001

National Total = 5,367 Cases*

ALPHA ORDER					RANK ORDER			
RANK	STATE		CASES	% of USA	RANK	STATE	CASES	% of USA
40	Alabama		24	0.4%	1	Minnesota	490	9.1%
49	Alaska		5	0.1%	2	California	462	8.6%
28	Arizona		54	1.0%	3	Ohio	385	7.2%
46	Arkansas		14	0.3%	4	New York	321	6.0%
2	California		462	8.6%	5	Wisconsin	304	5.7%
12	Colorado		143	2.7%	6	Illinois	298	5.6%
30	Connecticut		52	1.0%	7	Massachusetts	227	4.2%
47	Delaware		11	0.2%	8	Washington	197	3.7%
24	Florida		68	1.3%	9	Michigan	183	3.4%
32	Georgia		48	0.9%	10	Missouri	155	2.9%
36	Hawaii		29	0.5%	11	Oregon	145	2.7%
15	Idaho		120	2.2%	12	Colorado	143	2.7%
6	Illinois		298	5.6%	13	Iowa	141	2.6%
14	Indiana		128	2.4%	14	Indiana	128	2.4%
13	Iowa		141	2.6%	15	Idaho	120	2.2%
33	Kansas		41	0.8%	16	Kentucky	112	2.1%
16	Kentucky		112	2.1%	16	New Jersey	112	2.1%
35	Louisiana		30	0.6%	18	North Carolina	101	1.9%
28	Maine		54	1.0%	19	Texas	98	1.8%
36	Maryland		29	0.5%	20	Tennessee	94	1.8%
7	Massachusetts		227	4.2%	21	Virginia	92	1.7%
9	Michigan		183	3.4%	22	South Dakota	84	1.6%
1	Minnesota		490	9.1%	23	Utah	75	1.4%
43	Mississippi		19	0.4%	24	Florida	68	1.3%
10	Missouri		155	2.9%	25	New Hampshire	67	1.2%
42	Montana		20	0.4%	26	Oklahoma	64	1.2%
27	Nebraska		60	1.1%	27	Nebraska	60	1.1%
43	Nevada		19	0.4%	28	Arizona	54	1.0%
25	New Hampshire		67	1.2%	28	Maine	54	1.0%
16	New Jersey		112	2.1%	30	Connecticut	52	1.0%
38	New Mexico		28	0.5%	30	North Dakota	52	1.0%
4	New York		321	6.0%	32	Georgia	48	0.9%
18	North Carolina		101	1.9%	33	Kansas	41	0.8%
30	North Dakota		52	1.0%	34	South Carolina	34	0.6%
3	Ohio		385	7.2%	35	Louisiana	30	0.6%
26	Oklahoma		64	1.2%	36	Hawaii	29	0.5%
11	Oregon		145	2.7%	36	Maryland	29	0.5%
NA	Pennsylvania**		NA	NA	38	New Mexico	28	0.5%
38	Rhode Island		28	0.5%	38	Rhode Island	28	0.5%
34	South Carolina		34	0.6%	40	Alabama	24	0.4%
22	South Dakota		84	1.6%	40	Vermont	24	0.4%
20	Tennessee		94	1.8%	42	Montana	20	0.4%
19	Texas		98	1.8%	43	Mississippi	19	0.4%
23	Utah		75	1.4%	43	Nevada	19	0.4%
40	Vermont		24	0.4%	45	West Virginia	18	0.3%
21	Virginia		92	1.7%	46	Arkansas	14	0.3%
8	Washington		197	3.7%	47	Delaware	11	0.2%
45	West Virginia		18	0.3%	48	Wyoming	8	0.1%
5	Wisconsin		304	5.7%	49	Alaska	5	0.1%
48	Wyoming		8	0.1%	NA	Pennsylvania**	NA	NA
						District of Columbia**	NA	NA

Source: U.S. Department of Health and Human Services, National Center for Health Statistics
   "Morbidity and Mortality Weekly Report" (January 4, 2002, Vol. 50, No. 51)
*Individual cases may be reported through both the Public Health Laboratory Information System and the National Electronic Telecommunications System for Surveillance. Escherichia Coli is a common bacterium that normally inhabits the intestinal tracts of humans and animals but can cause infection in other parts of the body, especially the urinary tract. One strain, sometimes transmitted in hamburger meat, can cause serious infection resulting in sickness and death. **Not available.

E-Coli Rate in 2001

National Rate = 1.9 Cases per 100,000 Population*

ALPHA ORDER

RANK	STATE	RATE
45	Alabama	0.5
40	Alaska	0.8
37	Arizona	1.0
45	Arkansas	0.5
33	California	1.3
16	Colorado	3.2
29	Connecticut	1.5
32	Delaware	1.4
49	Florida	0.4
44	Georgia	0.6
20	Hawaii	2.4
3	Idaho	9.1
20	Illinois	2.4
23	Indiana	2.1
7	Iowa	4.8
29	Kansas	1.5
17	Kentucky	2.8
42	Louisiana	0.7
8	Maine	4.2
45	Maryland	0.5
11	Massachusetts	3.6
24	Michigan	1.8
2	Minnesota	9.9
42	Mississippi	0.7
17	Missouri	2.8
22	Montana	2.2
12	Nebraska	3.5
39	Nevada	0.9
6	New Hampshire	5.3
33	New Jersey	1.3
29	New Mexico	1.5
26	New York	1.7
36	North Carolina	1.2
4	North Dakota	8.2
13	Ohio	3.4
24	Oklahoma	1.8
8	Oregon	4.2
NA	Pennsylvania**	NA
19	Rhode Island	2.6
40	South Carolina	0.8
1	South Dakota	11.1
27	Tennessee	1.6
45	Texas	0.5
14	Utah	3.3
10	Vermont	3.9
33	Virginia	1.3
14	Washington	3.3
37	West Virginia	1.0
5	Wisconsin	5.6
27	Wyoming	1.6

RANK ORDER

RANK	STATE	RATE
1	South Dakota	11.1
2	Minnesota	9.9
3	Idaho	9.1
4	North Dakota	8.2
5	Wisconsin	5.6
6	New Hampshire	5.3
7	Iowa	4.8
8	Maine	4.2
8	Oregon	4.2
10	Vermont	3.9
11	Massachusetts	3.6
12	Nebraska	3.5
13	Ohio	3.4
14	Utah	3.3
14	Washington	3.3
16	Colorado	3.2
17	Kentucky	2.8
17	Missouri	2.8
19	Rhode Island	2.6
20	Hawaii	2.4
20	Illinois	2.4
22	Montana	2.2
23	Indiana	2.1
24	Michigan	1.8
24	Oklahoma	1.8
26	New York	1.7
27	Tennessee	1.6
27	Wyoming	1.6
29	Connecticut	1.5
29	Kansas	1.5
29	New Mexico	1.5
32	Delaware	1.4
33	California	1.3
33	New Jersey	1.3
33	Virginia	1.3
36	North Carolina	1.2
37	Arizona	1.0
37	West Virginia	1.0
39	Nevada	0.9
40	Alaska	0.8
40	South Carolina	0.8
42	Louisiana	0.7
42	Mississippi	0.7
44	Georgia	0.6
45	Alabama	0.5
45	Arkansas	0.5
45	Maryland	0.5
45	Texas	0.5
49	Florida	0.4
NA	Pennsylvania**	NA
	District of Columbia**	NA

Source: Morgan Quitno Press using data from U.S. Dept. of Health & Human Serv's, National Center for Health Statistics
"Morbidity and Mortality Weekly Report" (January 4, 2002, Vol. 50, No. 51)

*Individual cases may be reported through both the Public Health Laboratory Information System and the National Electronic Telecommunications System for Surveillance. Escherichia Coli is a common bacterium that normally inhabits the intestinal tracts of humans and animals but can cause infection in other parts of the body, especially the urinary tract. One strain, sometimes transmitted in hamburger meat, can cause serious infection resulting in sickness and death. **Not available.

German Measles (Rubella) Cases Reported in 2001

National Total = 19 Cases*

ALPHA ORDER

RANK	STATE	CASES	% of USA
13	Alabama	0	0.0%
13	Alaska	0	0.0%
13	Arizona	0	0.0%
13	Arkansas	0	0.0%
6	California	1	5.3%
13	Colorado	0	0.0%
13	Connecticut	0	0.0%
13	Delaware	0	0.0%
2	Florida	2	10.5%
6	Georgia	1	5.3%
6	Hawaii	1	5.3%
13	Idaho	0	0.0%
2	Illinois	2	10.5%
13	Indiana	0	0.0%
6	Iowa	1	5.3%
6	Kansas	1	5.3%
13	Kentucky	0	0.0%
13	Louisiana	0	0.0%
13	Maine	0	0.0%
13	Maryland	0	0.0%
13	Massachusetts	0	0.0%
13	Michigan	0	0.0%
13	Minnesota	0	0.0%
13	Mississippi	0	0.0%
6	Missouri	1	5.3%
13	Montana	0	0.0%
13	Nebraska	0	0.0%
13	Nevada	0	0.0%
13	New Hampshire	0	0.0%
6	New Jersey	1	5.3%
13	New Mexico	0	0.0%
1	New York	4	21.1%
13	North Carolina	0	0.0%
13	North Dakota	0	0.0%
13	Ohio	0	0.0%
13	Oklahoma	0	0.0%
13	Oregon	0	0.0%
13	Pennsylvania	0	0.0%
13	Rhode Island	0	0.0%
2	South Carolina	2	10.5%
13	South Dakota	0	0.0%
13	Tennessee	0	0.0%
2	Texas	2	10.5%
13	Utah	0	0.0%
13	Vermont	0	0.0%
13	Virginia	0	0.0%
13	Washington	0	0.0%
13	West Virginia	0	0.0%
13	Wisconsin	0	0.0%
13	Wyoming	0	0.0%

RANK ORDER

RANK	STATE	CASES	% of USA
1	New York	4	21.1%
2	Florida	2	10.5%
2	Illinois	2	10.5%
2	South Carolina	2	10.5%
2	Texas	2	10.5%
6	California	1	5.3%
6	Georgia	1	5.3%
6	Hawaii	1	5.3%
6	Iowa	1	5.3%
6	Kansas	1	5.3%
6	Missouri	1	5.3%
6	New Jersey	1	5.3%
13	Alabama	0	0.0%
13	Alaska	0	0.0%
13	Arizona	0	0.0%
13	Arkansas	0	0.0%
13	Colorado	0	0.0%
13	Connecticut	0	0.0%
13	Delaware	0	0.0%
13	Idaho	0	0.0%
13	Indiana	0	0.0%
13	Kentucky	0	0.0%
13	Louisiana	0	0.0%
13	Maine	0	0.0%
13	Maryland	0	0.0%
13	Massachusetts	0	0.0%
13	Michigan	0	0.0%
13	Minnesota	0	0.0%
13	Mississippi	0	0.0%
13	Montana	0	0.0%
13	Nebraska	0	0.0%
13	Nevada	0	0.0%
13	New Hampshire	0	0.0%
13	New Mexico	0	0.0%
13	North Carolina	0	0.0%
13	North Dakota	0	0.0%
13	Ohio	0	0.0%
13	Oklahoma	0	0.0%
13	Oregon	0	0.0%
13	Pennsylvania	0	0.0%
13	Rhode Island	0	0.0%
13	South Dakota	0	0.0%
13	Tennessee	0	0.0%
13	Utah	0	0.0%
13	Vermont	0	0.0%
13	Virginia	0	0.0%
13	Washington	0	0.0%
13	West Virginia	0	0.0%
13	Wisconsin	0	0.0%
13	Wyoming	0	0.0%
	District of Columbia	0	0.0%

Source: U.S. Department of Health and Human Services, National Center for Health Statistics
   "Morbidity and Mortality Weekly Report" (January 4, 2002, Vol. 50, No. 51)
*Provisional data. A mild, contagious, eruptive disease caused by a virus and capable of producing congenital
defects in infants born to mothers infected during the first three months of pregnancy.

German Measles (Rubella) Rate in 2001

National Rate = 0.01 Cases per 100,000 Population*

ALPHA ORDER			RANK ORDER		
RANK	STATE	RATE	RANK	STATE	RATE
12	Alabama	0.00	1	Hawaii	0.08
12	Alaska	0.00	2	South Carolina	0.05
12	Arizona	0.00	3	Kansas	0.04
12	Arkansas	0.00	4	Iowa	0.03
12	California	0.00	5	Illinois	0.02
12	Colorado	0.00	5	Missouri	0.02
12	Connecticut	0.00	5	New York	0.02
12	Delaware	0.00	8	Florida	0.01
8	Florida	0.01	8	Georgia	0.01
8	Georgia	0.01	8	New Jersey	0.01
1	Hawaii	0.08	8	Texas	0.01
12	Idaho	0.00	12	Alabama	0.00
5	Illinois	0.02	12	Alaska	0.00
12	Indiana	0.00	12	Arizona	0.00
4	Iowa	0.03	12	Arkansas	0.00
3	Kansas	0.04	12	California	0.00
12	Kentucky	0.00	12	Colorado	0.00
12	Louisiana	0.00	12	Connecticut	0.00
12	Maine	0.00	12	Delaware	0.00
12	Maryland	0.00	12	Idaho	0.00
12	Massachusetts	0.00	12	Indiana	0.00
12	Michigan	0.00	12	Kentucky	0.00
12	Minnesota	0.00	12	Louisiana	0.00
12	Mississippi	0.00	12	Maine	0.00
5	Missouri	0.02	12	Maryland	0.00
12	Montana	0.00	12	Massachusetts	0.00
12	Nebraska	0.00	12	Michigan	0.00
12	Nevada	0.00	12	Minnesota	0.00
12	New Hampshire	0.00	12	Mississippi	0.00
8	New Jersey	0.01	12	Montana	0.00
12	New Mexico	0.00	12	Nebraska	0.00
5	New York	0.02	12	Nevada	0.00
12	North Carolina	0.00	12	New Hampshire	0.00
12	North Dakota	0.00	12	New Mexico	0.00
12	Ohio	0.00	12	North Carolina	0.00
12	Oklahoma	0.00	12	North Dakota	0.00
12	Oregon	0.00	12	Ohio	0.00
12	Pennsylvania	0.00	12	Oklahoma	0.00
12	Rhode Island	0.00	12	Oregon	0.00
2	South Carolina	0.05	12	Pennsylvania	0.00
12	South Dakota	0.00	12	Rhode Island	0.00
12	Tennessee	0.00	12	South Dakota	0.00
8	Texas	0.01	12	Tennessee	0.00
12	Utah	0.00	12	Utah	0.00
12	Vermont	0.00	12	Vermont	0.00
12	Virginia	0.00	12	Virginia	0.00
12	Washington	0.00	12	Washington	0.00
12	West Virginia	0.00	12	West Virginia	0.00
12	Wisconsin	0.00	12	Wisconsin	0.00
12	Wyoming	0.00	12	Wyoming	0.00
				District of Columbia	0.00

Source: Morgan Quitno Press using data from U.S. Dept. of Health & Human Serv's, National Center for Health Statistics
"Morbidity and Mortality Weekly Report" (January 4, 2002, Vol. 50, No. 51)
*Provisional data. A mild, contagious, eruptive disease caused by a virus and capable of producing congenital defects in infants born to mothers infected during the first three months of pregnancy.

Hepatitis A and B Cases Reported in 2001

National Total = 17,495 Cases*

ALPHA ORDER

RANK	STATE	CASES	% of USA
26	Alabama	169	1.0%
43	Alaska	23	0.1%
9	Arizona	572	3.3%
25	Arkansas	170	1.0%
1	California	2,624	15.0%
23	Colorado	193	1.1%
18	Connecticut	265	1.5%
42	Delaware	26	0.1%
4	Florida	1,381	7.9%
3	Georgia	1,435	8.2%
43	Hawaii	23	0.1%
37	Idaho	68	0.4%
8	Illinois	610	3.5%
28	Indiana	152	0.9%
39	Iowa	58	0.3%
21	Kansas	201	1.1%
24	Kentucky	188	1.1%
31	Louisiana	109	0.6%
46	Maine	16	0.1%
10	Maryland	468	2.7%
16	Massachusetts	322	1.8%
6	Michigan	932	5.3%
35	Minnesota	73	0.4%
34	Mississippi	84	0.5%
20	Missouri	213	1.2%
46	Montana	16	0.1%
38	Nebraska	63	0.4%
29	Nevada	110	0.6%
41	New Hampshire	34	0.2%
7	New Jersey	739	4.2%
27	New Mexico	168	1.0%
5	New York	1,181	6.8%
11	North Carolina	464	2.7%
49	North Dakota	5	0.0%
14	Ohio	354	2.0%
19	Oklahoma	227	1.3%
21	Oregon	201	1.1%
12	Pennsylvania	450	2.6%
32	Rhode Island	105	0.6%
29	South Carolina	110	0.6%
50	South Dakota	4	0.0%
13	Tennessee	415	2.4%
2	Texas	1,506	8.6%
33	Utah	97	0.6%
45	Vermont	20	0.1%
15	Virginia	329	1.9%
17	Washington	304	1.7%
40	West Virginia	53	0.3%
36	Wisconsin	69	0.4%
48	Wyoming	10	0.1%

RANK ORDER

RANK	STATE	CASES	% of USA
1	California	2,624	15.0%
2	Texas	1,506	8.6%
3	Georgia	1,435	8.2%
4	Florida	1,381	7.9%
5	New York	1,181	6.8%
6	Michigan	932	5.3%
7	New Jersey	739	4.2%
8	Illinois	610	3.5%
9	Arizona	572	3.3%
10	Maryland	468	2.7%
11	North Carolina	464	2.7%
12	Pennsylvania	450	2.6%
13	Tennessee	415	2.4%
14	Ohio	354	2.0%
15	Virginia	329	1.9%
16	Massachusetts	322	1.8%
17	Washington	304	1.7%
18	Connecticut	265	1.5%
19	Oklahoma	227	1.3%
20	Missouri	213	1.2%
21	Kansas	201	1.1%
21	Oregon	201	1.1%
23	Colorado	193	1.1%
24	Kentucky	188	1.1%
25	Arkansas	170	1.0%
26	Alabama	169	1.0%
27	New Mexico	168	1.0%
28	Indiana	152	0.9%
29	Nevada	110	0.6%
29	South Carolina	110	0.6%
31	Louisiana	109	0.6%
32	Rhode Island	105	0.6%
33	Utah	97	0.6%
34	Mississippi	84	0.5%
35	Minnesota	73	0.4%
36	Wisconsin	69	0.4%
37	Idaho	68	0.4%
38	Nebraska	63	0.4%
39	Iowa	58	0.3%
40	West Virginia	53	0.3%
41	New Hampshire	34	0.2%
42	Delaware	26	0.1%
43	Alaska	23	0.1%
43	Hawaii	23	0.1%
45	Vermont	20	0.1%
46	Maine	16	0.1%
46	Montana	16	0.1%
48	Wyoming	10	0.1%
49	North Dakota	5	0.0%
50	South Dakota	4	0.0%
	District of Columbia	86	0.5%

Source: U.S. Department of Health and Human Services, National Center for Health Statistics
"Morbidity and Mortality Weekly Report" (January 4, 2002, Vol. 50, No. 51)
*Provisional data. An inflammation of the liver.

Hepatitis A and B Rate in 2001

National Rate = 6.1 Cases per 100,000 Population*

ALPHA ORDER

RANK	STATE	RATE
28	Alabama	3.8
32	Alaska	3.6
2	Arizona	10.8
15	Arkansas	6.3
10	California	7.6
26	Colorado	4.4
9	Connecticut	7.7
33	Delaware	3.3
8	Florida	8.4
1	Georgia	17.1
44	Hawaii	1.9
20	Idaho	5.1
23	Illinois	4.9
40	Indiana	2.5
42	Iowa	2.0
11	Kansas	7.5
24	Kentucky	4.6
41	Louisiana	2.4
48	Maine	1.2
6	Maryland	8.7
22	Massachusetts	5.0
4	Michigan	9.3
46	Minnesota	1.5
36	Mississippi	2.9
28	Missouri	3.8
45	Montana	1.8
30	Nebraska	3.7
19	Nevada	5.2
38	New Hampshire	2.7
6	New Jersey	8.7
5	New Mexico	9.2
16	New York	6.2
18	North Carolina	5.7
49	North Dakota	0.8
35	Ohio	3.1
14	Oklahoma	6.6
17	Oregon	5.8
30	Pennsylvania	3.7
3	Rhode Island	9.9
38	South Carolina	2.7
50	South Dakota	0.5
12	Tennessee	7.2
13	Texas	7.1
27	Utah	4.3
33	Vermont	3.3
24	Virginia	4.6
20	Washington	5.1
36	West Virginia	2.9
47	Wisconsin	1.3
42	Wyoming	2.0

RANK ORDER

RANK	STATE	RATE
1	Georgia	17.1
2	Arizona	10.8
3	Rhode Island	9.9
4	Michigan	9.3
5	New Mexico	9.2
6	Maryland	8.7
6	New Jersey	8.7
8	Florida	8.4
9	Connecticut	7.7
10	California	7.6
11	Kansas	7.5
12	Tennessee	7.2
13	Texas	7.1
14	Oklahoma	6.6
15	Arkansas	6.3
16	New York	6.2
17	Oregon	5.8
18	North Carolina	5.7
19	Nevada	5.2
20	Idaho	5.1
20	Washington	5.1
22	Massachusetts	5.0
23	Illinois	4.9
24	Kentucky	4.6
24	Virginia	4.6
26	Colorado	4.4
27	Utah	4.3
28	Alabama	3.8
28	Missouri	3.8
30	Nebraska	3.7
30	Pennsylvania	3.7
32	Alaska	3.6
33	Delaware	3.3
33	Vermont	3.3
35	Ohio	3.1
36	Mississippi	2.9
36	West Virginia	2.9
38	New Hampshire	2.7
38	South Carolina	2.7
40	Indiana	2.5
41	Louisiana	2.4
42	Iowa	2.0
42	Wyoming	2.0
44	Hawaii	1.9
45	Montana	1.8
46	Minnesota	1.5
47	Wisconsin	1.3
48	Maine	1.2
49	North Dakota	0.8
50	South Dakota	0.5

District of Columbia 15.0

Source: Morgan Quitno Press using data from U.S. Dept. of Health & Human Serv's, National Center for Health Statistics
    "Morbidity and Mortality Weekly Report" (January 4, 2002, Vol. 50, No. 51)
*Provisional data. An inflammation of the liver.

Hepatitis C Cases Reported in 2001

National Total = 3,227 Cases*

ALPHA ORDER

RANK	STATE	CASES	% of USA
32	Alabama	5	0.2%
41	Alaska	0	0.0%
24	Arizona	9	0.3%
33	Arkansas	4	0.1%
5	California	95	2.9%
17	Colorado	14	0.4%
41	Connecticut	0	0.0%
29	Delaware	7	0.2%
10	Florida	63	2.0%
38	Georgia	1	0.0%
41	Hawaii	0	0.0%
36	Idaho	2	0.1%
16	Illinois	15	0.5%
38	Indiana	1	0.0%
41	Iowa	0	0.0%
20	Kansas	12	0.4%
23	Kentucky	10	0.3%
6	Louisiana	90	2.8%
41	Maine	0	0.0%
15	Maryland	17	0.5%
12	Massachusetts	25	0.8%
3	Michigan	137	4.2%
18	Minnesota	13	0.4%
4	Mississippi	100	3.1%
2	Missouri	722	22.4%
38	Montana	1	0.0%
28	Nebraska	8	0.2%
22	Nevada	11	0.3%
41	New Hampshire	0	0.0%
1	New Jersey	1,473	45.6%
20	New Mexico	12	0.4%
11	New York	58	1.8%
14	North Carolina	22	0.7%
41	North Dakota	0	0.0%
24	Ohio	9	0.3%
33	Oklahoma	4	0.1%
18	Oregon	13	0.4%
8	Pennsylvania	67	2.1%
41	Rhode Island	0	0.0%
31	South Carolina	6	0.2%
41	South Dakota	0	0.0%
8	Tennessee	67	2.1%
7	Texas	81	2.5%
35	Utah	3	0.1%
29	Vermont	7	0.2%
36	Virginia	2	0.1%
13	Washington	23	0.7%
24	West Virginia	9	0.3%
41	Wisconsin	0	0.0%
24	Wyoming	9	0.3%

RANK ORDER

RANK	STATE	CASES	% of USA
1	New Jersey	1,473	45.6%
2	Missouri	722	22.4%
3	Michigan	137	4.2%
4	Mississippi	100	3.1%
5	California	95	2.9%
6	Louisiana	90	2.8%
7	Texas	81	2.5%
8	Pennsylvania	67	2.1%
8	Tennessee	67	2.1%
10	Florida	63	2.0%
11	New York	58	1.8%
12	Massachusetts	25	0.8%
13	Washington	23	0.7%
14	North Carolina	22	0.7%
15	Maryland	17	0.5%
16	Illinois	15	0.5%
17	Colorado	14	0.4%
18	Minnesota	13	0.4%
18	Oregon	13	0.4%
20	Kansas	12	0.4%
20	New Mexico	12	0.4%
22	Nevada	11	0.3%
23	Kentucky	10	0.3%
24	Arizona	9	0.3%
24	Ohio	9	0.3%
24	West Virginia	9	0.3%
24	Wyoming	9	0.3%
28	Nebraska	8	0.2%
29	Delaware	7	0.2%
29	Vermont	7	0.2%
31	South Carolina	6	0.2%
32	Alabama	5	0.2%
33	Arkansas	4	0.1%
33	Oklahoma	4	0.1%
35	Utah	3	0.1%
36	Idaho	2	0.1%
36	Virginia	2	0.1%
38	Georgia	1	0.0%
38	Indiana	1	0.0%
38	Montana	1	0.0%
41	Alaska	0	0.0%
41	Connecticut	0	0.0%
41	Hawaii	0	0.0%
41	Iowa	0	0.0%
41	Maine	0	0.0%
41	New Hampshire	0	0.0%
41	North Dakota	0	0.0%
41	Rhode Island	0	0.0%
41	South Dakota	0	0.0%
41	Wisconsin	0	0.0%
	District of Columbia	0	0.0%

Source: U.S. Department of Health and Human Services, National Center for Health Statistics
"Morbidity and Mortality Weekly Report" (January 4, 2002, Vol. 50, No. 51)
*Provisional data. An inflammation of the liver. It is the leading cause for liver transplantation and is transmitted by blood-to-blood contact. Most new cases of C are caused by high-risk drug behaviors.

Hepatitis C Rate in 2001

National Rate = 1.1 Cases per 100,000 Population*

ALPHA ORDER

RANK	STATE	RATE
32	Alabama	0.1
38	Alaska	0.0
28	Arizona	0.2
28	Arkansas	0.2
21	California	0.3
21	Colorado	0.3
38	Connecticut	0.0
9	Delaware	0.9
16	Florida	0.4
38	Georgia	0.0
38	Hawaii	0.0
28	Idaho	0.2
32	Illinois	0.1
38	Indiana	0.0
38	Iowa	0.0
12	Kansas	0.5
21	Kentucky	0.3
4	Louisiana	2.0
38	Maine	0.0
21	Maryland	0.3
16	Massachusetts	0.4
6	Michigan	1.4
21	Minnesota	0.3
3	Mississippi	3.5
2	Missouri	12.8
32	Montana	0.1
12	Nebraska	0.5
12	Nevada	0.5
38	New Hampshire	0.0
1	New Jersey	17.4
10	New Mexico	0.7
21	New York	0.3
21	North Carolina	0.3
38	North Dakota	0.0
32	Ohio	0.1
32	Oklahoma	0.1
16	Oregon	0.4
11	Pennsylvania	0.6
38	Rhode Island	0.0
28	South Carolina	0.2
38	South Dakota	0.0
7	Tennessee	1.2
16	Texas	0.4
32	Utah	0.1
8	Vermont	1.1
38	Virginia	0.0
16	Washington	0.4
12	West Virginia	0.5
38	Wisconsin	0.0
5	Wyoming	1.8

RANK ORDER

RANK	STATE	RATE
1	New Jersey	17.4
2	Missouri	12.8
3	Mississippi	3.5
4	Louisiana	2.0
5	Wyoming	1.8
6	Michigan	1.4
7	Tennessee	1.2
8	Vermont	1.1
9	Delaware	0.9
10	New Mexico	0.7
11	Pennsylvania	0.6
12	Kansas	0.5
12	Nebraska	0.5
12	Nevada	0.5
12	West Virginia	0.5
16	Florida	0.4
16	Massachusetts	0.4
16	Oregon	0.4
16	Texas	0.4
16	Washington	0.4
21	California	0.3
21	Colorado	0.3
21	Kentucky	0.3
21	Maryland	0.3
21	Minnesota	0.3
21	New York	0.3
21	North Carolina	0.3
28	Arizona	0.2
28	Arkansas	0.2
28	Idaho	0.2
28	South Carolina	0.2
32	Alabama	0.1
32	Illinois	0.1
32	Montana	0.1
32	Ohio	0.1
32	Oklahoma	0.1
32	Utah	0.1
38	Alaska	0.0
38	Connecticut	0.0
38	Georgia	0.0
38	Hawaii	0.0
38	Indiana	0.0
38	Iowa	0.0
38	Maine	0.0
38	New Hampshire	0.0
38	North Dakota	0.0
38	Rhode Island	0.0
38	South Dakota	0.0
38	Virginia	0.0
38	Wisconsin	0.0
	District of Columbia	0.0

Source: Morgan Quitno Press using data from U.S. Dept. of Health & Human Serv's, National Center for Health Statistics "Morbidity and Mortality Weekly Report" (January 4, 2002, Vol. 50, No. 51)

*Provisional data. An inflammation of the liver. It is the leading cause for liver transplantation and is transmitted by blood-to-blood contact. Most new cases of C are caused by high-risk drug behaviors.

Legionellosis Cases Reported in 2001

National Total = 1,085 Cases*

ALPHA ORDER

RANK	STATE	CASES	% of USA
20	Alabama	13	1.2%
46	Alaska	0	0.0%
13	Arizona	23	2.1%
46	Arkansas	0	0.0%
6	California	58	5.3%
16	Colorado	19	1.8%
18	Connecticut	14	1.3%
22	Delaware	12	1.1%
3	Florida	99	9.1%
26	Georgia	10	0.9%
34	Hawaii	4	0.4%
37	Idaho	3	0.3%
16	Illinois	19	1.8%
11	Indiana	25	2.3%
29	Iowa	8	0.7%
43	Kansas	1	0.1%
22	Kentucky	12	1.1%
41	Louisiana	2	0.2%
29	Maine	8	0.7%
7	Maryland	37	3.4%
15	Massachusetts	21	1.9%
5	Michigan	83	7.6%
28	Minnesota	9	0.8%
41	Mississippi	2	0.2%
13	Missouri	23	2.1%
46	Montana	0	0.0%
34	Nebraska	4	0.4%
34	Nevada	4	0.4%
22	New Hampshire	12	1.1%
11	New Jersey	25	2.3%
37	New Mexico	3	0.3%
2	New York	108	10.0%
25	North Carolina	11	1.0%
43	North Dakota	1	0.1%
1	Ohio	149	13.7%
37	Oklahoma	3	0.3%
NA	Oregon**	NA	NA
4	Pennsylvania	97	8.9%
20	Rhode Island	13	1.2%
18	South Carolina	14	1.3%
37	South Dakota	3	0.3%
9	Tennessee	30	2.8%
29	Texas	8	0.7%
32	Utah	7	0.6%
33	Vermont	5	0.5%
10	Virginia	28	2.6%
26	Washington	10	0.9%
NA	West Virginia**	NA	NA
8	Wisconsin	36	3.3%
43	Wyoming	1	0.1%

RANK ORDER

RANK	STATE	CASES	% of USA
1	Ohio	149	13.7%
2	New York	108	10.0%
3	Florida	99	9.1%
4	Pennsylvania	97	8.9%
5	Michigan	83	7.6%
6	California	58	5.3%
7	Maryland	37	3.4%
8	Wisconsin	36	3.3%
9	Tennessee	30	2.8%
10	Virginia	28	2.6%
11	Indiana	25	2.3%
11	New Jersey	25	2.3%
13	Arizona	23	2.1%
13	Missouri	23	2.1%
15	Massachusetts	21	1.9%
16	Colorado	19	1.8%
16	Illinois	19	1.8%
18	Connecticut	14	1.3%
18	South Carolina	14	1.3%
20	Alabama	13	1.2%
20	Rhode Island	13	1.2%
22	Delaware	12	1.1%
22	Kentucky	12	1.1%
22	New Hampshire	12	1.1%
25	North Carolina	11	1.0%
26	Georgia	10	0.9%
26	Washington	10	0.9%
28	Minnesota	9	0.8%
29	Iowa	8	0.7%
29	Maine	8	0.7%
29	Texas	8	0.7%
32	Utah	7	0.6%
33	Vermont	5	0.5%
34	Hawaii	4	0.4%
34	Nebraska	4	0.4%
34	Nevada	4	0.4%
37	Idaho	3	0.3%
37	New Mexico	3	0.3%
37	Oklahoma	3	0.3%
37	South Dakota	3	0.3%
41	Louisiana	2	0.2%
41	Mississippi	2	0.2%
43	Kansas	1	0.1%
43	North Dakota	1	0.1%
43	Wyoming	1	0.1%
46	Alaska	0	0.0%
46	Arkansas	0	0.0%
46	Montana	0	0.0%
NA	Oregon**	NA	NA
NA	West Virginia**	NA	NA
	District of Columbia	8	0.7%

Source: U.S. Department of Health and Human Services, National Center for Health Statistics
   "Morbidity and Mortality Weekly Report" (January 4, 2002, Vol. 50, No. 51)
*Provisional data. A pneumonia-like disease (Legionnaire's Disease).
**Not notifiable.

Legionellosis Rate in 2001

National Rate = 0.4 Cases per 100,000 Population*

ALPHA ORDER

RANK	STATE	RATE
21	Alabama	0.3
43	Alaska	0.0
14	Arizona	0.4
43	Arkansas	0.0
29	California	0.2
14	Colorado	0.4
14	Connecticut	0.4
1	Delaware	1.5
10	Florida	0.6
39	Georgia	0.1
21	Hawaii	0.3
29	Idaho	0.2
29	Illinois	0.2
14	Indiana	0.4
21	Iowa	0.3
43	Kansas	0.0
21	Kentucky	0.3
43	Louisiana	0.0
10	Maine	0.6
8	Maryland	0.7
21	Massachusetts	0.3
5	Michigan	0.8
29	Minnesota	0.2
39	Mississippi	0.1
14	Missouri	0.4
43	Montana	0.0
29	Nebraska	0.2
29	Nevada	0.2
4	New Hampshire	1.0
21	New Jersey	0.3
29	New Mexico	0.2
10	New York	0.6
39	North Carolina	0.1
29	North Dakota	0.2
2	Ohio	1.3
39	Oklahoma	0.1
NA	Oregon**	NA
5	Pennsylvania	0.8
3	Rhode Island	1.2
21	South Carolina	0.3
14	South Dakota	0.4
13	Tennessee	0.5
43	Texas	0.0
21	Utah	0.3
5	Vermont	0.8
14	Virginia	0.4
29	Washington	0.2
NA	West Virginia**	NA
8	Wisconsin	0.7
29	Wyoming	0.2

RANK ORDER

RANK	STATE	RATE
1	Delaware	1.5
2	Ohio	1.3
3	Rhode Island	1.2
4	New Hampshire	1.0
5	Michigan	0.8
5	Pennsylvania	0.8
5	Vermont	0.8
8	Maryland	0.7
8	Wisconsin	0.7
10	Florida	0.6
10	Maine	0.6
10	New York	0.6
13	Tennessee	0.5
14	Arizona	0.4
14	Colorado	0.4
14	Connecticut	0.4
14	Indiana	0.4
14	Missouri	0.4
14	South Dakota	0.4
14	Virginia	0.4
21	Alabama	0.3
21	Hawaii	0.3
21	Iowa	0.3
21	Kentucky	0.3
21	Massachusetts	0.3
21	New Jersey	0.3
21	South Carolina	0.3
21	Utah	0.3
29	California	0.2
29	Idaho	0.2
29	Illinois	0.2
29	Minnesota	0.2
29	Nebraska	0.2
29	Nevada	0.2
29	New Mexico	0.2
29	North Dakota	0.2
29	Washington	0.2
29	Wyoming	0.2
39	Georgia	0.1
39	Mississippi	0.1
39	North Carolina	0.1
39	Oklahoma	0.1
43	Alaska	0.0
43	Arkansas	0.0
43	Kansas	0.0
43	Louisiana	0.0
43	Montana	0.0
43	Texas	0.0
NA	Oregon**	NA
NA	West Virginia**	NA

District of Columbia   1.4

Source: Morgan Quitno Press using data from U.S. Dept. of Health & Human Serv's, National Center for Health Statistics
   "Morbidity and Mortality Weekly Report" (January 4, 2002, Vol. 50, No. 51)
*Provisional data. A pneumonia-like disease (Legionnaire's Disease).
**Not notifiable.

Lyme Disease Cases in 2001

National Total = 13,452 Cases*

ALPHA ORDER

RANK	STATE	CASES	% of USA
28	Alabama	10	0.1%
33	Alaska	2	0.0%
33	Arizona	2	0.0%
38	Arkansas	1	0.0%
14	California	104	0.8%
38	Colorado	1	0.0%
2	Connecticut	2,521	18.7%
10	Delaware	151	1.1%
16	Florida	54	0.4%
44	Georgia	0	0.0%
NA	Hawaii**	NA	NA
31	Idaho	5	0.0%
23	Illinois	22	0.2%
21	Indiana	23	0.2%
18	Iowa	36	0.3%
33	Kansas	2	0.0%
21	Kentucky	23	0.2%
33	Louisiana	2	0.0%
44	Maine	0	0.0%
6	Maryland	563	4.2%
5	Massachusetts	895	6.7%
25	Michigan	17	0.1%
9	Minnesota	333	2.5%
38	Mississippi	1	0.0%
20	Missouri	26	0.2%
44	Montana	0	0.0%
32	Nebraska	4	0.0%
33	Nevada	2	0.0%
12	New Hampshire	117	0.9%
3	New Jersey	1,854	13.8%
38	New Mexico	1	0.0%
1	New York	3,698	27.5%
17	North Carolina	41	0.3%
44	North Dakota	0	0.0%
13	Ohio	113	0.8%
44	Oklahoma	0	0.0%
26	Oregon	14	0.1%
4	Pennsylvania	1,525	11.3%
8	Rhode Island	493	3.7%
30	South Carolina	7	0.1%
44	South Dakota	0	0.0%
19	Tennessee	30	0.2%
15	Texas	79	0.6%
38	Utah	1	0.0%
24	Vermont	18	0.1%
11	Virginia	119	0.9%
29	Washington	9	0.1%
27	West Virginia	13	0.1%
7	Wisconsin	502	3.7%
38	Wyoming	1	0.0%

RANK ORDER

RANK	STATE	CASES	% of USA
1	New York	3,698	27.5%
2	Connecticut	2,521	18.7%
3	New Jersey	1,854	13.8%
4	Pennsylvania	1,525	11.3%
5	Massachusetts	895	6.7%
6	Maryland	563	4.2%
7	Wisconsin	502	3.7%
8	Rhode Island	493	3.7%
9	Minnesota	333	2.5%
10	Delaware	151	1.1%
11	Virginia	119	0.9%
12	New Hampshire	117	0.9%
13	Ohio	113	0.8%
14	California	104	0.8%
15	Texas	79	0.6%
16	Florida	54	0.4%
17	North Carolina	41	0.3%
18	Iowa	36	0.3%
19	Tennessee	30	0.2%
20	Missouri	26	0.2%
21	Indiana	23	0.2%
21	Kentucky	23	0.2%
23	Illinois	22	0.2%
24	Vermont	18	0.1%
25	Michigan	17	0.1%
26	Oregon	14	0.1%
27	West Virginia	13	0.1%
28	Alabama	10	0.1%
29	Washington	9	0.1%
30	South Carolina	7	0.1%
31	Idaho	5	0.0%
32	Nebraska	4	0.0%
33	Alaska	2	0.0%
33	Arizona	2	0.0%
33	Kansas	2	0.0%
33	Louisiana	2	0.0%
33	Nevada	2	0.0%
38	Arkansas	1	0.0%
38	Colorado	1	0.0%
38	Mississippi	1	0.0%
38	New Mexico	1	0.0%
38	Utah	1	0.0%
38	Wyoming	1	0.0%
44	Georgia	0	0.0%
44	Maine	0	0.0%
44	Montana	0	0.0%
44	North Dakota	0	0.0%
44	Oklahoma	0	0.0%
44	South Dakota	0	0.0%
NA	Hawaii**	NA	NA
	District of Columbia	17	0.1%

Source: U.S. Department of Health and Human Services, National Center for Health Statistics
"Morbidity and Mortality Weekly Report" (January 4, 2002, Vol. 50, No. 51)
*Provisional data. Caused by ticks-lesions, followed by arthritis of large joints, myalgia, malaise and neurologic and cardiac manifestations. Named after Old Lyme, CT, where the disease was first reported.
**Not notifiable.

Lyme Disease Rate in 2001

National Rate = 4.7 Cases per 100,000 Population*

ALPHA ORDER

RANK	STATE	RATE
28	Alabama	0.2
25	Alaska	0.3
38	Arizona	0.0
38	Arkansas	0.0
25	California	0.3
38	Colorado	0.0
1	Connecticut	73.6
5	Delaware	19.0
25	Florida	0.3
38	Georgia	0.0
NA	Hawaii**	NA
21	Idaho	0.4
28	Illinois	0.2
21	Indiana	0.4
14	Iowa	1.2
35	Kansas	0.1
17	Kentucky	0.6
38	Louisiana	0.0
38	Maine	0.0
8	Maryland	10.5
6	Massachusetts	14.0
28	Michigan	0.2
11	Minnesota	6.7
38	Mississippi	0.0
18	Missouri	0.5
38	Montana	0.0
28	Nebraska	0.2
35	Nevada	0.1
9	New Hampshire	9.3
3	New Jersey	21.9
35	New Mexico	0.1
4	New York	19.5
18	North Carolina	0.5
38	North Dakota	0.0
15	Ohio	1.0
38	Oklahoma	0.0
21	Oregon	0.4
7	Pennsylvania	12.4
2	Rhode Island	46.6
28	South Carolina	0.2
38	South Dakota	0.0
18	Tennessee	0.5
21	Texas	0.4
38	Utah	0.0
12	Vermont	2.9
13	Virginia	1.7
28	Washington	0.2
16	West Virginia	0.7
9	Wisconsin	9.3
28	Wyoming	0.2

RANK ORDER

RANK	STATE	RATE
1	Connecticut	73.6
2	Rhode Island	46.6
3	New Jersey	21.9
4	New York	19.5
5	Delaware	19.0
6	Massachusetts	14.0
7	Pennsylvania	12.4
8	Maryland	10.5
9	New Hampshire	9.3
9	Wisconsin	9.3
11	Minnesota	6.7
12	Vermont	2.9
13	Virginia	1.7
14	Iowa	1.2
15	Ohio	1.0
16	West Virginia	0.7
17	Kentucky	0.6
18	Missouri	0.5
18	North Carolina	0.5
18	Tennessee	0.5
21	Idaho	0.4
21	Indiana	0.4
21	Oregon	0.4
21	Texas	0.4
25	Alaska	0.3
25	California	0.3
25	Florida	0.3
28	Alabama	0.2
28	Illinois	0.2
28	Michigan	0.2
28	Nebraska	0.2
28	South Carolina	0.2
28	Washington	0.2
28	Wyoming	0.2
35	Kansas	0.1
35	Nevada	0.1
35	New Mexico	0.1
38	Arizona	0.0
38	Arkansas	0.0
38	Colorado	0.0
38	Georgia	0.0
38	Louisiana	0.0
38	Maine	0.0
38	Mississippi	0.0
38	Montana	0.0
38	North Dakota	0.0
38	Oklahoma	0.0
38	South Dakota	0.0
38	Utah	0.0
NA	Hawaii**	NA

District of Columbia 3.0

Source: Morgan Quitno Press using data from U.S. Dept. of Health & Human Serv's, National Center for Health Statistics
    "Morbidity and Mortality Weekly Report" (January 4, 2002, Vol. 50, No. 51)
*Provisional data. Caused by ticks-lesions, followed by arthritis of large joints, myalgia, malaise and neurologic
and cardiac manifestations. Named after Old Lyme, CT, where the disease was first reported.
**Not notifiable.

Malaria Cases Reported in 2001

National Total = 1,266 Cases*

ALPHA ORDER

RANK	STATE	CASES	% of USA
29	Alabama	6	0.5%
44	Alaska	1	0.1%
17	Arizona	17	1.3%
37	Arkansas	3	0.2%
2	California	174	13.7%
14	Colorado	23	1.8%
12	Connecticut	29	2.3%
41	Delaware	2	0.2%
5	Florida	61	4.8%
11	Georgia	30	2.4%
25	Hawaii	10	0.8%
34	Idaho	4	0.3%
9	Illinois	35	2.8%
18	Indiana	16	1.3%
26	Iowa	9	0.7%
31	Kansas	5	0.4%
23	Kentucky	12	0.9%
31	Louisiana	5	0.4%
31	Maine	5	0.4%
3	Maryland	113	8.9%
8	Massachusetts	38	3.0%
7	Michigan	42	3.3%
29	Minnesota	6	0.5%
34	Mississippi	4	0.3%
22	Missouri	13	1.0%
37	Montana	3	0.2%
41	Nebraska	2	0.2%
26	Nevada	9	0.7%
41	New Hampshire	2	0.2%
4	New Jersey	76	6.0%
37	New Mexico	3	0.2%
1	New York	270	21.3%
16	North Carolina	19	1.5%
48	North Dakota	0	0.0%
13	Ohio	27	2.1%
37	Oklahoma	3	0.2%
21	Oregon	14	1.1%
10	Pennsylvania	34	2.7%
18	Rhode Island	16	1.3%
28	South Carolina	8	0.6%
48	South Dakota	0	0.0%
23	Tennessee	12	0.9%
44	Texas	1	0.1%
34	Utah	4	0.3%
44	Vermont	1	0.1%
6	Virginia	49	3.9%
20	Washington	15	1.2%
44	West Virginia	1	0.1%
15	Wisconsin	21	1.7%
48	Wyoming	0	0.0%

RANK ORDER

RANK	STATE	CASES	% of USA
1	New York	270	21.3%
2	California	174	13.7%
3	Maryland	113	8.9%
4	New Jersey	76	6.0%
5	Florida	61	4.8%
6	Virginia	49	3.9%
7	Michigan	42	3.3%
8	Massachusetts	38	3.0%
9	Illinois	35	2.8%
10	Pennsylvania	34	2.7%
11	Georgia	30	2.4%
12	Connecticut	29	2.3%
13	Ohio	27	2.1%
14	Colorado	23	1.8%
15	Wisconsin	21	1.7%
16	North Carolina	19	1.5%
17	Arizona	17	1.3%
18	Indiana	16	1.3%
18	Rhode Island	16	1.3%
20	Washington	15	1.2%
21	Oregon	14	1.1%
22	Missouri	13	1.0%
23	Kentucky	12	0.9%
23	Tennessee	12	0.9%
25	Hawaii	10	0.8%
26	Iowa	9	0.7%
26	Nevada	9	0.7%
28	South Carolina	8	0.6%
29	Alabama	6	0.5%
29	Minnesota	6	0.5%
31	Kansas	5	0.4%
31	Louisiana	5	0.4%
31	Maine	5	0.4%
34	Idaho	4	0.3%
34	Mississippi	4	0.3%
34	Utah	4	0.3%
37	Arkansas	3	0.2%
37	Montana	3	0.2%
37	New Mexico	3	0.2%
37	Oklahoma	3	0.2%
41	Delaware	2	0.2%
41	Nebraska	2	0.2%
41	New Hampshire	2	0.2%
44	Alaska	1	0.1%
44	Texas	1	0.1%
44	Vermont	1	0.1%
44	West Virginia	1	0.1%
48	North Dakota	0	0.0%
48	South Dakota	0	0.0%
48	Wyoming	0	0.0%
	District of Columbia	13	1.0%

Source: U.S. Department of Health and Human Services, National Center for Health Statistics
"Morbidity and Mortality Weekly Report" (January 4, 2002, Vol. 50, No. 51)
*Provisional data. Infectious disease usually transmitted by bites of infected mosquitoes. Symptoms include high fever, shaking chills, sweating and anemia.

Malaria Rate in 2001

National Rate = 0.4 Cases per 100,000 Population*

ALPHA ORDER

RANK	STATE	RATE
39	Alabama	0.1
28	Alaska	0.2
18	Arizona	0.3
39	Arkansas	0.1
9	California	0.5
9	Colorado	0.5
4	Connecticut	0.9
18	Delaware	0.3
11	Florida	0.4
11	Georgia	0.4
6	Hawaii	0.8
18	Idaho	0.3
18	Illinois	0.3
18	Indiana	0.3
18	Iowa	0.3
28	Kansas	0.2
18	Kentucky	0.3
39	Louisiana	0.1
11	Maine	0.4
1	Maryland	2.1
8	Massachusetts	0.6
11	Michigan	0.4
39	Minnesota	0.1
39	Mississippi	0.1
28	Missouri	0.2
18	Montana	0.3
39	Nebraska	0.1
11	Nevada	0.4
28	New Hampshire	0.2
4	New Jersey	0.9
28	New Mexico	0.2
3	New York	1.4
28	North Carolina	0.2
47	North Dakota	0.0
28	Ohio	0.2
39	Oklahoma	0.1
11	Oregon	0.4
18	Pennsylvania	0.3
2	Rhode Island	1.5
28	South Carolina	0.2
47	South Dakota	0.0
28	Tennessee	0.2
47	Texas	0.0
28	Utah	0.2
28	Vermont	0.2
7	Virginia	0.7
18	Washington	0.3
39	West Virginia	0.1
11	Wisconsin	0.4
47	Wyoming	0.0

RANK ORDER

RANK	STATE	RATE
1	Maryland	2.1
2	Rhode Island	1.5
3	New York	1.4
4	Connecticut	0.9
4	New Jersey	0.9
6	Hawaii	0.8
7	Virginia	0.7
8	Massachusetts	0.6
9	California	0.5
9	Colorado	0.5
11	Florida	0.4
11	Georgia	0.4
11	Maine	0.4
11	Michigan	0.4
11	Nevada	0.4
11	Oregon	0.4
11	Wisconsin	0.4
18	Arizona	0.3
18	Delaware	0.3
18	Idaho	0.3
18	Illinois	0.3
18	Indiana	0.3
18	Iowa	0.3
18	Kentucky	0.3
18	Montana	0.3
18	Pennsylvania	0.3
18	Washington	0.3
28	Alaska	0.2
28	Kansas	0.2
28	Missouri	0.2
28	New Hampshire	0.2
28	New Mexico	0.2
28	North Carolina	0.2
28	Ohio	0.2
28	South Carolina	0.2
28	Tennessee	0.2
28	Utah	0.2
28	Vermont	0.2
39	Alabama	0.1
39	Arkansas	0.1
39	Louisiana	0.1
39	Minnesota	0.1
39	Mississippi	0.1
39	Nebraska	0.1
39	Oklahoma	0.1
39	West Virginia	0.1
47	North Dakota	0.0
47	South Dakota	0.0
47	Texas	0.0
47	Wyoming	0.0

District of Columbia — 2.3

Source: Morgan Quitno Press using data from U.S. Dept. of Health & Human Serv's, National Center for Health Statistics
"Morbidity and Mortality Weekly Report" (January 4, 2002, Vol. 50, No. 51)
*Provisional data. Infectious disease usually transmitted by bites of infected mosquitoes. Symptoms include high
fever, shaking chills, sweating and anemia.

Measles (Rubeola) Cases Reported in 2001

National Total = 108 Cases*

ALPHA ORDER

RANK	STATE	CASES	% of USA
23	Alabama	0	0.0%
23	Alaska	0	0.0%
15	Arizona	1	0.9%
23	Arkansas	0	0.0%
1	California	36	33.3%
23	Colorado	0	0.0%
15	Connecticut	1	0.9%
23	Delaware	0	0.0%
23	Florida	0	0.0%
15	Georgia	1	0.9%
4	Hawaii	7	6.5%
15	Idaho	1	0.9%
8	Illinois	3	2.8%
6	Indiana	4	3.7%
23	Iowa	0	0.0%
23	Kansas	0	0.0%
13	Kentucky	2	1.9%
23	Louisiana	0	0.0%
23	Maine	0	0.0%
8	Maryland	3	2.8%
8	Massachusetts	3	2.8%
23	Michigan	0	0.0%
8	Minnesota	3	2.8%
23	Mississippi	0	0.0%
13	Missouri	2	1.9%
23	Montana	0	0.0%
23	Nebraska	0	0.0%
23	Nevada	0	0.0%
23	New Hampshire	0	0.0%
15	New Jersey	1	0.9%
23	New Mexico	0	0.0%
3	New York	9	8.3%
23	North Carolina	0	0.0%
23	North Dakota	0	0.0%
8	Ohio	3	2.8%
23	Oklahoma	0	0.0%
6	Oregon	4	3.7%
5	Pennsylvania	6	5.6%
23	Rhode Island	0	0.0%
23	South Carolina	0	0.0%
23	South Dakota	0	0.0%
23	Tennessee	0	0.0%
15	Texas	1	0.9%
23	Utah	0	0.0%
15	Vermont	1	0.9%
15	Virginia	1	0.9%
2	Washington	15	13.9%
23	West Virginia	0	0.0%
23	Wisconsin	0	0.0%
23	Wyoming	0	0.0%

RANK ORDER

RANK	STATE	CASES	% of USA
1	California	36	33.3%
2	Washington	15	13.9%
3	New York	9	8.3%
4	Hawaii	7	6.5%
5	Pennsylvania	6	5.6%
6	Indiana	4	3.7%
6	Oregon	4	3.7%
8	Illinois	3	2.8%
8	Maryland	3	2.8%
8	Massachusetts	3	2.8%
8	Minnesota	3	2.8%
8	Ohio	3	2.8%
13	Kentucky	2	1.9%
13	Missouri	2	1.9%
15	Arizona	1	0.9%
15	Connecticut	1	0.9%
15	Georgia	1	0.9%
15	Idaho	1	0.9%
15	New Jersey	1	0.9%
15	Texas	1	0.9%
15	Vermont	1	0.9%
15	Virginia	1	0.9%
23	Alabama	0	0.0%
23	Alaska	0	0.0%
23	Arkansas	0	0.0%
23	Colorado	0	0.0%
23	Delaware	0	0.0%
23	Florida	0	0.0%
23	Iowa	0	0.0%
23	Kansas	0	0.0%
23	Louisiana	0	0.0%
23	Maine	0	0.0%
23	Michigan	0	0.0%
23	Mississippi	0	0.0%
23	Montana	0	0.0%
23	Nebraska	0	0.0%
23	Nevada	0	0.0%
23	New Hampshire	0	0.0%
23	New Mexico	0	0.0%
23	North Carolina	0	0.0%
23	North Dakota	0	0.0%
23	Oklahoma	0	0.0%
23	Rhode Island	0	0.0%
23	South Carolina	0	0.0%
23	South Dakota	0	0.0%
23	Tennessee	0	0.0%
23	Utah	0	0.0%
23	West Virginia	0	0.0%
23	Wisconsin	0	0.0%
23	Wyoming	0	0.0%
	District of Columbia	0	0.0%

*Source: U.S. Department of Health and Human Services, National Center for Health Statistics
"Morbidity and Mortality Weekly Report" (January 4, 2002, Vol. 50, No. 51)*
Provisional data. Includes indigenous and imported cases.

Measles (Rubeola) Rate in 2001

National Rate = 0.04 Cases per 100,000 Population*

ALPHA ORDER			RANK ORDER		
RANK	STATE	RATE	RANK	STATE	RATE
22	Alabama	0.00	1	Hawaii	0.57
22	Alaska	0.00	2	Washington	0.25
17	Arizona	0.02	3	Vermont	0.16
22	Arkansas	0.00	4	Oregon	0.12
5	California	0.10	5	California	0.10
22	Colorado	0.00	6	Idaho	0.08
15	Connecticut	0.03	7	Indiana	0.07
22	Delaware	0.00	8	Maryland	0.06
22	Florida	0.00	8	Minnesota	0.06
19	Georgia	0.01	10	Kentucky	0.05
1	Hawaii	0.57	10	Massachusetts	0.05
6	Idaho	0.08	10	New York	0.05
17	Illinois	0.02	10	Pennsylvania	0.05
7	Indiana	0.07	14	Missouri	0.04
22	Iowa	0.00	15	Connecticut	0.03
22	Kansas	0.00	15	Ohio	0.03
10	Kentucky	0.05	17	Arizona	0.02
22	Louisiana	0.00	17	Illinois	0.02
22	Maine	0.00	19	Georgia	0.01
8	Maryland	0.06	19	New Jersey	0.01
10	Massachusetts	0.05	19	Virginia	0.01
22	Michigan	0.00	22	Alabama	0.00
8	Minnesota	0.06	22	Alaska	0.00
22	Mississippi	0.00	22	Arkansas	0.00
14	Missouri	0.04	22	Colorado	0.00
22	Montana	0.00	22	Delaware	0.00
22	Nebraska	0.00	22	Florida	0.00
22	Nevada	0.00	22	Iowa	0.00
22	New Hampshire	0.00	22	Kansas	0.00
19	New Jersey	0.01	22	Louisiana	0.00
22	New Mexico	0.00	22	Maine	0.00
10	New York	0.05	22	Michigan	0.00
22	North Carolina	0.00	22	Mississippi	0.00
22	North Dakota	0.00	22	Montana	0.00
15	Ohio	0.03	22	Nebraska	0.00
22	Oklahoma	0.00	22	Nevada	0.00
4	Oregon	0.12	22	New Hampshire	0.00
10	Pennsylvania	0.05	22	New Mexico	0.00
22	Rhode Island	0.00	22	North Carolina	0.00
22	South Carolina	0.00	22	North Dakota	0.00
22	South Dakota	0.00	22	Oklahoma	0.00
22	Tennessee	0.00	22	Rhode Island	0.00
22	Texas	0.00	22	South Carolina	0.00
22	Utah	0.00	22	South Dakota	0.00
3	Vermont	0.16	22	Tennessee	0.00
19	Virginia	0.01	22	Texas	0.00
2	Washington	0.25	22	Utah	0.00
22	West Virginia	0.00	22	West Virginia	0.00
22	Wisconsin	0.00	22	Wisconsin	0.00
22	Wyoming	0.00	22	Wyoming	0.00
				District of Columbia	0.00

Source: Morgan Quitno Press using data from U.S. Dept. of Health & Human Serv's, National Center for Health Statistics
"Morbidity and Mortality Weekly Report" (January 4, 2002, Vol. 50, No. 51)
*Provisional data. Includes indigenous and imported cases.

Meningococcal Infections Reported in 2001

National Total = 2,255 Cases*

ALPHA ORDER

RANK	STATE	CASES	% of USA
23	Alabama	35	1.6%
50	Alaska	3	0.1%
32	Arizona	19	0.8%
31	Arkansas	21	0.9%
1	California	313	13.9%
22	Colorado	36	1.6%
28	Connecticut	25	1.1%
46	Delaware	5	0.2%
3	Florida	125	5.5%
16	Georgia	52	2.3%
37	Hawaii	13	0.6%
39	Idaho	8	0.4%
7	Illinois	72	3.2%
20	Indiana	43	1.9%
26	Iowa	31	1.4%
34	Kansas	15	0.7%
30	Kentucky	23	1.0%
9	Louisiana	66	2.9%
42	Maine	7	0.3%
21	Maryland	42	1.9%
13	Massachusetts	56	2.5%
8	Michigan	71	3.1%
27	Minnesota	27	1.2%
33	Mississippi	16	0.7%
13	Missouri	56	2.5%
49	Montana	4	0.2%
28	Nebraska	25	1.1%
39	Nevada	8	0.4%
35	New Hampshire	14	0.6%
5	New Jersey	93	4.1%
38	New Mexico	11	0.5%
4	New York	106	4.7%
11	North Carolina	63	2.8%
44	North Dakota	6	0.3%
6	Ohio	92	4.1%
25	Oklahoma	32	1.4%
18	Oregon	46	2.0%
13	Pennsylvania	56	2.5%
44	Rhode Island	6	0.3%
23	South Carolina	35	1.6%
46	South Dakota	5	0.2%
12	Tennessee	60	2.7%
2	Texas	221	9.8%
39	Utah	8	0.4%
42	Vermont	7	0.3%
19	Virginia	44	2.0%
9	Washington	66	2.9%
35	West Virginia	14	0.6%
17	Wisconsin	48	2.1%
46	Wyoming	5	0.2%

RANK ORDER

RANK	STATE	CASES	% of USA
1	California	313	13.9%
2	Texas	221	9.8%
3	Florida	125	5.5%
4	New York	106	4.7%
5	New Jersey	93	4.1%
6	Ohio	92	4.1%
7	Illinois	72	3.2%
8	Michigan	71	3.1%
9	Louisiana	66	2.9%
9	Washington	66	2.9%
11	North Carolina	63	2.8%
12	Tennessee	60	2.7%
13	Massachusetts	56	2.5%
13	Missouri	56	2.5%
13	Pennsylvania	56	2.5%
16	Georgia	52	2.3%
17	Wisconsin	48	2.1%
18	Oregon	46	2.0%
19	Virginia	44	2.0%
20	Indiana	43	1.9%
21	Maryland	42	1.9%
22	Colorado	36	1.6%
23	Alabama	35	1.6%
23	South Carolina	35	1.6%
25	Oklahoma	32	1.4%
26	Iowa	31	1.4%
27	Minnesota	27	1.2%
28	Connecticut	25	1.1%
28	Nebraska	25	1.1%
30	Kentucky	23	1.0%
31	Arkansas	21	0.9%
32	Arizona	19	0.8%
33	Mississippi	16	0.7%
34	Kansas	15	0.7%
35	New Hampshire	14	0.6%
35	West Virginia	14	0.6%
37	Hawaii	13	0.6%
38	New Mexico	11	0.5%
39	Idaho	8	0.4%
39	Nevada	8	0.4%
39	Utah	8	0.4%
42	Maine	7	0.3%
42	Vermont	7	0.3%
44	North Dakota	6	0.3%
44	Rhode Island	6	0.3%
46	Delaware	5	0.2%
46	South Dakota	5	0.2%
46	Wyoming	5	0.2%
49	Montana	4	0.2%
50	Alaska	3	0.1%
	District of Columbia	0	0.0%

Source: U.S. Department of Health and Human Services, National Center for Health Statistics
    "Morbidity and Mortality Weekly Report" (January 4, 2002, Vol. 50, No. 51)
*Provisional data. A bacterium (Neisseria meningitidis) that causes cerebrospinal meningitis.

Meningococcal Infection Rate in 2001

National Rate = 0.8 Cases per 100,000 Population*

<u>ALPHA ORDER</u>

RANK	STATE	RATE
20	Alabama	0.8
43	Alaska	0.5
47	Arizona	0.4
20	Arkansas	0.8
14	California	0.9
20	Colorado	0.8
28	Connecticut	0.7
32	Delaware	0.6
20	Florida	0.8
32	Georgia	0.6
4	Hawaii	1.1
32	Idaho	0.6
32	Illinois	0.6
28	Indiana	0.7
4	Iowa	1.1
32	Kansas	0.6
32	Kentucky	0.6
1	Louisiana	1.5
43	Maine	0.5
20	Maryland	0.8
14	Massachusetts	0.9
28	Michigan	0.7
43	Minnesota	0.5
32	Mississippi	0.6
10	Missouri	1.0
47	Montana	0.4
1	Nebraska	1.5
47	Nevada	0.4
4	New Hampshire	1.1
4	New Jersey	1.1
32	New Mexico	0.6
32	New York	0.6
20	North Carolina	0.8
14	North Dakota	0.9
20	Ohio	0.8
14	Oklahoma	0.9
3	Oregon	1.3
43	Pennsylvania	0.5
32	Rhode Island	0.6
14	South Carolina	0.9
28	South Dakota	0.7
10	Tennessee	1.0
10	Texas	1.0
47	Utah	0.4
4	Vermont	1.1
32	Virginia	0.6
4	Washington	1.1
20	West Virginia	0.8
14	Wisconsin	0.9
10	Wyoming	1.0

<u>RANK ORDER</u>

RANK	STATE	RATE
1	Louisiana	1.5
1	Nebraska	1.5
3	Oregon	1.3
4	Hawaii	1.1
4	Iowa	1.1
4	New Hampshire	1.1
4	New Jersey	1.1
4	Vermont	1.1
4	Washington	1.1
10	Missouri	1.0
10	Tennessee	1.0
10	Texas	1.0
10	Wyoming	1.0
14	California	0.9
14	Massachusetts	0.9
14	North Dakota	0.9
14	Oklahoma	0.9
14	South Carolina	0.9
14	Wisconsin	0.9
20	Alabama	0.8
20	Arkansas	0.8
20	Colorado	0.8
20	Florida	0.8
20	Maryland	0.8
20	North Carolina	0.8
20	Ohio	0.8
20	West Virginia	0.8
28	Connecticut	0.7
28	Indiana	0.7
28	Michigan	0.7
28	South Dakota	0.7
32	Delaware	0.6
32	Georgia	0.6
32	Idaho	0.6
32	Illinois	0.6
32	Kansas	0.6
32	Kentucky	0.6
32	Mississippi	0.6
32	New Mexico	0.6
32	New York	0.6
32	Rhode Island	0.6
32	Virginia	0.6
43	Alaska	0.5
43	Maine	0.5
43	Minnesota	0.5
43	Pennsylvania	0.5
47	Arizona	0.4
47	Montana	0.4
47	Nevada	0.4
47	Utah	0.4

District of Columbia   0.0

Source: Morgan Quitno Press using data from U.S. Dept. of Health & Human Serv's, National Center for Health Statistics "Morbidity and Mortality Weekly Report" (January 4, 2002, Vol. 50, No. 51)
*Provisional data. A bacterium (Neisseria meningitidis) that causes cerebrospinal meningitis.

Mumps Cases Reported in 2001

National Total = 231 Cases*

ALPHA ORDER

RANK ORDER

RANK	STATE	CASES	% of USA		RANK	STATE	CASES	% of USA
37	Alabama	0	0.0%		1	California	46	19.9%
28	Alaska	1	0.4%		2	Hawaii	41	17.7%
28	Arizona	1	0.4%		3	New York	16	6.9%
28	Arkansas	1	0.4%		4	Illinois	11	4.8%
1	California	46	19.9%		4	Texas	11	4.8%
19	Colorado	3	1.3%		6	Florida	8	3.5%
37	Connecticut	0	0.0%		6	Virginia	8	3.5%
37	Delaware	0	0.0%		8	Georgia	7	3.0%
6	Florida	8	3.5%		8	Maryland	7	3.0%
8	Georgia	7	3.0%		8	South Carolina	7	3.0%
2	Hawaii	41	17.7%		11	Kansas	6	2.6%
23	Idaho	2	0.9%		12	Michigan	5	2.2%
4	Illinois	11	4.8%		12	Minnesota	5	2.2%
19	Indiana	3	1.3%		12	Mississippi	5	2.2%
28	Iowa	1	0.4%		12	North Carolina	5	2.2%
11	Kansas	6	2.6%		16	Missouri	4	1.7%
19	Kentucky	3	1.3%		16	New Jersey	4	1.7%
23	Louisiana	2	0.9%		16	Pennsylvania	4	1.7%
37	Maine	0	0.0%		19	Colorado	3	1.3%
8	Maryland	7	3.0%		19	Indiana	3	1.3%
37	Massachusetts	0	0.0%		19	Kentucky	3	1.3%
12	Michigan	5	2.2%		19	Nevada	3	1.3%
12	Minnesota	5	2.2%		23	Idaho	2	0.9%
12	Mississippi	5	2.2%		23	Louisiana	2	0.9%
16	Missouri	4	1.7%		23	New Mexico	2	0.9%
28	Montana	1	0.4%		23	Washington	2	0.9%
28	Nebraska	1	0.4%		23	Wyoming	2	0.9%
19	Nevada	3	1.3%		28	Alaska	1	0.4%
37	New Hampshire	0	0.0%		28	Arizona	1	0.4%
16	New Jersey	4	1.7%		28	Arkansas	1	0.4%
23	New Mexico	2	0.9%		28	Iowa	1	0.4%
3	New York	16	6.9%		28	Montana	1	0.4%
12	North Carolina	5	2.2%		28	Nebraska	1	0.4%
37	North Dakota	0	0.0%		28	Ohio	1	0.4%
28	Ohio	1	0.4%		28	Tennessee	1	0.4%
37	Oklahoma	0	0.0%		28	Utah	1	0.4%
NA	Oregon**	NA	NA		37	Alabama	0	0.0%
16	Pennsylvania	4	1.7%		37	Connecticut	0	0.0%
37	Rhode Island	0	0.0%		37	Delaware	0	0.0%
8	South Carolina	7	3.0%		37	Maine	0	0.0%
37	South Dakota	0	0.0%		37	Massachusetts	0	0.0%
28	Tennessee	1	0.4%		37	New Hampshire	0	0.0%
4	Texas	11	4.8%		37	North Dakota	0	0.0%
28	Utah	1	0.4%		37	Oklahoma	0	0.0%
37	Vermont	0	0.0%		37	Rhode Island	0	0.0%
6	Virginia	8	3.5%		37	South Dakota	0	0.0%
23	Washington	2	0.9%		37	Vermont	0	0.0%
37	West Virginia	0	0.0%		37	West Virginia	0	0.0%
37	Wisconsin	0	0.0%		37	Wisconsin	0	0.0%
23	Wyoming	2	0.9%		NA	Oregon**	NA	NA
						District of Columbia	0	0.0%

Source: U.S. Department of Health and Human Services, National Center for Health Statistics
  "Morbidity and Mortality Weekly Report" (January 4, 2002, Vol. 50, No. 51)
*Provisional data. An acute, inflammatory, contagious disease caused by a paramyxovirus and characterized by swelling of the salivary glands, especially the parotids, and sometimes of the pancreas, ovaries, or testes. This disease, mainly affecting children, can be prevented by vaccination.
**Mumps is not a notifiable disease in Oregon.

Mumps Rate in 2001

National Rate = 0.08 Cases per 100,000 Population*

ALPHA ORDER

RANK ORDER

RANK	STATE	RATE		RANK	STATE	RATE
37	Alabama	0.00		1	Hawaii	3.35
6	Alaska	0.16		2	Wyoming	0.40
34	Arizona	0.02		3	Kansas	0.22
28	Arkansas	0.04		4	Mississippi	0.17
9	California	0.13		4	South Carolina	0.17
18	Colorado	0.07		6	Alaska	0.16
37	Connecticut	0.00		7	Idaho	0.15
37	Delaware	0.00		8	Nevada	0.14
23	Florida	0.05		9	California	0.13
16	Georgia	0.08		9	Maryland	0.13
1	Hawaii	3.35		11	Montana	0.11
7	Idaho	0.15		11	New Mexico	0.11
15	Illinois	0.09		11	Virginia	0.11
23	Indiana	0.05		14	Minnesota	0.10
31	Iowa	0.03		15	Illinois	0.09
3	Kansas	0.22		16	Georgia	0.08
18	Kentucky	0.07		16	New York	0.08
28	Louisiana	0.04		18	Colorado	0.07
37	Maine	0.00		18	Kentucky	0.07
9	Maryland	0.13		18	Missouri	0.07
37	Massachusetts	0.00		21	Nebraska	0.06
23	Michigan	0.05		21	North Carolina	0.06
14	Minnesota	0.10		23	Florida	0.05
4	Mississippi	0.17		23	Indiana	0.05
18	Missouri	0.07		23	Michigan	0.05
11	Montana	0.11		23	New Jersey	0.05
21	Nebraska	0.06		23	Texas	0.05
8	Nevada	0.14		28	Arkansas	0.04
37	New Hampshire	0.00		28	Louisiana	0.04
23	New Jersey	0.05		28	Utah	0.04
11	New Mexico	0.11		31	Iowa	0.03
16	New York	0.08		31	Pennsylvania	0.03
21	North Carolina	0.06		31	Washington	0.03
37	North Dakota	0.00		34	Arizona	0.02
36	Ohio	0.01		34	Tennessee	0.02
37	Oklahoma	0.00		36	Ohio	0.01
NA	Oregon**	NA		37	Alabama	0.00
31	Pennsylvania	0.03		37	Connecticut	0.00
37	Rhode Island	0.00		37	Delaware	0.00
4	South Carolina	0.17		37	Maine	0.00
37	South Dakota	0.00		37	Massachusetts	0.00
34	Tennessee	0.02		37	New Hampshire	0.00
23	Texas	0.05		37	North Dakota	0.00
28	Utah	0.04		37	Oklahoma	0.00
37	Vermont	0.00		37	Rhode Island	0.00
11	Virginia	0.11		37	South Dakota	0.00
31	Washington	0.03		37	Vermont	0.00
37	West Virginia	0.00		37	West Virginia	0.00
37	Wisconsin	0.00		37	Wisconsin	0.00
2	Wyoming	0.40		NA	Oregon**	NA

District of Columbia 0.00

Source: Morgan Quitno Press using data from U.S. Dept. of Health & Human Serv's, National Center for Health Statistics
"Morbidity and Mortality Weekly Report" (January 4, 2002, Vol. 50, No. 51)
*Provisional data. An acute, inflammatory, contagious disease caused by a paramyxovirus and characterized by swelling of the salivary glands, especially the parotids, and sometimes of the pancreas, ovaries, or testes. This disease, mainly affecting children, can be prevented by vaccination.
**Mumps is not a notifiable disease in Oregon.

Rabies (Animal) Cases Reported in 2001

National Total = 6,563 Cases*

ALPHA ORDER

ALPHA ORDER

RANK	STATE	CASES	% of USA	RANK	STATE	CASES	% of USA
21	Alabama	64	1.0%	1	Texas	962	14.7%
29	Alaska	40	0.6%	2	New York	807	12.3%
14	Arizona	116	1.8%	3	North Carolina	577	8.8%
37	Arkansas	20	0.3%	4	Virginia	485	7.4%
7	California	300	4.6%	5	Georgia	399	6.1%
48	Colorado	0	0.0%	6	Maryland	361	5.5%
9	Connecticut	240	3.7%	7	California	300	4.6%
32	Delaware	30	0.5%	8	Massachusetts	273	4.2%
10	Florida	204	3.1%	9	Connecticut	240	3.7%
5	Georgia	399	6.1%	10	Florida	204	3.1%
48	Hawaii	0	0.0%	11	New Jersey	192	2.9%
33	Idaho	28	0.4%	12	Pennsylvania	188	2.9%
35	Illinois	24	0.4%	13	West Virginia	140	2.1%
39	Indiana	15	0.2%	14	Arizona	116	1.8%
18	Iowa	82	1.2%	15	South Carolina	114	1.7%
17	Kansas	94	1.4%	16	Tennessee	106	1.6%
33	Kentucky	28	0.4%	17	Kansas	94	1.4%
45	Louisiana	3	0.0%	18	Iowa	82	1.2%
20	Maine	69	1.1%	19	Rhode Island	72	1.1%
6	Maryland	361	5.5%	20	Maine	69	1.1%
8	Massachusetts	273	4.2%	21	Alabama	64	1.0%
26	Michigan	46	0.7%	22	Vermont	62	0.9%
26	Minnesota	46	0.7%	23	Oklahoma	60	0.9%
43	Mississippi	4	0.1%	24	South Dakota	56	0.9%
29	Missouri	40	0.6%	25	Ohio	52	0.8%
31	Montana	38	0.6%	26	Michigan	46	0.7%
43	Nebraska	4	0.1%	26	Minnesota	46	0.7%
47	Nevada	1	0.0%	28	North Dakota	42	0.6%
36	New Hampshire	21	0.3%	29	Alaska	40	0.6%
11	New Jersey	192	2.9%	29	Missouri	40	0.6%
41	New Mexico	14	0.2%	31	Montana	38	0.6%
2	New York	807	12.3%	32	Delaware	30	0.5%
3	North Carolina	577	8.8%	33	Idaho	28	0.4%
28	North Dakota	42	0.6%	33	Kentucky	28	0.4%
25	Ohio	52	0.8%	35	Illinois	24	0.4%
23	Oklahoma	60	0.9%	36	New Hampshire	21	0.3%
45	Oregon	3	0.0%	37	Arkansas	20	0.3%
12	Pennsylvania	188	2.9%	37	Wyoming	20	0.3%
19	Rhode Island	72	1.1%	39	Indiana	15	0.2%
15	South Carolina	114	1.7%	39	Utah	15	0.2%
24	South Dakota	56	0.9%	41	New Mexico	14	0.2%
16	Tennessee	106	1.6%	42	Wisconsin	6	0.1%
1	Texas	962	14.7%	43	Mississippi	4	0.1%
39	Utah	15	0.2%	43	Nebraska	4	0.1%
22	Vermont	62	0.9%	45	Louisiana	3	0.0%
4	Virginia	485	7.4%	45	Oregon	3	0.0%
48	Washington	0	0.0%	47	Nevada	1	0.0%
13	West Virginia	140	2.1%	48	Colorado	0	0.0%
42	Wisconsin	6	0.1%	48	Hawaii	0	0.0%
37	Wyoming	20	0.3%	48	Washington	0	0.0%
					District of Columbia	0	0.0%

RANK ORDER

Source: U.S. Department of Health and Human Services, National Center for Health Statistics
"Morbidity and Mortality Weekly Report" (January 4, 2002, Vol. 50, No. 51)
Provisional data. An acute, infectious, often fatal viral disease of most warm-blooded animals, especially wolves, cats, and dogs, that attacks the central nervous system and is transmitted by the bite of infected animals.

Rabies (Animal) Rate in 2001

National Rate = 2.3 Cases per 100,000 Human Population*

ALPHA ORDER				RANK ORDER		
RANK	**STATE**	**RATE**		**RANK**	**STATE**	**RATE**
29	Alabama	1.4		1	Vermont	10.1
10	Alaska	6.3		2	West Virginia	7.8
23	Arizona	2.2		3	South Dakota	7.4
34	Arkansas	0.7		4	Connecticut	7.0
31	California	0.9		4	North Carolina	7.0
47	Colorado	0.0		6	Rhode Island	6.8
4	Connecticut	7.0		7	Maryland	6.7
18	Delaware	3.8		7	Virginia	6.7
30	Florida	1.2		9	North Dakota	6.6
12	Georgia	4.8		10	Alaska	6.3
47	Hawaii	0.0		11	Maine	5.4
24	Idaho	2.1		12	Georgia	4.8
40	Illinois	0.2		13	Texas	4.5
40	Indiana	0.2		14	Massachusetts	4.3
20	Iowa	2.8		15	Montana	4.2
19	Kansas	3.5		15	New York	4.2
34	Kentucky	0.7		17	Wyoming	4.0
43	Louisiana	0.1		18	Delaware	3.8
11	Maine	5.4		19	Kansas	3.5
7	Maryland	6.7		20	Iowa	2.8
14	Massachusetts	4.3		20	South Carolina	2.8
38	Michigan	0.5		22	New Jersey	2.3
31	Minnesota	0.9		23	Arizona	2.2
43	Mississippi	0.1		24	Idaho	2.1
34	Missouri	0.7		25	Tennessee	1.8
15	Montana	4.2		26	New Hampshire	1.7
40	Nebraska	0.2		26	Oklahoma	1.7
47	Nevada	0.0		28	Pennsylvania	1.5
26	New Hampshire	1.7		29	Alabama	1.4
22	New Jersey	2.3		30	Florida	1.2
33	New Mexico	0.8		31	California	0.9
15	New York	4.2		31	Minnesota	0.9
4	North Carolina	7.0		33	New Mexico	0.8
9	North Dakota	6.6		34	Arkansas	0.7
38	Ohio	0.5		34	Kentucky	0.7
26	Oklahoma	1.7		34	Missouri	0.7
43	Oregon	0.1		34	Utah	0.7
28	Pennsylvania	1.5		38	Michigan	0.5
6	Rhode Island	6.8		38	Ohio	0.5
20	South Carolina	2.8		40	Illinois	0.2
3	South Dakota	7.4		40	Indiana	0.2
25	Tennessee	1.8		40	Nebraska	0.2
13	Texas	4.5		43	Louisiana	0.1
34	Utah	0.7		43	Mississippi	0.1
1	Vermont	10.1		43	Oregon	0.1
7	Virginia	6.7		43	Wisconsin	0.1
47	Washington	0.0		47	Colorado	0.0
2	West Virginia	7.8		47	Hawaii	0.0
43	Wisconsin	0.1		47	Nevada	0.0
17	Wyoming	4.0		47	Washington	0.0
					District of Columbia	0.0

Source: Morgan Quitno Press using data from U.S. Dept. of Health & Human Serv's, National Center for Health Statistics "Morbidity and Mortality Weekly Report" (January 4, 2002, Vol. 50, No. 51)
Provisional data. An acute, infectious, often fatal viral disease of most warm-blooded animals, especially wolves, cats, and dogs, that attacks the central nervous system and is transmitted by the bite of infected animals.

Salmonellosis Cases Reported in 2001

National Total = 66,386 Cases*

ALPHA ORDER

RANK	STATE	CASES	% of USA
22	Alabama	1,222	1.8%
49	Alaska	79	0.1%
21	Arizona	1,286	1.9%
27	Arkansas	995	1.5%
1	California	6,685	10.1%
23	Colorado	1,169	1.8%
28	Connecticut	899	1.4%
43	Delaware	198	0.3%
3	Florida	3,756	5.7%
5	Georgia	2,871	4.3%
30	Hawaii	697	1.0%
42	Idaho	241	0.4%
8	Illinois	2,486	3.7%
26	Indiana	1,011	1.5%
31	Iowa	641	1.0%
34	Kansas	532	0.8%
32	Kentucky	613	0.9%
18	Louisiana	1,376	2.1%
38	Maine	318	0.5%
12	Maryland	1,665	2.5%
9	Massachusetts	2,430	3.7%
13	Michigan	1,630	2.5%
19	Minnesota	1,371	2.1%
24	Mississippi	1,144	1.7%
15	Missouri	1,579	2.4%
50	Montana	78	0.1%
46	Nebraska	153	0.2%
43	Nevada	198	0.3%
37	New Hampshire	319	0.5%
11	New Jersey	2,255	3.4%
35	New Mexico	515	0.8%
2	New York	4,944	7.4%
6	North Carolina	2,597	3.9%
47	North Dakota	144	0.2%
7	Ohio	2,524	3.8%
29	Oklahoma	857	1.3%
33	Oregon	557	0.8%
16	Pennsylvania	1,454	2.2%
39	Rhode Island	316	0.5%
14	South Carolina	1,622	2.4%
41	South Dakota	265	0.4%
17	Tennessee	1,439	2.2%
4	Texas	3,477	5.2%
36	Utah	417	0.6%
45	Vermont	154	0.2%
10	Virginia	2,361	3.6%
25	Washington	1,070	1.6%
40	West Virginia	282	0.4%
20	Wisconsin	1,304	2.0%
48	Wyoming	109	0.2%

RANK ORDER

RANK	STATE	CASES	% of USA
1	California	6,685	10.1%
2	New York	4,944	7.4%
3	Florida	3,756	5.7%
4	Texas	3,477	5.2%
5	Georgia	2,871	4.3%
6	North Carolina	2,597	3.9%
7	Ohio	2,524	3.8%
8	Illinois	2,486	3.7%
9	Massachusetts	2,430	3.7%
10	Virginia	2,361	3.6%
11	New Jersey	2,255	3.4%
12	Maryland	1,665	2.5%
13	Michigan	1,630	2.5%
14	South Carolina	1,622	2.4%
15	Missouri	1,579	2.4%
16	Pennsylvania	1,454	2.2%
17	Tennessee	1,439	2.2%
18	Louisiana	1,376	2.1%
19	Minnesota	1,371	2.1%
20	Wisconsin	1,304	2.0%
21	Arizona	1,286	1.9%
22	Alabama	1,222	1.8%
23	Colorado	1,169	1.8%
24	Mississippi	1,144	1.7%
25	Washington	1,070	1.6%
26	Indiana	1,011	1.5%
27	Arkansas	995	1.5%
28	Connecticut	899	1.4%
29	Oklahoma	857	1.3%
30	Hawaii	697	1.0%
31	Iowa	641	1.0%
32	Kentucky	613	0.9%
33	Oregon	557	0.8%
34	Kansas	532	0.8%
35	New Mexico	515	0.8%
36	Utah	417	0.6%
37	New Hampshire	319	0.5%
38	Maine	318	0.5%
39	Rhode Island	316	0.5%
40	West Virginia	282	0.4%
41	South Dakota	265	0.4%
42	Idaho	241	0.4%
43	Delaware	198	0.3%
43	Nevada	198	0.3%
45	Vermont	154	0.2%
46	Nebraska	153	0.2%
47	North Dakota	144	0.2%
48	Wyoming	109	0.2%
49	Alaska	79	0.1%
50	Montana	78	0.1%
	District of Columbia	81	0.1%

Source: U.S. Department of Health and Human Services, National Center for Health Statistics
    "Morbidity and Mortality Weekly Report" (January 4, 2002, Vol. 50, No. 51)
*Provisional data. Any disease caused by a salmonella infection, which may be manifested as food poisoning with acute gastroenteritis, vomiting and diarrhea. Reported through Public Health Laboratory Information System and the National Electronic Telecommunications System for Surveillance.

Salmonellosis Rate in 2001

National Rate = 23.3 Cases per 100,000 Population*

ALPHA ORDER				RANK ORDER		
RANK	**STATE**	**RATE**		**RANK**	**STATE**	**RATE**
16	Alabama	27.4		1	Hawaii	56.9
46	Alaska	12.4		2	Mississippi	40.0
27	Arizona	24.2		3	South Carolina	39.9
5	Arkansas	37.0		4	Massachusetts	38.1
36	California	19.4		5	Arkansas	37.0
18	Colorado	26.5		6	South Dakota	35.0
19	Connecticut	26.2		7	Georgia	34.2
24	Delaware	24.9		8	Virginia	32.8
29	Florida	22.9		9	North Carolina	31.7
7	Georgia	34.2		10	Maryland	31.0
1	Hawaii	56.9		11	Louisiana	30.8
38	Idaho	18.2		12	Rhode Island	29.8
34	Illinois	19.9		13	New Mexico	28.2
40	Indiana	16.5		14	Missouri	28.0
33	Iowa	21.9		15	Minnesota	27.6
35	Kansas	19.7		16	Alabama	27.4
45	Kentucky	15.1		17	New Jersey	26.6
11	Louisiana	30.8		18	Colorado	26.5
26	Maine	24.7		19	Connecticut	26.2
10	Maryland	31.0		20	New York	26.0
4	Massachusetts	38.1		21	New Hampshire	25.3
41	Michigan	16.3		22	Tennessee	25.1
15	Minnesota	27.6		22	Vermont	25.1
2	Mississippi	40.0		24	Delaware	24.9
14	Missouri	28.0		25	Oklahoma	24.8
50	Montana	8.6		26	Maine	24.7
49	Nebraska	8.9		27	Arizona	24.2
48	Nevada	9.4		28	Wisconsin	24.1
21	New Hampshire	25.3		29	Florida	22.9
17	New Jersey	26.6		30	North Dakota	22.7
13	New Mexico	28.2		31	Ohio	22.2
20	New York	26.0		32	Wyoming	22.0
9	North Carolina	31.7		33	Iowa	21.9
30	North Dakota	22.7		34	Illinois	19.9
31	Ohio	22.2		35	Kansas	19.7
25	Oklahoma	24.8		36	California	19.4
43	Oregon	16.0		37	Utah	18.4
47	Pennsylvania	11.8		38	Idaho	18.2
12	Rhode Island	29.8		39	Washington	17.9
3	South Carolina	39.9		40	Indiana	16.5
6	South Dakota	35.0		41	Michigan	16.3
22	Tennessee	25.1		41	Texas	16.3
41	Texas	16.3		43	Oregon	16.0
37	Utah	18.4		44	West Virginia	15.7
22	Vermont	25.1		45	Kentucky	15.1
8	Virginia	32.8		46	Alaska	12.4
39	Washington	17.9		47	Pennsylvania	11.8
44	West Virginia	15.7		48	Nevada	9.4
28	Wisconsin	24.1		49	Nebraska	8.9
32	Wyoming	22.0		50	Montana	8.6

District of Columbia 14.2

Source: Morgan Quitno Press using data from U.S. Dept. of Health & Human Serv's, National Center for Health Statistics "Morbidity and Mortality Weekly Report" (January 4, 2002, Vol. 50, No. 51)
*Provisional data. Any disease caused by a salmonella infection, which may be manifested as food poisoning with acute gastroenteritis, vomiting and diarrhea. Reported through Public Health Laboratory Information System and the National Electronic Telecommunications System for Surveillance.

Shigellosis Cases Reported in 2001

National Total = 26,400 Cases*

ALPHA ORDER					RANK ORDER			
RANK	STATE		CASES	% of USA	RANK	STATE	CASES	% of USA
24	Alabama		341	1.3%	1	Ohio	4,156	15.7%
45	Alaska		13	0.0%	2	Texas	2,490	9.4%
11	Arizona		734	2.8%	3	California	2,132	8.1%
12	Arkansas		698	2.6%	4	New York	1,307	5.0%
3	California		2,132	8.1%	5	Kentucky	1,140	4.3%
20	Colorado		504	1.9%	6	Florida	1,091	4.1%
38	Connecticut		82	0.3%	7	Virginia	908	3.4%
43	Delaware		31	0.1%	8	Minnesota	907	3.4%
6	Florida		1,091	4.1%	9	Illinois	904	3.4%
14	Georgia		581	2.2%	10	South Dakota	889	3.4%
35	Hawaii		119	0.5%	11	Arizona	734	2.8%
41	Idaho		55	0.2%	12	Arkansas	698	2.6%
9	Illinois		904	3.4%	13	Iowa	660	2.5%
27	Indiana		275	1.0%	14	Georgia	581	2.2%
13	Iowa		660	2.5%	15	Mississippi	557	2.1%
36	Kansas		114	0.4%	16	New Jersey	550	2.1%
5	Kentucky		1,140	4.3%	17	North Carolina	526	2.0%
25	Louisiana		315	1.2%	18	Missouri	525	2.0%
48	Maine		9	0.0%	19	Michigan	518	2.0%
29	Maryland		255	1.0%	20	Colorado	504	1.9%
22	Massachusetts		384	1.5%	21	Washington	385	1.5%
19	Michigan		518	2.0%	22	Massachusetts	384	1.5%
8	Minnesota		907	3.4%	23	South Carolina	374	1.4%
15	Mississippi		557	2.1%	24	Alabama	341	1.3%
18	Missouri		525	2.0%	25	Louisiana	315	1.2%
48	Montana		9	0.0%	26	Wisconsin	313	1.2%
37	Nebraska		98	0.4%	27	Indiana	275	1.0%
39	Nevada		75	0.3%	28	Pennsylvania	261	1.0%
47	New Hampshire		11	0.0%	29	Maryland	255	1.0%
16	New Jersey		550	2.1%	30	Tennessee	233	0.9%
32	New Mexico		200	0.8%	31	Oregon	207	0.8%
4	New York		1,307	5.0%	32	New Mexico	200	0.8%
17	North Carolina		526	2.0%	33	Oklahoma	145	0.5%
40	North Dakota		57	0.2%	34	Utah	120	0.5%
1	Ohio		4,156	15.7%	35	Hawaii	119	0.5%
33	Oklahoma		145	0.5%	36	Kansas	114	0.4%
31	Oregon		207	0.8%	37	Nebraska	98	0.4%
28	Pennsylvania		261	1.0%	38	Connecticut	82	0.3%
42	Rhode Island		50	0.2%	39	Nevada	75	0.3%
23	South Carolina		374	1.4%	40	North Dakota	57	0.2%
10	South Dakota		889	3.4%	41	Idaho	55	0.2%
30	Tennessee		233	0.9%	42	Rhode Island	50	0.2%
2	Texas		2,490	9.4%	43	Delaware	31	0.1%
34	Utah		120	0.5%	44	West Virginia	18	0.1%
45	Vermont		13	0.0%	45	Alaska	13	0.0%
7	Virginia		908	3.4%	45	Vermont	13	0.0%
21	Washington		385	1.5%	47	New Hampshire	11	0.0%
44	West Virginia		18	0.1%	48	Maine	9	0.0%
26	Wisconsin		313	1.2%	48	Montana	9	0.0%
50	Wyoming		8	0.0%	50	Wyoming	8	0.0%
						District of Columbia	53	0.2%

Source: U.S. Department of Health and Human Services, National Center for Health Statistics
   "Morbidity and Mortality Weekly Report" (January 4, 2002, Vol. 50, No. 51)
*Provisional data. Dysentery caused by any of various species of shigellae, occurring most frequently in areas where poor sanitation and malnutrition are prevalent and commonly affecting children and infants. Reported through Public Health Laboratory Information System and the National Electronic Telecommunications System for Surveillance.

Shigellosis Rate in 2001

National Rate = 9.3 Cases per 100,000 Population*

ALPHA ORDER

RANK	STATE	RATE
17	Alabama	7.6
45	Alaska	2.0
8	Arizona	13.8
4	Arkansas	25.9
26	California	6.2
11	Colorado	11.4
42	Connecticut	2.4
40	Delaware	3.9
22	Florida	6.7
20	Georgia	6.9
13	Hawaii	9.7
36	Idaho	4.2
18	Illinois	7.2
35	Indiana	4.5
5	Iowa	22.6
36	Kansas	4.2
3	Kentucky	28.0
19	Louisiana	7.1
50	Maine	0.7
33	Maryland	4.7
27	Massachusetts	6.0
32	Michigan	5.2
7	Minnesota	18.2
6	Mississippi	19.5
14	Missouri	9.3
47	Montana	1.0
30	Nebraska	5.7
41	Nevada	3.6
49	New Hampshire	0.9
23	New Jersey	6.5
12	New Mexico	10.9
20	New York	6.9
24	North Carolina	6.4
16	North Dakota	9.0
2	Ohio	36.5
36	Oklahoma	4.2
27	Oregon	6.0
43	Pennsylvania	2.1
33	Rhode Island	4.7
15	South Carolina	9.2
1	South Dakota	117.5
39	Tennessee	4.1
10	Texas	11.7
31	Utah	5.3
43	Vermont	2.1
9	Virginia	12.6
24	Washington	6.4
47	West Virginia	1.0
29	Wisconsin	5.8
46	Wyoming	1.6

RANK ORDER

RANK	STATE	RATE
1	South Dakota	117.5
2	Ohio	36.5
3	Kentucky	28.0
4	Arkansas	25.9
5	Iowa	22.6
6	Mississippi	19.5
7	Minnesota	18.2
8	Arizona	13.8
9	Virginia	12.6
10	Texas	11.7
11	Colorado	11.4
12	New Mexico	10.9
13	Hawaii	9.7
14	Missouri	9.3
15	South Carolina	9.2
16	North Dakota	9.0
17	Alabama	7.6
18	Illinois	7.2
19	Louisiana	7.1
20	Georgia	6.9
20	New York	6.9
22	Florida	6.7
23	New Jersey	6.5
24	North Carolina	6.4
24	Washington	6.4
26	California	6.2
27	Massachusetts	6.0
27	Oregon	6.0
29	Wisconsin	5.8
30	Nebraska	5.7
31	Utah	5.3
32	Michigan	5.2
33	Maryland	4.7
33	Rhode Island	4.7
35	Indiana	4.5
36	Idaho	4.2
36	Kansas	4.2
36	Oklahoma	4.2
39	Tennessee	4.1
40	Delaware	3.9
41	Nevada	3.6
42	Connecticut	2.4
43	Pennsylvania	2.1
43	Vermont	2.1
45	Alaska	2.0
46	Wyoming	1.6
47	Montana	1.0
47	West Virginia	1.0
49	New Hampshire	0.9
50	Maine	0.7

District of Columbia	9.3

Source: Morgan Quitno Press using data from U.S. Dept. of Health & Human Serv's, National Center for Health Statistics "Morbidity and Mortality Weekly Report" (January 4, 2002, Vol. 50, No. 51)
*Provisional data. Dysentery caused by any of various species of shigellae, occurring most frequently in areas where poor sanitation and malnutrition are prevalent and commonly affecting children and infants. Reported through Public Health Laboratory Information System and the National Electronic Telecommunications System for Surveillance.

Tuberculosis Cases Reported in 2001

National Total = 12,294 Cases*

ALPHA ORDER

RANK	STATE	CASES	% of USA
14	Alabama	265	2.2%
33	Alaska	51	0.4%
12	Arizona	269	2.2%
21	Arkansas	153	1.2%
1	California	2,493	20.3%
26	Colorado	120	1.0%
30	Connecticut	101	0.8%
41	Delaware	15	0.1%
3	Florida	952	7.7%
7	Georgia	445	3.6%
22	Hawaii	148	1.2%
44	Idaho	10	0.1%
4	Illinois	636	5.2%
28	Indiana	111	0.9%
36	Iowa	34	0.3%
49	Kansas	0	0.0%
27	Kentucky	115	0.9%
49	Louisiana	0	0.0%
47	Maine	3	0.0%
18	Maryland	232	1.9%
17	Massachusetts	246	2.0%
13	Michigan	268	2.2%
18	Minnesota	232	1.9%
24	Mississippi	136	1.1%
24	Missouri	136	1.1%
42	Montana	14	0.1%
37	Nebraska	32	0.3%
32	Nevada	69	0.6%
40	New Hampshire	17	0.1%
6	New Jersey	496	4.0%
39	New Mexico	25	0.2%
2	New York	1,475	12.0%
8	North Carolina	398	3.2%
45	North Dakota	4	0.0%
11	Ohio	273	2.2%
23	Oklahoma	138	1.1%
29	Oregon	108	0.9%
10	Pennsylvania	284	2.3%
34	Rhode Island	49	0.4%
20	South Carolina	207	1.7%
43	South Dakota	13	0.1%
9	Tennessee	294	2.4%
5	Texas	512	4.2%
35	Utah	35	0.3%
45	Vermont	4	0.0%
16	Virginia	256	2.1%
15	Washington	258	2.1%
38	West Virginia	28	0.2%
31	Wisconsin	80	0.7%
47	Wyoming	3	0.0%

RANK ORDER

RANK	STATE	CASES	% of USA
1	California	2,493	20.3%
2	New York	1,475	12.0%
3	Florida	952	7.7%
4	Illinois	636	5.2%
5	Texas	512	4.2%
6	New Jersey	496	4.0%
7	Georgia	445	3.6%
8	North Carolina	398	3.2%
9	Tennessee	294	2.4%
10	Pennsylvania	284	2.3%
11	Ohio	273	2.2%
12	Arizona	269	2.2%
13	Michigan	268	2.2%
14	Alabama	265	2.2%
15	Washington	258	2.1%
16	Virginia	256	2.1%
17	Massachusetts	246	2.0%
18	Maryland	232	1.9%
18	Minnesota	232	1.9%
20	South Carolina	207	1.7%
21	Arkansas	153	1.2%
22	Hawaii	148	1.2%
23	Oklahoma	138	1.1%
24	Mississippi	136	1.1%
24	Missouri	136	1.1%
26	Colorado	120	1.0%
27	Kentucky	115	0.9%
28	Indiana	111	0.9%
29	Oregon	108	0.9%
30	Connecticut	101	0.8%
31	Wisconsin	80	0.7%
32	Nevada	69	0.6%
33	Alaska	51	0.4%
34	Rhode Island	49	0.4%
35	Utah	35	0.3%
36	Iowa	34	0.3%
37	Nebraska	32	0.3%
38	West Virginia	28	0.2%
39	New Mexico	25	0.2%
40	New Hampshire	17	0.1%
41	Delaware	15	0.1%
42	Montana	14	0.1%
43	South Dakota	13	0.1%
44	Idaho	10	0.1%
45	North Dakota	4	0.0%
45	Vermont	4	0.0%
47	Maine	3	0.0%
47	Wyoming	3	0.0%
49	Kansas	0	0.0%
49	Louisiana	0	0.0%
	District of Columbia	51	0.4%

Source: U.S. Department of Health and Human Services, National Center for Health Statistics
   "Morbidity and Mortality Weekly Report" (January 4, 2002, Vol. 50, No. 51)
*Provisional data. An infectious disease caused by the tubercle bacillus and causing the formation of tubercles on the lungs and other tissues of the body, often developing long after the initial infection. Characterized by the coughing up of mucus and sputum, fever, weight loss, and chest pain.

Tuberculosis Rate in 2001

National Rate = 4.3 Cases per 100,00 Population*

ALPHA ORDER

RANK	STATE	RATE
5	Alabama	5.9
2	Alaska	8.0
10	Arizona	5.1
8	Arkansas	5.7
4	California	7.2
27	Colorado	2.7
25	Connecticut	2.9
33	Delaware	1.9
6	Florida	5.8
9	Georgia	5.3
1	Hawaii	12.1
44	Idaho	0.8
10	Illinois	5.1
35	Indiana	1.8
43	Iowa	1.2
49	Kansas	0.0
26	Kentucky	2.8
49	Louisiana	0.0
48	Maine	0.2
18	Maryland	4.3
21	Massachusetts	3.9
27	Michigan	2.7
16	Minnesota	4.7
15	Mississippi	4.8
29	Missouri	2.4
38	Montana	1.5
33	Nebraska	1.9
23	Nevada	3.3
41	New Hampshire	1.4
6	New Jersey	5.8
41	New Mexico	1.4
3	New York	7.8
14	North Carolina	4.9
46	North Dakota	0.6
29	Ohio	2.4
20	Oklahoma	4.0
24	Oregon	3.1
32	Pennsylvania	2.3
17	Rhode Island	4.6
10	South Carolina	5.1
36	South Dakota	1.7
10	Tennessee	5.1
29	Texas	2.4
38	Utah	1.5
45	Vermont	0.7
22	Virginia	3.6
18	Washington	4.3
37	West Virginia	1.6
38	Wisconsin	1.5
46	Wyoming	0.6

RANK ORDER

RANK	STATE	RATE
1	Hawaii	12.1
2	Alaska	8.0
3	New York	7.8
4	California	7.2
5	Alabama	5.9
6	Florida	5.8
6	New Jersey	5.8
8	Arkansas	5.7
9	Georgia	5.3
10	Arizona	5.1
10	Illinois	5.1
10	South Carolina	5.1
10	Tennessee	5.1
14	North Carolina	4.9
15	Mississippi	4.8
16	Minnesota	4.7
17	Rhode Island	4.6
18	Maryland	4.3
18	Washington	4.3
20	Oklahoma	4.0
21	Massachusetts	3.9
22	Virginia	3.6
23	Nevada	3.3
24	Oregon	3.1
25	Connecticut	2.9
26	Kentucky	2.8
27	Colorado	2.7
27	Michigan	2.7
29	Missouri	2.4
29	Ohio	2.4
29	Texas	2.4
32	Pennsylvania	2.3
33	Delaware	1.9
33	Nebraska	1.9
35	Indiana	1.8
36	South Dakota	1.7
37	West Virginia	1.6
38	Montana	1.5
38	Utah	1.5
38	Wisconsin	1.5
41	New Hampshire	1.4
41	New Mexico	1.4
43	Iowa	1.2
44	Idaho	0.8
45	Vermont	0.7
46	North Dakota	0.6
46	Wyoming	0.6
48	Maine	0.2
49	Kansas	0.0
49	Louisiana	0.0

District of Columbia   8.9

Source: Morgan Quitno Press using data from U.S. Dept. of Health & Human Serv's, National Center for Health Statistics
"Morbidity and Mortality Weekly Report" (January 4, 2002, Vol. 50, No. 51)
*Provisional data. An infectious disease caused by the tubercle bacillus and causing the formation of tubercles on
the lungs and other tissues of the body, often developing long after the initial infection. Characterized by the
coughing up of mucus and sputum, fever, weight loss, and chest pain.

Whooping Cough (Pertussis) Cases Reported in 2001

National Total = 5,396 Cases*

ALPHA ORDER

RANK	STATE	CASES	% of USA
32	Alabama	37	0.7%
41	Alaska	11	0.2%
1	Arizona	637	11.8%
27	Arkansas	47	0.9%
2	California	495	9.2%
5	Colorado	344	6.4%
40	Connecticut	17	0.3%
50	Delaware	0	0.0%
36	Florida	29	0.5%
37	Georgia	27	0.5%
29	Hawaii	43	0.8%
9	Idaho	171	3.2%
21	Illinois	80	1.5%
17	Indiana	96	1.8%
20	Iowa	81	1.5%
35	Kansas	30	0.6%
19	Kentucky	84	1.6%
48	Louisiana	3	0.1%
39	Maine	21	0.4%
28	Maryland	45	0.8%
4	Massachusetts	389	7.2%
13	Michigan	139	2.6%
7	Minnesota	207	3.8%
46	Mississippi	4	0.1%
14	Missouri	108	2.0%
25	Montana	54	1.0%
42	Nebraska	7	0.1%
30	Nevada	40	0.7%
31	New Hampshire	39	0.7%
38	New Jersey	22	0.4%
11	New Mexico	145	2.7%
8	New York	199	3.7%
23	North Carolina	74	1.4%
44	North Dakota	5	0.1%
6	Ohio	326	6.0%
34	Oklahoma	33	0.6%
26	Oregon	53	1.0%
18	Pennsylvania	86	1.6%
43	Rhode Island	6	0.1%
33	South Carolina	34	0.6%
44	South Dakota	5	0.1%
24	Tennessee	63	1.2%
3	Texas	460	8.5%
22	Utah	76	1.4%
15	Vermont	107	2.0%
12	Virginia	142	2.6%
9	Washington	171	3.2%
46	West Virginia	4	0.1%
16	Wisconsin	98	1.8%
49	Wyoming	1	0.0%

RANK ORDER

RANK	STATE	CASES	% of USA
1	Arizona	637	11.8%
2	California	495	9.2%
3	Texas	460	8.5%
4	Massachusetts	389	7.2%
5	Colorado	344	6.4%
6	Ohio	326	6.0%
7	Minnesota	207	3.8%
8	New York	199	3.7%
9	Idaho	171	3.2%
9	Washington	171	3.2%
11	New Mexico	145	2.7%
12	Virginia	142	2.6%
13	Michigan	139	2.6%
14	Missouri	108	2.0%
15	Vermont	107	2.0%
16	Wisconsin	98	1.8%
17	Indiana	96	1.8%
18	Pennsylvania	86	1.6%
19	Kentucky	84	1.6%
20	Iowa	81	1.5%
21	Illinois	80	1.5%
22	Utah	76	1.4%
23	North Carolina	74	1.4%
24	Tennessee	63	1.2%
25	Montana	54	1.0%
26	Oregon	53	1.0%
27	Arkansas	47	0.9%
28	Maryland	45	0.8%
29	Hawaii	43	0.8%
30	Nevada	40	0.7%
31	New Hampshire	39	0.7%
32	Alabama	37	0.7%
33	South Carolina	34	0.6%
34	Oklahoma	33	0.6%
35	Kansas	30	0.6%
36	Florida	29	0.5%
37	Georgia	27	0.5%
38	New Jersey	22	0.4%
39	Maine	21	0.4%
40	Connecticut	17	0.3%
41	Alaska	11	0.2%
42	Nebraska	7	0.1%
43	Rhode Island	6	0.1%
44	North Dakota	5	0.1%
44	South Dakota	5	0.1%
46	Mississippi	4	0.1%
46	West Virginia	4	0.1%
48	Louisiana	3	0.1%
49	Wyoming	1	0.0%
50	Delaware	0	0.0%
	District of Columbia	1	0.0%

Source: U.S. Department of Health and Human Services, National Center for Health Statistics
   "Morbidity and Mortality Weekly Report" (January 4, 2002, Vol. 50, No. 51)
*Provisional data. Acute, highly contagious infection of respiratory tract.

Whooping Cough (Pertussis) Rate in 2001

National Rate = 1.9 Cases per 100,000 Population*

<table>
<tr><td colspan="3">ALPHA ORDER</td><td colspan="3">RANK ORDER</td></tr>
<tr><td>RANK</td><td>STATE</td><td>RATE</td><td>RANK</td><td>STATE</td><td>RATE</td></tr>
<tr><td>33</td><td>Alabama</td><td>0.8</td><td>1</td><td>Vermont</td><td>17.5</td></tr>
<tr><td>21</td><td>Alaska</td><td>1.7</td><td>2</td><td>Idaho</td><td>12.9</td></tr>
<tr><td>3</td><td>Arizona</td><td>12.0</td><td>3</td><td>Arizona</td><td>12.0</td></tr>
<tr><td>21</td><td>Arkansas</td><td>1.7</td><td>4</td><td>New Mexico</td><td>7.9</td></tr>
<tr><td>26</td><td>California</td><td>1.4</td><td>5</td><td>Colorado</td><td>7.8</td></tr>
<tr><td>5</td><td>Colorado</td><td>7.8</td><td>6</td><td>Massachusetts</td><td>6.1</td></tr>
<tr><td>41</td><td>Connecticut</td><td>0.5</td><td>7</td><td>Montana</td><td>6.0</td></tr>
<tr><td>50</td><td>Delaware</td><td>0.0</td><td>8</td><td>Minnesota</td><td>4.2</td></tr>
<tr><td>45</td><td>Florida</td><td>0.2</td><td>9</td><td>Hawaii</td><td>3.5</td></tr>
<tr><td>43</td><td>Georgia</td><td>0.3</td><td>10</td><td>Utah</td><td>3.3</td></tr>
<tr><td>9</td><td>Hawaii</td><td>3.5</td><td>11</td><td>New Hampshire</td><td>3.1</td></tr>
<tr><td>2</td><td>Idaho</td><td>12.9</td><td>12</td><td>Ohio</td><td>2.9</td></tr>
<tr><td>39</td><td>Illinois</td><td>0.6</td><td>12</td><td>Washington</td><td>2.9</td></tr>
<tr><td>23</td><td>Indiana</td><td>1.6</td><td>14</td><td>Iowa</td><td>2.8</td></tr>
<tr><td>14</td><td>Iowa</td><td>2.8</td><td>15</td><td>Texas</td><td>2.2</td></tr>
<tr><td>28</td><td>Kansas</td><td>1.1</td><td>16</td><td>Kentucky</td><td>2.1</td></tr>
<tr><td>16</td><td>Kentucky</td><td>2.1</td><td>17</td><td>Virginia</td><td>2.0</td></tr>
<tr><td>48</td><td>Louisiana</td><td>0.1</td><td>18</td><td>Missouri</td><td>1.9</td></tr>
<tr><td>23</td><td>Maine</td><td>1.6</td><td>18</td><td>Nevada</td><td>1.9</td></tr>
<tr><td>33</td><td>Maryland</td><td>0.8</td><td>20</td><td>Wisconsin</td><td>1.8</td></tr>
<tr><td>6</td><td>Massachusetts</td><td>6.1</td><td>21</td><td>Alaska</td><td>1.7</td></tr>
<tr><td>26</td><td>Michigan</td><td>1.4</td><td>21</td><td>Arkansas</td><td>1.7</td></tr>
<tr><td>8</td><td>Minnesota</td><td>4.2</td><td>23</td><td>Indiana</td><td>1.6</td></tr>
<tr><td>48</td><td>Mississippi</td><td>0.1</td><td>23</td><td>Maine</td><td>1.6</td></tr>
<tr><td>18</td><td>Missouri</td><td>1.9</td><td>25</td><td>Oregon</td><td>1.5</td></tr>
<tr><td>7</td><td>Montana</td><td>6.0</td><td>26</td><td>California</td><td>1.4</td></tr>
<tr><td>42</td><td>Nebraska</td><td>0.4</td><td>26</td><td>Michigan</td><td>1.4</td></tr>
<tr><td>18</td><td>Nevada</td><td>1.9</td><td>28</td><td>Kansas</td><td>1.1</td></tr>
<tr><td>11</td><td>New Hampshire</td><td>3.1</td><td>28</td><td>Tennessee</td><td>1.1</td></tr>
<tr><td>43</td><td>New Jersey</td><td>0.3</td><td>30</td><td>New York</td><td>1.0</td></tr>
<tr><td>4</td><td>New Mexico</td><td>7.9</td><td>30</td><td>Oklahoma</td><td>1.0</td></tr>
<tr><td>30</td><td>New York</td><td>1.0</td><td>32</td><td>North Carolina</td><td>0.9</td></tr>
<tr><td>32</td><td>North Carolina</td><td>0.9</td><td>33</td><td>Alabama</td><td>0.8</td></tr>
<tr><td>33</td><td>North Dakota</td><td>0.8</td><td>33</td><td>Maryland</td><td>0.8</td></tr>
<tr><td>12</td><td>Ohio</td><td>2.9</td><td>33</td><td>North Dakota</td><td>0.8</td></tr>
<tr><td>30</td><td>Oklahoma</td><td>1.0</td><td>33</td><td>South Carolina</td><td>0.8</td></tr>
<tr><td>25</td><td>Oregon</td><td>1.5</td><td>37</td><td>Pennsylvania</td><td>0.7</td></tr>
<tr><td>37</td><td>Pennsylvania</td><td>0.7</td><td>37</td><td>South Dakota</td><td>0.7</td></tr>
<tr><td>39</td><td>Rhode Island</td><td>0.6</td><td>39</td><td>Illinois</td><td>0.6</td></tr>
<tr><td>33</td><td>South Carolina</td><td>0.8</td><td>39</td><td>Rhode Island</td><td>0.6</td></tr>
<tr><td>37</td><td>South Dakota</td><td>0.7</td><td>41</td><td>Connecticut</td><td>0.5</td></tr>
<tr><td>28</td><td>Tennessee</td><td>1.1</td><td>42</td><td>Nebraska</td><td>0.4</td></tr>
<tr><td>15</td><td>Texas</td><td>2.2</td><td>43</td><td>Georgia</td><td>0.3</td></tr>
<tr><td>10</td><td>Utah</td><td>3.3</td><td>43</td><td>New Jersey</td><td>0.3</td></tr>
<tr><td>1</td><td>Vermont</td><td>17.5</td><td>45</td><td>Florida</td><td>0.2</td></tr>
<tr><td>17</td><td>Virginia</td><td>2.0</td><td>45</td><td>West Virginia</td><td>0.2</td></tr>
<tr><td>12</td><td>Washington</td><td>2.9</td><td>45</td><td>Wyoming</td><td>0.2</td></tr>
<tr><td>45</td><td>West Virginia</td><td>0.2</td><td>48</td><td>Louisiana</td><td>0.1</td></tr>
<tr><td>20</td><td>Wisconsin</td><td>1.8</td><td>48</td><td>Mississippi</td><td>0.1</td></tr>
<tr><td>45</td><td>Wyoming</td><td>0.2</td><td>50</td><td>Delaware</td><td>0.0</td></tr>
<tr><td></td><td></td><td></td><td></td><td>District of Columbia</td><td>0.2</td></tr>
</table>

Source: Morgan Quitno Press using data from U.S. Dept. of Health & Human Serv's, National Center for Health Statistics
"Morbidity and Mortality Weekly Report" (January 4, 2002, Vol. 50, No. 51)
*Provisional data. Acute, highly contagious infection of respiratory tract.

Percent of Children Aged 19 to 35 Months Fully Immunized in 2000

National Percent = 72.8%*

ALPHA ORDER

RANK	STATE	PERCENT
17	Alabama	76.1
41	Alaska	70.6
47	Arizona	67.2
48	Arkansas	67.1
28	California	72.3
34	Colorado	71.6
4	Connecticut	81.6
42	Delaware	70.0
33	Florida	71.7
12	Georgia	77.7
26	Hawaii	72.8
39	Idaho	70.7
36	Illinois	71.2
30	Indiana	72.0
2	Iowa	82.5
35	Kansas	71.3
13	Kentucky	77.0
32	Louisiana	71.8
18	Maine	76.0
21	Maryland	75.4
5	Massachusetts	81.4
24	Michigan	73.7
3	Minnesota	82.4
19	Mississippi	75.9
15	Missouri	76.8
38	Montana	71.1
20	Nebraska	75.5
43	Nevada	69.1
8	New Hampshire	78.9
36	New Jersey	71.2
49	New Mexico	64.5
28	New York	72.3
1	North Carolina	82.8
7	North Dakota	80.3
44	Ohio	68.9
45	Oklahoma	68.3
22	Oregon	74.7
11	Pennsylvania	77.8
6	Rhode Island	80.5
9	South Carolina	78.5
25	South Dakota	73.6
15	Tennessee	76.8
50	Texas	63.5
46	Utah	68.2
13	Vermont	77.0
39	Virginia	70.7
27	Washington	72.5
31	West Virginia	71.9
23	Wisconsin	74.2
10	Wyoming	78.2

RANK ORDER

RANK	STATE	PERCENT
1	North Carolina	82.8
2	Iowa	82.5
3	Minnesota	82.4
4	Connecticut	81.6
5	Massachusetts	81.4
6	Rhode Island	80.5
7	North Dakota	80.3
8	New Hampshire	78.9
9	South Carolina	78.5
10	Wyoming	78.2
11	Pennsylvania	77.8
12	Georgia	77.7
13	Kentucky	77.0
13	Vermont	77.0
15	Missouri	76.8
15	Tennessee	76.8
17	Alabama	76.1
18	Maine	76.0
19	Mississippi	75.9
20	Nebraska	75.5
21	Maryland	75.4
22	Oregon	74.7
23	Wisconsin	74.2
24	Michigan	73.7
25	South Dakota	73.6
26	Hawaii	72.8
27	Washington	72.5
28	California	72.3
28	New York	72.3
30	Indiana	72.0
31	West Virginia	71.9
32	Louisiana	71.8
33	Florida	71.7
34	Colorado	71.6
35	Kansas	71.3
36	Illinois	71.2
36	New Jersey	71.2
38	Montana	71.1
39	Idaho	70.7
39	Virginia	70.7
41	Alaska	70.6
42	Delaware	70.0
43	Nevada	69.1
44	Ohio	68.9
45	Oklahoma	68.3
46	Utah	68.2
47	Arizona	67.2
48	Arkansas	67.1
49	New Mexico	64.5
50	Texas	63.5

| | District of Columbia | 66.2 |

Source: U.S. Department of Health and Human Services, Centers for Disease Control and Prevention
"State Vaccination Coverage Levels" (Morbidity and Mortality Weekly Report, Vol. 50, No. 30, August 3, 2001)
*Fully immunized children received four doses of DTP/DT/DTaP (Diphtheria, Tetanus, Pertussis (Whooping Cough), Acellular Pertussis), three doses of OPV (Oral Poliovirus Vaccine), one dose of MCV (Measles-Containing Vaccine) and three doses of Hib (Haemophilus influenzae type b).

Sexually Transmitted Diseases in 2000

National Total = 1,067,145 Cases*

ALPHA ORDER

RANK	STATE	CASES	% of USA
12	Alabama	27,510	2.6%
40	Alaska	2,930	0.3%
22	Arizona	16,910	1.6%
30	Arkansas	9,965	0.9%
1	California	117,339	11.0%
24	Colorado	15,124	1.4%
29	Connecticut	10,532	1.0%
37	Delaware	4,600	0.4%
3	Florida	56,584	5.3%
7	Georgia	50,026	4.7%
38	Hawaii	4,032	0.4%
44	Idaho	2,006	0.2%
4	Illinois	54,074	5.1%
19	Indiana	20,939	2.0%
33	Iowa	7,390	0.7%
31	Kansas	8,857	0.8%
27	Kentucky	11,650	1.1%
11	Louisiana	31,306	2.9%
45	Maine	1,565	0.1%
15	Maryland	24,670	2.3%
25	Massachusetts	14,082	1.3%
8	Michigan	44,749	4.2%
28	Minnesota	11,278	1.1%
18	Mississippi	22,051	2.1%
17	Missouri	22,360	2.1%
46	Montana	1,529	0.1%
36	Nebraska	5,327	0.5%
35	Nevada	5,577	0.5%
47	New Hampshire	1,242	0.1%
21	New Jersey	18,117	1.7%
34	New Mexico	6,372	0.6%
5	New York	51,766	4.9%
9	North Carolina	40,296	3.8%
48	North Dakota	982	0.1%
6	Ohio	50,563	4.7%
26	Oklahoma	13,676	1.3%
32	Oregon	8,157	0.8%
10	Pennsylvania	40,159	3.8%
39	Rhode Island	3,297	0.3%
20	South Carolina	18,572	1.7%
43	South Dakota	2,111	0.2%
13	Tennessee	27,477	2.6%
2	Texas	102,148	9.6%
42	Utah	2,423	0.2%
50	Vermont	591	0.1%
14	Virginia	25,655	2.4%
23	Washington	15,550	1.5%
41	West Virginia	2,792	0.3%
16	Wisconsin	23,428	2.2%
49	Wyoming	861	0.1%

RANK ORDER

RANK	STATE	CASES	% of USA
1	California	117,339	11.0%
2	Texas	102,148	9.6%
3	Florida	56,584	5.3%
4	Illinois	54,074	5.1%
5	New York	51,766	4.9%
6	Ohio	50,563	4.7%
7	Georgia	50,026	4.7%
8	Michigan	44,749	4.2%
9	North Carolina	40,296	3.8%
10	Pennsylvania	40,159	3.8%
11	Louisiana	31,306	2.9%
12	Alabama	27,510	2.6%
13	Tennessee	27,477	2.6%
14	Virginia	25,655	2.4%
15	Maryland	24,670	2.3%
16	Wisconsin	23,428	2.2%
17	Missouri	22,360	2.1%
18	Mississippi	22,051	2.1%
19	Indiana	20,939	2.0%
20	South Carolina	18,572	1.7%
21	New Jersey	18,117	1.7%
22	Arizona	16,910	1.6%
23	Washington	15,550	1.5%
24	Colorado	15,124	1.4%
25	Massachusetts	14,082	1.3%
26	Oklahoma	13,676	1.3%
27	Kentucky	11,650	1.1%
28	Minnesota	11,278	1.1%
29	Connecticut	10,532	1.0%
30	Arkansas	9,965	0.9%
31	Kansas	8,857	0.8%
32	Oregon	8,157	0.8%
33	Iowa	7,390	0.7%
34	New Mexico	6,372	0.6%
35	Nevada	5,577	0.5%
36	Nebraska	5,327	0.5%
37	Delaware	4,600	0.4%
38	Hawaii	4,032	0.4%
39	Rhode Island	3,297	0.3%
40	Alaska	2,930	0.3%
41	West Virginia	2,792	0.3%
42	Utah	2,423	0.2%
43	South Dakota	2,111	0.2%
44	Idaho	2,006	0.2%
45	Maine	1,565	0.1%
46	Montana	1,529	0.1%
47	New Hampshire	1,242	0.1%
48	North Dakota	982	0.1%
49	Wyoming	861	0.1%
50	Vermont	591	0.1%
	District of Columbia	5,948	0.6%

Source: Morgan Quitno Press using data from U.S. Dept. of Health and Human Services, Nat'l Center for Health Statistics "Sexually Transmitted Disease Surveillance 2000" (http://www.cdc.gov/nchstp/dstd/dstdp.html)
*Includes chancroid, chlamydia, gonorrhea and primary and secondary syphilis.

Sexually Transmitted Disease Rate in 2000

National Rate = 391.3 Cases per 100,000 Population*

ALPHA ORDER

RANK	STATE	RATE
4	Alabama	629.5
11	Alaska	473.0
24	Arizona	353.9
18	Arkansas	390.6
23	California	354.0
21	Colorado	372.8
30	Connecticut	320.9
5	Delaware	610.4
19	Florida	374.5
3	Georgia	642.4
26	Hawaii	340.1
44	Idaho	160.3
15	Illinois	445.8
25	Indiana	352.3
37	Iowa	257.5
28	Kansas	333.7
33	Kentucky	294.1
2	Louisiana	716.0
47	Maine	124.9
10	Maryland	477.0
40	Massachusetts	228.0
12	Michigan	453.6
39	Minnesota	236.2
1	Mississippi	796.4
16	Missouri	408.8
43	Montana	173.2
31	Nebraska	319.7
32	Nevada	308.2
49	New Hampshire	103.5
41	New Jersey	222.5
22	New Mexico	366.2
35	New York	284.4
6	North Carolina	526.8
45	North Dakota	155.0
13	Ohio	449.2
17	Oklahoma	407.3
38	Oregon	246.0
27	Pennsylvania	334.7
29	Rhode Island	332.7
9	South Carolina	478.0
34	South Dakota	288.0
8	Tennessee	501.1
7	Texas	509.6
48	Utah	113.7
50	Vermont	99.5
20	Virginia	373.2
36	Washington	270.1
46	West Virginia	154.6
14	Wisconsin	446.2
42	Wyoming	179.6

RANK ORDER

RANK	STATE	RATE
1	Mississippi	796.4
2	Louisiana	716.0
3	Georgia	642.4
4	Alabama	629.5
5	Delaware	610.4
6	North Carolina	526.8
7	Texas	509.6
8	Tennessee	501.1
9	South Carolina	478.0
10	Maryland	477.0
11	Alaska	473.0
12	Michigan	453.6
13	Ohio	449.2
14	Wisconsin	446.2
15	Illinois	445.8
16	Missouri	408.8
17	Oklahoma	407.3
18	Arkansas	390.6
19	Florida	374.5
20	Virginia	373.2
21	Colorado	372.8
22	New Mexico	366.2
23	California	354.0
24	Arizona	353.9
25	Indiana	352.3
26	Hawaii	340.1
27	Pennsylvania	334.7
28	Kansas	333.7
29	Rhode Island	332.7
30	Connecticut	320.9
31	Nebraska	319.7
32	Nevada	308.2
33	Kentucky	294.1
34	South Dakota	288.0
35	New York	284.4
36	Washington	270.1
37	Iowa	257.5
38	Oregon	246.0
39	Minnesota	236.2
40	Massachusetts	228.0
41	New Jersey	222.5
42	Wyoming	179.6
43	Montana	173.2
44	Idaho	160.3
45	North Dakota	155.0
46	West Virginia	154.6
47	Maine	124.9
48	Utah	113.7
49	New Hampshire	103.5
50	Vermont	99.5

District of Columbia   1,146.0

Source: Morgan Quitno Press using data from U.S. Dept. of Health and Human Services, Nat'l Center for Health Statistics "Sexually Transmitted Disease Surveillance 2000" (http://www.cdc.gov/nchstp/dstd/dstdp.html)
*Includes chancroid, chlamydia, gonorrhea and primary and secondary syphilis.

Chancroid Cases in 2000

National Total = 78 Cases*

ALPHA ORDER					RANK ORDER			
RANK	STATE	CASES	% of USA		RANK	STATE	CASES	% of USA
10	Alabama	1	1.3%		1	New York	26	33.3%
13	Alaska	0	0.0%		2	Texas	19	24.4%
13	Arizona	0	0.0%		3	South Carolina	10	12.8%
13	Arkansas	0	0.0%		4	Louisiana	6	7.7%
6	California	3	3.8%		5	North Carolina	5	6.4%
10	Colorado	1	1.3%		6	California	3	3.8%
13	Connecticut	0	0.0%		7	Massachusetts	2	2.6%
13	Delaware	0	0.0%		7	Virginia	2	2.6%
13	Florida	0	0.0%		7	Wisconsin	2	2.6%
13	Georgia	0	0.0%		10	Alabama	1	1.3%
13	Hawaii	0	0.0%		10	Colorado	1	1.3%
13	Idaho	0	0.0%		10	Ohio	1	1.3%
13	Illinois	0	0.0%		13	Alaska	0	0.0%
13	Indiana	0	0.0%		13	Arizona	0	0.0%
13	Iowa	0	0.0%		13	Arkansas	0	0.0%
13	Kansas	0	0.0%		13	Connecticut	0	0.0%
13	Kentucky	0	0.0%		13	Delaware	0	0.0%
4	Louisiana	6	7.7%		13	Florida	0	0.0%
13	Maine	0	0.0%		13	Georgia	0	0.0%
13	Maryland	0	0.0%		13	Hawaii	0	0.0%
7	Massachusetts	2	2.6%		13	Idaho	0	0.0%
13	Michigan	0	0.0%		13	Illinois	0	0.0%
13	Minnesota	0	0.0%		13	Indiana	0	0.0%
13	Mississippi	0	0.0%		13	Iowa	0	0.0%
13	Missouri	0	0.0%		13	Kansas	0	0.0%
13	Montana	0	0.0%		13	Kentucky	0	0.0%
13	Nebraska	0	0.0%		13	Maine	0	0.0%
13	Nevada	0	0.0%		13	Maryland	0	0.0%
13	New Hampshire	0	0.0%		13	Michigan	0	0.0%
13	New Jersey	0	0.0%		13	Minnesota	0	0.0%
13	New Mexico	0	0.0%		13	Mississippi	0	0.0%
1	New York	26	33.3%		13	Missouri	0	0.0%
5	North Carolina	5	6.4%		13	Montana	0	0.0%
13	North Dakota	0	0.0%		13	Nebraska	0	0.0%
10	Ohio	1	1.3%		13	Nevada	0	0.0%
13	Oklahoma	0	0.0%		13	New Hampshire	0	0.0%
13	Oregon	0	0.0%		13	New Jersey	0	0.0%
13	Pennsylvania	0	0.0%		13	New Mexico	0	0.0%
13	Rhode Island	0	0.0%		13	North Dakota	0	0.0%
3	South Carolina	10	12.8%		13	Oklahoma	0	0.0%
13	South Dakota	0	0.0%		13	Oregon	0	0.0%
13	Tennessee	0	0.0%		13	Pennsylvania	0	0.0%
2	Texas	19	24.4%		13	Rhode Island	0	0.0%
13	Utah	0	0.0%		13	South Dakota	0	0.0%
13	Vermont	0	0.0%		13	Tennessee	0	0.0%
7	Virginia	2	2.6%		13	Utah	0	0.0%
13	Washington	0	0.0%		13	Vermont	0	0.0%
13	West Virginia	0	0.0%		13	Washington	0	0.0%
7	Wisconsin	2	2.6%		13	West Virginia	0	0.0%
13	Wyoming	0	0.0%		13	Wyoming	0	0.0%
						District of Columbia	0	0.0%

Source: U.S. Department of Health and Human Services, National Center for Health Statistics
   "Sexually Transmitted Disease Surveillance 2000" (http://www.cdc.gov/nchstp/dstd/dstdp.html)
*A soft, highly infectious, nonsyphilitic venereal ulcer of the genital region, caused by the bacillus Hemophilus ducreyi. Also called soft chancre.

Chancroid Rate in 2000

National Rate = 0.0 Cases per 100,000 Population*

ALPHA ORDER

RANK	STATE	RATE
6	Alabama	0.0
6	Alaska	0.0
6	Arizona	0.0
6	Arkansas	0.0
6	California	0.0
6	Colorado	0.0
6	Connecticut	0.0
6	Delaware	0.0
6	Florida	0.0
6	Georgia	0.0
6	Hawaii	0.0
6	Idaho	0.0
6	Illinois	0.0
6	Indiana	0.0
6	Iowa	0.0
6	Kansas	0.0
6	Kentucky	0.0
2	Louisiana	0.1
6	Maine	0.0
6	Maryland	0.0
6	Massachusetts	0.0
6	Michigan	0.0
6	Minnesota	0.0
6	Mississippi	0.0
6	Missouri	0.0
6	Montana	0.0
6	Nebraska	0.0
6	Nevada	0.0
6	New Hampshire	0.0
6	New Jersey	0.0
6	New Mexico	0.0
2	New York	0.1
2	North Carolina	0.1
6	North Dakota	0.0
6	Ohio	0.0
6	Oklahoma	0.0
6	Oregon	0.0
6	Pennsylvania	0.0
6	Rhode Island	0.0
1	South Carolina	0.3
6	South Dakota	0.0
6	Tennessee	0.0
2	Texas	0.1
6	Utah	0.0
6	Vermont	0.0
6	Virginia	0.0
6	Washington	0.0
6	West Virginia	0.0
6	Wisconsin	0.0
6	Wyoming	0.0

RANK ORDER

RANK	STATE	RATE
1	South Carolina	0.3
2	Louisiana	0.1
2	New York	0.1
2	North Carolina	0.1
2	Texas	0.1
6	Alabama	0.0
6	Alaska	0.0
6	Arizona	0.0
6	Arkansas	0.0
6	California	0.0
6	Colorado	0.0
6	Connecticut	0.0
6	Delaware	0.0
6	Florida	0.0
6	Georgia	0.0
6	Hawaii	0.0
6	Idaho	0.0
6	Illinois	0.0
6	Indiana	0.0
6	Iowa	0.0
6	Kansas	0.0
6	Kentucky	0.0
6	Maine	0.0
6	Maryland	0.0
6	Massachusetts	0.0
6	Michigan	0.0
6	Minnesota	0.0
6	Mississippi	0.0
6	Missouri	0.0
6	Montana	0.0
6	Nebraska	0.0
6	Nevada	0.0
6	New Hampshire	0.0
6	New Jersey	0.0
6	New Mexico	0.0
6	North Dakota	0.0
6	Ohio	0.0
6	Oklahoma	0.0
6	Oregon	0.0
6	Pennsylvania	0.0
6	Rhode Island	0.0
6	South Dakota	0.0
6	Tennessee	0.0
6	Utah	0.0
6	Vermont	0.0
6	Virginia	0.0
6	Washington	0.0
6	West Virginia	0.0
6	Wisconsin	0.0
6	Wyoming	0.0
	District of Columbia	0.0

Source: U.S. Department of Health and Human Services, National Center for Health Statistics
"Sexually Transmitted Disease Surveillance 2000" (http://www.cdc.gov/nchstp/dstd/dstdp.html)
*A soft, highly infectious, nonsyphilitic venereal ulcer of the genital region, caused by the bacillus Hemophilus ducreyi. Also called soft chancre.

Chlamydia Cases Reported in 2000

National Total = 702,093 Cases*

ALPHA ORDER

RANK	STATE	CASES	% of USA
14	Alabama	15,323	2.2%
40	Alaska	2,569	0.4%
21	Arizona	12,591	1.8%
31	Arkansas	6,219	0.9%
1	California	95,392	13.6%
22	Colorado	12,000	1.7%
29	Connecticut	7,604	1.1%
38	Delaware	2,856	0.4%
3	Florida	33,390	4.8%
7	Georgia	29,359	4.2%
37	Hawaii	3,547	0.5%
43	Idaho	1,907	0.3%
4	Illinois	32,991	4.7%
17	Indiana	14,063	2.0%
33	Iowa	5,987	0.9%
32	Kansas	6,056	0.9%
28	Kentucky	8,063	1.1%
11	Louisiana	17,846	2.5%
45	Maine	1,474	0.2%
16	Maryland	14,533	2.1%
23	Massachusetts	10,967	1.6%
9	Michigan	26,237	3.7%
27	Minnesota	8,102	1.2%
20	Mississippi	12,697	1.8%
18	Missouri	13,448	1.9%
46	Montana	1,469	0.2%
36	Nebraska	3,791	0.5%
35	Nevada	4,019	0.6%
47	New Hampshire	1,130	0.2%
24	New Jersey	10,814	1.5%
34	New Mexico	5,204	0.7%
5	New York	31,494	4.5%
10	North Carolina	21,985	3.1%
48	North Dakota	909	0.1%
6	Ohio	31,190	4.4%
26	Oklahoma	9,331	1.3%
30	Oregon	7,107	1.0%
8	Pennsylvania	26,475	3.8%
39	Rhode Island	2,632	0.4%
25	South Carolina	9,950	1.4%
44	South Dakota	1,834	0.3%
15	Tennessee	15,069	2.1%
2	Texas	68,814	9.8%
41	Utah	2,190	0.3%
50	Vermont	526	0.1%
13	Virginia	15,352	2.2%
19	Washington	13,066	1.9%
42	West Virginia	2,144	0.3%
12	Wisconsin	16,365	2.3%
49	Wyoming	807	0.1%

RANK ORDER

RANK	STATE	CASES	% of USA
1	California	95,392	13.6%
2	Texas	68,814	9.8%
3	Florida	33,390	4.8%
4	Illinois	32,991	4.7%
5	New York	31,494	4.5%
6	Ohio	31,190	4.4%
7	Georgia	29,359	4.2%
8	Pennsylvania	26,475	3.8%
9	Michigan	26,237	3.7%
10	North Carolina	21,985	3.1%
11	Louisiana	17,846	2.5%
12	Wisconsin	16,365	2.3%
13	Virginia	15,352	2.2%
14	Alabama	15,323	2.2%
15	Tennessee	15,069	2.1%
16	Maryland	14,533	2.1%
17	Indiana	14,063	2.0%
18	Missouri	13,448	1.9%
19	Washington	13,066	1.9%
20	Mississippi	12,697	1.8%
21	Arizona	12,591	1.8%
22	Colorado	12,000	1.7%
23	Massachusetts	10,967	1.6%
24	New Jersey	10,814	1.5%
25	South Carolina	9,950	1.4%
26	Oklahoma	9,331	1.3%
27	Minnesota	8,102	1.2%
28	Kentucky	8,063	1.1%
29	Connecticut	7,604	1.1%
30	Oregon	7,107	1.0%
31	Arkansas	6,219	0.9%
32	Kansas	6,056	0.9%
33	Iowa	5,987	0.9%
34	New Mexico	5,204	0.7%
35	Nevada	4,019	0.6%
36	Nebraska	3,791	0.5%
37	Hawaii	3,547	0.5%
38	Delaware	2,856	0.4%
39	Rhode Island	2,632	0.4%
40	Alaska	2,569	0.4%
41	Utah	2,190	0.3%
42	West Virginia	2,144	0.3%
43	Idaho	1,907	0.3%
44	South Dakota	1,834	0.3%
45	Maine	1,474	0.2%
46	Montana	1,469	0.2%
47	New Hampshire	1,130	0.2%
48	North Dakota	909	0.1%
49	Wyoming	807	0.1%
50	Vermont	526	0.1%
	District of Columbia	3,205	0.5%

Source: U.S. Department of Health and Human Services, National Center for Health Statistics
   "Sexually Transmitted Disease Surveillance 2000" (http://www.cdc.gov/nchstp/dstd/dstdp.html)
*Any of several common, often asymptomatic, sexually transmitted diseases caused by the microorganism Chlamydia trachomatis, including nonspecific urethritis in men.

Chlamydia Rate in 2000

National Rate = 257.5 Cases per 100,000 Population*

ALPHA ORDER

RANK	STATE	RATE
6	Alabama	350.7
2	Alaska	414.7
21	Arizona	263.5
25	Arkansas	243.8
12	California	287.8
11	Colorado	295.8
27	Connecticut	231.7
4	Delaware	379.0
33	Florida	221.0
5	Georgia	377.0
9	Hawaii	299.2
43	Idaho	152.4
18	Illinois	272.0
26	Indiana	236.6
36	Iowa	208.6
28	Kansas	228.2
37	Kentucky	203.6
3	Louisiana	408.2
47	Maine	117.6
14	Maryland	281.0
38	Massachusetts	177.6
19	Michigan	266.0
40	Minnesota	169.7
1	Mississippi	458.6
24	Missouri	245.9
42	Montana	166.4
29	Nebraska	227.5
32	Nevada	222.1
49	New Hampshire	94.1
45	New Jersey	132.8
10	New Mexico	299.1
39	New York	173.1
13	North Carolina	287.4
44	North Dakota	143.5
16	Ohio	277.1
15	Oklahoma	277.9
35	Oregon	214.3
34	Pennsylvania	220.7
20	Rhode Island	265.6
22	South Carolina	256.1
23	South Dakota	250.2
17	Tennessee	274.8
7	Texas	343.3
48	Utah	102.8
50	Vermont	88.6
31	Virginia	223.4
30	Washington	227.0
46	West Virginia	118.7
8	Wisconsin	311.7
41	Wyoming	168.3

RANK ORDER

RANK	STATE	RATE
1	Mississippi	458.6
2	Alaska	414.7
3	Louisiana	408.2
4	Delaware	379.0
5	Georgia	377.0
6	Alabama	350.7
7	Texas	343.3
8	Wisconsin	311.7
9	Hawaii	299.2
10	New Mexico	299.1
11	Colorado	295.8
12	California	287.8
13	North Carolina	287.4
14	Maryland	281.0
15	Oklahoma	277.9
16	Ohio	277.1
17	Tennessee	274.8
18	Illinois	272.0
19	Michigan	266.0
20	Rhode Island	265.6
21	Arizona	263.5
22	South Carolina	256.1
23	South Dakota	250.2
24	Missouri	245.9
25	Arkansas	243.8
26	Indiana	236.6
27	Connecticut	231.7
28	Kansas	228.2
29	Nebraska	227.5
30	Washington	227.0
31	Virginia	223.4
32	Nevada	222.1
33	Florida	221.0
34	Pennsylvania	220.7
35	Oregon	214.3
36	Iowa	208.6
37	Kentucky	203.6
38	Massachusetts	177.6
39	New York	173.1
40	Minnesota	169.7
41	Wyoming	168.3
42	Montana	166.4
43	Idaho	152.4
44	North Dakota	143.5
45	New Jersey	132.8
46	West Virginia	118.7
47	Maine	117.6
48	Utah	102.8
49	New Hampshire	94.1
50	Vermont	88.6
	District of Columbia	617.5

Source: U.S. Department of Health and Human Services, National Center for Health Statistics
"Sexually Transmitted Disease Surveillance 2000" (http://www.cdc.gov/nchstp/dstd/dstdp.html)
*Any of several common, often asymptomatic, sexually transmitted diseases caused by the microorganism Chlamydia trachomatis, including nonspecific urethritis in men.

Gonorrhea Cases Reported in 2000

National Total = 358,995 Cases*

ALPHA ORDER

RANK	STATE	CASES	% of USA
12	Alabama	12,063	3.4%
41	Alaska	361	0.1%
23	Arizona	4,130	1.2%
24	Arkansas	3,642	1.0%
3	California	21,619	6.0%
27	Colorado	3,112	0.9%
29	Connecticut	2,912	0.8%
32	Delaware	1,735	0.5%
2	Florida	22,781	6.3%
5	Georgia	20,265	5.6%
40	Hawaii	483	0.1%
45	Idaho	98	0.0%
4	Illinois	20,671	5.8%
21	Indiana	6,525	1.8%
35	Iowa	1,392	0.4%
30	Kansas	2,795	0.8%
25	Kentucky	3,502	1.0%
11	Louisiana	13,245	3.7%
46	Maine	90	0.0%
15	Maryland	9,837	2.7%
28	Massachusetts	3,045	0.8%
8	Michigan	18,182	5.1%
26	Minnesota	3,160	0.9%
16	Mississippi	9,217	2.6%
17	Missouri	8,883	2.5%
49	Montana	60	0.0%
34	Nebraska	1,534	0.4%
33	Nevada	1,553	0.4%
44	New Hampshire	110	0.0%
19	New Jersey	7,232	2.0%
36	New Mexico	1,152	0.3%
6	New York	20,114	5.6%
9	North Carolina	17,823	5.0%
47	North Dakota	73	0.0%
7	Ohio	19,303	5.4%
22	Oklahoma	4,229	1.2%
37	Oregon	1,038	0.3%
10	Pennsylvania	13,607	3.8%
38	Rhode Island	661	0.2%
18	South Carolina	8,383	2.3%
42	South Dakota	277	0.1%
13	Tennessee	11,876	3.3%
1	Texas	32,919	9.2%
43	Utah	231	0.1%
48	Vermont	65	0.0%
14	Virginia	10,175	2.8%
31	Washington	2,418	0.7%
39	West Virginia	645	0.2%
20	Wisconsin	7,013	2.0%
50	Wyoming	53	0.0%

RANK ORDER

RANK	STATE	CASES	% of USA
1	Texas	32,919	9.2%
2	Florida	22,781	6.3%
3	California	21,619	6.0%
4	Illinois	20,671	5.8%
5	Georgia	20,265	5.6%
6	New York	20,114	5.6%
7	Ohio	19,303	5.4%
8	Michigan	18,182	5.1%
9	North Carolina	17,823	5.0%
10	Pennsylvania	13,607	3.8%
11	Louisiana	13,245	3.7%
12	Alabama	12,063	3.4%
13	Tennessee	11,876	3.3%
14	Virginia	10,175	2.8%
15	Maryland	9,837	2.7%
16	Mississippi	9,217	2.6%
17	Missouri	8,883	2.5%
18	South Carolina	8,383	2.3%
19	New Jersey	7,232	2.0%
20	Wisconsin	7,013	2.0%
21	Indiana	6,525	1.8%
22	Oklahoma	4,229	1.2%
23	Arizona	4,130	1.2%
24	Arkansas	3,642	1.0%
25	Kentucky	3,502	1.0%
26	Minnesota	3,160	0.9%
27	Colorado	3,112	0.9%
28	Massachusetts	3,045	0.8%
29	Connecticut	2,912	0.8%
30	Kansas	2,795	0.8%
31	Washington	2,418	0.7%
32	Delaware	1,735	0.5%
33	Nevada	1,553	0.4%
34	Nebraska	1,534	0.4%
35	Iowa	1,392	0.4%
36	New Mexico	1,152	0.3%
37	Oregon	1,038	0.3%
38	Rhode Island	661	0.2%
39	West Virginia	645	0.2%
40	Hawaii	483	0.1%
41	Alaska	361	0.1%
42	South Dakota	277	0.1%
43	Utah	231	0.1%
44	New Hampshire	110	0.0%
45	Idaho	98	0.0%
46	Maine	90	0.0%
47	North Dakota	73	0.0%
48	Vermont	65	0.0%
49	Montana	60	0.0%
50	Wyoming	53	0.0%
	District of Columbia	2,706	0.8%

Source: U.S. Department of Health and Human Services, National Center for Health Statistics
"Sexually Transmitted Disease Surveillance 2000" (http://www.cdc.gov/nchstp/dstd/dstdp.html)
*Gonorrhea is a sexually transmitted disease caused by gonococcal bacteria that affects the mucous membrane chiefly of the genital and urinary tracts and is characterized by an acute purulent discharge and painful or difficult urination, though women often have no symptoms.

Gonorrhea Rate in 2000

National Rate = 131.6 Cases per 100,000 Population*

ALPHA ORDER

RANK	STATE	RATE
3	Alabama	276.0
35	Alaska	58.3
28	Arizona	86.4
17	Arkansas	142.7
34	California	65.2
30	Colorado	76.7
26	Connecticut	88.7
6	Delaware	230.2
15	Florida	150.8
4	Georgia	260.2
39	Hawaii	40.7
48	Idaho	7.8
12	Illinois	170.4
22	Indiana	109.8
37	Iowa	48.5
23	Kansas	105.3
27	Kentucky	88.4
2	Louisiana	302.9
49	Maine	7.2
9	Maryland	190.2
36	Massachusetts	49.3
10	Michigan	184.3
32	Minnesota	66.2
1	Mississippi	332.9
14	Missouri	162.4
50	Montana	6.8
24	Nebraska	92.1
29	Nevada	85.8
47	New Hampshire	9.2
25	New Jersey	88.8
32	New Mexico	66.2
21	New York	110.5
5	North Carolina	233.0
43	North Dakota	11.5
11	Ohio	171.5
19	Oklahoma	125.9
42	Oregon	31.3
20	Pennsylvania	113.4
31	Rhode Island	66.7
8	South Carolina	215.7
40	South Dakota	37.8
7	Tennessee	216.6
13	Texas	164.2
46	Utah	10.8
45	Vermont	10.9
16	Virginia	148.0
38	Washington	42.0
41	West Virginia	35.7
18	Wisconsin	133.6
44	Wyoming	11.1

RANK ORDER

RANK	STATE	RATE
1	Mississippi	332.9
2	Louisiana	302.9
3	Alabama	276.0
4	Georgia	260.2
5	North Carolina	233.0
6	Delaware	230.2
7	Tennessee	216.6
8	South Carolina	215.7
9	Maryland	190.2
10	Michigan	184.3
11	Ohio	171.5
12	Illinois	170.4
13	Texas	164.2
14	Missouri	162.4
15	Florida	150.8
16	Virginia	148.0
17	Arkansas	142.7
18	Wisconsin	133.6
19	Oklahoma	125.9
20	Pennsylvania	113.4
21	New York	110.5
22	Indiana	109.8
23	Kansas	105.3
24	Nebraska	92.1
25	New Jersey	88.8
26	Connecticut	88.7
27	Kentucky	88.4
28	Arizona	86.4
29	Nevada	85.8
30	Colorado	76.7
31	Rhode Island	66.7
32	Minnesota	66.2
32	New Mexico	66.2
34	California	65.2
35	Alaska	58.3
36	Massachusetts	49.3
37	Iowa	48.5
38	Washington	42.0
39	Hawaii	40.7
40	South Dakota	37.8
41	West Virginia	35.7
42	Oregon	31.3
43	North Dakota	11.5
44	Wyoming	11.1
45	Vermont	10.9
46	Utah	10.8
47	New Hampshire	9.2
48	Idaho	7.8
49	Maine	7.2
50	Montana	6.8

| | District of Columbia | 521.4 |

Source: U.S. Department of Health and Human Services, National Center for Health Statistics
"Sexually Transmitted Disease Surveillance 2000" (http://www.cdc.gov/nchstp/dstd/dstdp.html)
*Gonorrhea is a sexually transmitted disease caused by gonococcal bacteria that affects the mucous membrane chiefly of the genital and urinary tracts and is characterized by an acute purulent discharge and painful or difficult urination, though women often have no symptoms.

Syphilis Cases Reported in 2000

National Total = 5,979 Cases*

ALPHA ORDER

RANK	STATE	CASES	% of USA
17	Alabama	123	2.1%
46	Alaska	0	0.0%
13	Arizona	189	3.2%
19	Arkansas	104	1.7%
9	California	325	5.4%
32	Colorado	11	0.2%
28	Connecticut	16	0.3%
34	Delaware	9	0.2%
3	Florida	413	6.9%
5	Georgia	402	6.7%
39	Hawaii	2	0.0%
43	Idaho	1	0.0%
4	Illinois	412	6.9%
7	Indiana	351	5.9%
32	Iowa	11	0.2%
35	Kansas	6	0.1%
20	Kentucky	85	1.4%
12	Louisiana	209	3.5%
43	Maine	1	0.0%
10	Maryland	300	5.0%
24	Massachusetts	68	1.1%
8	Michigan	330	5.5%
28	Minnesota	16	0.3%
14	Mississippi	137	2.3%
27	Missouri	29	0.5%
46	Montana	0	0.0%
39	Nebraska	2	0.0%
36	Nevada	5	0.1%
39	New Hampshire	2	0.0%
22	New Jersey	71	1.2%
28	New Mexico	16	0.3%
15	New York	132	2.2%
2	North Carolina	483	8.1%
46	North Dakota	0	0.0%
23	Ohio	69	1.2%
18	Oklahoma	116	1.9%
31	Oregon	12	0.2%
21	Pennsylvania	77	1.3%
37	Rhode Island	4	0.1%
11	South Carolina	229	3.8%
46	South Dakota	0	0.0%
1	Tennessee	532	8.9%
6	Texas	396	6.6%
39	Utah	2	0.0%
46	Vermont	0	0.0%
16	Virginia	126	2.1%
25	Washington	66	1.1%
38	West Virginia	3	0.1%
26	Wisconsin	48	0.8%
43	Wyoming	1	0.0%

RANK ORDER

RANK	STATE	CASES	% of USA
1	Tennessee	532	8.9%
2	North Carolina	483	8.1%
3	Florida	413	6.9%
4	Illinois	412	6.9%
5	Georgia	402	6.7%
6	Texas	396	6.6%
7	Indiana	351	5.9%
8	Michigan	330	5.5%
9	California	325	5.4%
10	Maryland	300	5.0%
11	South Carolina	229	3.8%
12	Louisiana	209	3.5%
13	Arizona	189	3.2%
14	Mississippi	137	2.3%
15	New York	132	2.2%
16	Virginia	126	2.1%
17	Alabama	123	2.1%
18	Oklahoma	116	1.9%
19	Arkansas	104	1.7%
20	Kentucky	85	1.4%
21	Pennsylvania	77	1.3%
22	New Jersey	71	1.2%
23	Ohio	69	1.2%
24	Massachusetts	68	1.1%
25	Washington	66	1.1%
26	Wisconsin	48	0.8%
27	Missouri	29	0.5%
28	Connecticut	16	0.3%
28	Minnesota	16	0.3%
28	New Mexico	16	0.3%
31	Oregon	12	0.2%
32	Colorado	11	0.2%
32	Iowa	11	0.2%
34	Delaware	9	0.2%
35	Kansas	6	0.1%
36	Nevada	5	0.1%
37	Rhode Island	4	0.1%
38	West Virginia	3	0.1%
39	Hawaii	2	0.0%
39	Nebraska	2	0.0%
39	New Hampshire	2	0.0%
39	Utah	2	0.0%
43	Idaho	1	0.0%
43	Maine	1	0.0%
43	Wyoming	1	0.0%
46	Alaska	0	0.0%
46	Montana	0	0.0%
46	North Dakota	0	0.0%
46	South Dakota	0	0.0%
46	Vermont	0	0.0%
	District of Columbia	37	0.6%

Source: U.S. Department of Health and Human Services, National Center for Health Statistics
"Sexually Transmitted Disease Surveillance 2000" (http://www.cdc.gov/nchstp/dstd/dstdp.html)
*Includes only primary and secondary cases. Does not include 25,596 cases in other stages. A chronic infectious disease caused by a spirochete (Treponema pallidum), either transmitted by direct contact, usually in sexual intercourse, or passed from mother to child in utero, and progressing through three stages characterized respectively by local formation of chancres, ulcerous skin eruptions, and systemic infection leading to general paresis.

Syphilis Rate in 2000

National Rate = 2.2 Cases per 100,000 Population*

ALPHA ORDER

RANK ORDER

RANK	STATE	RATE	RANK	STATE	RATE
14	Alabama	2.8	1	Tennessee	9.7
46	Alaska	0.0	2	North Carolina	6.3
10	Arizona	4.0	3	Indiana	5.9
9	Arkansas	4.1	3	South Carolina	5.9
22	California	1.0	5	Maryland	5.8
34	Colorado	0.3	6	Georgia	5.2
29	Connecticut	0.5	7	Mississippi	4.9
19	Delaware	1.2	8	Louisiana	4.8
15	Florida	2.7	9	Arkansas	4.1
6	Georgia	5.2	10	Arizona	4.0
37	Hawaii	0.2	11	Oklahoma	3.5
42	Idaho	0.1	12	Illinois	3.4
12	Illinois	3.4	13	Michigan	3.3
3	Indiana	5.9	14	Alabama	2.8
31	Iowa	0.4	15	Florida	2.7
37	Kansas	0.2	16	Kentucky	2.1
16	Kentucky	2.1	17	Texas	2.0
8	Louisiana	4.8	18	Virginia	1.8
42	Maine	0.1	19	Delaware	1.2
5	Maryland	5.8	20	Massachusetts	1.1
20	Massachusetts	1.1	20	Washington	1.1
13	Michigan	3.3	22	California	1.0
34	Minnesota	0.3	23	New Jersey	0.9
7	Mississippi	4.9	23	New Mexico	0.9
29	Missouri	0.5	23	Wisconsin	0.9
46	Montana	0.0	26	New York	0.7
42	Nebraska	0.1	27	Ohio	0.6
34	Nevada	0.3	27	Pennsylvania	0.6
37	New Hampshire	0.2	29	Connecticut	0.5
23	New Jersey	0.9	29	Missouri	0.5
23	New Mexico	0.9	31	Iowa	0.4
26	New York	0.7	31	Oregon	0.4
2	North Carolina	6.3	31	Rhode Island	0.4
46	North Dakota	0.0	34	Colorado	0.3
27	Ohio	0.6	34	Minnesota	0.3
11	Oklahoma	3.5	34	Nevada	0.3
31	Oregon	0.4	37	Hawaii	0.2
27	Pennsylvania	0.6	37	Kansas	0.2
31	Rhode Island	0.4	37	New Hampshire	0.2
3	South Carolina	5.9	37	West Virginia	0.2
46	South Dakota	0.0	37	Wyoming	0.2
1	Tennessee	9.7	42	Idaho	0.1
17	Texas	2.0	42	Maine	0.1
42	Utah	0.1	42	Nebraska	0.1
46	Vermont	0.0	42	Utah	0.1
18	Virginia	1.8	46	Alaska	0.0
20	Washington	1.1	46	Montana	0.0
37	West Virginia	0.2	46	North Dakota	0.0
23	Wisconsin	0.9	46	South Dakota	0.0
37	Wyoming	0.2	46	Vermont	0.0

District of Columbia		7.1

Source: U.S. Department of Health and Human Services, National Center for Health Statistics
   "Sexually Transmitted Disease Surveillance 2000" (http://www.cdc.gov/nchstp/dstd/dstdp.html)
*Includes only primary and secondary cases. Does not include 25,596 cases in other stages. A chronic infectious disease caused by a spirochete (Treponema pallidum), either transmitted by direct contact, usually in sexual intercourse, or passed from mother to child in utero, and progressing through three stages characterized respectively by local formation of chancres, ulcerous skin eruptions, and systemic infection leading to general paresis.

VI. PROVIDERS

422 Physicians in 2000
423 Male Physicians in 2000
424 Female Physicians in 2000
425 Percent of Physicians Who Are Female: 2000
426 Physicians Under 35 Years Old in 2000
427 Percent of Physicians Under 35 Years Old in 2000
428 Physicians 35 to 44 Years Old in 2000
429 Physicians 45 to 54 Years Old in 2000
430 Physicians 55 to 64 Years Old in 2000
431 Physicians 65 Years Old and Older in 2000
432 Percent of Physicians 65 Years Old and Older in 2000
433 Federal Physicians in 2000
434 Rate of Federal Physicians in 2000
435 Nonfederal Physicians in 2000
436 Rate of Nonfederal Physicians in 2000
437 Nonfederal Physicians in Patient Care in 2000
438 Rate of Nonfederal Physicians in Patient Care in 2000
439 Physicians in Primary Care in 2000
440 Rate of Physicians in Primary Care in 2000
441 Percent of Physicians in Primary Care in 2000
442 Percent of Population Lacking Access to Primary Care in 2001
443 Nonfederal Physicians in General/Family Practice in 2000
444 Rate of Nonfederal Physicians in General/Family Practice in 2000
445 Percent of Nonfederal Physicians Who Are Specialists in 2000
446 Nonfederal Physicians in Medical Specialties in 2000
447 Rate of Nonfederal Physicians in Medical Specialties in 2000
448 Nonfederal Physicians in Internal Medicine in 2000
449 Rate of Nonfederal Physicians in Internal Medicine in 2000
450 Nonfederal Physicians in Pediatrics in 2000
451 Rate of Nonfederal Physicians in Pediatrics in 2000
452 Nonfederal Physicians in Surgical Specialties in 2000
453 Rate of Nonfederal Physicians in Surgical Specialties in 2000
454 Nonfederal Physicians in General Surgery in 2000
455 Rate of Nonfederal Physicians in General Surgery in 2000
456 Nonfederal Physicians in Obstetrics and Gynecology in 2000
457 Rate of Nonfederal Physicians in Obstetrics and Gynecology in 2000
458 Nonfederal Physicians in Ophthalmology in 2000
459 Rate of Nonfederal Physicians in Ophthalmology in 2000
460 Nonfederal Physicians in Orthopedic Surgery in 2000
461 Rate of Nonfederal Physicians in Orthopedic Surgery in 2000
462 Nonfederal Physicians in Plastic Surgery in 2000
463 Rate of Nonfederal Physicians in Plastic Surgery in 2000
464 Nonfederal Physicians in Other Specialties in 2000
465 Rate of Nonfederal Physicians in Other Specialties in 2000
466 Nonfederal Physicians in Anesthesiology in 2000
467 Rate of Nonfederal Physicians in Anesthesiology in 2000
468 Nonfederal Physicians in Psychiatry in 2000
469 Rate of Nonfederal Physicians in Psychiatry in 2000
470 Percent of Population Lacking Access to Mental Health Care in 2001
471 International Medical School Graduates Practicing in the U.S. in 2000
472 Rate of International Medical School Graduates Practicing in the U.S. in 2000
473 International Medical School Graduates as a Percent of Nonfederal Physicians in 2000
474 Osteopathic Physicians in 2002
475 Rate of Osteopathic Physicians in 2002
476 Podiatric Physicians in 1999
477 Rate of Podiatric Physicians in 1999
478 Doctors of Chiropractic in 2000
479 Rate of Doctors of Chiropractic in 2000
480 Physician Assistants in Clinical Practice in 2002
481 Rate of Physician Assistants in Clinical Practice in 2002
482 Registered Nurses in 2000

VI. PROVIDERS (continued)

483 Rate of Registered Nurses in 2000
484 Dentists in 1998
485 Rate of Dentists in 1998
486 Percent of Population Lacking Access to Dental Care in 2001
487 Employment in Health Care in 1999

Physicians in 2000

National Total = 802,156 Physicians*

<table>
<tr><td colspan="4">ALPHA ORDER</td><td colspan="4">RANK ORDER</td></tr>
<tr><td>RANK</td><td>STATE</td><td>PHYSICIANS</td><td>% of USA</td><td>RANK</td><td>STATE</td><td>PHYSICIANS</td><td>% of USA</td></tr>
<tr><td>25</td><td>Alabama</td><td>9,887</td><td>1.2%</td><td>1</td><td>California</td><td>97,213</td><td>12.1%</td></tr>
<tr><td>49</td><td>Alaska</td><td>1,362</td><td>0.2%</td><td>2</td><td>New York</td><td>78,524</td><td>9.8%</td></tr>
<tr><td>22</td><td>Arizona</td><td>12,250</td><td>1.5%</td><td>3</td><td>Texas</td><td>46,904</td><td>5.8%</td></tr>
<tr><td>32</td><td>Arkansas</td><td>5,711</td><td>0.7%</td><td>4</td><td>Florida</td><td>46,013</td><td>5.7%</td></tr>
<tr><td>1</td><td>California</td><td>97,213</td><td>12.1%</td><td>5</td><td>Pennsylvania</td><td>39,603</td><td>4.9%</td></tr>
<tr><td>24</td><td>Colorado</td><td>11,692</td><td>1.5%</td><td>6</td><td>Illinois</td><td>35,943</td><td>4.5%</td></tr>
<tr><td>21</td><td>Connecticut</td><td>13,279</td><td>1.7%</td><td>7</td><td>Ohio</td><td>30,229</td><td>3.8%</td></tr>
<tr><td>46</td><td>Delaware</td><td>2,099</td><td>0.3%</td><td>8</td><td>Massachusetts</td><td>28,886</td><td>3.6%</td></tr>
<tr><td>4</td><td>Florida</td><td>46,013</td><td>5.7%</td><td>9</td><td>New Jersey</td><td>27,462</td><td>3.4%</td></tr>
<tr><td>14</td><td>Georgia</td><td>19,324</td><td>2.4%</td><td>10</td><td>Michigan</td><td>25,209</td><td>3.1%</td></tr>
<tr><td>39</td><td>Hawaii</td><td>3,887</td><td>0.5%</td><td>11</td><td>Maryland</td><td>23,449</td><td>2.9%</td></tr>
<tr><td>43</td><td>Idaho</td><td>2,370</td><td>0.3%</td><td>12</td><td>North Carolina</td><td>21,118</td><td>2.6%</td></tr>
<tr><td>6</td><td>Illinois</td><td>35,943</td><td>4.5%</td><td>13</td><td>Virginia</td><td>20,362</td><td>2.5%</td></tr>
<tr><td>20</td><td>Indiana</td><td>13,461</td><td>1.7%</td><td>14</td><td>Georgia</td><td>19,324</td><td>2.4%</td></tr>
<tr><td>31</td><td>Iowa</td><td>5,927</td><td>0.7%</td><td>15</td><td>Washington</td><td>16,693</td><td>2.1%</td></tr>
<tr><td>30</td><td>Kansas</td><td>6,486</td><td>0.8%</td><td>16</td><td>Tennessee</td><td>15,360</td><td>1.9%</td></tr>
<tr><td>27</td><td>Kentucky</td><td>9,468</td><td>1.2%</td><td>17</td><td>Minnesota</td><td>14,257</td><td>1.8%</td></tr>
<tr><td>23</td><td>Louisiana</td><td>12,207</td><td>1.5%</td><td>18</td><td>Missouri</td><td>14,061</td><td>1.8%</td></tr>
<tr><td>41</td><td>Maine</td><td>3,598</td><td>0.4%</td><td>19</td><td>Wisconsin</td><td>13,954</td><td>1.7%</td></tr>
<tr><td>11</td><td>Maryland</td><td>23,449</td><td>2.9%</td><td>20</td><td>Indiana</td><td>13,461</td><td>1.7%</td></tr>
<tr><td>8</td><td>Massachusetts</td><td>28,886</td><td>3.6%</td><td>21</td><td>Connecticut</td><td>13,279</td><td>1.7%</td></tr>
<tr><td>10</td><td>Michigan</td><td>25,209</td><td>3.1%</td><td>22</td><td>Arizona</td><td>12,250</td><td>1.5%</td></tr>
<tr><td>17</td><td>Minnesota</td><td>14,257</td><td>1.8%</td><td>23</td><td>Louisiana</td><td>12,207</td><td>1.5%</td></tr>
<tr><td>33</td><td>Mississippi</td><td>5,399</td><td>0.7%</td><td>24</td><td>Colorado</td><td>11,692</td><td>1.5%</td></tr>
<tr><td>18</td><td>Missouri</td><td>14,061</td><td>1.8%</td><td>25</td><td>Alabama</td><td>9,887</td><td>1.2%</td></tr>
<tr><td>45</td><td>Montana</td><td>2,188</td><td>0.3%</td><td>26</td><td>South Carolina</td><td>9,689</td><td>1.2%</td></tr>
<tr><td>37</td><td>Nebraska</td><td>4,300</td><td>0.5%</td><td>27</td><td>Kentucky</td><td>9,468</td><td>1.2%</td></tr>
<tr><td>38</td><td>Nevada</td><td>4,025</td><td>0.5%</td><td>28</td><td>Oregon</td><td>9,312</td><td>1.2%</td></tr>
<tr><td>42</td><td>New Hampshire</td><td>3,438</td><td>0.4%</td><td>29</td><td>Oklahoma</td><td>6,565</td><td>0.8%</td></tr>
<tr><td>9</td><td>New Jersey</td><td>27,462</td><td>3.4%</td><td>30</td><td>Kansas</td><td>6,486</td><td>0.8%</td></tr>
<tr><td>35</td><td>New Mexico</td><td>4,565</td><td>0.6%</td><td>31</td><td>Iowa</td><td>5,927</td><td>0.7%</td></tr>
<tr><td>2</td><td>New York</td><td>78,524</td><td>9.8%</td><td>32</td><td>Arkansas</td><td>5,711</td><td>0.7%</td></tr>
<tr><td>12</td><td>North Carolina</td><td>21,118</td><td>2.6%</td><td>33</td><td>Mississippi</td><td>5,399</td><td>0.7%</td></tr>
<tr><td>48</td><td>North Dakota</td><td>1,603</td><td>0.2%</td><td>34</td><td>Utah</td><td>5,041</td><td>0.6%</td></tr>
<tr><td>7</td><td>Ohio</td><td>30,229</td><td>3.8%</td><td>35</td><td>New Mexico</td><td>4,565</td><td>0.6%</td></tr>
<tr><td>29</td><td>Oklahoma</td><td>6,565</td><td>0.8%</td><td>36</td><td>West Virginia</td><td>4,442</td><td>0.6%</td></tr>
<tr><td>28</td><td>Oregon</td><td>9,312</td><td>1.2%</td><td>37</td><td>Nebraska</td><td>4,300</td><td>0.5%</td></tr>
<tr><td>5</td><td>Pennsylvania</td><td>39,603</td><td>4.9%</td><td>38</td><td>Nevada</td><td>4,025</td><td>0.5%</td></tr>
<tr><td>40</td><td>Rhode Island</td><td>3,814</td><td>0.5%</td><td>39</td><td>Hawaii</td><td>3,887</td><td>0.5%</td></tr>
<tr><td>26</td><td>South Carolina</td><td>9,689</td><td>1.2%</td><td>40</td><td>Rhode Island</td><td>3,814</td><td>0.5%</td></tr>
<tr><td>47</td><td>South Dakota</td><td>1,708</td><td>0.2%</td><td>41</td><td>Maine</td><td>3,598</td><td>0.4%</td></tr>
<tr><td>16</td><td>Tennessee</td><td>15,360</td><td>1.9%</td><td>42</td><td>New Hampshire</td><td>3,438</td><td>0.4%</td></tr>
<tr><td>3</td><td>Texas</td><td>46,904</td><td>5.8%</td><td>43</td><td>Idaho</td><td>2,370</td><td>0.3%</td></tr>
<tr><td>34</td><td>Utah</td><td>5,041</td><td>0.6%</td><td>44</td><td>Vermont</td><td>2,318</td><td>0.3%</td></tr>
<tr><td>44</td><td>Vermont</td><td>2,318</td><td>0.3%</td><td>45</td><td>Montana</td><td>2,188</td><td>0.3%</td></tr>
<tr><td>13</td><td>Virginia</td><td>20,362</td><td>2.5%</td><td>46</td><td>Delaware</td><td>2,099</td><td>0.3%</td></tr>
<tr><td>15</td><td>Washington</td><td>16,693</td><td>2.1%</td><td>47</td><td>South Dakota</td><td>1,708</td><td>0.2%</td></tr>
<tr><td>36</td><td>West Virginia</td><td>4,442</td><td>0.6%</td><td>48</td><td>North Dakota</td><td>1,603</td><td>0.2%</td></tr>
<tr><td>19</td><td>Wisconsin</td><td>13,954</td><td>1.7%</td><td>49</td><td>Alaska</td><td>1,362</td><td>0.2%</td></tr>
<tr><td>50</td><td>Wyoming</td><td>1,013</td><td>0.1%</td><td>50</td><td>Wyoming</td><td>1,013</td><td>0.1%</td></tr>
<tr><td></td><td></td><td></td><td></td><td></td><td>District of Columbia</td><td>4,488</td><td>0.6%</td></tr>
</table>

Source: American Medical Association (Chicago, Illinois)
  "Physician Characteristics and Distribution in the U.S." (2002-2003 Edition)
*As of December 31, 2000. Comprised of federal and nonfederal physicians. Total does not include 11,614 physicians in the U.S. territories and possessions, at APO's and FPO's and whose addresses are unknown.

Male Physicians in 2000

National Total = 609,781 Physicians*

ALPHA ORDER

RANK	STATE	PHYSICIANS	% of USA
25	Alabama	8,056	1.3%
49	Alaska	1,001	0.2%
22	Arizona	9,619	1.6%
32	Arkansas	4,658	0.8%
1	California	73,834	12.1%
24	Colorado	8,831	1.4%
21	Connecticut	9,946	1.6%
46	Delaware	1,578	0.3%
3	Florida	37,839	6.2%
14	Georgia	15,073	2.5%
39	Hawaii	2,992	0.5%
43	Idaho	2,016	0.3%
6	Illinois	25,892	4.2%
20	Indiana	10,632	1.7%
31	Iowa	4,749	0.8%
30	Kansas	5,074	0.8%
27	Kentucky	7,471	1.2%
23	Louisiana	9,524	1.6%
40	Maine	2,768	0.5%
11	Maryland	16,847	2.8%
8	Massachusetts	20,305	3.3%
10	Michigan	18,780	3.1%
18	Minnesota	10,771	1.8%
33	Mississippi	4,439	0.7%
17	Missouri	10,801	1.8%
44	Montana	1,826	0.3%
36	Nebraska	3,448	0.6%
38	Nevada	3,281	0.5%
42	New Hampshire	2,689	0.4%
9	New Jersey	19,902	3.3%
37	New Mexico	3,295	0.5%
2	New York	56,311	9.2%
12	North Carolina	16,358	2.7%
48	North Dakota	1,330	0.2%
7	Ohio	22,857	3.7%
29	Oklahoma	5,284	0.9%
28	Oregon	7,153	1.2%
5	Pennsylvania	29,844	4.9%
41	Rhode Island	2,765	0.5%
26	South Carolina	7,810	1.3%
47	South Dakota	1,417	0.2%
16	Tennessee	12,286	2.0%
4	Texas	36,295	6.0%
34	Utah	4,183	0.7%
45	Vermont	1,704	0.3%
13	Virginia	15,311	2.5%
15	Washington	12,705	2.1%
35	West Virginia	3,530	0.6%
19	Wisconsin	10,750	1.8%
50	Wyoming	857	0.1%

RANK ORDER

RANK	STATE	PHYSICIANS	% of USA
1	California	73,834	12.1%
2	New York	56,311	9.2%
3	Florida	37,839	6.2%
4	Texas	36,295	6.0%
5	Pennsylvania	29,844	4.9%
6	Illinois	25,892	4.2%
7	Ohio	22,857	3.7%
8	Massachusetts	20,305	3.3%
9	New Jersey	19,902	3.3%
10	Michigan	18,780	3.1%
11	Maryland	16,847	2.8%
12	North Carolina	16,358	2.7%
13	Virginia	15,311	2.5%
14	Georgia	15,073	2.5%
15	Washington	12,705	2.1%
16	Tennessee	12,286	2.0%
17	Missouri	10,801	1.8%
18	Minnesota	10,771	1.8%
19	Wisconsin	10,750	1.8%
20	Indiana	10,632	1.7%
21	Connecticut	9,946	1.6%
22	Arizona	9,619	1.6%
23	Louisiana	9,524	1.6%
24	Colorado	8,831	1.4%
25	Alabama	8,056	1.3%
26	South Carolina	7,810	1.3%
27	Kentucky	7,471	1.2%
28	Oregon	7,153	1.2%
29	Oklahoma	5,284	0.9%
30	Kansas	5,074	0.8%
31	Iowa	4,749	0.8%
32	Arkansas	4,658	0.8%
33	Mississippi	4,439	0.7%
34	Utah	4,183	0.7%
35	West Virginia	3,530	0.6%
36	Nebraska	3,448	0.6%
37	New Mexico	3,295	0.5%
38	Nevada	3,281	0.5%
39	Hawaii	2,992	0.5%
40	Maine	2,768	0.5%
41	Rhode Island	2,765	0.5%
42	New Hampshire	2,689	0.4%
43	Idaho	2,016	0.3%
44	Montana	1,826	0.3%
45	Vermont	1,704	0.3%
46	Delaware	1,578	0.3%
47	South Dakota	1,417	0.2%
48	North Dakota	1,330	0.2%
49	Alaska	1,001	0.2%
50	Wyoming	857	0.1%
	District of Columbia	3,094	0.5%

Source: American Medical Association (Chicago, Illinois)
  "Physician Characteristics and Distribution in the U.S." (2002-2003 Edition)
As of December 31, 2000. Comprised of federal and nonfederal physicians. Total does not include 8,452 male physicians in the U.S. territories and possessions, at APO's and FPO's and whose addresses are unknown.

Female Physicians in 2000

National Total = 192,375 Physicians*

ALPHA ORDER				RANK ORDER			
RANK	STATE	PHYSICIANS	% of USA	RANK	STATE	PHYSICIANS	% of USA
28	Alabama	1,831	1.0%	1	California	23,379	12.2%
46	Alaska	361	0.2%	2	New York	22,213	11.5%
24	Arizona	2,631	1.4%	3	Texas	10,609	5.5%
33	Arkansas	1,053	0.5%	4	Illinois	10,051	5.2%
1	California	23,379	12.2%	5	Pennsylvania	9,759	5.1%
21	Colorado	2,861	1.5%	6	Massachusetts	8,581	4.5%
17	Connecticut	3,333	1.7%	7	Florida	8,174	4.2%
44	Delaware	521	0.3%	8	New Jersey	7,560	3.9%
7	Florida	8,174	4.2%	9	Ohio	7,372	3.8%
14	Georgia	4,251	2.2%	10	Maryland	6,602	3.4%
37	Hawaii	895	0.5%	11	Michigan	6,429	3.3%
47	Idaho	354	0.2%	12	Virginia	5,051	2.6%
4	Illinois	10,051	5.2%	13	North Carolina	4,760	2.5%
22	Indiana	2,829	1.5%	14	Georgia	4,251	2.2%
32	Iowa	1,178	0.6%	15	Washington	3,988	2.1%
29	Kansas	1,412	0.7%	16	Minnesota	3,486	1.8%
26	Kentucky	1,997	1.0%	17	Connecticut	3,333	1.7%
23	Louisiana	2,683	1.4%	18	Missouri	3,260	1.7%
40	Maine	830	0.4%	19	Wisconsin	3,204	1.7%
10	Maryland	6,602	3.4%	20	Tennessee	3,074	1.6%
6	Massachusetts	8,581	4.5%	21	Colorado	2,861	1.5%
11	Michigan	6,429	3.3%	22	Indiana	2,829	1.5%
16	Minnesota	3,486	1.8%	23	Louisiana	2,683	1.4%
35	Mississippi	960	0.5%	24	Arizona	2,631	1.4%
18	Missouri	3,260	1.7%	25	Oregon	2,159	1.1%
45	Montana	362	0.2%	26	Kentucky	1,997	1.0%
39	Nebraska	852	0.4%	27	South Carolina	1,879	1.0%
42	Nevada	744	0.4%	28	Alabama	1,831	1.0%
41	New Hampshire	749	0.4%	29	Kansas	1,412	0.7%
8	New Jersey	7,560	3.9%	30	Oklahoma	1,281	0.7%
31	New Mexico	1,270	0.7%	31	New Mexico	1,270	0.7%
2	New York	22,213	11.5%	32	Iowa	1,178	0.6%
13	North Carolina	4,760	2.5%	33	Arkansas	1,053	0.5%
49	North Dakota	273	0.1%	34	Rhode Island	1,049	0.5%
9	Ohio	7,372	3.8%	35	Mississippi	960	0.5%
30	Oklahoma	1,281	0.7%	36	West Virginia	912	0.5%
25	Oregon	2,159	1.1%	37	Hawaii	895	0.5%
5	Pennsylvania	9,759	5.1%	38	Utah	858	0.4%
34	Rhode Island	1,049	0.5%	39	Nebraska	852	0.4%
27	South Carolina	1,879	1.0%	40	Maine	830	0.4%
48	South Dakota	291	0.2%	41	New Hampshire	749	0.4%
20	Tennessee	3,074	1.6%	42	Nevada	744	0.4%
3	Texas	10,609	5.5%	43	Vermont	614	0.3%
38	Utah	858	0.4%	44	Delaware	521	0.3%
43	Vermont	614	0.3%	45	Montana	362	0.2%
12	Virginia	5,051	2.6%	46	Alaska	361	0.2%
15	Washington	3,988	2.1%	47	Idaho	354	0.2%
36	West Virginia	912	0.5%	48	South Dakota	291	0.2%
19	Wisconsin	3,204	1.7%	49	North Dakota	273	0.1%
50	Wyoming	156	0.1%	50	Wyoming	156	0.1%
					District of Columbia	1,394	0.7%

Source: American Medical Association (Chicago, Illinois)
"Physician Characteristics and Distribution in the U.S." (2002-2003 Edition)
As of December 31, 2000. Comprised of federal and nonfederal physicians. Total does not include 3,162 female physicians in the U.S. territories and possessions, at APO's and FPO's and whose addresses are unknown.

Percent of Physicians Who Are Female: 2000

National Percent = 24.0% of Physicians*

ALPHA ORDER

RANK	STATE	PERCENT
40	Alabama	18.5
8	Alaska	26.5
31	Arizona	21.5
42	Arkansas	18.4
18	California	24.0
15	Colorado	24.5
11	Connecticut	25.1
12	Delaware	24.8
43	Florida	17.8
27	Georgia	22.0
23	Hawaii	23.0
50	Idaho	14.9
4	Illinois	28.0
33	Indiana	21.0
36	Iowa	19.9
29	Kansas	21.8
32	Kentucky	21.1
27	Louisiana	22.0
22	Maine	23.1
3	Maryland	28.2
1	Massachusetts	29.7
10	Michigan	25.5
15	Minnesota	24.5
43	Mississippi	17.8
20	Missouri	23.2
48	Montana	16.5
37	Nebraska	19.8
40	Nevada	18.5
29	New Hampshire	21.8
6	New Jersey	27.5
5	New Mexico	27.8
2	New York	28.3
26	North Carolina	22.5
45	North Dakota	17.0
17	Ohio	24.4
38	Oklahoma	19.5
20	Oregon	23.2
14	Pennsylvania	24.6
6	Rhode Island	27.5
39	South Carolina	19.4
45	South Dakota	17.0
35	Tennessee	20.0
25	Texas	22.6
45	Utah	17.0
8	Vermont	26.5
12	Virginia	24.8
19	Washington	23.9
34	West Virginia	20.5
23	Wisconsin	23.0
49	Wyoming	15.4

RANK ORDER

RANK	STATE	PERCENT
1	Massachusetts	29.7
2	New York	28.3
3	Maryland	28.2
4	Illinois	28.0
5	New Mexico	27.8
6	New Jersey	27.5
6	Rhode Island	27.5
8	Alaska	26.5
8	Vermont	26.5
10	Michigan	25.5
11	Connecticut	25.1
12	Delaware	24.8
12	Virginia	24.8
14	Pennsylvania	24.6
15	Colorado	24.5
15	Minnesota	24.5
17	Ohio	24.4
18	California	24.0
19	Washington	23.9
20	Missouri	23.2
20	Oregon	23.2
22	Maine	23.1
23	Hawaii	23.0
23	Wisconsin	23.0
25	Texas	22.6
26	North Carolina	22.5
27	Georgia	22.0
27	Louisiana	22.0
29	Kansas	21.8
29	New Hampshire	21.8
31	Arizona	21.5
32	Kentucky	21.1
33	Indiana	21.0
34	West Virginia	20.5
35	Tennessee	20.0
36	Iowa	19.9
37	Nebraska	19.8
38	Oklahoma	19.5
39	South Carolina	19.4
40	Alabama	18.5
40	Nevada	18.5
42	Arkansas	18.4
43	Florida	17.8
43	Mississippi	17.8
45	North Dakota	17.0
45	South Dakota	17.0
45	Utah	17.0
48	Montana	16.5
49	Wyoming	15.4
50	Idaho	14.9

District of Columbia — 31.1

Source: Morgan Quitno Press using data from American Medical Association (Chicago, Illinois)
"Physician Characteristics and Distribution in the U.S." (2002-2003 Edition)
*As of December 31, 2000. Comprised of federal and nonfederal physicians. National percent does not include physicians in the U.S. territories and possessions, at APO's and FPO's and whose addresses are unknown.

Physicians Under 35 Years Old in 2000

National Total = 135,024 Physicians*

ALPHA ORDER

RANK	STATE	PHYSICIANS	% of USA
24	Alabama	1,661	1.2%
48	Alaska	156	0.1%
26	Arizona	1,635	1.2%
32	Arkansas	941	0.7%
2	California	13,629	10.1%
25	Colorado	1,646	1.2%
19	Connecticut	2,212	1.6%
43	Delaware	368	0.3%
9	Florida	4,657	3.4%
14	Georgia	3,214	2.4%
39	Hawaii	499	0.4%
46	Idaho	206	0.2%
4	Illinois	7,728	5.7%
22	Indiana	2,129	1.6%
30	Iowa	996	0.7%
29	Kansas	1,046	0.8%
27	Kentucky	1,531	1.1%
18	Louisiana	2,514	1.9%
42	Maine	372	0.3%
11	Maryland	4,020	3.0%
7	Massachusetts	5,865	4.3%
8	Michigan	5,155	3.8%
17	Minnesota	2,551	1.9%
33	Mississippi	824	0.6%
15	Missouri	2,780	2.1%
49	Montana	140	0.1%
35	Nebraska	780	0.6%
40	Nevada	466	0.3%
41	New Hampshire	428	0.3%
10	New Jersey	4,065	3.0%
38	New Mexico	598	0.4%
1	New York	15,899	11.8%
12	North Carolina	3,901	2.9%
45	North Dakota	213	0.2%
6	Ohio	6,057	4.5%
31	Oklahoma	969	0.7%
28	Oregon	1,079	0.8%
5	Pennsylvania	7,357	5.4%
34	Rhode Island	821	0.6%
23	South Carolina	1,671	1.2%
47	South Dakota	183	0.1%
16	Tennessee	2,630	1.9%
3	Texas	8,571	6.3%
36	Utah	770	0.6%
44	Vermont	360	0.3%
13	Virginia	3,547	2.6%
21	Washington	2,140	1.6%
37	West Virginia	734	0.5%
20	Wisconsin	2,199	1.6%
50	Wyoming	110	0.1%

RANK ORDER

RANK	STATE	PHYSICIANS	% of USA
1	New York	15,899	11.8%
2	California	13,629	10.1%
3	Texas	8,571	6.3%
4	Illinois	7,728	5.7%
5	Pennsylvania	7,357	5.4%
6	Ohio	6,057	4.5%
7	Massachusetts	5,865	4.3%
8	Michigan	5,155	3.8%
9	Florida	4,657	3.4%
10	New Jersey	4,065	3.0%
11	Maryland	4,020	3.0%
12	North Carolina	3,901	2.9%
13	Virginia	3,547	2.6%
14	Georgia	3,214	2.4%
15	Missouri	2,780	2.1%
16	Tennessee	2,630	1.9%
17	Minnesota	2,551	1.9%
18	Louisiana	2,514	1.9%
19	Connecticut	2,212	1.6%
20	Wisconsin	2,199	1.6%
21	Washington	2,140	1.6%
22	Indiana	2,129	1.6%
23	South Carolina	1,671	1.2%
24	Alabama	1,661	1.2%
25	Colorado	1,646	1.2%
26	Arizona	1,635	1.2%
27	Kentucky	1,531	1.1%
28	Oregon	1,079	0.8%
29	Kansas	1,046	0.8%
30	Iowa	996	0.7%
31	Oklahoma	969	0.7%
32	Arkansas	941	0.7%
33	Mississippi	824	0.6%
34	Rhode Island	821	0.6%
35	Nebraska	780	0.6%
36	Utah	770	0.6%
37	West Virginia	734	0.5%
38	New Mexico	598	0.4%
39	Hawaii	499	0.4%
40	Nevada	466	0.3%
41	New Hampshire	428	0.3%
42	Maine	372	0.3%
43	Delaware	368	0.3%
44	Vermont	360	0.3%
45	North Dakota	213	0.2%
46	Idaho	206	0.2%
47	South Dakota	183	0.1%
48	Alaska	156	0.1%
49	Montana	140	0.1%
50	Wyoming	110	0.1%
	District of Columbia	1,001	0.7%

Source: American Medical Association (Chicago, Illinois)
  "Physician Characteristics and Distribution in the U.S." (2002-2003 Edition)
As of December 31, 2000. Comprised of federal and nonfederal physicians. Total does not include 1,680 physicians in the U.S. territories and possessions, at APO's and FPO's and whose addresses are unknown.

Percent of Physicians Under 35 Years Old in 2000

National Percent = 16.8% of Physicians*

ALPHA ORDER

RANK	STATE	PERCENT
19	Alabama	16.8
44	Alaska	11.5
36	Arizona	13.3
23	Arkansas	16.5
35	California	14.0
34	Colorado	14.1
21	Connecticut	16.7
14	Delaware	17.5
48	Florida	10.1
22	Georgia	16.6
39	Hawaii	12.8
49	Idaho	8.7
1	Illinois	21.5
27	Indiana	15.8
19	Iowa	16.8
26	Kansas	16.1
25	Kentucky	16.2
3	Louisiana	20.6
47	Maine	10.3
17	Maryland	17.1
5	Massachusetts	20.3
4	Michigan	20.4
13	Minnesota	17.9
30	Mississippi	15.3
8	Missouri	19.8
50	Montana	6.4
12	Nebraska	18.1
42	Nevada	11.6
41	New Hampshire	12.4
32	New Jersey	14.8
38	New Mexico	13.1
6	New York	20.2
10	North Carolina	18.5
36	North Dakota	13.3
7	Ohio	20.0
32	Oklahoma	14.8
42	Oregon	11.6
9	Pennsylvania	18.6
1	Rhode Island	21.5
16	South Carolina	17.2
46	South Dakota	10.7
17	Tennessee	17.1
11	Texas	18.3
30	Utah	15.3
29	Vermont	15.5
15	Virginia	17.4
39	Washington	12.8
23	West Virginia	16.5
27	Wisconsin	15.8
45	Wyoming	10.9

RANK ORDER

RANK	STATE	PERCENT
1	Illinois	21.5
1	Rhode Island	21.5
3	Louisiana	20.6
4	Michigan	20.4
5	Massachusetts	20.3
6	New York	20.2
7	Ohio	20.0
8	Missouri	19.8
9	Pennsylvania	18.6
10	North Carolina	18.5
11	Texas	18.3
12	Nebraska	18.1
13	Minnesota	17.9
14	Delaware	17.5
15	Virginia	17.4
16	South Carolina	17.2
17	Maryland	17.1
17	Tennessee	17.1
19	Alabama	16.8
19	Iowa	16.8
21	Connecticut	16.7
22	Georgia	16.6
23	Arkansas	16.5
23	West Virginia	16.5
25	Kentucky	16.2
26	Kansas	16.1
27	Indiana	15.8
27	Wisconsin	15.8
29	Vermont	15.5
30	Mississippi	15.3
30	Utah	15.3
32	New Jersey	14.8
32	Oklahoma	14.8
34	Colorado	14.1
35	California	14.0
36	Arizona	13.3
36	North Dakota	13.3
38	New Mexico	13.1
39	Hawaii	12.8
39	Washington	12.8
41	New Hampshire	12.4
42	Nevada	11.6
42	Oregon	11.6
44	Alaska	11.5
45	Wyoming	10.9
46	South Dakota	10.7
47	Maine	10.3
48	Florida	10.1
49	Idaho	8.7
50	Montana	6.4

| | District of Columbia | 22.3 |

Source: Morgan Quitno Press using data from American Medical Association (Chicago, Illinois)
   "Physician Characteristics and Distribution in the U.S." (2002-2003 Edition)
*As of December 31, 2000. Comprised of federal and nonfederal physicians. National percent does not include
physicians in the U.S. territories and possessions, at APO's and FPO's and whose addresses are unknown.

Physicians 35 to 44 Years Old in 2000

National Total = 208,602 Physicians*

ALPHA ORDER

RANK	STATE	PHYSICIANS	% of USA
26	Alabama	2,815	1.3%
49	Alaska	420	0.2%
24	Arizona	3,092	1.5%
33	Arkansas	1,496	0.7%
1	California	21,685	10.4%
23	Colorado	3,099	1.5%
21	Connecticut	3,355	1.6%
46	Delaware	546	0.3%
4	Florida	11,388	5.5%
13	Georgia	5,592	2.7%
40	Hawaii	962	0.5%
43	Idaho	641	0.3%
6	Illinois	9,305	4.5%
20	Indiana	3,703	1.8%
31	Iowa	1,560	0.7%
29	Kansas	1,677	0.8%
27	Kentucky	2,679	1.3%
22	Louisiana	3,140	1.5%
41	Maine	909	0.4%
12	Maryland	6,187	3.0%
8	Massachusetts	7,944	3.8%
10	Michigan	6,577	3.2%
18	Minnesota	4,014	1.9%
32	Mississippi	1,529	0.7%
19	Missouri	3,925	1.9%
45	Montana	558	0.3%
35	Nebraska	1,241	0.6%
36	Nevada	1,179	0.6%
42	New Hampshire	860	0.4%
9	New Jersey	7,233	3.5%
37	New Mexico	1,124	0.5%
2	New York	19,913	9.5%
11	North Carolina	6,212	3.0%
48	North Dakota	464	0.2%
7	Ohio	8,062	3.9%
30	Oklahoma	1,641	0.8%
28	Oregon	2,243	1.1%
5	Pennsylvania	10,219	4.9%
39	Rhode Island	989	0.5%
25	South Carolina	2,824	1.4%
47	South Dakota	492	0.2%
15	Tennessee	4,316	2.1%
3	Texas	13,076	6.3%
34	Utah	1,468	0.7%
44	Vermont	574	0.3%
14	Virginia	5,232	2.5%
16	Washington	4,158	2.0%
38	West Virginia	1,077	0.5%
17	Wisconsin	4,029	1.9%
50	Wyoming	227	0.1%

RANK ORDER

RANK	STATE	PHYSICIANS	% of USA
1	California	21,685	10.4%
2	New York	19,913	9.5%
3	Texas	13,076	6.3%
4	Florida	11,388	5.5%
5	Pennsylvania	10,219	4.9%
6	Illinois	9,305	4.5%
7	Ohio	8,062	3.9%
8	Massachusetts	7,944	3.8%
9	New Jersey	7,233	3.5%
10	Michigan	6,577	3.2%
11	North Carolina	6,212	3.0%
12	Maryland	6,187	3.0%
13	Georgia	5,592	2.7%
14	Virginia	5,232	2.5%
15	Tennessee	4,316	2.1%
16	Washington	4,158	2.0%
17	Wisconsin	4,029	1.9%
18	Minnesota	4,014	1.9%
19	Missouri	3,925	1.9%
20	Indiana	3,703	1.8%
21	Connecticut	3,355	1.6%
22	Louisiana	3,140	1.5%
23	Colorado	3,099	1.5%
24	Arizona	3,092	1.5%
25	South Carolina	2,824	1.4%
26	Alabama	2,815	1.3%
27	Kentucky	2,679	1.3%
28	Oregon	2,243	1.1%
29	Kansas	1,677	0.8%
30	Oklahoma	1,641	0.8%
31	Iowa	1,560	0.7%
32	Mississippi	1,529	0.7%
33	Arkansas	1,496	0.7%
34	Utah	1,468	0.7%
35	Nebraska	1,241	0.6%
36	Nevada	1,179	0.6%
37	New Mexico	1,124	0.5%
38	West Virginia	1,077	0.5%
39	Rhode Island	989	0.5%
40	Hawaii	962	0.5%
41	Maine	909	0.4%
42	New Hampshire	860	0.4%
43	Idaho	641	0.3%
44	Vermont	574	0.3%
45	Montana	558	0.3%
46	Delaware	546	0.3%
47	South Dakota	492	0.2%
48	North Dakota	464	0.2%
49	Alaska	420	0.2%
50	Wyoming	227	0.1%
	District of Columbia	951	0.5%

Source: American Medical Association (Chicago, Illinois)
   "Physician Characteristics and Distribution in the U.S." (2002-2003 Edition)
As of December 31, 2000. Comprised of federal and nonfederal physicians. Total does not include 3,271 physicians in the U.S. territories and possessions, at APO's and FPO's and whose addresses are unknown.

Physicians 45 to 54 Years Old in 2000

National Total = 198,661 Physicians*

ALPHA ORDER

RANK	STATE	PHYSICIANS	% of USA
26	Alabama	2,558	1.3%
49	Alaska	392	0.2%
24	Arizona	2,930	1.5%
32	Arkansas	1,517	0.8%
1	California	24,588	12.4%
22	Colorado	3,133	1.6%
21	Connecticut	3,381	1.7%
48	Delaware	453	0.2%
4	Florida	11,117	5.6%
14	Georgia	4,952	2.5%
38	Hawaii	1,020	0.5%
43	Idaho	653	0.3%
6	Illinois	8,469	4.3%
18	Indiana	3,549	1.8%
31	Iowa	1,536	0.8%
30	Kansas	1,605	0.8%
27	Kentucky	2,492	1.3%
23	Louisiana	3,045	1.5%
40	Maine	992	0.5%
11	Maryland	5,858	2.9%
9	Massachusetts	6,829	3.4%
10	Michigan	5,885	3.0%
17	Minnesota	3,702	1.9%
35	Mississippi	1,299	0.7%
20	Missouri	3,416	1.7%
44	Montana	623	0.3%
36	Nebraska	1,085	0.5%
39	Nevada	993	0.5%
41	New Hampshire	961	0.5%
7	New Jersey	7,145	3.6%
33	New Mexico	1,318	0.7%
2	New York	17,970	9.0%
12	North Carolina	5,095	2.6%
47	North Dakota	459	0.2%
8	Ohio	6,967	3.5%
29	Oklahoma	1,749	0.9%
25	Oregon	2,587	1.3%
5	Pennsylvania	9,749	4.9%
42	Rhode Island	808	0.4%
28	South Carolina	2,347	1.2%
46	South Dakota	520	0.3%
16	Tennessee	4,066	2.0%
3	Texas	11,437	5.8%
34	Utah	1,302	0.7%
45	Vermont	587	0.3%
13	Virginia	5,039	2.5%
15	Washington	4,661	2.3%
36	West Virginia	1,085	0.5%
19	Wisconsin	3,542	1.8%
50	Wyoming	286	0.1%

RANK ORDER

RANK	STATE	PHYSICIANS	% of USA
1	California	24,588	12.4%
2	New York	17,970	9.0%
3	Texas	11,437	5.8%
4	Florida	11,117	5.6%
5	Pennsylvania	9,749	4.9%
6	Illinois	8,469	4.3%
7	New Jersey	7,145	3.6%
8	Ohio	6,967	3.5%
9	Massachusetts	6,829	3.4%
10	Michigan	5,885	3.0%
11	Maryland	5,858	2.9%
12	North Carolina	5,095	2.6%
13	Virginia	5,039	2.5%
14	Georgia	4,952	2.5%
15	Washington	4,661	2.3%
16	Tennessee	4,066	2.0%
17	Minnesota	3,702	1.9%
18	Indiana	3,549	1.8%
19	Wisconsin	3,542	1.8%
20	Missouri	3,416	1.7%
21	Connecticut	3,381	1.7%
22	Colorado	3,133	1.6%
23	Louisiana	3,045	1.5%
24	Arizona	2,930	1.5%
25	Oregon	2,587	1.3%
26	Alabama	2,558	1.3%
27	Kentucky	2,492	1.3%
28	South Carolina	2,347	1.2%
29	Oklahoma	1,749	0.9%
30	Kansas	1,605	0.8%
31	Iowa	1,536	0.8%
32	Arkansas	1,517	0.8%
33	New Mexico	1,318	0.7%
34	Utah	1,302	0.7%
35	Mississippi	1,299	0.7%
36	Nebraska	1,085	0.5%
36	West Virginia	1,085	0.5%
38	Hawaii	1,020	0.5%
39	Nevada	993	0.5%
40	Maine	992	0.5%
41	New Hampshire	961	0.5%
42	Rhode Island	808	0.4%
43	Idaho	653	0.3%
44	Montana	623	0.3%
45	Vermont	587	0.3%
46	South Dakota	520	0.3%
47	North Dakota	459	0.2%
48	Delaware	453	0.2%
49	Alaska	392	0.2%
50	Wyoming	286	0.1%
	District of Columbia	909	0.5%

Source: American Medical Association (Chicago, Illinois)
  "Physician Characteristics and Distribution in the U.S." (2002-2003 Edition)
*As of December 31, 2000. Comprised of federal and nonfederal physicians. Total does not include 2,985
physicians in the U.S. territories and possessions, at APO's and FPO's and whose addresses are unknown.

Physicians 55 to 64 Years Old in 2000

National Total = 117,070 Physicians*

ALPHA ORDER

RANK	STATE	PHYSICIANS	% of USA
26	Alabama	1,403	1.2%
47	Alaska	246	0.2%
20	Arizona	1,831	1.6%
33	Arkansas	797	0.7%
1	California	16,393	14.0%
22	Colorado	1,786	1.5%
19	Connecticut	1,890	1.6%
45	Delaware	341	0.3%
3	Florida	6,976	6.0%
13	Georgia	2,727	2.3%
37	Hawaii	633	0.5%
44	Idaho	387	0.3%
5	Illinois	5,292	4.5%
21	Indiana	1,810	1.5%
31	Iowa	820	0.7%
30	Kansas	943	0.8%
27	Kentucky	1,370	1.2%
24	Louisiana	1,644	1.4%
39	Maine	550	0.5%
11	Maryland	3,543	3.0%
9	Massachusetts	3,785	3.2%
10	Michigan	3,572	3.1%
23	Minnesota	1,763	1.5%
34	Mississippi	778	0.7%
17	Missouri	1,940	1.7%
43	Montana	410	0.4%
40	Nebraska	513	0.4%
38	Nevada	596	0.5%
42	New Hampshire	451	0.4%
7	New Jersey	4,384	3.7%
35	New Mexico	745	0.6%
2	New York	10,967	9.4%
15	North Carolina	2,566	2.2%
49	North Dakota	227	0.2%
8	Ohio	4,128	3.5%
29	Oklahoma	1,023	0.9%
25	Oregon	1,564	1.3%
6	Pennsylvania	5,291	4.5%
41	Rhode Island	492	0.4%
28	South Carolina	1,243	1.1%
48	South Dakota	236	0.2%
16	Tennessee	2,033	1.7%
4	Texas	6,656	5.7%
36	Utah	712	0.6%
46	Vermont	320	0.3%
12	Virginia	2,970	2.5%
14	Washington	2,607	2.2%
32	West Virginia	814	0.7%
18	Wisconsin	1,892	1.6%
50	Wyoming	183	0.2%

RANK ORDER

RANK	STATE	PHYSICIANS	% of USA
1	California	16,393	14.0%
2	New York	10,967	9.4%
3	Florida	6,976	6.0%
4	Texas	6,656	5.7%
5	Illinois	5,292	4.5%
6	Pennsylvania	5,291	4.5%
7	New Jersey	4,384	3.7%
8	Ohio	4,128	3.5%
9	Massachusetts	3,785	3.2%
10	Michigan	3,572	3.1%
11	Maryland	3,543	3.0%
12	Virginia	2,970	2.5%
13	Georgia	2,727	2.3%
14	Washington	2,607	2.2%
15	North Carolina	2,566	2.2%
16	Tennessee	2,033	1.7%
17	Missouri	1,940	1.7%
18	Wisconsin	1,892	1.6%
19	Connecticut	1,890	1.6%
20	Arizona	1,831	1.6%
21	Indiana	1,810	1.5%
22	Colorado	1,786	1.5%
23	Minnesota	1,763	1.5%
24	Louisiana	1,644	1.4%
25	Oregon	1,564	1.3%
26	Alabama	1,403	1.2%
27	Kentucky	1,370	1.2%
28	South Carolina	1,243	1.1%
29	Oklahoma	1,023	0.9%
30	Kansas	943	0.8%
31	Iowa	820	0.7%
32	West Virginia	814	0.7%
33	Arkansas	797	0.7%
34	Mississippi	778	0.7%
35	New Mexico	745	0.6%
36	Utah	712	0.6%
37	Hawaii	633	0.5%
38	Nevada	596	0.5%
39	Maine	550	0.5%
40	Nebraska	513	0.4%
41	Rhode Island	492	0.4%
42	New Hampshire	451	0.4%
43	Montana	410	0.4%
44	Idaho	387	0.3%
45	Delaware	341	0.3%
46	Vermont	320	0.3%
47	Alaska	246	0.2%
48	South Dakota	236	0.2%
49	North Dakota	227	0.2%
50	Wyoming	183	0.2%
	District of Columbia	827	0.7%

Source: American Medical Association (Chicago, Illinois)
"Physician Characteristics and Distribution in the U.S." (2002-2003 Edition)
*As of December 31, 2000. Comprised of federal and nonfederal physicians. Total does not include 1,538 physicians in the U.S. territories and possessions, at APO's and FPO's and whose addresses are unknown.

Physicians 65 Years Old and Older in 2000

National Total = 142,799 Physicians*

<table>
<tr><th colspan="4">ALPHA ORDER</th><th colspan="4">RANK ORDER</th></tr>
<tr><th>RANK</th><th>STATE</th><th>PHYSICIANS</th><th>% of USA</th><th>RANK</th><th>STATE</th><th>PHYSICIANS</th><th>% of USA</th></tr>
<tr><td>27</td><td>Alabama</td><td>1,450</td><td>1.0%</td><td>1</td><td>California</td><td>20,918</td><td>14.6%</td></tr>
<tr><td>50</td><td>Alaska</td><td>148</td><td>0.1%</td><td>2</td><td>New York</td><td>13,775</td><td>9.6%</td></tr>
<tr><td>16</td><td>Arizona</td><td>2,762</td><td>1.9%</td><td>3</td><td>Florida</td><td>11,875</td><td>8.3%</td></tr>
<tr><td>33</td><td>Arkansas</td><td>960</td><td>0.7%</td><td>4</td><td>Texas</td><td>7,164</td><td>5.0%</td></tr>
<tr><td>1</td><td>California</td><td>20,918</td><td>14.6%</td><td>5</td><td>Pennsylvania</td><td>6,987</td><td>4.9%</td></tr>
<tr><td>22</td><td>Colorado</td><td>2,028</td><td>1.4%</td><td>6</td><td>Illinois</td><td>5,149</td><td>3.6%</td></tr>
<tr><td>17</td><td>Connecticut</td><td>2,441</td><td>1.7%</td><td>7</td><td>Ohio</td><td>5,015</td><td>3.5%</td></tr>
<tr><td>46</td><td>Delaware</td><td>391</td><td>0.3%</td><td>8</td><td>New Jersey</td><td>4,635</td><td>3.2%</td></tr>
<tr><td>3</td><td>Florida</td><td>11,875</td><td>8.3%</td><td>9</td><td>Massachusetts</td><td>4,463</td><td>3.1%</td></tr>
<tr><td>15</td><td>Georgia</td><td>2,839</td><td>2.0%</td><td>10</td><td>Michigan</td><td>4,020</td><td>2.8%</td></tr>
<tr><td>38</td><td>Hawaii</td><td>773</td><td>0.5%</td><td>11</td><td>Maryland</td><td>3,841</td><td>2.7%</td></tr>
<tr><td>43</td><td>Idaho</td><td>483</td><td>0.3%</td><td>12</td><td>Virginia</td><td>3,574</td><td>2.5%</td></tr>
<tr><td>6</td><td>Illinois</td><td>5,149</td><td>3.6%</td><td>13</td><td>North Carolina</td><td>3,344</td><td>2.3%</td></tr>
<tr><td>20</td><td>Indiana</td><td>2,270</td><td>1.6%</td><td>14</td><td>Washington</td><td>3,127</td><td>2.2%</td></tr>
<tr><td>31</td><td>Iowa</td><td>1,015</td><td>0.7%</td><td>15</td><td>Georgia</td><td>2,839</td><td>2.0%</td></tr>
<tr><td>29</td><td>Kansas</td><td>1,215</td><td>0.9%</td><td>16</td><td>Arizona</td><td>2,762</td><td>1.9%</td></tr>
<tr><td>28</td><td>Kentucky</td><td>1,396</td><td>1.0%</td><td>17</td><td>Connecticut</td><td>2,441</td><td>1.7%</td></tr>
<tr><td>24</td><td>Louisiana</td><td>1,864</td><td>1.3%</td><td>18</td><td>Tennessee</td><td>2,315</td><td>1.6%</td></tr>
<tr><td>37</td><td>Maine</td><td>775</td><td>0.5%</td><td>19</td><td>Wisconsin</td><td>2,292</td><td>1.6%</td></tr>
<tr><td>11</td><td>Maryland</td><td>3,841</td><td>2.7%</td><td>20</td><td>Indiana</td><td>2,270</td><td>1.6%</td></tr>
<tr><td>9</td><td>Massachusetts</td><td>4,463</td><td>3.1%</td><td>21</td><td>Minnesota</td><td>2,227</td><td>1.6%</td></tr>
<tr><td>10</td><td>Michigan</td><td>4,020</td><td>2.8%</td><td>22</td><td>Colorado</td><td>2,028</td><td>1.4%</td></tr>
<tr><td>21</td><td>Minnesota</td><td>2,227</td><td>1.6%</td><td>23</td><td>Missouri</td><td>2,000</td><td>1.4%</td></tr>
<tr><td>32</td><td>Mississippi</td><td>969</td><td>0.7%</td><td>24</td><td>Louisiana</td><td>1,864</td><td>1.3%</td></tr>
<tr><td>23</td><td>Missouri</td><td>2,000</td><td>1.4%</td><td>25</td><td>Oregon</td><td>1,839</td><td>1.3%</td></tr>
<tr><td>45</td><td>Montana</td><td>457</td><td>0.3%</td><td>26</td><td>South Carolina</td><td>1,604</td><td>1.1%</td></tr>
<tr><td>42</td><td>Nebraska</td><td>681</td><td>0.5%</td><td>27</td><td>Alabama</td><td>1,450</td><td>1.0%</td></tr>
<tr><td>34</td><td>Nevada</td><td>791</td><td>0.6%</td><td>28</td><td>Kentucky</td><td>1,396</td><td>1.0%</td></tr>
<tr><td>39</td><td>New Hampshire</td><td>738</td><td>0.5%</td><td>29</td><td>Kansas</td><td>1,215</td><td>0.9%</td></tr>
<tr><td>8</td><td>New Jersey</td><td>4,635</td><td>3.2%</td><td>30</td><td>Oklahoma</td><td>1,183</td><td>0.8%</td></tr>
<tr><td>36</td><td>New Mexico</td><td>780</td><td>0.5%</td><td>31</td><td>Iowa</td><td>1,015</td><td>0.7%</td></tr>
<tr><td>2</td><td>New York</td><td>13,775</td><td>9.6%</td><td>32</td><td>Mississippi</td><td>969</td><td>0.7%</td></tr>
<tr><td>13</td><td>North Carolina</td><td>3,344</td><td>2.3%</td><td>33</td><td>Arkansas</td><td>960</td><td>0.7%</td></tr>
<tr><td>48</td><td>North Dakota</td><td>240</td><td>0.2%</td><td>34</td><td>Nevada</td><td>791</td><td>0.6%</td></tr>
<tr><td>7</td><td>Ohio</td><td>5,015</td><td>3.5%</td><td>35</td><td>Utah</td><td>789</td><td>0.6%</td></tr>
<tr><td>30</td><td>Oklahoma</td><td>1,183</td><td>0.8%</td><td>36</td><td>New Mexico</td><td>780</td><td>0.5%</td></tr>
<tr><td>25</td><td>Oregon</td><td>1,839</td><td>1.3%</td><td>37</td><td>Maine</td><td>775</td><td>0.5%</td></tr>
<tr><td>5</td><td>Pennsylvania</td><td>6,987</td><td>4.9%</td><td>38</td><td>Hawaii</td><td>773</td><td>0.5%</td></tr>
<tr><td>41</td><td>Rhode Island</td><td>704</td><td>0.5%</td><td>39</td><td>New Hampshire</td><td>738</td><td>0.5%</td></tr>
<tr><td>26</td><td>South Carolina</td><td>1,604</td><td>1.1%</td><td>40</td><td>West Virginia</td><td>732</td><td>0.5%</td></tr>
<tr><td>47</td><td>South Dakota</td><td>277</td><td>0.2%</td><td>41</td><td>Rhode Island</td><td>704</td><td>0.5%</td></tr>
<tr><td>18</td><td>Tennessee</td><td>2,315</td><td>1.6%</td><td>42</td><td>Nebraska</td><td>681</td><td>0.5%</td></tr>
<tr><td>4</td><td>Texas</td><td>7,164</td><td>5.0%</td><td>43</td><td>Idaho</td><td>483</td><td>0.3%</td></tr>
<tr><td>35</td><td>Utah</td><td>789</td><td>0.6%</td><td>44</td><td>Vermont</td><td>477</td><td>0.3%</td></tr>
<tr><td>44</td><td>Vermont</td><td>477</td><td>0.3%</td><td>45</td><td>Montana</td><td>457</td><td>0.3%</td></tr>
<tr><td>12</td><td>Virginia</td><td>3,574</td><td>2.5%</td><td>46</td><td>Delaware</td><td>391</td><td>0.3%</td></tr>
<tr><td>14</td><td>Washington</td><td>3,127</td><td>2.2%</td><td>47</td><td>South Dakota</td><td>277</td><td>0.2%</td></tr>
<tr><td>40</td><td>West Virginia</td><td>732</td><td>0.5%</td><td>48</td><td>North Dakota</td><td>240</td><td>0.2%</td></tr>
<tr><td>19</td><td>Wisconsin</td><td>2,292</td><td>1.6%</td><td>49</td><td>Wyoming</td><td>207</td><td>0.1%</td></tr>
<tr><td>49</td><td>Wyoming</td><td>207</td><td>0.1%</td><td>50</td><td>Alaska</td><td>148</td><td>0.1%</td></tr>
<tr><td></td><td></td><td></td><td></td><td></td><td>District of Columbia</td><td>800</td><td>0.6%</td></tr>
</table>

Source: American Medical Association (Chicago, Illinois)
"Physician Characteristics and Distribution in the U.S." (2002-2003 Edition)
As of December 31, 2000. Comprised of federal and nonfederal physicians. Total does not include 2,140 physicians in the U.S. territories and possessions, at APO's and FPO's and whose addresses are unknown.

Percent of Physicians 65 Years Old and Older in 2000

National Percent = 17.8% of Physicians*

<table>
<tr><td colspan="3">ALPHA ORDER</td><td colspan="3">RANK ORDER</td></tr>
<tr><th>RANK</th><th>STATE</th><th>PERCENT</th><th>RANK</th><th>STATE</th><th>PERCENT</th></tr>
<tr><td>45</td><td>Alabama</td><td>14.7</td><td>1</td><td>Florida</td><td>25.8</td></tr>
<tr><td>50</td><td>Alaska</td><td>10.9</td><td>2</td><td>Arizona</td><td>22.5</td></tr>
<tr><td>2</td><td>Arizona</td><td>22.5</td><td>3</td><td>California</td><td>21.5</td></tr>
<tr><td>28</td><td>Arkansas</td><td>16.8</td><td>3</td><td>Maine</td><td>21.5</td></tr>
<tr><td>3</td><td>California</td><td>21.5</td><td>3</td><td>New Hampshire</td><td>21.5</td></tr>
<tr><td>23</td><td>Colorado</td><td>17.3</td><td>6</td><td>Montana</td><td>20.9</td></tr>
<tr><td>17</td><td>Connecticut</td><td>18.4</td><td>7</td><td>Vermont</td><td>20.6</td></tr>
<tr><td>15</td><td>Delaware</td><td>18.6</td><td>8</td><td>Idaho</td><td>20.4</td></tr>
<tr><td>1</td><td>Florida</td><td>25.8</td><td>8</td><td>Wyoming</td><td>20.4</td></tr>
<tr><td>45</td><td>Georgia</td><td>14.7</td><td>10</td><td>Hawaii</td><td>19.9</td></tr>
<tr><td>10</td><td>Hawaii</td><td>19.9</td><td>11</td><td>Nevada</td><td>19.7</td></tr>
<tr><td>8</td><td>Idaho</td><td>20.4</td><td>11</td><td>Oregon</td><td>19.7</td></tr>
<tr><td>48</td><td>Illinois</td><td>14.3</td><td>13</td><td>Kansas</td><td>18.7</td></tr>
<tr><td>26</td><td>Indiana</td><td>16.9</td><td>13</td><td>Washington</td><td>18.7</td></tr>
<tr><td>24</td><td>Iowa</td><td>17.1</td><td>15</td><td>Delaware</td><td>18.6</td></tr>
<tr><td>13</td><td>Kansas</td><td>18.7</td><td>16</td><td>Rhode Island</td><td>18.5</td></tr>
<tr><td>45</td><td>Kentucky</td><td>14.7</td><td>17</td><td>Connecticut</td><td>18.4</td></tr>
<tr><td>41</td><td>Louisiana</td><td>15.3</td><td>18</td><td>Oklahoma</td><td>18.0</td></tr>
<tr><td>3</td><td>Maine</td><td>21.5</td><td>19</td><td>Mississippi</td><td>17.9</td></tr>
<tr><td>32</td><td>Maryland</td><td>16.4</td><td>20</td><td>Pennsylvania</td><td>17.6</td></tr>
<tr><td>40</td><td>Massachusetts</td><td>15.5</td><td>20</td><td>Virginia</td><td>17.6</td></tr>
<tr><td>35</td><td>Michigan</td><td>15.9</td><td>22</td><td>New York</td><td>17.5</td></tr>
<tr><td>39</td><td>Minnesota</td><td>15.6</td><td>23</td><td>Colorado</td><td>17.3</td></tr>
<tr><td>19</td><td>Mississippi</td><td>17.9</td><td>24</td><td>Iowa</td><td>17.1</td></tr>
<tr><td>49</td><td>Missouri</td><td>14.2</td><td>24</td><td>New Mexico</td><td>17.1</td></tr>
<tr><td>6</td><td>Montana</td><td>20.9</td><td>26</td><td>Indiana</td><td>16.9</td></tr>
<tr><td>36</td><td>Nebraska</td><td>15.8</td><td>26</td><td>New Jersey</td><td>16.9</td></tr>
<tr><td>11</td><td>Nevada</td><td>19.7</td><td>28</td><td>Arkansas</td><td>16.8</td></tr>
<tr><td>3</td><td>New Hampshire</td><td>21.5</td><td>29</td><td>Ohio</td><td>16.6</td></tr>
<tr><td>26</td><td>New Jersey</td><td>16.9</td><td>29</td><td>South Carolina</td><td>16.6</td></tr>
<tr><td>24</td><td>New Mexico</td><td>17.1</td><td>31</td><td>West Virginia</td><td>16.5</td></tr>
<tr><td>22</td><td>New York</td><td>17.5</td><td>32</td><td>Maryland</td><td>16.4</td></tr>
<tr><td>36</td><td>North Carolina</td><td>15.8</td><td>32</td><td>Wisconsin</td><td>16.4</td></tr>
<tr><td>44</td><td>North Dakota</td><td>15.0</td><td>34</td><td>South Dakota</td><td>16.2</td></tr>
<tr><td>29</td><td>Ohio</td><td>16.6</td><td>35</td><td>Michigan</td><td>15.9</td></tr>
<tr><td>18</td><td>Oklahoma</td><td>18.0</td><td>36</td><td>Nebraska</td><td>15.8</td></tr>
<tr><td>11</td><td>Oregon</td><td>19.7</td><td>36</td><td>North Carolina</td><td>15.8</td></tr>
<tr><td>20</td><td>Pennsylvania</td><td>17.6</td><td>38</td><td>Utah</td><td>15.7</td></tr>
<tr><td>16</td><td>Rhode Island</td><td>18.5</td><td>39</td><td>Minnesota</td><td>15.6</td></tr>
<tr><td>29</td><td>South Carolina</td><td>16.6</td><td>40</td><td>Massachusetts</td><td>15.5</td></tr>
<tr><td>34</td><td>South Dakota</td><td>16.2</td><td>41</td><td>Louisiana</td><td>15.3</td></tr>
<tr><td>43</td><td>Tennessee</td><td>15.1</td><td>41</td><td>Texas</td><td>15.3</td></tr>
<tr><td>41</td><td>Texas</td><td>15.3</td><td>43</td><td>Tennessee</td><td>15.1</td></tr>
<tr><td>38</td><td>Utah</td><td>15.7</td><td>44</td><td>North Dakota</td><td>15.0</td></tr>
<tr><td>7</td><td>Vermont</td><td>20.6</td><td>45</td><td>Alabama</td><td>14.7</td></tr>
<tr><td>20</td><td>Virginia</td><td>17.6</td><td>45</td><td>Georgia</td><td>14.7</td></tr>
<tr><td>13</td><td>Washington</td><td>18.7</td><td>45</td><td>Kentucky</td><td>14.7</td></tr>
<tr><td>31</td><td>West Virginia</td><td>16.5</td><td>48</td><td>Illinois</td><td>14.3</td></tr>
<tr><td>32</td><td>Wisconsin</td><td>16.4</td><td>49</td><td>Missouri</td><td>14.2</td></tr>
<tr><td>8</td><td>Wyoming</td><td>20.4</td><td>50</td><td>Alaska</td><td>10.9</td></tr>
<tr><td></td><td></td><td></td><td></td><td>District of Columbia</td><td>17.8</td></tr>
</table>

Source: Morgan Quitno Press using data from American Medical Association (Chicago, Illinois)
"Physician Characteristics and Distribution in the U.S." (2002-2003 Edition)
*As of December 31, 2000. Comprised of federal and nonfederal physicians. National percent does not include physicians in the U.S. territories and possessions, at APO's and FPO's and whose addresses are unknown.

Federal Physicians in 2000

National Total = 20,242 Physicians*

ALPHA ORDER

RANK	STATE	PHYSICIANS	% of USA
28	Alabama	211	1.0%
35	Alaska	150	0.7%
13	Arizona	459	2.3%
34	Arkansas	153	0.8%
1	California	2,175	10.7%
16	Colorado	362	1.8%
31	Connecticut	184	0.9%
47	Delaware	55	0.3%
4	Florida	1,266	6.3%
7	Georgia	881	4.4%
23	Hawaii	256	1.3%
43	Idaho	72	0.4%
8	Illinois	583	2.9%
33	Indiana	179	0.9%
39	Iowa	102	0.5%
30	Kansas	192	0.9%
32	Kentucky	182	0.9%
26	Louisiana	230	1.1%
45	Maine	70	0.3%
2	Maryland	1,921	9.5%
14	Massachusetts	429	2.1%
17	Michigan	308	1.5%
21	Minnesota	267	1.3%
22	Mississippi	262	1.3%
19	Missouri	285	1.4%
46	Montana	67	0.3%
41	Nebraska	80	0.4%
37	Nevada	132	0.7%
43	New Hampshire	72	0.4%
18	New Jersey	307	1.5%
25	New Mexico	238	1.2%
6	New York	988	4.9%
9	North Carolina	575	2.8%
48	North Dakota	53	0.3%
12	Ohio	484	2.4%
27	Oklahoma	212	1.0%
24	Oregon	248	1.2%
10	Pennsylvania	551	2.7%
42	Rhode Island	73	0.4%
20	South Carolina	283	1.4%
40	South Dakota	97	0.5%
15	Tennessee	406	2.0%
3	Texas	1,585	7.8%
38	Utah	113	0.6%
50	Vermont	38	0.2%
5	Virginia	1,107	5.5%
11	Washington	539	2.7%
36	West Virginia	146	0.7%
29	Wisconsin	194	1.0%
49	Wyoming	40	0.2%

RANK ORDER

RANK	STATE	PHYSICIANS	% of USA
1	California	2,175	10.7%
2	Maryland	1,921	9.5%
3	Texas	1,585	7.8%
4	Florida	1,266	6.3%
5	Virginia	1,107	5.5%
6	New York	988	4.9%
7	Georgia	881	4.4%
8	Illinois	583	2.9%
9	North Carolina	575	2.8%
10	Pennsylvania	551	2.7%
11	Washington	539	2.7%
12	Ohio	484	2.4%
13	Arizona	459	2.3%
14	Massachusetts	429	2.1%
15	Tennessee	406	2.0%
16	Colorado	362	1.8%
17	Michigan	308	1.5%
18	New Jersey	307	1.5%
19	Missouri	285	1.4%
20	South Carolina	283	1.4%
21	Minnesota	267	1.3%
22	Mississippi	262	1.3%
23	Hawaii	256	1.3%
24	Oregon	248	1.2%
25	New Mexico	238	1.2%
26	Louisiana	230	1.1%
27	Oklahoma	212	1.0%
28	Alabama	211	1.0%
29	Wisconsin	194	1.0%
30	Kansas	192	0.9%
31	Connecticut	184	0.9%
32	Kentucky	182	0.9%
33	Indiana	179	0.9%
34	Arkansas	153	0.8%
35	Alaska	150	0.7%
36	West Virginia	146	0.7%
37	Nevada	132	0.7%
38	Utah	113	0.6%
39	Iowa	102	0.5%
40	South Dakota	97	0.5%
41	Nebraska	80	0.4%
42	Rhode Island	73	0.4%
43	Idaho	72	0.4%
43	New Hampshire	72	0.4%
45	Maine	70	0.3%
46	Montana	67	0.3%
47	Delaware	55	0.3%
48	North Dakota	53	0.3%
49	Wyoming	40	0.2%
50	Vermont	38	0.2%
	District of Columbia	380	1.9%

Source: American Medical Association (Chicago, Illinois)
"Physician Characteristics and Distribution in the U.S." (2002-2003 Edition)
*As of December 31, 2000. Total does not include 317 physicians in U.S. territories and possessions.

Rate of Federal Physicians in 2000

National Rate = 7.2 Physicians per 100,000 Population*

ALPHA ORDER			RANK ORDER		
RANK	STATE	RATE	RANK	STATE	RATE
40	Alabama	4.7	1	Maryland	36.2
2	Alaska	23.9	2	Alaska	23.9
10	Arizona	8.9	3	Hawaii	21.1
31	Arkansas	5.7	4	Virginia	15.6
27	California	6.4	5	New Mexico	13.1
11	Colorado	8.4	6	South Dakota	12.8
34	Connecticut	5.4	7	Georgia	10.7
22	Delaware	7.0	8	Mississippi	9.2
15	Florida	7.9	9	Washington	9.1
7	Georgia	10.7	10	Arizona	8.9
3	Hawaii	21.1	11	Colorado	8.4
32	Idaho	5.5	12	North Dakota	8.3
40	Illinois	4.7	13	West Virginia	8.1
50	Indiana	2.9	13	Wyoming	8.1
48	Iowa	3.5	15	Florida	7.9
19	Kansas	7.1	16	Texas	7.6
43	Kentucky	4.5	17	Montana	7.4
37	Louisiana	5.1	18	Oregon	7.2
32	Maine	5.5	19	Kansas	7.1
1	Maryland	36.2	19	North Carolina	7.1
25	Massachusetts	6.7	19	Tennessee	7.1
49	Michigan	3.1	22	Delaware	7.0
34	Minnesota	5.4	22	Rhode Island	7.0
8	Mississippi	9.2	22	South Carolina	7.0
37	Missouri	5.1	25	Massachusetts	6.7
17	Montana	7.4	26	Nevada	6.5
40	Nebraska	4.7	27	California	6.4
26	Nevada	6.5	28	Vermont	6.2
30	New Hampshire	5.8	29	Oklahoma	6.1
46	New Jersey	3.6	30	New Hampshire	5.8
5	New Mexico	13.1	31	Arkansas	5.7
36	New York	5.2	32	Idaho	5.5
19	North Carolina	7.1	32	Maine	5.5
12	North Dakota	8.3	34	Connecticut	5.4
45	Ohio	4.3	34	Minnesota	5.4
29	Oklahoma	6.1	36	New York	5.2
18	Oregon	7.2	37	Louisiana	5.1
43	Pennsylvania	4.5	37	Missouri	5.1
22	Rhode Island	7.0	39	Utah	5.0
22	South Carolina	7.0	40	Alabama	4.7
6	South Dakota	12.8	40	Illinois	4.7
19	Tennessee	7.1	40	Nebraska	4.7
16	Texas	7.6	43	Kentucky	4.5
39	Utah	5.0	43	Pennsylvania	4.5
28	Vermont	6.2	45	Ohio	4.3
4	Virginia	15.6	46	New Jersey	3.6
9	Washington	9.1	46	Wisconsin	3.6
13	West Virginia	8.1	48	Iowa	3.5
46	Wisconsin	3.6	49	Michigan	3.1
13	Wyoming	8.1	50	Indiana	2.9
				District of Columbia	66.5

Source: Morgan Quitno Press using data from American Medical Association (Chicago, Illinois)
"Physician Characteristics and Distribution in the U.S." (2002-2003 Edition)
As of December 31, 2000. National rate does not include physicians in U.S. territories and possessions.

Nonfederal Physicians in 2000

National Total = 781,914 Physicians*

ALPHA ORDER

RANK	STATE	PHYSICIANS	% of USA
25	Alabama	9,676	1.2%
49	Alaska	1,212	0.2%
23	Arizona	11,791	1.5%
32	Arkansas	5,558	0.7%
1	California	95,038	12.2%
24	Colorado	11,330	1.4%
21	Connecticut	13,095	1.7%
46	Delaware	2,044	0.3%
4	Florida	44,747	5.7%
14	Georgia	18,443	2.4%
40	Hawaii	3,631	0.5%
43	Idaho	2,298	0.3%
6	Illinois	35,360	4.5%
20	Indiana	13,282	1.7%
31	Iowa	5,825	0.7%
30	Kansas	6,294	0.8%
27	Kentucky	9,286	1.2%
22	Louisiana	11,977	1.5%
41	Maine	3,528	0.5%
11	Maryland	21,528	2.8%
8	Massachusetts	28,457	3.6%
10	Michigan	24,901	3.2%
17	Minnesota	13,990	1.8%
33	Mississippi	5,137	0.7%
18	Missouri	13,776	1.8%
45	Montana	2,121	0.3%
37	Nebraska	4,220	0.5%
38	Nevada	3,893	0.5%
42	New Hampshire	3,366	0.4%
9	New Jersey	27,155	3.5%
35	New Mexico	4,327	0.6%
2	New York	77,536	9.9%
12	North Carolina	20,543	2.6%
48	North Dakota	1,550	0.2%
7	Ohio	29,745	3.8%
29	Oklahoma	6,353	0.8%
28	Oregon	9,064	1.2%
5	Pennsylvania	39,052	5.0%
39	Rhode Island	3,741	0.5%
26	South Carolina	9,406	1.2%
47	South Dakota	1,611	0.2%
16	Tennessee	14,954	1.9%
3	Texas	45,319	5.8%
34	Utah	4,928	0.6%
44	Vermont	2,280	0.3%
13	Virginia	19,255	2.5%
15	Washington	16,154	2.1%
36	West Virginia	4,296	0.5%
19	Wisconsin	13,760	1.8%
50	Wyoming	973	0.1%

RANK ORDER

RANK	STATE	PHYSICIANS	% of USA
1	California	95,038	12.2%
2	New York	77,536	9.9%
3	Texas	45,319	5.8%
4	Florida	44,747	5.7%
5	Pennsylvania	39,052	5.0%
6	Illinois	35,360	4.5%
7	Ohio	29,745	3.8%
8	Massachusetts	28,457	3.6%
9	New Jersey	27,155	3.5%
10	Michigan	24,901	3.2%
11	Maryland	21,528	2.8%
12	North Carolina	20,543	2.6%
13	Virginia	19,255	2.5%
14	Georgia	18,443	2.4%
15	Washington	16,154	2.1%
16	Tennessee	14,954	1.9%
17	Minnesota	13,990	1.8%
18	Missouri	13,776	1.8%
19	Wisconsin	13,760	1.8%
20	Indiana	13,282	1.7%
21	Connecticut	13,095	1.7%
22	Louisiana	11,977	1.5%
23	Arizona	11,791	1.5%
24	Colorado	11,330	1.4%
25	Alabama	9,676	1.2%
26	South Carolina	9,406	1.2%
27	Kentucky	9,286	1.2%
28	Oregon	9,064	1.2%
29	Oklahoma	6,353	0.8%
30	Kansas	6,294	0.8%
31	Iowa	5,825	0.7%
32	Arkansas	5,558	0.7%
33	Mississippi	5,137	0.7%
34	Utah	4,928	0.6%
35	New Mexico	4,327	0.6%
36	West Virginia	4,296	0.5%
37	Nebraska	4,220	0.5%
38	Nevada	3,893	0.5%
39	Rhode Island	3,741	0.5%
40	Hawaii	3,631	0.5%
41	Maine	3,528	0.5%
42	New Hampshire	3,366	0.4%
43	Idaho	2,298	0.3%
44	Vermont	2,280	0.3%
45	Montana	2,121	0.3%
46	Delaware	2,044	0.3%
47	South Dakota	1,611	0.2%
48	North Dakota	1,550	0.2%
49	Alaska	1,212	0.2%
50	Wyoming	973	0.1%
	District of Columbia	4,108	0.5%

Source: American Medical Association (Chicago, Illinois)
"Physician Characteristics and Distribution in the U.S." (2002-2003 Edition)
*As of December 31, 2000. Total does not include 11,297 nonfederal physicians in U.S. territories and possessions.

Rate of Nonfederal Physicians in 2000

National Rate = 277 Physicians per 100,000 Population*

ALPHA ORDER

RANK	STATE	RATE
40	Alabama	217
46	Alaska	193
36	Arizona	228
43	Arkansas	208
12	California	280
20	Colorado	262
4	Connecticut	384
23	Delaware	260
13	Florida	279
37	Georgia	224
9	Hawaii	300
50	Idaho	177
10	Illinois	284
39	Indiana	218
44	Iowa	199
33	Kansas	234
35	Kentucky	229
18	Louisiana	268
14	Maine	276
3	Maryland	405
1	Massachusetts	448
26	Michigan	250
10	Minnesota	284
49	Mississippi	180
27	Missouri	246
32	Montana	235
27	Nebraska	246
46	Nevada	193
16	New Hampshire	271
7	New Jersey	322
30	New Mexico	238
2	New York	408
25	North Carolina	254
29	North Dakota	242
20	Ohio	262
48	Oklahoma	184
19	Oregon	264
8	Pennsylvania	318
6	Rhode Island	356
33	South Carolina	234
42	South Dakota	213
20	Tennessee	262
41	Texas	216
38	Utah	220
5	Vermont	374
16	Virginia	271
15	Washington	273
30	West Virginia	238
24	Wisconsin	256
45	Wyoming	197

RANK ORDER

RANK	STATE	RATE
1	Massachusetts	448
2	New York	408
3	Maryland	405
4	Connecticut	384
5	Vermont	374
6	Rhode Island	356
7	New Jersey	322
8	Pennsylvania	318
9	Hawaii	300
10	Illinois	284
10	Minnesota	284
12	California	280
13	Florida	279
14	Maine	276
15	Washington	273
16	New Hampshire	271
16	Virginia	271
18	Louisiana	268
19	Oregon	264
20	Colorado	262
20	Ohio	262
20	Tennessee	262
23	Delaware	260
24	Wisconsin	256
25	North Carolina	254
26	Michigan	250
27	Missouri	246
27	Nebraska	246
29	North Dakota	242
30	New Mexico	238
30	West Virginia	238
32	Montana	235
33	Kansas	234
33	South Carolina	234
35	Kentucky	229
36	Arizona	228
37	Georgia	224
38	Utah	220
39	Indiana	218
40	Alabama	217
41	Texas	216
42	South Dakota	213
43	Arkansas	208
44	Iowa	199
45	Wyoming	197
46	Alaska	193
46	Nevada	193
48	Oklahoma	184
49	Mississippi	180
50	Idaho	177

	District of Columbia	719

Source: Morgan Quitno Press using data from American Medical Association (Chicago, Illinois)
"Physician Characteristics and Distribution in the U.S." (2002-2003 Edition)
*As of December 31, 2000. National rate does not include population or physicians in U.S. territories and possessions.

Nonfederal Physicians in Patient Care in 2000

National Total = 623,247 Physicians*

ALPHA ORDER

RANK	STATE	PHYSICIANS	% of USA
25	Alabama	8,103	1.3%
49	Alaska	1,022	0.2%
23	Arizona	9,014	1.4%
31	Arkansas	4,632	0.7%
1	California	73,277	11.8%
24	Colorado	9,000	1.4%
21	Connecticut	10,306	1.7%
46	Delaware	1,648	0.3%
4	Florida	33,903	5.4%
14	Georgia	15,247	2.4%
40	Hawaii	2,901	0.5%
43	Idaho	1,858	0.3%
6	Illinois	28,730	4.6%
20	Indiana	10,932	1.8%
32	Iowa	4,534	0.7%
30	Kansas	5,044	0.8%
27	Kentucky	7,708	1.2%
22	Louisiana	10,030	1.6%
41	Maine	2,759	0.4%
11	Maryland	16,487	2.6%
9	Massachusetts	21,868	3.5%
10	Michigan	20,063	3.2%
18	Minnesota	11,293	1.8%
33	Mississippi	4,317	0.7%
17	Missouri	11,326	1.8%
45	Montana	1,692	0.3%
36	Nebraska	3,444	0.6%
38	Nevada	3,170	0.5%
42	New Hampshire	2,677	0.4%
8	New Jersey	22,041	3.5%
37	New Mexico	3,366	0.5%
2	New York	61,256	9.8%
12	North Carolina	16,466	2.6%
48	North Dakota	1,271	0.2%
7	Ohio	24,211	3.9%
29	Oklahoma	5,123	0.8%
28	Oregon	7,028	1.1%
5	Pennsylvania	31,230	5.0%
39	Rhode Island	3,019	0.5%
26	South Carolina	7,777	1.2%
47	South Dakota	1,333	0.2%
16	Tennessee	12,406	2.0%
3	Texas	37,363	6.0%
34	Utah	3,969	0.6%
44	Vermont	1,753	0.3%
13	Virginia	15,538	2.5%
15	Washington	12,485	2.0%
35	West Virginia	3,525	0.6%
19	Wisconsin	11,210	1.8%
50	Wyoming	773	0.1%

RANK ORDER

RANK	STATE	PHYSICIANS	% of USA
1	California	73,277	11.8%
2	New York	61,256	9.8%
3	Texas	37,363	6.0%
4	Florida	33,903	5.4%
5	Pennsylvania	31,230	5.0%
6	Illinois	28,730	4.6%
7	Ohio	24,211	3.9%
8	New Jersey	22,041	3.5%
9	Massachusetts	21,868	3.5%
10	Michigan	20,063	3.2%
11	Maryland	16,487	2.6%
12	North Carolina	16,466	2.6%
13	Virginia	15,538	2.5%
14	Georgia	15,247	2.4%
15	Washington	12,485	2.0%
16	Tennessee	12,406	2.0%
17	Missouri	11,326	1.8%
18	Minnesota	11,293	1.8%
19	Wisconsin	11,210	1.8%
20	Indiana	10,932	1.8%
21	Connecticut	10,306	1.7%
22	Louisiana	10,030	1.6%
23	Arizona	9,014	1.4%
24	Colorado	9,000	1.4%
25	Alabama	8,103	1.3%
26	South Carolina	7,777	1.2%
27	Kentucky	7,708	1.2%
28	Oregon	7,028	1.1%
29	Oklahoma	5,123	0.8%
30	Kansas	5,044	0.8%
31	Arkansas	4,632	0.7%
32	Iowa	4,534	0.7%
33	Mississippi	4,317	0.7%
34	Utah	3,969	0.6%
35	West Virginia	3,525	0.6%
36	Nebraska	3,444	0.6%
37	New Mexico	3,366	0.5%
38	Nevada	3,170	0.5%
39	Rhode Island	3,019	0.5%
40	Hawaii	2,901	0.5%
41	Maine	2,759	0.4%
42	New Hampshire	2,677	0.4%
43	Idaho	1,858	0.3%
44	Vermont	1,753	0.3%
45	Montana	1,692	0.3%
46	Delaware	1,648	0.3%
47	South Dakota	1,333	0.2%
48	North Dakota	1,271	0.2%
49	Alaska	1,022	0.2%
50	Wyoming	773	0.1%
	District of Columbia	3,119	0.5%

Source: *American Medical Association (Chicago, Illinois)*
"Physician Characteristics and Distribution in the U.S." (2002-2003 Edition)
*As of December 31, 2000. Total does not include 8,184 physicians in U.S. territories and possessions.

Rate of Nonfederal Physicians in Patient Care in 2000

National Rate = 221 Physicians per 100,000 Population*

ALPHA ORDER

RANK	STATE	RATE
37	Alabama	182
44	Alaska	163
42	Arizona	175
43	Arkansas	173
15	California	216
23	Colorado	208
4	Connecticut	302
21	Delaware	210
19	Florida	211
35	Georgia	185
9	Hawaii	239
50	Idaho	143
10	Illinois	231
38	Indiana	180
47	Iowa	155
33	Kansas	187
32	Kentucky	190
12	Louisiana	224
15	Maine	216
3	Maryland	310
1	Massachusetts	344
26	Michigan	202
11	Minnesota	229
48	Mississippi	152
26	Missouri	202
33	Montana	187
28	Nebraska	201
45	Nevada	157
15	New Hampshire	216
7	New Jersey	261
35	New Mexico	185
2	New York	323
25	North Carolina	204
29	North Dakota	198
18	Ohio	213
49	Oklahoma	148
24	Oregon	205
8	Pennsylvania	254
6	Rhode Island	287
31	South Carolina	193
41	South Dakota	176
14	Tennessee	218
39	Texas	178
40	Utah	177
5	Vermont	288
13	Virginia	219
19	Washington	211
30	West Virginia	195
22	Wisconsin	209
46	Wyoming	156

RANK ORDER

RANK	STATE	RATE
1	Massachusetts	344
2	New York	323
3	Maryland	310
4	Connecticut	302
5	Vermont	288
6	Rhode Island	287
7	New Jersey	261
8	Pennsylvania	254
9	Hawaii	239
10	Illinois	231
11	Minnesota	229
12	Louisiana	224
13	Virginia	219
14	Tennessee	218
15	California	216
15	Maine	216
15	New Hampshire	216
18	Ohio	213
19	Florida	211
19	Washington	211
21	Delaware	210
22	Wisconsin	209
23	Colorado	208
24	Oregon	205
25	North Carolina	204
26	Michigan	202
26	Missouri	202
28	Nebraska	201
29	North Dakota	198
30	West Virginia	195
31	South Carolina	193
32	Kentucky	190
33	Kansas	187
33	Montana	187
35	Georgia	185
35	New Mexico	185
37	Alabama	182
38	Indiana	180
39	Texas	178
40	Utah	177
41	South Dakota	176
42	Arizona	175
43	Arkansas	173
44	Alaska	163
45	Nevada	157
46	Wyoming	156
47	Iowa	155
48	Mississippi	152
49	Oklahoma	148
50	Idaho	143

	District of Columbia	546

Source: Morgan Quitno Press using data from American Medical Association (Chicago, Illinois)
"Physician Characteristics and Distribution in the U.S." (2002-2003 Edition)
*As of December 31, 2000. National rate does not include physicians in U.S. territories and possessions.

Physicians in Primary Care in 2000

National Total = 270,058 Physicians*

ALPHA ORDER

RANK	STATE	PHYSICIANS	% of USA
25	Alabama	3,628	1.3%
49	Alaska	593	0.2%
24	Arizona	3,911	1.4%
31	Arkansas	2,133	0.8%
1	California	32,237	11.9%
23	Colorado	3,938	1.5%
21	Connecticut	4,278	1.6%
46	Delaware	687	0.3%
4	Florida	13,737	5.1%
14	Georgia	6,931	2.6%
39	Hawaii	1,379	0.5%
43	Idaho	839	0.3%
5	Illinois	13,098	4.9%
19	Indiana	4,785	1.8%
32	Iowa	2,027	0.8%
29	Kansas	2,328	0.9%
27	Kentucky	3,330	1.2%
22	Louisiana	4,073	1.5%
41	Maine	1,234	0.5%
11	Maryland	7,283	2.7%
9	Massachusetts	8,700	3.2%
10	Michigan	8,622	3.2%
17	Minnesota	5,257	1.9%
33	Mississippi	1,947	0.7%
20	Missouri	4,643	1.7%
45	Montana	745	0.3%
35	Nebraska	1,621	0.6%
38	Nevada	1,387	0.5%
42	New Hampshire	1,166	0.4%
8	New Jersey	9,514	3.5%
37	New Mexico	1,610	0.6%
2	New York	25,668	9.5%
12	North Carolina	7,200	2.7%
48	North Dakota	635	0.2%
7	Ohio	10,415	3.9%
30	Oklahoma	2,321	0.9%
28	Oregon	3,173	1.2%
6	Pennsylvania	12,602	4.7%
40	Rhode Island	1,298	0.5%
26	South Carolina	3,483	1.3%
47	South Dakota	667	0.2%
16	Tennessee	5,316	2.0%
3	Texas	15,895	5.9%
34	Utah	1,664	0.6%
44	Vermont	823	0.3%
13	Virginia	7,177	2.7%
15	Washington	5,708	2.1%
35	West Virginia	1,621	0.6%
18	Wisconsin	5,030	1.9%
50	Wyoming	398	0.1%

RANK ORDER

RANK	STATE	PHYSICIANS	% of USA
1	California	32,237	11.9%
2	New York	25,668	9.5%
3	Texas	15,895	5.9%
4	Florida	13,737	5.1%
5	Illinois	13,098	4.9%
6	Pennsylvania	12,602	4.7%
7	Ohio	10,415	3.9%
8	New Jersey	9,514	3.5%
9	Massachusetts	8,700	3.2%
10	Michigan	8,622	3.2%
11	Maryland	7,283	2.7%
12	North Carolina	7,200	2.7%
13	Virginia	7,177	2.7%
14	Georgia	6,931	2.6%
15	Washington	5,708	2.1%
16	Tennessee	5,316	2.0%
17	Minnesota	5,257	1.9%
18	Wisconsin	5,030	1.9%
19	Indiana	4,785	1.8%
20	Missouri	4,643	1.7%
21	Connecticut	4,278	1.6%
22	Louisiana	4,073	1.5%
23	Colorado	3,938	1.5%
24	Arizona	3,911	1.4%
25	Alabama	3,628	1.3%
26	South Carolina	3,483	1.3%
27	Kentucky	3,330	1.2%
28	Oregon	3,173	1.2%
29	Kansas	2,328	0.9%
30	Oklahoma	2,321	0.9%
31	Arkansas	2,133	0.8%
32	Iowa	2,027	0.8%
33	Mississippi	1,947	0.7%
34	Utah	1,664	0.6%
35	Nebraska	1,621	0.6%
35	West Virginia	1,621	0.6%
37	New Mexico	1,610	0.6%
38	Nevada	1,387	0.5%
39	Hawaii	1,379	0.5%
40	Rhode Island	1,298	0.5%
41	Maine	1,234	0.5%
42	New Hampshire	1,166	0.4%
43	Idaho	839	0.3%
44	Vermont	823	0.3%
45	Montana	745	0.3%
46	Delaware	687	0.3%
47	South Dakota	667	0.2%
48	North Dakota	635	0.2%
49	Alaska	593	0.2%
50	Wyoming	398	0.1%
	District of Columbia	1,303	0.5%

Source: American Medical Association (Chicago, Illinois)
"Physician Characteristics and Distribution in the U.S." (2002-2003 Edition)
*Federal and nonfederal physicians as of December 31, 2000. National total does not include 4,595 physicians in U.S. territories and possessions. Primary Care Specialties include Family Practice, General Practice, Internal Medicine, Obstetrics/Gynecology and Pediatrics excluding subspecialties within each category.

Rate of Physicians in Primary Care in 2000

National Rate = 96 Physicians per 100,000 Population*

ALPHA ORDER			RANK ORDER		
RANK	STATE	RATE	RANK	STATE	RATE
37	Alabama	82	1	Maryland	137
18	Alaska	94	1	Massachusetts	137
43	Arizona	76	3	New York	135
41	Arkansas	80	3	Vermont	135
16	California	95	5	Connecticut	125
24	Colorado	91	6	Rhode Island	124
5	Connecticut	125	7	Hawaii	114
30	Delaware	87	8	New Jersey	113
33	Florida	86	9	Minnesota	107
35	Georgia	84	10	Illinois	105
7	Hawaii	114	11	Pennsylvania	103
50	Idaho	65	12	Virginia	101
10	Illinois	105	13	North Dakota	99
42	Indiana	79	14	Maine	97
46	Iowa	69	14	Washington	97
33	Kansas	86	16	California	95
37	Kentucky	82	16	Nebraska	95
24	Louisiana	91	18	Alaska	94
14	Maine	97	18	New Hampshire	94
1	Maryland	137	18	Wisconsin	94
1	Massachusetts	137	21	Oregon	93
30	Michigan	87	21	Tennessee	93
9	Minnesota	107	23	Ohio	92
48	Mississippi	68	24	Colorado	91
36	Missouri	83	24	Louisiana	91
37	Montana	82	26	West Virginia	90
16	Nebraska	95	27	North Carolina	89
46	Nevada	69	28	New Mexico	88
18	New Hampshire	94	28	South Dakota	88
8	New Jersey	113	30	Delaware	87
28	New Mexico	88	30	Michigan	87
3	New York	135	30	South Carolina	87
27	North Carolina	89	33	Florida	86
13	North Dakota	99	33	Kansas	86
23	Ohio	92	35	Georgia	84
49	Oklahoma	67	36	Missouri	83
21	Oregon	93	37	Alabama	82
11	Pennsylvania	103	37	Kentucky	82
6	Rhode Island	124	37	Montana	82
30	South Carolina	87	40	Wyoming	81
28	South Dakota	88	41	Arkansas	80
21	Tennessee	93	42	Indiana	79
43	Texas	76	43	Arizona	76
45	Utah	74	43	Texas	76
3	Vermont	135	45	Utah	74
12	Virginia	101	46	Iowa	69
14	Washington	97	46	Nevada	69
26	West Virginia	90	48	Mississippi	68
18	Wisconsin	94	49	Oklahoma	67
40	Wyoming	81	50	Idaho	65
				District of Columbia	228

Source: Morgan Quitno Press using data from American Medical Association (Chicago, Illinois)
"Physician Characteristics and Distribution in the U.S." (2002-2003 Edition)
*Federal and nonfederal physicians as of December 31, 2000. National rate does not include physicians in U.S. territories and possessions. Primary Care Specialties include Family Practice, General Practice, Internal Medicine, Obstetrics/Gynecology and Pediatrics excluding subspecialties within each category.

Percent of Physicians in Primary Care in 2000

National Percent = 33.7% of Physicians*

ALPHA ORDER

RANK	STATE	PERCENT
8	Alabama	36.7
1	Alaska	43.5
46	Arizona	31.9
6	Arkansas	37.3
40	California	33.2
38	Colorado	33.7
45	Connecticut	32.2
43	Delaware	32.7
50	Florida	29.9
13	Georgia	35.9
16	Hawaii	35.5
19	Idaho	35.4
10	Illinois	36.4
16	Indiana	35.5
29	Iowa	34.2
13	Kansas	35.9
22	Kentucky	35.2
39	Louisiana	33.4
28	Maine	34.3
48	Maryland	31.1
49	Massachusetts	30.1
29	Michigan	34.2
7	Minnesota	36.9
11	Mississippi	36.1
41	Missouri	33.0
34	Montana	34.0
5	Nebraska	37.7
26	Nevada	34.5
36	New Hampshire	33.9
24	New Jersey	34.6
21	New Mexico	35.3
43	New York	32.7
32	North Carolina	34.1
2	North Dakota	39.6
26	Ohio	34.5
19	Oklahoma	35.4
32	Oregon	34.1
47	Pennsylvania	31.8
34	Rhode Island	34.0
13	South Carolina	35.9
4	South Dakota	39.1
24	Tennessee	34.6
36	Texas	33.9
41	Utah	33.0
16	Vermont	35.5
22	Virginia	35.2
29	Washington	34.2
9	West Virginia	36.5
12	Wisconsin	36.0
3	Wyoming	39.3

RANK ORDER

RANK	STATE	PERCENT
1	Alaska	43.5
2	North Dakota	39.6
3	Wyoming	39.3
4	South Dakota	39.1
5	Nebraska	37.7
6	Arkansas	37.3
7	Minnesota	36.9
8	Alabama	36.7
9	West Virginia	36.5
10	Illinois	36.4
11	Mississippi	36.1
12	Wisconsin	36.0
13	Georgia	35.9
13	Kansas	35.9
13	South Carolina	35.9
16	Hawaii	35.5
16	Indiana	35.5
16	Vermont	35.5
19	Idaho	35.4
19	Oklahoma	35.4
21	New Mexico	35.3
22	Kentucky	35.2
22	Virginia	35.2
24	New Jersey	34.6
24	Tennessee	34.6
26	Nevada	34.5
26	Ohio	34.5
28	Maine	34.3
29	Iowa	34.2
29	Michigan	34.2
29	Washington	34.2
32	North Carolina	34.1
32	Oregon	34.1
34	Montana	34.0
34	Rhode Island	34.0
36	New Hampshire	33.9
36	Texas	33.9
38	Colorado	33.7
39	Louisiana	33.4
40	California	33.2
41	Missouri	33.0
41	Utah	33.0
43	Delaware	32.7
43	New York	32.7
45	Connecticut	32.2
46	Arizona	31.9
47	Pennsylvania	31.8
48	Maryland	31.1
49	Massachusetts	30.1
50	Florida	29.9

District of Columbia — 29.0

Source: Morgan Quitno Press using data from American Medical Association (Chicago, Illinois)
    "Physician Characteristics and Distribution in the U.S." (2002-2003 Edition)
*Federal and nonfederal physicians as of December 31, 2000. National percent does not include physicians in U.S. territories and possessions. Primary Care Specialties include Family Practice, General Practice, Internal Medicine, Obstetrics/Gynecology and Pediatrics excluding subspecialties within each category.

Percent of Population Lacking Access to Primary Care in 2001

National Percent = 10.9% of Population*

ALPHA ORDER

RANK	STATE	PERCENT
3	Alabama	23.3
18	Alaska	12.4
30	Arizona	9.4
24	Arkansas	11.0
40	California	7.4
29	Colorado	9.5
44	Connecticut	5.9
45	Delaware	5.1
19	Florida	12.2
10	Georgia	16.8
49	Hawaii	3.2
5	Idaho	20.1
19	Illinois	12.2
34	Indiana	8.9
35	Iowa	8.6
17	Kansas	13.1
14	Kentucky	15.1
6	Louisiana	19.6
36	Maine	8.4
39	Maryland	7.5
46	Massachusetts	4.8
25	Michigan	10.7
23	Minnesota	11.2
1	Mississippi	27.5
2	Missouri	24.5
11	Montana	16.7
38	Nebraska	7.6
27	Nevada	10.1
47	New Hampshire	4.2
50	New Jersey	3.1
9	New Mexico	17.6
30	New York	9.4
26	North Carolina	10.4
13	North Dakota	16.6
43	Ohio	7.0
33	Oklahoma	9.1
37	Oregon	8.0
41	Pennsylvania	7.2
32	Rhode Island	9.3
11	South Carolina	16.7
7	South Dakota	19.5
21	Tennessee	11.3
15	Texas	14.1
4	Utah	20.3
48	Vermont	3.9
42	Virginia	7.1
21	Washington	11.3
15	West Virginia	14.1
28	Wisconsin	9.7
8	Wyoming	18.2

RANK ORDER

RANK	STATE	PERCENT
1	Mississippi	27.5
2	Missouri	24.5
3	Alabama	23.3
4	Utah	20.3
5	Idaho	20.1
6	Louisiana	19.6
7	South Dakota	19.5
8	Wyoming	18.2
9	New Mexico	17.6
10	Georgia	16.8
11	Montana	16.7
11	South Carolina	16.7
13	North Dakota	16.6
14	Kentucky	15.1
15	Texas	14.1
15	West Virginia	14.1
17	Kansas	13.1
18	Alaska	12.4
19	Florida	12.2
19	Illinois	12.2
21	Tennessee	11.3
21	Washington	11.3
23	Minnesota	11.2
24	Arkansas	11.0
25	Michigan	10.7
26	North Carolina	10.4
27	Nevada	10.1
28	Wisconsin	9.7
29	Colorado	9.5
30	Arizona	9.4
30	New York	9.4
32	Rhode Island	9.3
33	Oklahoma	9.1
34	Indiana	8.9
35	Iowa	8.6
36	Maine	8.4
37	Oregon	8.0
38	Nebraska	7.6
39	Maryland	7.5
40	California	7.4
41	Pennsylvania	7.2
42	Virginia	7.1
43	Ohio	7.0
44	Connecticut	5.9
45	Delaware	5.1
46	Massachusetts	4.8
47	New Hampshire	4.2
48	Vermont	3.9
49	Hawaii	3.2
50	New Jersey	3.1

District of Columbia 15.2

Source: Morgan Quitno Press using data from U.S. Dept. of Health and Human Services, Div. of Shortage Designation
"Selected Statistics on Health Professional Shortage Areas, As of December 31, 2001"
*Percent of population considered under-served by primary medical practitioners (Family & General Practice doctors, Internists, Ob/Gyns and Pediatricians). An under-served population does not have primary medical care within reasonable economic and geographic bounds.

Nonfederal Physicians in General/Family Practice in 2000

National Total = 82,866 Physicians*

ALPHA ORDER

RANK	STATE	PHYSICIANS	% of USA
23	Alabama	1,242	1.5%
46	Alaska	282	0.3%
20	Arizona	1,302	1.6%
28	Arkansas	1,122	1.4%
1	California	9,979	12.0%
18	Colorado	1,550	1.9%
37	Connecticut	592	0.7%
49	Delaware	217	0.3%
3	Florida	4,448	5.4%
15	Georgia	1,979	2.4%
45	Hawaii	319	0.4%
39	Idaho	470	0.6%
6	Illinois	3,677	4.4%
13	Indiana	2,275	2.7%
27	Iowa	1,125	1.4%
30	Kansas	1,067	1.3%
21	Kentucky	1,274	1.5%
24	Louisiana	1,235	1.5%
38	Maine	525	0.6%
22	Maryland	1,264	1.5%
26	Massachusetts	1,198	1.4%
8	Michigan	2,574	3.1%
10	Minnesota	2,511	3.0%
33	Mississippi	741	0.9%
25	Missouri	1,219	1.5%
42	Montana	362	0.4%
32	Nebraska	838	1.0%
40	Nevada	432	0.5%
41	New Hampshire	414	0.5%
17	New Jersey	1,606	1.9%
35	New Mexico	635	0.8%
5	New York	3,853	4.6%
11	North Carolina	2,458	3.0%
44	North Dakota	344	0.4%
7	Ohio	3,349	4.0%
31	Oklahoma	989	1.2%
29	Oregon	1,093	1.3%
4	Pennsylvania	3,930	4.7%
50	Rhode Island	210	0.3%
19	South Carolina	1,430	1.7%
43	South Dakota	357	0.4%
16	Tennessee	1,757	2.1%
2	Texas	5,662	6.8%
36	Utah	625	0.8%
47	Vermont	275	0.3%
12	Virginia	2,294	2.8%
9	Washington	2,560	3.1%
34	West Virginia	665	0.8%
14	Wisconsin	2,168	2.6%
48	Wyoming	218	0.3%

RANK ORDER

RANK	STATE	PHYSICIANS	% of USA
1	California	9,979	12.0%
2	Texas	5,662	6.8%
3	Florida	4,448	5.4%
4	Pennsylvania	3,930	4.7%
5	New York	3,853	4.6%
6	Illinois	3,677	4.4%
7	Ohio	3,349	4.0%
8	Michigan	2,574	3.1%
9	Washington	2,560	3.1%
10	Minnesota	2,511	3.0%
11	North Carolina	2,458	3.0%
12	Virginia	2,294	2.8%
13	Indiana	2,275	2.7%
14	Wisconsin	2,168	2.6%
15	Georgia	1,979	2.4%
16	Tennessee	1,757	2.1%
17	New Jersey	1,606	1.9%
18	Colorado	1,550	1.9%
19	South Carolina	1,430	1.7%
20	Arizona	1,302	1.6%
21	Kentucky	1,274	1.5%
22	Maryland	1,264	1.5%
23	Alabama	1,242	1.5%
24	Louisiana	1,235	1.5%
25	Missouri	1,219	1.5%
26	Massachusetts	1,198	1.4%
27	Iowa	1,125	1.4%
28	Arkansas	1,122	1.4%
29	Oregon	1,093	1.3%
30	Kansas	1,067	1.3%
31	Oklahoma	989	1.2%
32	Nebraska	838	1.0%
33	Mississippi	741	0.9%
34	West Virginia	665	0.8%
35	New Mexico	635	0.8%
36	Utah	625	0.8%
37	Connecticut	592	0.7%
38	Maine	525	0.6%
39	Idaho	470	0.6%
40	Nevada	432	0.5%
41	New Hampshire	414	0.5%
42	Montana	362	0.4%
43	South Dakota	357	0.4%
44	North Dakota	344	0.4%
45	Hawaii	319	0.4%
46	Alaska	282	0.3%
47	Vermont	275	0.3%
48	Wyoming	218	0.3%
49	Delaware	217	0.3%
50	Rhode Island	210	0.3%
	District of Columbia	155	0.2%

Source: American Medical Association (Chicago, Illinois)
"Physician Characteristics and Distribution in the U.S." (2002-2003 Edition)
As of December 31, 2000. Total does not include 2,037 physicians in U.S. territories and possessions.

Rate of Nonfederal Physicians in General/Family Practice in 2000

National Rate = 29 Physicians per 100,000 Population*

ALPHA ORDER

RANK	STATE	RATE
32	Alabama	28
5	Alaska	45
41	Arizona	25
9	Arkansas	42
29	California	29
17	Colorado	36
50	Connecticut	17
32	Delaware	28
32	Florida	28
42	Georgia	24
38	Hawaii	26
17	Idaho	36
27	Illinois	30
15	Indiana	37
14	Iowa	38
11	Kansas	40
25	Kentucky	31
32	Louisiana	28
10	Maine	41
42	Maryland	24
48	Massachusetts	19
38	Michigan	26
2	Minnesota	51
38	Mississippi	26
44	Missouri	22
11	Montana	40
3	Nebraska	49
45	Nevada	21
21	New Hampshire	33
48	New Jersey	19
20	New Mexico	35
46	New York	20
27	North Carolina	30
1	North Dakota	54
29	Ohio	29
29	Oklahoma	29
22	Oregon	32
22	Pennsylvania	32
46	Rhode Island	20
17	South Carolina	36
4	South Dakota	47
25	Tennessee	31
37	Texas	27
32	Utah	28
5	Vermont	45
22	Virginia	32
8	Washington	43
15	West Virginia	37
11	Wisconsin	40
7	Wyoming	44

RANK ORDER

RANK	STATE	RATE
1	North Dakota	54
2	Minnesota	51
3	Nebraska	49
4	South Dakota	47
5	Alaska	45
5	Vermont	45
7	Wyoming	44
8	Washington	43
9	Arkansas	42
10	Maine	41
11	Kansas	40
11	Montana	40
11	Wisconsin	40
14	Iowa	38
15	Indiana	37
15	West Virginia	37
17	Colorado	36
17	Idaho	36
17	South Carolina	36
20	New Mexico	35
21	New Hampshire	33
22	Oregon	32
22	Pennsylvania	32
22	Virginia	32
25	Kentucky	31
25	Tennessee	31
27	Illinois	30
27	North Carolina	30
29	California	29
29	Ohio	29
29	Oklahoma	29
32	Alabama	28
32	Delaware	28
32	Florida	28
32	Louisiana	28
32	Utah	28
37	Texas	27
38	Hawaii	26
38	Michigan	26
38	Mississippi	26
41	Arizona	25
42	Georgia	24
42	Maryland	24
44	Missouri	22
45	Nevada	21
46	New York	20
46	Rhode Island	20
48	Massachusetts	19
48	New Jersey	19
50	Connecticut	17

District of Columbia	27

Source: Morgan Quitno Press using data from American Medical Association (Chicago, Illinois)
"Physician Characteristics and Distribution in the U.S." (2002-2003 Edition)
*As of December 31, 2000. National rate does not include physicians in U.S. territories and possessions.

Percent of Nonfederal Physicians Who Are Specialists in 2000

National Percent = 74.4% of Physicians*

ALPHA ORDER

RANK ORDER

RANK	STATE	PERCENT	RANK	STATE	PERCENT
14	Alabama	75.4	1	Connecticut	81.4
45	Alaska	64.9	2	Rhode Island	80.9
33	Arizona	69.8	3	New Jersey	80.6
42	Arkansas	66.9	4	Massachusetts	80.5
25	California	71.9	5	New York	80.1
28	Colorado	71.2	6	Maryland	79.2
1	Connecticut	81.4	7	Missouri	78.9
16	Delaware	74.7	8	Louisiana	77.6
35	Florida	69.6	9	Georgia	76.4
9	Georgia	76.4	10	Pennsylvania	76.1
13	Hawaii	75.6	11	Illinois	75.9
49	Idaho	62.6	12	Tennessee	75.7
11	Illinois	75.9	13	Hawaii	75.6
34	Indiana	69.7	14	Alabama	75.4
46	Iowa	63.7	15	Michigan	75.3
40	Kansas	67.4	16	Delaware	74.7
23	Kentucky	73.2	16	Ohio	74.7
8	Louisiana	77.6	18	Texas	74.6
38	Maine	68.1	19	North Carolina	73.8
6	Maryland	79.2	20	Nevada	73.5
4	Massachusetts	80.5	21	Utah	73.4
15	Michigan	75.3	21	Virginia	73.4
39	Minnesota	67.9	23	Kentucky	73.2
24	Mississippi	72.8	24	Mississippi	72.8
7	Missouri	78.9	25	California	71.9
44	Montana	65.6	26	South Carolina	71.8
43	Nebraska	66.2	27	New Hampshire	71.6
20	Nevada	73.5	28	Colorado	71.2
27	New Hampshire	71.6	29	Vermont	71.0
3	New Jersey	80.6	30	West Virginia	70.9
37	New Mexico	68.7	31	Wisconsin	70.6
5	New York	80.1	32	Oregon	69.9
19	North Carolina	73.8	33	Arizona	69.8
47	North Dakota	63.4	34	Indiana	69.7
16	Ohio	74.7	35	Florida	69.6
36	Oklahoma	69.2	36	Oklahoma	69.2
32	Oregon	69.9	37	New Mexico	68.7
10	Pennsylvania	76.1	38	Maine	68.1
2	Rhode Island	80.9	39	Minnesota	67.9
26	South Carolina	71.8	40	Kansas	67.4
47	South Dakota	63.4	41	Washington	67.0
12	Tennessee	75.7	42	Arkansas	66.9
18	Texas	74.6	43	Nebraska	66.2
21	Utah	73.4	44	Montana	65.6
29	Vermont	71.0	45	Alaska	64.9
21	Virginia	73.4	46	Iowa	63.7
41	Washington	67.0	47	North Dakota	63.4
30	West Virginia	70.9	47	South Dakota	63.4
31	Wisconsin	70.6	49	Idaho	62.6
50	Wyoming	60.8	50	Wyoming	60.8

District of Columbia   82.5

Source: Morgan Quitno Press using data from American Medical Association (Chicago, Illinois)
    "Physician Characteristics and Distribution in the U.S." (2002-2003 Edition)
*As of December 31, 2000. National percent does not include physicians in U.S. territories and possessions.
Includes physicians in medical, surgical and other specialties.

Nonfederal Physicians in Medical Specialties in 2000

National Total = 242,460 Physicians*

ALPHA ORDER

RANK	STATE	PHYSICIANS	% of USA
25	Alabama	3,026	1.2%
49	Alaska	258	0.1%
23	Arizona	3,175	1.3%
32	Arkansas	1,389	0.6%
2	California	28,061	11.6%
24	Colorado	3,077	1.3%
15	Connecticut	4,816	2.0%
44	Delaware	617	0.3%
4	Florida	12,987	5.4%
14	Georgia	5,626	2.3%
38	Hawaii	1,139	0.5%
46	Idaho	441	0.2%
6	Illinois	11,891	4.9%
22	Indiana	3,496	1.4%
35	Iowa	1,351	0.6%
30	Kansas	1,576	0.7%
26	Kentucky	2,649	1.1%
21	Louisiana	3,694	1.5%
42	Maine	899	0.4%
11	Maryland	7,571	3.1%
7	Massachusetts	10,594	4.4%
10	Michigan	7,825	3.2%
19	Minnesota	3,949	1.6%
33	Mississippi	1,385	0.6%
17	Missouri	4,599	1.9%
45	Montana	459	0.2%
40	Nebraska	1,042	0.4%
39	Nevada	1,136	0.5%
41	New Hampshire	923	0.4%
8	New Jersey	10,320	4.3%
37	New Mexico	1,159	0.5%
1	New York	28,756	11.9%
12	North Carolina	6,130	2.5%
48	North Dakota	361	0.1%
9	Ohio	9,251	3.8%
29	Oklahoma	1,700	0.7%
28	Oregon	2,443	1.0%
5	Pennsylvania	12,203	5.0%
31	Rhode Island	1,434	0.6%
27	South Carolina	2,466	1.0%
47	South Dakota	367	0.2%
16	Tennessee	4,684	1.9%
3	Texas	13,173	5.4%
34	Utah	1,352	0.6%
43	Vermont	653	0.3%
13	Virginia	5,719	2.4%
18	Washington	4,066	1.7%
36	West Virginia	1,185	0.5%
20	Wisconsin	3,786	1.6%
50	Wyoming	164	0.1%

RANK ORDER

RANK	STATE	PHYSICIANS	% of USA
1	New York	28,756	11.9%
2	California	28,061	11.6%
3	Texas	13,173	5.4%
4	Florida	12,987	5.4%
5	Pennsylvania	12,203	5.0%
6	Illinois	11,891	4.9%
7	Massachusetts	10,594	4.4%
8	New Jersey	10,320	4.3%
9	Ohio	9,251	3.8%
10	Michigan	7,825	3.2%
11	Maryland	7,571	3.1%
12	North Carolina	6,130	2.5%
13	Virginia	5,719	2.4%
14	Georgia	5,626	2.3%
15	Connecticut	4,816	2.0%
16	Tennessee	4,684	1.9%
17	Missouri	4,599	1.9%
18	Washington	4,066	1.7%
19	Minnesota	3,949	1.6%
20	Wisconsin	3,786	1.6%
21	Louisiana	3,694	1.5%
22	Indiana	3,496	1.4%
23	Arizona	3,175	1.3%
24	Colorado	3,077	1.3%
25	Alabama	3,026	1.2%
26	Kentucky	2,649	1.1%
27	South Carolina	2,466	1.0%
28	Oregon	2,443	1.0%
29	Oklahoma	1,700	0.7%
30	Kansas	1,576	0.7%
31	Rhode Island	1,434	0.6%
32	Arkansas	1,389	0.6%
33	Mississippi	1,385	0.6%
34	Utah	1,352	0.6%
35	Iowa	1,351	0.6%
36	West Virginia	1,185	0.5%
37	New Mexico	1,159	0.5%
38	Hawaii	1,139	0.5%
39	Nevada	1,136	0.5%
40	Nebraska	1,042	0.4%
41	New Hampshire	923	0.4%
42	Maine	899	0.4%
43	Vermont	653	0.3%
44	Delaware	617	0.3%
45	Montana	459	0.2%
46	Idaho	441	0.2%
47	South Dakota	367	0.2%
48	North Dakota	361	0.1%
49	Alaska	258	0.1%
50	Wyoming	164	0.1%
	District of Columbia	1,437	0.6%

Source: American Medical Association (Chicago, Illinois)
  "Physician Characteristics and Distribution in the U.S." (2002-2003 Edition)
*As of December 31, 2000. Total does not include 2,816 physicians in U.S. territories and possessions. Medical Specialties are Allergy/Immunology, Cardiovascular Diseases, Dermatology, Gastroenterology, Internal Medicine, Pediatrics, Pediatric Cardiology and Pulmonary Diseases.

Rate of Nonfederal Physicians in Medical Specialties in 2000

National Rate = 86 Physicians per 100,000 Population*

ALPHA ORDER

RANK ORDER

RANK	STATE	RATE
28	Alabama	68
48	Alaska	41
34	Arizona	61
42	Arkansas	52
11	California	83
23	Colorado	71
4	Connecticut	141
20	Delaware	78
15	Florida	81
28	Georgia	68
10	Hawaii	94
49	Idaho	34
9	Illinois	96
39	Indiana	57
47	Iowa	46
38	Kansas	59
31	Kentucky	65
11	Louisiana	83
25	Maine	70
3	Maryland	143
1	Massachusetts	167
19	Michigan	79
18	Minnesota	80
44	Mississippi	49
13	Missouri	82
43	Montana	51
34	Nebraska	61
40	Nevada	56
22	New Hampshire	74
6	New Jersey	122
32	New Mexico	64
2	New York	151
21	North Carolina	76
40	North Dakota	56
15	Ohio	81
44	Oklahoma	49
23	Oregon	71
8	Pennsylvania	99
5	Rhode Island	137
34	South Carolina	61
44	South Dakota	49
13	Tennessee	82
33	Texas	63
37	Utah	60
7	Vermont	107
15	Virginia	81
27	Washington	69
30	West Virginia	66
25	Wisconsin	70
50	Wyoming	33

RANK	STATE	RATE
1	Massachusetts	167
2	New York	151
3	Maryland	143
4	Connecticut	141
5	Rhode Island	137
6	New Jersey	122
7	Vermont	107
8	Pennsylvania	99
9	Illinois	96
10	Hawaii	94
11	California	83
11	Louisiana	83
13	Missouri	82
13	Tennessee	82
15	Florida	81
15	Ohio	81
15	Virginia	81
18	Minnesota	80
19	Michigan	79
20	Delaware	78
21	North Carolina	76
22	New Hampshire	74
23	Colorado	71
23	Oregon	71
25	Maine	70
25	Wisconsin	70
27	Washington	69
28	Alabama	68
28	Georgia	68
30	West Virginia	66
31	Kentucky	65
32	New Mexico	64
33	Texas	63
34	Arizona	61
34	Nebraska	61
34	South Carolina	61
37	Utah	60
38	Kansas	59
39	Indiana	57
40	Nevada	56
40	North Dakota	56
42	Arkansas	52
43	Montana	51
44	Mississippi	49
44	Oklahoma	49
44	South Dakota	49
47	Iowa	46
48	Alaska	41
49	Idaho	34
50	Wyoming	33

| | District of Columbia | 252 |

Source: Morgan Quitno Press using data from American Medical Association (Chicago, Illinois)
    "Physician Characteristics and Distribution in the U.S." (2002-2003 Edition)

*As of December 31, 2000. National rate does not include physicians in U.S. territories and possessions. Medical Specialties are Allergy/Immunology, Cardiovascular Diseases, Dermatology, Gastroenterology, Internal Medicine, Pediatrics, Pediatric Cardiology and Pulmonary Diseases.

Nonfederal Physicians in Internal Medicine in 2000

National Total = 128,409 Physicians*

ALPHA ORDER

RANK	STATE	PHYSICIANS	% of USA
23	Alabama	1,631	1.3%
49	Alaska	124	0.1%
25	Arizona	1,548	1.2%
38	Arkansas	594	0.5%
2	California	14,686	11.4%
24	Colorado	1,565	1.2%
15	Connecticut	2,797	2.2%
44	Delaware	297	0.2%
6	Florida	6,303	4.9%
14	Georgia	2,955	2.3%
34	Hawaii	631	0.5%
47	Idaho	207	0.2%
3	Illinois	6,704	5.2%
22	Indiana	1,722	1.3%
36	Iowa	621	0.5%
30	Kansas	825	0.6%
27	Kentucky	1,294	1.0%
21	Louisiana	1,811	1.4%
41	Maine	489	0.4%
11	Maryland	4,202	3.3%
7	Massachusetts	6,154	4.8%
10	Michigan	4,291	3.3%
19	Minnesota	2,127	1.7%
32	Mississippi	706	0.5%
16	Missouri	2,433	1.9%
45	Montana	247	0.2%
40	Nebraska	504	0.4%
35	Nevada	625	0.5%
42	New Hampshire	476	0.4%
8	New Jersey	5,476	4.3%
37	New Mexico	600	0.5%
1	New York	16,322	12.7%
12	North Carolina	3,062	2.4%
46	North Dakota	213	0.2%
9	Ohio	4,706	3.7%
29	Oklahoma	866	0.7%
26	Oregon	1,433	1.1%
4	Pennsylvania	6,637	5.2%
31	Rhode Island	790	0.6%
28	South Carolina	1,209	0.9%
48	South Dakota	204	0.2%
17	Tennessee	2,379	1.9%
5	Texas	6,345	4.9%
39	Utah	577	0.4%
43	Vermont	364	0.3%
13	Virginia	2,989	2.3%
18	Washington	2,150	1.7%
33	West Virginia	638	0.5%
20	Wisconsin	2,021	1.6%
50	Wyoming	85	0.1%

RANK ORDER

RANK	STATE	PHYSICIANS	% of USA
1	New York	16,322	12.7%
2	California	14,686	11.4%
3	Illinois	6,704	5.2%
4	Pennsylvania	6,637	5.2%
5	Texas	6,345	4.9%
6	Florida	6,303	4.9%
7	Massachusetts	6,154	4.8%
8	New Jersey	5,476	4.3%
9	Ohio	4,706	3.7%
10	Michigan	4,291	3.3%
11	Maryland	4,202	3.3%
12	North Carolina	3,062	2.4%
13	Virginia	2,989	2.3%
14	Georgia	2,955	2.3%
15	Connecticut	2,797	2.2%
16	Missouri	2,433	1.9%
17	Tennessee	2,379	1.9%
18	Washington	2,150	1.7%
19	Minnesota	2,127	1.7%
20	Wisconsin	2,021	1.6%
21	Louisiana	1,811	1.4%
22	Indiana	1,722	1.3%
23	Alabama	1,631	1.3%
24	Colorado	1,565	1.2%
25	Arizona	1,548	1.2%
26	Oregon	1,433	1.1%
27	Kentucky	1,294	1.0%
28	South Carolina	1,209	0.9%
29	Oklahoma	866	0.7%
30	Kansas	825	0.6%
31	Rhode Island	790	0.6%
32	Mississippi	706	0.5%
33	West Virginia	638	0.5%
34	Hawaii	631	0.5%
35	Nevada	625	0.5%
36	Iowa	621	0.5%
37	New Mexico	600	0.5%
38	Arkansas	594	0.5%
39	Utah	577	0.4%
40	Nebraska	504	0.4%
41	Maine	489	0.4%
42	New Hampshire	476	0.4%
43	Vermont	364	0.3%
44	Delaware	297	0.2%
45	Montana	247	0.2%
46	North Dakota	213	0.2%
47	Idaho	207	0.2%
48	South Dakota	204	0.2%
49	Alaska	124	0.1%
50	Wyoming	85	0.1%
	District of Columbia	774	0.6%

Source: American Medical Association (Chicago, Illinois)
   "Physician Characteristics and Distribution in the U.S." (2002-2003 Edition)
*As of December 31, 2000. Total does not include 1,284 physicians in U.S. territories and possessions. Internal Medicine includes Diabetes, Endocrinology, Geriatrics, Hematology, Infectious Diseases, Nephrology, Nutrition, Medical Oncology and Rheumatology.

Rate of Nonfederal Physicians in Internal Medicine in 2000

National Rate = 46 Physicians per 100,000 Population*

ALPHA ORDER

RANK	STATE	RATE
26	Alabama	37
48	Alaska	20
36	Arizona	30
46	Arkansas	22
11	California	43
27	Colorado	36
3	Connecticut	82
21	Delaware	38
20	Florida	39
27	Georgia	36
10	Hawaii	52
50	Idaho	16
8	Illinois	54
40	Indiana	28
47	Iowa	21
34	Kansas	31
33	Kentucky	32
18	Louisiana	41
21	Maine	38
4	Maryland	79
1	Massachusetts	97
11	Michigan	43
11	Minnesota	43
44	Mississippi	25
11	Missouri	43
41	Montana	27
39	Nebraska	29
34	Nevada	31
21	New Hampshire	38
6	New Jersey	65
31	New Mexico	33
2	New York	86
21	North Carolina	38
31	North Dakota	33
18	Ohio	41
44	Oklahoma	25
15	Oregon	42
8	Pennsylvania	54
5	Rhode Island	75
36	South Carolina	30
41	South Dakota	27
15	Tennessee	42
36	Texas	30
43	Utah	26
7	Vermont	60
15	Virginia	42
27	Washington	36
30	West Virginia	35
21	Wisconsin	38
49	Wyoming	17

RANK ORDER

RANK	STATE	RATE
1	Massachusetts	97
2	New York	86
3	Connecticut	82
4	Maryland	79
5	Rhode Island	75
6	New Jersey	65
7	Vermont	60
8	Illinois	54
8	Pennsylvania	54
10	Hawaii	52
11	California	43
11	Michigan	43
11	Minnesota	43
11	Missouri	43
15	Oregon	42
15	Tennessee	42
15	Virginia	42
18	Louisiana	41
18	Ohio	41
20	Florida	39
21	Delaware	38
21	Maine	38
21	New Hampshire	38
21	North Carolina	38
21	Wisconsin	38
26	Alabama	37
27	Colorado	36
27	Georgia	36
27	Washington	36
30	West Virginia	35
31	New Mexico	33
31	North Dakota	33
33	Kentucky	32
34	Kansas	31
34	Nevada	31
36	Arizona	30
36	South Carolina	30
36	Texas	30
39	Nebraska	29
40	Indiana	28
41	Montana	27
41	South Dakota	27
43	Utah	26
44	Mississippi	25
44	Oklahoma	25
46	Arkansas	22
47	Iowa	21
48	Alaska	20
49	Wyoming	17
50	Idaho	16

| | District of Columbia | 136 |

Source: Morgan Quitno Press using data from American Medical Association (Chicago, Illinois)
"Physician Characteristics and Distribution in the U.S." (2002-2003 Edition)

*As of December 31, 2000. National rate does not include physicians in U.S. territories and possessions. Internal Medicine includes Diabetes, Endocrinology, Geriatrics, Hematology, Infectious Diseases, Nephrology, Nutrition, Medical Oncology and Rheumatology.

Nonfederal Physicians in Pediatrics in 2000

National Total = 60,456 Physicians*

<table>
<tr><td colspan="4">ALPHA ORDER</td><td colspan="4">RANK ORDER</td></tr>
<tr><td>RANK</td><td>STATE</td><td>PHYSICIANS</td><td>% of USA</td><td>RANK</td><td>STATE</td><td>PHYSICIANS</td><td>% of USA</td></tr>
<tr><td>26</td><td>Alabama</td><td>729</td><td>1.2%</td><td>1</td><td>California</td><td>7,237</td><td>12.0%</td></tr>
<tr><td>47</td><td>Alaska</td><td>92</td><td>0.2%</td><td>2</td><td>New York</td><td>6,887</td><td>11.4%</td></tr>
<tr><td>23</td><td>Arizona</td><td>835</td><td>1.4%</td><td>3</td><td>Texas</td><td>3,675</td><td>6.1%</td></tr>
<tr><td>30</td><td>Arkansas</td><td>425</td><td>0.7%</td><td>4</td><td>Florida</td><td>3,068</td><td>5.1%</td></tr>
<tr><td>1</td><td>California</td><td>7,237</td><td>12.0%</td><td>5</td><td>Illinois</td><td>2,837</td><td>4.7%</td></tr>
<tr><td>24</td><td>Colorado</td><td>792</td><td>1.3%</td><td>6</td><td>New Jersey</td><td>2,626</td><td>4.3%</td></tr>
<tr><td>17</td><td>Connecticut</td><td>1,022</td><td>1.7%</td><td>7</td><td>Pennsylvania</td><td>2,621</td><td>4.3%</td></tr>
<tr><td>43</td><td>Delaware</td><td>195</td><td>0.3%</td><td>8</td><td>Ohio</td><td>2,553</td><td>4.2%</td></tr>
<tr><td>4</td><td>Florida</td><td>3,068</td><td>5.1%</td><td>9</td><td>Massachusetts</td><td>2,339</td><td>3.9%</td></tr>
<tr><td>14</td><td>Georgia</td><td>1,452</td><td>2.4%</td><td>10</td><td>Michigan</td><td>1,924</td><td>3.2%</td></tr>
<tr><td>36</td><td>Hawaii</td><td>322</td><td>0.5%</td><td>11</td><td>Maryland</td><td>1,855</td><td>3.1%</td></tr>
<tr><td>45</td><td>Idaho</td><td>99</td><td>0.2%</td><td>12</td><td>North Carolina</td><td>1,620</td><td>2.7%</td></tr>
<tr><td>5</td><td>Illinois</td><td>2,837</td><td>4.7%</td><td>13</td><td>Virginia</td><td>1,508</td><td>2.5%</td></tr>
<tr><td>21</td><td>Indiana</td><td>894</td><td>1.5%</td><td>14</td><td>Georgia</td><td>1,452</td><td>2.4%</td></tr>
<tr><td>35</td><td>Iowa</td><td>340</td><td>0.6%</td><td>15</td><td>Tennessee</td><td>1,273</td><td>2.1%</td></tr>
<tr><td>32</td><td>Kansas</td><td>395</td><td>0.7%</td><td>16</td><td>Missouri</td><td>1,111</td><td>1.8%</td></tr>
<tr><td>25</td><td>Kentucky</td><td>737</td><td>1.2%</td><td>17</td><td>Connecticut</td><td>1,022</td><td>1.7%</td></tr>
<tr><td>19</td><td>Louisiana</td><td>1,006</td><td>1.7%</td><td>18</td><td>Washington</td><td>1,015</td><td>1.7%</td></tr>
<tr><td>42</td><td>Maine</td><td>212</td><td>0.4%</td><td>19</td><td>Louisiana</td><td>1,006</td><td>1.7%</td></tr>
<tr><td>11</td><td>Maryland</td><td>1,855</td><td>3.1%</td><td>20</td><td>Wisconsin</td><td>943</td><td>1.6%</td></tr>
<tr><td>9</td><td>Massachusetts</td><td>2,339</td><td>3.9%</td><td>21</td><td>Indiana</td><td>894</td><td>1.5%</td></tr>
<tr><td>10</td><td>Michigan</td><td>1,924</td><td>3.2%</td><td>22</td><td>Minnesota</td><td>889</td><td>1.5%</td></tr>
<tr><td>22</td><td>Minnesota</td><td>889</td><td>1.5%</td><td>23</td><td>Arizona</td><td>835</td><td>1.4%</td></tr>
<tr><td>34</td><td>Mississippi</td><td>356</td><td>0.6%</td><td>24</td><td>Colorado</td><td>792</td><td>1.3%</td></tr>
<tr><td>16</td><td>Missouri</td><td>1,111</td><td>1.8%</td><td>25</td><td>Kentucky</td><td>737</td><td>1.2%</td></tr>
<tr><td>46</td><td>Montana</td><td>94</td><td>0.2%</td><td>26</td><td>Alabama</td><td>729</td><td>1.2%</td></tr>
<tr><td>39</td><td>Nebraska</td><td>283</td><td>0.5%</td><td>27</td><td>South Carolina</td><td>640</td><td>1.1%</td></tr>
<tr><td>41</td><td>Nevada</td><td>229</td><td>0.4%</td><td>28</td><td>Oregon</td><td>519</td><td>0.9%</td></tr>
<tr><td>40</td><td>New Hampshire</td><td>233</td><td>0.4%</td><td>29</td><td>Utah</td><td>429</td><td>0.7%</td></tr>
<tr><td>6</td><td>New Jersey</td><td>2,626</td><td>4.3%</td><td>30</td><td>Arkansas</td><td>425</td><td>0.7%</td></tr>
<tr><td>37</td><td>New Mexico</td><td>305</td><td>0.5%</td><td>31</td><td>Oklahoma</td><td>417</td><td>0.7%</td></tr>
<tr><td>2</td><td>New York</td><td>6,887</td><td>11.4%</td><td>32</td><td>Kansas</td><td>395</td><td>0.7%</td></tr>
<tr><td>12</td><td>North Carolina</td><td>1,620</td><td>2.7%</td><td>33</td><td>Rhode Island</td><td>362</td><td>0.6%</td></tr>
<tr><td>48</td><td>North Dakota</td><td>78</td><td>0.1%</td><td>34</td><td>Mississippi</td><td>356</td><td>0.6%</td></tr>
<tr><td>8</td><td>Ohio</td><td>2,553</td><td>4.2%</td><td>35</td><td>Iowa</td><td>340</td><td>0.6%</td></tr>
<tr><td>31</td><td>Oklahoma</td><td>417</td><td>0.7%</td><td>36</td><td>Hawaii</td><td>322</td><td>0.5%</td></tr>
<tr><td>28</td><td>Oregon</td><td>519</td><td>0.9%</td><td>37</td><td>New Mexico</td><td>305</td><td>0.5%</td></tr>
<tr><td>7</td><td>Pennsylvania</td><td>2,621</td><td>4.3%</td><td>38</td><td>West Virginia</td><td>304</td><td>0.5%</td></tr>
<tr><td>33</td><td>Rhode Island</td><td>362</td><td>0.6%</td><td>39</td><td>Nebraska</td><td>283</td><td>0.5%</td></tr>
<tr><td>27</td><td>South Carolina</td><td>640</td><td>1.1%</td><td>40</td><td>New Hampshire</td><td>233</td><td>0.4%</td></tr>
<tr><td>49</td><td>South Dakota</td><td>68</td><td>0.1%</td><td>41</td><td>Nevada</td><td>229</td><td>0.4%</td></tr>
<tr><td>15</td><td>Tennessee</td><td>1,273</td><td>2.1%</td><td>42</td><td>Maine</td><td>212</td><td>0.4%</td></tr>
<tr><td>3</td><td>Texas</td><td>3,675</td><td>6.1%</td><td>43</td><td>Delaware</td><td>195</td><td>0.3%</td></tr>
<tr><td>29</td><td>Utah</td><td>429</td><td>0.7%</td><td>44</td><td>Vermont</td><td>181</td><td>0.3%</td></tr>
<tr><td>44</td><td>Vermont</td><td>181</td><td>0.3%</td><td>45</td><td>Idaho</td><td>99</td><td>0.2%</td></tr>
<tr><td>13</td><td>Virginia</td><td>1,508</td><td>2.5%</td><td>46</td><td>Montana</td><td>94</td><td>0.2%</td></tr>
<tr><td>18</td><td>Washington</td><td>1,015</td><td>1.7%</td><td>47</td><td>Alaska</td><td>92</td><td>0.2%</td></tr>
<tr><td>38</td><td>West Virginia</td><td>304</td><td>0.5%</td><td>48</td><td>North Dakota</td><td>78</td><td>0.1%</td></tr>
<tr><td>20</td><td>Wisconsin</td><td>943</td><td>1.6%</td><td>49</td><td>South Dakota</td><td>68</td><td>0.1%</td></tr>
<tr><td>50</td><td>Wyoming</td><td>44</td><td>0.1%</td><td>50</td><td>Wyoming</td><td>44</td><td>0.1%</td></tr>
<tr><td></td><td></td><td></td><td></td><td></td><td>District of Columbia</td><td>386</td><td>0.6%</td></tr>
</table>

Source: American Medical Association (Chicago, Illinois)
    "Physician Characteristics and Distribution in the U.S." (2002-2003 Edition)
*As of December 31, 2000. Total does not include 1,019 physicians in U.S. territories and possessions. Pediatrics includes Adolescent Medicine, Neonatal-Perinatal, Pediatric Allergy, Pediatric Endocrinology, Pediatric Pulmonology, Pediatric Hematology-Oncology and Pediatric Nephrology.

Rate of Nonfederal Physicians in Pediatrics in 2000

National Rate = 84 Physicians per 100,000 Population 17 Years and Younger*

ALPHA ORDER

RANK	STATE	RATE
30	Alabama	65
41	Alaska	48
35	Arizona	61
33	Arkansas	62
18	California	78
24	Colorado	72
7	Connecticut	121
9	Delaware	100
15	Florida	84
28	Georgia	67
8	Hawaii	109
50	Idaho	27
13	Illinois	87
39	Indiana	57
44	Iowa	46
40	Kansas	55
22	Kentucky	74
16	Louisiana	82
25	Maine	70
4	Maryland	137
1	Massachusetts	156
22	Michigan	74
26	Minnesota	69
44	Mississippi	46
18	Missouri	78
47	Montana	41
31	Nebraska	63
46	Nevada	45
21	New Hampshire	75
5	New Jersey	126
37	New Mexico	60
2	New York	147
16	North Carolina	82
41	North Dakota	48
12	Ohio	88
43	Oklahoma	47
35	Oregon	61
11	Pennsylvania	90
3	Rhode Island	146
31	South Carolina	63
48	South Dakota	34
10	Tennessee	91
33	Texas	62
37	Utah	60
6	Vermont	123
13	Virginia	87
28	Washington	67
20	West Virginia	76
26	Wisconsin	69
48	Wyoming	34

RANK ORDER

RANK	STATE	RATE
1	Massachusetts	156
2	New York	147
3	Rhode Island	146
4	Maryland	137
5	New Jersey	126
6	Vermont	123
7	Connecticut	121
8	Hawaii	109
9	Delaware	100
10	Tennessee	91
11	Pennsylvania	90
12	Ohio	88
13	Illinois	87
13	Virginia	87
15	Florida	84
16	Louisiana	82
16	North Carolina	82
18	California	78
18	Missouri	78
20	West Virginia	76
21	New Hampshire	75
22	Kentucky	74
22	Michigan	74
24	Colorado	72
25	Maine	70
26	Minnesota	69
26	Wisconsin	69
28	Georgia	67
28	Washington	67
30	Alabama	65
31	Nebraska	63
31	South Carolina	63
33	Arkansas	62
33	Texas	62
35	Arizona	61
35	Oregon	61
37	New Mexico	60
37	Utah	60
39	Indiana	57
40	Kansas	55
41	Alaska	48
41	North Dakota	48
43	Oklahoma	47
44	Iowa	46
44	Mississippi	46
46	Nevada	45
47	Montana	41
48	South Dakota	34
48	Wyoming	34
50	Idaho	27

District of Columbia	336

Source: Morgan Quitno Press using data from American Medical Association (Chicago, Illinois)
    "Physician Characteristics and Distribution in the U.S." (2002-2003 Edition)
*As of December 31, 2000. National rate does not include physicians in U.S. territories and possessions. Pediatrics includes Adolescent Medicine, Neonatal-Perinatal, Pediatric Allergy, Pediatric Endocrinology, Pediatric Pulmonology, Pediatric Hematology-Oncology and Pediatric Nephrology.

Nonfederal Physicians in Surgical Specialties in 2000

National Total = 149,873 Physicians*

ALPHA ORDER				RANK ORDER			
RANK	STATE	PHYSICIANS	% of USA	RANK	STATE	PHYSICIANS	% of USA
24	Alabama	2,176	1.5%	1	California	17,211	11.5%
49	Alaska	240	0.2%	2	New York	13,763	9.2%
23	Arizona	2,247	1.5%	3	Texas	9,526	6.4%
33	Arkansas	1,094	0.7%	4	Florida	8,497	5.7%
1	California	17,211	11.5%	5	Pennsylvania	7,503	5.0%
25	Colorado	2,128	1.4%	6	Illinois	6,446	4.3%
21	Connecticut	2,458	1.6%	7	Ohio	5,907	3.9%
45	Delaware	398	0.3%	8	New Jersey	5,211	3.5%
4	Florida	8,497	5.7%	9	Michigan	4,780	3.2%
12	Georgia	4,077	2.7%	10	Massachusetts	4,532	3.0%
39	Hawaii	726	0.5%	11	North Carolina	4,247	2.8%
43	Idaho	531	0.4%	12	Georgia	4,077	2.7%
6	Illinois	6,446	4.3%	13	Maryland	3,887	2.6%
20	Indiana	2,519	1.7%	14	Virginia	3,862	2.6%
32	Iowa	1,111	0.7%	15	Tennessee	3,240	2.2%
31	Kansas	1,178	0.8%	16	Missouri	2,928	2.0%
27	Kentucky	1,930	1.3%	17	Washington	2,805	1.9%
18	Louisiana	2,796	1.9%	18	Louisiana	2,796	1.9%
42	Maine	622	0.4%	19	Wisconsin	2,528	1.7%
13	Maryland	3,887	2.6%	20	Indiana	2,519	1.7%
10	Massachusetts	4,532	3.0%	21	Connecticut	2,458	1.6%
9	Michigan	4,780	3.2%	22	Minnesota	2,397	1.6%
22	Minnesota	2,397	1.6%	23	Arizona	2,247	1.5%
30	Mississippi	1,214	0.8%	24	Alabama	2,176	1.5%
16	Missouri	2,928	2.0%	25	Colorado	2,128	1.4%
44	Montana	431	0.3%	26	South Carolina	2,050	1.4%
36	Nebraska	842	0.6%	27	Kentucky	1,930	1.3%
37	Nevada	797	0.5%	28	Oregon	1,704	1.1%
41	New Hampshire	657	0.4%	29	Oklahoma	1,266	0.8%
8	New Jersey	5,211	3.5%	30	Mississippi	1,214	0.8%
38	New Mexico	744	0.5%	31	Kansas	1,178	0.8%
2	New York	13,763	9.2%	32	Iowa	1,111	0.7%
11	North Carolina	4,247	2.8%	33	Arkansas	1,094	0.7%
48	North Dakota	284	0.2%	34	Utah	1,050	0.7%
7	Ohio	5,907	3.9%	35	West Virginia	880	0.6%
29	Oklahoma	1,266	0.8%	36	Nebraska	842	0.6%
28	Oregon	1,704	1.1%	37	Nevada	797	0.5%
5	Pennsylvania	7,503	5.0%	38	New Mexico	744	0.5%
40	Rhode Island	721	0.5%	39	Hawaii	726	0.5%
26	South Carolina	2,050	1.4%	40	Rhode Island	721	0.5%
47	South Dakota	322	0.2%	41	New Hampshire	657	0.4%
15	Tennessee	3,240	2.2%	42	Maine	622	0.4%
3	Texas	9,526	6.4%	43	Idaho	531	0.4%
34	Utah	1,050	0.7%	44	Montana	431	0.3%
46	Vermont	387	0.3%	45	Delaware	398	0.3%
14	Virginia	3,862	2.6%	46	Vermont	387	0.3%
17	Washington	2,805	1.9%	47	South Dakota	322	0.2%
35	West Virginia	880	0.6%	48	North Dakota	284	0.2%
19	Wisconsin	2,528	1.7%	49	Alaska	240	0.2%
50	Wyoming	213	0.1%	50	Wyoming	213	0.1%
					District of Columbia	810	0.5%

Source: American Medical Association (Chicago, Illinois)
    "Physician Characteristics and Distribution in the U.S." (2002-2003 Edition)
*As of December 31, 2000. Total does not include 1,575 physicians in U.S. territories and possessions. Surgical Specialties include Colon and Rectal, General, Neurological, Obstetrics & Gynecology, Ophthalmology, Orthopedic, Otolaryngology, Plastic, Thoracic and Urological Surgeries.

Rate of Nonfederal Physicians in Surgical Specialties in 2000

National Rate = 53 Physicians per 100,000 Population*

ALPHA ORDER

RANK	STATE	RATE
24	Alabama	49
48	Alaska	38
37	Arizona	44
43	Arkansas	41
19	California	51
24	Colorado	49
2	Connecticut	72
19	Delaware	51
13	Florida	53
22	Georgia	50
10	Hawaii	60
43	Idaho	41
16	Illinois	52
43	Indiana	41
48	Iowa	38
37	Kansas	44
30	Kentucky	48
6	Louisiana	63
24	Maine	49
1	Maryland	73
4	Massachusetts	71
30	Michigan	48
24	Minnesota	49
40	Mississippi	43
16	Missouri	52
30	Montana	48
24	Nebraska	49
47	Nevada	39
13	New Hampshire	53
8	New Jersey	62
43	New Mexico	41
2	New York	72
13	North Carolina	53
37	North Dakota	44
16	Ohio	52
50	Oklahoma	37
22	Oregon	50
9	Pennsylvania	61
5	Rhode Island	69
19	South Carolina	51
40	South Dakota	43
11	Tennessee	57
36	Texas	45
33	Utah	47
6	Vermont	63
12	Virginia	54
33	Washington	47
24	West Virginia	49
33	Wisconsin	47
40	Wyoming	43

RANK ORDER

RANK	STATE	RATE
1	Maryland	73
2	Connecticut	72
2	New York	72
4	Massachusetts	71
5	Rhode Island	69
6	Louisiana	63
6	Vermont	63
8	New Jersey	62
9	Pennsylvania	61
10	Hawaii	60
11	Tennessee	57
12	Virginia	54
13	Florida	53
13	New Hampshire	53
13	North Carolina	53
16	Illinois	52
16	Missouri	52
16	Ohio	52
19	California	51
19	Delaware	51
19	South Carolina	51
22	Georgia	50
22	Oregon	50
24	Alabama	49
24	Colorado	49
24	Maine	49
24	Minnesota	49
24	Nebraska	49
24	West Virginia	49
30	Kentucky	48
30	Michigan	48
30	Montana	48
33	Utah	47
33	Washington	47
33	Wisconsin	47
36	Texas	45
37	Arizona	44
37	Kansas	44
37	North Dakota	44
40	Mississippi	43
40	South Dakota	43
40	Wyoming	43
43	Arkansas	41
43	Idaho	41
43	Indiana	41
43	New Mexico	41
47	Nevada	39
48	Alaska	38
48	Iowa	38
50	Oklahoma	37

District of Columbia   142

Source: Morgan Quitno Press using data from American Medical Association (Chicago, Illinois)
   "Physician Characteristics and Distribution in the U.S." (2002-2003 Edition)

*As of December 31, 2000. National rate does not include physicians in U.S. territories and possessions. Surgical Specialties include Colon and Rectal, General, Neurological, Obstetrics & Gynecology, Ophthalmology, Orthopedic, Otolaryngology, Plastic, Thoracic and Urological Surgeries.

Nonfederal Physicians in General Surgery in 2000

National Total = 35,528 Physicians*

ALPHA ORDER					RANK ORDER			
RANK	STATE		PHYSICIANS	% of USA	RANK	STATE	PHYSICIANS	% of USA
25	Alabama		504	1.4%	1	California	3,603	10.2%
49	Alaska		51	0.1%	2	New York	3,522	10.0%
23	Arizona		521	1.5%	3	Texas	2,138	6.1%
33	Arkansas		258	0.7%	4	Pennsylvania	1,926	5.5%
1	California		3,603	10.2%	5	Florida	1,717	4.9%
27	Colorado		464	1.3%	6	Illinois	1,557	4.4%
20	Connecticut		562	1.6%	7	Ohio	1,495	4.2%
45	Delaware		102	0.3%	8	New Jersey	1,236	3.5%
5	Florida		1,717	4.9%	9	Michigan	1,212	3.4%
12	Georgia		945	2.7%	10	Massachusetts	1,195	3.4%
41	Hawaii		162	0.5%	11	North Carolina	991	2.8%
43	Idaho		123	0.3%	12	Georgia	945	2.7%
6	Illinois		1,557	4.4%	13	Maryland	912	2.6%
21	Indiana		557	1.6%	14	Virginia	899	2.5%
32	Iowa		281	0.8%	15	Tennessee	798	2.3%
29	Kansas		299	0.8%	16	Missouri	700	2.0%
26	Kentucky		497	1.4%	17	Louisiana	646	1.8%
17	Louisiana		646	1.8%	18	Washington	601	1.7%
42	Maine		161	0.5%	19	Wisconsin	596	1.7%
13	Maryland		912	2.6%	20	Connecticut	562	1.6%
10	Massachusetts		1,195	3.4%	21	Indiana	557	1.6%
9	Michigan		1,212	3.4%	22	Minnesota	551	1.6%
22	Minnesota		551	1.6%	23	Arizona	521	1.5%
30	Mississippi		291	0.8%	24	South Carolina	508	1.4%
16	Missouri		700	2.0%	25	Alabama	504	1.4%
46	Montana		91	0.3%	26	Kentucky	497	1.4%
35	Nebraska		228	0.6%	27	Colorado	464	1.3%
40	Nevada		168	0.5%	28	Oregon	371	1.1%
39	New Hampshire		170	0.5%	29	Kansas	299	0.8%
8	New Jersey		1,236	3.5%	30	Mississippi	291	0.8%
37	New Mexico		188	0.5%	31	Oklahoma	286	0.8%
2	New York		3,522	10.0%	32	Iowa	281	0.8%
11	North Carolina		991	2.8%	33	Arkansas	258	0.7%
48	North Dakota		78	0.2%	34	West Virginia	251	0.7%
7	Ohio		1,495	4.2%	35	Nebraska	228	0.6%
31	Oklahoma		286	0.8%	36	Utah	210	0.6%
28	Oregon		371	1.1%	37	New Mexico	188	0.5%
4	Pennsylvania		1,926	5.5%	38	Rhode Island	177	0.5%
38	Rhode Island		177	0.5%	39	New Hampshire	170	0.5%
24	South Carolina		508	1.4%	40	Nevada	168	0.5%
47	South Dakota		84	0.2%	41	Hawaii	162	0.5%
15	Tennessee		798	2.3%	42	Maine	161	0.5%
3	Texas		2,138	6.1%	43	Idaho	123	0.3%
36	Utah		210	0.6%	44	Vermont	112	0.3%
44	Vermont		112	0.3%	45	Delaware	102	0.3%
14	Virginia		899	2.5%	46	Montana	91	0.3%
18	Washington		601	1.7%	47	South Dakota	84	0.2%
34	West Virginia		251	0.7%	48	North Dakota	78	0.2%
19	Wisconsin		596	1.7%	49	Alaska	51	0.1%
50	Wyoming		48	0.1%	50	Wyoming	48	0.1%
						District of Columbia	215	0.6%

Source: American Medical Association (Chicago, Illinois)
   "Physician Characteristics and Distribution in the U.S." (2002-2003 Edition)
*As of December 31, 2000. Total does not include 414 physicians in U.S. territories and possessions. General Surgery includes Abdominal, Cardiovascular, Hand, Head and Neck, Pediatric, Traumatic and Vascular Surgeries.

Rate of Nonfederal Physicians in General Surgery in 2000

National Rate = 12.5 Physicians per 100,000 Population*

ALPHA ORDER

RANK	STATE	RATE
27	Alabama	11.3
50	Alaska	8.1
40	Arizona	10.1
43	Arkansas	9.6
35	California	10.6
33	Colorado	10.7
6	Connecticut	16.5
16	Delaware	13.0
33	Florida	10.7
26	Georgia	11.5
13	Hawaii	13.4
45	Idaho	9.5
20	Illinois	12.5
47	Indiana	9.1
43	Iowa	9.6
29	Kansas	11.1
22	Kentucky	12.3
9	Louisiana	14.5
18	Maine	12.6
4	Maryland	17.2
1	Massachusetts	18.8
24	Michigan	12.2
28	Minnesota	11.2
37	Mississippi	10.2
20	Missouri	12.5
40	Montana	10.1
14	Nebraska	13.3
48	Nevada	8.3
12	New Hampshire	13.7
8	New Jersey	14.7
36	New Mexico	10.3
2	New York	18.5
22	North Carolina	12.3
24	North Dakota	12.2
15	Ohio	13.2
48	Oklahoma	8.3
32	Oregon	10.8
7	Pennsylvania	15.7
5	Rhode Island	16.9
18	South Carolina	12.6
29	South Dakota	11.1
10	Tennessee	14.0
37	Texas	10.2
46	Utah	9.4
3	Vermont	18.4
17	Virginia	12.7
37	Washington	10.2
11	West Virginia	13.9
29	Wisconsin	11.1
42	Wyoming	9.7

RANK ORDER

RANK	STATE	RATE
1	Massachusetts	18.8
2	New York	18.5
3	Vermont	18.4
4	Maryland	17.2
5	Rhode Island	16.9
6	Connecticut	16.5
7	Pennsylvania	15.7
8	New Jersey	14.7
9	Louisiana	14.5
10	Tennessee	14.0
11	West Virginia	13.9
12	New Hampshire	13.7
13	Hawaii	13.4
14	Nebraska	13.3
15	Ohio	13.2
16	Delaware	13.0
17	Virginia	12.7
18	Maine	12.6
18	South Carolina	12.6
20	Illinois	12.5
20	Missouri	12.5
22	Kentucky	12.3
22	North Carolina	12.3
24	Michigan	12.2
24	North Dakota	12.2
26	Georgia	11.5
27	Alabama	11.3
28	Minnesota	11.2
29	Kansas	11.1
29	South Dakota	11.1
29	Wisconsin	11.1
32	Oregon	10.8
33	Colorado	10.7
33	Florida	10.7
35	California	10.6
36	New Mexico	10.3
37	Mississippi	10.2
37	Texas	10.2
37	Washington	10.2
40	Arizona	10.1
40	Montana	10.1
42	Wyoming	9.7
43	Arkansas	9.6
43	Iowa	9.6
45	Idaho	9.5
46	Utah	9.4
47	Indiana	9.1
48	Nevada	8.3
48	Oklahoma	8.3
50	Alaska	8.1

District of Columbia	37.6

Source: Morgan Quitno Press using data from American Medical Association (Chicago, Illinois)
"Physician Characteristics and Distribution in the U.S." (2002-2003 Edition)
*As of December 31, 2000. National rate does not include physicians in U.S. territories and possessions. General Surgery includes Abdominal, Cardiovascular, Hand, Head and Neck, Pediatric, Traumatic and Vascular Surgeries.

Nonfederal Physicians in Obstetrics and Gynecology in 2000

National Total = 39,110 Physicians*

<table>
<tr><td colspan="4">ALPHA ORDER</td><td colspan="4">RANK ORDER</td></tr>
<tr><td>RANK</td><td>STATE</td><td>PHYSICIANS</td><td>% of USA</td><td>RANK</td><td>STATE</td><td>PHYSICIANS</td><td>% of USA</td></tr>
<tr><td>25</td><td>Alabama</td><td>545</td><td>1.4%</td><td>1</td><td>California</td><td>4,597</td><td>11.8%</td></tr>
<tr><td>47</td><td>Alaska</td><td>64</td><td>0.2%</td><td>2</td><td>New York</td><td>3,637</td><td>9.3%</td></tr>
<tr><td>21</td><td>Arizona</td><td>608</td><td>1.6%</td><td>3</td><td>Texas</td><td>2,629</td><td>6.7%</td></tr>
<tr><td>33</td><td>Arkansas</td><td>244</td><td>0.6%</td><td>4</td><td>Florida</td><td>2,048</td><td>5.2%</td></tr>
<tr><td>1</td><td>California</td><td>4,597</td><td>11.8%</td><td>5</td><td>Illinois</td><td>1,857</td><td>4.7%</td></tr>
<tr><td>22</td><td>Colorado</td><td>558</td><td>1.4%</td><td>6</td><td>Pennsylvania</td><td>1,791</td><td>4.6%</td></tr>
<tr><td>19</td><td>Connecticut</td><td>669</td><td>1.7%</td><td>7</td><td>New Jersey</td><td>1,526</td><td>3.9%</td></tr>
<tr><td>44</td><td>Delaware</td><td>101</td><td>0.3%</td><td>8</td><td>Ohio</td><td>1,519</td><td>3.9%</td></tr>
<tr><td>4</td><td>Florida</td><td>2,048</td><td>5.2%</td><td>9</td><td>Michigan</td><td>1,320</td><td>3.4%</td></tr>
<tr><td>10</td><td>Georgia</td><td>1,256</td><td>3.2%</td><td>10</td><td>Georgia</td><td>1,256</td><td>3.2%</td></tr>
<tr><td>35</td><td>Hawaii</td><td>230</td><td>0.6%</td><td>11</td><td>North Carolina</td><td>1,152</td><td>2.9%</td></tr>
<tr><td>43</td><td>Idaho</td><td>116</td><td>0.3%</td><td>12</td><td>Massachusetts</td><td>1,127</td><td>2.9%</td></tr>
<tr><td>5</td><td>Illinois</td><td>1,857</td><td>4.7%</td><td>13</td><td>Maryland</td><td>1,086</td><td>2.8%</td></tr>
<tr><td>20</td><td>Indiana</td><td>623</td><td>1.6%</td><td>14</td><td>Virginia</td><td>1,080</td><td>2.8%</td></tr>
<tr><td>36</td><td>Iowa</td><td>211</td><td>0.5%</td><td>15</td><td>Tennessee</td><td>818</td><td>2.1%</td></tr>
<tr><td>31</td><td>Kansas</td><td>279</td><td>0.7%</td><td>16</td><td>Missouri</td><td>728</td><td>1.9%</td></tr>
<tr><td>27</td><td>Kentucky</td><td>471</td><td>1.2%</td><td>17</td><td>Louisiana</td><td>727</td><td>1.9%</td></tr>
<tr><td>17</td><td>Louisiana</td><td>727</td><td>1.9%</td><td>18</td><td>Washington</td><td>693</td><td>1.8%</td></tr>
<tr><td>42</td><td>Maine</td><td>141</td><td>0.4%</td><td>19</td><td>Connecticut</td><td>669</td><td>1.7%</td></tr>
<tr><td>13</td><td>Maryland</td><td>1,086</td><td>2.8%</td><td>20</td><td>Indiana</td><td>623</td><td>1.6%</td></tr>
<tr><td>12</td><td>Massachusetts</td><td>1,127</td><td>2.9%</td><td>21</td><td>Arizona</td><td>608</td><td>1.6%</td></tr>
<tr><td>9</td><td>Michigan</td><td>1,320</td><td>3.4%</td><td>22</td><td>Colorado</td><td>558</td><td>1.4%</td></tr>
<tr><td>26</td><td>Minnesota</td><td>526</td><td>1.3%</td><td>23</td><td>Wisconsin</td><td>556</td><td>1.4%</td></tr>
<tr><td>29</td><td>Mississippi</td><td>314</td><td>0.8%</td><td>24</td><td>South Carolina</td><td>546</td><td>1.4%</td></tr>
<tr><td>16</td><td>Missouri</td><td>728</td><td>1.9%</td><td>25</td><td>Alabama</td><td>545</td><td>1.4%</td></tr>
<tr><td>46</td><td>Montana</td><td>85</td><td>0.2%</td><td>26</td><td>Minnesota</td><td>526</td><td>1.3%</td></tr>
<tr><td>41</td><td>Nebraska</td><td>171</td><td>0.4%</td><td>27</td><td>Kentucky</td><td>471</td><td>1.2%</td></tr>
<tr><td>34</td><td>Nevada</td><td>241</td><td>0.6%</td><td>28</td><td>Oregon</td><td>432</td><td>1.1%</td></tr>
<tr><td>40</td><td>New Hampshire</td><td>174</td><td>0.4%</td><td>29</td><td>Mississippi</td><td>314</td><td>0.8%</td></tr>
<tr><td>7</td><td>New Jersey</td><td>1,526</td><td>3.9%</td><td>30</td><td>Oklahoma</td><td>293</td><td>0.7%</td></tr>
<tr><td>39</td><td>New Mexico</td><td>191</td><td>0.5%</td><td>31</td><td>Kansas</td><td>279</td><td>0.7%</td></tr>
<tr><td>2</td><td>New York</td><td>3,637</td><td>9.3%</td><td>32</td><td>Utah</td><td>260</td><td>0.7%</td></tr>
<tr><td>11</td><td>North Carolina</td><td>1,152</td><td>2.9%</td><td>33</td><td>Arkansas</td><td>244</td><td>0.6%</td></tr>
<tr><td>50</td><td>North Dakota</td><td>48</td><td>0.1%</td><td>34</td><td>Nevada</td><td>241</td><td>0.6%</td></tr>
<tr><td>8</td><td>Ohio</td><td>1,519</td><td>3.9%</td><td>35</td><td>Hawaii</td><td>230</td><td>0.6%</td></tr>
<tr><td>30</td><td>Oklahoma</td><td>293</td><td>0.7%</td><td>36</td><td>Iowa</td><td>211</td><td>0.5%</td></tr>
<tr><td>28</td><td>Oregon</td><td>432</td><td>1.1%</td><td>37</td><td>West Virginia</td><td>199</td><td>0.5%</td></tr>
<tr><td>6</td><td>Pennsylvania</td><td>1,791</td><td>4.6%</td><td>38</td><td>Rhode Island</td><td>193</td><td>0.5%</td></tr>
<tr><td>38</td><td>Rhode Island</td><td>193</td><td>0.5%</td><td>39</td><td>New Mexico</td><td>191</td><td>0.5%</td></tr>
<tr><td>24</td><td>South Carolina</td><td>546</td><td>1.4%</td><td>40</td><td>New Hampshire</td><td>174</td><td>0.4%</td></tr>
<tr><td>48</td><td>South Dakota</td><td>62</td><td>0.2%</td><td>41</td><td>Nebraska</td><td>171</td><td>0.4%</td></tr>
<tr><td>15</td><td>Tennessee</td><td>818</td><td>2.1%</td><td>42</td><td>Maine</td><td>141</td><td>0.4%</td></tr>
<tr><td>3</td><td>Texas</td><td>2,629</td><td>6.7%</td><td>43</td><td>Idaho</td><td>116</td><td>0.3%</td></tr>
<tr><td>32</td><td>Utah</td><td>260</td><td>0.7%</td><td>44</td><td>Delaware</td><td>101</td><td>0.3%</td></tr>
<tr><td>45</td><td>Vermont</td><td>91</td><td>0.2%</td><td>45</td><td>Vermont</td><td>91</td><td>0.2%</td></tr>
<tr><td>14</td><td>Virginia</td><td>1,080</td><td>2.8%</td><td>46</td><td>Montana</td><td>85</td><td>0.2%</td></tr>
<tr><td>18</td><td>Washington</td><td>693</td><td>1.8%</td><td>47</td><td>Alaska</td><td>64</td><td>0.2%</td></tr>
<tr><td>37</td><td>West Virginia</td><td>199</td><td>0.5%</td><td>48</td><td>South Dakota</td><td>62</td><td>0.2%</td></tr>
<tr><td>23</td><td>Wisconsin</td><td>556</td><td>1.4%</td><td>49</td><td>Wyoming</td><td>52</td><td>0.1%</td></tr>
<tr><td>49</td><td>Wyoming</td><td>52</td><td>0.1%</td><td>50</td><td>North Dakota</td><td>48</td><td>0.1%</td></tr>
<tr><td></td><td></td><td></td><td></td><td></td><td>District of Columbia</td><td>225</td><td>0.6%</td></tr>
</table>

Source: American Medical Association (Chicago, Illinois)
"Physician Characteristics and Distribution in the U.S." (2002-2003 Edition)
*As of December 31, 2000. Total does not include 578 physicians in U.S. territories and possessions. Obstetrics and Gynecology includes Gynecology and Oncology, Maternal and Fetal Medicine and Reproductive Endocrinology.

Rate of Nonfederal Physicians in Obstetrics and Gynecology in 2000

National Rate = 27 Physicians per 100,000 Female Population*

ALPHA ORDER

RANK	STATE	RATE
28	Alabama	24
34	Alaska	21
28	Arizona	24
45	Arkansas	18
17	California	27
18	Colorado	26
2	Connecticut	38
22	Delaware	25
22	Florida	25
9	Georgia	30
2	Hawaii	38
45	Idaho	18
11	Illinois	29
41	Indiana	20
50	Iowa	14
34	Kansas	21
30	Kentucky	23
8	Louisiana	32
33	Maine	22
1	Maryland	40
7	Massachusetts	34
18	Michigan	26
34	Minnesota	21
34	Mississippi	21
22	Missouri	25
44	Montana	19
41	Nebraska	20
22	Nevada	25
13	New Hampshire	28
5	New Jersey	35
34	New Mexico	21
4	New York	37
13	North Carolina	28
49	North Dakota	15
18	Ohio	26
47	Oklahoma	17
22	Oregon	25
13	Pennsylvania	28
5	Rhode Island	35
18	South Carolina	26
48	South Dakota	16
13	Tennessee	28
22	Texas	25
30	Utah	23
11	Vermont	29
9	Virginia	30
30	Washington	23
34	West Virginia	21
41	Wisconsin	20
34	Wyoming	21

RANK ORDER

RANK	STATE	RATE
1	Maryland	40
2	Connecticut	38
2	Hawaii	38
4	New York	37
5	New Jersey	35
5	Rhode Island	35
7	Massachusetts	34
8	Louisiana	32
9	Georgia	30
9	Virginia	30
11	Illinois	29
11	Vermont	29
13	New Hampshire	28
13	North Carolina	28
13	Pennsylvania	28
13	Tennessee	28
17	California	27
18	Colorado	26
18	Michigan	26
18	Ohio	26
18	South Carolina	26
22	Delaware	25
22	Florida	25
22	Missouri	25
22	Nevada	25
22	Oregon	25
22	Texas	25
28	Alabama	24
28	Arizona	24
30	Kentucky	23
30	Utah	23
30	Washington	23
33	Maine	22
34	Alaska	21
34	Kansas	21
34	Minnesota	21
34	Mississippi	21
34	New Mexico	21
34	West Virginia	21
34	Wyoming	21
41	Indiana	20
41	Nebraska	20
41	Wisconsin	20
44	Montana	19
45	Arkansas	18
45	Idaho	18
47	Oklahoma	17
48	South Dakota	16
49	North Dakota	15
50	Iowa	14

| | District of Columbia | 74 |

Source: Morgan Quitno Press using data from American Medical Association (Chicago, Illinois)
"Physician Characteristics and Distribution in the U.S." (2002-2003 Edition)

*As of December 31, 2000. National rate does not include physicians in U.S. territories and possessions. Obstetrics and Gynecology includes Gynecology and Oncology, Maternal and Fetal Medicine and Reproductive Endocrinology.

Nonfederal Physicians in Ophthalmology in 2000

National Total = 17,664 Physicians*

ALPHA ORDER

RANK	STATE	PHYSICIANS	% of USA
27	Alabama	215	1.2%
49	Alaska	28	0.2%
23	Arizona	273	1.5%
32	Arkansas	138	0.8%
1	California	2,152	12.2%
24	Colorado	262	1.5%
21	Connecticut	306	1.7%
46	Delaware	45	0.3%
3	Florida	1,121	6.3%
14	Georgia	393	2.2%
37	Hawaii	90	0.5%
43	Idaho	62	0.4%
6	Illinois	709	4.0%
22	Indiana	276	1.6%
29	Iowa	151	0.9%
30	Kansas	149	0.8%
28	Kentucky	197	1.1%
18	Louisiana	327	1.9%
41	Maine	74	0.4%
11	Maryland	510	2.9%
10	Massachusetts	531	3.0%
9	Michigan	565	3.2%
20	Minnesota	308	1.7%
32	Mississippi	138	0.8%
16	Missouri	332	1.9%
44	Montana	49	0.3%
35	Nebraska	99	0.6%
38	Nevada	83	0.5%
42	New Hampshire	66	0.4%
7	New Jersey	644	3.6%
40	New Mexico	76	0.4%
2	New York	1,743	9.9%
13	North Carolina	418	2.4%
47	North Dakota	39	0.2%
8	Ohio	643	3.6%
30	Oklahoma	149	0.8%
26	Oregon	216	1.2%
5	Pennsylvania	909	5.1%
39	Rhode Island	77	0.4%
25	South Carolina	241	1.4%
48	South Dakota	36	0.2%
15	Tennessee	340	1.9%
4	Texas	1,034	5.9%
34	Utah	118	0.7%
45	Vermont	48	0.3%
12	Virginia	419	2.4%
19	Washington	326	1.8%
36	West Virginia	98	0.6%
16	Wisconsin	332	1.9%
50	Wyoming	17	0.1%

RANK ORDER

RANK	STATE	PHYSICIANS	% of USA
1	California	2,152	12.2%
2	New York	1,743	9.9%
3	Florida	1,121	6.3%
4	Texas	1,034	5.9%
5	Pennsylvania	909	5.1%
6	Illinois	709	4.0%
7	New Jersey	644	3.6%
8	Ohio	643	3.6%
9	Michigan	565	3.2%
10	Massachusetts	531	3.0%
11	Maryland	510	2.9%
12	Virginia	419	2.4%
13	North Carolina	418	2.4%
14	Georgia	393	2.2%
15	Tennessee	340	1.9%
16	Missouri	332	1.9%
16	Wisconsin	332	1.9%
18	Louisiana	327	1.9%
19	Washington	326	1.8%
20	Minnesota	308	1.7%
21	Connecticut	306	1.7%
22	Indiana	276	1.6%
23	Arizona	273	1.5%
24	Colorado	262	1.5%
25	South Carolina	241	1.4%
26	Oregon	216	1.2%
27	Alabama	215	1.2%
28	Kentucky	197	1.1%
29	Iowa	151	0.9%
30	Kansas	149	0.8%
30	Oklahoma	149	0.8%
32	Arkansas	138	0.8%
32	Mississippi	138	0.8%
34	Utah	118	0.7%
35	Nebraska	99	0.6%
36	West Virginia	98	0.6%
37	Hawaii	90	0.5%
38	Nevada	83	0.5%
39	Rhode Island	77	0.4%
40	New Mexico	76	0.4%
41	Maine	74	0.4%
42	New Hampshire	66	0.4%
43	Idaho	62	0.4%
44	Montana	49	0.3%
45	Vermont	48	0.3%
46	Delaware	45	0.3%
47	North Dakota	39	0.2%
48	South Dakota	36	0.2%
49	Alaska	28	0.2%
50	Wyoming	17	0.1%
	District of Columbia	92	0.5%

Source: American Medical Association (Chicago, Illinois)
    "Physician Characteristics and Distribution in the U.S." (2002-2003 Edition)
As of December 31, 2000. Total does not include 182 physicians in U.S. territories and possessions.
Ophthalmology is the branch of medicine dealing with the anatomy, functions and diseases of the eye.

Rate of Nonfederal Physicians in Ophthalmology in 2000

National Rate = 6.3 Physicians per 100,000 Population*

ALPHA ORDER

RANK	STATE	RATE
40	Alabama	4.8
45	Alaska	4.5
32	Arizona	5.3
35	Arkansas	5.2
12	California	6.3
16	Colorado	6.1
3	Connecticut	9.0
24	Delaware	5.7
11	Florida	7.0
40	Georgia	4.8
7	Hawaii	7.4
40	Idaho	4.8
24	Illinois	5.7
45	Indiana	4.5
35	Iowa	5.2
28	Kansas	5.5
38	Kentucky	4.9
9	Louisiana	7.3
22	Maine	5.8
1	Maryland	9.6
4	Massachusetts	8.4
24	Michigan	5.7
14	Minnesota	6.2
40	Mississippi	4.8
20	Missouri	5.9
30	Montana	5.4
22	Nebraska	5.8
49	Nevada	4.1
32	New Hampshire	5.3
6	New Jersey	7.6
48	New Mexico	4.2
2	New York	9.2
35	North Carolina	5.2
16	North Dakota	6.1
24	Ohio	5.7
47	Oklahoma	4.3
12	Oregon	6.3
7	Pennsylvania	7.4
9	Rhode Island	7.3
18	South Carolina	6.0
40	South Dakota	4.8
18	Tennessee	6.0
38	Texas	4.9
32	Utah	5.3
5	Vermont	7.9
20	Virginia	5.9
28	Washington	5.5
30	West Virginia	5.4
14	Wisconsin	6.2
50	Wyoming	3.4

RANK ORDER

RANK	STATE	RATE
1	Maryland	9.6
2	New York	9.2
3	Connecticut	9.0
4	Massachusetts	8.4
5	Vermont	7.9
6	New Jersey	7.6
7	Hawaii	7.4
7	Pennsylvania	7.4
9	Louisiana	7.3
9	Rhode Island	7.3
11	Florida	7.0
12	California	6.3
12	Oregon	6.3
14	Minnesota	6.2
14	Wisconsin	6.2
16	Colorado	6.1
16	North Dakota	6.1
18	South Carolina	6.0
18	Tennessee	6.0
20	Missouri	5.9
20	Virginia	5.9
22	Maine	5.8
22	Nebraska	5.8
24	Delaware	5.7
24	Illinois	5.7
24	Michigan	5.7
24	Ohio	5.7
28	Kansas	5.5
28	Washington	5.5
30	Montana	5.4
30	West Virginia	5.4
32	Arizona	5.3
32	New Hampshire	5.3
32	Utah	5.3
35	Arkansas	5.2
35	Iowa	5.2
35	North Carolina	5.2
38	Kentucky	4.9
38	Texas	4.9
40	Alabama	4.8
40	Georgia	4.8
40	Idaho	4.8
40	Mississippi	4.8
40	South Dakota	4.8
45	Alaska	4.5
45	Indiana	4.5
47	Oklahoma	4.3
48	New Mexico	4.2
49	Nevada	4.1
50	Wyoming	3.4

District of Columbia 16.1

Source: Morgan Quitno Press using data from American Medical Association (Chicago, Illinois)
    "Physician Characteristics and Distribution in the U.S." (2002-2003 Edition)
*As of December 31, 2000. National rate does not include physicians in U.S. territories and possessions.
Ophthalmology is the branch of medicine dealing with the anatomy, functions and diseases of the eye.

Nonfederal Physicians in Orthopedic Surgery in 2000

National Total = 21,744 Physicians*

ALPHA ORDER | | | | | RANK ORDER

RANK	STATE	PHYSICIANS	% of USA
24	Alabama	327	1.5%
49	Alaska	48	0.2%
25	Arizona	324	1.5%
33	Arkansas	175	0.8%
1	California	2,672	12.3%
23	Colorado	353	1.6%
22	Connecticut	363	1.7%
46	Delaware	58	0.3%
4	Florida	1,240	5.7%
13	Georgia	548	2.5%
43	Hawaii	100	0.5%
42	Idaho	105	0.5%
6	Illinois	866	4.0%
20	Indiana	404	1.9%
32	Iowa	177	0.8%
30	Kansas	185	0.9%
27	Kentucky	277	1.3%
21	Louisiana	386	1.8%
39	Maine	113	0.5%
14	Maryland	510	2.3%
8	Massachusetts	673	3.1%
10	Michigan	601	2.8%
19	Minnesota	411	1.9%
34	Mississippi	164	0.8%
18	Missouri	415	1.9%
44	Montana	94	0.4%
35	Nebraska	140	0.6%
41	Nevada	108	0.5%
40	New Hampshire	111	0.5%
9	New Jersey	662	3.0%
35	New Mexico	140	0.6%
2	New York	1,731	8.0%
10	North Carolina	601	2.8%
50	North Dakota	39	0.2%
7	Ohio	845	3.9%
29	Oklahoma	197	0.9%
28	Oregon	267	1.2%
5	Pennsylvania	1,067	4.9%
37	Rhode Island	120	0.6%
26	South Carolina	296	1.4%
47	South Dakota	56	0.3%
16	Tennessee	476	2.2%
3	Texas	1,328	6.1%
31	Utah	178	0.8%
45	Vermont	65	0.3%
12	Virginia	552	2.5%
15	Washington	486	2.2%
38	West Virginia	114	0.5%
17	Wisconsin	427	2.0%
48	Wyoming	51	0.2%

RANK	STATE	PHYSICIANS	% of USA
1	California	2,672	12.3%
2	New York	1,731	8.0%
3	Texas	1,328	6.1%
4	Florida	1,240	5.7%
5	Pennsylvania	1,067	4.9%
6	Illinois	866	4.0%
7	Ohio	845	3.9%
8	Massachusetts	673	3.1%
9	New Jersey	662	3.0%
10	Michigan	601	2.8%
10	North Carolina	601	2.8%
12	Virginia	552	2.5%
13	Georgia	548	2.5%
14	Maryland	510	2.3%
15	Washington	486	2.2%
16	Tennessee	476	2.2%
17	Wisconsin	427	2.0%
18	Missouri	415	1.9%
19	Minnesota	411	1.9%
20	Indiana	404	1.9%
21	Louisiana	386	1.8%
22	Connecticut	363	1.7%
23	Colorado	353	1.6%
24	Alabama	327	1.5%
25	Arizona	324	1.5%
26	South Carolina	296	1.4%
27	Kentucky	277	1.3%
28	Oregon	267	1.2%
29	Oklahoma	197	0.9%
30	Kansas	185	0.9%
31	Utah	178	0.8%
32	Iowa	177	0.8%
33	Arkansas	175	0.8%
34	Mississippi	164	0.8%
35	Nebraska	140	0.6%
35	New Mexico	140	0.6%
37	Rhode Island	120	0.6%
38	West Virginia	114	0.5%
39	Maine	113	0.5%
40	New Hampshire	111	0.5%
41	Nevada	108	0.5%
42	Idaho	105	0.5%
43	Hawaii	100	0.5%
44	Montana	94	0.4%
45	Vermont	65	0.3%
46	Delaware	58	0.3%
47	South Dakota	56	0.3%
48	Wyoming	51	0.2%
49	Alaska	48	0.2%
50	North Dakota	39	0.2%
	District of Columbia	98	0.5%

Source: American Medical Association (Chicago, Illinois)
   "Physician Characteristics and Distribution in the U.S." (2002-2003 Edition)
*As of December 31, 2000. Total does not include 122 physicians in U.S. territories and possessions.
Orthopedics is the branch of medicine dealing with the skeletal system.

Rate of Nonfederal Physicians in Orthopedic Surgery in 2000

National Rate = 7.7 Physicians per 100,000 Population*

ALPHA ORDER

RANK	STATE	RATE
35	Alabama	7.3
28	Alaska	7.6
42	Arizona	6.3
41	Arkansas	6.5
20	California	7.9
15	Colorado	8.2
3	Connecticut	10.6
29	Delaware	7.4
26	Florida	7.7
39	Georgia	6.7
15	Hawaii	8.2
19	Idaho	8.1
36	Illinois	7.0
40	Indiana	6.6
46	Iowa	6.0
37	Kansas	6.9
38	Kentucky	6.8
12	Louisiana	8.6
10	Maine	8.8
7	Maryland	9.6
3	Massachusetts	10.6
46	Michigan	6.0
13	Minnesota	8.3
48	Mississippi	5.8
29	Missouri	7.4
5	Montana	10.4
15	Nebraska	8.2
50	Nevada	5.3
9	New Hampshire	9.0
20	New Jersey	7.9
26	New Mexico	7.7
8	New York	9.1
29	North Carolina	7.4
45	North Dakota	6.1
29	Ohio	7.4
49	Oklahoma	5.7
24	Oregon	7.8
11	Pennsylvania	8.7
1	Rhode Island	11.4
29	South Carolina	7.4
29	South Dakota	7.4
13	Tennessee	8.3
42	Texas	6.3
20	Utah	7.9
2	Vermont	10.7
24	Virginia	7.8
15	Washington	8.2
42	West Virginia	6.3
20	Wisconsin	7.9
6	Wyoming	10.3

RANK ORDER

RANK	STATE	RATE
1	Rhode Island	11.4
2	Vermont	10.7
3	Connecticut	10.6
3	Massachusetts	10.6
5	Montana	10.4
6	Wyoming	10.3
7	Maryland	9.6
8	New York	9.1
9	New Hampshire	9.0
10	Maine	8.8
11	Pennsylvania	8.7
12	Louisiana	8.6
13	Minnesota	8.3
13	Tennessee	8.3
15	Colorado	8.2
15	Hawaii	8.2
15	Nebraska	8.2
15	Washington	8.2
19	Idaho	8.1
20	California	7.9
20	New Jersey	7.9
20	Utah	7.9
20	Wisconsin	7.9
24	Oregon	7.8
24	Virginia	7.8
26	Florida	7.7
26	New Mexico	7.7
28	Alaska	7.6
29	Delaware	7.4
29	Missouri	7.4
29	North Carolina	7.4
29	Ohio	7.4
29	South Carolina	7.4
29	South Dakota	7.4
35	Alabama	7.3
36	Illinois	7.0
37	Kansas	6.9
38	Kentucky	6.8
39	Georgia	6.7
40	Indiana	6.6
41	Arkansas	6.5
42	Arizona	6.3
42	Texas	6.3
42	West Virginia	6.3
45	North Dakota	6.1
46	Iowa	6.0
46	Michigan	6.0
48	Mississippi	5.8
49	Oklahoma	5.7
50	Nevada	5.3

District of Columbia	17.2

Source: Morgan Quitno Press using data from American Medical Association (Chicago, Illinois)
"Physician Characteristics and Distribution in the U.S." (2002-2003 Edition)
*As of December 31, 2000. National rate does not include physicians in U.S. territories and possessions.
Orthopedics is the branch of medicine dealing with the skeletal system.

Nonfederal Physicians in Plastic Surgery in 2000

National Total = 6,104 Physicians*

ALPHA ORDER

RANK	STATE	PHYSICIANS	% of USA
22	Alabama	84	1.4%
49	Alaska	6	0.1%
17	Arizona	122	2.0%
35	Arkansas	29	0.5%
1	California	902	14.8%
19	Colorado	92	1.5%
19	Connecticut	92	1.5%
42	Delaware	16	0.3%
3	Florida	468	7.7%
12	Georgia	152	2.5%
34	Hawaii	31	0.5%
40	Idaho	23	0.4%
6	Illinois	221	3.6%
21	Indiana	88	1.4%
38	Iowa	24	0.4%
30	Kansas	47	0.8%
25	Kentucky	81	1.3%
23	Louisiana	83	1.4%
45	Maine	13	0.2%
14	Maryland	147	2.4%
10	Massachusetts	164	2.7%
9	Michigan	188	3.1%
26	Minnesota	76	1.2%
33	Mississippi	37	0.6%
16	Missouri	129	2.1%
42	Montana	16	0.3%
36	Nebraska	27	0.4%
32	Nevada	41	0.7%
42	New Hampshire	16	0.3%
8	New Jersey	195	3.2%
38	New Mexico	24	0.4%
2	New York	590	9.7%
10	North Carolina	164	2.7%
46	North Dakota	10	0.2%
7	Ohio	199	3.3%
31	Oklahoma	42	0.7%
29	Oregon	58	1.0%
5	Pennsylvania	246	4.0%
41	Rhode Island	20	0.3%
28	South Carolina	60	1.0%
48	South Dakota	8	0.1%
15	Tennessee	139	2.3%
4	Texas	453	7.4%
27	Utah	66	1.1%
46	Vermont	10	0.2%
12	Virginia	152	2.5%
18	Washington	110	1.8%
37	West Virginia	26	0.4%
23	Wisconsin	83	1.4%
50	Wyoming	3	0.0%

RANK ORDER

RANK	STATE	PHYSICIANS	% of USA
1	California	902	14.8%
2	New York	590	9.7%
3	Florida	468	7.7%
4	Texas	453	7.4%
5	Pennsylvania	246	4.0%
6	Illinois	221	3.6%
7	Ohio	199	3.3%
8	New Jersey	195	3.2%
9	Michigan	188	3.1%
10	Massachusetts	164	2.7%
10	North Carolina	164	2.7%
12	Georgia	152	2.5%
12	Virginia	152	2.5%
14	Maryland	147	2.4%
15	Tennessee	139	2.3%
16	Missouri	129	2.1%
17	Arizona	122	2.0%
18	Washington	110	1.8%
19	Colorado	92	1.5%
19	Connecticut	92	1.5%
21	Indiana	88	1.4%
22	Alabama	84	1.4%
23	Louisiana	83	1.4%
23	Wisconsin	83	1.4%
25	Kentucky	81	1.3%
26	Minnesota	76	1.2%
27	Utah	66	1.1%
28	South Carolina	60	1.0%
29	Oregon	58	1.0%
30	Kansas	47	0.8%
31	Oklahoma	42	0.7%
32	Nevada	41	0.7%
33	Mississippi	37	0.6%
34	Hawaii	31	0.5%
35	Arkansas	29	0.5%
36	Nebraska	27	0.4%
37	West Virginia	26	0.4%
38	Iowa	24	0.4%
38	New Mexico	24	0.4%
40	Idaho	23	0.4%
41	Rhode Island	20	0.3%
42	Delaware	16	0.3%
42	Montana	16	0.3%
42	New Hampshire	16	0.3%
45	Maine	13	0.2%
46	North Dakota	10	0.2%
46	Vermont	10	0.2%
48	South Dakota	8	0.1%
49	Alaska	6	0.1%
50	Wyoming	3	0.0%
	District of Columbia	31	0.5%

Source: American Medical Association (Chicago, Illinois)
"Physician Characteristics and Distribution in the U.S." (2002-2003 Edition)
*As of December 31, 2000. Total does not include 36 physicians in U.S. territories and possessions.

Rate of Nonfederal Physicians in Plastic Surgery in 2000

National Rate = 2.2 Physicians per 100,000 Population*

ALPHA ORDER

RANK	STATE	RATE
21	Alabama	1.9
47	Alaska	1.0
9	Arizona	2.4
45	Arkansas	1.1
5	California	2.7
14	Colorado	2.1
5	Connecticut	2.7
16	Delaware	2.0
2	Florida	2.9
26	Georgia	1.8
7	Hawaii	2.6
26	Idaho	1.8
26	Illinois	1.8
39	Indiana	1.4
49	Iowa	0.8
31	Kansas	1.7
16	Kentucky	2.0
21	Louisiana	1.9
47	Maine	1.0
4	Maryland	2.8
7	Massachusetts	2.6
21	Michigan	1.9
36	Minnesota	1.5
41	Mississippi	1.3
11	Missouri	2.3
26	Montana	1.8
33	Nebraska	1.6
16	Nevada	2.0
41	New Hampshire	1.3
11	New Jersey	2.3
41	New Mexico	1.3
1	New York	3.1
16	North Carolina	2.0
33	North Dakota	1.6
26	Ohio	1.8
44	Oklahoma	1.2
31	Oregon	1.7
16	Pennsylvania	2.0
21	Rhode Island	1.9
36	South Carolina	1.5
45	South Dakota	1.1
9	Tennessee	2.4
13	Texas	2.2
2	Utah	2.9
33	Vermont	1.6
14	Virginia	2.1
21	Washington	1.9
39	West Virginia	1.4
36	Wisconsin	1.5
50	Wyoming	0.6

RANK ORDER

RANK	STATE	RATE
1	New York	3.1
2	Florida	2.9
2	Utah	2.9
4	Maryland	2.8
5	California	2.7
5	Connecticut	2.7
7	Hawaii	2.6
7	Massachusetts	2.6
9	Arizona	2.4
9	Tennessee	2.4
11	Missouri	2.3
11	New Jersey	2.3
13	Texas	2.2
14	Colorado	2.1
14	Virginia	2.1
16	Delaware	2.0
16	Kentucky	2.0
16	Nevada	2.0
16	North Carolina	2.0
16	Pennsylvania	2.0
21	Alabama	1.9
21	Louisiana	1.9
21	Michigan	1.9
21	Rhode Island	1.9
21	Washington	1.9
26	Georgia	1.8
26	Idaho	1.8
26	Illinois	1.8
26	Montana	1.8
26	Ohio	1.8
31	Kansas	1.7
31	Oregon	1.7
33	Nebraska	1.6
33	North Dakota	1.6
33	Vermont	1.6
36	Minnesota	1.5
36	South Carolina	1.5
36	Wisconsin	1.5
39	Indiana	1.4
39	West Virginia	1.4
41	Mississippi	1.3
41	New Hampshire	1.3
41	New Mexico	1.3
44	Oklahoma	1.2
45	Arkansas	1.1
45	South Dakota	1.1
47	Alaska	1.0
47	Maine	1.0
49	Iowa	0.8
50	Wyoming	0.6

District of Columbia   5.4

Source: Morgan Quitno Press using data from American Medical Association (Chicago, Illinois)
    "Physician Characteristics and Distribution in the U.S." (2002-2003 Edition)
*As of December 31, 2000. National rate does not include physicians in U.S. territories and possessions.

Nonfederal Physicians in Other Specialties in 2000

National Total = 189,201 Physicians*

ALPHA ORDER

RANK	STATE	PHYSICIANS	% of USA
28	Alabama	2,091	1.1%
49	Alaska	288	0.2%
24	Arizona	2,804	1.5%
32	Arkansas	1,234	0.7%
1	California	23,047	12.2%
22	Colorado	2,865	1.5%
18	Connecticut	3,383	1.8%
44	Delaware	511	0.3%
5	Florida	9,641	5.1%
14	Georgia	4,391	2.3%
39	Hawaii	880	0.5%
46	Idaho	467	0.2%
6	Illinois	8,501	4.5%
20	Indiana	3,240	1.7%
31	Iowa	1,247	0.7%
29	Kansas	1,489	0.8%
26	Kentucky	2,220	1.2%
23	Louisiana	2,810	1.5%
39	Maine	880	0.5%
11	Maryland	5,592	3.0%
7	Massachusetts	7,787	4.1%
10	Michigan	6,134	3.2%
21	Minnesota	3,151	1.7%
34	Mississippi	1,140	0.6%
19	Missouri	3,336	1.8%
45	Montana	501	0.3%
38	Nebraska	908	0.5%
37	Nevada	929	0.5%
42	New Hampshire	830	0.4%
9	New Jersey	6,365	3.4%
35	New Mexico	1,071	0.6%
2	New York	19,613	10.4%
12	North Carolina	4,782	2.5%
47	North Dakota	338	0.2%
8	Ohio	7,072	3.7%
30	Oklahoma	1,432	0.8%
27	Oregon	2,190	1.2%
4	Pennsylvania	10,031	5.3%
41	Rhode Island	870	0.5%
25	South Carolina	2,237	1.2%
48	South Dakota	332	0.2%
17	Tennessee	3,401	1.8%
3	Texas	11,128	5.9%
33	Utah	1,214	0.6%
43	Vermont	579	0.3%
13	Virginia	4,552	2.4%
15	Washington	3,959	2.1%
36	West Virginia	980	0.5%
16	Wisconsin	3,402	1.8%
50	Wyoming	215	0.1%

RANK ORDER

RANK	STATE	PHYSICIANS	% of USA
1	California	23,047	12.2%
2	New York	19,613	10.4%
3	Texas	11,128	5.9%
4	Pennsylvania	10,031	5.3%
5	Florida	9,641	5.1%
6	Illinois	8,501	4.5%
7	Massachusetts	7,787	4.1%
8	Ohio	7,072	3.7%
9	New Jersey	6,365	3.4%
10	Michigan	6,134	3.2%
11	Maryland	5,592	3.0%
12	North Carolina	4,782	2.5%
13	Virginia	4,552	2.4%
14	Georgia	4,391	2.3%
15	Washington	3,959	2.1%
16	Wisconsin	3,402	1.8%
17	Tennessee	3,401	1.8%
18	Connecticut	3,383	1.8%
19	Missouri	3,336	1.8%
20	Indiana	3,240	1.7%
21	Minnesota	3,151	1.7%
22	Colorado	2,865	1.5%
23	Louisiana	2,810	1.5%
24	Arizona	2,804	1.5%
25	South Carolina	2,237	1.2%
26	Kentucky	2,220	1.2%
27	Oregon	2,190	1.2%
28	Alabama	2,091	1.1%
29	Kansas	1,489	0.8%
30	Oklahoma	1,432	0.8%
31	Iowa	1,247	0.7%
32	Arkansas	1,234	0.7%
33	Utah	1,214	0.6%
34	Mississippi	1,140	0.6%
35	New Mexico	1,071	0.6%
36	West Virginia	980	0.5%
37	Nevada	929	0.5%
38	Nebraska	908	0.5%
39	Hawaii	880	0.5%
39	Maine	880	0.5%
41	Rhode Island	870	0.5%
42	New Hampshire	830	0.4%
43	Vermont	579	0.3%
44	Delaware	511	0.3%
45	Montana	501	0.3%
46	Idaho	467	0.2%
47	North Dakota	338	0.2%
48	South Dakota	332	0.2%
49	Alaska	288	0.2%
50	Wyoming	215	0.1%
	District of Columbia	1,141	0.6%

Source: American Medical Association (Chicago, Illinois)
"Physician Characteristics and Distribution in the U.S." (2002-2003 Edition)
As of December 31, 2000. Total does not include 2,159 physicians in U.S. territories and possessions. Other Specialties include Aerospace Medicine, Anesthesiology, Child Psychiatry, Diagnostic Radiology, Emergency Medicine, Forensic Pathology, Nuclear Medicine, Occupational Medicine, Neurology, Psychiatry, Public Health, Anatomic/Clinical Pathology, Radiology, Radiation Oncology and other specialties.

Rate of Nonfederal Physicians in Other Specialties in 2000

National Rate = 67 Physicians per 100,000 Population*

ALPHA ORDER

RANK	STATE	RATE
41	Alabama	47
42	Alaska	46
33	Arizona	54
42	Arkansas	46
11	California	68
15	Colorado	66
4	Connecticut	99
16	Delaware	65
24	Florida	60
36	Georgia	53
9	Hawaii	73
50	Idaho	36
11	Illinois	68
36	Indiana	53
47	Iowa	43
30	Kansas	55
30	Kentucky	55
20	Louisiana	63
10	Maine	69
2	Maryland	105
1	Massachusetts	122
22	Michigan	62
17	Minnesota	64
49	Mississippi	40
24	Missouri	60
30	Montana	55
36	Nebraska	53
42	Nevada	46
13	New Hampshire	67
8	New Jersey	76
27	New Mexico	59
3	New York	103
27	North Carolina	59
36	North Dakota	53
22	Ohio	62
48	Oklahoma	41
17	Oregon	64
7	Pennsylvania	82
6	Rhode Island	83
29	South Carolina	56
45	South Dakota	44
24	Tennessee	60
36	Texas	53
33	Utah	54
5	Vermont	95
17	Virginia	64
13	Washington	67
33	West Virginia	54
20	Wisconsin	63
45	Wyoming	44

RANK ORDER

RANK	STATE	RATE
1	Massachusetts	122
2	Maryland	105
3	New York	103
4	Connecticut	99
5	Vermont	95
6	Rhode Island	83
7	Pennsylvania	82
8	New Jersey	76
9	Hawaii	73
10	Maine	69
11	California	68
11	Illinois	68
13	New Hampshire	67
13	Washington	67
15	Colorado	66
16	Delaware	65
17	Minnesota	64
17	Oregon	64
17	Virginia	64
20	Louisiana	63
20	Wisconsin	63
22	Michigan	62
22	Ohio	62
24	Florida	60
24	Missouri	60
24	Tennessee	60
27	New Mexico	59
27	North Carolina	59
29	South Carolina	56
30	Kansas	55
30	Kentucky	55
30	Montana	55
33	Arizona	54
33	Utah	54
33	West Virginia	54
36	Georgia	53
36	Indiana	53
36	Nebraska	53
36	North Dakota	53
36	Texas	53
41	Alabama	47
42	Alaska	46
42	Arkansas	46
42	Nevada	46
45	South Dakota	44
45	Wyoming	44
47	Iowa	43
48	Oklahoma	41
49	Mississippi	40
50	Idaho	36

| | District of Columbia | 200 |

Source: Morgan Quitno Press using data from American Medical Association (Chicago, Illinois)
"Physician Characteristics and Distribution in the U.S." (2002-2003 Edition)
*As of December 31, 2000. National rate does not include physicians in U.S. territories and possessions. Other Specialties include Aerospace Medicine, Anesthesiology, Child Psychiatry, Diagnostic Radiology, Emergency Medicine, Forensic Pathology, Nuclear Medicine, Occupational Medicine, Neurology, Psychiatry, Public Health, Anatomic/Clinical Pathology, Radiology, Radiation Oncology and other specialties.

Nonfederal Physicians in Anesthesiology in 2000

National Total = 34,813 Physicians*

ALPHA ORDER

RANK	STATE	PHYSICIANS	% of USA
27	Alabama	421	1.2%
47	Alaska	58	0.2%
19	Arizona	621	1.8%
33	Arkansas	257	0.7%
1	California	4,325	12.4%
21	Colorado	553	1.6%
22	Connecticut	515	1.5%
46	Delaware	62	0.2%
4	Florida	2,117	6.1%
13	Georgia	831	2.4%
41	Hawaii	135	0.4%
44	Idaho	84	0.2%
5	Illinois	1,642	4.7%
15	Indiana	779	2.2%
32	Iowa	277	0.8%
30	Kansas	285	0.8%
26	Kentucky	441	1.3%
24	Louisiana	464	1.3%
39	Maine	148	0.4%
10	Maryland	902	2.6%
9	Massachusetts	1,216	3.5%
12	Michigan	843	2.4%
23	Minnesota	493	1.4%
34	Mississippi	248	0.7%
20	Missouri	585	1.7%
42	Montana	111	0.3%
36	Nebraska	186	0.5%
35	Nevada	243	0.7%
40	New Hampshire	140	0.4%
8	New Jersey	1,280	3.7%
37	New Mexico	182	0.5%
2	New York	3,108	8.9%
14	North Carolina	795	2.3%
49	North Dakota	50	0.1%
7	Ohio	1,297	3.7%
29	Oklahoma	305	0.9%
25	Oregon	443	1.3%
6	Pennsylvania	1,598	4.6%
43	Rhode Island	102	0.3%
28	South Carolina	397	1.1%
48	South Dakota	52	0.1%
18	Tennessee	692	2.0%
3	Texas	2,557	7.3%
31	Utah	281	0.8%
45	Vermont	75	0.2%
16	Virginia	754	2.2%
11	Washington	855	2.5%
38	West Virginia	163	0.5%
17	Wisconsin	693	2.0%
50	Wyoming	45	0.1%

RANK ORDER

RANK	STATE	PHYSICIANS	% of USA
1	California	4,325	12.4%
2	New York	3,108	8.9%
3	Texas	2,557	7.3%
4	Florida	2,117	6.1%
5	Illinois	1,642	4.7%
6	Pennsylvania	1,598	4.6%
7	Ohio	1,297	3.7%
8	New Jersey	1,280	3.7%
9	Massachusetts	1,216	3.5%
10	Maryland	902	2.6%
11	Washington	855	2.5%
12	Michigan	843	2.4%
13	Georgia	831	2.4%
14	North Carolina	795	2.3%
15	Indiana	779	2.2%
16	Virginia	754	2.2%
17	Wisconsin	693	2.0%
18	Tennessee	692	2.0%
19	Arizona	621	1.8%
20	Missouri	585	1.7%
21	Colorado	553	1.6%
22	Connecticut	515	1.5%
23	Minnesota	493	1.4%
24	Louisiana	464	1.3%
25	Oregon	443	1.3%
26	Kentucky	441	1.3%
27	Alabama	421	1.2%
28	South Carolina	397	1.1%
29	Oklahoma	305	0.9%
30	Kansas	285	0.8%
31	Utah	281	0.8%
32	Iowa	277	0.8%
33	Arkansas	257	0.7%
34	Mississippi	248	0.7%
35	Nevada	243	0.7%
36	Nebraska	186	0.5%
37	New Mexico	182	0.5%
38	West Virginia	163	0.5%
39	Maine	148	0.4%
40	New Hampshire	140	0.4%
41	Hawaii	135	0.4%
42	Montana	111	0.3%
43	Rhode Island	102	0.3%
44	Idaho	84	0.2%
45	Vermont	75	0.2%
46	Delaware	62	0.2%
47	Alaska	58	0.2%
48	South Dakota	52	0.1%
49	North Dakota	50	0.1%
50	Wyoming	45	0.1%
	District of Columbia	107	0.3%

Source: American Medical Association (Chicago, Illinois)
   "Physician Characteristics and Distribution in the U.S." (2002-2003 Edition)
As of December 31, 2000. Total does not include 226 physicians in U.S. territories and possessions.

Rate of Nonfederal Physicians in Anesthesiology in 2000

National Rate = 12.3 Physicians per 100,000 Population*

ALPHA ORDER

RANK	STATE	RATE
39	Alabama	9.5
41	Alaska	9.2
20	Arizona	12.0
38	Arkansas	9.6
14	California	12.7
12	Colorado	12.8
5	Connecticut	15.1
47	Delaware	7.9
7	Florida	13.2
32	Georgia	10.1
25	Hawaii	11.1
50	Idaho	6.5
7	Illinois	13.2
12	Indiana	12.8
39	Iowa	9.5
28	Kansas	10.6
26	Kentucky	10.9
30	Louisiana	10.4
22	Maine	11.6
2	Maryland	17.0
1	Massachusetts	19.1
46	Michigan	8.5
33	Minnesota	10.0
45	Mississippi	8.7
30	Missouri	10.4
16	Montana	12.3
26	Nebraska	10.9
20	Nevada	12.0
24	New Hampshire	11.3
4	New Jersey	15.2
33	New Mexico	10.0
3	New York	16.4
36	North Carolina	9.8
48	North Dakota	7.8
23	Ohio	11.4
44	Oklahoma	8.8
10	Oregon	12.9
9	Pennsylvania	13.0
37	Rhode Island	9.7
35	South Carolina	9.9
49	South Dakota	6.9
19	Tennessee	12.1
18	Texas	12.2
15	Utah	12.5
16	Vermont	12.3
28	Virginia	10.6
6	Washington	14.5
43	West Virginia	9.0
10	Wisconsin	12.9
42	Wyoming	9.1

RANK ORDER

RANK	STATE	RATE
1	Massachusetts	19.1
2	Maryland	17.0
3	New York	16.4
4	New Jersey	15.2
5	Connecticut	15.1
6	Washington	14.5
7	Florida	13.2
7	Illinois	13.2
9	Pennsylvania	13.0
10	Oregon	12.9
10	Wisconsin	12.9
12	Colorado	12.8
12	Indiana	12.8
14	California	12.7
15	Utah	12.5
16	Montana	12.3
16	Vermont	12.3
18	Texas	12.2
19	Tennessee	12.1
20	Arizona	12.0
20	Nevada	12.0
22	Maine	11.6
23	Ohio	11.4
24	New Hampshire	11.3
25	Hawaii	11.1
26	Kentucky	10.9
26	Nebraska	10.9
28	Kansas	10.6
28	Virginia	10.6
30	Louisiana	10.4
30	Missouri	10.4
32	Georgia	10.1
33	Minnesota	10.0
33	New Mexico	10.0
35	South Carolina	9.9
36	North Carolina	9.8
37	Rhode Island	9.7
38	Arkansas	9.6
39	Alabama	9.5
39	Iowa	9.5
41	Alaska	9.2
42	Wyoming	9.1
43	West Virginia	9.0
44	Oklahoma	8.8
45	Mississippi	8.7
46	Michigan	8.5
47	Delaware	7.9
48	North Dakota	7.8
49	South Dakota	6.9
50	Idaho	6.5

	District of Columbia	18.7

Source: Morgan Quitno Press using data from American Medical Association (Chicago, Illinois)
    "Physician Characteristics and Distribution in the U.S." (2002-2003 Edition)
*As of December 31, 2000. National rate does not include physicians in U.S. territories and possessions.

Nonfederal Physicians in Psychiatry in 2000

National Total = 37,100 Physicians*

ALPHA ORDER

RANK	STATE	PHYSICIANS	% of USA
28	Alabama	305	0.8%
49	Alaska	56	0.2%
23	Arizona	470	1.3%
36	Arkansas	185	0.5%
2	California	5,046	13.6%
18	Colorado	540	1.5%
14	Connecticut	879	2.4%
44	Delaware	87	0.2%
6	Florida	1,554	4.2%
15	Georgia	799	2.2%
34	Hawaii	192	0.5%
46	Idaho	60	0.2%
7	Illinois	1,511	4.1%
24	Indiana	444	1.2%
37	Iowa	178	0.5%
29	Kansas	304	0.8%
27	Kentucky	368	1.0%
21	Louisiana	501	1.4%
33	Maine	204	0.5%
9	Maryland	1,249	3.4%
3	Massachusetts	1,975	5.3%
11	Michigan	1,052	2.8%
22	Minnesota	495	1.3%
38	Mississippi	164	0.4%
19	Missouri	537	1.4%
45	Montana	77	0.2%
41	Nebraska	153	0.4%
43	Nevada	127	0.3%
35	New Hampshire	191	0.5%
8	New Jersey	1,340	3.6%
31	New Mexico	224	0.6%
1	New York	5,347	14.4%
13	North Carolina	901	2.4%
47	North Dakota	59	0.2%
10	Ohio	1,094	2.9%
30	Oklahoma	248	0.7%
26	Oregon	389	1.0%
4	Pennsylvania	1,935	5.2%
32	Rhode Island	205	0.6%
25	South Carolina	439	1.2%
48	South Dakota	57	0.2%
20	Tennessee	515	1.4%
5	Texas	1,676	4.5%
38	Utah	164	0.4%
40	Vermont	161	0.4%
12	Virginia	910	2.5%
16	Washington	686	1.8%
42	West Virginia	143	0.4%
17	Wisconsin	556	1.5%
50	Wyoming	29	0.1%

RANK ORDER

RANK	STATE	PHYSICIANS	% of USA
1	New York	5,347	14.4%
2	California	5,046	13.6%
3	Massachusetts	1,975	5.3%
4	Pennsylvania	1,935	5.2%
5	Texas	1,676	4.5%
6	Florida	1,554	4.2%
7	Illinois	1,511	4.1%
8	New Jersey	1,340	3.6%
9	Maryland	1,249	3.4%
10	Ohio	1,094	2.9%
11	Michigan	1,052	2.8%
12	Virginia	910	2.5%
13	North Carolina	901	2.4%
14	Connecticut	879	2.4%
15	Georgia	799	2.2%
16	Washington	686	1.8%
17	Wisconsin	556	1.5%
18	Colorado	540	1.5%
19	Missouri	537	1.4%
20	Tennessee	515	1.4%
21	Louisiana	501	1.4%
22	Minnesota	495	1.3%
23	Arizona	470	1.3%
24	Indiana	444	1.2%
25	South Carolina	439	1.2%
26	Oregon	389	1.0%
27	Kentucky	368	1.0%
28	Alabama	305	0.8%
29	Kansas	304	0.8%
30	Oklahoma	248	0.7%
31	New Mexico	224	0.6%
32	Rhode Island	205	0.6%
33	Maine	204	0.5%
34	Hawaii	192	0.5%
35	New Hampshire	191	0.5%
36	Arkansas	185	0.5%
37	Iowa	178	0.5%
38	Mississippi	164	0.4%
38	Utah	164	0.4%
40	Vermont	161	0.4%
41	Nebraska	153	0.4%
42	West Virginia	143	0.4%
43	Nevada	127	0.3%
44	Delaware	87	0.2%
45	Montana	77	0.2%
46	Idaho	60	0.2%
47	North Dakota	59	0.2%
48	South Dakota	57	0.2%
49	Alaska	56	0.2%
50	Wyoming	29	0.1%
	District of Columbia	319	0.9%

Source: American Medical Association (Chicago, Illinois)
   "Physician Characteristics and Distribution in the U.S." (2002-2003 Edition)
*As of December 31, 2000. Total does not include 372 physicians in U.S. territories and possessions. Psychiatry includes psychoanalysis.

Rate of Nonfederal Physicians in Psychiatry in 2000

National Rate = 13.2 Physicians per 100,000 Population*

<u>ALPHA ORDER</u>

RANK	STATE	RATE
44	Alabama	6.9
35	Alaska	8.9
32	Arizona	9.1
44	Arkansas	6.9
12	California	14.8
14	Colorado	12.5
4	Connecticut	25.8
22	Delaware	11.1
27	Florida	9.7
27	Georgia	9.7
9	Hawaii	15.8
50	Idaho	4.6
16	Illinois	12.2
41	Indiana	7.3
47	Iowa	6.1
18	Kansas	11.3
32	Kentucky	9.1
20	Louisiana	11.2
7	Maine	16.0
5	Maryland	23.5
1	Massachusetts	31.1
24	Michigan	10.6
26	Minnesota	10.0
49	Mississippi	5.8
29	Missouri	9.6
37	Montana	8.5
35	Nebraska	8.9
46	Nevada	6.3
11	New Hampshire	15.4
8	New Jersey	15.9
15	New Mexico	12.3
2	New York	28.2
20	North Carolina	11.2
31	North Dakota	9.2
29	Ohio	9.6
43	Oklahoma	7.2
18	Oregon	11.3
9	Pennsylvania	15.8
6	Rhode Island	19.5
23	South Carolina	10.9
40	South Dakota	7.5
34	Tennessee	9.0
38	Texas	8.0
41	Utah	7.3
3	Vermont	26.4
13	Virginia	12.8
17	Washington	11.6
39	West Virginia	7.9
25	Wisconsin	10.3
48	Wyoming	5.9

<u>RANK ORDER</u>

RANK	STATE	RATE
1	Massachusetts	31.1
2	New York	28.2
3	Vermont	26.4
4	Connecticut	25.8
5	Maryland	23.5
6	Rhode Island	19.5
7	Maine	16.0
8	New Jersey	15.9
9	Hawaii	15.8
9	Pennsylvania	15.8
11	New Hampshire	15.4
12	California	14.8
13	Virginia	12.8
14	Colorado	12.5
15	New Mexico	12.3
16	Illinois	12.2
17	Washington	11.6
18	Kansas	11.3
18	Oregon	11.3
20	Louisiana	11.2
20	North Carolina	11.2
22	Delaware	11.1
23	South Carolina	10.9
24	Michigan	10.6
25	Wisconsin	10.3
26	Minnesota	10.0
27	Florida	9.7
27	Georgia	9.7
29	Missouri	9.6
29	Ohio	9.6
31	North Dakota	9.2
32	Arizona	9.1
32	Kentucky	9.1
34	Tennessee	9.0
35	Alaska	8.9
35	Nebraska	8.9
37	Montana	8.5
38	Texas	8.0
39	West Virginia	7.9
40	South Dakota	7.5
41	Indiana	7.3
41	Utah	7.3
43	Oklahoma	7.2
44	Alabama	6.9
44	Arkansas	6.9
46	Nevada	6.3
47	Iowa	6.1
48	Wyoming	5.9
49	Mississippi	5.8
50	Idaho	4.6

	District of Columbia	55.9

Source: Morgan Quitno Press using data from American Medical Association (Chicago, Illinois)
"Physician Characteristics and Distribution in the U.S." (2002-2003 Edition)
*As of December 31, 2000. National rate does not include physicians in U.S. territories and possessions.
Psychiatry includes psychoanalysis.

Percent of Population Lacking Access to Mental Health Care in 2001

National Percent = 12.5% of Population*

ALPHA ORDER				RANK ORDER		
RANK	STATE	PERCENT		RANK	STATE	PERCENT
1	Alabama	46.8		1	Alabama	46.8
11	Alaska	33.0		2	Idaho	44.7
27	Arizona	10.1		3	Montana	42.2
4	Arkansas	41.7		4	Arkansas	41.7
40	California	5.1		5	New Mexico	38.7
42	Colorado	2.8		6	Wyoming	37.3
47	Connecticut	0.6		7	Iowa	36.0
49	Delaware	0.0		7	North Dakota	36.0
37	Florida	5.9		9	South Carolina	34.6
22	Georgia	17.0		10	Nebraska	33.4
34	Hawaii	7.6		11	Alaska	33.0
2	Idaho	44.7		12	Kansas	29.5
29	Illinois	9.7		13	Oklahoma	28.9
41	Indiana	4.8		14	Texas	22.4
7	Iowa	36.0		15	Kentucky	22.1
12	Kansas	29.5		16	Wisconsin	21.3
15	Kentucky	22.1		17	Utah	19.5
46	Louisiana	1.1		18	Mississippi	19.2
32	Maine	9.1		19	Missouri	19.0
43	Maryland	1.9		20	Oregon	17.3
45	Massachusetts	1.2		21	Michigan	17.1
21	Michigan	17.1		22	Georgia	17.0
22	Minnesota	17.0		22	Minnesota	17.0
18	Mississippi	19.2		24	Tennessee	16.9
19	Missouri	19.0		25	Washington	13.6
3	Montana	42.2		26	Vermont	12.6
10	Nebraska	33.4		27	Arizona	10.1
31	Nevada	9.6		28	North Carolina	10.0
38	New Hampshire	5.8		29	Illinois	9.7
47	New Jersey	0.6		29	Pennsylvania	9.7
5	New Mexico	38.7		31	Nevada	9.6
39	New York	5.5		32	Maine	9.1
28	North Carolina	10.0		33	West Virginia	7.8
7	North Dakota	36.0		34	Hawaii	7.6
35	Ohio	7.2		35	Ohio	7.2
13	Oklahoma	28.9		36	South Dakota	6.1
20	Oregon	17.3		37	Florida	5.9
29	Pennsylvania	9.7		38	New Hampshire	5.8
49	Rhode Island	0.0		39	New York	5.5
9	South Carolina	34.6		40	California	5.1
36	South Dakota	6.1		41	Indiana	4.8
24	Tennessee	16.9		42	Colorado	2.8
14	Texas	22.4		43	Maryland	1.9
17	Utah	19.5		44	Virginia	1.5
26	Vermont	12.6		45	Massachusetts	1.2
44	Virginia	1.5		46	Louisiana	1.1
25	Washington	13.6		47	Connecticut	0.6
33	West Virginia	7.8		47	New Jersey	0.6
16	Wisconsin	21.3		49	Delaware	0.0
6	Wyoming	37.3		49	Rhode Island	0.0
					District of Columbia	0.7

Source: Morgan Quitno Press using data from U.S. Dept. of Health and Human Services, Div. of Shortage Designation
"Selected Statistics on Health Professional Shortage Areas, As of December 31, 2001"
*Percent of population considered under-served by mental health practitioners. An under-served population does
not have primary medical care within reasonable economic and geographic bounds.

International Medical School Graduates Practicing in the U.S. in 2000

National Total = 186,724 Nonfederal Physicians*

ALPHA ORDER

RANK	STATE	PHYSICIANS	% of USA
26	Alabama	1,343	0.7%
48	Alaska	84	0.0%
20	Arizona	1,978	1.1%
34	Arkansas	657	0.4%
2	California	20,783	11.1%
33	Colorado	684	0.4%
13	Connecticut	3,576	1.9%
36	Delaware	576	0.3%
3	Florida	15,383	8.2%
14	Georgia	3,115	1.7%
38	Hawaii	558	0.3%
49	Idaho	57	0.0%
5	Illinois	11,972	6.4%
16	Indiana	2,416	1.3%
31	Iowa	935	0.5%
28	Kansas	1,049	0.6%
23	Kentucky	1,775	1.0%
21	Louisiana	1,915	1.0%
42	Maine	407	0.2%
10	Maryland	6,025	3.2%
11	Massachusetts	5,762	3.1%
9	Michigan	7,833	4.2%
22	Minnesota	1,789	1.0%
39	Mississippi	547	0.3%
15	Missouri	2,813	1.5%
47	Montana	86	0.0%
40	Nebraska	451	0.2%
32	Nevada	878	0.5%
41	New Hampshire	421	0.2%
4	New Jersey	12,090	6.5%
37	New Mexico	568	0.3%
1	New York	32,338	17.3%
18	North Carolina	2,209	1.2%
43	North Dakota	315	0.2%
8	Ohio	7,847	4.2%
27	Oklahoma	1,055	0.6%
35	Oregon	633	0.3%
7	Pennsylvania	9,018	4.8%
30	Rhode Island	983	0.5%
29	South Carolina	997	0.5%
46	South Dakota	185	0.1%
19	Tennessee	2,109	1.1%
6	Texas	10,033	5.4%
44	Utah	299	0.2%
45	Vermont	189	0.1%
12	Virginia	3,965	2.1%
24	Washington	1,552	0.8%
25	West Virginia	1,457	0.8%
17	Wisconsin	2,215	1.2%
50	Wyoming	52	0.0%

RANK ORDER

RANK	STATE	PHYSICIANS	% of USA
1	New York	32,338	17.3%
2	California	20,783	11.1%
3	Florida	15,383	8.2%
4	New Jersey	12,090	6.5%
5	Illinois	11,972	6.4%
6	Texas	10,033	5.4%
7	Pennsylvania	9,018	4.8%
8	Ohio	7,847	4.2%
9	Michigan	7,833	4.2%
10	Maryland	6,025	3.2%
11	Massachusetts	5,762	3.1%
12	Virginia	3,965	2.1%
13	Connecticut	3,576	1.9%
14	Georgia	3,115	1.7%
15	Missouri	2,813	1.5%
16	Indiana	2,416	1.3%
17	Wisconsin	2,215	1.2%
18	North Carolina	2,209	1.2%
19	Tennessee	2,109	1.1%
20	Arizona	1,978	1.1%
21	Louisiana	1,915	1.0%
22	Minnesota	1,789	1.0%
23	Kentucky	1,775	1.0%
24	Washington	1,552	0.8%
25	West Virginia	1,457	0.8%
26	Alabama	1,343	0.7%
27	Oklahoma	1,055	0.6%
28	Kansas	1,049	0.6%
29	South Carolina	997	0.5%
30	Rhode Island	983	0.5%
31	Iowa	935	0.5%
32	Nevada	878	0.5%
33	Colorado	684	0.4%
34	Arkansas	657	0.4%
35	Oregon	633	0.3%
36	Delaware	576	0.3%
37	New Mexico	568	0.3%
38	Hawaii	558	0.3%
39	Mississippi	547	0.3%
40	Nebraska	451	0.2%
41	New Hampshire	421	0.2%
42	Maine	407	0.2%
43	North Dakota	315	0.2%
44	Utah	299	0.2%
45	Vermont	189	0.1%
46	South Dakota	185	0.1%
47	Montana	86	0.0%
48	Alaska	84	0.0%
49	Idaho	57	0.0%
50	Wyoming	52	0.0%
	District of Columbia	747	0.4%

Source: American Medical Association (Chicago, Illinois)
    "Physician Characteristics and Distribution in the U.S." (2002-2003 Edition)
*Nonfederal physicians as of December 31, 2000. Total does not include 5,417 physicians in U.S. territories and possessions.

Rate of International Medical School Graduates Practicing in the U.S. in 2000

National Rate = 66 Nonfederal Physicians per 100,000 Population*

ALPHA ORDER

RANK	STATE	RATE
36	Alabama	30
46	Alaska	13
26	Arizona	38
40	Arkansas	25
14	California	61
45	Colorado	16
4	Connecticut	105
11	Delaware	73
5	Florida	96
26	Georgia	38
19	Hawaii	46
50	Idaho	4
5	Illinois	96
24	Indiana	40
31	Iowa	32
25	Kansas	39
20	Kentucky	44
21	Louisiana	43
31	Maine	32
3	Maryland	113
8	Massachusetts	91
10	Michigan	79
29	Minnesota	36
43	Mississippi	19
16	Missouri	50
49	Montana	10
38	Nebraska	26
21	Nevada	43
30	New Hampshire	34
2	New Jersey	143
33	New Mexico	31
1	New York	170
37	North Carolina	27
17	North Dakota	49
13	Ohio	69
33	Oklahoma	31
44	Oregon	18
11	Pennsylvania	73
7	Rhode Island	94
40	South Carolina	25
42	South Dakota	24
28	Tennessee	37
18	Texas	48
46	Utah	13
33	Vermont	31
15	Virginia	56
38	Washington	26
9	West Virginia	81
23	Wisconsin	41
48	Wyoming	11

RANK ORDER

RANK	STATE	RATE
1	New York	170
2	New Jersey	143
3	Maryland	113
4	Connecticut	105
5	Florida	96
5	Illinois	96
7	Rhode Island	94
8	Massachusetts	91
9	West Virginia	81
10	Michigan	79
11	Delaware	73
11	Pennsylvania	73
13	Ohio	69
14	California	61
15	Virginia	56
16	Missouri	50
17	North Dakota	49
18	Texas	48
19	Hawaii	46
20	Kentucky	44
21	Louisiana	43
21	Nevada	43
23	Wisconsin	41
24	Indiana	40
25	Kansas	39
26	Arizona	38
26	Georgia	38
28	Tennessee	37
29	Minnesota	36
30	New Hampshire	34
31	Iowa	32
31	Maine	32
33	New Mexico	31
33	Oklahoma	31
33	Vermont	31
36	Alabama	30
37	North Carolina	27
38	Nebraska	26
38	Washington	26
40	Arkansas	25
40	South Carolina	25
42	South Dakota	24
43	Mississippi	19
44	Oregon	18
45	Colorado	16
46	Alaska	13
46	Utah	13
48	Wyoming	11
49	Montana	10
50	Idaho	4

District of Columbia 131

Source: Morgan Quitno Press using data from American Medical Association (Chicago, Illinois)
"Physician Characteristics and Distribution in the U.S." (2002-2003 Edition)
*As of December 31, 2000. National rate does not include physicians in U.S. territories and possessions.

International Medical School Graduates
As a Percent of Nonfederal Physicians in 2000
National Percent = 23.9% of Nonfederal Physicians*

ALPHA ORDER			RANK ORDER		
RANK	**STATE**	**PERCENT**	**RANK**	**STATE**	**PERCENT**
31	Alabama	13.9	1	New Jersey	44.5
45	Alaska	6.9	2	New York	41.7
23	Arizona	16.8	3	Florida	34.4
35	Arkansas	11.8	4	Illinois	33.9
15	California	21.9	4	West Virginia	33.9
47	Colorado	6.0	6	Michigan	31.5
9	Connecticut	27.3	7	Delaware	28.2
7	Delaware	28.2	8	Maryland	28.0
3	Florida	34.4	9	Connecticut	27.3
22	Georgia	16.9	10	Ohio	26.4
29	Hawaii	15.4	11	Rhode Island	26.3
50	Idaho	2.5	12	Pennsylvania	23.1
4	Illinois	33.9	13	Nevada	22.6
21	Indiana	18.2	14	Texas	22.1
26	Iowa	16.1	15	California	21.9
24	Kansas	16.7	16	Virginia	20.6
20	Kentucky	19.1	17	Missouri	20.4
28	Louisiana	16.0	18	North Dakota	20.3
36	Maine	11.5	19	Massachusetts	20.2
8	Maryland	28.0	20	Kentucky	19.1
19	Massachusetts	20.2	21	Indiana	18.2
6	Michigan	31.5	22	Georgia	16.9
33	Minnesota	12.8	23	Arizona	16.8
40	Mississippi	10.6	24	Kansas	16.7
17	Missouri	20.4	25	Oklahoma	16.6
49	Montana	4.1	26	Iowa	16.1
39	Nebraska	10.7	26	Wisconsin	16.1
13	Nevada	22.6	28	Louisiana	16.0
34	New Hampshire	12.5	29	Hawaii	15.4
1	New Jersey	44.5	30	Tennessee	14.1
32	New Mexico	13.1	31	Alabama	13.9
2	New York	41.7	32	New Mexico	13.1
38	North Carolina	10.8	33	Minnesota	12.8
18	North Dakota	20.3	34	New Hampshire	12.5
10	Ohio	26.4	35	Arkansas	11.8
25	Oklahoma	16.6	36	Maine	11.5
44	Oregon	7.0	36	South Dakota	11.5
12	Pennsylvania	23.1	38	North Carolina	10.8
11	Rhode Island	26.3	39	Nebraska	10.7
40	South Carolina	10.6	40	Mississippi	10.6
36	South Dakota	11.5	40	South Carolina	10.6
30	Tennessee	14.1	42	Washington	9.6
14	Texas	22.1	43	Vermont	8.3
46	Utah	6.1	44	Oregon	7.0
43	Vermont	8.3	45	Alaska	6.9
16	Virginia	20.6	46	Utah	6.1
42	Washington	9.6	47	Colorado	6.0
4	West Virginia	33.9	48	Wyoming	5.3
26	Wisconsin	16.1	49	Montana	4.1
48	Wyoming	5.3	50	Idaho	2.5
			District of Columbia		18.2

Source: Morgan Quitno Press using data from American Medical Association (Chicago, Illinois)
"Physician Characteristics and Distribution in the U.S." (2002-2003 Edition)
*As of December 31, 2000. National percent does not include physicians in U.S. territories and possessions.

Osteopathic Physicians in 2002

National Total = 41,402 Osteopathic Physicians*

ALPHA ORDER

RANK	STATE	OSTEOPATHS	% of USA
28	Alabama	287	0.7%
44	Alaska	91	0.2%
12	Arizona	1,059	2.6%
37	Arkansas	167	0.4%
8	California	2,244	5.4%
14	Colorado	649	1.6%
31	Connecticut	231	0.6%
35	Delaware	179	0.4%
4	Florida	2,689	6.5%
16	Georgia	577	1.4%
40	Hawaii	127	0.3%
41	Idaho	123	0.3%
9	Illinois	1,822	4.4%
15	Indiana	610	1.5%
13	Iowa	923	2.2%
17	Kansas	523	1.3%
34	Kentucky	222	0.5%
45	Louisiana	89	0.2%
22	Maine	458	1.1%
23	Maryland	443	1.1%
25	Massachusetts	378	0.9%
2	Michigan	4,346	10.5%
30	Minnesota	255	0.6%
33	Mississippi	226	0.5%
10	Missouri	1,590	3.8%
46	Montana	79	0.2%
43	Nebraska	92	0.2%
29	Nevada	279	0.7%
42	New Hampshire	120	0.3%
7	New Jersey	2,411	5.8%
36	New Mexico	177	0.4%
5	New York	2,647	6.4%
26	North Carolina	350	0.8%
48	North Dakota	55	0.1%
3	Ohio	3,071	7.4%
11	Oklahoma	1,215	2.9%
24	Oregon	379	0.9%
1	Pennsylvania	4,688	11.3%
38	Rhode Island	165	0.4%
32	South Carolina	228	0.6%
47	South Dakota	65	0.2%
27	Tennessee	322	0.8%
6	Texas	2,545	6.1%
39	Utah	137	0.3%
49	Vermont	45	0.1%
20	Virginia	482	1.2%
18	Washington	515	1.2%
19	West Virginia	492	1.2%
21	Wisconsin	461	1.1%
50	Wyoming	43	0.1%

RANK ORDER

RANK	STATE	OSTEOPATHS	% of USA
1	Pennsylvania	4,688	11.3%
2	Michigan	4,346	10.5%
3	Ohio	3,071	7.4%
4	Florida	2,689	6.5%
5	New York	2,647	6.4%
6	Texas	2,545	6.1%
7	New Jersey	2,411	5.8%
8	California	2,244	5.4%
9	Illinois	1,822	4.4%
10	Missouri	1,590	3.8%
11	Oklahoma	1,215	2.9%
12	Arizona	1,059	2.6%
13	Iowa	923	2.2%
14	Colorado	649	1.6%
15	Indiana	610	1.5%
16	Georgia	577	1.4%
17	Kansas	523	1.3%
18	Washington	515	1.2%
19	West Virginia	492	1.2%
20	Virginia	482	1.2%
21	Wisconsin	461	1.1%
22	Maine	458	1.1%
23	Maryland	443	1.1%
24	Oregon	379	0.9%
25	Massachusetts	378	0.9%
26	North Carolina	350	0.8%
27	Tennessee	322	0.8%
28	Alabama	287	0.7%
29	Nevada	279	0.7%
30	Minnesota	255	0.6%
31	Connecticut	231	0.6%
32	South Carolina	228	0.6%
33	Mississippi	226	0.5%
34	Kentucky	222	0.5%
35	Delaware	179	0.4%
36	New Mexico	177	0.4%
37	Arkansas	167	0.4%
38	Rhode Island	165	0.4%
39	Utah	137	0.3%
40	Hawaii	127	0.3%
41	Idaho	123	0.3%
42	New Hampshire	120	0.3%
43	Nebraska	92	0.2%
44	Alaska	91	0.2%
45	Louisiana	89	0.2%
46	Montana	79	0.2%
47	South Dakota	65	0.2%
48	North Dakota	55	0.1%
49	Vermont	45	0.1%
50	Wyoming	43	0.1%
	District of Columbia	31	0.1%

Source: American Osteopathic Association
"Fact Sheet: Active D.O.'s by State" (February 2002, http://www.aoa.net/AOAGeneral/facts202.pdf)
Excludes retired, disabled, foreign and federal osteopaths. Osteopaths practice a system of medicine based on the theory that disturbances in the musculoskeletal system affect other body parts, causing many disorders that can be corrected by various manipulative techniques in conjunction with conventional medical, surgical, pharmacological, and other therapeutic procedures.

Rate of Osteopathic Physicians in 2002

National Rate = 15 Osteopaths per 100,000 Population*

ALPHA ORDER

RANK	STATE	RATE
40	Alabama	6
17	Alaska	14
11	Arizona	20
40	Arkansas	6
35	California	7
15	Colorado	15
35	Connecticut	7
10	Delaware	22
13	Florida	16
35	Georgia	7
22	Hawaii	10
26	Idaho	9
15	Illinois	15
22	Indiana	10
5	Iowa	32
12	Kansas	19
46	Kentucky	5
50	Louisiana	2
3	Maine	36
33	Maryland	8
40	Massachusetts	6
1	Michigan	43
46	Minnesota	5
33	Mississippi	8
6	Missouri	28
26	Montana	9
46	Nebraska	5
19	Nevada	13
22	New Hampshire	10
6	New Jersey	28
22	New Mexico	10
17	New York	14
49	North Carolina	4
26	North Dakota	9
8	Ohio	27
4	Oklahoma	35
21	Oregon	11
2	Pennsylvania	38
13	Rhode Island	16
40	South Carolina	6
26	South Dakota	9
40	Tennessee	6
20	Texas	12
40	Utah	6
35	Vermont	7
35	Virginia	7
26	Washington	9
8	West Virginia	27
26	Wisconsin	9
26	Wyoming	9

RANK ORDER

RANK	STATE	RATE
1	Michigan	43
2	Pennsylvania	38
3	Maine	36
4	Oklahoma	35
5	Iowa	32
6	Missouri	28
6	New Jersey	28
8	Ohio	27
8	West Virginia	27
10	Delaware	22
11	Arizona	20
12	Kansas	19
13	Florida	16
13	Rhode Island	16
15	Colorado	15
15	Illinois	15
17	Alaska	14
17	New York	14
19	Nevada	13
20	Texas	12
21	Oregon	11
22	Hawaii	10
22	Indiana	10
22	New Hampshire	10
22	New Mexico	10
26	Idaho	9
26	Montana	9
26	North Dakota	9
26	South Dakota	9
26	Washington	9
26	Wisconsin	9
26	Wyoming	9
33	Maryland	8
33	Mississippi	8
35	California	7
35	Connecticut	7
35	Georgia	7
35	Vermont	7
35	Virginia	7
40	Alabama	6
40	Arkansas	6
40	Massachusetts	6
40	South Carolina	6
40	Tennessee	6
40	Utah	6
46	Kentucky	5
46	Minnesota	5
46	Nebraska	5
49	North Carolina	4
50	Louisiana	2
	District of Columbia	5

Source: Morgan Quitno Press using data from American Osteopathic Association
"Fact Sheet: Active D.O.'s by State" (February 2002, http://www.aoa.net/AOAGeneral/facts202.pdf)
*Calculated using 2001 population estimates. Excludes retired, disabled, foreign and federal osteopaths.
Osteopaths practice a system of medicine based on the theory that disturbances in the musculoskeletal system affect other body parts, causing many disorders that can be corrected by various manipulative techniques in conjunction with conventional medical, surgical, pharmacological, and other therapeutic procedures.

Podiatric Physicians in 1999

National Total = 13,318 Podiatric Physicians*

ALPHA ORDER

RANK	STATE	PODIATRISTS	% of USA
27	Alabama	97	0.7%
46	Alaska	24	0.2%
17	Arizona	198	1.5%
38	Arkansas	55	0.4%
2	California	1,522	11.4%
24	Colorado	128	1.0%
12	Connecticut	269	2.0%
43	Delaware	36	0.3%
4	Florida	914	6.9%
14	Georgia	241	1.8%
47	Hawaii	22	0.2%
42	Idaho	39	0.3%
5	Illinois	863	6.5%
14	Indiana	241	1.8%
21	Iowa	152	1.1%
28	Kansas	90	0.7%
30	Kentucky	82	0.6%
26	Louisiana	103	0.8%
36	Maine	59	0.4%
11	Maryland	290	2.2%
10	Massachusetts	439	3.3%
9	Michigan	530	4.0%
22	Minnesota	134	1.0%
43	Mississippi	36	0.3%
20	Missouri	171	1.3%
41	Montana	41	0.3%
35	Nebraska	60	0.5%
38	Nevada	55	0.4%
40	New Hampshire	54	0.4%
6	New Jersey	744	5.6%
36	New Mexico	59	0.4%
1	New York	1,602	12.0%
18	North Carolina	195	1.5%
47	North Dakota	22	0.2%
7	Ohio	688	5.2%
31	Oklahoma	81	0.6%
29	Oregon	85	0.6%
3	Pennsylvania	1,120	8.4%
32	Rhode Island	77	0.6%
33	South Carolina	66	0.5%
45	South Dakota	27	0.2%
22	Tennessee	134	1.0%
8	Texas	569	4.3%
25	Utah	113	0.8%
49	Vermont	16	0.1%
13	Virginia	248	1.9%
19	Washington	192	1.4%
34	West Virginia	65	0.5%
16	Wisconsin	201	1.5%
50	Wyoming	11	0.1%

RANK ORDER

RANK	STATE	PODIATRISTS	% of USA
1	New York	1,602	12.0%
2	California	1,522	11.4%
3	Pennsylvania	1,120	8.4%
4	Florida	914	6.9%
5	Illinois	863	6.5%
6	New Jersey	744	5.6%
7	Ohio	688	5.2%
8	Texas	569	4.3%
9	Michigan	530	4.0%
10	Massachusetts	439	3.3%
11	Maryland	290	2.2%
12	Connecticut	269	2.0%
13	Virginia	248	1.9%
14	Georgia	241	1.8%
14	Indiana	241	1.8%
16	Wisconsin	201	1.5%
17	Arizona	198	1.5%
18	North Carolina	195	1.5%
19	Washington	192	1.4%
20	Missouri	171	1.3%
21	Iowa	152	1.1%
22	Minnesota	134	1.0%
22	Tennessee	134	1.0%
24	Colorado	128	1.0%
25	Utah	113	0.8%
26	Louisiana	103	0.8%
27	Alabama	97	0.7%
28	Kansas	90	0.7%
29	Oregon	85	0.6%
30	Kentucky	82	0.6%
31	Oklahoma	81	0.6%
32	Rhode Island	77	0.6%
33	South Carolina	66	0.5%
34	West Virginia	65	0.5%
35	Nebraska	60	0.5%
36	Maine	59	0.4%
36	New Mexico	59	0.4%
38	Arkansas	55	0.4%
38	Nevada	55	0.4%
40	New Hampshire	54	0.4%
41	Montana	41	0.3%
42	Idaho	39	0.3%
43	Delaware	36	0.3%
43	Mississippi	36	0.3%
45	South Dakota	27	0.2%
46	Alaska	24	0.2%
47	Hawaii	22	0.2%
47	North Dakota	22	0.2%
49	Vermont	16	0.1%
50	Wyoming	11	0.1%
	District of Columbia	58	0.4%

Source: American Podiatric Medical Association, Inc.
   "Podiatric Physicians in Active Practice"
As of Fall 1999. Includes only Podiatric physicians considered in "active practice." Podiatry deals with the diagnosis, treatment, and prevention of diseases of the human foot. National total does not include four podiatrists in Puerto Rico.

Rate of Podiatric Physicians in 1999

National Rate = 4.9 Podiatrists per 100,000 Population*

ALPHA ORDER

RANK	STATE	RATE
45	Alabama	2.2
21	Alaska	3.9
19	Arizona	4.1
45	Arkansas	2.2
16	California	4.6
31	Colorado	3.2
4	Connecticut	8.2
14	Delaware	4.8
9	Florida	6.0
32	Georgia	3.1
48	Hawaii	1.9
32	Idaho	3.1
6	Illinois	7.1
19	Indiana	4.1
12	Iowa	5.3
28	Kansas	3.4
47	Kentucky	2.1
41	Louisiana	2.4
15	Maine	4.7
10	Maryland	5.6
6	Massachusetts	7.1
11	Michigan	5.4
36	Minnesota	2.8
50	Mississippi	1.3
32	Missouri	3.1
16	Montana	4.6
24	Nebraska	3.6
35	Nevada	3.0
18	New Hampshire	4.5
2	New Jersey	9.1
28	New Mexico	3.4
3	New York	8.8
40	North Carolina	2.5
27	North Dakota	3.5
8	Ohio	6.1
41	Oklahoma	2.4
39	Oregon	2.6
1	Pennsylvania	9.3
5	Rhode Island	7.8
49	South Carolina	1.7
23	South Dakota	3.7
41	Tennessee	2.4
36	Texas	2.8
12	Utah	5.3
38	Vermont	2.7
24	Virginia	3.6
30	Washington	3.3
24	West Virginia	3.6
22	Wisconsin	3.8
44	Wyoming	2.3

RANK ORDER

RANK	STATE	RATE
1	Pennsylvania	9.3
2	New Jersey	9.1
3	New York	8.8
4	Connecticut	8.2
5	Rhode Island	7.8
6	Illinois	7.1
6	Massachusetts	7.1
8	Ohio	6.1
9	Florida	6.0
10	Maryland	5.6
11	Michigan	5.4
12	Iowa	5.3
12	Utah	5.3
14	Delaware	4.8
15	Maine	4.7
16	California	4.6
16	Montana	4.6
18	New Hampshire	4.5
19	Arizona	4.1
19	Indiana	4.1
21	Alaska	3.9
22	Wisconsin	3.8
23	South Dakota	3.7
24	Nebraska	3.6
24	Virginia	3.6
24	West Virginia	3.6
27	North Dakota	3.5
28	Kansas	3.4
28	New Mexico	3.4
30	Washington	3.3
31	Colorado	3.2
32	Georgia	3.1
32	Idaho	3.1
32	Missouri	3.1
35	Nevada	3.0
36	Minnesota	2.8
36	Texas	2.8
38	Vermont	2.7
39	Oregon	2.6
40	North Carolina	2.5
41	Louisiana	2.4
41	Oklahoma	2.4
41	Tennessee	2.4
44	Wyoming	2.3
45	Alabama	2.2
45	Arkansas	2.2
47	Kentucky	2.1
48	Hawaii	1.9
49	South Carolina	1.7
50	Mississippi	1.3

| | District of Columbia | 11.2 |

Source: Morgan Quitno Press using data from American Podiatric Medical Association, Inc.
        "Podiatric Physicians in Active Practice"
*Includes only Podiatric physicians considered in "active practice." Podiatry deals with the diagnosis, treatment,
and prevention of diseases of the human foot. National rate does not include podiatrists in Puerto Rico.

Doctors of Chiropractic in 2000

National Total = 81,011 Chiropractors*

ALPHA ORDER

RANK ORDER

RANK	STATE	CHIROPRACTOR	% of USA
30	Alabama	759	0.9%
48	Alaska	175	0.2%
10	Arizona	2,488	3.1%
33	Arkansas	557	0.7%
1	California	12,600	15.6%
11	Colorado	2,063	2.5%
27	Connecticut	893	1.1%
45	Delaware	242	0.3%
3	Florida	4,335	5.4%
6	Georgia	3,552	4.4%
34	Hawaii	521	0.6%
38	Idaho	363	0.4%
8	Illinois	2,925	3.6%
25	Indiana	964	1.2%
21	Iowa	1,309	1.6%
26	Kansas	932	1.2%
24	Kentucky	1,121	1.4%
22	Louisiana	1,289	1.6%
39	Maine	355	0.4%
32	Maryland	587	0.7%
15	Massachusetts	1,934	2.4%
9	Michigan	2,755	3.4%
13	Minnesota	1,960	2.4%
41	Mississippi	339	0.4%
16	Missouri	1,917	2.4%
43	Montana	302	0.4%
42	Nebraska	324	0.4%
37	Nevada	427	0.5%
36	New Hampshire	449	0.6%
7	New Jersey	3,383	4.2%
35	New Mexico	493	0.6%
2	New York	5,885	7.3%
17	North Carolina	1,628	2.0%
46	North Dakota	240	0.3%
12	Ohio	2,015	2.5%
28	Oklahoma	867	1.1%
19	Oregon	1,396	1.7%
5	Pennsylvania	3,704	4.6%
NA	Rhode Island**	NA	NA
23	South Carolina	1,263	1.6%
40	South Dakota	346	0.4%
29	Tennessee	802	1.0%
4	Texas	4,268	5.3%
31	Utah	754	0.9%
47	Vermont	215	0.3%
20	Virginia	1,311	1.6%
14	Washington	1,938	2.4%
44	West Virginia	276	0.3%
18	Wisconsin	1,584	2.0%
49	Wyoming	171	0.2%

RANK	STATE	CHIROPRACTOR	% of USA
1	California	12,600	15.6%
2	New York	5,885	7.3%
3	Florida	4,335	5.4%
4	Texas	4,268	5.3%
5	Pennsylvania	3,704	4.6%
6	Georgia	3,552	4.4%
7	New Jersey	3,383	4.2%
8	Illinois	2,925	3.6%
9	Michigan	2,755	3.4%
10	Arizona	2,488	3.1%
11	Colorado	2,063	2.5%
12	Ohio	2,015	2.5%
13	Minnesota	1,960	2.4%
14	Washington	1,938	2.4%
15	Massachusetts	1,934	2.4%
16	Missouri	1,917	2.4%
17	North Carolina	1,628	2.0%
18	Wisconsin	1,584	2.0%
19	Oregon	1,396	1.7%
20	Virginia	1,311	1.6%
21	Iowa	1,309	1.6%
22	Louisiana	1,289	1.6%
23	South Carolina	1,263	1.6%
24	Kentucky	1,121	1.4%
25	Indiana	964	1.2%
26	Kansas	932	1.2%
27	Connecticut	893	1.1%
28	Oklahoma	867	1.1%
29	Tennessee	802	1.0%
30	Alabama	759	0.9%
31	Utah	754	0.9%
32	Maryland	587	0.7%
33	Arkansas	557	0.7%
34	Hawaii	521	0.6%
35	New Mexico	493	0.6%
36	New Hampshire	449	0.6%
37	Nevada	427	0.5%
38	Idaho	363	0.4%
39	Maine	355	0.4%
40	South Dakota	346	0.4%
41	Mississippi	339	0.4%
42	Nebraska	324	0.4%
43	Montana	302	0.4%
44	West Virginia	276	0.3%
45	Delaware	242	0.3%
46	North Dakota	240	0.3%
47	Vermont	215	0.3%
48	Alaska	175	0.2%
49	Wyoming	171	0.2%
NA	Rhode Island**	NA	NA
	District of Columbia	35	0.0%

Source: Federation of Chiropractic Licensing Boards
"Official Directory" (http://www.fclb.org/directory/index.htm)
*As of December 2000. Licensed active doctors. There is some duplication as some doctors are licensed in more than one state.
**Not available.

Rate of Doctors of Chiropractic in 2000

National Rate = 29 Chiropractors per 100,000 Population*

ALPHA ORDER				RANK ORDER		
RANK	STATE	RATE		RANK	STATE	RATE
44	Alabama	17		1	Arizona	48
27	Alaska	28		1	Colorado	48
1	Arizona	48		3	South Dakota	46
37	Arkansas	21		4	Iowa	45
10	California	37		5	Georgia	43
1	Colorado	48		5	Hawaii	43
34	Connecticut	26		7	Oregon	41
20	Delaware	31		8	Minnesota	40
32	Florida	27		8	New Jersey	40
5	Georgia	43		10	California	37
5	Hawaii	43		10	North Dakota	37
27	Idaho	28		12	New Hampshire	36
36	Illinois	24		13	Kansas	35
45	Indiana	16		13	Vermont	35
4	Iowa	45		13	Wyoming	35
13	Kansas	35		16	Missouri	34
27	Kentucky	28		16	Utah	34
25	Louisiana	29		18	Montana	33
27	Maine	28		18	Washington	33
49	Maryland	11		20	Delaware	31
23	Massachusetts	30		20	New York	31
27	Michigan	28		20	South Carolina	31
8	Minnesota	40		23	Massachusetts	30
48	Mississippi	12		23	Pennsylvania	30
16	Missouri	34		25	Louisiana	29
18	Montana	33		25	Wisconsin	29
41	Nebraska	19		27	Alaska	28
37	Nevada	21		27	Idaho	28
12	New Hampshire	36		27	Kentucky	28
8	New Jersey	40		27	Maine	28
32	New Mexico	27		27	Michigan	28
20	New York	31		32	Florida	27
39	North Carolina	20		32	New Mexico	27
10	North Dakota	37		34	Connecticut	26
42	Ohio	18		35	Oklahoma	25
35	Oklahoma	25		36	Illinois	24
7	Oregon	41		37	Arkansas	21
23	Pennsylvania	30		37	Nevada	21
NA	Rhode Island**	NA		39	North Carolina	20
20	South Carolina	31		39	Texas	20
3	South Dakota	46		41	Nebraska	19
47	Tennessee	14		42	Ohio	18
39	Texas	20		42	Virginia	18
16	Utah	34		44	Alabama	17
13	Vermont	35		45	Indiana	16
42	Virginia	18		46	West Virginia	15
18	Washington	33		47	Tennessee	14
46	West Virginia	15		48	Mississippi	12
25	Wisconsin	29		49	Maryland	11
13	Wyoming	35		NA	Rhode Island**	NA
					District of Columbia	6

Source: Morgan Quitno Press using data from Federation of Chiropractic Licensing Boards
"Official Directory" (http://www.fclb.org/directory/index.htm)
*As of December 2000. Licensed active doctors. There is some duplication as some doctors are licensed in more than one state.
**Not available.

Physician Assistants in Clinical Practice in 2002

National Total = 42,220 Physician Assistants*

ALPHA ORDER

RANK	STATE	PA'S	% of USA
37	Alabama	254	0.6%
39	Alaska	237	0.6%
17	Arizona	786	1.9%
49	Arkansas	56	0.1%
2	California	4,108	9.7%
12	Colorado	1,050	2.5%
16	Connecticut	823	1.9%
48	Delaware	96	0.2%
5	Florida	2,322	5.5%
8	Georgia	1,408	3.3%
47	Hawaii	100	0.2%
37	Idaho	254	0.6%
13	Illinois	1,021	2.4%
33	Indiana	312	0.7%
24	Iowa	519	1.2%
27	Kansas	465	1.1%
21	Kentucky	593	1.4%
34	Louisiana	297	0.7%
29	Maine	397	0.9%
10	Maryland	1,225	2.9%
14	Massachusetts	898	2.1%
7	Michigan	1,760	4.2%
19	Minnesota	641	1.5%
50	Mississippi	37	0.1%
35	Missouri	291	0.7%
42	Montana	200	0.5%
25	Nebraska	507	1.2%
40	Nevada	229	0.5%
41	New Hampshire	221	0.5%
22	New Jersey	560	1.3%
31	New Mexico	367	0.9%
1	New York	5,097	12.1%
6	North Carolina	2,121	5.0%
43	North Dakota	186	0.4%
11	Ohio	1,200	2.8%
20	Oklahoma	640	1.5%
28	Oregon	407	1.0%
4	Pennsylvania	2,425	5.7%
44	Rhode Island	139	0.3%
32	South Carolina	352	0.8%
36	South Dakota	271	0.6%
23	Tennessee	523	1.2%
3	Texas	2,678	6.3%
30	Utah	369	0.9%
45	Vermont	130	0.3%
18	Virginia	724	1.7%
9	Washington	1,248	3.0%
26	West Virginia	491	1.2%
15	Wisconsin	877	2.1%
46	Wyoming	123	0.3%

RANK ORDER

RANK	STATE	PA'S	% of USA
1	New York	5,097	12.1%
2	California	4,108	9.7%
3	Texas	2,678	6.3%
4	Pennsylvania	2,425	5.7%
5	Florida	2,322	5.5%
6	North Carolina	2,121	5.0%
7	Michigan	1,760	4.2%
8	Georgia	1,408	3.3%
9	Washington	1,248	3.0%
10	Maryland	1,225	2.9%
11	Ohio	1,200	2.8%
12	Colorado	1,050	2.5%
13	Illinois	1,021	2.4%
14	Massachusetts	898	2.1%
15	Wisconsin	877	2.1%
16	Connecticut	823	1.9%
17	Arizona	786	1.9%
18	Virginia	724	1.7%
19	Minnesota	641	1.5%
20	Oklahoma	640	1.5%
21	Kentucky	593	1.4%
22	New Jersey	560	1.3%
23	Tennessee	523	1.2%
24	Iowa	519	1.2%
25	Nebraska	507	1.2%
26	West Virginia	491	1.2%
27	Kansas	465	1.1%
28	Oregon	407	1.0%
29	Maine	397	0.9%
30	Utah	369	0.9%
31	New Mexico	367	0.9%
32	South Carolina	352	0.8%
33	Indiana	312	0.7%
34	Louisiana	297	0.7%
35	Missouri	291	0.7%
36	South Dakota	271	0.6%
37	Alabama	254	0.6%
37	Idaho	254	0.6%
39	Alaska	237	0.6%
40	Nevada	229	0.5%
41	New Hampshire	221	0.5%
42	Montana	200	0.5%
43	North Dakota	186	0.4%
44	Rhode Island	139	0.3%
45	Vermont	130	0.3%
46	Wyoming	123	0.3%
47	Hawaii	100	0.2%
48	Delaware	96	0.2%
49	Arkansas	56	0.1%
50	Mississippi	37	0.1%
	District of Columbia	185	0.4%

Source: The American Academy of Physician Assistants
 "Projected Number of PAs in Clinical Practice as of January 1, 2002"
 (http://www.aapa.org/research/clinprac2002.html)
Projected. National total does not include 488 physician assistants who work outside the United States or whose location is unknown.

Rate of Physician Assistants in Clinical Practice in 2002

National Rate = 14.8 PA's per 100,000 Population*

ALPHA ORDER			RANK ORDER		
RANK	STATE	RATE	RANK	STATE	RATE
46	Alabama	5.7	1	Alaska	37.3
1	Alaska	37.3	2	South Dakota	35.8
27	Arizona	14.8	3	Maine	30.9
49	Arkansas	2.1	4	Nebraska	29.6
35	California	11.9	5	North Dakota	29.3
11	Colorado	23.8	6	West Virginia	27.2
10	Connecticut	24.0	7	New York	26.8
34	Delaware	12.1	8	North Carolina	25.9
29	Florida	14.2	9	Wyoming	24.9
24	Georgia	16.8	10	Connecticut	24.0
42	Hawaii	8.2	11	Colorado	23.8
18	Idaho	19.2	12	Maryland	22.8
42	Illinois	8.2	13	Montana	22.1
48	Indiana	5.1	14	Vermont	21.2
20	Iowa	17.8	15	Washington	20.8
23	Kansas	17.3	16	New Mexico	20.1
28	Kentucky	14.6	17	Pennsylvania	19.7
44	Louisiana	6.7	18	Idaho	19.2
3	Maine	30.9	19	Oklahoma	18.5
12	Maryland	22.8	20	Iowa	17.8
30	Massachusetts	14.1	21	Michigan	17.6
21	Michigan	17.6	21	New Hampshire	17.6
32	Minnesota	12.9	23	Kansas	17.3
50	Mississippi	1.3	24	Georgia	16.8
47	Missouri	5.2	25	Utah	16.3
13	Montana	22.1	26	Wisconsin	16.2
4	Nebraska	29.6	27	Arizona	14.8
37	Nevada	10.9	28	Kentucky	14.6
21	New Hampshire	17.6	29	Florida	14.2
45	New Jersey	6.6	30	Massachusetts	14.1
16	New Mexico	20.1	31	Rhode Island	13.1
7	New York	26.8	32	Minnesota	12.9
8	North Carolina	25.9	33	Texas	12.6
5	North Dakota	29.3	34	Delaware	12.1
38	Ohio	10.6	35	California	11.9
19	Oklahoma	18.5	36	Oregon	11.7
36	Oregon	11.7	37	Nevada	10.9
17	Pennsylvania	19.7	38	Ohio	10.6
31	Rhode Island	13.1	39	Virginia	10.1
41	South Carolina	8.7	40	Tennessee	9.1
2	South Dakota	35.8	41	South Carolina	8.7
40	Tennessee	9.1	42	Hawaii	8.2
33	Texas	12.6	42	Illinois	8.2
25	Utah	16.3	44	Louisiana	6.7
14	Vermont	21.2	45	New Jersey	6.6
39	Virginia	10.1	46	Alabama	5.7
15	Washington	20.8	47	Missouri	5.2
6	West Virginia	27.2	48	Indiana	5.1
26	Wisconsin	16.2	49	Arkansas	2.1
9	Wyoming	24.9	50	Mississippi	1.3
				District of Columbia	32.4

Source: Morgan Quitno Press using data from The American Academy of Physician Assistants
    "Projected Number of PAs in Clinical Practice as of January 1, 2002"
     (http://www.aapa.org/research/clinprac2002.html)
*Projected. Rates calculated using 2001 Census population figures.

Registered Nurses in 2000

National Total = 2,201,813 Registered Nurses*

ALPHA ORDER

RANK	STATE	NURSES	% of USA
22	Alabama	34,073	1.5%
49	Alaska	4,914	0.2%
24	Arizona	32,222	1.5%
33	Arkansas	18,752	0.9%
1	California	184,329	8.4%
26	Colorado	31,695	1.4%
25	Connecticut	32,073	1.5%
45	Delaware	7,337	0.3%
4	Florida	125,439	5.7%
12	Georgia	55,881	2.5%
42	Hawaii	8,518	0.4%
44	Idaho	8,230	0.4%
6	Illinois	101,660	4.6%
18	Indiana	46,244	2.1%
27	Iowa	31,020	1.4%
30	Kansas	23,779	1.1%
23	Kentucky	33,655	1.5%
21	Louisiana	37,275	1.7%
37	Maine	13,072	0.6%
19	Maryland	45,323	2.1%
9	Massachusetts	75,795	3.4%
8	Michigan	79,353	3.6%
17	Minnesota	47,102	2.1%
32	Mississippi	21,338	1.0%
13	Missouri	53,730	2.4%
46	Montana	7,327	0.3%
34	Nebraska	16,399	0.7%
41	Nevada	10,384	0.5%
40	New Hampshire	11,321	0.5%
11	New Jersey	67,280	3.1%
38	New Mexico	11,932	0.5%
2	New York	160,009	7.3%
10	North Carolina	69,057	3.1%
47	North Dakota	7,039	0.3%
7	Ohio	100,144	4.5%
31	Oklahoma	21,905	1.0%
29	Oregon	27,121	1.2%
5	Pennsylvania	123,997	5.6%
39	Rhode Island	11,542	0.5%
28	South Carolina	29,226	1.3%
43	South Dakota	8,511	0.4%
15	Tennessee	49,626	2.3%
3	Texas	126,436	5.7%
36	Utah	13,229	0.6%
48	Vermont	5,829	0.3%
14	Virginia	50,359	2.3%
20	Washington	43,482	2.0%
35	West Virginia	15,523	0.7%
16	Wisconsin	47,895	2.2%
50	Wyoming	3,849	0.2%

RANK ORDER

RANK	STATE	NURSES	% of USA
1	California	184,329	8.4%
2	New York	160,009	7.3%
3	Texas	126,436	5.7%
4	Florida	125,439	5.7%
5	Pennsylvania	123,997	5.6%
6	Illinois	101,660	4.6%
7	Ohio	100,144	4.5%
8	Michigan	79,353	3.6%
9	Massachusetts	75,795	3.4%
10	North Carolina	69,057	3.1%
11	New Jersey	67,280	3.1%
12	Georgia	55,881	2.5%
13	Missouri	53,730	2.4%
14	Virginia	50,359	2.3%
15	Tennessee	49,626	2.3%
16	Wisconsin	47,895	2.2%
17	Minnesota	47,102	2.1%
18	Indiana	46,244	2.1%
19	Maryland	45,323	2.1%
20	Washington	43,482	2.0%
21	Louisiana	37,275	1.7%
22	Alabama	34,073	1.5%
23	Kentucky	33,655	1.5%
24	Arizona	32,222	1.5%
25	Connecticut	32,073	1.5%
26	Colorado	31,695	1.4%
27	Iowa	31,020	1.4%
28	South Carolina	29,226	1.3%
29	Oregon	27,121	1.2%
30	Kansas	23,779	1.1%
31	Oklahoma	21,905	1.0%
32	Mississippi	21,338	1.0%
33	Arkansas	18,752	0.9%
34	Nebraska	16,399	0.7%
35	West Virginia	15,523	0.7%
36	Utah	13,229	0.6%
37	Maine	13,072	0.6%
38	New Mexico	11,932	0.5%
39	Rhode Island	11,542	0.5%
40	New Hampshire	11,321	0.5%
41	Nevada	10,384	0.5%
42	Hawaii	8,518	0.4%
43	South Dakota	8,511	0.4%
44	Idaho	8,230	0.4%
45	Delaware	7,337	0.3%
46	Montana	7,327	0.3%
47	North Dakota	7,039	0.3%
48	Vermont	5,829	0.3%
49	Alaska	4,914	0.2%
50	Wyoming	3,849	0.2%
	District of Columbia	9,583	0.4%

Source: U.S. Department of Health and Human Services, Health Resources and Services Administration "The Registered Nurse Population" (February 2001)
*Preliminary as of March 2000. Does not include 494,727 registered nurses not employed in nursing.

Rate of Registered Nurses in 2000

National Rate = 782 Nurses per 100,000 Population*

ALPHA ORDER

RANK ORDER

RANK	STATE	RATE		RANK	STATE	RATE
33	Alabama	766		1	Massachusetts	1,194
31	Alaska	784		2	South Dakota	1,128
46	Arizona	628		3	Rhode Island	1,101
41	Arkansas	701		4	North Dakota	1,096
49	California	544		5	Iowa	1,060
37	Colorado	737		6	Maine	1,025
12	Connecticut	942		7	Pennsylvania	1,010
13	Delaware	936		8	Missouri	960
30	Florida	785		9	Nebraska	958
42	Georgia	683		10	Minnesota	957
40	Hawaii	703		10	Vermont	957
44	Idaho	636		12	Connecticut	942
25	Illinois	819		13	Delaware	936
34	Indiana	761		14	New Hampshire	916
5	Iowa	1,060		15	Wisconsin	893
16	Kansas	885		16	Kansas	885
24	Kentucky	833		17	Ohio	882
23	Louisiana	834		18	Tennessee	872
6	Maine	1,025		19	North Carolina	858
21	Maryland	856		19	West Virginia	858
1	Massachusetts	1,194		21	Maryland	856
28	Michigan	798		22	New York	843
10	Minnesota	957		23	Louisiana	834
35	Mississippi	750		24	Kentucky	833
8	Missouri	960		25	Illinois	819
26	Montana	812		26	Montana	812
9	Nebraska	958		27	New Jersey	800
50	Nevada	520		28	Michigan	798
14	New Hampshire	916		29	Oregon	793
27	New Jersey	800		30	Florida	785
43	New Mexico	656		31	Alaska	784
22	New York	843		32	Wyoming	780
19	North Carolina	858		33	Alabama	766
4	North Dakota	1,096		34	Indiana	761
17	Ohio	882		35	Mississippi	750
45	Oklahoma	635		36	Washington	738
29	Oregon	793		37	Colorado	737
7	Pennsylvania	1,010		38	South Carolina	728
3	Rhode Island	1,101		39	Virginia	711
38	South Carolina	728		40	Hawaii	703
2	South Dakota	1,128		41	Arkansas	701
18	Tennessee	872		42	Georgia	683
47	Texas	606		43	New Mexico	656
48	Utah	592		44	Idaho	636
10	Vermont	957		45	Oklahoma	635
39	Virginia	711		46	Arizona	628
36	Washington	738		47	Texas	606
19	West Virginia	858		48	Utah	592
15	Wisconsin	893		49	California	544
32	Wyoming	780		50	Nevada	520

District of Columbia 1,675

Source: U.S. Department of Health and Human Services, Health Resources and Services Administration
"The Registered Nurse Population" (February 2001)
*Preliminary as of March 2000. Rates do not include registered nurses not employed in nursing.

Dentists in 1998

National Total = 149,350 Dentists*

ALPHA ORDER

RANK ORDER

RANK	STATE	DENTISTS	% of USA		RANK	STATE	DENTISTS	% of USA
27	Alabama	1,785	1.2%		1	California	20,404	13.7%
45	Alaska	427	0.3%		2	New York	13,189	8.8%
25	Arizona	2,036	1.4%		3	Texas	8,656	5.8%
35	Arkansas	1,004	0.7%		4	Illinois	7,475	5.0%
1	California	20,404	13.7%		5	Pennsylvania	7,295	4.9%
21	Colorado	2,516	1.7%		6	Florida	7,084	4.7%
22	Connecticut	2,400	1.6%		7	New Jersey	5,837	3.9%
48	Delaware	331	0.2%		8	Ohio	5,712	3.8%
6	Florida	7,084	4.7%		9	Michigan	5,511	3.7%
14	Georgia	3,126	2.1%		10	Massachusetts	4,393	2.9%
36	Hawaii	941	0.6%		11	Virginia	3,649	2.4%
40	Idaho	637	0.4%		12	Maryland	3,477	2.3%
4	Illinois	7,475	5.0%		13	Washington	3,434	2.3%
18	Indiana	2,693	1.8%		14	Georgia	3,126	2.1%
30	Iowa	1,499	1.0%		15	North Carolina	3,036	2.0%
31	Kansas	1,258	0.8%		16	Wisconsin	2,890	1.9%
24	Kentucky	2,042	1.4%		17	Minnesota	2,798	1.9%
26	Louisiana	1,983	1.3%		18	Indiana	2,693	1.8%
42	Maine	585	0.4%		19	Tennessee	2,632	1.8%
12	Maryland	3,477	2.3%		20	Missouri	2,538	1.7%
10	Massachusetts	4,393	2.9%		21	Colorado	2,516	1.7%
9	Michigan	5,511	3.7%		22	Connecticut	2,400	1.6%
17	Minnesota	2,798	1.9%		23	Oregon	2,068	1.4%
34	Mississippi	1,017	0.7%		24	Kentucky	2,042	1.4%
20	Missouri	2,538	1.7%		25	Arizona	2,036	1.4%
44	Montana	457	0.3%		26	Louisiana	1,983	1.3%
33	Nebraska	1,034	0.7%		27	Alabama	1,785	1.2%
41	Nevada	628	0.4%		28	South Carolina	1,592	1.1%
39	New Hampshire	647	0.4%		29	Oklahoma	1,548	1.0%
7	New Jersey	5,837	3.9%		30	Iowa	1,499	1.0%
38	New Mexico	690	0.5%		31	Kansas	1,258	0.8%
2	New York	13,189	8.8%		32	Utah	1,238	0.8%
15	North Carolina	3,036	2.0%		33	Nebraska	1,034	0.7%
49	North Dakota	309	0.2%		34	Mississippi	1,017	0.7%
8	Ohio	5,712	3.8%		35	Arkansas	1,004	0.7%
29	Oklahoma	1,548	1.0%		36	Hawaii	941	0.6%
23	Oregon	2,068	1.4%		37	West Virginia	781	0.5%
5	Pennsylvania	7,295	4.9%		38	New Mexico	690	0.5%
43	Rhode Island	547	0.4%		39	New Hampshire	647	0.4%
28	South Carolina	1,592	1.1%		40	Idaho	637	0.4%
46	South Dakota	339	0.2%		41	Nevada	628	0.4%
19	Tennessee	2,632	1.8%		42	Maine	585	0.4%
3	Texas	8,656	5.8%		43	Rhode Island	547	0.4%
32	Utah	1,238	0.8%		44	Montana	457	0.3%
47	Vermont	336	0.2%		45	Alaska	427	0.3%
11	Virginia	3,649	2.4%		46	South Dakota	339	0.2%
13	Washington	3,434	2.3%		47	Vermont	336	0.2%
37	West Virginia	781	0.5%		48	Delaware	331	0.2%
16	Wisconsin	2,890	1.9%		49	North Dakota	309	0.2%
50	Wyoming	240	0.2%		50	Wyoming	240	0.2%
						District of Columbia	592	0.4%

Source: American Dental Association
    "Distribution of Dentists, by Region and State, 1998"
*Professionally active dentists. Total does not include 1,714 dentists in territories nor dentists in the Armed Forces stationed overseas.

Rate of Dentists in 1998

National Rate = 55 Dentists per 100,000 Population*

ALPHA ORDER				RANK ORDER		
RANK	STATE	RATE		RANK	STATE	RATE
43	Alabama	41		1	Hawaii	79
6	Alaska	69		2	Connecticut	73
39	Arizona	44		2	New York	73
46	Arkansas	40		4	New Jersey	72
10	California	62		5	Massachusetts	71
8	Colorado	63		6	Alaska	69
2	Connecticut	73		7	Maryland	68
39	Delaware	44		8	Colorado	63
29	Florida	48		8	Oregon	63
43	Georgia	41		10	California	62
1	Hawaii	79		10	Illinois	62
23	Idaho	52		10	Nebraska	62
10	Illinois	62		13	Pennsylvania	61
35	Indiana	46		14	Washington	60
23	Iowa	52		15	Minnesota	59
29	Kansas	48		15	Utah	59
23	Kentucky	52		17	Vermont	57
38	Louisiana	45		18	Michigan	56
33	Maine	47		19	New Hampshire	55
7	Maryland	68		19	Rhode Island	55
5	Massachusetts	71		19	Wisconsin	55
18	Michigan	56		22	Virginia	54
15	Minnesota	59		23	Idaho	52
49	Mississippi	37		23	Iowa	52
33	Missouri	47		23	Kentucky	52
23	Montana	52		23	Montana	52
10	Nebraska	62		27	Ohio	51
50	Nevada	36		28	Wyoming	50
19	New Hampshire	55		29	Florida	48
4	New Jersey	72		29	Kansas	48
46	New Mexico	40		29	North Dakota	48
2	New York	73		29	Tennessee	48
46	North Carolina	40		33	Maine	47
29	North Dakota	48		33	Missouri	47
27	Ohio	51		35	Indiana	46
35	Oklahoma	46		35	Oklahoma	46
8	Oregon	63		35	South Dakota	46
13	Pennsylvania	61		38	Louisiana	45
19	Rhode Island	55		39	Arizona	44
43	South Carolina	41		39	Delaware	44
35	South Dakota	46		39	Texas	44
29	Tennessee	48		42	West Virginia	43
39	Texas	44		43	Alabama	41
15	Utah	59		43	Georgia	41
17	Vermont	57		43	South Carolina	41
22	Virginia	54		46	Arkansas	40
14	Washington	60		46	New Mexico	40
42	West Virginia	43		46	North Carolina	40
19	Wisconsin	55		49	Mississippi	37
28	Wyoming	50		50	Nevada	36
					District of Columbia	114

Source: Morgan Quitno Press using data from American Dental Association
      "Distribution of Dentists, by Region and State, 1998"
*Professionally active dentists. Total does not include 1,714 dentists in territories nor dentists in the Armed Forces
stationed overseas.

Percent of Population Lacking Access to Dental Care in 2001

National Percent = 8.6% of Population*

RANK	STATE	PERCENT
1	Alabama	33.0
14	Alaska	13.1
33	Arizona	6.0
38	Arkansas	4.8
47	California	1.6
44	Colorado	3.1
42	Connecticut	3.9
9	Delaware	16.4
21	Florida	9.9
23	Georgia	9.2
40	Hawaii	4.4
12	Idaho	14.5
27	Illinois	8.1
45	Indiana	2.8
8	Iowa	17.0
15	Kansas	12.9
31	Kentucky	6.3
30	Louisiana	6.4
5	Maine	21.3
37	Maryland	5.2
41	Massachusetts	4.0
18	Michigan	11.7
43	Minnesota	3.4
10	Mississippi	15.6
4	Missouri	22.5
13	Montana	14.0
49	Nebraska	1.3
15	Nevada	12.9
35	New Hampshire	5.4
48	New Jersey	1.5
3	New Mexico	22.7
33	New York	6.0
17	North Carolina	11.9
28	North Dakota	7.1
29	Ohio	6.9
39	Oklahoma	4.5
11	Oregon	15.1
22	Pennsylvania	9.5
24	Rhode Island	8.9
2	South Carolina	24.3
25	South Dakota	8.7
6	Tennessee	20.3
19	Texas	10.9
7	Utah	18.5
46	Vermont	2.3
31	Virginia	6.3
20	Washington	10.1
35	West Virginia	5.4
26	Wisconsin	8.5
50	Wyoming	0.5

RANK	STATE	PERCENT
1	Alabama	33.0
2	South Carolina	24.3
3	New Mexico	22.7
4	Missouri	22.5
5	Maine	21.3
6	Tennessee	20.3
7	Utah	18.5
8	Iowa	17.0
9	Delaware	16.4
10	Mississippi	15.6
11	Oregon	15.1
12	Idaho	14.5
13	Montana	14.0
14	Alaska	13.1
15	Kansas	12.9
15	Nevada	12.9
17	North Carolina	11.9
18	Michigan	11.7
19	Texas	10.9
20	Washington	10.1
21	Florida	9.9
22	Pennsylvania	9.5
23	Georgia	9.2
24	Rhode Island	8.9
25	South Dakota	8.7
26	Wisconsin	8.5
27	Illinois	8.1
28	North Dakota	7.1
29	Ohio	6.9
30	Louisiana	6.4
31	Kentucky	6.3
31	Virginia	6.3
33	Arizona	6.0
33	New York	6.0
35	New Hampshire	5.4
35	West Virginia	5.4
37	Maryland	5.2
38	Arkansas	4.8
39	Oklahoma	4.5
40	Hawaii	4.4
41	Massachusetts	4.0
42	Connecticut	3.9
43	Minnesota	3.4
44	Colorado	3.1
45	Indiana	2.8
46	Vermont	2.3
47	California	1.6
48	New Jersey	1.5
49	Nebraska	1.3
50	Wyoming	0.5

District of Columbia 1.1

Source: Morgan Quitno Press using data from U.S. Dept. of Health and Human Services, Div. of Shortage Designation
"Selected Statistics on Health Professional Shortage Areas, As of December 31, 2001"
*Percent of population considered under-served by dental practitioners. An under-served population does not have primary medical care within reasonable economic and geographic bounds.

Employment in Health Care in 1999

National Total = 12,034,676 Employees*

ALPHA ORDER

RANK	STATE	EMPLOYEES	% of USA
22	Alabama	184,161	1.5%
46	Alaska	23,171	0.2%
25	Arizona	167,295	1.4%
33	Arkansas	111,098	0.9%
1	California	1,111,777	9.2%
26	Colorado	160,400	1.3%
23	Connecticut	183,227	1.5%
45	Delaware	34,482	0.3%
4	Florida	653,321	5.4%
12	Georgia	293,026	2.4%
43	Hawaii	41,522	0.3%
42	Idaho	44,840	0.4%
7	Illinois	535,687	4.5%
14	Indiana	276,702	2.3%
27	Iowa	152,776	1.3%
30	Kansas	130,942	1.1%
24	Kentucky	174,230	1.4%
21	Louisiana	203,643	1.7%
37	Maine	69,207	0.6%
20	Maryland	223,101	1.9%
9	Massachusetts	378,156	3.1%
8	Michigan	434,472	3.6%
15	Minnesota	265,474	2.2%
32	Mississippi	111,617	0.9%
13	Missouri	277,543	2.3%
44	Montana	39,213	0.3%
34	Nebraska	87,203	0.7%
41	Nevada	53,842	0.4%
39	New Hampshire	56,294	0.5%
10	New Jersey	361,302	3.0%
38	New Mexico	62,060	0.5%
2	New York	980,077	8.1%
11	North Carolina	338,114	2.8%
NA	North Dakota**	NA	NA
6	Ohio	558,587	4.6%
29	Oklahoma	142,877	1.2%
31	Oregon	129,108	1.1%
5	Pennsylvania	640,071	5.3%
40	Rhode Island	54,990	0.5%
28	South Carolina	148,659	1.2%
NA	South Dakota**	NA	NA
18	Tennessee	249,446	2.1%
3	Texas	815,619	6.8%
36	Utah	75,246	0.6%
NA	Vermont**	NA	NA
16	Virginia	254,171	2.1%
19	Washington	230,655	1.9%
35	West Virginia	85,929	0.7%
17	Wisconsin	251,117	2.1%
NA	Wyoming**	NA	NA

RANK ORDER

RANK	STATE	EMPLOYEES	% of USA
1	California	1,111,777	9.2%
2	New York	980,077	8.1%
3	Texas	815,619	6.8%
4	Florida	653,321	5.4%
5	Pennsylvania	640,071	5.3%
6	Ohio	558,587	4.6%
7	Illinois	535,687	4.5%
8	Michigan	434,472	3.6%
9	Massachusetts	378,156	3.1%
10	New Jersey	361,302	3.0%
11	North Carolina	338,114	2.8%
12	Georgia	293,026	2.4%
13	Missouri	277,543	2.3%
14	Indiana	276,702	2.3%
15	Minnesota	265,474	2.2%
16	Virginia	254,171	2.1%
17	Wisconsin	251,117	2.1%
18	Tennessee	249,446	2.1%
19	Washington	230,655	1.9%
20	Maryland	223,101	1.9%
21	Louisiana	203,643	1.7%
22	Alabama	184,161	1.5%
23	Connecticut	183,227	1.5%
24	Kentucky	174,230	1.4%
25	Arizona	167,295	1.4%
26	Colorado	160,400	1.3%
27	Iowa	152,776	1.3%
28	South Carolina	148,659	1.2%
29	Oklahoma	142,877	1.2%
30	Kansas	130,942	1.1%
31	Oregon	129,108	1.1%
32	Mississippi	111,617	0.9%
33	Arkansas	111,098	0.9%
34	Nebraska	87,203	0.7%
35	West Virginia	85,929	0.7%
36	Utah	75,246	0.6%
37	Maine	69,207	0.6%
38	New Mexico	62,060	0.5%
39	New Hampshire	56,294	0.5%
40	Rhode Island	54,990	0.5%
41	Nevada	53,842	0.4%
42	Idaho	44,840	0.4%
43	Hawaii	41,522	0.3%
44	Montana	39,213	0.3%
45	Delaware	34,482	0.3%
46	Alaska	23,171	0.2%
NA	North Dakota**	NA	NA
NA	South Dakota**	NA	NA
NA	Vermont**	NA	NA
NA	Wyoming**	NA	NA
	District of Columbia	47,469	0.4%

Source: U.S. Bureau of the Census
  "County Business Patterns 1999 (NAICS)" (http://tier2.census.gov/cbp_naics/index.html)
*Includes employees at establishments exempt from as well as subject to the federal income tax. Includes
employees at those establishments within the North American Industry Classification System (NAICS) classifications
621 (ambulatory health care services), 622 (hospitals) and 623 (nursing and residential care facilities). See
Facilities Chapter for establishments. **Not available.

VII. PHYSICAL FITNESS

488 Users of Exercise Equipment in 2000
489 Participants in Golf in 2000
490 Participants in Running/Jogging in 2000
491 Participants in Swimming in 2000
492 Participants in Tennis in 2000
493 Alcohol Consumption in 1998
494 Adult Per Capita Alcohol Consumption in 1998
495 Apparent Beer Consumption in 1998
496 Adult Per Capita Beer Consumption in 1998
497 Wine Consumption in 1998
498 Adult Per Capita Wine Consumption in 1998
499 Distilled Spirits Consumption in 1998
500 Adult Per Capita Apparent Distilled Spirits Consumption in 1998
501 Percent of Adults Who Are Binge Drinkers: 1999
502 Percent of Adults Who Drink and Drive: 1999
503 Percent of Adults Who Smoke: 2000
504 Percent of Males Who Smoke: 2000
505 Percent of Women Who Smoke: 2000
506 Percent of Adults Overweight or Obese: 2000
507 Percent of Adults Who Have Not Had Their Blood Pressure Checked in the Past Two Years: 1999
508 Percent of Adults Who Have Not Been Tested in Past Year for HIV: 2000
509 Number of Days in Past Month When Physical Health was "Not Good": 2000
510 Number of Days in Past Month When Mental Health was "Not Good": 2000
511 Percent of Population Who are Illicit Drug Users: 1999
512 Safety Belt Usage Rate in 2000

Users of Exercise Equipment in 2000

National Total = 44,820,000 Users

ALPHA ORDER

RANK	STATE	USERS	% of USA
24	Alabama	637,000	1.4%
NA	Alaska*	NA	NA
19	Arizona	870,000	1.9%
32	Arkansas	433,000	1.0%
1	California	6,483,000	14.5%
22	Colorado	734,000	1.6%
23	Connecticut	700,000	1.6%
44	Delaware	93,000	0.2%
5	Florida	1,998,000	4.5%
11	Georgia	1,198,000	2.7%
NA	Hawaii*	NA	NA
39	Idaho	223,000	0.5%
6	Illinois	1,822,000	4.1%
18	Indiana	884,000	2.0%
29	Iowa	520,000	1.2%
30	Kansas	499,000	1.1%
33	Kentucky	391,000	0.9%
25	Louisiana	618,000	1.4%
37	Maine	269,000	0.6%
12	Maryland	1,121,000	2.5%
14	Massachusetts	1,052,000	2.3%
8	Michigan	1,601,000	3.6%
17	Minnesota	904,000	2.0%
35	Mississippi	345,000	0.8%
15	Missouri	1,028,000	2.3%
42	Montana	145,000	0.3%
36	Nebraska	315,000	0.7%
40	Nevada	203,000	0.5%
41	New Hampshire	156,000	0.3%
13	New Jersey	1,054,000	2.4%
38	New Mexico	256,000	0.6%
2	New York	3,386,000	7.6%
10	North Carolina	1,244,000	2.8%
48	North Dakota	68,000	0.2%
7	Ohio	1,652,000	3.7%
27	Oklahoma	550,000	1.2%
31	Oregon	486,000	1.1%
4	Pennsylvania	2,109,000	4.7%
46	Rhode Island	86,000	0.2%
26	South Carolina	609,000	1.4%
45	South Dakota	87,000	0.2%
21	Tennessee	774,000	1.7%
3	Texas	2,985,000	6.7%
28	Utah	524,000	1.2%
47	Vermont	84,000	0.2%
9	Virginia	1,297,000	2.9%
16	Washington	957,000	2.1%
34	West Virginia	381,000	0.9%
20	Wisconsin	791,000	1.8%
43	Wyoming	110,000	0.2%

RANK ORDER

RANK	STATE	USERS	% of USA
1	California	6,483,000	14.5%
2	New York	3,386,000	7.6%
3	Texas	2,985,000	6.7%
4	Pennsylvania	2,109,000	4.7%
5	Florida	1,998,000	4.5%
6	Illinois	1,822,000	4.1%
7	Ohio	1,652,000	3.7%
8	Michigan	1,601,000	3.6%
9	Virginia	1,297,000	2.9%
10	North Carolina	1,244,000	2.8%
11	Georgia	1,198,000	2.7%
12	Maryland	1,121,000	2.5%
13	New Jersey	1,054,000	2.4%
14	Massachusetts	1,052,000	2.3%
15	Missouri	1,028,000	2.3%
16	Washington	957,000	2.1%
17	Minnesota	904,000	2.0%
18	Indiana	884,000	2.0%
19	Arizona	870,000	1.9%
20	Wisconsin	791,000	1.8%
21	Tennessee	774,000	1.7%
22	Colorado	734,000	1.6%
23	Connecticut	700,000	1.6%
24	Alabama	637,000	1.4%
25	Louisiana	618,000	1.4%
26	South Carolina	609,000	1.4%
27	Oklahoma	550,000	1.2%
28	Utah	524,000	1.2%
29	Iowa	520,000	1.2%
30	Kansas	499,000	1.1%
31	Oregon	486,000	1.1%
32	Arkansas	433,000	1.0%
33	Kentucky	391,000	0.9%
34	West Virginia	381,000	0.9%
35	Mississippi	345,000	0.8%
36	Nebraska	315,000	0.7%
37	Maine	269,000	0.6%
38	New Mexico	256,000	0.6%
39	Idaho	223,000	0.5%
40	Nevada	203,000	0.5%
41	New Hampshire	156,000	0.3%
42	Montana	145,000	0.3%
43	Wyoming	110,000	0.2%
44	Delaware	93,000	0.2%
45	South Dakota	87,000	0.2%
46	Rhode Island	86,000	0.2%
47	Vermont	84,000	0.2%
48	North Dakota	68,000	0.2%
NA	Alaska*	NA	NA
NA	Hawaii*	NA	NA
	District of Columbia*	NA	NA

Source: The National Sporting Goods Association
"NSGA Sports Participation Survey, January-December 2000 (Copyright 2001, reprinted with permission)
*Not available.

Participants in Golf in 2000

National Total = 26,401,000 Golfers

<u>ALPHA ORDER</u>

RANK	STATE	GOLFERS	% of USA
33	Alabama	256,000	1.0%
NA	Alaska*	NA	NA
19	Arizona	503,000	1.9%
31	Arkansas	265,000	1.0%
1	California	2,417,000	9.2%
24	Colorado	365,000	1.4%
26	Connecticut	356,000	1.3%
45	Delaware	67,000	0.3%
5	Florida	1,399,000	5.3%
15	Georgia	676,000	2.6%
NA	Hawaii*	NA	NA
38	Idaho	146,000	0.6%
7	Illinois	1,285,000	4.9%
20	Indiana	458,000	1.7%
23	Iowa	383,000	1.5%
35	Kansas	172,000	0.7%
28	Kentucky	316,000	1.2%
30	Louisiana	274,000	1.0%
34	Maine	221,000	0.8%
21	Maryland	450,000	1.7%
13	Massachusetts	746,000	2.8%
6	Michigan	1,353,000	5.1%
9	Minnesota	978,000	3.7%
46	Mississippi	52,000	0.2%
14	Missouri	703,000	2.7%
41	Montana	113,000	0.4%
32	Nebraska	261,000	1.0%
36	Nevada	168,000	0.6%
39	New Hampshire	138,000	0.5%
17	New Jersey	571,000	2.2%
36	New Mexico	168,000	0.6%
2	New York	1,685,000	6.4%
16	North Carolina	634,000	2.4%
42	North Dakota	103,000	0.4%
8	Ohio	1,191,000	4.5%
22	Oklahoma	384,000	1.5%
29	Oregon	304,000	1.2%
4	Pennsylvania	1,432,000	5.4%
44	Rhode Island	97,000	0.4%
18	South Carolina	527,000	2.0%
40	South Dakota	121,000	0.5%
24	Tennessee	365,000	1.4%
3	Texas	1,462,000	5.5%
27	Utah	323,000	1.2%
47	Vermont	48,000	0.2%
11	Virginia	761,000	2.9%
10	Washington	833,000	3.2%
43	West Virginia	98,000	0.4%
12	Wisconsin	756,000	2.9%
48	Wyoming	19,000	0.1%

<u>RANK ORDER</u>

RANK	STATE	GOLFERS	% of USA
1	California	2,417,000	9.2%
2	New York	1,685,000	6.4%
3	Texas	1,462,000	5.5%
4	Pennsylvania	1,432,000	5.4%
5	Florida	1,399,000	5.3%
6	Michigan	1,353,000	5.1%
7	Illinois	1,285,000	4.9%
8	Ohio	1,191,000	4.5%
9	Minnesota	978,000	3.7%
10	Washington	833,000	3.2%
11	Virginia	761,000	2.9%
12	Wisconsin	756,000	2.9%
13	Massachusetts	746,000	2.8%
14	Missouri	703,000	2.7%
15	Georgia	676,000	2.6%
16	North Carolina	634,000	2.4%
17	New Jersey	571,000	2.2%
18	South Carolina	527,000	2.0%
19	Arizona	503,000	1.9%
20	Indiana	458,000	1.7%
21	Maryland	450,000	1.7%
22	Oklahoma	384,000	1.5%
23	Iowa	383,000	1.5%
24	Colorado	365,000	1.4%
24	Tennessee	365,000	1.4%
26	Connecticut	356,000	1.3%
27	Utah	323,000	1.2%
28	Kentucky	316,000	1.2%
29	Oregon	304,000	1.2%
30	Louisiana	274,000	1.0%
31	Arkansas	265,000	1.0%
32	Nebraska	261,000	1.0%
33	Alabama	256,000	1.0%
34	Maine	221,000	0.8%
35	Kansas	172,000	0.7%
36	Nevada	168,000	0.6%
36	New Mexico	168,000	0.6%
38	Idaho	146,000	0.6%
39	New Hampshire	138,000	0.5%
40	South Dakota	121,000	0.5%
41	Montana	113,000	0.4%
42	North Dakota	103,000	0.4%
43	West Virginia	98,000	0.4%
44	Rhode Island	97,000	0.4%
45	Delaware	67,000	0.3%
46	Mississippi	52,000	0.2%
47	Vermont	48,000	0.2%
48	Wyoming	19,000	0.1%
NA	Alaska*	NA	NA
NA	Hawaii*	NA	NA
	District of Columbia*	NA	NA

Source: The National Sporting Goods Association
   "NSGA Sports Participation Survey, January-December 2000 (Copyright 2001, reprinted with permission)
Not available.

Participants in Running/Jogging in 2000

National Total = 22,812,000 Runners/Joggers

ALPHA ORDER					RANK ORDER			
RANK	STATE	RUNNERS	% of USA		RANK	STATE	RUNNERS	% of USA
22	Alabama	390,000	1.7%		1	California	3,153,000	13.8%
NA	Alaska*	NA	NA		2	Texas	1,724,000	7.6%
14	Arizona	581,000	2.5%		3	New York	1,547,000	6.8%
35	Arkansas	173,000	0.8%		4	Illinois	1,085,000	4.8%
1	California	3,153,000	13.8%		5	Pennsylvania	986,000	4.3%
15	Colorado	527,000	2.3%		6	Florida	887,000	3.9%
29	Connecticut	278,000	1.2%		7	Virginia	708,000	3.1%
46	Delaware	44,000	0.2%		8	North Carolina	683,000	3.0%
6	Florida	887,000	3.9%		9	New Jersey	664,000	2.9%
11	Georgia	609,000	2.7%		10	Michigan	657,000	2.9%
NA	Hawaii*	NA	NA		11	Georgia	609,000	2.7%
38	Idaho	122,000	0.5%		12	Indiana	593,000	2.6%
4	Illinois	1,085,000	4.8%		13	Ohio	582,000	2.6%
12	Indiana	593,000	2.6%		14	Arizona	581,000	2.5%
30	Iowa	244,000	1.1%		15	Colorado	527,000	2.3%
25	Kansas	341,000	1.5%		16	Maryland	524,000	2.3%
27	Kentucky	304,000	1.3%		17	Oklahoma	477,000	2.1%
26	Louisiana	309,000	1.4%		18	South Carolina	449,000	2.0%
43	Maine	103,000	0.5%		19	Washington	422,000	1.8%
16	Maryland	524,000	2.3%		20	Massachusetts	414,000	1.8%
20	Massachusetts	414,000	1.8%		21	Tennessee	396,000	1.7%
10	Michigan	657,000	2.9%		22	Alabama	390,000	1.7%
24	Minnesota	368,000	1.6%		23	Missouri	379,000	1.7%
34	Mississippi	196,000	0.9%		24	Minnesota	368,000	1.6%
23	Missouri	379,000	1.7%		25	Kansas	341,000	1.5%
40	Montana	109,000	0.5%		26	Louisiana	309,000	1.4%
32	Nebraska	217,000	1.0%		27	Kentucky	304,000	1.3%
44	Nevada	68,000	0.3%		28	Oregon	297,000	1.3%
42	New Hampshire	107,000	0.5%		29	Connecticut	278,000	1.2%
9	New Jersey	664,000	2.9%		30	Iowa	244,000	1.1%
39	New Mexico	116,000	0.5%		31	Wisconsin	231,000	1.0%
3	New York	1,547,000	6.8%		32	Nebraska	217,000	1.0%
8	North Carolina	683,000	3.0%		33	Utah	206,000	0.9%
47	North Dakota	39,000	0.2%		34	Mississippi	196,000	0.9%
13	Ohio	582,000	2.6%		35	Arkansas	173,000	0.8%
17	Oklahoma	477,000	2.1%		36	West Virginia	162,000	0.7%
28	Oregon	297,000	1.3%		37	Wyoming	125,000	0.5%
5	Pennsylvania	986,000	4.3%		38	Idaho	122,000	0.5%
41	Rhode Island	108,000	0.5%		39	New Mexico	116,000	0.5%
18	South Carolina	449,000	2.0%		40	Montana	109,000	0.5%
48	South Dakota	31,000	0.1%		41	Rhode Island	108,000	0.5%
21	Tennessee	396,000	1.7%		42	New Hampshire	107,000	0.5%
2	Texas	1,724,000	7.6%		43	Maine	103,000	0.5%
33	Utah	206,000	0.9%		44	Nevada	68,000	0.3%
45	Vermont	49,000	0.2%		45	Vermont	49,000	0.2%
7	Virginia	708,000	3.1%		46	Delaware	44,000	0.2%
19	Washington	422,000	1.8%		47	North Dakota	39,000	0.2%
36	West Virginia	162,000	0.7%		48	South Dakota	31,000	0.1%
31	Wisconsin	231,000	1.0%		NA	Alaska*	NA	NA
37	Wyoming	125,000	0.5%		NA	Hawaii*	NA	NA
						District of Columbia*	NA	NA

Source: The National Sporting Goods Association
"NSGA Sports Participation Survey, January-December 2000 (Copyright 2001, reprinted with permission)
*Not available.

Participants in Swimming in 2000

National Total = 60,758,000 Swimmers

ALPHA ORDER				RANK ORDER			
RANK	STATE	SWIMMERS	% of USA	RANK	STATE	SWIMMERS	% of USA
19	Alabama	1,174,000	1.9%	1	California	6,205,000	10.2%
NA	Alaska*	NA	NA	2	Florida	4,065,000	6.7%
13	Arizona	1,592,000	2.6%	3	New York	3,909,000	6.4%
27	Arkansas	712,000	1.2%	4	Texas	3,642,000	6.0%
1	California	6,205,000	10.2%	5	Pennsylvania	3,082,000	5.1%
29	Colorado	661,000	1.1%	6	Ohio	2,707,000	4.5%
26	Connecticut	749,000	1.2%	7	Illinois	2,413,000	4.0%
46	Delaware	149,000	0.2%	8	North Carolina	2,270,000	3.7%
2	Florida	4,065,000	6.7%	9	Georgia	2,035,000	3.3%
9	Georgia	2,035,000	3.3%	10	Michigan	1,864,000	3.1%
NA	Hawaii*	NA	NA	11	New Jersey	1,862,000	3.1%
38	Idaho	432,000	0.7%	12	Maryland	1,747,000	2.9%
7	Illinois	2,413,000	4.0%	13	Arizona	1,592,000	2.6%
16	Indiana	1,316,000	2.2%	14	Missouri	1,430,000	2.4%
35	Iowa	455,000	0.7%	15	Virginia	1,338,000	2.2%
30	Kansas	537,000	0.9%	16	Indiana	1,316,000	2.2%
28	Kentucky	684,000	1.1%	17	Massachusetts	1,292,000	2.1%
23	Louisiana	1,020,000	1.7%	18	Washington	1,253,000	2.1%
37	Maine	436,000	0.7%	19	Alabama	1,174,000	1.9%
12	Maryland	1,747,000	2.9%	20	Wisconsin	1,116,000	1.8%
17	Massachusetts	1,292,000	2.1%	21	Tennessee	1,046,000	1.7%
10	Michigan	1,864,000	3.1%	22	South Carolina	1,033,000	1.7%
25	Minnesota	818,000	1.3%	23	Louisiana	1,020,000	1.7%
36	Mississippi	450,000	0.7%	24	Oklahoma	884,000	1.5%
14	Missouri	1,430,000	2.4%	25	Minnesota	818,000	1.3%
43	Montana	260,000	0.4%	26	Connecticut	749,000	1.2%
33	Nebraska	520,000	0.9%	27	Arkansas	712,000	1.2%
34	Nevada	516,000	0.8%	28	Kentucky	684,000	1.1%
42	New Hampshire	262,000	0.4%	29	Colorado	661,000	1.1%
11	New Jersey	1,862,000	3.1%	30	Kansas	537,000	0.9%
40	New Mexico	403,000	0.7%	31	Oregon	529,000	0.9%
3	New York	3,909,000	6.4%	32	West Virginia	523,000	0.9%
8	North Carolina	2,270,000	3.7%	33	Nebraska	520,000	0.9%
45	North Dakota	175,000	0.3%	34	Nevada	516,000	0.8%
6	Ohio	2,707,000	4.5%	35	Iowa	455,000	0.7%
24	Oklahoma	884,000	1.5%	36	Mississippi	450,000	0.7%
31	Oregon	529,000	0.9%	37	Maine	436,000	0.7%
5	Pennsylvania	3,082,000	5.1%	38	Idaho	432,000	0.7%
41	Rhode Island	308,000	0.5%	39	Utah	414,000	0.7%
22	South Carolina	1,033,000	1.7%	40	New Mexico	403,000	0.7%
47	South Dakota	120,000	0.2%	41	Rhode Island	308,000	0.5%
21	Tennessee	1,046,000	1.7%	42	New Hampshire	262,000	0.4%
4	Texas	3,642,000	6.0%	43	Montana	260,000	0.4%
39	Utah	414,000	0.7%	44	Vermont	205,000	0.3%
44	Vermont	205,000	0.3%	45	North Dakota	175,000	0.3%
15	Virginia	1,338,000	2.2%	46	Delaware	149,000	0.2%
18	Washington	1,253,000	2.1%	47	South Dakota	120,000	0.2%
32	West Virginia	523,000	0.9%	48	Wyoming	41,000	0.1%
20	Wisconsin	1,116,000	1.8%	NA	Alaska*	NA	NA
48	Wyoming	41,000	0.1%	NA	Hawaii*	NA	NA
					District of Columbia*	NA	NA

Source: The National Sporting Goods Association
"NSGA Sports Participation Survey, January-December 2000 (Copyright 2001, reprinted with permission)
*Not available.

Participants in Tennis in 2000

National Total = 10,032,000 Tennis Players

ALPHA ORDER

RANK	STATE	PLAYERS	% of USA
26	Alabama	108,000	1.1%
NA	Alaska*	NA	NA
34	Arizona	66,000	0.7%
34	Arkansas	66,000	0.7%
1	California	1,314,000	13.1%
28	Colorado	95,000	0.9%
36	Connecticut	65,000	0.6%
40	Delaware	42,000	0.4%
6	Florida	406,000	4.0%
8	Georgia	333,000	3.3%
NA	Hawaii*	NA	NA
39	Idaho	48,000	0.5%
5	Illinois	536,000	5.3%
13	Indiana	287,000	2.9%
20	Iowa	163,000	1.6%
32	Kansas	79,000	0.8%
22	Kentucky	141,000	1.4%
27	Louisiana	107,000	1.1%
30	Maine	80,000	0.8%
12	Maryland	305,000	3.0%
11	Massachusetts	307,000	3.1%
7	Michigan	367,000	3.7%
15	Minnesota	256,000	2.6%
24	Mississippi	123,000	1.2%
21	Missouri	148,000	1.5%
45	Montana	19,000	0.2%
47	Nebraska	7,000	0.1%
42	Nevada	29,000	0.3%
41	New Hampshire	33,000	0.3%
9	New Jersey	332,000	3.3%
29	New Mexico	85,000	0.8%
2	New York	846,000	8.4%
16	North Carolina	210,000	2.1%
46	North Dakota	9,000	0.1%
10	Ohio	310,000	3.1%
30	Oklahoma	80,000	0.8%
19	Oregon	175,000	1.7%
4	Pennsylvania	575,000	5.7%
33	Rhode Island	76,000	0.8%
25	South Carolina	116,000	1.2%
43	South Dakota	22,000	0.2%
17	Tennessee	197,000	2.0%
3	Texas	748,000	7.5%
38	Utah	55,000	0.5%
43	Vermont	22,000	0.2%
23	Virginia	136,000	1.4%
18	Washington	187,000	1.9%
37	West Virginia	60,000	0.6%
14	Wisconsin	263,000	2.6%
NA	Wyoming*	NA	NA

RANK ORDER

RANK	STATE	PLAYERS	% of USA
1	California	1,314,000	13.1%
2	New York	846,000	8.4%
3	Texas	748,000	7.5%
4	Pennsylvania	575,000	5.7%
5	Illinois	536,000	5.3%
6	Florida	406,000	4.0%
7	Michigan	367,000	3.7%
8	Georgia	333,000	3.3%
9	New Jersey	332,000	3.3%
10	Ohio	310,000	3.1%
11	Massachusetts	307,000	3.1%
12	Maryland	305,000	3.0%
13	Indiana	287,000	2.9%
14	Wisconsin	263,000	2.6%
15	Minnesota	256,000	2.6%
16	North Carolina	210,000	2.1%
17	Tennessee	197,000	2.0%
18	Washington	187,000	1.9%
19	Oregon	175,000	1.7%
20	Iowa	163,000	1.6%
21	Missouri	148,000	1.5%
22	Kentucky	141,000	1.4%
23	Virginia	136,000	1.4%
24	Mississippi	123,000	1.2%
25	South Carolina	116,000	1.2%
26	Alabama	108,000	1.1%
27	Louisiana	107,000	1.1%
28	Colorado	95,000	0.9%
29	New Mexico	85,000	0.8%
30	Maine	80,000	0.8%
30	Oklahoma	80,000	0.8%
32	Kansas	79,000	0.8%
33	Rhode Island	76,000	0.8%
34	Arizona	66,000	0.7%
34	Arkansas	66,000	0.7%
36	Connecticut	65,000	0.6%
37	West Virginia	60,000	0.6%
38	Utah	55,000	0.5%
39	Idaho	48,000	0.5%
40	Delaware	42,000	0.4%
41	New Hampshire	33,000	0.3%
42	Nevada	29,000	0.3%
43	South Dakota	22,000	0.2%
43	Vermont	22,000	0.2%
45	Montana	19,000	0.2%
46	North Dakota	9,000	0.1%
47	Nebraska	7,000	0.1%
NA	Alaska*	NA	NA
NA	Hawaii*	NA	NA
NA	Wyoming*	NA	NA
	District of Columbia*	NA	NA

Source: The National Sporting Goods Association
  "NSGA Sports Participation Survey, January-December 2000 (Copyright 2001, reprinted with permission)
Not available.

Alcohol Consumption in 1998

National Total = 472,066,000 Gallons*

ALPHA ORDER

RANK ORDER

RANK	STATE	GALLONS	% of USA	RANK	STATE	GALLONS	% of USA
25	Alabama	6,448,000	1.4%	1	California	55,755,000	11.8%
47	Alaska	1,288,000	0.3%	2	Texas	35,222,000	7.5%
17	Arizona	9,436,000	2.0%	3	Florida	31,351,000	6.6%
35	Arkansas	3,641,000	0.8%	4	New York	28,142,000	6.0%
1	California	55,755,000	11.8%	5	Illinois	21,980,000	4.7%
22	Colorado	8,339,000	1.8%	6	Pennsylvania	18,570,000	3.9%
27	Connecticut	5,912,000	1.3%	7	Ohio	17,900,000	3.8%
45	Delaware	1,733,000	0.4%	8	Michigan	16,587,000	3.5%
3	Florida	31,351,000	6.6%	9	New Jersey	14,140,000	3.0%
10	Georgia	13,381,000	2.8%	10	Georgia	13,381,000	2.8%
41	Hawaii	2,180,000	0.5%	11	Massachusetts	12,176,000	2.6%
40	Idaho	2,204,000	0.5%	12	North Carolina	11,802,000	2.5%
5	Illinois	21,980,000	4.7%	13	Wisconsin	11,292,000	2.4%
18	Indiana	9,215,000	2.0%	14	Virginia	10,793,000	2.3%
32	Iowa	4,457,000	0.9%	15	Washington	10,053,000	2.1%
34	Kansas	3,785,000	0.8%	16	Missouri	9,652,000	2.0%
28	Kentucky	5,549,000	1.2%	17	Arizona	9,436,000	2.0%
21	Louisiana	8,512,000	1.8%	18	Indiana	9,215,000	2.0%
39	Maine	2,222,000	0.5%	19	Minnesota	9,085,000	1.9%
20	Maryland	8,633,000	1.8%	20	Maryland	8,633,000	1.8%
11	Massachusetts	12,176,000	2.6%	21	Louisiana	8,512,000	1.8%
8	Michigan	16,587,000	3.5%	22	Colorado	8,339,000	1.8%
19	Minnesota	9,085,000	1.9%	23	Tennessee	8,278,000	1.8%
30	Mississippi	4,607,000	1.0%	24	South Carolina	7,386,000	1.6%
16	Missouri	9,652,000	2.0%	25	Alabama	6,448,000	1.4%
44	Montana	1,753,000	0.4%	26	Oregon	6,095,000	1.3%
37	Nebraska	2,922,000	0.6%	27	Connecticut	5,912,000	1.3%
29	Nevada	5,353,000	1.1%	28	Kentucky	5,549,000	1.2%
33	New Hampshire	3,851,000	0.8%	29	Nevada	5,353,000	1.1%
9	New Jersey	14,140,000	3.0%	30	Mississippi	4,607,000	1.0%
36	New Mexico	3,200,000	0.7%	31	Oklahoma	4,559,000	1.0%
4	New York	28,142,000	6.0%	32	Iowa	4,457,000	0.9%
12	North Carolina	11,802,000	2.5%	33	New Hampshire	3,851,000	0.8%
48	North Dakota	1,249,000	0.3%	34	Kansas	3,785,000	0.8%
7	Ohio	17,900,000	3.8%	35	Arkansas	3,641,000	0.8%
31	Oklahoma	4,559,000	1.0%	36	New Mexico	3,200,000	0.7%
26	Oregon	6,095,000	1.3%	37	Nebraska	2,922,000	0.6%
6	Pennsylvania	18,570,000	3.9%	38	West Virginia	2,457,000	0.5%
43	Rhode Island	1,886,000	0.4%	39	Maine	2,222,000	0.5%
24	South Carolina	7,386,000	1.6%	40	Idaho	2,204,000	0.5%
46	South Dakota	1,323,000	0.3%	41	Hawaii	2,180,000	0.5%
23	Tennessee	8,278,000	1.8%	42	Utah	1,952,000	0.4%
2	Texas	35,222,000	7.5%	43	Rhode Island	1,886,000	0.4%
42	Utah	1,952,000	0.4%	44	Montana	1,753,000	0.4%
49	Vermont	1,141,000	0.2%	45	Delaware	1,733,000	0.4%
14	Virginia	10,793,000	2.3%	46	South Dakota	1,323,000	0.3%
15	Washington	10,053,000	2.1%	47	Alaska	1,288,000	0.3%
38	West Virginia	2,457,000	0.5%	48	North Dakota	1,249,000	0.3%
13	Wisconsin	11,292,000	2.4%	49	Vermont	1,141,000	0.2%
50	Wyoming	941,000	0.2%	50	Wyoming	941,000	0.2%
					District of Columbia	1,676,000	0.4%

Source: U.S. Department of Health and Human Services, National Institute on Alcohol Abuse and Alcoholism
"Volume Beverage and Ethanol Consumption for States" (http://silk.nih.gov/silk/niaaa1/database/consum02.txt)

This is apparent consumption of actual alcohol, not entire volume of an alcoholic beverage (e.g. wine is roughly 11% absolute alcohol content). Apparent consumption is based on several sources which together approximate sales but do not actually measure consumption. Accordingly, figures for some states may be skewed by purchases by nonresidents.

Adult Per Capita Alcohol Consumption in 1998

National Per Capita = 2.5 Gallons Consumed per Adult Age 21 & Older*

ALPHA ORDER

RANK ORDER

RANK	STATE	PER CAPITA
42	Alabama	2.1
3	Alaska	3.3
6	Arizona	3.0
42	Arkansas	2.1
26	California	2.5
6	Colorado	3.0
26	Connecticut	2.5
4	Delaware	3.2
8	Florida	2.9
26	Georgia	2.5
21	Hawaii	2.6
15	Idaho	2.7
21	Illinois	2.6
37	Indiana	2.2
37	Iowa	2.2
42	Kansas	2.1
47	Kentucky	2.0
8	Louisiana	2.9
26	Maine	2.5
33	Maryland	2.4
15	Massachusetts	2.7
33	Michigan	2.4
12	Minnesota	2.8
26	Mississippi	2.5
26	Missouri	2.5
8	Montana	2.9
21	Nebraska	2.6
2	Nevada	4.4
1	New Hampshire	4.6
33	New Jersey	2.4
12	New Mexico	2.8
37	New York	2.2
37	North Carolina	2.2
12	North Dakota	2.8
36	Ohio	2.3
47	Oklahoma	2.0
21	Oregon	2.6
42	Pennsylvania	2.1
21	Rhode Island	2.6
15	South Carolina	2.7
15	South Dakota	2.7
42	Tennessee	2.1
15	Texas	2.7
50	Utah	1.5
15	Vermont	2.7
37	Virginia	2.2
26	Washington	2.5
49	West Virginia	1.9
5	Wisconsin	3.1
8	Wyoming	2.9

RANK	STATE	PER CAPITA
1	New Hampshire	4.6
2	Nevada	4.4
3	Alaska	3.3
4	Delaware	3.2
5	Wisconsin	3.1
6	Arizona	3.0
6	Colorado	3.0
8	Florida	2.9
8	Louisiana	2.9
8	Montana	2.9
8	Wyoming	2.9
12	Minnesota	2.8
12	New Mexico	2.8
12	North Dakota	2.8
15	Idaho	2.7
15	Massachusetts	2.7
15	South Carolina	2.7
15	South Dakota	2.7
15	Texas	2.7
15	Vermont	2.7
21	Hawaii	2.6
21	Illinois	2.6
21	Nebraska	2.6
21	Oregon	2.6
21	Rhode Island	2.6
26	California	2.5
26	Connecticut	2.5
26	Georgia	2.5
26	Maine	2.5
26	Mississippi	2.5
26	Missouri	2.5
26	Washington	2.5
33	Maryland	2.4
33	Michigan	2.4
33	New Jersey	2.4
36	Ohio	2.3
37	Indiana	2.2
37	Iowa	2.2
37	New York	2.2
37	North Carolina	2.2
37	Virginia	2.2
42	Alabama	2.1
42	Arkansas	2.1
42	Kansas	2.1
42	Pennsylvania	2.1
42	Tennessee	2.1
47	Kentucky	2.0
47	Oklahoma	2.0
49	West Virginia	1.9
50	Utah	1.5

District of Columbia   4.1

Source: Morgan Quitno Press using data from U.S. Dept. of HHS, National Institute on Alcohol Abuse and Alcoholism "Volume Beverage and Ethanol Consumption for States" (http://silk.nih.gov/silk/niaaa1/database/consum02.txt)
*This is apparent consumption of actual alcohol, not entire volume of an alcoholic beverage (e.g. wine is roughly 11% absolute alcohol content). Apparent consumption is based on several sources which together approximate sales but do not actually measure consumption. Accordingly, figures for some states may be skewed by purchases by nonresidents.

Apparent Beer Consumption in 1998

National Total = 5,979,047,000 Gallons of Beer Consumed*

ALPHA ORDER

RANK	STATE	GALLONS	% of USA
25	Alabama	92,082,000	1.5%
48	Alaska	14,315,000	0.2%
16	Arizona	124,001,000	2.1%
33	Arkansas	51,525,000	0.9%
1	California	630,458,000	10.5%
23	Colorado	97,093,000	1.6%
32	Connecticut	58,076,000	1.0%
46	Delaware	18,602,000	0.3%
3	Florida	366,863,000	6.1%
9	Georgia	167,681,000	2.8%
39	Hawaii	28,745,000	0.5%
42	Idaho	25,096,000	0.4%
5	Illinois	276,800,000	4.6%
17	Indiana	119,242,000	2.0%
29	Iowa	68,458,000	1.1%
34	Kansas	51,428,000	0.9%
26	Kentucky	76,272,000	1.3%
19	Louisiana	116,816,000	2.0%
41	Maine	26,046,000	0.4%
24	Maryland	96,852,000	1.6%
15	Massachusetts	129,459,000	2.2%
8	Michigan	208,797,000	3.5%
21	Minnesota	108,143,000	1.8%
28	Mississippi	68,686,000	1.1%
14	Missouri	130,325,000	2.2%
43	Montana	24,093,000	0.4%
36	Nebraska	41,857,000	0.7%
31	Nevada	59,159,000	1.0%
38	New Hampshire	36,896,000	0.6%
13	New Jersey	144,840,000	2.4%
35	New Mexico	45,918,000	0.8%
4	New York	315,657,000	5.3%
10	North Carolina	158,927,000	2.7%
47	North Dakota	17,349,000	0.3%
7	Ohio	265,079,000	4.4%
30	Oklahoma	67,617,000	1.1%
27	Oregon	72,528,000	1.2%
6	Pennsylvania	269,034,000	4.5%
44	Rhode Island	21,330,000	0.4%
22	South Carolina	99,267,000	1.7%
45	South Dakota	18,655,000	0.3%
18	Tennessee	119,222,000	2.0%
2	Texas	531,579,000	8.9%
40	Utah	26,418,000	0.4%
49	Vermont	13,515,000	0.2%
12	Virginia	145,634,000	2.4%
20	Washington	114,627,000	1.9%
37	West Virginia	39,246,000	0.7%
11	Wisconsin	152,275,000	2.5%
50	Wyoming	12,063,000	0.2%

RANK ORDER

RANK	STATE	GALLONS	% of USA
1	California	630,458,000	10.5%
2	Texas	531,579,000	8.9%
3	Florida	366,863,000	6.1%
4	New York	315,657,000	5.3%
5	Illinois	276,800,000	4.6%
6	Pennsylvania	269,034,000	4.5%
7	Ohio	265,079,000	4.4%
8	Michigan	208,797,000	3.5%
9	Georgia	167,681,000	2.8%
10	North Carolina	158,927,000	2.7%
11	Wisconsin	152,275,000	2.5%
12	Virginia	145,634,000	2.4%
13	New Jersey	144,840,000	2.4%
14	Missouri	130,325,000	2.2%
15	Massachusetts	129,459,000	2.2%
16	Arizona	124,001,000	2.1%
17	Indiana	119,242,000	2.0%
18	Tennessee	119,222,000	2.0%
19	Louisiana	116,816,000	2.0%
20	Washington	114,627,000	1.9%
21	Minnesota	108,143,000	1.8%
22	South Carolina	99,267,000	1.7%
23	Colorado	97,093,000	1.6%
24	Maryland	96,852,000	1.6%
25	Alabama	92,082,000	1.5%
26	Kentucky	76,272,000	1.3%
27	Oregon	72,528,000	1.2%
28	Mississippi	68,686,000	1.1%
29	Iowa	68,458,000	1.1%
30	Oklahoma	67,617,000	1.1%
31	Nevada	59,159,000	1.0%
32	Connecticut	58,076,000	1.0%
33	Arkansas	51,525,000	0.9%
34	Kansas	51,428,000	0.9%
35	New Mexico	45,918,000	0.8%
36	Nebraska	41,857,000	0.7%
37	West Virginia	39,246,000	0.7%
38	New Hampshire	36,896,000	0.6%
39	Hawaii	28,745,000	0.5%
40	Utah	26,418,000	0.4%
41	Maine	26,046,000	0.4%
42	Idaho	25,096,000	0.4%
43	Montana	24,093,000	0.4%
44	Rhode Island	21,330,000	0.4%
45	South Dakota	18,655,000	0.3%
46	Delaware	18,602,000	0.3%
47	North Dakota	17,349,000	0.3%
48	Alaska	14,315,000	0.2%
49	Vermont	13,515,000	0.2%
50	Wyoming	12,063,000	0.2%
	District of Columbia	14,401,000	0.2%

Source: U.S. Department of Health and Human Services, National Institute on Alcohol Abuse and Alcoholism
"Volume Beverage and Ethanol Consumption for States" (http://silk.nih.gov/silk/niaaa1/database/consum02.txt)
*This is apparent consumption and is based on several sources which together approximate sales but do not actually measure consumption. Reported state volumes reflect only in-state purchases. Accordingly, figures for some states may be skewed by purchases by nonresidents.

Adult Per Capita Beer Consumption in 1998

National Per Capita = 31.7 Gallons Consumed per Adult 21 Years and Older*

ALPHA ORDER

RANK ORDER

RANK	STATE	PER CAPITA	RANK	STATE	PER CAPITA
33	Alabama	29.9	1	Nevada	48.9
13	Alaska	36.8	2	New Hampshire	43.9
8	Arizona	39.1	3	Wisconsin	41.9
38	Arkansas	29.2	4	Texas	40.5
44	California	28.2	5	New Mexico	39.9
16	Colorado	35.3	6	Louisiana	39.7
48	Connecticut	24.7	7	Montana	39.4
17	Delaware	34.9	8	Arizona	39.1
21	Florida	33.8	8	North Dakota	39.1
25	Georgia	31.8	10	South Dakota	37.8
19	Hawaii	34.2	11	Wyoming	37.1
29	Idaho	30.9	12	Mississippi	37.0
24	Illinois	33.0	13	Alaska	36.8
40	Indiana	28.9	13	Nebraska	36.8
20	Iowa	34.1	15	South Carolina	36.6
43	Kansas	28.3	16	Colorado	35.3
45	Kentucky	27.5	17	Delaware	34.9
6	Louisiana	39.7	18	Missouri	34.3
42	Maine	28.8	19	Hawaii	34.2
46	Maryland	26.6	20	Iowa	34.1
39	Massachusetts	29.0	21	Florida	33.8
31	Michigan	30.5	22	Ohio	33.5
23	Minnesota	33.2	23	Minnesota	33.2
12	Mississippi	37.0	24	Illinois	33.0
18	Missouri	34.3	25	Georgia	31.8
7	Montana	39.4	25	Vermont	31.8
13	Nebraska	36.8	27	Oregon	31.3
1	Nevada	48.9	28	Pennsylvania	31.0
2	New Hampshire	43.9	29	Idaho	30.9
47	New Jersey	25.0	30	Tennessee	30.8
5	New Mexico	39.9	31	Michigan	30.5
49	New York	24.3	32	Virginia	30.0
33	North Carolina	29.9	33	Alabama	29.9
8	North Dakota	39.1	33	North Carolina	29.9
22	Ohio	33.5	33	Rhode Island	29.9
37	Oklahoma	29.4	36	West Virginia	29.8
27	Oregon	31.3	37	Oklahoma	29.4
28	Pennsylvania	31.0	38	Arkansas	29.2
33	Rhode Island	29.9	39	Massachusetts	29.0
15	South Carolina	36.6	40	Indiana	28.9
10	South Dakota	37.8	40	Washington	28.9
30	Tennessee	30.8	42	Maine	28.8
4	Texas	40.5	43	Kansas	28.3
50	Utah	20.9	44	California	28.2
25	Vermont	31.8	45	Kentucky	27.5
32	Virginia	30.0	46	Maryland	26.6
40	Washington	28.9	47	New Jersey	25.0
36	West Virginia	29.8	48	Connecticut	24.7
3	Wisconsin	41.9	49	New York	24.3
11	Wyoming	37.1	50	Utah	20.9
				District of Columbia	35.6

Source: Morgan Quitno Press using data from U.S. Dept. of HHS, National Institute on Alcohol Abuse and Alcoholism "Volume Beverage and Ethanol Consumption for States" (http://silk.nih.gov/silk/niaaa1/database/consum02.txt)
*This is apparent consumption and is based on several sources which together approximate sales but do not actually measure consumption. Reported state volumes reflect only in-state purchases. Accordingly, figures for some states may be skewed by purchases by nonresidents.

Wine Consumption in 1998

National Total = 514,672,000 Gallons of Wine Consumed*

ALPHA ORDER

RANK ORDER

RANK	STATE	GALLONS	% of USA	RANK	STATE	GALLONS	% of USA
30	Alabama	3,943,000	0.8%	1	California	90,647,000	17.6%
45	Alaska	1,412,000	0.3%	2	New York	42,856,000	8.3%
18	Arizona	9,520,000	1.8%	3	Florida	37,218,000	7.2%
41	Arkansas	1,899,000	0.4%	4	Texas	27,455,000	5.3%
1	California	90,647,000	17.6%	5	Illinois	25,612,000	5.0%
17	Colorado	9,544,000	1.9%	6	New Jersey	23,567,000	4.6%
15	Connecticut	10,039,000	2.0%	7	Massachusetts	19,556,000	3.8%
38	Delaware	2,253,000	0.4%	8	Washington	15,398,000	3.0%
3	Florida	37,218,000	7.2%	9	Pennsylvania	14,946,000	2.9%
13	Georgia	11,470,000	2.2%	10	Michigan	13,660,000	2.7%
33	Hawaii	2,797,000	0.5%	11	Ohio	13,022,000	2.5%
28	Idaho	4,479,000	0.9%	12	Virginia	12,382,000	2.4%
5	Illinois	25,612,000	5.0%	13	Georgia	11,470,000	2.2%
23	Indiana	7,060,000	1.4%	14	North Carolina	11,324,000	2.2%
39	Iowa	2,228,000	0.4%	15	Connecticut	10,039,000	2.0%
37	Kansas	2,503,000	0.5%	16	Maryland	9,584,000	1.9%
31	Kentucky	3,213,000	0.6%	17	Colorado	9,544,000	1.9%
25	Louisiana	6,184,000	1.2%	18	Arizona	9,520,000	1.8%
34	Maine	2,718,000	0.5%	19	Oregon	9,052,000	1.8%
16	Maryland	9,584,000	1.9%	20	Wisconsin	8,481,000	1.6%
7	Massachusetts	19,556,000	3.8%	21	Minnesota	7,990,000	1.6%
10	Michigan	13,660,000	2.7%	22	Missouri	7,809,000	1.5%
21	Minnesota	7,990,000	1.6%	23	Indiana	7,060,000	1.4%
44	Mississippi	1,546,000	0.3%	24	Nevada	6,703,000	1.3%
22	Missouri	7,809,000	1.5%	25	Louisiana	6,184,000	1.2%
43	Montana	1,579,000	0.3%	26	Tennessee	5,279,000	1.0%
40	Nebraska	1,926,000	0.4%	27	South Carolina	5,008,000	1.0%
24	Nevada	6,703,000	1.3%	28	Idaho	4,479,000	0.9%
29	New Hampshire	4,043,000	0.8%	29	New Hampshire	4,043,000	0.8%
6	New Jersey	23,567,000	4.6%	30	Alabama	3,943,000	0.8%
36	New Mexico	2,532,000	0.5%	31	Kentucky	3,213,000	0.6%
2	New York	42,856,000	8.3%	32	Rhode Island	3,066,000	0.6%
14	North Carolina	11,324,000	2.2%	33	Hawaii	2,797,000	0.5%
50	North Dakota	520,000	0.1%	34	Maine	2,718,000	0.5%
11	Ohio	13,022,000	2.5%	35	Oklahoma	2,610,000	0.5%
35	Oklahoma	2,610,000	0.5%	36	New Mexico	2,532,000	0.5%
19	Oregon	9,052,000	1.8%	37	Kansas	2,503,000	0.5%
9	Pennsylvania	14,946,000	2.9%	38	Delaware	2,253,000	0.4%
32	Rhode Island	3,066,000	0.6%	39	Iowa	2,228,000	0.4%
27	South Carolina	5,008,000	1.0%	40	Nebraska	1,926,000	0.4%
49	South Dakota	613,000	0.1%	41	Arkansas	1,899,000	0.4%
26	Tennessee	5,279,000	1.0%	42	Vermont	1,786,000	0.3%
4	Texas	27,455,000	5.3%	43	Montana	1,579,000	0.3%
46	Utah	1,224,000	0.2%	44	Mississippi	1,546,000	0.3%
42	Vermont	1,786,000	0.3%	45	Alaska	1,412,000	0.3%
12	Virginia	12,382,000	2.4%	46	Utah	1,224,000	0.2%
8	Washington	15,398,000	3.0%	47	West Virginia	1,111,000	0.2%
47	West Virginia	1,111,000	0.2%	48	Wyoming	619,000	0.1%
20	Wisconsin	8,481,000	1.6%	49	South Dakota	613,000	0.1%
48	Wyoming	619,000	0.1%	50	North Dakota	520,000	0.1%
					District of Columbia	2,685,000	0.5%

Source: U.S. Department of Health and Human Services, National Institute on Alcohol Abuse and Alcoholism
"Volume Beverage and Ethanol Consumption for States" (http://silk.nih.gov/silk/niaaa1/database/consum02.txt)
*This is apparent consumption and is based on several sources which together approximate sales but do not
actually measure consumption. Reported state volumes reflect only in-state purchases. Accordingly, figures for
some states may be skewed by purchases by nonresidents.

Adult Per Capita Wine Consumption in 1998

National Per Capita = 2.7 Gallons Consumed per Adult 21 Years and Older*

ALPHA ORDER

RANK	STATE	PER CAPITA
41	Alabama	1.3
13	Alaska	3.6
19	Arizona	3.0
45	Arkansas	1.1
9	California	4.1
14	Colorado	3.5
5	Connecticut	4.3
7	Delaware	4.2
15	Florida	3.4
26	Georgia	2.2
16	Hawaii	3.3
1	Idaho	5.5
18	Illinois	3.1
35	Indiana	1.7
45	Iowa	1.1
39	Kansas	1.4
42	Kentucky	1.2
28	Louisiana	2.1
19	Maine	3.0
21	Maryland	2.6
4	Massachusetts	4.4
32	Michigan	2.0
24	Minnesota	2.5
49	Mississippi	0.8
28	Missouri	2.1
21	Montana	2.6
35	Nebraska	1.7
1	Nevada	5.5
3	New Hampshire	4.8
9	New Jersey	4.1
26	New Mexico	2.2
16	New York	3.3
28	North Carolina	2.1
42	North Dakota	1.2
38	Ohio	1.6
45	Oklahoma	1.1
11	Oregon	3.9
35	Pennsylvania	1.7
5	Rhode Island	4.3
34	South Carolina	1.8
42	South Dakota	1.2
39	Tennessee	1.4
28	Texas	2.1
48	Utah	1.0
7	Vermont	4.2
21	Virginia	2.6
11	Washington	3.9
49	West Virginia	0.8
25	Wisconsin	2.3
33	Wyoming	1.9

RANK ORDER

RANK	STATE	PER CAPITA
1	Idaho	5.5
1	Nevada	5.5
3	New Hampshire	4.8
4	Massachusetts	4.4
5	Connecticut	4.3
5	Rhode Island	4.3
7	Delaware	4.2
7	Vermont	4.2
9	California	4.1
9	New Jersey	4.1
11	Oregon	3.9
11	Washington	3.9
13	Alaska	3.6
14	Colorado	3.5
15	Florida	3.4
16	Hawaii	3.3
16	New York	3.3
18	Illinois	3.1
19	Arizona	3.0
19	Maine	3.0
21	Maryland	2.6
21	Montana	2.6
21	Virginia	2.6
24	Minnesota	2.5
25	Wisconsin	2.3
26	Georgia	2.2
26	New Mexico	2.2
28	Louisiana	2.1
28	Missouri	2.1
28	North Carolina	2.1
28	Texas	2.1
32	Michigan	2.0
33	Wyoming	1.9
34	South Carolina	1.8
35	Indiana	1.7
35	Nebraska	1.7
35	Pennsylvania	1.7
38	Ohio	1.6
39	Kansas	1.4
39	Tennessee	1.4
41	Alabama	1.3
42	Kentucky	1.2
42	North Dakota	1.2
42	South Dakota	1.2
45	Arkansas	1.1
45	Iowa	1.1
45	Oklahoma	1.1
48	Utah	1.0
49	Mississippi	0.8
49	West Virginia	0.8
	District of Columbia	6.6

Source: Morgan Quitno Press using data from U.S. Dept. of HHS, National Institute on Alcohol Abuse and Alcoholism
"Volume Beverage and Ethanol Consumption for States" (http://silk.nih.gov/silk/niaaa1/database/consum02.txt)
*This is apparent consumption and is based on several sources which together approximate sales but do not
actually measure consumption. Reported state volumes reflect only in-state purchases. Accordingly, figures for
some states may be skewed by purchases by nonresidents.

Distilled Spirits Consumption in 1998

National Total = 332,400,000 Gallons of Distilled Spirits Consumed*

ALPHA ORDER

RANK	STATE	GALLONS	% of USA
27	Alabama	4,370,000	1.3%
46	Alaska	1,122,000	0.3%
21	Arizona	6,393,000	1.9%
35	Arkansas	2,622,000	0.8%
1	California	38,176,000	11.5%
19	Colorado	6,664,000	2.0%
25	Connecticut	4,875,000	1.5%
39	Delaware	1,473,000	0.4%
2	Florida	24,432,000	7.4%
9	Georgia	10,598,000	3.2%
43	Hawaii	1,280,000	0.4%
44	Idaho	1,208,000	0.4%
5	Illinois	15,134,000	4.6%
16	Indiana	7,150,000	2.2%
34	Iowa	2,649,000	0.8%
33	Kansas	2,794,000	0.8%
28	Kentucky	4,143,000	1.2%
22	Louisiana	5,980,000	1.8%
38	Maine	1,701,000	0.5%
15	Maryland	7,393,000	2.2%
11	Massachusetts	9,313,000	2.8%
6	Michigan	13,210,000	4.0%
14	Minnesota	7,755,000	2.3%
31	Mississippi	3,203,000	1.0%
18	Missouri	6,763,000	2.0%
45	Montana	1,133,000	0.3%
37	Nebraska	1,923,000	0.6%
26	Nevada	4,444,000	1.3%
29	New Hampshire	4,061,000	1.2%
7	New Jersey	11,149,000	3.4%
36	New Mexico	1,964,000	0.6%
3	New York	20,459,000	6.2%
13	North Carolina	7,759,000	2.3%
48	North Dakota	977,000	0.3%
10	Ohio	10,442,000	3.1%
32	Oklahoma	2,869,000	0.9%
30	Oregon	4,047,000	1.2%
8	Pennsylvania	11,036,000	3.3%
42	Rhode Island	1,292,000	0.4%
23	South Carolina	5,530,000	1.7%
47	South Dakota	984,000	0.3%
24	Tennessee	5,432,000	1.6%
4	Texas	18,879,000	5.7%
40	Utah	1,472,000	0.4%
50	Vermont	736,000	0.2%
20	Virginia	6,428,000	1.9%
17	Washington	7,075,000	2.1%
41	West Virginia	1,333,000	0.4%
12	Wisconsin	8,141,000	2.4%
49	Wyoming	775,000	0.2%

RANK ORDER

RANK	STATE	GALLONS	% of USA
1	California	38,176,000	11.5%
2	Florida	24,432,000	7.4%
3	New York	20,459,000	6.2%
4	Texas	18,879,000	5.7%
5	Illinois	15,134,000	4.6%
6	Michigan	13,210,000	4.0%
7	New Jersey	11,149,000	3.4%
8	Pennsylvania	11,036,000	3.3%
9	Georgia	10,598,000	3.2%
10	Ohio	10,442,000	3.1%
11	Massachusetts	9,313,000	2.8%
12	Wisconsin	8,141,000	2.4%
13	North Carolina	7,759,000	2.3%
14	Minnesota	7,755,000	2.3%
15	Maryland	7,393,000	2.2%
16	Indiana	7,150,000	2.2%
17	Washington	7,075,000	2.1%
18	Missouri	6,763,000	2.0%
19	Colorado	6,664,000	2.0%
20	Virginia	6,428,000	1.9%
21	Arizona	6,393,000	1.9%
22	Louisiana	5,980,000	1.8%
23	South Carolina	5,530,000	1.7%
24	Tennessee	5,432,000	1.6%
25	Connecticut	4,875,000	1.5%
26	Nevada	4,444,000	1.3%
27	Alabama	4,370,000	1.3%
28	Kentucky	4,143,000	1.2%
29	New Hampshire	4,061,000	1.2%
30	Oregon	4,047,000	1.2%
31	Mississippi	3,203,000	1.0%
32	Oklahoma	2,869,000	0.9%
33	Kansas	2,794,000	0.8%
34	Iowa	2,649,000	0.8%
35	Arkansas	2,622,000	0.8%
36	New Mexico	1,964,000	0.6%
37	Nebraska	1,923,000	0.6%
38	Maine	1,701,000	0.5%
39	Delaware	1,473,000	0.4%
40	Utah	1,472,000	0.4%
41	West Virginia	1,333,000	0.4%
42	Rhode Island	1,292,000	0.4%
43	Hawaii	1,280,000	0.4%
44	Idaho	1,208,000	0.4%
45	Montana	1,133,000	0.3%
46	Alaska	1,122,000	0.3%
47	South Dakota	984,000	0.3%
48	North Dakota	977,000	0.3%
49	Wyoming	775,000	0.2%
50	Vermont	736,000	0.2%
	District of Columbia	1,660,000	0.5%

*Source: U.S. Department of Health and Human Services, National Institute on Alcohol Abuse and Alcoholism
"Volume Beverage and Ethanol Consumption for States" (http://silk.nih.gov/silk/niaaa1/database/consum02.txt)
*This is apparent consumption and is based on several sources which together approximate sales but do not
actually measure consumption. Reported state volumes reflect only in-state purchases. Accordingly, figures for
some states may be skewed by purchases by nonresidents.*

Adult Per Capita Apparent Distilled Spirits Consumption in 1998

National Per Capita = 1.8 Gallons Consumed per Adult 21 Years and Older*

ALPHA ORDER

RANK ORDER

RANK	STATE	PER CAPITA		RANK	STATE	PER CAPITA
41	Alabama	1.4		1	New Hampshire	4.8
3	Alaska	2.9		2	Nevada	3.7
13	Arizona	2.0		3	Alaska	2.9
35	Arkansas	1.5		4	Delaware	2.8
27	California	1.7		5	Colorado	2.4
5	Colorado	2.4		5	Minnesota	2.4
11	Connecticut	2.1		5	Wyoming	2.4
4	Delaware	2.8		8	Florida	2.3
8	Florida	2.3		9	North Dakota	2.2
13	Georgia	2.0		9	Wisconsin	2.2
35	Hawaii	1.5		11	Connecticut	2.1
35	Idaho	1.5		11	Massachusetts	2.1
23	Illinois	1.8		13	Arizona	2.0
27	Indiana	1.7		13	Georgia	2.0
44	Iowa	1.3		13	Louisiana	2.0
35	Kansas	1.5		13	Maryland	2.0
35	Kentucky	1.5		13	South Carolina	2.0
13	Louisiana	2.0		13	South Dakota	2.0
19	Maine	1.9		19	Maine	1.9
13	Maryland	2.0		19	Michigan	1.9
11	Massachusetts	2.1		19	Montana	1.9
19	Michigan	1.9		19	New Jersey	1.9
5	Minnesota	2.4		23	Illinois	1.8
27	Mississippi	1.7		23	Missouri	1.8
23	Missouri	1.8		23	Rhode Island	1.8
19	Montana	1.9		23	Washington	1.8
27	Nebraska	1.7		27	California	1.7
2	Nevada	3.7		27	Indiana	1.7
1	New Hampshire	4.8		27	Mississippi	1.7
19	New Jersey	1.9		27	Nebraska	1.7
27	New Mexico	1.7		27	New Mexico	1.7
34	New York	1.6		27	Oregon	1.7
35	North Carolina	1.5		27	Vermont	1.7
9	North Dakota	2.2		34	New York	1.6
44	Ohio	1.3		35	Arkansas	1.5
48	Oklahoma	1.2		35	Hawaii	1.5
27	Oregon	1.7		35	Idaho	1.5
44	Pennsylvania	1.3		35	Kansas	1.5
23	Rhode Island	1.8		35	Kentucky	1.5
13	South Carolina	2.0		35	North Carolina	1.5
13	South Dakota	2.0		41	Alabama	1.4
41	Tennessee	1.4		41	Tennessee	1.4
41	Texas	1.4		41	Texas	1.4
48	Utah	1.2		44	Iowa	1.3
27	Vermont	1.7		44	Ohio	1.3
44	Virginia	1.3		44	Pennsylvania	1.3
23	Washington	1.8		44	Virginia	1.3
50	West Virginia	1.0		48	Oklahoma	1.2
9	Wisconsin	2.2		48	Utah	1.2
5	Wyoming	2.4		50	West Virginia	1.0
					District of Columbia	4.1

Source: Morgan Quitno Press using data from U.S. Dept. of HHS, National Institute on Alcohol Abuse and Alcoholism "Volume Beverage and Ethanol Consumption for States" (http://silk.nih.gov/silk/niaaa1/database/consum02.txt)
*This is apparent consumption and is based on several sources which together approximate sales but do not actually measure consumption. Reported state volumes reflect only in-state purchases. Accordingly, figures for some states may be skewed by purchases by nonresidents.

Percent of Adults Who Are Binge Drinkers: 1999

National Median = 14.9% of Adults*

ALPHA ORDER

RANK	STATE	PERCENT
43	Alabama	11.7
8	Alaska	18.9
47	Arizona	8.8
44	Arkansas	10.3
24	California	15.5
17	Colorado	17.2
31	Connecticut	14.0
8	Delaware	18.9
34	Florida	12.9
36	Georgia	12.5
31	Hawaii	14.0
29	Idaho	14.7
4	Illinois	19.7
6	Indiana	19.1
10	Iowa	18.3
42	Kansas	11.8
46	Kentucky	9.8
25	Louisiana	15.0
28	Maine	14.8
21	Maryland	15.9
12	Massachusetts	17.4
7	Michigan	19.0
20	Minnesota	16.3
39	Mississippi	12.1
19	Missouri	16.4
11	Montana	17.6
18	Nebraska	16.6
2	Nevada	21.0
3	New Hampshire	20.0
37	New Jersey	12.3
25	New Mexico	15.0
33	New York	13.9
41	North Carolina	12.0
4	North Dakota	19.7
39	Ohio	12.1
49	Oklahoma	8.1
27	Oregon	14.9
21	Pennsylvania	15.9
23	Rhode Island	15.6
37	South Carolina	12.3
12	South Dakota	17.4
50	Tennessee	7.7
15	Texas	17.3
45	Utah	10.2
12	Vermont	17.4
35	Virginia	12.7
30	Washington	14.4
48	West Virginia	8.6
1	Wisconsin	27.0
15	Wyoming	17.3

RANK ORDER

RANK	STATE	PERCENT
1	Wisconsin	27.0
2	Nevada	21.0
3	New Hampshire	20.0
4	Illinois	19.7
4	North Dakota	19.7
6	Indiana	19.1
7	Michigan	19.0
8	Alaska	18.9
8	Delaware	18.9
10	Iowa	18.3
11	Montana	17.6
12	Massachusetts	17.4
12	South Dakota	17.4
12	Vermont	17.4
15	Texas	17.3
15	Wyoming	17.3
17	Colorado	17.2
18	Nebraska	16.6
19	Missouri	16.4
20	Minnesota	16.3
21	Maryland	15.9
21	Pennsylvania	15.9
23	Rhode Island	15.6
24	California	15.5
25	Louisiana	15.0
25	New Mexico	15.0
27	Oregon	14.9
28	Maine	14.8
29	Idaho	14.7
30	Washington	14.4
31	Connecticut	14.0
31	Hawaii	14.0
33	New York	13.9
34	Florida	12.9
35	Virginia	12.7
36	Georgia	12.5
37	New Jersey	12.3
37	South Carolina	12.3
39	Mississippi	12.1
39	Ohio	12.1
41	North Carolina	12.0
42	Kansas	11.8
43	Alabama	11.7
44	Arkansas	10.3
45	Utah	10.2
46	Kentucky	9.8
47	Arizona	8.8
48	West Virginia	8.6
49	Oklahoma	8.1
50	Tennessee	7.7
	District of Columbia	13.0

Source: U.S. Department of Health and Human Services, Centers for Disease Control and Prevention
"1999 Behavioral Risk Factor Surveillance Summary Prevalence Report" (June 23, 2000)
*Persons 18 and older reporting consumption of five or more alcoholic drinks on one or more occasions during the previous month.

Percent of Adults Who Drink and Drive: 1999

National Median = 2.4% of Adults*

ALPHA ORDER

RANK ORDER

RANK	STATE	PERCENT		RANK	STATE	PERCENT
35	Alabama	1.9		1	Nevada	5.5
32	Alaska	2.1		2	Wisconsin	4.9
37	Arizona	1.8		3	Illinois	4.4
43	Arkansas	1.5		3	North Dakota	4.4
29	California	2.3		5	Minnesota	4.1
10	Colorado	3.6		5	South Dakota	4.1
17	Connecticut	2.9		7	Iowa	3.9
13	Delaware	3.2		8	New Hampshire	3.8
34	Florida	2.0		9	Nebraska	3.7
43	Georgia	1.5		10	Colorado	3.6
29	Hawaii	2.3		10	Louisiana	3.6
37	Idaho	1.8		12	Montana	3.4
3	Illinois	4.4		13	Delaware	3.2
13	Indiana	3.2		13	Indiana	3.2
7	Iowa	3.9		15	Michigan	3.1
18	Kansas	2.8		16	Missouri	3.0
41	Kentucky	1.6		17	Connecticut	2.9
10	Louisiana	3.6		18	Kansas	2.8
49	Maine	1.1		18	Massachusetts	2.8
24	Maryland	2.4		18	Texas	2.8
18	Massachusetts	2.8		21	Mississippi	2.7
15	Michigan	3.1		22	Rhode Island	2.6
5	Minnesota	4.1		23	Oklahoma	2.5
21	Mississippi	2.7		24	Maryland	2.4
16	Missouri	3.0		24	Pennsylvania	2.4
12	Montana	3.4		24	Vermont	2.4
9	Nebraska	3.7		24	Virginia	2.4
1	Nevada	5.5		24	Wyoming	2.4
8	New Hampshire	3.8		29	California	2.3
46	New Jersey	1.3		29	Hawaii	2.3
29	New Mexico	2.3		29	New Mexico	2.3
41	New York	1.6		32	Alaska	2.1
39	North Carolina	1.7		32	South Carolina	2.1
3	North Dakota	4.4		34	Florida	2.0
47	Ohio	1.2		35	Alabama	1.9
23	Oklahoma	2.5		35	Oregon	1.9
35	Oregon	1.9		37	Arizona	1.8
24	Pennsylvania	2.4		37	Idaho	1.8
22	Rhode Island	2.6		39	North Carolina	1.7
32	South Carolina	2.1		39	Washington	1.7
5	South Dakota	4.1		41	Kentucky	1.6
43	Tennessee	1.5		41	New York	1.6
18	Texas	2.8		43	Arkansas	1.5
47	Utah	1.2		43	Georgia	1.5
24	Vermont	2.4		43	Tennessee	1.5
24	Virginia	2.4		46	New Jersey	1.3
39	Washington	1.7		47	Ohio	1.2
49	West Virginia	1.1		47	Utah	1.2
2	Wisconsin	4.9		49	Maine	1.1
24	Wyoming	2.4		49	West Virginia	1.1
					District of Columbia	1.4

Source: U.S. Department of Health and Human Services, Centers for Disease Control and Prevention
"1999 Behavioral Risk Factor Surveillance Summary Prevalence Report" (June 23, 2000)
*Persons 18 and over who "drive after having too much to drink, one or more times in the past month."

Percent of Adults Who Smoke: 2000

National Median = 23.2% of Adults*

ALPHA ORDER				RANK ORDER		
RANK	STATE	PERCENT		RANK	STATE	PERCENT
10	Alabama	25.2		1	Kentucky	30.5
12	Alaska	25.0		2	Nevada	29.0
48	Arizona	18.6		3	Missouri	27.2
11	Arkansas	25.1		4	Indiana	26.9
49	California	17.2		5	Ohio	26.2
42	Colorado	20.0		6	North Carolina	26.1
44	Connecticut	19.9		6	West Virginia	26.1
28	Delaware	22.9		8	Tennessee	25.7
25	Florida	23.2		9	New Hampshire	25.3
21	Georgia	23.5		10	Alabama	25.2
46	Hawaii	19.7		11	Arkansas	25.1
29	Idaho	22.3		12	Alaska	25.0
29	Illinois	22.3		13	South Carolina	24.9
4	Indiana	26.9		14	Pennsylvania	24.3
25	Iowa	23.2		15	Louisiana	24.1
37	Kansas	21.1		15	Michigan	24.1
1	Kentucky	30.5		15	Wisconsin	24.1
15	Louisiana	24.1		18	Maine	23.8
18	Maine	23.8		18	Wyoming	23.8
41	Maryland	20.5		20	New Mexico	23.6
42	Massachusetts	20.0		21	Georgia	23.5
15	Michigan	24.1		21	Mississippi	23.5
45	Minnesota	19.8		23	Rhode Island	23.4
21	Mississippi	23.5		24	Oklahoma	23.3
3	Missouri	27.2		25	Florida	23.2
47	Montana	18.8		25	Iowa	23.2
36	Nebraska	21.2		25	North Dakota	23.2
2	Nevada	29.0		28	Delaware	22.9
9	New Hampshire	25.3		29	Idaho	22.3
38	New Jersey	21.0		29	Illinois	22.3
20	New Mexico	23.6		31	South Dakota	21.9
33	New York	21.6		31	Texas	21.9
6	North Carolina	26.1		33	New York	21.6
25	North Dakota	23.2		34	Vermont	21.5
5	Ohio	26.2		35	Virginia	21.4
24	Oklahoma	23.3		36	Nebraska	21.2
39	Oregon	20.8		37	Kansas	21.1
14	Pennsylvania	24.3		38	New Jersey	21.0
23	Rhode Island	23.4		39	Oregon	20.8
13	South Carolina	24.9		40	Washington	20.7
31	South Dakota	21.9		41	Maryland	20.5
8	Tennessee	25.7		42	Colorado	20.0
31	Texas	21.9		42	Massachusetts	20.0
50	Utah	12.9		44	Connecticut	19.9
34	Vermont	21.5		45	Minnesota	19.8
35	Virginia	21.4		46	Hawaii	19.7
40	Washington	20.7		47	Montana	18.8
6	West Virginia	26.1		48	Arizona	18.6
15	Wisconsin	24.1		49	California	17.2
18	Wyoming	23.8		50	Utah	12.9
					District of Columbia	20.9

Source: U.S. Department of Health and Human Services, Centers for Disease Control and Prevention
"2000 Behavioral Risk Factor Surveillance Summary Prevalence Report" (May 3, 2001)
*Persons 18 and older who smoke everyday or some days.

Percent of Males Who Smoke: 2000

National Median = 24.4% of Men*

ALPHA ORDER				RANK ORDER		
RANK	**STATE**	**PERCENT**		**RANK**	**STATE**	**PERCENT**
3	Alabama	28.9		1	Kentucky	33.4
11	Alaska	26.8		2	Missouri	30.1
48	Arizona	18.3		3	Alabama	28.9
16	Arkansas	26.1		4	South Carolina	28.7
46	California	20.1		5	Nevada	28.6
47	Colorado	19.5		6	Indiana	28.4
44	Connecticut	20.4		6	North Carolina	28.4
18	Delaware	25.7		8	West Virginia	27.7
26	Florida	24.5		9	Tennessee	27.6
14	Georgia	26.3		10	New Hampshire	27.0
34	Hawaii	22.9		11	Alaska	26.8
35	Idaho	22.8		11	Louisiana	26.8
24	Illinois	24.9		13	Ohio	26.6
6	Indiana	28.4		14	Georgia	26.3
18	Iowa	25.7		15	New Mexico	26.2
28	Kansas	24.2		16	Arkansas	26.1
1	Kentucky	33.4		17	Michigan	26.0
11	Louisiana	26.8		18	Delaware	25.7
25	Maine	24.6		18	Iowa	25.7
39	Maryland	22.0		18	North Dakota	25.7
45	Massachusetts	20.2		21	Pennsylvania	25.5
17	Michigan	26.0		22	Mississippi	25.2
43	Minnesota	20.7		22	Texas	25.2
22	Mississippi	25.2		24	Illinois	24.9
2	Missouri	30.1		25	Maine	24.6
49	Montana	18.0		26	Florida	24.5
40	Nebraska	21.9		27	Wisconsin	24.4
5	Nevada	28.6		28	Kansas	24.2
10	New Hampshire	27.0		28	Virginia	24.2
32	New Jersey	23.6		30	Rhode Island	23.8
15	New Mexico	26.2		31	Oklahoma	23.7
36	New York	22.6		32	New Jersey	23.6
6	North Carolina	28.4		33	Wyoming	23.2
18	North Dakota	25.7		34	Hawaii	22.9
13	Ohio	26.6		35	Idaho	22.8
31	Oklahoma	23.7		36	New York	22.6
38	Oregon	22.2		37	South Dakota	22.5
21	Pennsylvania	25.5		38	Oregon	22.2
30	Rhode Island	23.8		39	Maryland	22.0
4	South Carolina	28.7		40	Nebraska	21.9
37	South Dakota	22.5		41	Washington	21.8
9	Tennessee	27.6		42	Vermont	21.7
22	Texas	25.2		43	Minnesota	20.7
50	Utah	14.5		44	Connecticut	20.4
42	Vermont	21.7		45	Massachusetts	20.2
28	Virginia	24.2		46	California	20.1
41	Washington	21.8		47	Colorado	19.5
8	West Virginia	27.7		48	Arizona	18.3
27	Wisconsin	24.4		49	Montana	18.0
33	Wyoming	23.2		50	Utah	14.5
					District of Columbia	22.1

*Source: U.S. Department of Health and Human Services, Centers for Disease Control and Prevention
"2000 Behavioral Risk Factor Surveillance Summary Prevalence Report" (May 3, 2001)
Persons 18 and older who smoke everyday or some days.

Percent of Women Who Smoke: 2000

National Median = 21.2% of Women*

ALPHA ORDER

RANK	STATE	PERCENT
20	Alabama	22.0
14	Alaska	23.1
42	Arizona	19.0
8	Arkansas	24.1
49	California	14.4
33	Colorado	20.5
39	Connecticut	19.4
34	Delaware	20.3
19	Florida	22.1
28	Georgia	20.9
48	Hawaii	16.4
22	Idaho	21.8
35	Illinois	20.0
4	Indiana	25.5
28	Iowa	20.9
47	Kansas	18.1
2	Kentucky	27.9
23	Louisiana	21.7
14	Maine	23.1
41	Maryland	19.1
36	Massachusetts	19.7
18	Michigan	22.4
43	Minnesota	18.9
21	Mississippi	21.9
6	Missouri	24.5
36	Montana	19.7
32	Nebraska	20.6
1	Nevada	29.4
12	New Hampshire	23.7
46	New Jersey	18.6
26	New Mexico	21.2
31	New York	20.7
9	North Carolina	23.9
30	North Dakota	20.8
3	Ohio	25.9
17	Oklahoma	22.9
39	Oregon	19.4
13	Pennsylvania	23.3
16	Rhode Island	23.0
24	South Carolina	21.5
25	South Dakota	21.3
9	Tennessee	23.9
45	Texas	18.7
50	Utah	11.3
26	Vermont	21.2
44	Virginia	18.8
36	Washington	19.7
5	West Virginia	24.7
9	Wisconsin	23.9
7	Wyoming	24.3

RANK ORDER

RANK	STATE	PERCENT
1	Nevada	29.4
2	Kentucky	27.9
3	Ohio	25.9
4	Indiana	25.5
5	West Virginia	24.7
6	Missouri	24.5
7	Wyoming	24.3
8	Arkansas	24.1
9	North Carolina	23.9
9	Tennessee	23.9
9	Wisconsin	23.9
12	New Hampshire	23.7
13	Pennsylvania	23.3
14	Alaska	23.1
14	Maine	23.1
16	Rhode Island	23.0
17	Oklahoma	22.9
18	Michigan	22.4
19	Florida	22.1
20	Alabama	22.0
21	Mississippi	21.9
22	Idaho	21.8
23	Louisiana	21.7
24	South Carolina	21.5
25	South Dakota	21.3
26	New Mexico	21.2
26	Vermont	21.2
28	Georgia	20.9
28	Iowa	20.9
30	North Dakota	20.8
31	New York	20.7
32	Nebraska	20.6
33	Colorado	20.5
34	Delaware	20.3
35	Illinois	20.0
36	Massachusetts	19.7
36	Montana	19.7
36	Washington	19.7
39	Connecticut	19.4
39	Oregon	19.4
41	Maryland	19.1
42	Arizona	19.0
43	Minnesota	18.9
44	Virginia	18.8
45	Texas	18.7
46	New Jersey	18.6
47	Kansas	18.1
48	Hawaii	16.4
49	California	14.4
50	Utah	11.3
	District of Columbia	19.9

Source: U.S. Department of Health and Human Services, Centers for Disease Control and Prevention
"2000 Behavioral Risk Factor Surveillance Summary Prevalence Report" (May 3, 2001)
*Persons 18 and older who smoke everyday or some days.

Percent of Adults Overweight or Obese: 2000

National Median = 57.1% of Adults*

ALPHA ORDER

RANK	STATE	PERCENT
4	Alabama	60.8
13	Alaska	59.2
33	Arizona	55.9
8	Arkansas	59.9
24	California	57.3
50	Colorado	48.0
44	Connecticut	53.7
34	Delaware	55.8
42	Florida	53.9
11	Georgia	59.4
49	Hawaii	50.2
35	Idaho	55.7
16	Illinois	58.9
20	Indiana	58.4
6	Iowa	60.0
18	Kansas	58.7
2	Kentucky	61.0
6	Louisiana	60.0
30	Maine	56.3
27	Maryland	56.7
47	Massachusetts	52.8
2	Michigan	61.0
39	Minnesota	55.0
1	Mississippi	61.7
29	Missouri	56.4
46	Montana	53.1
19	Nebraska	58.5
45	Nevada	53.2
40	New Hampshire	54.6
27	New Jersey	56.7
36	New Mexico	55.5
26	New York	56.9
13	North Carolina	59.2
5	North Dakota	60.4
24	Ohio	57.3
30	Oklahoma	56.3
23	Oregon	57.6
22	Pennsylvania	57.7
43	Rhode Island	53.8
15	South Carolina	59.0
17	South Dakota	58.8
11	Tennessee	59.4
9	Texas	59.8
41	Utah	54.1
47	Vermont	52.8
32	Virginia	56.1
37	Washington	55.1
9	West Virginia	59.8
21	Wisconsin	57.8
37	Wyoming	55.1

RANK ORDER

RANK	STATE	PERCENT
1	Mississippi	61.7
2	Kentucky	61.0
2	Michigan	61.0
4	Alabama	60.8
5	North Dakota	60.4
6	Iowa	60.0
6	Louisiana	60.0
8	Arkansas	59.9
9	Texas	59.8
9	West Virginia	59.8
11	Georgia	59.4
11	Tennessee	59.4
13	Alaska	59.2
13	North Carolina	59.2
15	South Carolina	59.0
16	Illinois	58.9
17	South Dakota	58.8
18	Kansas	58.7
19	Nebraska	58.5
20	Indiana	58.4
21	Wisconsin	57.8
22	Pennsylvania	57.7
23	Oregon	57.6
24	California	57.3
24	Ohio	57.3
26	New York	56.9
27	Maryland	56.7
27	New Jersey	56.7
29	Missouri	56.4
30	Maine	56.3
30	Oklahoma	56.3
32	Virginia	56.1
33	Arizona	55.9
34	Delaware	55.8
35	Idaho	55.7
36	New Mexico	55.5
37	Washington	55.1
37	Wyoming	55.1
39	Minnesota	55.0
40	New Hampshire	54.6
41	Utah	54.1
42	Florida	53.9
43	Rhode Island	53.8
44	Connecticut	53.7
45	Nevada	53.2
46	Montana	53.1
47	Massachusetts	52.8
47	Vermont	52.8
49	Hawaii	50.2
50	Colorado	48.0
	District of Columbia	53.3

Source: U.S. Department of Health and Human Services, Centers for Disease Control and Prevention
"2000 Behavioral Risk Factor Surveillance Summary Prevalence Report" (May 3, 2001)
*Persons 18 and older. This table reflects a revised definition of overweight and differs from previous years. It is now defined as a Body Mass Index (BMI) of 25.0 to 29.9 and obese is defined as a BMI of 30.0 or more regardless of sex. BMI is a ratio of height to weight. As an example, a person 5' 8" and weighing 185 pounds has a BMI of 28. See http://www.cdc.gov/nccdphp/dnpa/bmi/bmi-adult.htm.

Percent of Adults Who Have Not Had Their Blood Pressure Checked in the Past Two Years: 1999
National Median = 5.4% of Adults*

<table>
<tr><td colspan="3">ALPHA ORDER</td><td colspan="3">RANK ORDER</td></tr>
<tr><td>RANK</td><td>STATE</td><td>PERCENT</td><td>RANK</td><td>STATE</td><td>PERCENT</td></tr>
<tr><td>33</td><td>Alabama</td><td>4.8</td><td>1</td><td>New Mexico</td><td>9.7</td></tr>
<tr><td>19</td><td>Alaska</td><td>6.2</td><td>2</td><td>Idaho</td><td>9.4</td></tr>
<tr><td>12</td><td>Arizona</td><td>7.2</td><td>3</td><td>Texas</td><td>8.7</td></tr>
<tr><td>14</td><td>Arkansas</td><td>6.7</td><td>4</td><td>Oregon</td><td>8.5</td></tr>
<tr><td>6</td><td>California</td><td>8.0</td><td>5</td><td>Nevada</td><td>8.1</td></tr>
<tr><td>7</td><td>Colorado</td><td>7.8</td><td>6</td><td>California</td><td>8.0</td></tr>
<tr><td>33</td><td>Connecticut</td><td>4.8</td><td>7</td><td>Colorado</td><td>7.8</td></tr>
<tr><td>46</td><td>Delaware</td><td>3.8</td><td>8</td><td>Indiana</td><td>7.7</td></tr>
<tr><td>26</td><td>Florida</td><td>5.4</td><td>8</td><td>Wyoming</td><td>7.7</td></tr>
<tr><td>40</td><td>Georgia</td><td>4.4</td><td>10</td><td>Utah</td><td>7.6</td></tr>
<tr><td>48</td><td>Hawaii</td><td>3.5</td><td>11</td><td>Wisconsin</td><td>7.4</td></tr>
<tr><td>2</td><td>Idaho</td><td>9.4</td><td>12</td><td>Arizona</td><td>7.2</td></tr>
<tr><td>16</td><td>Illinois</td><td>6.5</td><td>13</td><td>Washington</td><td>7.1</td></tr>
<tr><td>8</td><td>Indiana</td><td>7.7</td><td>14</td><td>Arkansas</td><td>6.7</td></tr>
<tr><td>26</td><td>Iowa</td><td>5.4</td><td>14</td><td>Montana</td><td>6.7</td></tr>
<tr><td>38</td><td>Kansas</td><td>4.5</td><td>16</td><td>Illinois</td><td>6.5</td></tr>
<tr><td>23</td><td>Kentucky</td><td>5.6</td><td>17</td><td>New York</td><td>6.4</td></tr>
<tr><td>41</td><td>Louisiana</td><td>4.2</td><td>17</td><td>Virginia</td><td>6.4</td></tr>
<tr><td>29</td><td>Maine</td><td>5.2</td><td>19</td><td>Alaska</td><td>6.2</td></tr>
<tr><td>49</td><td>Maryland</td><td>3.4</td><td>19</td><td>West Virginia</td><td>6.2</td></tr>
<tr><td>42</td><td>Massachusetts</td><td>4.1</td><td>21</td><td>South Dakota</td><td>5.7</td></tr>
<tr><td>31</td><td>Michigan</td><td>4.9</td><td>21</td><td>Vermont</td><td>5.7</td></tr>
<tr><td>23</td><td>Minnesota</td><td>5.6</td><td>23</td><td>Kentucky</td><td>5.6</td></tr>
<tr><td>37</td><td>Mississippi</td><td>4.7</td><td>23</td><td>Minnesota</td><td>5.6</td></tr>
<tr><td>31</td><td>Missouri</td><td>4.9</td><td>25</td><td>New Hampshire</td><td>5.5</td></tr>
<tr><td>14</td><td>Montana</td><td>6.7</td><td>26</td><td>Florida</td><td>5.4</td></tr>
<tr><td>26</td><td>Nebraska</td><td>5.4</td><td>26</td><td>Iowa</td><td>5.4</td></tr>
<tr><td>5</td><td>Nevada</td><td>8.1</td><td>26</td><td>Nebraska</td><td>5.4</td></tr>
<tr><td>25</td><td>New Hampshire</td><td>5.5</td><td>29</td><td>Maine</td><td>5.2</td></tr>
<tr><td>30</td><td>New Jersey</td><td>5.0</td><td>30</td><td>New Jersey</td><td>5.0</td></tr>
<tr><td>1</td><td>New Mexico</td><td>9.7</td><td>31</td><td>Michigan</td><td>4.9</td></tr>
<tr><td>17</td><td>New York</td><td>6.4</td><td>31</td><td>Missouri</td><td>4.9</td></tr>
<tr><td>46</td><td>North Carolina</td><td>3.8</td><td>33</td><td>Alabama</td><td>4.8</td></tr>
<tr><td>38</td><td>North Dakota</td><td>4.5</td><td>33</td><td>Connecticut</td><td>4.8</td></tr>
<tr><td>44</td><td>Ohio</td><td>3.9</td><td>33</td><td>Oklahoma</td><td>4.8</td></tr>
<tr><td>33</td><td>Oklahoma</td><td>4.8</td><td>33</td><td>South Carolina</td><td>4.8</td></tr>
<tr><td>4</td><td>Oregon</td><td>8.5</td><td>37</td><td>Mississippi</td><td>4.7</td></tr>
<tr><td>44</td><td>Pennsylvania</td><td>3.9</td><td>38</td><td>Kansas</td><td>4.5</td></tr>
<tr><td>50</td><td>Rhode Island</td><td>3.3</td><td>38</td><td>North Dakota</td><td>4.5</td></tr>
<tr><td>33</td><td>South Carolina</td><td>4.8</td><td>40</td><td>Georgia</td><td>4.4</td></tr>
<tr><td>21</td><td>South Dakota</td><td>5.7</td><td>41</td><td>Louisiana</td><td>4.2</td></tr>
<tr><td>42</td><td>Tennessee</td><td>4.1</td><td>42</td><td>Massachusetts</td><td>4.1</td></tr>
<tr><td>3</td><td>Texas</td><td>8.7</td><td>42</td><td>Tennessee</td><td>4.1</td></tr>
<tr><td>10</td><td>Utah</td><td>7.6</td><td>44</td><td>Ohio</td><td>3.9</td></tr>
<tr><td>21</td><td>Vermont</td><td>5.7</td><td>44</td><td>Pennsylvania</td><td>3.9</td></tr>
<tr><td>17</td><td>Virginia</td><td>6.4</td><td>46</td><td>Delaware</td><td>3.8</td></tr>
<tr><td>13</td><td>Washington</td><td>7.1</td><td>46</td><td>North Carolina</td><td>3.8</td></tr>
<tr><td>19</td><td>West Virginia</td><td>6.2</td><td>48</td><td>Hawaii</td><td>3.5</td></tr>
<tr><td>11</td><td>Wisconsin</td><td>7.4</td><td>49</td><td>Maryland</td><td>3.4</td></tr>
<tr><td>8</td><td>Wyoming</td><td>7.7</td><td>50</td><td>Rhode Island</td><td>3.3</td></tr>
<tr><td></td><td></td><td></td><td></td><td>District of Columbia</td><td>3.9</td></tr>
</table>

Source: U.S. Department of Health and Human Services, Centers for Disease Control and Prevention
"1999 Behavioral Risk Factor Surveillance Summary Prevalence Report" (June 23, 2000)
*Persons 18 and older.

Percent of Adults Who Have Not Been Tested in Past Year for HIV: 2000

National Median = 64.3% Have Not Been Tested in Past Year*

ALPHA ORDER

RANK	STATE	PERCENT
28	Alabama	63.3
23	Alaska	64.8
22	Arizona	64.9
20	Arkansas	65.0
5	California	68.9
3	Colorado	69.3
27	Connecticut	63.4
45	Delaware	57.9
42	Florida	59.0
46	Georgia	56.4
50	Hawaii	49.8
6	Idaho	68.7
14	Illinois	66.4
8	Indiana	68.4
11	Iowa	67.3
41	Kansas	59.2
33	Kentucky	62.5
34	Louisiana	62.2
3	Maine	69.3
36	Maryland	61.0
26	Massachusetts	64.1
18	Michigan	65.5
6	Minnesota	68.7
49	Mississippi	52.9
42	Missouri	59.0
10	Montana	67.4
40	Nebraska	59.9
2	Nevada	71.8
20	New Hampshire	65.0
31	New Jersey	62.9
11	New Mexico	67.3
39	New York	60.0
35	North Carolina	61.7
44	North Dakota	58.0
38	Ohio	60.2
16	Oklahoma	65.9
15	Oregon	66.2
17	Pennsylvania	65.7
29	Rhode Island	63.0
47	South Carolina	54.4
19	South Dakota	65.2
32	Tennessee	62.7
37	Texas	60.9
29	Utah	63.0
1	Vermont	73.6
48	Virginia	54.2
25	Washington	64.6
13	West Virginia	66.8
24	Wisconsin	64.7
9	Wyoming	67.8

RANK ORDER

RANK	STATE	PERCENT
1	Vermont	73.6
2	Nevada	71.8
3	Colorado	69.3
3	Maine	69.3
5	California	68.9
6	Idaho	68.7
6	Minnesota	68.7
8	Indiana	68.4
9	Wyoming	67.8
10	Montana	67.4
11	Iowa	67.3
11	New Mexico	67.3
13	West Virginia	66.8
14	Illinois	66.4
15	Oregon	66.2
16	Oklahoma	65.9
17	Pennsylvania	65.7
18	Michigan	65.5
19	South Dakota	65.2
20	Arkansas	65.0
20	New Hampshire	65.0
22	Arizona	64.9
23	Alaska	64.8
24	Wisconsin	64.7
25	Washington	64.6
26	Massachusetts	64.1
27	Connecticut	63.4
28	Alabama	63.3
29	Rhode Island	63.0
29	Utah	63.0
31	New Jersey	62.9
32	Tennessee	62.7
33	Kentucky	62.5
34	Louisiana	62.2
35	North Carolina	61.7
36	Maryland	61.0
37	Texas	60.9
38	Ohio	60.2
39	New York	60.0
40	Nebraska	59.9
41	Kansas	59.2
42	Florida	59.0
42	Missouri	59.0
44	North Dakota	58.0
45	Delaware	57.9
46	Georgia	56.4
47	South Carolina	54.4
48	Virginia	54.2
49	Mississippi	52.9
50	Hawaii	49.8
	District of Columbia	53.7

Source: U.S. Department of Health and Human Services, Centers for Disease Control and Prevention "2000 Behavioral Risk Factor Surveillance Summary Prevalence Report" (May 3, 2001)
Persons 18 to 64 years old. Does not include HIV testing for blood donations.

Number of Days in Past Month When Physical Health was "Not Good": 2000

National Median = 3.3 Days*

ALPHA ORDER			RANK ORDER		
RANK	STATE	DAYS	RANK	STATE	DAYS
4	Alabama	3.9	1	West Virginia	5.2
43	Alaska	2.8	2	Arkansas	4.1
20	Arizona	3.3	3	Kentucky	4.0
2	Arkansas	4.1	4	Alabama	3.9
11	California	3.5	5	North Carolina	3.7
20	Colorado	3.3	5	Oregon	3.7
28	Connecticut	3.2	7	Nevada	3.6
20	Delaware	3.3	7	New York	3.6
17	Florida	3.4	7	Rhode Island	3.6
28	Georgia	3.2	7	Wisconsin	3.6
49	Hawaii	2.6	11	California	3.5
28	Idaho	3.2	11	Indiana	3.5
39	Illinois	3.0	11	Maine	3.5
11	Indiana	3.5	11	Mississippi	3.5
41	Iowa	2.9	11	New Mexico	3.5
41	Kansas	2.9	11	Utah	3.5
3	Kentucky	4.0	17	Florida	3.4
28	Louisiana	3.2	17	Massachusetts	3.4
11	Maine	3.5	17	Texas	3.4
20	Maryland	3.3	20	Arizona	3.3
17	Massachusetts	3.4	20	Colorado	3.3
20	Michigan	3.3	20	Delaware	3.3
49	Minnesota	2.6	20	Maryland	3.3
11	Mississippi	3.5	20	Michigan	3.3
28	Missouri	3.2	20	Ohio	3.3
45	Montana	2.7	20	South Carolina	3.3
45	Nebraska	2.7	20	Tennessee	3.3
7	Nevada	3.6	28	Connecticut	3.2
35	New Hampshire	3.1	28	Georgia	3.2
35	New Jersey	3.1	28	Idaho	3.2
11	New Mexico	3.5	28	Louisiana	3.2
7	New York	3.6	28	Missouri	3.2
5	North Carolina	3.7	28	Pennsylvania	3.2
45	North Dakota	2.7	28	Washington	3.2
20	Ohio	3.3	35	New Hampshire	3.1
35	Oklahoma	3.1	35	New Jersey	3.1
5	Oregon	3.7	35	Oklahoma	3.1
28	Pennsylvania	3.2	35	Vermont	3.1
7	Rhode Island	3.6	39	Illinois	3.0
20	South Carolina	3.3	39	Wyoming	3.0
43	South Dakota	2.8	41	Iowa	2.9
20	Tennessee	3.3	41	Kansas	2.9
17	Texas	3.4	43	Alaska	2.8
11	Utah	3.5	43	South Dakota	2.8
35	Vermont	3.1	45	Montana	2.7
45	Virginia	2.7	45	Nebraska	2.7
28	Washington	3.2	45	North Dakota	2.7
1	West Virginia	5.2	45	Virginia	2.7
7	Wisconsin	3.6	49	Hawaii	2.6
39	Wyoming	3.0	49	Minnesota	2.6
				District of Columbia	3.2

Source: U.S. Department of Health and Human Services, Centers for Disease Control and Prevention
"2000 Behavioral Risk Factor Surveillance Summary Prevalence Report" (May 3, 2001)
*Persons 18 and older.

Number of Days in Past Month When Mental Health was "Not Good": 2000

National Median = 3.2 Days*

ALPHA ORDER				RANK ORDER		
RANK	STATE	DAYS		RANK	STATE	DAYS
9	Alabama	3.4		1	Kentucky	4.4
37	Alaska	2.8		2	West Virginia	4.1
40	Arizona	2.7		3	Oregon	3.7
17	Arkansas	3.3		3	Wisconsin	3.7
21	California	3.2		5	Michigan	3.6
29	Colorado	3.1		5	Mississippi	3.6
34	Connecticut	2.9		5	Texas	3.6
29	Delaware	3.1		8	New Mexico	3.5
21	Florida	3.2		9	Alabama	3.4
9	Georgia	3.4		9	Georgia	3.4
48	Hawaii	2.3		9	Idaho	3.4
9	Idaho	3.4		9	Indiana	3.4
37	Illinois	2.8		9	Nevada	3.4
9	Indiana	3.4		9	Ohio	3.4
45	Iowa	2.5		9	Rhode Island	3.4
37	Kansas	2.8		9	Utah	3.4
1	Kentucky	4.4		17	Arkansas	3.3
33	Louisiana	3.0		17	Massachusetts	3.3
21	Maine	3.2		17	Virginia	3.3
29	Maryland	3.1		17	Wyoming	3.3
17	Massachusetts	3.3		21	California	3.2
5	Michigan	3.6		21	Florida	3.2
40	Minnesota	2.7		21	Maine	3.2
5	Mississippi	3.6		21	Missouri	3.2
21	Missouri	3.2		21	New Jersey	3.2
48	Montana	2.3		21	New York	3.2
47	Nebraska	2.4		21	Pennsylvania	3.2
9	Nevada	3.4		21	Washington	3.2
45	New Hampshire	2.5		29	Colorado	3.1
21	New Jersey	3.2		29	Delaware	3.1
8	New Mexico	3.5		29	Maryland	3.1
21	New York	3.2		29	South Carolina	3.1
34	North Carolina	2.9		33	Louisiana	3.0
43	North Dakota	2.6		34	Connecticut	2.9
9	Ohio	3.4		34	North Carolina	2.9
50	Oklahoma	2.2		34	Vermont	2.9
3	Oregon	3.7		37	Alaska	2.8
21	Pennsylvania	3.2		37	Illinois	2.8
9	Rhode Island	3.4		37	Kansas	2.8
29	South Carolina	3.1		40	Arizona	2.7
43	South Dakota	2.6		40	Minnesota	2.7
40	Tennessee	2.7		40	Tennessee	2.7
5	Texas	3.6		43	North Dakota	2.6
9	Utah	3.4		43	South Dakota	2.6
34	Vermont	2.9		45	Iowa	2.5
17	Virginia	3.3		45	New Hampshire	2.5
21	Washington	3.2		47	Nebraska	2.4
2	West Virginia	4.1		48	Hawaii	2.3
3	Wisconsin	3.7		48	Montana	2.3
17	Wyoming	3.3		50	Oklahoma	2.2
					District of Columbia	3.5

Source: U.S. Department of Health and Human Services, Centers for Disease Control and Prevention
"2000 Behavioral Risk Factor Surveillance Summary Prevalence Report" (May 3, 2001)
*Persons 18 and older.

Percent of Population Who are Illicit Drug Users: 1999

National Percent = 6.9% of Population*

<table>
<tr><td colspan="3">ALPHA ORDER</td><td colspan="3">RANK ORDER</td></tr>
<tr><td>RANK</td><td>STATE</td><td>PERCENT</td><td>RANK</td><td>STATE</td><td>PERCENT</td></tr>
<tr><td>46</td><td>Alabama</td><td>5.1</td><td>1</td><td>Alaska</td><td>10.7</td></tr>
<tr><td>1</td><td>Alaska</td><td>10.7</td><td>2</td><td>Massachusetts</td><td>10.1</td></tr>
<tr><td>17</td><td>Arizona</td><td>7.1</td><td>3</td><td>Nevada</td><td>9.6</td></tr>
<tr><td>49</td><td>Arkansas</td><td>5.0</td><td>4</td><td>Colorado</td><td>9.3</td></tr>
<tr><td>9</td><td>California</td><td>8.3</td><td>5</td><td>New Mexico</td><td>8.9</td></tr>
<tr><td>4</td><td>Colorado</td><td>9.3</td><td>6</td><td>Rhode Island</td><td>8.7</td></tr>
<tr><td>11</td><td>Connecticut</td><td>7.7</td><td>7</td><td>Delaware</td><td>8.5</td></tr>
<tr><td>7</td><td>Delaware</td><td>8.5</td><td>8</td><td>Washington</td><td>8.4</td></tr>
<tr><td>25</td><td>Florida</td><td>6.8</td><td>9</td><td>California</td><td>8.3</td></tr>
<tr><td>36</td><td>Georgia</td><td>5.8</td><td>10</td><td>Michigan</td><td>8.0</td></tr>
<tr><td>17</td><td>Hawaii</td><td>7.1</td><td>11</td><td>Connecticut</td><td>7.7</td></tr>
<tr><td>30</td><td>Idaho</td><td>6.4</td><td>11</td><td>Montana</td><td>7.7</td></tr>
<tr><td>24</td><td>Illinois</td><td>6.9</td><td>11</td><td>New Jersey</td><td>7.7</td></tr>
<tr><td>15</td><td>Indiana</td><td>7.5</td><td>11</td><td>Oregon</td><td>7.7</td></tr>
<tr><td>40</td><td>Iowa</td><td>5.5</td><td>15</td><td>Indiana</td><td>7.5</td></tr>
<tr><td>35</td><td>Kansas</td><td>5.9</td><td>16</td><td>Wyoming</td><td>7.3</td></tr>
<tr><td>33</td><td>Kentucky</td><td>6.0</td><td>17</td><td>Arizona</td><td>7.1</td></tr>
<tr><td>38</td><td>Louisiana</td><td>5.7</td><td>17</td><td>Hawaii</td><td>7.1</td></tr>
<tr><td>17</td><td>Maine</td><td>7.1</td><td>17</td><td>Maine</td><td>7.1</td></tr>
<tr><td>45</td><td>Maryland</td><td>5.3</td><td>20</td><td>New Hampshire</td><td>7.0</td></tr>
<tr><td>2</td><td>Massachusetts</td><td>10.1</td><td>20</td><td>New York</td><td>7.0</td></tr>
<tr><td>10</td><td>Michigan</td><td>8.0</td><td>20</td><td>Pennsylvania</td><td>7.0</td></tr>
<tr><td>27</td><td>Minnesota</td><td>6.7</td><td>20</td><td>Wisconsin</td><td>7.0</td></tr>
<tr><td>36</td><td>Mississippi</td><td>5.8</td><td>24</td><td>Illinois</td><td>6.9</td></tr>
<tr><td>28</td><td>Missouri</td><td>6.6</td><td>25</td><td>Florida</td><td>6.8</td></tr>
<tr><td>11</td><td>Montana</td><td>7.7</td><td>25</td><td>Vermont</td><td>6.8</td></tr>
<tr><td>39</td><td>Nebraska</td><td>5.6</td><td>27</td><td>Minnesota</td><td>6.7</td></tr>
<tr><td>3</td><td>Nevada</td><td>9.6</td><td>28</td><td>Missouri</td><td>6.6</td></tr>
<tr><td>20</td><td>New Hampshire</td><td>7.0</td><td>29</td><td>Ohio</td><td>6.5</td></tr>
<tr><td>11</td><td>New Jersey</td><td>7.7</td><td>30</td><td>Idaho</td><td>6.4</td></tr>
<tr><td>5</td><td>New Mexico</td><td>8.9</td><td>31</td><td>North Carolina</td><td>6.3</td></tr>
<tr><td>20</td><td>New York</td><td>7.0</td><td>32</td><td>Utah</td><td>6.2</td></tr>
<tr><td>31</td><td>North Carolina</td><td>6.3</td><td>33</td><td>Kentucky</td><td>6.0</td></tr>
<tr><td>42</td><td>North Dakota</td><td>5.4</td><td>33</td><td>South Dakota</td><td>6.0</td></tr>
<tr><td>29</td><td>Ohio</td><td>6.5</td><td>35</td><td>Kansas</td><td>5.9</td></tr>
<tr><td>46</td><td>Oklahoma</td><td>5.1</td><td>36</td><td>Georgia</td><td>5.8</td></tr>
<tr><td>11</td><td>Oregon</td><td>7.7</td><td>36</td><td>Mississippi</td><td>5.8</td></tr>
<tr><td>20</td><td>Pennsylvania</td><td>7.0</td><td>38</td><td>Louisiana</td><td>5.7</td></tr>
<tr><td>6</td><td>Rhode Island</td><td>8.7</td><td>39</td><td>Nebraska</td><td>5.6</td></tr>
<tr><td>42</td><td>South Carolina</td><td>5.4</td><td>40</td><td>Iowa</td><td>5.5</td></tr>
<tr><td>33</td><td>South Dakota</td><td>6.0</td><td>40</td><td>Tennessee</td><td>5.5</td></tr>
<tr><td>40</td><td>Tennessee</td><td>5.5</td><td>42</td><td>North Dakota</td><td>5.4</td></tr>
<tr><td>42</td><td>Texas</td><td>5.4</td><td>42</td><td>South Carolina</td><td>5.4</td></tr>
<tr><td>32</td><td>Utah</td><td>6.2</td><td>42</td><td>Texas</td><td>5.4</td></tr>
<tr><td>25</td><td>Vermont</td><td>6.8</td><td>45</td><td>Maryland</td><td>5.3</td></tr>
<tr><td>50</td><td>Virginia</td><td>4.7</td><td>46</td><td>Alabama</td><td>5.1</td></tr>
<tr><td>8</td><td>Washington</td><td>8.4</td><td>46</td><td>Oklahoma</td><td>5.1</td></tr>
<tr><td>46</td><td>West Virginia</td><td>5.1</td><td>46</td><td>West Virginia</td><td>5.1</td></tr>
<tr><td>20</td><td>Wisconsin</td><td>7.0</td><td>49</td><td>Arkansas</td><td>5.0</td></tr>
<tr><td>16</td><td>Wyoming</td><td>7.3</td><td>50</td><td>Virginia</td><td>4.7</td></tr>
<tr><td></td><td></td><td></td><td></td><td>District of Columbia</td><td>7.6</td></tr>
</table>

Source: U.S. Department of Health and Human Services, Substance Abuse and Mental Health Services Administration
   "National Household Survey on Drug Abuse, 1999"
*Population 12 years old and over who used any illicit drug at least once within month of survey.

Safety Belt Usage Rate in 2000

National Rate = 71.0% Use Safety Belts*

ALPHA ORDER				RANK ORDER		
RANK	STATE	PERCENT		RANK	STATE	PERCENT
22	Alabama	70.6		1	California	88.9
39	Alaska	61.0		2	New Mexico	86.6
16	Arizona	75.2		3	Maryland	85.0
45	Arkansas	52.4		4	Oregon	83.6
1	California	88.9		5	Michigan	83.5
33	Colorado	65.1		6	Washington	81.6
13	Connecticut	76.3		7	North Carolina	80.5
30	Delaware	66.1		8	Hawaii	80.4
34	Florida	64.8		9	Nevada	78.5
19	Georgia	73.6		10	Iowa	78.0
8	Hawaii	80.4		11	New York	77.3
43	Idaho	58.6		12	Texas	76.6
24	Illinois	70.2		13	Connecticut	76.3
36	Indiana	62.1		14	Utah	75.7
10	Iowa	78.0		15	Montana	75.6
37	Kansas	61.6		16	Arizona	75.2
41	Kentucky	60.0		17	New Jersey	74.2
26	Louisiana	68.2		18	South Carolina	73.9
40	Maine	60.4		19	Georgia	73.6
3	Maryland	85.0		20	Minnesota	73.4
47	Massachusetts	50.0		21	Pennsylvania	70.7
5	Michigan	83.5		22	Alabama	70.6
20	Minnesota	73.4		23	Nebraska	70.5
46	Mississippi	50.4		24	Illinois	70.2
27	Missouri	67.7		25	Virginia	69.9
15	Montana	75.6		26	Louisiana	68.2
23	Nebraska	70.5		27	Missouri	67.7
9	Nevada	78.5		28	Oklahoma	67.5
49	New Hampshire	48.2		29	Wyoming	66.8
17	New Jersey	74.2		30	Delaware	66.1
2	New Mexico	86.6		31	Wisconsin	65.4
11	New York	77.3		32	Ohio	65.3
7	North Carolina	80.5		33	Colorado	65.1
50	North Dakota	47.7		34	Florida	64.8
32	Ohio	65.3		35	Rhode Island	64.4
28	Oklahoma	67.5		36	Indiana	62.1
4	Oregon	83.6		37	Kansas	61.6
21	Pennsylvania	70.7		37	Vermont	61.6
35	Rhode Island	64.4		39	Alaska	61.0
18	South Carolina	73.9		40	Maine	60.4
44	South Dakota	53.4		41	Kentucky	60.0
42	Tennessee	59.0		42	Tennessee	59.0
12	Texas	76.6		43	Idaho	58.6
14	Utah	75.7		44	South Dakota	53.4
37	Vermont	61.6		45	Arkansas	52.4
25	Virginia	69.9		46	Mississippi	50.4
6	Washington	81.6		47	Massachusetts	50.0
48	West Virginia	49.5		48	West Virginia	49.5
31	Wisconsin	65.4		49	New Hampshire	48.2
29	Wyoming	66.8		50	North Dakota	47.7
					District of Columbia	82.6

Source: U.S. Department of Transportation, National Highway Traffic Safety Administration
"Traffic Safety Facts 2000" (http://www-nrd.nhtsa.dot.gov/pdf/nrd-30/ncsa/tsf2000/2000stdfacts.pdf)
*As of December 2000.

VIII. APPENDIX

Population Charts

A-1   Population in 2001
A-2   Population in 2000 Census
A-3   Male Population in 2000
A-4   Female Population in 2000
A-5   Population in 1998

Population in 2001

National Total = 284,796,887*

RANK	STATE	POPULATION	% of USA
23	Alabama	4,464,356	1.6%
47	Alaska	634,892	0.2%
20	Arizona	5,307,331	1.9%
33	Arkansas	2,692,090	0.9%
1	California	34,501,130	12.1%
24	Colorado	4,417,714	1.6%
29	Connecticut	3,425,074	1.2%
45	Delaware	796,165	0.3%
4	Florida	16,396,515	5.8%
10	Georgia	8,383,915	2.9%
42	Hawaii	1,224,398	0.4%
39	Idaho	1,321,006	0.5%
5	Illinois	12,482,301	4.4%
14	Indiana	6,114,745	2.1%
30	Iowa	2,923,179	1.0%
32	Kansas	2,694,641	0.9%
25	Kentucky	4,065,556	1.4%
22	Louisiana	4,465,430	1.6%
40	Maine	1,286,670	0.5%
19	Maryland	5,375,156	1.9%
13	Massachusetts	6,379,304	2.2%
8	Michigan	9,990,817	3.5%
21	Minnesota	4,972,294	1.7%
31	Mississippi	2,858,029	1.0%
17	Missouri	5,629,707	2.0%
44	Montana	904,433	0.3%
38	Nebraska	1,713,235	0.6%
35	Nevada	2,106,074	0.7%
41	New Hampshire	1,259,181	0.4%
9	New Jersey	8,484,431	3.0%
36	New Mexico	1,829,146	0.6%
3	New York	19,011,378	6.7%
11	North Carolina	8,186,268	2.9%
48	North Dakota	634,448	0.2%
7	Ohio	11,373,541	4.0%
28	Oklahoma	3,460,097	1.2%
27	Oregon	3,472,867	1.2%
6	Pennsylvania	12,287,150	4.3%
43	Rhode Island	1,058,920	0.4%
26	South Carolina	4,063,011	1.4%
46	South Dakota	756,600	0.3%
16	Tennessee	5,740,021	2.0%
2	Texas	21,325,018	7.5%
34	Utah	2,269,789	0.8%
49	Vermont	613,090	0.2%
12	Virginia	7,187,734	2.5%
15	Washington	5,987,973	2.1%
37	West Virginia	1,801,916	0.6%
18	Wisconsin	5,401,906	1.9%
50	Wyoming	494,423	0.2%

RANK	STATE	POPULATION	% of USA
1	California	34,501,130	12.1%
2	Texas	21,325,018	7.5%
3	New York	19,011,378	6.7%
4	Florida	16,396,515	5.8%
5	Illinois	12,482,301	4.4%
6	Pennsylvania	12,287,150	4.3%
7	Ohio	11,373,541	4.0%
8	Michigan	9,990,817	3.5%
9	New Jersey	8,484,431	3.0%
10	Georgia	8,383,915	2.9%
11	North Carolina	8,186,268	2.9%
12	Virginia	7,187,734	2.5%
13	Massachusetts	6,379,304	2.2%
14	Indiana	6,114,745	2.1%
15	Washington	5,987,973	2.1%
16	Tennessee	5,740,021	2.0%
17	Missouri	5,629,707	2.0%
18	Wisconsin	5,401,906	1.9%
19	Maryland	5,375,156	1.9%
20	Arizona	5,307,331	1.9%
21	Minnesota	4,972,294	1.7%
22	Louisiana	4,465,430	1.6%
23	Alabama	4,464,356	1.6%
24	Colorado	4,417,714	1.6%
25	Kentucky	4,065,556	1.4%
26	South Carolina	4,063,011	1.4%
27	Oregon	3,472,867	1.2%
28	Oklahoma	3,460,097	1.2%
29	Connecticut	3,425,074	1.2%
30	Iowa	2,923,179	1.0%
31	Mississippi	2,858,029	1.0%
32	Kansas	2,694,641	0.9%
33	Arkansas	2,692,090	0.9%
34	Utah	2,269,789	0.8%
35	Nevada	2,106,074	0.7%
36	New Mexico	1,829,146	0.6%
37	West Virginia	1,801,916	0.6%
38	Nebraska	1,713,235	0.6%
39	Idaho	1,321,006	0.5%
40	Maine	1,286,670	0.5%
41	New Hampshire	1,259,181	0.4%
42	Hawaii	1,224,398	0.4%
43	Rhode Island	1,058,920	0.4%
44	Montana	904,433	0.3%
45	Delaware	796,165	0.3%
46	South Dakota	756,600	0.3%
47	Alaska	634,892	0.2%
48	North Dakota	634,448	0.2%
49	Vermont	613,090	0.2%
50	Wyoming	494,423	0.2%
	District of Columbia	571,822	0.2%

Source: U.S. Bureau of the Census
    "States" (December 27, 2001, http://eire.census.gov/popest/data/states.php)
*Resident population.

Population in 2000 Census

National Total = 281,421,906*

ALPHA ORDER

RANK	STATE	POPULATION	% of USA
23	Alabama	4,447,100	1.6%
48	Alaska	626,932	0.2%
20	Arizona	5,130,632	1.8%
33	Arkansas	2,673,400	0.9%
1	California	33,871,648	12.0%
24	Colorado	4,301,261	1.5%
29	Connecticut	3,405,565	1.2%
45	Delaware	783,600	0.3%
4	Florida	15,982,378	5.7%
10	Georgia	8,186,453	2.9%
42	Hawaii	1,211,537	0.4%
39	Idaho	1,293,953	0.5%
5	Illinois	12,419,293	4.4%
14	Indiana	6,080,485	2.2%
30	Iowa	2,926,324	1.0%
32	Kansas	2,688,418	1.0%
25	Kentucky	4,041,769	1.4%
22	Louisiana	4,468,976	1.6%
40	Maine	1,274,923	0.5%
19	Maryland	5,296,486	1.9%
13	Massachusetts	6,349,097	2.3%
8	Michigan	9,938,444	3.5%
21	Minnesota	4,919,479	1.7%
31	Mississippi	2,844,658	1.0%
17	Missouri	5,595,211	2.0%
44	Montana	902,195	0.3%
38	Nebraska	1,711,263	0.6%
35	Nevada	1,998,257	0.7%
41	New Hampshire	1,235,786	0.4%
9	New Jersey	8,414,350	3.0%
36	New Mexico	1,819,046	0.6%
3	New York	18,976,457	6.7%
11	North Carolina	8,049,313	2.9%
47	North Dakota	642,200	0.2%
7	Ohio	11,353,140	4.0%
27	Oklahoma	3,450,654	1.2%
28	Oregon	3,421,399	1.2%
6	Pennsylvania	12,281,054	4.4%
43	Rhode Island	1,048,319	0.4%
26	South Carolina	4,012,012	1.4%
46	South Dakota	754,844	0.3%
16	Tennessee	5,689,283	2.0%
2	Texas	20,851,820	7.4%
34	Utah	2,233,169	0.8%
49	Vermont	608,827	0.2%
12	Virginia	7,078,515	2.5%
15	Washington	5,894,121	2.1%
37	West Virginia	1,808,344	0.6%
18	Wisconsin	5,363,675	1.9%
50	Wyoming	493,782	0.2%

RANK ORDER

RANK	STATE	POPULATION	% of USA
1	California	33,871,648	12.0%
2	Texas	20,851,820	7.4%
3	New York	18,976,457	6.7%
4	Florida	15,982,378	5.7%
5	Illinois	12,419,293	4.4%
6	Pennsylvania	12,281,054	4.4%
7	Ohio	11,353,140	4.0%
8	Michigan	9,938,444	3.5%
9	New Jersey	8,414,350	3.0%
10	Georgia	8,186,453	2.9%
11	North Carolina	8,049,313	2.9%
12	Virginia	7,078,515	2.5%
13	Massachusetts	6,349,097	2.3%
14	Indiana	6,080,485	2.2%
15	Washington	5,894,121	2.1%
16	Tennessee	5,689,283	2.0%
17	Missouri	5,595,211	2.0%
18	Wisconsin	5,363,675	1.9%
19	Maryland	5,296,486	1.9%
20	Arizona	5,130,632	1.8%
21	Minnesota	4,919,479	1.7%
22	Louisiana	4,468,976	1.6%
23	Alabama	4,447,100	1.6%
24	Colorado	4,301,261	1.5%
25	Kentucky	4,041,769	1.4%
26	South Carolina	4,012,012	1.4%
27	Oklahoma	3,450,654	1.2%
28	Oregon	3,421,399	1.2%
29	Connecticut	3,405,565	1.2%
30	Iowa	2,926,324	1.0%
31	Mississippi	2,844,658	1.0%
32	Kansas	2,688,418	1.0%
33	Arkansas	2,673,400	0.9%
34	Utah	2,233,169	0.8%
35	Nevada	1,998,257	0.7%
36	New Mexico	1,819,046	0.6%
37	West Virginia	1,808,344	0.6%
38	Nebraska	1,711,263	0.6%
39	Idaho	1,293,953	0.5%
40	Maine	1,274,923	0.5%
41	New Hampshire	1,235,786	0.4%
42	Hawaii	1,211,537	0.4%
43	Rhode Island	1,048,319	0.4%
44	Montana	902,195	0.3%
45	Delaware	783,600	0.3%
46	South Dakota	754,844	0.3%
47	North Dakota	642,200	0.2%
48	Alaska	626,932	0.2%
49	Vermont	608,827	0.2%
50	Wyoming	493,782	0.2%
	District of Columbia	572,059	0.2%

Source: U.S. Bureau of the Census
"First Census 2000 Results" (December 28, 2000, http://www.census.gov/main/www/cen2000.html)
*Resident population as of April 2000 Census.

Male Population in 2000

National Total = 138,053,563 Males

ALPHA ORDER

RANK	STATE	MALES	% of USA
24	Alabama	2,146,504	1.6%
47	Alaska	324,112	0.2%
19	Arizona	2,561,057	1.9%
33	Arkansas	1,304,693	0.9%
1	California	16,874,892	12.2%
22	Colorado	2,165,983	1.6%
29	Connecticut	1,649,319	1.2%
45	Delaware	380,541	0.3%
4	Florida	7,797,715	5.6%
10	Georgia	4,027,113	2.9%
41	Hawaii	608,671	0.4%
39	Idaho	648,660	0.5%
5	Illinois	6,080,336	4.4%
14	Indiana	2,982,474	2.2%
30	Iowa	1,435,515	1.0%
32	Kansas	1,328,474	1.0%
25	Kentucky	1,975,368	1.4%
23	Louisiana	2,162,903	1.6%
40	Maine	620,309	0.4%
20	Maryland	2,557,794	1.9%
13	Massachusetts	3,058,816	2.2%
8	Michigan	4,873,095	3.5%
21	Minnesota	2,435,631	1.8%
31	Mississippi	1,373,554	1.0%
17	Missouri	2,720,177	2.0%
44	Montana	449,480	0.3%
38	Nebraska	843,351	0.6%
35	Nevada	1,018,051	0.7%
42	New Hampshire	607,687	0.4%
9	New Jersey	4,082,813	3.0%
36	New Mexico	894,317	0.6%
3	New York	9,146,748	6.6%
11	North Carolina	3,942,695	2.9%
48	North Dakota	320,524	0.2%
7	Ohio	5,512,262	4.0%
28	Oklahoma	1,695,895	1.2%
27	Oregon	1,696,550	1.2%
6	Pennsylvania	5,929,663	4.3%
43	Rhode Island	503,635	0.4%
26	South Carolina	1,948,929	1.4%
46	South Dakota	374,558	0.3%
16	Tennessee	2,770,275	2.0%
2	Texas	10,352,910	7.5%
34	Utah	1,119,031	0.8%
49	Vermont	298,337	0.2%
12	Virginia	3,471,895	2.5%
15	Washington	2,934,300	2.1%
37	West Virginia	879,170	0.6%
18	Wisconsin	2,649,041	1.9%
50	Wyoming	248,374	0.2%

RANK ORDER

RANK	STATE	MALES	% of USA
1	California	16,874,892	12.2%
2	Texas	10,352,910	7.5%
3	New York	9,146,748	6.6%
4	Florida	7,797,715	5.6%
5	Illinois	6,080,336	4.4%
6	Pennsylvania	5,929,663	4.3%
7	Ohio	5,512,262	4.0%
8	Michigan	4,873,095	3.5%
9	New Jersey	4,082,813	3.0%
10	Georgia	4,027,113	2.9%
11	North Carolina	3,942,695	2.9%
12	Virginia	3,471,895	2.5%
13	Massachusetts	3,058,816	2.2%
14	Indiana	2,982,474	2.2%
15	Washington	2,934,300	2.1%
16	Tennessee	2,770,275	2.0%
17	Missouri	2,720,177	2.0%
18	Wisconsin	2,649,041	1.9%
19	Arizona	2,561,057	1.9%
20	Maryland	2,557,794	1.9%
21	Minnesota	2,435,631	1.8%
22	Colorado	2,165,983	1.6%
23	Louisiana	2,162,903	1.6%
24	Alabama	2,146,504	1.6%
25	Kentucky	1,975,368	1.4%
26	South Carolina	1,948,929	1.4%
27	Oregon	1,696,550	1.2%
28	Oklahoma	1,695,895	1.2%
29	Connecticut	1,649,319	1.2%
30	Iowa	1,435,515	1.0%
31	Mississippi	1,373,554	1.0%
32	Kansas	1,328,474	1.0%
33	Arkansas	1,304,693	0.9%
34	Utah	1,119,031	0.8%
35	Nevada	1,018,051	0.7%
36	New Mexico	894,317	0.6%
37	West Virginia	879,170	0.6%
38	Nebraska	843,351	0.6%
39	Idaho	648,660	0.5%
40	Maine	620,309	0.4%
41	Hawaii	608,671	0.4%
42	New Hampshire	607,687	0.4%
43	Rhode Island	503,635	0.4%
44	Montana	449,480	0.3%
45	Delaware	380,541	0.3%
46	South Dakota	374,558	0.3%
47	Alaska	324,112	0.2%
48	North Dakota	320,524	0.2%
49	Vermont	298,337	0.2%
50	Wyoming	248,374	0.2%
	District of Columbia	269,366	0.2%

Source: U.S. Bureau of the Census
"Census 2000 Summary File 1"

Female Population in 2000

National Total = 143,368,343 Females

ALPHA ORDER

RANK	STATE	FEMALES	% of USA
23	Alabama	2,300,596	1.6%
49	Alaska	302,820	0.2%
20	Arizona	2,569,575	1.8%
32	Arkansas	1,368,707	1.0%
1	California	16,996,756	11.9%
24	Colorado	2,135,278	1.5%
27	Connecticut	1,756,246	1.2%
45	Delaware	403,059	0.3%
4	Florida	8,184,663	5.7%
10	Georgia	4,159,340	2.9%
42	Hawaii	602,866	0.4%
40	Idaho	645,293	0.5%
6	Illinois	6,338,957	4.4%
14	Indiana	3,098,011	2.2%
30	Iowa	1,490,809	1.0%
33	Kansas	1,359,944	0.9%
25	Kentucky	2,066,401	1.4%
22	Louisiana	2,306,073	1.6%
39	Maine	654,614	0.5%
18	Maryland	2,738,692	1.9%
13	Massachusetts	3,290,281	2.3%
8	Michigan	5,065,349	3.5%
21	Minnesota	2,483,848	1.7%
31	Mississippi	1,471,104	1.0%
17	Missouri	2,875,034	2.0%
44	Montana	452,715	0.3%
38	Nebraska	867,912	0.6%
35	Nevada	980,206	0.7%
41	New Hampshire	628,099	0.4%
9	New Jersey	4,331,537	3.0%
37	New Mexico	924,729	0.6%
3	New York	9,829,709	6.9%
11	North Carolina	4,106,618	2.9%
47	North Dakota	321,676	0.2%
7	Ohio	5,840,878	4.1%
28	Oklahoma	1,754,759	1.2%
29	Oregon	1,724,849	1.2%
5	Pennsylvania	6,351,391	4.4%
43	Rhode Island	544,684	0.4%
26	South Carolina	2,063,083	1.4%
46	South Dakota	380,286	0.3%
16	Tennessee	2,919,008	2.0%
2	Texas	10,498,910	7.3%
34	Utah	1,114,138	0.8%
48	Vermont	310,490	0.2%
12	Virginia	3,606,620	2.5%
15	Washington	2,959,821	2.1%
36	West Virginia	929,174	0.6%
19	Wisconsin	2,714,634	1.9%
50	Wyoming	245,408	0.2%

RANK ORDER

RANK	STATE	FEMALES	% of USA
1	California	16,996,756	11.9%
2	Texas	10,498,910	7.3%
3	New York	9,829,709	6.9%
4	Florida	8,184,663	5.7%
5	Pennsylvania	6,351,391	4.4%
6	Illinois	6,338,957	4.4%
7	Ohio	5,840,878	4.1%
8	Michigan	5,065,349	3.5%
9	New Jersey	4,331,537	3.0%
10	Georgia	4,159,340	2.9%
11	North Carolina	4,106,618	2.9%
12	Virginia	3,606,620	2.5%
13	Massachusetts	3,290,281	2.3%
14	Indiana	3,098,011	2.2%
15	Washington	2,959,821	2.1%
16	Tennessee	2,919,008	2.0%
17	Missouri	2,875,034	2.0%
18	Maryland	2,738,692	1.9%
19	Wisconsin	2,714,634	1.9%
20	Arizona	2,569,575	1.8%
21	Minnesota	2,483,848	1.7%
22	Louisiana	2,306,073	1.6%
23	Alabama	2,300,596	1.6%
24	Colorado	2,135,278	1.5%
25	Kentucky	2,066,401	1.4%
26	South Carolina	2,063,083	1.4%
27	Connecticut	1,756,246	1.2%
28	Oklahoma	1,754,759	1.2%
29	Oregon	1,724,849	1.2%
30	Iowa	1,490,809	1.0%
31	Mississippi	1,471,104	1.0%
32	Arkansas	1,368,707	1.0%
33	Kansas	1,359,944	0.9%
34	Utah	1,114,138	0.8%
35	Nevada	980,206	0.7%
36	West Virginia	929,174	0.6%
37	New Mexico	924,729	0.6%
38	Nebraska	867,912	0.6%
39	Maine	654,614	0.5%
40	Idaho	645,293	0.5%
41	New Hampshire	628,099	0.4%
42	Hawaii	602,866	0.4%
43	Rhode Island	544,684	0.4%
44	Montana	452,715	0.3%
45	Delaware	403,059	0.3%
46	South Dakota	380,286	0.3%
47	North Dakota	321,676	0.2%
48	Vermont	310,490	0.2%
49	Alaska	302,820	0.2%
50	Wyoming	245,408	0.2%
	District of Columbia	302,693	0.2%

Source: U.S. Bureau of the Census
"Census 2000 Summary File 1"

Population in 1998

National Total = 270,248,003*

RANK	STATE	POPULATION	% of USA	RANK	STATE	POPULATION	% of USA
23	Alabama	4,351,037	1.6%	1	California	32,682,794	12.1%
48	Alaska	615,205	0.2%	2	Texas	19,712,389	7.3%
21	Arizona	4,667,277	1.7%	3	New York	18,159,175	6.7%
33	Arkansas	2,538,202	0.9%	4	Florida	14,908,230	5.5%
1	California	32,682,794	12.1%	5	Illinois	12,069,774	4.5%
24	Colorado	3,968,967	1.5%	6	Pennsylvania	12,002,329	4.4%
29	Connecticut	3,272,563	1.2%	7	Ohio	11,237,752	4.2%
45	Delaware	744,066	0.3%	8	Michigan	9,820,231	3.6%
4	Florida	14,908,230	5.5%	9	New Jersey	8,095,542	3.0%
10	Georgia	7,636,522	2.8%	10	Georgia	7,636,522	2.8%
41	Hawaii	1,190,472	0.4%	11	North Carolina	7,545,828	2.8%
40	Idaho	1,230,923	0.5%	12	Virginia	6,789,225	2.5%
5	Illinois	12,069,774	4.5%	13	Massachusetts	6,144,407	2.3%
14	Indiana	5,907,617	2.2%	14	Indiana	5,907,617	2.2%
30	Iowa	2,861,025	1.1%	15	Washington	5,687,832	2.1%
32	Kansas	2,638,667	1.0%	16	Missouri	5,437,562	2.0%
25	Kentucky	3,934,310	1.5%	17	Tennessee	5,432,679	2.0%
22	Louisiana	4,362,758	1.6%	18	Wisconsin	5,222,124	1.9%
39	Maine	1,247,554	0.5%	19	Maryland	5,130,072	1.9%
19	Maryland	5,130,072	1.9%	20	Minnesota	4,726,411	1.7%
13	Massachusetts	6,144,407	2.3%	21	Arizona	4,667,277	1.7%
8	Michigan	9,820,231	3.6%	22	Louisiana	4,362,758	1.6%
20	Minnesota	4,726,411	1.7%	23	Alabama	4,351,037	1.6%
31	Mississippi	2,751,335	1.0%	24	Colorado	3,968,967	1.5%
16	Missouri	5,437,562	2.0%	25	Kentucky	3,934,310	1.5%
44	Montana	879,533	0.3%	26	South Carolina	3,839,578	1.4%
38	Nebraska	1,660,772	0.6%	27	Oklahoma	3,339,478	1.2%
36	Nevada	1,743,772	0.6%	28	Oregon	3,282,055	1.2%
42	New Hampshire	1,185,823	0.4%	29	Connecticut	3,272,563	1.2%
9	New Jersey	8,095,542	3.0%	30	Iowa	2,861,025	1.1%
37	New Mexico	1,733,535	0.6%	31	Mississippi	2,751,335	1.0%
3	New York	18,159,175	6.7%	32	Kansas	2,638,667	1.0%
11	North Carolina	7,545,828	2.8%	33	Arkansas	2,538,202	0.9%
47	North Dakota	637,808	0.2%	34	Utah	2,100,562	0.8%
7	Ohio	11,237,752	4.2%	35	West Virginia	1,811,688	0.7%
27	Oklahoma	3,339,478	1.2%	36	Nevada	1,743,772	0.6%
28	Oregon	3,282,055	1.2%	37	New Mexico	1,733,535	0.6%
6	Pennsylvania	12,002,329	4.4%	38	Nebraska	1,660,772	0.6%
43	Rhode Island	987,704	0.4%	39	Maine	1,247,554	0.5%
26	South Carolina	3,839,578	1.4%	40	Idaho	1,230,923	0.5%
46	South Dakota	730,789	0.3%	41	Hawaii	1,190,472	0.4%
17	Tennessee	5,432,679	2.0%	42	New Hampshire	1,185,823	0.4%
2	Texas	19,712,389	7.3%	43	Rhode Island	987,704	0.4%
34	Utah	2,100,562	0.8%	44	Montana	879,533	0.3%
49	Vermont	590,579	0.2%	45	Delaware	744,066	0.3%
12	Virginia	6,789,225	2.5%	46	South Dakota	730,789	0.3%
15	Washington	5,687,832	2.1%	47	North Dakota	637,808	0.2%
35	West Virginia	1,811,688	0.7%	48	Alaska	615,205	0.2%
18	Wisconsin	5,222,124	1.9%	49	Vermont	590,579	0.2%
50	Wyoming	480,045	0.2%	50	Wyoming	480,045	0.2%
					District of Columbia	521,426	0.2%

Source: U.S. Bureau of the Census
    "State Population Estimates" (December 29, 1999, http://www.census.gov/population/estimates/state/st-99-3.txt)
*Includes armed forces residing in each state. This updates earlier 1998 population estimates.

IX. SOURCES

American Academy of Physicians Assistants
950 North Washington Street
Alexandria, VA 22314-1552
703-836-2272
Internet: www.aapa.org

American Cancer Society, Inc.
1599 Clifton Road, NE.
Atlanta, GA 30329-4251
800-227-2345
Internet: http://www.cancer.org

American Dental Association
211 E. Chicago Ave.
Chicago, IL 60611
312-440-2500
Internet: www.ada.org

American Hospital Association
One North Franklin
Chicago, IL 60606-3421
312-422-3000
Internet: www.aha.org

American Medical Association
515 North State Street
Chicago, IL 60610
312-464-5000
Internet: http://www.ama-assn.org

American Osteopathic Association
142 East Ontario Street
Chicago, IL 60611
800-621-1773
Internet: www.aoa-net.org

American Podiatric Medical Association
9312 Old Georgetown Road
Bethesda, MD 20814-1698
301-581-9221
Internet: www.apma.org

Bureau of Labor Statistics
Census of Fatal Occupational Injuries
2 Massachusetts Ave., NE
Washington, DC 20212
202-691-6175
Internet: http://stats.bls.gov/oshhome.htm

Census Bureau
4700 Silver Hill Road
Suitland, MD 20746
301-457-2800
Internet: http://www.census.gov

Centers for Disease Control and Prevention
1600 Clifton Road, NE.
Atlanta, GA 30333
404-639-3534 (Public Affairs)
800-458-5231 (AIDS Clearinghouse)
Internet: http://www.cdc.gov

Centers for Medicare and Medicaid Services
(Formerly Health Care Financing Administration)
7500 Security Boulevard
Baltimore, MD 21244
410-786-3000
Internet: http://www.cms.gov

Federation of Chiropractic Licensing Boards
901 54th Ave., Ste. 101
Greeley, CO 80634-4400
970-356-3500
Internet: www.fclb.org

Health Care Financing Administration
See Centers for Medicare and Medicaid Services

InterStudy
P.O. Box 4366
St. Paul, MN 55104
800-844-3351
Internet: www.hmodata.com

National Center for Health Statistics
U.S. Department of Health and Human Services
6525 Belcrest Road
Hyattsville, MD 20782-2003
301-458-4636
Internet: http://www.cdc.gov/nchswww/

**National Institute on Alcohol Abuse
and Alcoholism**
National Institutes of Health
6000 Executive Boulevard
Bethesda, MD 20892-7003
301-443-9970
Internet: www.niaaa.nih.gov/

National Highway Traffic Safety Admin.
400 Seventh Street, SW
Washington, DC 20590
202-366-9550
Internet: www.nhtsa.dot.gov

National Sporting Goods Association
1601 Feehanville Drive, Ste 300
Mt. Prospect, IL 60056-6035
847-296-6742
Internet: www.nsga.org

Smoking and Health Office
Centers for Disease Control and Prevention
4770 Buford Hwy, NE., Mail Stop K-50
Atlanta, GA 30341-3724
770-488-5701
www.cdc.gov/nccdphp/

X. INDEX

Abortion 59-75
Abortion, rates 60, 61
Abortions, by age of woman 67-71
Abortions, by stage of gestation 72-75
Abortions to out-of-state residents 62
Abortions to teenagers 67-71
Accidents, deaths by 165-167
Alcohol-induced deaths 183-185
Admissions to community hospitals 204
AIDS, cases 377-380
AIDS, children cases 380
AIDS, deaths 104-107
AIDS, testing for 508
Alcohol consumption 493, 494
Anesthesiologists 466, 467
Alzheimer's Disease, deaths by 132-134
Atherosclerosis, deaths by 135-137
Beds, average number per hospital 203
Beds, children's hospital 216
Beds, community hospital 201-203
Beds, hospital 201-203, 214, 216, 218, 220
Beds, psychiatric hospital 220
Beds, rehabilitation hospital 218
Beds, nursing home 228, 229
Beer consumption 495, 496
Binge drinkers 501
Births, 1-49, 58
Births, black 10, 11, 16, 17, 22, 23, 32-34
Births, by age of mother 24-43
Births, by method of delivery 46-49
Births, by race of mother 8-11, 14-17, 20-23, 29-34
Births, low birthweight 12-17
Births, number of 1, 3
Births, rates 2, 4
Births, white 8, 9, 14, 15, 20, 21, 29-31
Births to death ratio 78
Births to teenagers 24-41
Births to unmarried women 18-23
Bladder cancer, cases 357, 358
Blood pressure, check 507
Brain cancer, deaths by 130, 131
Breast cancer cases 359, 360
Breast cancer deaths 112, 113
Cancer, bladder cases 357, 358
Cancer, brain deaths 130, 131
Cancer, breast (female) cases 359, 360
Cancer, breast (female) deaths 112, 113
Cancer, cases 353-375
Cancer, cervical cases 374, 375
Cancer, colon and rectum cases 362, 363
Cancer, colon and rectum deaths 114, 115
Cancer, death rates 109-111, 113, 115, 117, 119, 121, 123, 125, 127, 129, 131
Cancer, death rates, by sex 110, 111
Cancer, deaths by 108-131

Cancer, deaths (number) 108, 112, 114, 116, 118, 120, 122, 124, 126, 128, 130
Cancer, leukemia deaths 116, 117
Cancer, liver deaths 118, 119
Cancer, lung cases 366, 367
Cancer, lung deaths 120, 121
Cancer, lymphoma cases 368, 369
Cancer, lymphoma deaths 122, 123
Cancer, ovarian deaths 128, 129
Cancer, pancreatic deaths 125, 126
Cancer, prostate cases 370, 371
Cancer, prostate deaths 126, 127
Cancer, skin melanoma cases 372, 373
Cerebrovascular disease, deaths by 138-140
Cervical cancer cases 374, 375
Cesarean births 46-48
Chancroid cases 414, 415
Children's hospitals 215, 216
Children's insurance 246-248, 270
Chiropractors 478, 479
Chlamydia cases 416, 417
Chronic liver disease, deaths by 141-143
Chronic lower respiratory disease, deaths by 144-146
Colon and rectum cancer deaths 114, 115
Community hospitals, per square miles 193
Community hospitals, rate of 192
Community hospitals 191-211
Community mental health centers 221
Deaths 76-190
Deaths, age-adjusted rates 81, 107, 110, 111, 134, 137, 140, 143, 146, 149, 152, 155, 158, 161, 164, 167, 170, 173, 176, 185, 188
Deaths, alcohol-induced 183-185
Deaths, by cause 104-176, 183-190
Deaths, drug-induced 186-188
Deaths, infant 84-97
Deaths, infant by race 92-97
Deaths, infant (number of) 84, 86, 92, 94
Deaths, infant (rate) 85, 87-91, 93, 95-97
Deaths, leukemia 116, 117
Deaths, neonatal 98-103
Deaths, numbers of 76, 79
Deaths, occupational 189, 190
Deaths, premature 177-182
Deaths, rate of 77, 80, 81
Dental care, access to 486
Dental services, expenditures for 313-317
Dentists 484, 485
Dentists, offices 235
Dentists, receipts of 352
Diabetes mellitus, deaths by 147-149
Distilled spirits, consumption of 499, 500
Doctors of medicine 422-473
Doctors, receipts per office 351
Drinking and driving, incidence of 502

X. INDEX (continued)

Drinkers, binge 501
Drugs, expenditures for 306-312, 328-331
Drugs, use of illicit 511
Drug-induced deaths 186-188
Emergency outpatient visits 210
Expenditures, health care 279-341
Employment, health industries 487
Exercise equipment, use of 488
Fatalities, occupational 189, 190
Federal physicians (M.D.) 433, 434
Fee for service plans, Medicare 265
Fertility, rate of 7
Finance, health care 236-352
For-profit hospitals 199
General surgeons 454, 455
General/family practice physicians 443, 444
German measles, cases and rates 383, 384
Golf, participants in 489
Gonorrhea, cases and rates 418, 419
Government health insurance 251
Government, state health expenditures 343-346
Graduates of international medical schools
 471-473
Gynecologists and obstetricians 456, 457
Health Maintenance Organizations (HMOs)
 253-257
Health programs, state expenditures for 343, 344
Health services, employment in 487
Health services, establishments 233
Heart disease, deaths by 150-152
Hepatitis, cases and rates 385-388
HMOs 253-257
Home health agencies 224
Home health care, expenditures for 322-327
Homicide, deaths by 171-173, 180
Hospices 225, 226
Hospital admissions 204
Hospital beds, rate of 202
Hospital beds 201-203, 214, 216, 218, 220, 228
Hospital care, expenditures for 288-296
Hospital, receipt per 350
Hospitals 191-220
Hospitals, average stay in 207
Hospitals, community 191-211
Hospitals, for-profit 199
Hospitals, nongovernment not-for-profit 198
Hospitals, occupancy rate 208
Hospitals, psychiatric 219, 220
Hospitals, receipts of 350
Hospitals, state and local government-owned
 200
Hospitals, state expenditures for 345, 346
Immunizations 411
Infant deaths 84-97
Influenza and pneumonia, deaths by 156-158
Injury, deaths by 162-164, 182

Inpatient days, community hospitals 205
Insurance, children's health 246-248, 270
Insurance, employment-based 250
Insurance, government 251
Insurance, health 236-278
Insurance, military health 252
Insurance, private health 249
Insured persons 238, 239
Internal medicine physicians 448, 449
International medical school graduates 471, 473
Investor-owned hospitals 199
Jogging/running, participants in 490
Legionellosis, cases and rates 389, 390
Leukemia, deaths 116, 117
Liquor, consumption of 499, 500
Liver cancer, deaths by 118, 119
Liver disease, deaths by 141-143
Low birth weight births 12-17
Lung cancer cases 366, 367
Lung cancer deaths 120, 121
Lyme disease, cases and rates 391, 392
Malaria, cases and rates 393, 394
Managed care 253-257, 263, 264, 276, 277
Mammograms, prevalence of 361
Measles, cases and rates 383, 384, 395, 396
Medicaid 268-278, 287, 296, 305, 327
Medicaid enrollees 268-271, 274-277
Medicaid expenditures 272, 274, 287, 296, 305,
 327
Medicaid facilities 212-229
Medicaid, federal match 278
Medicare 258-267, 286, 295, 304, 326, 340
Medicare enrollees 258, 260-263
Medicare managed care enrollees 263, 264
Medicare-certified facilities 212-229
Medicare payments 259, 260
Melanoma (skin) cases 372, 373
Meningitis, cases and rates 397, 398
Mental health, quality of 510
Mental health, community centers 224
Mental health care, access to 470
Midwives, deliveries by 58
Military health insurance 252
Mortality 76-190
Mothers, teenage 24-41
Motor vehicle accidents, deaths by 168-170
Mumps, cases and rates 399, 400
Natality 1-58
Neonatal deaths 98-103
Neonatal deaths, by race 100-103
Neonatal deaths, number of 98, 100, 102
Neonatal deaths, rate 99, 101, 103
Nonfederal physicians (M.D.) 435-469
Nongovernment not-for-profit hospitals 198
Nurses 482, 483
Nursing care facilities 227-229

X. INDEX (continued)

Nursing home care, expenditures for 336-341
Nursing home occupancy 230
Nursing home resident rate 231
Nursing home population 232
Nursing homes 227
Obese adults 506
Obstetricians and gynecologists 456, 457
Occupancy rates, hospital 208
Occupational fatalities 189, 190
Operations, surgical 211
Ophthalmologists 458, 459
Osteopathic physicians 474, 475
Over-the-counter drugs, expenditures for 328-331
Outpatient visits 209
Ovarian cancer deaths 128, 129
Overweight adults 506
Pap smears, frequency of 376
Pediatric physicians 450, 451
Personnel, health care 487
Pertussis, cases and rates 409, 410
Physical health, quality of 509
Physical therapy facilities 222
Physician assistants 480, 481
Physician services, expenditures for 297-305
Physicians 422-477
Physicians, Chiropractic 478, 479
Physicians (M.D.) 422-473
Physicians (M.D.), by age 426-432
Physicians (M.D.), by sex 423-425
Physicians (M.D.), by specialty 437-469
Physicians (M.D.), federal 433, 434
Physicians (M.D.), nonfederal 435-469
Physicians, Medicare participation 266, 267
Physicians, Osteopathic 474, 475
Physicians, Podiatric 476, 477
Plastic surgeons 462, 463
Pneumonia and influenza, deaths by 156-158
Podiatrists 476, 477
Population, of states A1-A5
Pregnancy rate, teenage 35
Premature deaths, by cause 177-182
Prenatal care 50-57
Prescription drugs, expenditures for 306-312
Primary care, physicians in 439-441
Primary care, access to 442
Private health insurance 249, 250
Prostate cancer cases 370, 371

Prostate cancer deaths 126, 127
Providers, health care 422-487
Psychiatric hospitals 219, 220
Psychiatrists 468, 469
Rabies (animal), cases and rates 401, 402
Rectum and colon cancer cases 362, 363
Rectum and colon cancer deaths 114, 115
Rehabilitation hospitals 217, 218
Registered nurses 482, 483
Rubella, cases and rates 383, 384
Rubeola, cases and rates 395, 396
Running/jogging, participants 490
Rural health clinics 223
Salmonellosis, cases and rates 403, 404
SCHIP 246-249
Sexually transmitted diseases 412-421
Seatbelt use 512
Shigellosis, cases and rates 405, 406
Skin melanoma cases 372, 373
Smokers 503-505
Smokers, by sex 504, 505
Smoking during pregnancy 57
Smoking deaths 184, 185
Specialists, medical 437-469
Sports participation 488-492
State government expenditures for health 343-346
State and local government-owned hospitals 200
Suicide, deaths by 174-176, 181
Surgeons 452-463
Surgical operations 211
Swimming, participants 491
Syphilis, cases and rates 420, 421
Teenagers, births to 24-41
Teenagers, births to by race 29-34
Tennis, participants 492
Tobacco settlement, state funds from 342
Tuberculosis, cases and rates 407, 408
Tuberculosis, deaths by 159, 160
Uninsured 236, 237, 240-245
Unmarried women, births to 18-23
Vaccinations 411
Vaginal births 44, 45, 49
Vaginal births after cesareans (VBACs) 49
Vision products, expenditures for 332-335
Whooping cough, cases and rates 409, 410
Wine consumption 497, 498

Births and Reproductive Health

Deaths

Facilities

Finance

Incidence of Disease

Providers

Physical Fitness

CHAPTER INDEX